DRAIN'S

PERIANESTHESIA NURSING

A CRITICAL CARE APPROACH

DRAIN'S

PERIANESTHESIA NURSING

A CRITICAL CARE APPROACH

SIXTH EDITION

JAN ODOM-FORREN, PhD, RN, CPAN, FAAN

Assistant Professor, College of Nursing
University of Kentucky
Lexington, Kentucky
Perianesthesia/Perioperative Consultant
Co-Editor, Journal of PeriAnesthesia Nursing
Louisville, Kentucky

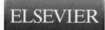

3251 Riverport Lane
St. Louis, Missouri 63043

DRAIN'S PERIANESTHESIA NURSING:
A CRITICAL CARE APPROACH, SIXTH EDITION

ISBN: 978-1-4377-1894-2

Notices

Knowledge and best practice in this field are constantly changing. As new research and experience broaden our understanding, changes in research methods, professional practices, or medical treatment may become necessary.

Practitioners and researchers must always rely on their own experience and knowledge in evaluating and using any information, methods, compounds, or experiments described herein. In using such information or methods they should be mindful of their own safety and the safety of others, including parties for whom they have a professional responsibility.

With respect to any drug or pharmaceutical products identified, readers are advised to check the most current information provided (i) on procedures featured or (ii) by the manufacturer of each product to be administered, to verify the recommended dose or formula, the method and duration of administration, and contraindications. It is the responsibility of practitioners, relying on their own experience and knowledge of their patients, to make diagnoses, to determine dosages and the best treatment for each individual patient, and to take all appropriate safety precautions.

To the fullest extent of the law, neither the Publisher nor the authors, contributors, or editors, assume any liability for any injury and/or damage to persons or property as a matter of products liability, negligence or otherwise, or from any use or operation of any methods, products, instructions, or ideas contained in the material herein.

Library of Congress Cataloging-in-Publication Data

Drain's perianesthesia nursing : a critical care approach / [edited by] Jan Odom-Forren. -- 6th ed.
  p. ; cm.
Perianesthesia nursing
Rev. ed. of: Perianesthesia nursing / [edited by] Cecil B. Drain, Jan Odom-Forren. c2009.
Includes bibliographical references and index.
ISBN 978-1-4377-1894-2 (hardcover : alk. paper)
I. Odom-Forren, Jan. II. Drain, Cecil B. III. Perianesthesia nursing. IV. Title: Perianesthesia nursing.
[DNLM: 1. Postanesthesia Nursing--methods. 2. Anesthesia--nursing. 3. Anesthesia Recovery Period.
4. Perioperative Nursing--methods. 5. Postoperative Care--nursing. 6. Recovery Room. WY 161]

617.9'6--dc23

2012018366

Executive Content Strategist: Teri Hines Burnham
Senior Content Development Specialist: Laura M. Selkirk
Publishing Services Manager: Jeff Patterson
Project Manager: Megan Isenberg
Designer: Ashley Eberts

Printed in the United States of America

Last digit is the print number: 9 8 7 6 5 4 3 2 1

*This edition of Drain's Perianesthesia Nursing
is dedicated to Dr. Cecil Drain, who has been a friend
and a mentor for many years—both to me and to all
nurses who have chosen this fascinating specialty
of perianesthesia nursing. This book is your legacy to us all.*

*Special thanks goes to my family, who share
me willingly with this profession that I so love.
Gary, Kelsey, Brittny, Andrew, and Patrick—you keep
me grounded, and I love you.*

Jan Odom-Forren

Contributors

Susan M. Andrews, BAN, MA, RN, CAPA
Perioperative Manager
Georgia Health Sciences Medical Center
Augusta, Georgia
Chapter 2: Perianesthesia Nursing as a Specialty
Chapter 3: Management and Policies

Carolyn G. Baddeley, BSN, MSN, APN, CRNA
Nurse Anesthetist, Department of Anesthesia
Delta Medical Center
Memphis, Tennessee
Chapter 33: Care of the Ophthalmic Surgical Patient

Kay Ball, BSN, MSA, PhD, RN, CNOR, FAAN
Associate Professor, Nursing Department
Otterbein University
Westerville, Ohio
Consultant, K & D Medical Inc.
Lewis Center, Ohio
Chapter 26: Transition from the Operating Room to the PACU
Chapter 47: Care of the Laser/Laparoscopic Surgical Patient

Andrea Bianco, BSN, MSN, RN
Registered Nurse, Post Anesthesia Care Unit
UCSD Medical Center, Hillcrest
San Diego, California
Chapter 15: The Endocrine System

Robin Blixt, BSN, MS, RN, CNOR
LTC, Army Nurse Corps
Education Department
Landstuhl Regional Medical Center
Landstuhl, Germany
Chapter 56: Bioterrorism and Its Impact on the PACU

Joni M. Brady, MSN, RN, CAPA, CLC
Pain Management Nurse, Nursing Administration
INOVA Alexandria Hospital
Alexandria, Virginia
Chapter 39: Care of the Thyroid and Parathyroid Surgical Patient
Chapter 44: Care of the Plastic and Reconstructive Surgical Patient

Beverly Breyette, MSN, RN, CDE
Clinical Specialist/Diabetes Educator
Baptist Hospital East
Louisville, Kentucky
Chapter 48: Care of the Patient with Chronic Disorders

Nancy Burden, MS, RN, CPAN, CAPA
Director of Ambulatory Surgery
BayCare Health System
Tampa Bay, Florida
Chapter 46: Care of the Ambulatory Surgical Patient

Joseph F. Burkard, DNSc, CRNA
Associate Professor
University of San Diego, School of Nursing
Saint Paul, Minnesota
Chapter 11: The Cardiovascular System
Chapter 15: The Endocrine System
Chapter 51: Care of the Pregnant Patient

Matthew D. Byrne, PhD, RN, CPAN
Assistant Professor
Saint Catherine University
Saint Paul, Minnesota
Chapter 39: Care of the Thyroid and Parathyroid Surgical Patient
Chapter 44: Care of the Plastic and Reconstructive Surgical Patient

Sarah M. I. Cartwright, BA, RN, CAPA
Senior Staff Nurse
Georgia Health Sciences Medical Center
Augusta, Georgia
Chapter 2: Perianesthesia Nursing as a Specialty
Chapter 3: Management and Policies

Zohn Centimole, MSN, CRNA
Certified Registered Nurse Anesthetist
University of Kentucky, Department of Anesthesiology
Lexington, Kentucky
Chapter 18: The Immune System

Theresa L. Clifford, MSN, RN, CPAN
PACU Resource Nurse
Mercy Hospital
Portland, Maine
Cherry Hill, New Jersey
Chapter 45: Care of the Obese Patient Undergoing Bariatric Surgery

Lindsay Cosco, BSN, RN
Assistant Nurse Manager
Thornton Perioperative Services
University of California San Diego
San Diego, California
Chapter 11: The Cardiovascular System

Mallorie Croal, BS, MSN, CLE
Registered Nurse, Oncology
Orange Coast Memorial Medical Center
Fountain Valley, California
Chapter 51: Care of the Pregnant Patient

Cecil B. Drain, PhD, RN, CRNA, FAAN, FASAHP
Professor and Dean
School of Allied Health Professions
Virginia Commonwealth University, MCV Campus
Richmond, Virginia
Chapter 12: The Respiratory System
Chapter 20: Inhalation Anesthesia
Chapter 21: Nonopioid Intravenous Anesthetics
Chapter 22: Opioid Intravenous Anesthetics
Chapter 23: Neuromuscular Blocking Agents
Chapter 48: Care of the Patient with Chronic Disorders
Chapter 52: Care of the Substance-Using Patient

Michael D. Fallacaro, DNS, CRNA
Professor and Chair, Nurse Anesthesia
Virginia Commonwealth University
Richmond, Virginia
Chapter 4: Crisis Resource Management in the PACU

Ken Faulkner, MA, MDiv
Assistant Professor, Department of Patient Counseling
Virginia Commonwealth University
Richmond, Virginia
Chapter 8: Ethics in Perianesthesia Nursing

Susan J. Fetzer, BA, BSN, MSN, MBA, PhD, CNL
Professor, Department of Nursing
University of New Hampshire, College of Health and Human Services
Durham, New Hampshire
Chapter 13: The Renal System

Tracey Gendron, MSG
Assistant Professor, Gerontology
Virginia Commonwealth University
Richmond, Virginia
Chapter 50: Care of the Older Patient

William Hartland, Jr., PhD, CRNA
Director of Education
Associate Professor, Nurse Anesthesia
School of Allied Health Professions
Virginia Commonwealth University
Richmond, Virginia
Chapter 57: Cardiopulmonary Resuscitation in the PACU

Melody Heffline, MSN, RN, ACNS-BC, ACNP-BC
Acute Care Nurse Practitioner
Lexington Medical Center, Southern Surgical Group
West Columbia, South Carolina
Chapter 36: Care of the Vascular Surgical Patient

Vallire D. Hooper, PhD, RN, CPAN, FAAN
Manager, Nursing Practice, Education, and Research
Mission Hospital
Asheville, North Carolina
Chapter 9: Evidence-Based Practice and Research
Chapter 53: Care of the Patient with Thermal Imbalance

Elizabeth Howell, BS, BSN, CRNA
Assistant Professor and Director of Professional Development
Nurse Anesthesia
Virginia Commonwealth University
Richmond, Virginia
Chapter 49: Care of the Pediatric Patient

Xinliang Liu, MBBS, MSc
Research Assistant
Virginia Commonwealth University
Richmond, Virginia
Chapter 6: The Changing Health Care System and Its Implications for the PACU

Mary Beth Flynn Makic, PhD, RN, CNS, CCNS, CCRN
Research Nurse Scientist, Critical Care
University of Colorado Hospital
Assistant Professor, Adjoint
College of Nursing
University of Colorado
Aurora, Colorado
Chapter 55: Care of the Intensive Care Unit Patient in the PACU

Debra Pecka Malina, DNSc, MBA, CRNA
Assistant Professor, Anesthesiology Program Assistant Director for Clinical Education
Barry University
Malina Anesthesia and Consulting Services
Hollywood, Florida
Chapter 14: Fluid and Electrolytes
Chapter 17: The Integumentary System

Myrna E. Mamaril, MS, RN, CPAN, CAPA, FAAN
Nurse Manager, Pediatric PACU
Johns Hopkins Hospital
Baltimore, Maryland
Chapter 54: Care of the Shock Trauma Patient
Chapter 55: Care of the Intensive Care Unit Patient in the PACU

Daniel D. Moos, MS, EdD, CRNA
Staff Anesthetist, Kearney Anesthesia Associates, PC
Kearney, Nebraska
Adjunct Faculty, School of Nurse Anesthesia
Bryan/LGH College of Health Sciences
Lincoln, Nebraska
Chapter 24: Local Anesthetics
Chapter 25: Regional Anesthesia

John J. Nagelhout, PhD, CRNA, FAAN
Director, Kaiser Permanente School of Anesthesia
California State University Fullerton
Pasadena, California
Chapter 19: Basic Principles of Pharmacology

Denise O'Brien, DNP, RN, ACNS-BC, CPAN, CAPA, FAAN
Perianesthesia Clinical Nurse Specialist
Department of Operating Rooms/PACU
University of Michigan Health System
Clinical Adjunct Faculty, School of Nursing
University of Michigan
Ann Arbor, Michigan
Chapter 1: Space Planning and Basic Equipment Systems
Chapter 28: Patient Education and Care of the Perianesthesia Patient
Chapter 29: Postanesthesia Care Complications
Chapter 40: Care of the Gastrointestinal, Abdominal, and Anorectal Surgical Patient

Chris Pasero, MS, RN-BC, FAAN
Pain Management Educator and Clinical Consultant
El Dorado Hills, California
Chapter 31: Pain Management

Corey R. Peterson, DNP, CRNA
Assistant Professor
Georgia Health Sciences University
Augusta, Georgia
Chapter 10: The Nervous System
Chapter 16: The Hepatobiliary and Gastrointestinal System

Audrey R. Roberson, MS, RN, CPAN, CNS-BC
Nurse Clinician, Clinical Nurse Specialist
Department of Medical Nursing
Medical Respiratory Intensive Care Unit
Adjunct Clinical Faculty-VCU School of Nursing
Virginia Commonwealth University Health Systems
Richmond, Virginia
Chapter 8: Ethics in Perianesthesia Nursing

Jacqueline Ross, PhD, RN, CPAN
Perianesthesia Nursing Research Consultant
Patient Safety Analyst
The Doctors Company
Napa, California
Chapter 7: Patient Safety and Legal Issues in the PACU

Nancy M. Saufl, MS, RN, CPAN, CAPA
Manager, Preadmission Testing Department
Florida Hospital Memorial Medical Center
Daytona Beach, Florida
Chapter 37: Care of the Orthopedic Surgical Patient
Chapter 43: Care of the Breast Surgical Patient

Lois Schick, MBA, MN, RN, CPAN, CAPA
Perianesthesia Nurse Consultant
Per Diem Staff Nurse, PACU
Exempla Lutheran Medical Center
Wheatridge, Colorado
Chapter 27: Assessment and Monitoring of the Perianesthesia Patient

Patricia C. Seifert, MSN, RN, CNOR, CRNFA, FAAN
Staff Nurse, Cardiovascular Operating Room
Inova Heart and Vascular Institute
Falls Church, Virginia
Chapter 35: Care of the Cardiac Surgical Patient

Beverly A. Smith, BSN, RN, CPAN, CAPA
Nurse Manager
University of Michigan Hospitals and Health Centers
Ann Arbor, Michigan
Chapter 1: Space Planning and Basic Equipment Systems

Lisa Sturm, MPH, CIC
Supervisor, Infection Control & Epidemiology
University of Michigan Hospitals and Health
    Centers
Ann Arbor, Michigan
*Chapter 5: Infection Prevention and Control in the
    PACU*

**Alexander Tartaglia, MA, MDiv, DMin, BCC,
    ACPE Supervisor,**
Senior Associate Dean, School of Allied Health
    Professions
Katherine I. Lantz Professor, Patient Counseling
Virginia Commonwealth University
Richmond, Virginia
Chapter 8: Ethics in Perianesthesia Nursing

Candace N. Taylor, BSN, RN, CPAN
PACU Supervisor
Cedar Oaks Surgery Center
Warrensburg, Missouri
*Chapter 32: Care of the Ear, Nose, Throat, Neck, and
    Maxillofacial Surgical Patient*
*Chapter 41: Care of the Genitourinary Surgical
    Patient*

Melissa Thomas, BSN, RN, CAPA
Perioperative Education Coordinator, Surgical
    Services
Baptist Hospital East
Louisville, Kentucky
Chapter 38: Care of the Neurosurgical Patient

Carolyn A. Watts, PhD
Professor and Chair
Department of Health Administration
Virginia Commonwealth University
Richmond, Virginia
*Chapter 6: The Changing Health Care System and
    Its Implications for the PACU*

E. Ayn Welleford, MSG, PhD, AGHEF
Gerontologist
Chair & Associate Professor
Department of Gerontology
Virginia Commonwealth University
Richmond, Virginia
Chapter 50: Care of the Older Patient

**Kenneth R. White, MSN, PhD, RN, MPH,
    FACHE**
Sentara Professor, Department of Health Admin-
    istration
Virginia Commonwealth University
Richmond, Virginia
*Chapter 6: The Changing Health Care System and
    Its Implications for the PACU*

Wendy K. Winer, BSN, RN, CNOR
Endoscopic Surgery Specialist
Director of Research and Technology Development
Center for Endometriosis Care
Atlanta, Georgia
*Chapter 42: Care of the Obstetric and Gynecologic
    Surgical Patient*

Suzanne M. Wright, PhD, CRNA
Assistant Professor, Nurse Anesthesia
Director, The Center for Research in Human
    Simulation
Virginia Commonwealth University
Richmond, Virginia
*Chapter 4: Crisis Resource Management in the
    PACU*
*Chapter 30: Assessment and Management of the
    Airway*

Reviewers

Michael D. Aldridge, MSN, RN, CCRN, CNS
Assistant Professor of Nursing
Concordia University
Austin, Texas

Joy Don Baker, PhD, RN-BC, CNE, CNOR, NEA-BC
Clinical Associate Professor, College of Nursing
University of Texas at Arlington
Arlington, Texas

Marcia Bixby, MS, RN, APRN-BC, CCRN
Critical Care Clinical Nurse Specialist
Boston, Massachusetts

Shari M. Burns, MSN, CRNA, EdD
Interim Program Director/Associate Professor
Midwestern University, Nurse Anesthesia Program
Glendale, Arizona

Martha L. Clark, MSN, RN, CPAN
Staff Nurse
UC Health Surgical Hospital
West Chester, Ohio

Theresa L. Clifford, MSN, RN, CPAN
PACU Resource Nurse
Mercy Hospital
Portland, Maine
ASPAN Past President 2009-2010
Cherry Hill, New Jersey

Donna DeFazio Quinn, BSN, MBA, RN, CPAN, CAPA
Director
Orthopaedic Surgery Center
Concord, New Hampshire

Marjorie A. Geisz-Everson, PhD, CRNA
Instructor and Staff Anesthetist
Nurse Anesthesia Program
Louisiana State University Health Sciences Center
New Orleans, Louisiana

Becki L. Hoyle, BSN, RN, CPAN, CAPA
Registered Nurse, Patient Care Coordinator
Medical Center of the Rockies
Poudre Valley Health Systems
Loveland, Colorado

Dolly Ireland, MSN, RN, CAPA, CPN
Assistant Clinical Manager/Educator
PACU/PAT/ENDO
McLaren Macomb Medical Center
Mount Clemens, Michigan
Area Chair, College of Nursing
University of Phoenix, Detroit Metro Campus
Troy, Michigan

Joseph A. Joyce, BS, CRNA
Staff CRNA
Moses Cone Health System
Greensboro, North Carolina

Janice Lopez, BSN, RN, CPAN, CAPA
Registered Nurse, IV
KCMO Hospitals
Kansas City, Missouri

Kandace K. Maier, BSN, RN, NP, CPAN
SkyRidge Medical Center
Lone Tree, Colorado

Kathleen J. Menard, MS, RN, CPAN, CAPA
Perianesthesia Nurse Education Specialist
University of Massachusetts Memorial Medical Center, University Campus PACU/SACU
Worcester, Massachusetts

Daniel D. Moos, MS, EdD, CRNA
Staff Anesthetist, Kearney Anesthesia Associates, PC
Kearney, Nebraska
Adjunct Faculty, School of Nurse Anesthesia
Bryan/LGH College of Health Sciences
Lincoln, Nebraska

John J. Nagelhout, PhD, CRNA, FAAN
Director, Kaiser Permanente School of Anesthesia
California State University Fullerton
Pasadena, California

Janice D. Nunnelee, PhD, RN
Associate Professor
University of Missouri, St. Louis
St. Louis, Missouri

Denise O'Brien, DNP, RN, ACNS-BC, CPAN, CAPA, FAAN
Perianesthesia Clinical Nurse Specialist
Department of Operating Rooms/PACU
University of Michigan Health System
Clinical Adjunct Faculty, School of Nursing
University of Michigan
Ann Arbor, Michigan

Ellen L. Poole, PhD, RN, CNE, CPAN
Professor
Chamberlain College of Nursing
Phoenix, Arizona

Christine M. Price, MSN, RN, CPAN, CAPA
Director of Perioperative Services
Bayhealth Medical Center
Dover, Delaware
ASPAN Vice President/President Elect 2010-2011
Cherry Hill, New Jersey

Wanda Rodriguez, MA, RN, CCRN, CPAN
Clinical Nurse Specialist, PACU
Memorial Sloan-Kettering Cancer Center
New York, New York

Paul St. Jacques, MD
Associate Professor of Anesthesiology
Vanderbilt University School of Medicine
Nashville, Tennessee

Nancy M. Saufl, MS, RN, CPAN, CAPA
Manager, Preadmission Testing Department
Florida Hospital Memorial Medical Center
Daytona Beach, Florida

Lois Schick, MBA, MN, RN, CPAN, CAPA
Perianesthesia Nurse Consultant
Per Diem Staff Nurse, PACU
Exempla Lutheran Medical Center
Wheatridge, Colorado

Twilla Shrout, BSN, MBA, CPAN, CAPA
Staff Nurse, Same Day Surgery
Harry S. Truman Memorial Veterans Hospital
Columbia, Missouri

Candace N. Taylor, BSN, RN, CPAN
PACU Supervisor
Cedar Oaks Surgery Center
Warrensburg, Missouri

Terri Voepel-Lewis, MS, RN
Research Lead
University of Michigan
Ann Arbor, Michigan

Valerie S. Watkins, BSN, RN, CAPA
Clinical Nurse IV
Denver, Colorado

Pamela E. Windle, MS, RN, NE-BC, CPAN, CAPA, FAAN
Nurse Manager
St. Luke's Episcopal Hospital
Houston, Texas

Preface

Dr. Drain wrote the first edition of this book, then titled *The Recovery Room*, after working with "recovery room" nurses who had many questions about care of the anesthetized patient. He discovered that there were no texts that offered this kind of information to nurses in this specialty. So after working all day, Dr. Drain would write until the wee hours of the morning. First published in 1979, *The Recovery Room* has since become known as the standard textbook for perianesthesia nurses. Known unofficially as "the blue book", the title has evolved as the specialty has progressed, changing from *The Recovery Room* to *The Post Anesthesia Care Unit: A Critical Care Approach* to *Post Anesthesia Nursing* to *Perianesthesia Nursing: A Critical Care Approach*. This sixth edition is a significant milestone because it will be the first edition without Cecil Drain, PhD, RN, CRNA, FAAN, FASAHP, listed as an editor. However, it continues the tradition of excellence established by Dr. Drain, providing the perianesthesia nurse with the most comprehensive knowledge base for this nursing specialty available under one cover. The title of the sixth edition, *Drain's Perianesthesia Nursing: A Critical Care Approach*, not only reflects the evolving professionalism of this advanced nursing practice specialty, but reflects the time and effort of Dr. Drain in his pursuit to provide a textbook with comprehensive information about the complete nursing care of the patient who undergoes a surgical procedure.

All the chapters in this sixth edition contain an opening paragraph introducing the reader to the topic to be discussed. After the introduction, a complete section on the definitions of terms particular to the chapter topic is provided, and then the chapter topic is presented in detail. The final portion of the chapter contains a summary of the material and, in some chapters, a list of resources the reader can use to facilitate further reading about the topic. New in this edition are Evidence-Based Practice boxes that will alert the reader to new evidence related to the chapter topic.

This book is organized into five major sections. Section I, "The Postanesthesia Care Unit," focuses on the postanesthesia facilities and equipment, the specialty of perianesthesia nursing, and management and policy issues. The chapter on crisis resource management in the PACU covers the newest techniques in the care of the patient with use of technology such as anesthesia simulators and provides the most up-to-date concepts in regard to patient safety. The health care system continues to change, particularly in the PACU, so a chapter is devoted to those changes and the impact on the PACU. The chapter on research has been revised to explore the basic concepts of evidence-based practice (EBP) and their relationship to research as well as to explore the application of EBP in the perianesthesia setting.

Section II deals with physiologic considerations in the PACU. All chapters have been revised to reflect current concepts in anatomy and physiology. Section III, "Concepts in Anesthetic Agents," presents the reader with up-to-date pharmacologic considerations of postanesthesia care, including an extensive update of the chapters on regional and local anesthesia.

Section IV addresses nursing care in the PACU for various surgical specialties. Chapter 31, "Pain Management in the PACU," which includes discussions on related physiology and pharmacology, has been extensively revised and updated. The previous chapter on the care of the burn patient was incorporated into Chapter 55, "Care of the Intensive Care Unit Patient in the PACU." Added to this section was a chapter entitled "Care of the Obese Patient Undergoing Bariatric Surgery." This chapter discusses caring for the patient with bariatric concerns and addresses the challenges for the perianesthesia nurse in caring for this population.

Section V, "Special Considerations," has been revised and updated in this edition. This section offers up-to-date information on the special needs and concerns of perianesthesia nurses. Chapter 53, "Care of the Patient with Thermal Imbalance," provides a complete discussion of the care of patients with hyperthermia and hypothermia. Chapter 54 addresses the needs and care of the shock trauma patient. The chapter "Care of the Intensive Care Patient in the PACU" was extensively amended to include additional information on the patient with burns. The chapter focusing on bioterrorism and its impact on the PACU reflects the most current thinking in regard to this public health concern. The chapter "Cardiopulmonary Resuscitation in the PACU" features current information based on the 2010 AHA guidelines for CPR and ECC as it applies to the PACU.

The success of any multi-authored book is in large part dependent on the expertise and commitment of the contributors. I am grateful to all past contributors, including Dr. Susan Christoph, who was enlisted by Dr. Drain to assist with the first two editions of this book. These contributors have helped to build this book into the comprehensive text that it is. I am grateful to all the returning and new contributors who offer their knowledge and expertise to the reader. The contributors to this book were invited because they are acknowledged authorities in their fields. With their help, it is hoped that this book will continue to inform and guide students, teachers, and clinicians in the critical care specialty of perianesthesia nursing.

It is impossible to produce a book of quality without an able and expert publisher. I would like to particularly thank Laura Selkirk, who kept me on task and reasonably sane during the writing process, and Megan Isenberg, whose contributions to the final project resulted in the book you now see. Thank you both for your guidance and support.

Jan Odom-Forren

Contents

SECTION IV: NURSING CARE IN THE PACU, 342

SECTION V: SPECIAL CONSIDERATIONS, 674

Section I
THE POSTANESTHESIA CARE UNIT

1 Space Planning and Basic Equipment Systems

Beverly A. Smith, BSN, RN, CPAN, CAPA, and
Denise O'Brien, DNP, RN, ACNS-BC, CPAN, CAPA, FAAN

From the birth of the recovery room in the 1940s to the postanesthesia care unit (PACU) of the twenty-first century, the look and function of this room (or unit) have been in a state of continual evolution.[1] Throughout the last six decades, surgical procedures have become more extensive and complex and thus require more specially prepared nursing staff and equipment for care of the patients.

The first recovery rooms were established for centralization of patients and personnel. The PACUs of today have evolved from general care to intensive care specialty units that provide a spectrum of nursing care, from neonatal to geriatric and from outpatient or same-day surgery to inpatient surgery. The modern PACU must be flexible to serve all perianesthesia phases and patient acuities. The design of the space is critical to the ability of the staff to care safely and efficiently for a variety of patients.[2]

SPACE

Many factors are considered in the design of a PACU. Before the architect or design firm is consulted, the users of the space (i.e., perianesthesia nurses, anesthesia providers, clerical staff) should meet to answer the following questions regarding the function of the space:
- Is this new construction or is the current space to be remodeled?
- How will the space be used?
- Will a separate preoperative holding area be created, or will preoperative functions be carried out in this space?
- Is this space used for PACU Phase I level of care, PACU Phase II level of care, or both?
- What patient population will be served (i.e., outpatient, same-day admission, inpatient)?

- What patient age groups will be served (i.e., neonatal, pediatric, adult only, combined age groups)?

Current and future programs in the Department of Surgery and the institutional demographics are also important considerations. The following questions should be answered:
- How many operating rooms (ORs) will this area serve?
- How many surgeries will be done per day?
- How many different surgical services will be served?
- What types of procedures will be done?
- Will some patients need prolonged monitoring or observation?
- What type of anesthesia practices will impact this area (i.e., regional anesthesia program, acute or chronic pain service)?
- What is the average patient acuity (i.e., American Society of Anesthesiologists' physical status classification)?
- Will nonsurgical or procedural patients who need anesthesia undergo recovery in this same space?

Purpose of the Space

Flexibility is an important consideration. One of the first factors for consideration is how the space will be used. Will the bays be used strictly for postoperative care, or will the unit need the flexibility of preoperative use? Many institutions have a separate area dedicated to preadmission testing or screening. This area is best located near the surgical clinics and testing areas (i.e., blood draw station, radiology and cardiology [electrocardiography] departments). However, consideration should be given to how the preoperative holding area will be designed and used. Because

1

of the cost of construction and the limited hours of use, many administrators are reluctant to build space that has only a single function and that does not lend itself to change as the users or programs evolve. Therefore all disciplines that use or expect to use the area need to engage in the discussion related to space usage so that future needs can be anticipated.

Perianesthesia nurses have knowledge of the entire process from preadmission testing to discharge the day of surgery. The staff members in the surgery department need to have input regarding types of operations, new surgical techniques, and the need for prolonged observation before discharge. The anesthesiology department medical staff members will have input regarding preoperative needs (e.g., a preadmission testing or screening area, day-of-surgery preoperative procedures area). Clerical services personnel should have input related to the flow of patients and record and paperwork systems. Input from environmental services personnel is related to needs of janitorial space and house cleaning supplies and equipment. Central supply personnel should be consulted regarding the space needed for storage of disposable supplies and linen for ready availability on the unit. Patient equipment personnel should give input regarding space needed to deliver and store reusable equipment, such as stretchers, beds, wheelchairs, infusion pumps, intermittent or sequential pneumatic compression devices, patient-controlled analgesia pumps (intravenous [IV] or epidural), and implantable cardioverter defibrillators.

Adequate time for consultation with all of the potential users and ancillary personnel who will use or provide services in the space is wise. One needs only a brief conversation with staff who have had to work in a poorly designed space to understand the importance of this first step in the design process.

Determine the Location

The same factors that influence the building of a housing development or retail shops in one place versus another can be applied to this discussion of perianesthesia space needs. A new construction design typically offers greater probability of optimization of design than remodeling does. The first consideration before construction should be ease of access for the patients and families. Parking should be easily accessible and plentiful, and the entrance should be located adjacent to the parking garage or lot. The patient reception and waiting area should be near the entrance to decrease the patient anxiety and frustration that results from searching for an area.

The second consideration should be egress. A logical patient flow—with adjacent areas that naturally follow the patients' transit through the unit—should be established for maximization of staff efficiency and decreased steps between areas. The waiting area should be adjacent to the preoperative holding area. PACU Phase I and PACU Phase II should be adjacent but with separate entrances from the ORs for safety and efficiency. In an inpatient setting, a separate elevator is ideal for patients of the OR to be transported to general care and intensive care units (ICUs). This separate elevator is a matter of safety for patients going to an ICU, and it maximizes staff efficiency for patients going to general care. With remodeling, great care should be taken to determine that the design shows consideration of these factors and incorporation whenever possible.

Components of the Space

Several key components must be incorporated into the design of the space. The first element that needs determination is the number of patient bays. Before this number can be calculated, consideration must be given to several key factors that influence that number.[2,3]

- How are the bays to be used? Will they be used for preoperative care only, PACU only, PACU Phase II only? Or will they be used interchangeably for all levels of care?
- Are they to be used for preoperative care, or is a separate space available for that function?
- How many ORs does the preoperative area and PACU service, and how many cases are done per day?
- Does the PACU service other procedure areas of the hospital (i.e., cardiac catheterization, electrophysiology laboratory, electroconvulsive therapy treatments, medical procedures [endoscopy, bronchoscopy], radiology and angiography, anesthesia pain service [chronic and acute])? If so, how many cases per day and at what time of day?
- Are the patients adults, children, or both?
- What is the scheduling method used by the department of surgery? How many different surgical services are served?
- What is the hospital bed capacity and usual census?
- Do patients wait long periods for inpatient beds?
- Is the PACU used for ICU, telemetry, or general care overflow? If so, how often and for how many patients at one time?

- Does the department of anesthesia have a regional anesthesia program? Does it need space for these services?
- What is the average patient acuity (i.e., American Society of Anesthesiologists' physical status classification)?
- What is the average length of surgical procedures?
- What is the average length of stay for different patient types (i.e., outpatient, inpatient, same-day admission)?

For an inpatient hospital PACU that services a combined patient population of inpatients and same-day admission patients, a ratio of 1.5 to 2 PACU bays per OR is necessary to safely care for the patients and not back up the OR. For an ambulatory surgery center with a limited number of surgical services and types of procedures, 2.5 to 3 PACU Phase I and PACU Phase II (combined) bays are necessary. The shorter surgical procedures necessitate an increased number of PACU slots because the recovery time may be two to three times the length of the procedure. If pediatric patients receive care in either setting, the number of bays may need to be increased, because this patient population necessitates 1:1 nursing care for a longer time than does a solely adult population.

Cases of antibiotic-resistant organisms and tuberculosis infections have been on the rise over the past several years. As a result, the need for negative pressure isolation or body substance isolation should be considered in the design. Geographic location and patient population demographics should be reviewed to determine the number of isolation rooms needed. Every PACU should have at least one negative pressure room. However, more rooms may be necessary if the institution services a more susceptible population. Consultation with the institution's infectious diseases department is advisable to ensure that the design meets institutional policy and is prepared to serve the patient population.[4]

Another consideration in the design of patient bays is size and means of separation. Most states have building codes that define the minimum square footage of each bay (e.g., *Minimum Design Standards for Health Care Facilities in Michigan* requirement is 80 square feet).[5] However, consideration should be given to how the bays are to be used. If they are strictly for patients requiring a PACU Phase I level of care, the minimum required square footage may be adequate. If the bays are to be used for anesthesia preoperative procedures or anesthesia pain procedures that necessitate equipment such as fluoroscopy or bronchoscopy, the size may need to be increased

(to as much as 150 square feet). Also, if the bays are to be used alternatively as PACU Phase I or PACU Phase II levels of care and then as observation for 23-hour admissions, they may need to be large enough to accommodate a patient bed, table, lounge chair, or other equipment. Building some of the bays larger to accommodate these future needs may also be wise, but it is important to realize that the size of the bays affects the configuration of the space.

Patient privacy needs to be considered in determination of the means of separation between patient bays. Typically, PACU bays are open spaces defined only by a curtain that can be pulled for privacy. The open floor plan maximizes patient safety and staff efficiency in the higher acuity PACU Phase I setting. With preoperative and PACU Phase II care, patient acuity is typically lower and continual observation of patients is usually not necessary. Patients are more alert and families are generally present; therefore the need for privacy is increased. Half walls may be considered in these spaces. A half wall (i.e., floor-to-ceiling wall one third to half the depth of the bay) gives more privacy to the patient and family from the sights and sounds of the adjacent bays. However, this configuration still allows the clinicians to observe patients and be readily available for acute needs.

The bays should be carefully arranged for maximized staffing efficiency within the constraints of the American Society of PeriAnesthesia Nurses (ASPAN) staffing resource guidelines.[4] The PACU Phase I staffing recommendation is a maximum of two patients per registered nurse (RN)—less for an unstable condition or a pediatric patient. For PACU Phase II staffing, the recommendation is a maximum of three patients to one RN—less for a patient with an unstable condition who needs transfer or a pediatric patient without family or staff support. Grouping of slots in multiples of two or three allows the most efficient, safe staffing. Careful consideration should be given to how the space will be used (i.e., as preoperative care, PACU Phase I or PACU Phase II, or interchangeably).

The ASPAN *Perianesthesia Nursing Standards and Practice Recommendations* do not define staffing ratios for preoperative cases.[4] Ideal safe staffing ratios are determined by individual institutions on the basis of the particular patient population, the number of ORs, the OR turnover time, and the number of preoperative procedures performed with anesthesia. The amount of nursing time necessary to prepare for surgery depends on the patient's age, the amount of preparation done in the surgery clinic, and the patient's knowledge and anxiety level. Patients who are well prepared when they arrive for surgery may require less preoperative nursing time. The number of ORs, the average length of procedures, and turnover time affect how many patients are in the preoperative area at one time and how much time they wait before going into the OR. In a small ambulatory surgery center, one or more rooms may be used for quick procedures that necessitate little equipment or cleaning to ready the OR for the next patient. In this case, two patients for that same OR may need to be in the preoperative area at the same time. Another factor that affects preoperative staffing is the number and type of anesthesia preoperative procedures. Again, in a small ambulatory surgery center, most procedures can be performed with a general anesthetic or sedation; therefore the preparation time is shorter. Conversely, a teaching institution may have a patient population with significant comorbid conditions that necessitate monitoring lines (e.g., pulmonary artery catheters, arterial lines, central lines). In addition, many institutions have a pain service that offers patients epidural catheters or extremity blocks for postoperative pain management. These patients occupy the preoperative holding area bay for a longer period and may need nursing assistance for sedation or monitoring during and after the procedure until they go into the OR. In these situations, a ratio of three to five patients to one RN is safe and efficient. However, staffing should be flexible to decrease the number of patients per RN as the patient acuity rises or the need for nursing care and monitoring increases.

For space that is flexible for any need, preoperative or postoperative care, all the headwalls should be designed uniformly to allow flexibility day-to-day or in the future as institutional needs change. During new construction, when the walls are open, the addition of piped-in medical gases and vacuum for suction at each bay is simple and cost effective. For the care of critically ill patients in PACU Phase I, each bay should have a minimum of two oxygen outlets, one air outlet, and three vacuum outlets for suction. In a freestanding ambulatory surgery center that never serves a critically ill inpatient population, it may be more prudent to decrease the number of oxygen and vacuum outlets. However, consideration should be given to the possibility of a patient with a surgical or anesthesia complication that necessitates more intensive care. The other elements of the headwall design include electrical outlets and data and telephone jacks. Again, whether the unit is new construction or renovation, a plan for maximum care and future needs is wise. Each bay should have adequate electrical outlets to service a variety of pieces of equipment, including a patient bed, a forced air warming and cooling device, multiple infusion pumps, a ventilator, a physiologic monitor, a computer, a compression device, and a patient-controlled analgesia machine. Telephone and data jacks should be installed to service the current standard of practice and future needs. Most physiologic monitors are computers that need a data jack. Technology development has brought online data entry to the bedside. Planning for adequate data jacks to support this need is wise and necessary. In addition, wireless networking capability should be considered when designing the space to allow for the use of smartphones, wireless local area network–enabled computers, and other technology in the unit.

Another important component of the design of the patient care bay is lighting. Adequate light needs to be available for admission assessment and emergency situations. Large overhead lights provide the best source of light to meet this safety need. Consideration should be given to the patient in stable condition for whom bright lighting is not a safety concern. Wall-mounted lights, overhead canned lights on a dimmer, or low-wattage lighting provide the appropriate ambience for the patient and still allow the nurse to provide safe care.

Storage in the patient bay is also essential. Some emergency equipment must be stored at each bay for ready availability to the practitioners. However, careful planning should occur to avoid clutter that would hamper the nurses' ability to quickly access equipment. Many different systems are available to service this need. Before any system is purchased, the items to be stored and the space needed must be assessed. Another point for consideration is what constitutes emergent equipment and what is at the bedside for convenience.[4] Figure 1-1 shows one example of a bedside cart storage system. The carts are mobile, are stocked with essential bedside supplies, and contain an interior locked space. A larger storage cart complements this system; it contains items that need to be readily available for efficiency but are not needed emergently. The ability to care for patients in the PACU safely and efficiently depends on the layout of the room. Beyond the confines of the patient bay and its components, immediate access to supplies, equipment, and service areas is essential. Box 1-1 contains a list of the space and service areas needed for the function of the preoperative holding area and PACU. Many of the supplies, pieces of equipment, and service areas overlap, which should be considered in the design. If service areas are strategically placed, they can service two units and thus increase staff

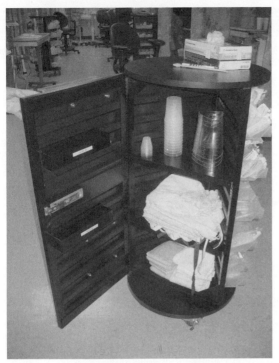

FIG. 1-1 Example of perianesthesia bedside supply carts with exterior open storage and interior locked storage capacity.

efficiency while decreasing the cost of building and maintenance.

The amount of duplication can be decreased with determination of the components that may be shared. These spaces should be placed between two units or in close proximity to one another. This thoughtful, careful planning allows for safe, efficient care and minimization of duplication and cost.

Staff needs are an important consideration in the design. Staff lounge and toilets adjacent to the unit are essential and allow staff members the opportunity to take breaks consistent with the workflow. Because of the dynamic nature of the preoperative holding area and PACU, scheduling of breaks consistent with staff members' requests is sometimes difficult. Facilities that are immediately adjacent to the unit allow flexibility of scheduling and ensure the availability of staff members in an emergency.

Ergonomics and efficiency are important elements in the design of the space and the equipment. For patient safety, the nurse must be able to visualize the patient from every point in the room. Essential equipment should be in the room so the nurse can constantly monitor the patient while obtaining and using the equipment. A bedside

table and chair should be available for every staff member for sitting at the patient's bedside and documenting during observation. Tables, chairs, and computer monitors and keyboards should be adjustable to fit multiple users. With an aging workforce, the lack of adequate adjustable furnishings could lead to increased injury and exacerbate the growing nursing shortage.

Another component of the space is the reception and waiting area, which varies depending on the location (i.e., inpatient hospital-based versus freestanding ambulatory surgery center). In either location, several items need to be incorporated. If possible, preoperative patients and their families should wait in a separate location from the families of patients in the OR or PACU. Preoperative patient anxiety can increase when a physician is seen with another family or a family is visibly upset. Also, the sight and smell of food and drink are inconsiderate to a patient who has been fasting. Conversely, families of patients in the OR or PACU want to stay in close proximity to their loved ones and need to be readily available to clinical staff; therefore they need to be able to eat and drink in the waiting area. In addition, the waiting areas should accommodate a variety of needs so that waiting patients and families can be entertained or distracted or work, if necessary. Some considerations are: an area dedicated to Internet access with computer work stations and data connections for laptops; a television area; a quiet area for reading; a children's play area with toys; and furniture appropriate to the patient population being served. Consultation rooms should be available for private consultation with physicians, patients, and families.

STANDARD EQUIPMENT

The type and amount of equipment needed for the safe care of preoperative and postanesthesia patients vary to some extent on the basis of environment and patient population. However, some basic items are essential in any setting.

Types of equipment can be divided into three categories: emergent, readily available, and necessary. Emergency cases in the PACU typically start as a result of airway compromise; therefore the availability of supplies (e.g., resuscitation bag, oral and nasal airways, suction catheters, lubricant) at the bedside is prudent. Intubation equipment should be readily available as part of the emergency cart or as a separate container or bag of anesthesia supplies. Box 1-2 provides a list of suggested items to be stocked in an anesthesia PACU emergency bag. In addition, the ASPAN *Perianesthesia Nursing Standards and Practice*

BOX 1-1   Support Areas and Equipment*

PREOPERATIVE HOLDING AREA
- Clean storage
- Dirty or soiled utility
- Patient toilet
- Equipment storage (e.g., stretchers, beds, wheelchairs, infusion pumps, transducer setups)
- Procedure cart
- Blanket warmer
- Emergency cart
- Automated medication dispensing unit (e.g., Pyxis, Omnicell)
- Point-of-care testing (blood gas laboratory)
- Medical records storage
- Radiograph view box
- Bulletin board for patient education material
- Computers (stationery and mobile)
- Nursing station

PACU PHASE I
- Clean storage
- Dirty or soiled utility
- Automated medication dispensing unit (e.g., Pyxis, Omnicell)
- Blanket warmer
- Emergency cart
- Equipment storage (e.g., stretchers, beds, wheelchairs, infusion pumps, patient warming devices, patient-controlled analgesia pumps, implantable cardioverter defibrillators)
- Point-of-care testing (blood gas laboratory)

- Radiographic view box
- Patient toilet
- Patient nourishment
- Medical records storage
- Computers (stationery and mobile)
- Procedure cart
- Patient education bulletin board
- Nursing station
- Physician dictation
- Staff toilet
- Staff lounge
- Staff locker room

PACU PHASE II
- Clean storage
- Dirty or soiled utility
- Medication dispensing unit (e.g., Pyxis, Omnicell)
- Patient toilet
- Emergency cart
- Equipment storage (e.g., stretchers, beds, wheelchairs)
- Blanket warmer
- Patient nourishment
- Patient education bulletin board
- Computers (stationery and mobile)
- Nursing station
- Physician dictation
- Staff toilet
- Staff lounge
- Staff locker room

*This list is not meant to be all inclusive. It should serve as a guide to help determine the needs of the institution.

Recommendations 2010-2012 Practice Recommendation 3 provides a list of suggested equipment for a preoperative holding area, PACU Phase I, and PACU Phase II.[4]

Malignant hyperthermia (MH) is a rare but potentially fatal complication of anesthesia. An MH box or cart or the equivalent supplies in the PACU Phase I is essential. The Malignant Hyperthermia Association of the United States has a recommended list of supplies for MH emergency cases (Box 1-3; see also Chapter 53).[6]

Institutions where intensive care patients recover in the PACU should have an emergency or "travel box" of medications and supplies available for use in transportation. Each institution may choose to have a dedicated travel box or use the standard emergency drug box, which can be secured in a medication room or automated medication dispensing cabinet.

Readily available bedside supplies may vary between institutions depending on the types of patients and volume. However, some essential supplies should be at every patient bedside. In addition to the aforementioned airway supplies, several means of oxygen delivery (see Chapter 28), suction catheters and tubing, gloves, emesis basins, and tissues should be immediately available at the bedside. Bedside supplies should be limited to only essential items to ensure that they are stocked and easily retrieved by all personnel.

Other supplies that need to be readily available can be stored in a variety of ways. If the clean storage room is in close proximity to all patient bays and has a user-friendly system, equipment can be left there and retrieved at the time it is needed. If the room design does not allow for quick retrieval of supplies from the clean storage room, consideration should be given to a storage system located in the immediate proximity of patient bays. This system could be a cart that would be moved from bay to bay or built-in cupboards that would service several bays. It is essential that staff members

---

BOX 1-2   Contents of Anesthesia PACU Emergency Bag

MAIN COMPARTMENT
- ET tubes with stylet and syringe (6.0, 7.0, 8.0)
- Extra ET tube (5.0, 5.5, 6.0, 6.5, 7.0, 7.5, 8.0)
- Light wand with ET tube
- Bougie
- Laryngoscope with blades (MacIntosh 3 and 4, Miller 2 and 4)
- Face mask, clear (2)
- Pediatric ET tubes (2.5, 3.0, 3.5, 4.0)
- Succinylcholine
- Sodium pentothal

FRONT COMPARTMENT
- Guedel airway (red, green, yellow)
- Disposable airway
- Yankauer suction
- Breathing circuit
- Nasopharyngeal airway (6.5, 7.5, 8.5)

SIDE POCKET
- Syringes
- Alcohol pads

BACK POCKET EMERGENCY KIT
- Cricothyrotomy
- Nasal cannula
- Laryngeal mask airway 3, 4, 5
- 60-mL syringes (2)

PACU, Postanesthesia care unit; *ET*, endotracheal.

---

are involved in the choice of a storage system so their needs are met.

Institutions that have 24-hour equipment delivery service, which allows for just-in-time delivery, may not need to store such items as IV pumps, pneumatic compression devices, forced air warming devices, and IV poles for transport. However, if these items are not readily available, they should be stored on the unit.

Pain management is an essential part of the patient care delivered in the PACU. If the institution uses IV patient-controlled analgesia pumps and epidural pumps for patient-controlled analgesia, a supply of this equipment should be kept in the PACU for ready availability. The PACU is a critical care unit and should therefore have a ventilator available at all times. Individual institutional policy governs which department is responsible for setting up and maintaining of any ventilators.

SUMMARY

Many changes in the care of perianesthesia patients have occurred in the last 60 years, and continued change is inevitable. Thoughtful planning and interdisciplinary communication are essential for the space and equipment to continue to meet the patient care needs in PACUs.

BOX 1-3   Malignant Hyperthermia Cart or Kit Supplies

An MH cart or kit that contains the following drugs, equipment, supplies, and forms should be immediately accessible to ORs and the PACU.

DRUGS
- Dantrolene sodium IV, 36 vials (each diluted with 60-mL sterile water)
- Sterile water for injection USP (without a bacteriostatic agent) to reconstitute dantrolene, 1000 mL (2)
- Sodium bicarbonate (8.4%), 50 mL (5)
- Furosemide, 40 mg/ampule (4 ampules)
- D50%, 50-mL vials (2)
- Calcium chloride (10%; 2)
- Regular insulin, 100 units/mL (1; refrigerated)
- Lidocaine HCl (2%), 1 box (2 g) or 20 mL vials (5)

GENERAL EQUIPMENT
- Syringes (60 mL; 5) to dilute dantrolene
- Mini spike IV additive pins (2) and Multi-Ad fluid transfer sets (2; to reconstitute dantrolene)

- IV catheters: 16-gauge, 18-gauge, 20-gauge, 2-inch; 22-gauge, 1-inch; 24-gauge, ¾-inch (4 each; for IV access and arterial line)
- NG tubes: sizes appropriate for the patient population
- Blood pump
- Irrigation tray with piston syringe (1) for NG irrigation
- Toomey irrigation syringes (60 mL; 2) for NG irrigation
- Large clear plastic bags for ice
- Bucket for ice
- Disposable cold packs (4)

MONITORING EQUIPMENT
- Esophageal or other core temperature probes
- Central venous pressure kits (sizes appropriate to the patient population)
- Transducer kit

Continued

BOX 1-3   Malignant Hyperthermia Cart or Kit Supplies—cont'd

DRIP SUPPLIES
- D$_5$W, 250 mL (1)
- Microdrip IV set (1)

NURSING SUPPLIES
- Large sterile Steri-Drape (for rapid drape of wound)
- Three-way irrigating urinary catheters: sizes appropriate for the patient population
- Urine meter (1)
- Toomey irrigation syringe (60 mL; 2)
- Rectal tubes: sizes (Malecot drain) 14F, 16F, 32F, 34F
- Large clear plastic bags for ice (4)
- Small plastic bags for ice (4)
- Tray for ice

LABORATORY TESTING SUPPLIES
- Syringes (3 mL) or arterial blood gas kits (6)
- Blood specimen tubes (each test should have two pediatric and two large tubes): (A) creatine kinase, myoglobin, sequential multiple analysis (SMA 19 [lactate dehydrogenase, electrolytes, thyroid studies]); (B) prothrombin time/partial thromboplastin time, fibrinogen, fibrin split products; (C) complete blood cell count, platelets; (D) blood gas syringe (lactic acid level)
- Urine cup (2), myoglobin level
- Urine dipstick, hemoglobin

FORMS (OR ORDER SETS IN COMPUTERIZED PROVIDER ORDER ENTRY APPLICATION)
- Laboratory request forms: arterial blood gas form (6), hematology form (2), chemistry form (2), coagulation form (2), urinalysis form (2), physician order form (2)
- Adverse Metabolic Reaction to Anesthesia report form (obtained from the Malignant Hyperthermia Association of United States)
- Consult form

MH, Malignant hyperthermia; *OR*, operating room; *PACU*, postanesthesia care unit; *IV*, intravenous; *NG*, nasogastric.

REFERENCES

1. American Society of PeriAnesthesia Nurses: *ASPAN's history timeline*, available at www.aspan.org/AboutUs/History/tabid/3146/Default.aspx. Accessed August 15, 2011.
2. Israel JS, DeKornfeld TJ: *Recovery room care*, ed 2, Chicago, 1987, Year Book Medical Publishers.
3. Nicholau D: The postanesthesia care unit. In Miller RD, editor: *Miller's anesthesia*, ed 7, Philadelphia, 2009, Churchill Livingstone.
4. American Society of PeriAnesthesia Nurses: *Perianesthesia nursing standards and practice recommendations 2010–2012*, Cherry Hill, NJ, 2010, ASPAN.
5. Michigan Department of Community Health: *The 2007 minimum design standards for health care facilities in Michigan*, available at www.michigan.gov/documents/mdch/bhs_2007_Minimum_Design_Standards_Final_PDF_Doc._198958_7.pdf. Accessed February 10, 2012.
6. Malignant Hyperthermia Association of the United States: *Drugs, equipment, and Dantrolene—managing MH*, available at http://medical.mhaus.org/index.cfm/fuseaction/Online-Brochures.Display/BrochurePK/B5DBDF12-20C3-4537-948C098DAB0777E3.cfm. Accessed December 4, 2011.

2 Perianesthesia Nursing as a Specialty

Sarah M. I. Cartwright, BA, RN, CAPA, and
Susan M. Andrews, BAN, MA, RN, CAPA

Perianesthesia nursing is a diverse field that encompasses patient care in a variety of settings. Recognition of perianesthesia nursing as a critical care specialty is well established. The main goal of the perianesthesia nurse is to provide competent, efficient care to patients and their families who are experiencing an anesthetic event. This care can be given in a traditional care setting, such as the hospital setting, or in a nontraditional care environment, such as a physician's office. Where there is an opportunity for a patient to experience anesthesia—from moderate sedation to general anesthesia—there is an opportunity for a perianesthesia nurse to provide care.

Recent history has been witness to a number of significant factors that have influenced the practice of perianesthesia nursing. Among these factors are the emphasis on cost containment in health care; declining reimbursement for medical services; the aging and increased acuity level of the population; advances in technology; advances in pharmaceutical therapy; and fast-tracking of patients through the postanesthesia recovery process.

The American Society of PeriAnesthesia Nurses (ASPAN) is the professional organization that represents the professional interests of perianesthesia nurses and sets the clinical standards of care in this specialty in the United States and its territories. In an effort to define the role of the perianesthesia nurse, ASPAN has published a formal *Scope of Practice* document (Box 2-1) that addresses the core, dimensions, boundaries, and intersections of perianesthesia nursing practice.[1] The members and governing bodies partner to establish practice standards, guidelines, and evidenced-based practices to promote safe patient care. These standards encourage competent practice through their use, as vetted through peer review processes and member representation. The guidelines define practice issues such as evaluation of patient condition, practice statements for staffing patterns, use of unlicensed care personnel, and overflow of intensive care patients. ASPAN also partners with other nursing professional organizations to establish professional nursing standards advocating for safe conditions for both the patient and the caregiver.[1]

Perianesthesia nursing is practiced in multiple modalities, both inpatient and outpatient, within the hospital setting and in free-standing practice settings (Box 2-2). The continued emphasis on cost containment has stimulated the regionalization of health care and the development of tertiary care centers in major cities, while primary care has increasingly moved to ambulatory settings.[2] As a consequence, perianesthesia nursing is practiced in a variety of traditional and nontraditional settings, from the physician's office to recovery care centers to highly specialized postanesthesia care units (PACUs) in dedicated medical centers, such as eye institutes and surgical hospitals as well as practice sites that include dental clinics, ambulatory surgery centers, office-based procedure areas, endoscopy suites, and pain management centers.

The traditional hospital-based approach is most prevalent with perianesthesia nurses practicing in areas from preoperative evaluation and pretesting to the PACU and beyond. As patient care evolves, the nontraditional perianesthesia environments are becoming more frequently used and in demand. The care provided by the perianesthesia nurse is similar in fashion regardless of the location. The use of outstanding assessment skills, monitoring, and use of specific specialized knowledge are needed regardless of the physical site and setting. The patient experiences this care initially in the pretesting and evaluation area, followed by the immediate pre-procedure evaluation, monitoring of the patient during and immediately after anesthesia, during phase II recovery, and through extended observation as necessary. The detail and care required during each one of these phases depends on the patient, procedure, anesthetic agent, and care environment.

The perianesthesia environment is delineated by the following phases: preanesthesia phase (preanesthetic evaluation and preanesthesia on the day of procedure), postanesthesia phase I, postanesthesia phase II, and extended observation (formerly known as phase III).[1] Care during all

BOX 2-1   Scope of Practice: Perianesthesia Nursing

The American Society of PeriAnesthesia Nurses (ASPAN), the professional organization for the specialty of perianesthesia nursing, is responsible for the defining and establishing of the scope of perianesthesia nursing. In doing so, ASPAN recognizes the role of the American Nurses Association (ANA) in defining the scope of practice for the nursing profession as a whole.

ASPAN supports the ANA Social Policy Statement 2003.[1,2] This statement charges specialty nursing organizations with definition of their individual scope of practice and identification of the characteristics within their unique specialty areas.

Evolving professional and societal demands have necessitated a statement clarifying the scope of perianesthesia nursing practice. Given rapid changes in health care delivery, trends, and technologies, the task of definition of this scope is complex. This document allows for flexibility in response to emerging issues and technologies in health care delivery and the practice of perianesthesia nursing.

The Scope of Perianesthesia Nursing Practice involves the age-specific assessment, diagnosis, intervention, and evaluation of individuals within the perianesthesia continuum. Those individuals have had or will have sedation/analgesia and/or anesthesia for surgical, diagnostic, or therapeutic procedures. Our practice is systematic, integrative, and holistic and involves critical thinking, clinical decision making and inquiry. ASPAN strives to promote an environment in which the perianesthesia nurse can deliver quality care among a diverse population within a multidisciplinary healthcare team.

This scope of practice includes, but is not limited to:
- Preanesthesia Level of Care
  - Preadmission
  - Day of Surgery/Procedure
- Postanesthesia Levels of Care
  - Phase I
  - Phase II
  - Extended Observation

The delivery of care includes, but is not limited to, the following environments:
- Hospitals
- Ambulatory Surgery Units/Centers
- Procedural Areas (e.g., Cardiology, ECT, GI/Endoscopy, Interventional and Diagnostic Radiology, Oncology, Pain Management, etc.)
- Obstetrical Units
- Office Based Settings

This specialty of perianesthesia nursing encompasses the care of the patient and family/significant other along the perianesthesia continuum of care—Preanesthesia, Postanesthesia Phase I, Phase II, and Extended Observation. Characteristics unique to perianesthesia practice are:

PREANESTHESIA PHASE
PREADMISSION
The nursing roles in this phase focus on physical, psychological, sociocultural and spiritual preparation for the experience. Interview and assessment techniques are used to identify potential or actual problems. Education and interventions are initiated to optimize positive outcomes.
DAY OF SURGERY/PROCEDURE
The nursing roles in this phase focus on validating existing information, reinforcing preoperative teaching, reviewing discharge instructions and providing nursing care to complete preparation for the experience.

POSTANESTHESIA PHASE
POSTANESTHESIA PHASE I
The nursing roles in this phase focus on providing postanesthesia nursing in the immediate postanesthesia period, transitioning to Phase II, the in-patient setting, or to an intensive care setting for continued care. Basic life-sustaining needs are of the highest priority. Constant vigilance is required during this phase.
POSTANESTHESIA PHASE II
The nursing roles in this phase focus on preparation for care in the home or an extended care environment.
EXTENDED CARE
The nursing roles in this phase focus on providing care when extended observation/intervention after discharge from Phase I or Phase II is required.

Perianesthesia nursing roles include those of patient care, research, administration, management, education, consultation, and advocacy. The specialty practice of perianesthesia nursing is defined through the implementation

BOX 2-1   Scope of Practice: Perianesthesia Nursing—cont'd

of specific role functions that are delineated in documents including *ASPAN's Perianesthesia Nursing Core Curriculum: Preoperative, Phase I and Phase II PACU Nursing*[3] and the *Standards of Perianesthesia Nursing Practice.*[4] The scope of perianesthesia nursing practice is also regulated by policies and procedures dictated by the hospital/facility, state and federal regulatory agencies, and national accreditation bodies.

Professional behaviors inherent in perianesthesia practice are the acquisition and application of a specialized body of knowledge and skills, accountability and responsibility, communication, autonomy, and collaborative relationships with others. Resources to support this defined body of knowledge and nursing practice include ASPAN's *Perianesthesia Nursing Core Curriculum: Preoperative, Phase I and Phase II PACU Nursing,*[3] *Standards of Perianesthesia Nursing Practice,*[4] and *Competency Based Orientation and Credentialing Program for the Registered Nurse in the Perianesthesia Setting.*[5] Certification in perianesthesia nursing (Certified Post Anesthesia Nurse: CPAN® and Certified Ambulatory Perianesthesia Nurse: CAPA®) is recognized by ASPAN as it validates the defined body of knowledge for perianesthesia nursing practice.

ASPAN interacts with other professional groups to advance the delivery of quality care. These include but may not be limited to:

- Ambulatory Surgery Center Association (ACS)
- American Association of Anesthesia Assistants (AAAA)
- American Association of Clinical Directors (AACD)
- American Association of Colleges of Nursing (AACN)
- American Association of Critical Care Nurses (AACN)
- American Association of Nurse Anesthetists (AANA)
- American Board of Perianesthesia Nursing Certification (ABPANC)
- American Nurses Association (ANA)
- American Society of Anesthesiologists (ASA)
- American Society of Pain Management Nurses (ASPMN)
- American Society of Plastic Surgical Nurses (ASPSN)
- Anesthesia Patient Safety Foundation (APSF)
- Association of periOperative Registered Nurses (AORN)
- Association of Radiologic and Imaging Nurses (ARIN)
- Association of Women's Health, Obstetric and Neonatal Nurses (AWHONN)
- British Anaesthetic & Recovery Nurses Association (BARNA)
- Council of Surgical and Perioperative Safety (CSPS)
- Irish Anaesthetic and Recovery Nurses Association (IARNA)
- National Association of Clinical Nurse Specialists (NACNS)
- National Association of Perianesthesia Nurses of Canada (NAPANc)
- National League for Nursing (NLN)
- National Student Nurses Association (NSNA)
- Nursing Organizations Alliance (NOA)
- Society for Ambulatory Anesthesia (SAMBA)
- Society for Perioperative Assessment and Quality Improvement (SPAQI)
- Society of Gastroenterology Nurses and Associates (SGNA)
- Society of Office Based Anesthesia (SOBA)

This *Scope of Perianesthesia Nursing Practice* document defines the specialty practice of perianesthesia nursing. The intent of this document is to conceptualize practice and provide education to practitioners, educators, researchers, and administrators, and to inform other health professions, legislators and the public about perianesthesia nursing's participation in and contribution to health care.

REFERENCES:
1. American Nurses Association: *Nursing's social policy statement: second edition*, Washington, DC, 2003, available at nursesbooks.org.
2. American Nurses Association: *Nursing scope and standards of practice*, Washington, DC, 2004, available at nursesbooks.org.
3. Schick L, Windle PE, editors: *Perianesthesia nursing core curriculum: preoperative, phase I, and phase II nursing*, Philadelphia, 2010, Saunders.
4. American Society of PeriAnesthesia Nurses: *Standards of perianesthesia nursing practice 2008–2010*, Cherry Hill, NJ, 2008, ASPAN.
5. American Society of PeriAnesthesia Nurses: *Competency based orientation and credentialing program for the registered nurse in the perianesthesia setting*, Cherry Hill, NJ, 2009, ASPAN.

From The American Society of PeriAnesthesia Nurses: *Perianesthesia nursing standards and practice recommendations 2010–2012*, Cherry Hill, NJ, 2010, ASPAN. Reprinted with permission.
ECT, Electroconvulsive therapy; *GI,* gastrointestinal.

BOX 2-2   Perianesthesia Practice Settings

- Hospital (inpatient and outpatient units)
  - Postanesthesia care unit
  - Ambulatory surgery unit
  - Endoscopy unit
  - Radiology unit
  - Obstetric unit
  - Cardiology unit
  - Oncology unit
  - Pain management unit
  - Special care unit
- Surgical hospital
- Free-standing ambulatory surgery unit
- Recovery care center
- Office-based setting
  - Physician (medical or surgical)
  - Dental
  - Plastic surgery

phases assists the patient with transition through the perianesthetic event. The care provided to the perianesthesia patient by the perianesthesia nurse must be delivered with the understanding that it is critical care requiring critical thinking. The perianesthesia patient is most vulnerable during and immediately after anesthesia when the most basic functions are controlled by the providers.[3] Perianesthesia nurses advocate for their patients during this most vulnerable time. This advocacy begins with the preanesthetic evaluation, in which system reviews identify potential complications and continues through the postanesthesia experience with specific and individualized discharge teaching.[3]

ROLES OF PERIANESTHESIA NURSES THROUGH THE CONTINUUM OF CARE

Role of the Perianesthesia Nurse in the Preoperative Evaluation, Preadmission Testing, and Preanesthesia Evaluation Setting

The preanesthesia evaluation establishes the initial contact of the perianesthesia nurse with the patient and the patient's support persons. This initial contact is crucial because it establishes the baseline trust the patient will have in the care provided to them during this vulnerable time. The purpose of this preoperative evaluation is to identify potential complications that can arise during the scheduled event, provide an opportunity for patient education, and establish guidelines in preparation for the procedure. The goal of the

preoperative phase is to provide a complete picture of the patient relevant to the procedure while providing education that will allow the patient to have decreased anxiety regarding the perianesthesia care.[1]

The preanesthesia evaluation can occur in several ways depending on the clinical enterprise from which the patient is receiving care. The assessment is a historical assessment that can be conducted in person, by telephone interview, or via a computer-based patient questionnaire application. This historical assessment is a full system review, psychosocial assessment, functional assessment, as well as medication reconciliation and learning needs assessment. A brief physical examination of heart and lung sounds as well as airway evaluation can also occur if the interview is conducted in person. Preanesthetic testing to include laboratory studies, cardiac studies, radiology examinations, and other tests, as deemed necessary per patient condition and physician orders, can also be completed at this time.

The perianesthesia nurse, in the preanesthesia evaluation period, acts as a liaison between multiple providers to obtain data that provide a complete picture of the patient's clinical presentation. The nurse can work with offsite physician offices to obtain referral records and test results. Competency-based orientation programs provide the perianesthesia nurse the judgment to complete the initial review of the documentation and send for further review or recommend additional testing as necessary. Partnering with other providers allows for the optimization of the risk stratification of the preanesthetic patient while reducing costs associated with redundant testing.

The patient population that the perianesthesia nurse encounters during this phase depends on the area of practice. Each specialty patient population brings challenges to the perianesthesia nurse and allows for further specialization within the field of perianesthesia nursing. The patient population can vary from pediatric to geriatric. Pediatric perianesthesia nurses face challenges with their patient populations that are different from, but just as challenging as, the geriatric population. Perianesthesia nurses in the nontraditional care areas also face challenges of limited resources and specialized assessments. For example, perianesthesia nurses in the pain management clinic area may be more aware of patient coping mechanisms related to chronic pain conditions that are not expressed in the general population.

The effects of the preanesthesia evaluation are multifaceted. The patient who is adequately prepared for the procedure has a better postprocedure outcome.[4] Information gathered during this phase is communicated forward to the next phase of care, which allows each subsequent perianesthesia care provider to follow the established plan of care while adapting the plan to meet each patient's individual circumstance or concern.[4] For example, patients identified in the preanesthesia evaluation as having a family history of malignant hyperthermia will have their anesthesia plans altered to reflect that information. Likewise, patients identified as having risk factors for postoperative nausea and vomiting will be given appropriate premedication to prevent nausea postprocedure. The effects of the preanesthesia evaluation are evidenced by patient readiness for the operative experience and further evidenced by limited incidences of patient complications during subsequent phases of perianesthesia care. Verifying historical assessment information with current physical status potentiates patient safety by addressing needs such as medication reconciliation, fall risk assessments and interventions, side or site verification of planned procedure, potential for compliance of instructions, and discharge planning assessments.[1]

Role of the Perianesthesia Nurse in Ambulatory Surgery and Preoperative Holding

The ambulatory surgery unit and preoperative holding areas provide the perianesthesia nurse the opportunity to interact with the patient and the patient's family or other support persons before the procedure. This time period may be surreal for the patient and the family with heightened anxiety as the level of vulnerability increases.[3] The perianesthesia nurse in this phase provides competent care including an assessment to identify any changes from the preanesthetic evaluation, pain and anxiety control, advocacy, and clinical skills such as intravenous line insertion and medication management. The perianesthesia nurse uses therapeutic communication skills with the patients and their families to ensure a calming environment and patient readiness for the scheduled procedure.

This phase of perianesthesia care can occur in any clinical practice site before the procedure. Hospital-based ambulatory settings can provide care for patients from same-day outpatient procedures to complex cases requiring lengthy postoperative admissions. The preprocedure perianesthesia nurse can promote the safety of the patient by verifying patient compliance and identifying any alteration from preanesthetic instructions, such as validation of NPO status. The perianesthesia nurse also reviews relevant preoperative testing results, current orders, completion of medication reconciliation to include last dose date and time

verification, comfort and safety needs, and verification of discharge planning such as validation of the postprocedure driver and care provider.[1]

The patient population under the care of the perianesthesia nurse depends on the provider's scope of care. In addition to the patient, this care period will include the patient's support structure of family members, friends, clergy, and other support providers. These additional support persons (e.g., family or friends) can provide relief from anxiety for the patient and may be able to provide the perianesthesia nurse with additional information the patient is unable to share because of heightened anxiety. It is important to note that, during all interactions with the patient and the patient's support system, the perianesthesia nurse's interaction must maintain patient privacy and respect.

After obtaining the day-of-procedure assessment update and initiating patient care preparation orders, the perianesthesia nurse hands off care. The critical thinking and interpretation of the assessment by the perianesthesia nurse is essential, as is the communication of this assessment along with any changes or concerns, to the procedure nurse who will be involved with the immediate care of the patient during the procedure. This vital communication provides the patient with the best opportunity for a safe, successful anesthetic event. While the patient is receiving care, the perianesthesia nurse continues to support the patient's family.

Role of the Perianesthesia Nurse in the Post Anesthesia Care Unit Phase I Recovery

The perianesthesia nurse in phase I recovery cares for patients in the PACU and provides care for patients who have completed their anesthetic event. The PACU is a critical care environment; therefore it is designed to provide active line-of-sight monitoring of patients who have undergone a general anesthetic. Phase I recovery is available in all areas for care after a general anesthetic, such as hospital-based surgery units, ambulatory surgery clinics, and office-based procedure areas. Because these patients have had their basic life-sustaining reflexes suppressed during their anesthetics, it is imperative for the perianesthesia nurse in this setting to be acutely aware of changes in the patient's status, such as a sudden oxygen desaturation possibly indicating a loss of airway. Phase I status is determined by the patient condition, rather than location of care.[1]

During this critical care period, the patient is acutely monitored and evaluated for subtle changes indicating a change in homeostasis. As the patient recovers from the anesthetic, the patient is vulnerable, uncertain of location, and often in pain. The perianesthesia nurse offers reassurance; assesses for pain and other physical indicators; and provides medication, monitoring, and additional comfort measures. Using therapeutic communication techniques, the perianesthesia nurse guides the patient through the experience, allowing the patient to express any needs. The perianesthesia nurse communicates frequently with the patient's support members, providing condition updates. The perianesthesia nurse also communicates frequently with the physician or anesthesia care provider to ensure an optimal continuum of care.

The perianesthesia nursing assessment includes integration of relevant preoperative information, such as patient comorbidities. Understanding the patient's anesthetic technique and potential consequences, such as airway management or resedation potential is critical to the patient's safe recovery. The perianesthesia nurse obtains information from the anesthesia provider regarding technique, length, and drugs administered to include reversal agents. Cardiovascular, pulmonary, and neurologic assessments are completed to validate return to baseline values following the administration of anesthetic agents. The critical aspect of this assessment cannot be understated. The PACU nurse is the primary care provider who uses critical care skills and training to detect early subtle changes that could become catastrophic without intervention. The PACU nurse assesses the patient for pain and discomfort using a variety of pain scales from an observational scale for sedated patients to the numeric scale for those who are more alert and able to answer questions. The patient's procedure will dictate additional assessments for wound assessment, potential for hypovolemia owing to hemorrhage, alteration in maintenance of normothermia, as well as additional physical assessments such as peripheral pulse verification. A thorough skin integrity assessment should also be performed to verify continued integrity of skin structures or identify concerns with skin integrity from the operative procedure or positioning.[1]

As in any critical care nursing unit, the PACU nurse may care for patients who need a ventilator, requiring hemodynamic intravenous medication administration and intensive cardiac monitoring. If the requirements of the phase I recovery for the institution includes care and management of these most critical patients, appropriate competencies—to include patient assessment and intervention, advanced cardiac monitoring skills, advanced hemodynamic medication administration, and advanced pulmonary care, such as ventilator management

skills—must be included in the competency-based orientation program for the phase I PACU nurse.

Communication with the anesthesia care team to understand the patient's emotional status pre-procedure will allow the perianesthesia nurse to provide the appropriate emotional support to the emerging patient who will have anxiety because of the surgical event, surgical findings, and general loss of control. Patients who experience pre-procedure heightened levels of anxiety often emerge from anesthesia in the PACU with continued expressions of anxiety and may lash out as a result of anxiety, fear, or pain.

The patient population receiving care by the perianesthesia nurse in the PACU depends on the organization's scope of care and can include patients from the pediatric age group to patients in the geriatric population. Changing dynamics toward open visitation in the PACU allow for this care period to include the patient's support structure of family members, friends, clergy, and other support providers. These individuals may give the perianesthesia nurse additional support by helping to relieve patient anxiety during this postanesthesia experience and sharing an understanding of the patient's normal response to pain and other stimuli, as these responses may still be depressed from the anesthetic (see Chapter 3). ASPAN has developed a position statement specifically targeting patient visitation in the PACU.[1]

The acuity of inpatient cases has increased significantly. In addition, the increasing age of the population in the United States means that many surgical patients have a number of concomitant chronic problems, such as chronic obstructive lung disease, diabetes mellitus, and chronic heart conditions. The provision of quality care in the PACU necessitates a strong, knowledgeable clinician with excellent skills using critical thinking to the fullest while supporting patients, their families, and other caregivers.

In many institutions, discharge from PACU Phase I occurs when the patient has met predetermined discharge criteria established in conjunction with the anesthesia providers and medical staff in lieu of individual orders.[1] The phase I perianesthesia nurse's critical judgment and skill is crucial because many patients are not seen and evaluated by a physician or anesthesia provider before leaving this intense monitoring setting. Items for consideration to determine discharge eligibility include airway patency, independent and dependent respiratory function, and gas exchange as validated by oxygen saturation. The patient's ability to maintain cardiac and hemodynamic stability, normothermia, expected level of consciousness, and sensory–motor function should be assessed. Further assessments include pain and comfort status, postoperative nausea and vomiting, and emotional status.[1] Patency of lines, completion of medication administration, and wound integrity are also considered when determining discharge eligibility. When the patient is deemed eligible for discharge to the next level of care, the patient is discharged from phase I to either an inpatient hospital bed or to phase II recovery in anticipation of discharge to home.[1]

In an effort at cost containment, hospitals have increased the use of the PACU. In the critical care setting, highly skilled perianesthesia nursing staff and proximity to anesthesia providers has made the PACU a prime location for special procedures, such as electroconvulsive therapy (ECT), elective cardioversion, and endoscopic examination.[1] In addition, the PACU is often used for services such as pain clinics for block placement; as preoperative holding areas (for both inpatient and outpatient services); as a recovery area for remote procedure patients from areas such as interventional radiology and cardiology; and as an overflow unit when intensive care unit or inpatient beds are full.[1] Although some of these changes seem to create less than optimal conditions for patient care, the creative collaboration of all health care practitioners can meet the challenges of the rapidly changing health care environment. PACUs have the unique opportunity to be innovative and creative in implementation of methods to meet these challenges while continuing to support the operating room schedule and surgical PACU patients within the organizational and operational structure of the unit.[1]

Role of the Perianesthesia Nurse in the Postanesthesia Phase II Recovery

Patients who have met discharge criteria for phase I recovery are transferred to phase II recovery where they continue to respond to interventions aimed at recovering from the anesthetic agents. Assessment of the phase II patient continues as with the phase I patient. Validation of hemodynamic stability is monitored as the patient's activity level increases. Thermoregulation monitoring continues. Verification of the patient's ability to swallow before the administration of diet or medications by mouth is completed. Of note, the patients in this phase of recovery may have less fluctuation in their vital signs as their condition stabilizes toward baseline. They may be more vocal regarding pain management needs or postoperative nausea. Their families are more involved with their care as they are more alert and responsive to stimuli. These patients often alter their position from lying to sitting and consume clear liquids.[1]

The patients in phase II recovery are preparing for discharge to home following their anesthesia event. Verification of emotional readiness for discharge of both the patient and caregiver is to be completed by the phase II perianesthesia nurse, because concerns not previously identified can occur in this postoperative period. Continued discharge teaching that includes home care instructions are given to both the patient and the care provider, to include contact numbers for further information. Should the perianesthesia nurse encounter any concerns with a safe discharge, the perianesthesia nurse should escalate the concerns to the physician provider for additional intervention.[1]

The phase II setting may be present in an ambulatory surgery setting, or it may be a chair recovery area in an office-based procedure suite. As with phase I recovery, the patient's condition dictates the level of recovery more than the physical location.[1] Monitoring needs in phase II care are less intense because the patient should be at or near baseline before leaving the phase I setting.

As with previous areas, the patient population receiving care from the perianesthesia nurse is dependent on the provider's scope of care, pediatric through geriatric. In the phase II setting, discharge education and validation of understanding is completed with the patient and their support structure of family members, friends, clergy, and other support providers.

Role of the Perianesthesia Nurse in the Fast-Tracking of Recovery Patients to Phase II

Fast-tracking has become a popular concept in the PACU. Fast-tracking involves admission of patients from the operating room directly to phase II and the bypass of phase I for both the ambulatory and inpatient.[1] These patients must meet discharge criteria for phase I before leaving the operating room, and as such, policies and procedures on fast-tracking should be developed collaboratively with the involvement of nursing and anesthesia personnel.[1] Policies should address patient selection and criteria for direct admission to phase II (inpatient floor), patient monitoring, and outpatient discharge. Nurses in the phase II unit must be competent to handle any unexpected outcome that may be a direct result of fast-tracking.

ASPAN supports the use of fast-tracking within the bounds of safe patient care.[1] Patient selection before fast-tracking is vital to decrease potential complications. Appropriate candidates include those who have motivation to progress the postoperative care, short-acting anesthetic agents, limited preexisting comorbidities, and collaborative care teams who communicate well with one another. Criteria for discharge from the operating room should include level of consciousness (awake or easily aroused), hemodynamic stability (towards baseline), appropriate gas exchange (patient maintaining oxygen saturation on room air), limited pain, nausea, and stable wound site (no active bleeding). Phase II is a level of care, not a physical place. As a result, before fast-tracking the patient needs clinical assessments, and potential outcomes should be assessed and honored.[1]

Role of the Perianesthesia Nurse in Extended Observation

Following the assessment of the patient in phase II, some patients do not meet discharge criteria related to continued pain or nausea management needs or social indications, such as no appropriate transportation available. These patients can receive care in an extended observation unit maintained under the perianesthesia department. In this setting, the patient continues to be monitored for hemodynamics, respiratory and circulatory stability, and pain control. Additional assessment for skin integrity to include the surgical site and dressing are completed and documented. The perianesthesia nurse provides emotional support and communication with the patient and any support members present. Administration of medications, diet, and treatments can occur. The patient's safety is maintained through fall risk assessments and additional risk identifiers. These patients continue to have their discharge needs managed by the perianesthesia nurse, who then contacts appropriate resources to help facilitate discharge to the next level of care.[1]

NONTRADITIONAL PERIANESTHESIA NURSE SETTINGS

The increasingly competitive business environment for health care and technologic advances has significantly increased the use of ambulatory surgical settings. The emergence of surgical hospitals has added to the equation. These multispecialty facilities provide both inpatient and outpatient surgical services. By functioning much the same as an ambulatory surgery center (ASC), the surgical hospital operates in a cost-effective mode. The focus is on quick turnovers and a user-friendly atmosphere—hallmarks that make the ASC successful.

Additional areas of perianesthesia nursing include pain management centers; dental sedation sites; physician surgical centers such as vascular, ophthalmology, and plastic surgery centers; and endoscopy suites. Radiology practice sites that administer sedation have roles for perianesthesia nurses, from diagnostic testing to interventional radiology services.

Perianesthesia nurses may adapt their clinical skills to the management of sedation sites and staff. Using their unique perspective on patients and care needs, these nurses help to develop outpatient service centers where anesthesia is administered at various levels.

AREAS FOR GROWTH WITHIN PERIANESTHESIA NURSING

The American Board of Perianesthesia Nursing Certification (ABPANC)[5] was created in 1985 by ASPAN to sponsor certification programs for qualified registered nurses who care for patients who have experienced sedation, analgesia, and anesthesia. The perianesthesia nurse who meets current eligibility requirements is able to complete a comprehensive examination to detail advanced competency in the role of a perianesthesia nurse. The credentials are divided into two specialties, Certified Post Anesthesia Nurse (CPAN) and Certified Ambulatory PeriAnesthesia (CAPA) nurse, to differentiate between the roles of the perianesthesia nurse. Both credentials require the nurse to have 1800 hours of qualified experience before the examination period. Continued credentialing is determined by the completion of continuing education via contact hours through approved providers or re-examination every 3 years.[5]

The CPAN credential is most appropriate for the perianesthesia nurse whose care is focused in the Phase I PACU. This examination concentrates on the physiologic needs of the patient with emphasis on critical care applications. The examination also includes patient safety, advocacy, and cognitive or behavioral needs.[5]

The CAPA credential is most appropriate for the perianesthesia nurse who functions in roles outside of the Phase I PACU, such as preadmission testing, day surgery phase II, and office-based settings. This examination also focuses on the physiologic needs of the patient, but with emphasis on the needs of an ambulatory patient environment, such as patient teaching and noncritical care monitoring. Also included on the examination are questions on patient advocacy, cognitive and behavioral needs, and patient safety.[5]

The goal of advanced certification is to validate the specialty knowledge of the perianesthesia nurse. The certification verifies the perianesthesia nurse's knowledge of prerequisites, such as anatomy and physiology, medication administration and complications, anesthesia techniques and complication management, advanced assessment skills, critical care evaluations, and the ability to adapt to changing patient conditions.[5]

SUMMARY

The perianesthesia environment can be both challenging and rewarding for nurses who choose to work in this specialty area. Nurses who enjoy a fast pace and unexpected emergencies, balanced with critical independent decision-making skills, thrive in one of the many different opportunities that perianesthesia nursing provides. There are multiple opportunities during the perianesthesia continuum of care for the perianesthesia nurse to learn, grow, adapt, and interact with a diverse patient population. The opportunity to advocate for the patient population from completion of the initial assessment through discharge planning is a hallmark of this specialty nursing care.

REFERENCES

1. American Society of PeriAnesthesia Nurses: *Perianesthesia nursing standards and practice recommendations 2010–2012,* Cherry Hill, NJ, 2010, ASPAN.
2. Manchikanti L, et al: *Ambulatory surgery centers and interventional techniques: a look at long-term survival,* available at www.painphysicianjournal.com/2011/march/2011;14;E177-E215.pdf. Accessed June 26, 2011.
3. Shafer A, et al: *Preoperative anxiety and fear: a comparison of assessments by patients and anesthesia and surgery residents,* available at www.anesthesia-analgesia.org/content/83/6/1285.full.pdf. Accessed June 26, 2011.
4. Schoofs Hundt A, et al: *Outpatient surgery and patient safety—the patient's voice,* available at www.ncbi.nlm.nih.gov/books/NBK20595/. Accessed June 26, 2011.
5. American Board of PeriAnesthesia Nursing: *CPAN and CAPA certification: nursing passion in action,* available at www.cpancapa.org. Accessed June 26, 2011.

THE POSTANESTHESIA CARE UNIT

Management and Policies

Susan M. Andrews, BAN, MA, RN, CAPA, and
Sarah M. I. Cartwright, BA, RN, CAPA

All management procedures and policies of the postanesthesia care unit (PACU) should be established through joint efforts of the PACU staff, the nurse manager, and the medical director of the unit. These procedures and policies should be written and readily available to all staff working in the PACU and all advanced practice nurses or physicians using the area for care of patients.

Policies are guidelines that give direction and have been approved by the administration of the institution. Procedures specify how a policy is to be implemented and are either managerial in scope or specific to clinical nursing methods. The PACU policies and procedures should be reviewed periodically, so that appropriate changes can be made when necessary. Policies and procedures must always reflect the actual practice of the unit.

PURPOSE OF THE PACU

The PACU is designed and staffed for intensive observation and care of patients after a procedure for which an anesthetic agent is necessary. Criteria for admission to the PACU should be clearly outlined, and exceptions to the policy should be explicitly delineated.

The effects on staffing and the use of PACU beds for a multitude of services—such as cardiac catheterization, arteriography or specialized radiologic tests, electroshock therapy, other special procedures, or observation of patients who have undergone special procedures—have created special concerns in the management of the PACU. Another recent development is the use of the PACU for patients of the intensive care unit, telemetry, or emergency departments when no beds are available in those areas of the hospital. A shortage of hospital medical and surgical beds has also turned the PACU into a holding area for surgical patients awaiting inpatient bed availability. Specific policies and procedures that address any special procedures performed in the PACU and nursing care of these nonsurgical and post-PACU patients need to be developed and in place before these situations arise. A list of potential PACU policy and procedure titles can be found in Box 3-1.

ORGANIZATIONAL STRUCTURE

One person should have ultimate responsibility for the management of the PACU. Typically, the title of this role is nurse manager, director, supervisor, clinical leader, or head nurse. For the purpose of clarity, this person with direct responsibility will be referred to as the *nurse manager*. The nurse manager is responsible for the administrative control of the PACU and typically reports directly to the surgical service, although it is possible that in an ambulatory surgery center the nurse manager will report to anesthesia services or a combination of surgery and anesthesia services. The reporting structure depends on the institution's organizational structure.

The chief of anesthesiology is usually the medical director of the PACU. In large institutions, if the chief of anesthesiology cannot fill this role because of other duties, the chief may appoint a designee to this position. The medical director works closely with the nurse manager to develop policies and procedures and to assist with continuing education activities for the nursing staff. The director may also be involved in the development and implementation of continuous quality improvement activities in the unit. Maintenance of a good working relationship between the perianesthesia nurse manager and the medical director of the unit is essential so that areas of concern can be addressed in a collaborative and productive fashion.

Patient Classification

Most PACUs have some type of patient classification system (PCS) either formal or informal. The most accurate PCSs are those that base the patient classification on length of stay in the PACU and intensity of the care required. The PCS can be used to justify budget for staffing and supplies as well as space requirements and charges for the PACU stay. For example, a patient with a classification of 1 has a lower charge than a patient with a classification of 3.

BOX 3-1   Suggested Policies and Procedures for the PACU

- Purpose and structure of the unit
  - Facility and unit philosophy and objectives
  - Scope of service (patient population)
  - Mission, vision, and values statements
- Administrative
  - Administrative organizational chart
  - Chain of command
  - Governing body
  - Job descriptions
  - Staffing patterns
  - Hours of operation
  - Standards of care
- Medical staff
  - Physician privileges
  - Physician credentialing procedure
  - Medical advisory committee
- Patient rights
  - Rights and responsibility statement
  - Ethical treatment
  - Patient grievance process
  - Advance directives
  - Health Insurance Portability and Accountability Act (HIPAA) privacy notice
- Admission
  - Criteria
  - Population served
  - Preoperative assessment
- Discharge
  - Criteria and scoring system
  - Patient instructions
  - Responsible adult escort
- Anesthesia requirements
  - Anesthesia consent
  - Monitoring of patients who receive anesthesia
  - Fast-tracking guidelines
- Consents
  - Informed consent
  - Minors
  - Power of attorney
  - Sterilization
  - Administration of blood products
  - Do not resuscitate (DNR) orders
  - Experimental treatment
  - Procurement of forensic evidence
  - Electroconvulsive therapy
  - Cardioversion
  - Hepatitis B immunization
  - Release of medical information
- Emergency procedures
  - Emergency eye wash station
  - CPR, basic cardiac life support (BCLS), and advanced cardiac life support (ACLS) standards
  - Malignant hyperthermia crisis
  - Cardiac arrest
- Equipment
  - Operative
  - Emergency

- Preventative maintenance program
- Repairs
- Medical device reporting
- Biomedical engineering requests
- Facilities management
  - Emergency generator protocol
  - Maintenance of fire warning system
  - Preventative maintenance program
  - Occupational Safety and Health Administration (OSHA) regulations
- Environment of care plans
  - Safety management
  - Utilities management
  - Life safety management
  - Medical equipment management
  - Employee safety
  - Security management
  - Hazardous materials management
  - Emergency preparedness
- Infection control
  - Universal precautions
  - Personal protective equipment
  - Disposal of contaminated needles and sharps
  - Transmission-based precautions
  - Hepatitis B vaccine
  - Handwashing
  - Housekeeping procedures
  - Operating room attire
  - Traffic patterns
  - Visitors
  - Restricted areas
- Information systems
  - Description and use of systems
  - Confidentiality and security agreements
  - System backup and retention policy
  - System access and password policy
- Employee health
  - Annual requirements
  - Tuberculosis testing requirements
  - Sick leave
  - Worker's compensation
- Patient care
  - PACU standards of care
  - National, state, and facility standards of care
  - Nurse:patient ratios
  - Preoperative testing requirements
  - Moderate sedation and analgesia guidelines
  - Postoperative monitoring procedures
  - Patient education requirements
- Physician orders
  - Standing preoperative orders
  - Standing anesthesia orders
  - Standing orders for specialty services (e.g., ophthalmology, total joint)

Continued

BOX 3-1	Suggested Policies and Procedures for the PACU—cont'd

- Quality management and performance improvement
  - Overview of quality management and performance improvement program
  - Goals of quality management and performance improvement program
  - Description of indicators and benchmarks
- Patient records
  - Consents
  - Confidentiality and HIPAA requirements
  - Electronic documentation
  - Order of medical record
  - Medical record retention
  - Release of information
- Safety
  - Fire safety
  - Electrical safety
  - Hazardous material training
  - Emergency preparedness training
  - Glutaraldehyde exposure monitoring
- Waste gas monitoring
- Exposure control plan
- Postexposure follow-up
- Bomb threat
- Violence in the workplace
- Body mechanics
- Radiation safety
- Control of radioactive materials
- Staff member rules and responsibilities
  - Orientation
  - Confidentiality
  - Security
  - Competency requirements
  - Performance appraisals
  - Required education and certification
  - Conflict of interest statement
- Supplies
  - Procurement and ordering
  - Sterilization
  - Storage
  - Annual inventory

Adapted from Shick L, Windle PE: *ASPAN's perianesthesia core curriculum: preprocedure, phase I and phase II PACU nursing,* ed 2, St. Louis, 2010, Saunders.

Developing a PCS for the PACU is difficult. Many variables must be considered and addressed when developing a PCS. Length of stay and anesthesia patient classification are starting points for PCS, but length of stay of each patient may vary significantly, and the acuity of a patient can change within a short period of time. Moreover, patient populations can range from pediatric to geriatric and can include minor to extensive surgical procedures, depending on the makeup and mission of the institution.

The advantages of a PCS include a more accurate assessment of the nursing time and energy needed for each patient, which helps a manager to estimate staffing requirements on the basis of the next day's schedule. Other advantages can include knowledge of the highest workload time periods each day, allowing the manager to flex staff accordingly. This allows PACU nurses the knowledge that the type of workload in the PACU, with its peaks and valleys, is acknowledged and management is responsive to their unique staffing needs.

Visitors

The merits and benefits of visitation in the PACU are well documented. Patient visitation lowers anxiety and decreases stress for both the patient and the family. The result is an increase in patient and family satisfaction and increased adherence to the recovery plan.[1,2] In the past, PACU visitation was restricted for reasons such as the lack of privacy, the acuity of the patients, and the fast turnover that is common to the PACU. Visitation may have been allowed only if staffing and the physical structure of the unit permitted. In many institutions a change in culture surrounding PACU visitation has shown that the positive outcomes from visitation have outweighed the real and perceived drawbacks. A main catalyst behind the change has been the lack of available postoperative beds, thus extending the stay in the PACU for many patients. Some patients may have a prolonged stay in the PACU while they await critical care, telemetry, or surgical beds in the nursing unit. As the frequency of morning admissions increases, the incidence rate of extended PACU stays also increases because of lack of postoperative bed availability.[1,3]

Part of the challenge with a change in the organizational culture to allow visitation in the PACU is that nursing care historically has concentrated on the care of the patient only. However, many family members also need nursing interventions, such as explanations of the PACU care provided to their loved ones, and require time and effort on the part of the nurses. However, PACU visitation can provide an excellent opportunity to start postoperative education with families.

Visitation times vary greatly, with some PACUs that still do not allow visitation and others that have adopted policies originally designed for other critical care units. Some PACUs may include a 5-minute visit each hour or a 20-minute visit every 4 hours, whereas other institutions have open visitation that is restricted only during the timeframe when a critical event is occurring in the PACU. Other criteria may include a limited number of family members at one time, the patient's desire for visitors, the unit needs, and the patient's condition. Privacy of other patients in the PACU must always be a consideration and priority.

Situations in which visitation should be encouraged include the following:
- Death of the patient may be imminent.
- The patient must return to surgery.
- The patient is a child whose physical and emotional well being may depend on the calming effect of the parent's presence.
- The patient's well being depends on the presence of a significant other. Patients in this category include persons with mental disabilities, mental illnesses, or profound sensory deficits.
- The patient needs a translator because of language differences.

As facilities renovate or build new surgical suites, the design of the perianesthesia area should accommodate patients and families. In addition, patient privacy and visitation must be considered. The PACU needs to allow for the comfort and privacy of the patient population who may need an extended PACU stay, including the ability to allow for family members to have extended visits in the PACU setting.

Patient Records

The postanesthesia care record is essential for every patient admitted to the PACU. Many institutions have evolved to total electronic documentation or a hybrid of computerized and paper documentation. Whether traditional paper documentation or electronic format is used, the record should be an accurate account of the patient's postanesthesia stay and the care that was provided. Anecdotal notes should detail admission observations. The assessment, planning, and implementation phases of the nursing process should be documented, and an evaluation of the patient's response to the care should be provided. A discharge summary should also be included.

The trend in many institutions is toward a fully electronic medical record, which allows multiple users in remote locations to have access to the medical record at the same time. The fully computerized record for the surgical patient begins in the preoperative evaluation phase and follows the patient through the PACU period to the ambulatory surgery unit or an inpatient unit. One of the important advantages of a computerized medical record includes immediate access by other health care practitioners involved in the patient's care. It can also be a time saver for nurses, because data entry is often accomplished with drop-down menus much like a checklist as well as documentation prompts for critical areas that must be completed before the record is closed, thus ensuring all required documentation has been completed. Disadvantages include the cost of installation and education and the time necessary to orient the staff to the system, as well as staff resistance to change from paper to computer charting.

Discharge of the Patient from the PACU

Written criteria for discharge of the patient from PACU must be available. At a minimum the criteria should include:
- The patient regained consciousness and is oriented to time and place (or return to baseline cognitive function).
- The patient's airway is clear and danger of vomiting and aspiration passed.
- The patient's circulatory and respiratory vital signs are stabilized.

The criteria for discharge of a patient from the PACU vary by the unit, location of transfer, anesthetic technique, and physiologic status. Ultimately the physician is in charge of the patient's discharge from the PACU. Predetermined criteria can be applied if the criteria have been approved by the physician staff members.

The use of a numeric scoring system for assessment of the patient's recovery from anesthesia is common. Many institutions have incorporated the postanesthesia recovery score as part of the discharge criteria. Box 3-2 shows an example of two discharge scoring systems. The Aldrete Scoring System was introduced by Aldrete and Kroulik in 1970 and was later modified by Dr. Aldrete to reflect oxygen saturation instead of color. Clinical assessment must also be used in the determination of a patient's readiness for discharge from the PACU. This scoring system does not include detailed observations such as urinary output, bleeding or other drainage, changing requirements for hemodynamic support, temperature trends, or patient's pain management needs. All these criteria should be considered in the determination of readiness for discharge. The unit policy and the

BOX 3-2   Discharge Scoring Systems

ALDRETE SCORING SYSTEM

RESPIRATION
- Ability to take deep breath and cough = 2
- Dyspnea/shallow breathing = 1
- Apnea = 0

O_2 SATURATION
- Maintenance of O_2 saturation greater than 92% on room air = 2
- O_2 inhalation needed to maintain O_2 saturation greater than 90% = 1
- O_2 saturation less than 90% even with supplemental oxygen = 0

CONSCIOUSNESS
- Fully awake = 2
- Arousable on calling = 1
- Not responding = 0

CIRCULATION
- BP ± 20 mm Hg preoperative value = 2
- BP ± 20 to 50 mm Hg preoperative value = 1
- BP ± 50 mm Hg preoperative value = 0

ACTIVITY
- Ability to move four extremities = 2
- Ability to move three extremities = 1
- Ability to move no extremities = 0

POST ANESTHETIC DISCHARGE SCORING SYSTEM

VITAL SIGNS
- BP and pulse within 20% preoperative value = 2
- BP and pulse within 20% to 40% preoperative value = 1
- BP and pulse greater than 40% preoperative value = 0

ACTIVITY
- Steady gait, no dizziness, or preoperative level met = 2
- Assistance needed = 1
- Inability to ambulate = 0

NAUSEA AND VOMITING
- Minimal or treated with oral medication = 2
- Moderate or treated with parenteral medication = 1
- Severe or continues despite treatment = 0

PAIN
- Controlled with oral analgesics and acceptable to patient:
  - Yes = 2
  - No = 1

SURGICAL BLEEDING
- Minimal or no dressing changes = 2
- Moderate or up to two dressing changes needed = 1
- Severe or more than three dressing changes needed = 0

From Ead H: From Aldrete to PADSS: reviewing discharge criteria after ambulatory surgery, *J Perianesth Nurs* 21(4): 259–267, 2006.
BP, Blood pressure.

established PACU discharge criteria determine the appropriate postanesthesia recovery score and physical condition for discharge from the PACU. The patient must have a preestablished score to be discharged from the PACU. Scores or conditions lower than the preestablished level necessitate evaluation by the anesthesia provider or surgeon and can result in an extension of the PACU stay or possible disposition to a special care or critical care unit.

Because patient conditions vary with surgical procedure, anesthesia used, use of analgesics, and patient response, no specific time requirements for the PACU stay can be stated. Professional judgment is needed to determine when the patient is ready for discharge from the PACU. A complete accurate report is required from the PACU nurse to the nurse who will be responsible for the care of the patient. Hand-off communication has been identified as an area in which patient safety can be compromised if not performed accurately.

When ambulatory surgical patients are discharged to home, other criteria should be assessed. These criteria may include the following: pain control to an acceptable level for the patient, control of nausea, ambulation in a manner consistent with the procedure and previous ability, and a responsible adult present to accompany the patient home. Some Phase II PACUs require the patient to void or tolerate oral fluids before discharge to home. The Post Anesthetic Discharge Scoring System is often used for assessing the readiness of the patient to be discharged home or to an extended observation area.[4]

Phase II patients should receive a follow-up visit by the anesthesia provider and be released as appropriate, or as in phase I where the nursing staff of the Phase II PACU are appropriately educated, a discharge by criteria policy that defines discharge parameters and allows the nurse to discharge the patient may be in effect. Discharge criteria should be developed to meet appropriate standards, but should be individualized to each PACU.

Home care instructions should be taught to the patient and responsible adult, both of whom should verbalize an understanding of the instructions. Written instructions should be given to the patient to take home. Information on what to do if a problem or question arises should be addressed, and emergency and routine telephone numbers must be included in the instructions.

Standards of Care

Every profession has the responsibility to identify and define its practice to protect consumers by ensuring the delivery of quality service.[1] The

American Society of PeriAnesthesia Nurses (ASPAN) *Perianesthesia Nursing Standards and Practice Recommendations* provides a basic framework for nurses who practice in all phases of the perianesthesia care specialty.[1] These standards have been devised to stand alone or be used in conjunction with other health care standards and are monitored, reviewed, revised, and updated regularly. A copy of these standards can be obtained from the ASPAN National Office, 90 Frontage Road, Cherry Hill, NJ 08034-1424, or ordered via the ASPAN website at www.aspan.org.

All preanesthesia, postanesthesia, and ambulatory surgical nurses should be familiar with their professional organization's standards of practice, and a copy of these standards should be available in each unit. The PACU may develop its own standards specific to the hospital, using the ASPAN standards as a reference, or adopt the ASPAN standards for use. If the PACU adopts the ASPAN standards, they must be adopted in their entirety or a policy must be added to note any exceptions. Any written standards must be attainable reflections of the actual practice.

Nurses must possess a minimum level of knowledge and ability. Standards are objective and are the same for all staff members, which means that an inexperienced nurse in the PACU is held to the same standard of practice as an experienced nurse. Standards are commonly used today in legal proceedings to measure the care a patient received. The ASPAN standards have been used in court proceedings, and many medical malpractice attorneys have the latest copy of the ASPAN *Perianesthesia Nursing Standards and Practice Recommendations* in their libraries.

Quality Management and Performance Improvement

A multidisciplinary team to address quality management process improvement in the PACU is essential to basic operations. The quality management team's composition should encompass management and staff level personnel. Members should at a minimum include the medical director, nurse manager, staff from both areas, and surgeons. Others to consider as either permanent or as ad hoc team members are: pharmacy, central distribution, the operating room manager and staff members, radiology, and respiratory therapy staff members. This quality team's mission should focus on current practices and processes that require improvement, as well as review and critique any events. They should also have the goal of discovering how and where systems might have failed and what changes or improvements can be initiated to prevent future occurrences. The goal

of this team is to improve processes thereby improving outcomes. Process improvement programs differ from the quality management programs of the past in that the emphasis on inspection has changed to an emphasis on continuous improvement. When excellent patient care is put first, departmental boundaries fade. The common, seamless focus becomes providing the patient with the best possible care.

The Centers for Medicare and Medicaid Services and the Centers for Disease Control and Prevention initiated the Surgical Care Improvement Project. This project is a multiple-year national campaign and partnership of leading public and private healthcare organizations aimed at reducing surgical complications. PACU staff members have a major role in partnering with both the surgeon and anesthesia providers to ensure that many of these measures are addressed appropriately.[5] Every nurse is responsible for quality management and performance improvement. The result is an effective program that has a positive effect on the process and outcome of care where patient care problems can be prevented, or where basic operating procedures or systems can be changed and improved.

Monitoring and evaluation are still important elements of the quality management process. The trend is no longer one of just data collection, but of using the collected data to improve systems and processes. These system improvements may affect only the PACU area or may be far reaching into the institution. Examples of performance improvement activities might include reduction in the time the pharmacy takes to respond to PACU needs, improvement in the system to decrease the length of time patients remain in the PACU waiting for beds, a change in staffing patterns in the PACU or ambulatory care areas to meet patient care needs, or a patient education program written for all outpatients discharged with a venous access device to ensure that all patients receive the same quality education.

COLLABORATIVE MANAGEMENT

The PACU setting is a multifaceted, complex area. It encompasses the PACU staff and requires close working relations with the entire perioperative team to ensure the safest care and best outcome for the patient. The anesthesia providers have a key role in the functioning of the PACU. The partnerships between PACU and the anesthesia staff members must be strong because it is the anesthesia provider who is the first line of defense for addressing patient issues in the

PACU. In addition to anesthesia providers, the PACU and operating room staff, along with the surgeon and their team, must work in tandem to provide safe care. All who work in the PACU need to exhibit excellent communication skills, mutual respect, and the ability to collaborate effectively with different personalities and people of different cultures.

ROLE DELINEATION

Nurse Manager

Each institution identifies the qualifications needed for a nurse manager position. It generally includes a baccalaureate degree in nursing and preferably a master's degree in nursing or another health-related field, with an emphasis on administration and business. The nurse manager for a PACU should have a minimum of 5 years of strong medical-surgical and perianesthesia background, or critical care experience. It is also preferable that the nurse manager have previous managerial experience. Another prerequisite of the position should be national certification, either as a certified postanesthesia nurse (CPAN) or a certified ambulatory perianesthesia nurse (CAPA), or the requirement to obtain it within a specified timeframe. Active involvement in professional organizations such as ASPAN should be an expectation of any perianesthesia manager. This membership assists the manager with networking and keeping abreast of the latest professional developments within the specialty.

The nurse manager of the PACU is responsible for planning, organizing, implementing, and evaluating the activities of both the nursing staff and the patient care functions. In addition, the manager is responsible for staff scheduling, assignments, performance evaluation, counseling, hiring, firing, educational program coordination (including the development and implementation of a unit-specific orientation program), and the unit budget formulation and monitoring. The nurse manager is also responsible for developing and implementing standards of care and the unit's quality improvement program; for evaluating and monitoring their effectiveness; as well as for the professional growth of the assigned staff.

The perianesthesia nurse manager should be skilled in time management, decision making, organization, financial management, communication, interpersonal relations, and conflict resolution. In addition, the manager should have the ability to negotiate and collaborate with other departments and health care team members. The nurse manager should also project a positive nursing image and with the clinical nurse specialist should have clinical expertise related to the PACU.

Clinical Nurse Specialist

The clinical nurse specialist (CNS) in the PACU can be identified by a number of titles, including advanced practice nurse, nurse practitioner, clinical leader, resource nurse, nurse educator, and nurse consultant. For the purpose of this discussion, the nurse in this role is referred to as the *CNS*.

Qualifications of the CNS include strong leadership skills, clinical expertise in the perianesthesia setting, excellent communication skills, the ability to share knowledge and ensure understanding, the ability to work in a collaborative manner with all members of the health care team, the capability to incorporate nursing research into practice, and the ability to multitask. The CNS usually is a master's-prepared nurse or may be doctorally prepared (e.g., doctorate of nursing practice [DNP]). The nurse in this role should possess advanced clinical expertise in perianesthesia nursing. The CNS should also have CPAN or CAPA certification. Each institution develops role requirements for the CNS. Examples of activities that may involve the CNS are included in Box 3-3.

The CNS works closely with the nurse manager to achieve the mission and goals of the PACU. In addition, the CNS is involved in ensuring the clinical competencies of each perianesthesia nurse and provides in-service training and education to the staff on health care regulatory requirements and standards.

BOX 3-3   Examples of CNS Activities

- Education of PACU clinical staff (RNs, LPNs, UAPs)
- Education of hospital and facility staff who receive patients from the PACU
- Development and implementation of new programs and services
- Development and implementation of patient and family education programs
- Quality improvement activities
- Liaison between management and staff nurses
- Liaison between departments (e.g., anesthesia, operating room, surgical units, critical care units)
- Evaluation of clinical staff members outside the PACU (e.g., surgical units, critical care units)

PACU, Postanesthesia care unit; *RN,* registered nurse; *LPN,* licensed practical nurse; *UAP,* unlicensed assistive personnel.

The CNS role should be part of the PACU's quality team and plays an important part in the development of an effective monitoring and evaluation programs. This nurse is instrumental in implementing corrective action to rectify deficiencies and improve patient outcomes. The CNS can be invaluable in assisting staff members to develop and implement evidence-based practice (EBP) projects. EBP activities should be ongoing in the PACU. EBP can serve to strengthen the identity of perianesthesia nursing as a specialty and give the staff nurse direct input into their practice, which results in greater staff buy-in to changes resulting from the data.

The CNS is also the resource person for clinical problem solving and dissemination of information of an advanced nature. In addition, the CNS can ensure that standards of practice are implemented consistently throughout the organization. As a liaison, the CNS can work closely with units outside the PACU that are involved in patient recovery. These areas include labor and delivery, endoscopy, and special procedure units. The CNS can also be instrumental in collaborating with free-standing ambulatory surgery centers if the hospital is so affiliated.

The role of the CNS is an important one, but because of cost constraints it is a position that is not always budgeted for in the PACU setting. Through skill and expertise, the CNS can offer support and encouragement to staff members, thereby promoting satisfaction and teamwork in the PACU and improved patient outcomes. These factors ultimately lead to continued individual and professional growth among team members.

Staff Nurses

The selection of quality nursing personnel for the PACU is of the utmost importance. The nurse manager, in conjunction with the institution's human resource department and the CNS, should establish qualifications for PACU nursing personnel. These qualifications along with requirements such as shift rotation, weekend, and call expectations should be written and used in all employment proceedings. This practice tends to preclude, or at least minimize, subsequent problems such as job dissatisfaction, unsatisfactory work performance, and staff turnover; it also helps to ensure a smoothly functioning PACU.

The following qualifications should be considered in establishing selection criteria. The nurse who considers employment in the PACU must have an interest in perianesthesia nursing. The nurse needs a solid foundation in the care required for preanesthesia and postanesthesia patients[1] and should be committed to providing high-quality,

individualized patient care. The candidate should also demonstrate exceptional communications skills and communicate in a positive manner with all members of the health care team. The nurse should have the ability to form good working relationships and be a positive team player. The perianesthesia nurse should be capable of making intelligent independent decisions and initiating appropriate action as necessary, and willing to accept the responsibility that accompanies working in a critical care unit. In addition, the nurse must have excellent patient teaching skills, the ability to coordinate care being rendered by a variety of health care team members, and the ability to function effectively in a crisis situation. The ability to be flexible is of the utmost importance for nurses working in the PACU.

The nurse who seeks employment in the PACU should also express an interest in and have the ability to learn the scientific principles and theory underlying patient care and the technologic aspects of perianesthesia nursing. The person should be in good health, dependable, and motivated and should express an intention to stay at least 1 year in the PACU after completing the unit orientation. The orientation and training of a perianesthesia nurse requires significant time, energy, and money. Temporary assignment to the PACU is not worthwhile, except as a student learning experience.

The cross-training of nurses to the PACU may be a feasible solution in hospitals or facilities where staffing is a concern. The nurse who is cross-trained to the PACU should fulfill the required competencies of competent support staff as outlined in the ASPAN *Perianesthesia Nursing Standards and Practice Recommendations*.[1]

Ideally the PACU nurse should have at least 1 year of general medical-surgical nursing. Critical care experience may be an advantage. The perianesthesia nurse must also be able to adapt to changes in the health care setting. Continuous restructuring and reengineering of hospital practices has led to turmoil in some institutions. Nurses must be able to accept and adapt to the constantly changing environment of the future.

Membership in professional organizations as well as national certification by one of the professional nursing associations (Table 3-1) shows commitment to professional excellence and should be considered positively in the selection of perianesthesia nurses. If everything else is equal, ideally, candidates for PACU positions who have attained a CPAN or CAPA credential should be given preference in hiring. Commitments to other professional nursing organizations should also help the candidate to be considered for a PACU position.

Table 3-1	Certification by Professional Nursing Associations
PROFESSIONAL ASSOCIATION	**CREDENTIAL**
American Nurses Association	Medical-surgical certification
American Association of Critical Care Nurses	CCRN
American Society of PeriAnesthesia Nurses	CPAN or CAPA
Association of peri-Operative Registered Nurses	CNOR
Emergency Nurses Association	CEN

CPAN, Certified Post Anesthesia Nurse; *CAPA,* Certified Ambulatory Perianesthesia Nurse; *CEN,* Certified Emergency Nurse; *CCRN,* Critical Care Registered Nurse; *CNOR,* a certification of competency in the field of perioperative nursing.

Certification in basic cardiac life support (BCLS) and advanced cardiac life support (ACLS) is required of all nurses who work in the PACU.[1] For units with a high volume of pediatric patients, certification in pediatric advanced life support (PALS) is also required. Application of BCLS in the PACU or ambulatory surgical unit helps to sustain a patient's condition in a crisis until ACLS techniques can be instituted. ACLS includes training in dysrhythmia recognition, intravenous infusion, blood gas interpretation, defibrillation, intubation, and emergency drug administration. If the perianesthesia nurse responds quickly and efficiently during crisis situations, the patient's chance of survival increases.

Perianesthesia nurses take pride in their competence to deliver safe patient care. Opportunities to broaden and expand the perianesthesia nurse's knowledge base should be fostered. The knowledge necessary for direct patient care is provided by working with staff members individually to ensure the vital training, support, and guidance that eventually enables the nurse to function efficiently and competently. This process allows for consistent teaching and evaluation on an individual level.

The ultimate goal of the PACU nurse is delivery of quality patient care. To accomplish this goal, continuous professional nursing judgment is necessary; therefore only professional registered nurses should be assigned patient care.

Ancillary Personnel

Minimal numbers of ancillary personnel should be assigned to the unit to support the registered nurses. Licensed practical nurses (LPNs) or licensed vocational nurses (LVNs) assigned to the PACU are restricted in their roles. A registered nurse must be the primary nursing care provider in the PACU, thereby limiting the role of the practical nurse in the PACU setting to one that does not allow functioning at their fullest capacity. This situation often causes dissatisfaction for the LPN/LVN and is not a cost effective use of limited budget dollars. Some PACUs have effectively used the LPN/LVN as a transport nurse to deliver appropriate patients safely to the unit after discharge. The PACU may employ unlicensed assistive personnel (UAP). When working with UAPs, the registered nurse (RN) is responsible for knowing the policies and procedures as set forth by the individual institution. UAPs can be a valuable asset to the PACU, but the RN should remain cognizant of the fact that nursing assessment, diagnosis, outcome identification, planning, implementation and evaluation cannot be delegated to UAPs. UAPs can assist the nurse by performing tasks that the perianesthesia RN supervises and determine the appropriate use of UAP providing direct patient care in accordance with state regulations.[1] Ultimately, the RN is responsible and accountable for the safe delivery of nursing care.

A skilled secretary clerk is a definite asset to the PACU. A person who is adept at handling and redirecting the numerous phone calls to the PACU and is proficient in clerical duties makes the job of the perianesthesia nurse much easier. A proficient secretary can assist the unit by acting as the liaison to family members. Frequent updates on the status of the patient help to reassure family members that the recovery is progressing as planned. The secretary clerk should possess excellent communication skills because this person communicates to a wide spectrum of individuals—from patient and family members to physicians and other health care workers. Often the first contact the family has with the PACU, either by phone or in person, is with the secretary clerk. As a result, this person must possess exceptional customer service skills. An individual who gives the impression that the patient is the most important contact of the day is certainly the individual wanted on the front line.

TALENT RECRUITMENT, RETENTION, AND REVIEW CONSIDERATIONS

Retaining Nursing Staff in the PACU

As demand continues to outweigh supply, the existing nursing shortage only worsens over time. Regrettably, perianesthesia nursing is not immune to this shortage. Many nurses have found the perianesthesia specialty to be where they want to focus their careers. This group of experienced, dedicated staff members is an exceptional bonus to institutions lucky enough to have them. Unfortunately, many of these nurses are from the baby boomer generation and are looking to retire in the near future. At the same time, fewer nurses are graduating and demand for nurses is growing. Simultaneously, many colleges and universities have seen the recent number of nursing applicants increase, only to be turned away because of the lack of qualified nursing educators.[6]

In order to recruit and retain the dedicated and talented nurses needed in the perianesthesia setting, institutions must look at factors that influence job satisfaction and retainability. Recruitment into nursing and into specific hospitals is a widely discussed topic. After nurses are recruited into the perianesthesia setting, retention of these experienced staff members becomes a major challenge. Although salary is a factor, studies show that it is not the top reason for dissatisfaction and turnover.[7] Items such as a workplace environment free from ongoing conflict, where staff has autonomy and where their ideas and opinions are valued, play a big role in job satisfaction. Other issues such as inflexible working hours and mandatory overtime are also major causes of dissatisfaction. Some research has defined that the nurse manager leadership behaviors and relations with staff members had the most influence on retention of hospital staff nurses (Box 3-4).

Retention of qualified nurses is fast becoming a priority for nursing administration. In exit interviews, nurses cite an unhealthy work environment as the reason they leave the workplace. The treatment of nurses toward each other continues to be challenge. Some reasons given for nurses who leave the workplace include lack of support, mentoring, and clear direction.[8] Nurses are not exempt from conflict in the workplace. As trite as it may seem, women are generally expected to work harmoniously together in a sisterlike fashion. This belief could not be farther from the truth. When issues of conflict arise, some individuals may find it difficult to confront the situation and establish a resolution. As a result, an ongoing underlying current of tension may exist on the unit. Box 3-5 identifies some strategies that the nurse manager may use to build a supportive workplace.

Creation of an environment conducive to staff growth and development is the manager's responsibility. A survey conducted by the American Academy of Nursing in 1982 identified variables in nursing that attracted and retained quality

---

BOX 3-4　Retention Practices for Nurse Managers

- Peer interviews
  - Use appropriately educated staff to collaborate in the interview process.
- Use of preceptors for new hires
  - Provide support for new hire and positive reinforcement for preceptor.
- High-risk retention monitoring
  - Develop specific plans of action to retain those nurses at high risk for transfer.
- Supplies and resources available to do the job
  - Find out from staff any barriers to doing their jobs (e.g., supplies) and take action.
- Individual career plan with each employee
  - Each employee should have an individualized career development plan.
- Regular feedback
  - Guarantee formal feedback to staff at least twice a year.
- Open communication in unit
  - Make open communication a priority—staff with staff and manager with staff.
- Unit as a team
  - Make outside activities available for the unit; rely on staff input into unit goals.

Modified from The Advisory Board Company: *Becoming a chief retention officer*, Washington, DC, 2001, The Advisory Board Company: Nursing Executive Center.

BOX 3-5　Management Strategies to Build a Supportive Workplace

- Forge honest and open relationships.
- Set realistic expectations.
- Demonstrate how to deal effectively with colleagues who disagree or disapprove.
- Recognize when being "nice" prevents discussion and resolution of issues.
- Acknowledge conflicts and find solutions.
- Recognize that some competitive tensions will always exist and talk them through.
- Openly discuss how dealing with the issues can lead to optimism, movement, and growth.
- Lead with respect for each person and empathy for the inevitable workplace tensions that will arise.

From Vestal K: Conflict and competition in the workplace, *Nurs Leader* 4(6):6–7, 2006.

---

nurses. These variables include nursing autonomy and personal and job satisfaction, and nursing practice that resulted in excellence. As a result of this survey, the Magnet Recognition Program was established for recognizing health care organizations that provide nursing excellence.[9] Facilities that strive for recognition as a Magnet facility have identified that the nurses employed at the facility provide quality patient care. Nurses who believe they have the support and resources needed to provide quality patient care are more likely to be satisfied in the workplace.

Nurse managers need to be cognizant of the workplace environment. When strife is evident in the unit, the issues need to be identified and addressed immediately to avoid a deluge of conflict, which can soon translate to discord among the staff.

Other factors linked to job satisfaction and retention have been flexible work schedules, appropriate pay scales, and shared governance. Flexible schedules and a shared governance philosophy are created and overseen by the manager.

Shared Governance

Many units use a participative type of management. It is a well-documented fact that nurses want to be treated as professionals and desire autonomy and participation. A concept used by many hospitals to meet these needs is shared governance. In this form of management, the PACU nurse assumes more authority and responsibility and shares management skills and duties with peers. The overall structure is that of self management, with staff involvement in the decision-making processes that affect their nursing practice.

Committees that address the needs of the unit, the employees, and the patients are established. Usually a nursing practice committee is in charge of any decisions about policies and procedures or practice issues; a quality management committee is in charge of quality management and performance improvement activities for the unit; and an educational committee is responsible for meeting the educational needs of the unit. Other unit-specific committees that have been used are equipment and supply, budget and finance, communications, and statistics.

The nurse manager becomes a facilitator and a resource person for the staff. Most nurse managers retain responsibilities such as employee evaluations, interviews, and liaison with administration or physicians. The challenge for the nurse manager within this system of management is to maintain a vision and to impart that vision to the staff. In addition, the nurse manager must learn how to relinquish control and to support the decisions of the staff and the staff members must accept ownership and accountability of their practice and unit.

Self-Scheduling

Managers need to reassess age-old beliefs that nurses must work set shifts. The 7:00 AM to 3:30 PM shift is a thing of the past. A creative manager works with the nursing staff to accommodate individual work schedules whenever possible. The mother who needs to put her children on the school bus before work may prefer to work 8:00 AM to 4:30 PM instead of the traditional 7:00 AM to 3:30 PM. For mothers or fathers who work the evening shift, a 5:00 PM to 1:00 AM shift may be a better fit to accommodate childcare issues. Implementation of a 10- or 12-hour shift or a split shift may assist in covering the gaps. Supporting creative scheduling solutions, which are key to staff retention and employee satisfaction, can become a juggling act for the manager who must also provide for safe patient care and stay within the staffing budget.

One option for scheduling of staff is a system that is completely coordinated by the staff nurses that also recognizes professional nurses as capable of making crucial decisions about their practices. The schedule is developed and implemented by nurses and other staff in the unit. The nurses are given preestablished requirements that must be filled. They can be as creative and flexible as they want in developing the staffing schedule. Advantages include decreased amount of time spent by the nurse manager on scheduling, increased team building by the staff, increased job satisfaction, increased staff autonomy, and decreased staff turnover. The manager must have final review and approval of the schedule to ensure that an overall fairness exists and all the preestablished requirements are met.

Basic Staff Orientation Program

The orientation program for the PACU should be designed to specifically meet the needs of the nurse who works in the PACU. The program should include formal lectures and discussions and informal demonstrations and supervised practice. The orientation program should be structured to include objectives, content, resources, and the method used to evaluate the orientee's progress. The orientee should be provided with materials that clearly delineate the structure of the orientation program. The expectations the orientee faces should be absolutely clear to everyone.

Each nurse who undergoes orientation to the PACU should have an individually assigned preceptor. The preceptor works closely with the CNS and orientee to ensure that individual needs are met and deficiencies are addressed promptly. In addition, anesthesia providers, surgeons, the CNS, and other nurses in the PACU should be involved in the orientation program. Fostering of seasoned nurses to prepare and present short lectures or skill demonstrations not only recognizes the nurse for individual expertise but also displays the manager's confidence in the individual's ability to provide quality patient care. Lectures and presentations should be geared toward the specific needs of the orientee.

Experienced staff members should support and encourage new staff members. Nurses who are made to feel a part of a team are certainly more likely to stay, whereas nurses who are unhappy leave. Orientation of a new staff nurse is costly and time consuming; therefore implementation of all possible measures to limit staff turnover is essential. Working to create a stable cohesive staff helps with staff morale. This process begins at orientation.

Objectives should be clearly stated, and methods for evaluation of the achievement of the objectives should be clearly outlined. A notebook of the objectives, resources, evaluation forms, pertinent PACU policies and procedures, and other valuable resources should be given to each orientee. The notebook should be carefully reviewed with each orientee. A clear understanding of objectives and expectations in the beginning avoids problems in the long term.

Competency-based orientation focuses on acquiring the knowledge necessary to perform the job and additionally encompasses applying that knowledge to real-life situations. Competency-based orientation is effective because it allows an expert clinician to transfer knowledge and skills to the novice learner. The learner then becomes responsible for the progress and the preceptor facilitates and guides the learner.

Content of the Orientation Program

The length of the orientation program should be tailored to meet the individual needs and previous experience of the orientee. Consideration should be given to the expectations placed on the orientee. Will they be expected to perform in a "call" situation at the conclusion of the orientation period, or will an experienced perianesthesia nurse be working with them for an indefinite period? The orientation period should be customized and adjusted as needed based on the orientee's ability to grasp, understand, and process the information and situations encountered. During the orientation time, the orientee should work full time. An experienced perianesthesia nurse will require a much shorter orientation phase than an inexperienced PACU nurse. Suggested topics and content of the PACU orientation program are presented in Box 3-6. Additional material, as appropriate to the practice setting, should also be included.

During the orientation period, careful and constant communication must be maintained between the nurse manager, the orientee, the preceptor, and

---

BOX 3-6 Suggested Topics for a PACU Orientation Program

REVIEW OF THE ANATOMY AND PHYSIOLOGY OF THE CARDIORESPIRATORY SYSTEM
- Pathophysiologic processes of the cardiorespiratory system
- Factors that alter circulatory or respiratory function after surgery and anesthesia
- Position
- Type of incision
- Medication
- Blood loss and replacement; intake and output
- Anesthetic agent used
- Type of operative procedure
- Monitoring techniques
- Hemodynamic monitoring
- Pulse oximetry
- Cardiac dysrhythmias
- Identification and treatment
- ACLS or PALS certification
- Airway maintenance, equipment, and techniques, pharmacologic and nonpharmacologic
  - Evaluation of treatment
  - Techniques for maintenance of a patent airway

- Administration of oxygen
- Use of suction equipment
- Ventilatory support, equipment, and procedures
  - Bag-valve mask
  - Airway insertion
- Cardiorespiratory arrest and its management
  - Use of monitor-defibrillator
  - Emergency medications
- Pain management
  - Assessment of patient's pain level in all age groups
  - Use of pain scales
  - Documentation of pain level
  - Treatment methods, including patient education
- Treatment of hypotension or hypertension
- Interpretation of laboratory values
- Identification and treatment of malignant hyperthermia

REVIEW OF OTHER PHYSIOLOGIC CONSIDERATIONS IN THE PACU
- Neurologic system
- Musculoskeletal system

Continued

BOX 3-6   Suggested Topics for a PACU Orientation Program—cont'd

- Genitourinary system
  - Fluid and electrolyte balance
  - Fluid and electrolyte imbalance
- Gastrointestinal system
- Integumentary system
  - Identification of risk factors
  - Preventive measures
- Pediatric-adolescent physiology
  - Age-specific competencies
  - Patient education strategies
- Geriatric physiology
  - Age-specific competencies
  - Patient education strategies
- Physiology of pregnancy

ANESTHESIA
- Administration and properties of selected agents (include all agents routinely used in the institution)
  - Intravenous agents
  - Muscle relaxants
  - Conduction anesthesia
  - Reversal agents
- Intravenous moderate sedation
  - Policies and procedures
  - Medications used
- Nursing implications

CARE OF THE PATIENT IN THE PACU
- Preoperative preparation
  - Physical assessment
  - Implementation of comfort measures
  - Nursing interventions to decrease anxiety
- Consent (surgical and anesthesia)
- Intravenous insertion
- Correct site policy (facility specific)
- Postoperative care
  - Physical assessment of the patient after surgery
  - General PACU care
    - Psychologic considerations
    - Anxiety
    - Coping responses
- The stir-up regimen
- Intravenous therapy and blood transfusion

- Infection control
  - Universal precautions
  - Occupational Safety and Health Administration regulations
- General comfort and safety measures
- Specific care needed after surgical procedures
  - Ear, nose, and throat surgery
  - Ocular surgery
  - Cardiothoracic surgery
  - Neurosurgery
  - Orthopedic surgery
  - Genitourinary surgery
  - Gastrointestinal surgery
  - Gynecologic and obstetric surgery
  - Plastic surgery
  - Vascular surgery
  - Special considerations for the pediatric-adolescent patient
  - Special procedures, such as electroconvulsive therapy and pain blocks
- Postoperative medications
  - Pain control medications (intravenous, intramuscular, oral, epidural, patient-controlled analgesia, and pain pumps)
  - Age-dependent assessment measures
  - Numeric, visual analog, or faces scale
  - Antiemetics
  - Others (antihypertensives, antiarrhythmics)
- Patient and family teaching
  - Preprocedure
  - Postprocedure
- Thermoregulation
  - Hypothermia
  - Hyperthermia (malignant hyperthermia)
- Department specifics
  - Layout
  - Policies and procedures
  - Preparation of patient units
- Documentation
  - Policies and procedures
  - Electronic charting
- Orientation program
  - Goals and expectations
  - Performance evaluation
  - Competency assessment

From American Society of PeriAnesthesia Nurses: *Perianesthesia nursing standards and practice recommendations 2010–2012*, Cherry Hill, NJ, 2010, ASPAN.
PACU, Postanesthesia care unit; *ACLS*, advanced cardiac life support; *PALS*, pediatric advanced life support.

the CNS. Evaluation by the nurse manager and preceptor should be ongoing, and the orientee should receive a formal written evaluation at the end of the orientation. The orientee should clearly understand the expectations as set forth by the perianesthesia nurse manager, and the orientee and preceptor should discuss progress daily. If issues arise, the manager or the CNS may need to step in and clearly review progress and expectations with the orientee. In some cases, an orientee might clearly not fit into the perianesthesia environment. In these circumstances, the best solution is to assist the orientee in gaining the required prerequisite skills or explore employment opportunities in another area rather than allowing the orientee to flounder in an environment in which success is not possible.

Development of Expertise

Expertise in nursing involves the overlapping of the following three basic components of nursing: knowledge, skill, and experience. Mastering any one or two of these components never equates with expertise. The expert nurse uses a complex linkage of knowledge, experience, skill, clue identification, gut feelings, logic, and intuition in problem-solving and the nursing process. As the nurse gains knowledge and experience through formal and informal programs, nursing intuition begins to develop. Intuition may be thought of as identification of a deviation from the expected or the feeling that "something just doesn't seem right." Over time, with experience and practice, the nurse becomes proficient. The accumulation of knowledge, along with the chance to practice the skills acquired, leads to competence.[10]

When the nurse finishes the formal PACU orientation program, the nurse should work continuously on improving background theory and skills. This improvement can be accomplished with active participation in on-the-job training, nursing in-service programs presented on the unit, outside reading, membership in ASPAN and other state and local professional nursing organizations, and attendance at both in-house and outside-sponsored seminars and educational offerings. Constant review of basic knowledge and procedures is essential. Keeping abreast of new scientific information and innovations is necessary to ensure quality care.

After the orientee has worked in the perianesthesia environment for at least 1 year and believes that sufficient knowledge and experience have been gained, certification as a CPAN or CAPA should be considered. Certification is one method of demonstrating to patients and families that the quality of services they receive is enhanced because the nurses caring for them have attained a CPAN or CAPA credential.

An investment made to stimulate the professional development of the nursing staff is directly reflected in the level of nursing care provided to the patient. Inclusion of funds in budgeting to send nurses to important educational and information-sharing meetings for the unit is essential. In addition, the individual nurse should be willing to finance some of the costs associated with advancement of their professional growth and practice.

Competency Assessment

When the orientation period has ended, the assurance that staff members remain competent is essential. Integration of a competency checklist with the annual performance evaluation is one method to ensure competency. Assessment of competency on an annual basis provides a number of benefits. Staff members are forced to review procedures and equipment that might not be routinely used.

Assessment of competency can be divided into two aspects. The first aspect of staff competence assessment relates to policies and procedures and could include facility standards and national standards as set forth by organizations such as ASPAN. Some competencies that managers may want to address include:

- Unit-specific administrative policies and procedures
- Patient confidentiality and patient rights
- Fire safety and patient safety issues, including The Joint Commission's National Patient Safety Goals[11]
- Environment of care issues
- Infection control practices
- Thermoregulation, including normothermia[1] and hyperthermia
- Variance and occurrence reporting
- Compliance policies
- Medications commonly administered in the practice setting, including intravenous moderate sedation, anesthetic agents, antiemetics, and analgesics
- Age-specific competencies (pediatric, adolescent, adult, geriatric)

A complete list of Recommended Competencies for the Perianesthesia Nurse can be found in the ASPAN *Perianesthesia Nursing Standards and Practice Recommendations*.[1]

The second aspect of assessing staff competence relates to equipment. Evaluation of staff members is essential to ensure that their skills and knowledge in the operation of and caring for equipment used in the practice setting is proficient. Specific equipment competencies include:

- Monitors, including electrocardiography, pulse oximetry, capnography, and noninvasive blood pressure
- Defibrillator (defibrillation, cardioversion, external pacing)
- Warming devices
- Intravenous and epidural infusion pumps
- Ventilators

Managers should develop processes to assess the previously named activities. For assessment of equipment competence, employees must be able to appropriately demonstrate proper use of the specific piece of equipment. Unit-specific tests can be developed to assess competence of policies and procedures.

In an effort to streamline processes, assessment of competence of the new orientee and of senior staff members should follow the same path. Competency assessment methods differ. The new orientee may be required to demonstrate the step-by-step process of defibrillation and to verbalize the rationale for each step. In contrast, the seasoned nurse may be required to just demonstrate the process.

Incorporation of competency assessments into monthly staff meetings may also be helpful. One method is the assignment of a staff member to present a short in-service on a specific piece of equipment or a specific policy to the staff members. Competence can then be assessed with a follow-up posttest or return demonstration from the staff members. Documentation can be a checklist that outlines the step-by-step return demonstration or the posttest that is filed electronically or in employee personnel files to document competence in the specific skill.

Quality management and improvement activities may uncover a specific deficiency. In this instance, development of a program to educate staff on the proper skills needed is important. After completion of the education, the nurse manager can follow up with a competency assessment of the problem-prone activity.

Perianesthesia nursing is unique in that the nurse has only a small amount of time to assess the patient, identify a plan of care, implement the plan, and then evaluate the effectiveness of the plan before care is turned over to someone else, be it another nursing professional, a family member, or the patient. The skill and expertise needed to provide quality care in the fast-paced environment takes time to obtain. Nurses who are motivated to learn, like a fast-paced environment, and work well in teams enjoy the challenges of the PACU work environment.

STAFFING

Assignment of nursing personnel to the PACU should be permanent, and staff members should not be routinely rotated to other units. Staffing in the PACU is dependent on volume, patient acuity, patient flow processes, and the physical layout of the unit. Two registered nurses, one of whom is competent in perianesthesia nursing, should be in attendance at all times when a patient is receiving care. ASPAN provides detailed information concerning staffing requirements for phase I, phase II, and extended observation.[1]

Student nurses should not be used to staff the PACU. Students are assigned to the PACU primarily for observation. Any patient care delivered by student nurses should occur only under the direct supervision of a permanent staff nurse. No private duty or "float" nurses should be used to staff the PACU unless they have been oriented and possess current PACU competencies.

SUMMARY

All management procedures, clinical practices, and policies of the PACU should be established through joint efforts of the PACU staff, the nurse manager, CNS, and the medical director of the unit. These procedures and policies should be written and readily available to all staff members working in the PACU and all physicians using the area for care of patients. Changes in the clinical situation of the facility and advances in science and technology make revision of policies and procedures a continuous challenge.

REFERENCES

1. American Society of PeriAnesthesia Nurses: *Perianesthesia nursing standards and practice recommendations 2010–2012*, Cherry Hill, NJ, 2010, ASPAN.
2. Dewitt L, Albert N: Preferences for visitation in the PACU, *J Perianesth Nurs* 25(5):296–301, 2010.
3. Price C, et al: Reducing boarding in a post-anesthesia care unit, *Production and Operations Management* 20(3):431–441, 2011.
4. Chung F, et al: A post-anesthetic discharge scoring system for home readiness after ambulatory surgery, *J Clin Anesth* 7(6):500–506, 1995.
5. Anesthesia Business Consultants: *Using post-anesthesia data to improve and demonstrate value*, available at www.anesthesiallc.com/about-abc/ealerts/194-using-post-anesthesia-data-to-improve-and-demonstrate-value. Accessed April 5, 2011.
6. American Association of Colleges of Nursing: *Nursing shortage fact sheet*, available at www.centerfornursing.org/nursemanpower/NursingShortageFactSheet.pdf. Accessed April 10, 2011.
7. Simmons B: *Does pay level affect job satisfaction?* available at www.bretlsimmons.com/2010-09/does-pay-level-affect-job-satisfaction. Accessed April 10, 2011.
8. The College Network Blog: *Five reasons why new nurses quit*, available at http://blog.collegenetwork.com/blog/the-future-of-distance-education/five-reasons-why-new-nurses-quit. Accessed April 15, 2011.
9. American Nurses Credentialing Center: *ANCC magnet recognition program*, available at http://nursingworld.org/ancc/magnet/index.html. Accessed April 15, 2011.
10. Dracup K, Bryan-Brown C: From novice to expert to mentor: shaping the future, *Am J Crit Care* 13(6):448–450, 2004.
11. The Joint Commission: *National patient safety goals*, available at www.jointcommission.org/standards_information/npsgs.aspx. Accessed April 15, 2011.

4   Crisis Resource Management in the PACU

Suzanne M. Wright, PhD, CRNA, and
Michael D. Fallacaro, DNS, CRNA

Perianesthesia nurses perform a vast proportion of their work in a complex environment where keen awareness of each patient's situation and a high level of vigilance throughout the perianesthesia period are essential to ensure positive patient outcomes. Postanesthesia care units (PACUs) are error-prone environments where opportunities for egregious mistakes are inherent because of high cognitive burdens and stress loads, high noise levels, demands on attention, and time pressures. Each day, perianesthesia nurses must ensure the proper functioning of highly technical equipment, perform a detailed postanesthesia assessment on each patient, calculate and administer proper doses of potent medications, monitor multiple patients simultaneously, perceive and understand individualized patient responses to medications and surgical interventions, troubleshoot ambiguous patient conditions, make complex decisions under times of distress, and respond appropriately and accurately under production pressure. Patient, surgical, and anesthesia factors can all contribute to critical incidents during the perianesthesia period.

The dynamic nature of delivering care and a recent explosion of technology affect the educational needs of perianesthesia nurses. Technologic advances such as electronic charting, computer monitoring systems, and complex procedural equipment have altered the skills necessary to care for patients immediately after surgery. Given the high workload and an environment rich with distractions, perianesthesia nurses must anticipate and be quick to respond to critical situations in the PACU. Academic programs responsible for preparing adept perianesthesia nurses are continuously challenged because of a limited number of actual emergencies in the PACU during student clinical training.

Although routine nursing practice involves a set of basic skills, complex technical and nontechnical skills are essential for an effective response to urgent and emergent situations occurring in the PACU. Technologic advancements in human simulation are currently used in many fields of health care to enhance traditional educational methods by allowing an opportunity for educators to recreate critical, but rare, events. Crisis resource management (CRM) training—which incorporates the basic principles of human factors design, domain-specific expertise, and human patient simulators—has the potential, in theory, to improve the way health care providers respond to and manage emergencies.

Since World War II, the field of aviation has used flight simulators as a safe yet realistic training method for all types of pilots. Investigations of airline disasters have demonstrated that a pilot's technical skills are not usually the cause of accidents.[1] Instead, poor teamwork and inadequate communication were found to be commonly associated with these adverse incidents. In response to this discovery, airline crew team training was born in the 1980s to promote effective collaboration among cockpit and cabin crews, ground personnel, and air traffic controllers. Although the practice has never been validated empirically, simulation techniques have become the mainstay of aviation training. Pilots train extensively in all emergency procedures in simulated environments to become proficient in crisis management before encountering similar situations on actual flights.

Training in health care is now possible with the introduction of full-sized human patient simulators in the early 1990s. Gaba and colleagues, at Stanford University in Palo Alto, California, adapted the principles of CRM training to the medical domain.[2] They found that the principles were as applicable to health care as they were to aviation. Both fields are characterized as dynamic, necessitate rapid decision making under stress, and require teams of individuals to work together effectively to prevent loss of life. Critical care medicine, emergency medicine, and trauma teams use simulation technology and CRM training. Although the initial emphasis was to educate physicians, the technique is now used to educate nurse anesthetists, nurse practitioners, critical care nurses, paramedics, and other allied health personnel. Simulation has also been incorporated into many curricula for health care providers and continues to expand its role in education and training to improve health care delivery.

HUMAN FACTORS TRAINING AND THE SYSTEMS APPROACH TO REDUCING MEDICAL ERROR

Everyone has made a mistake such as locking his or her keys in the car or calling someone by the wrong name. These unintended events, although seemingly significant at the time, pale in comparison to a nurse who accidentally administers the wrong medication or forgets to deliver the proper concentration of oxygen to a patient. In principle, the fundamental human nature of these errors of omission is the same. Nothing is more concerning to a patient than the possibility of becoming a victim of medical error. CRM training addresses the management of critical events in health care with a strong emphasis on human factors. The primary focus is on improvement of human performance in complex work environments to facilitate better decision making under stress, more effective teamwork, and improved patient outcomes.

Human error is an inevitable part of complex and rapidly changing work domains, such as aviation, anesthesiology, and critical care medicine.[3] Human error in any discipline can lead to catastrophic outcomes. Major incidents in any industry, such as the crash of the Concorde jet in 2000, gain media interest and prompt public attention and action primarily because of the drama and scope of the event in terms of lives altered or lost. Until recently, human error–related accidents in health care tended to be less visible to the public, primarily because these events usually affect one patient at a time.

Theorists in human factors have identified particular circumstances and error types that can help to train individuals to recognize the signs of errant problem solving. Although human error can never be eradicated, it can certainly be minimized.[4] Aviation, for example, favors teaching error management techniques rather than an aiming for human perfection. Numerous organizations are dedicated to improving patient safety by funding research endeavors in this area. One such organization, the Anesthesia Patient Safety Foundation, has funded many studies examining human factors and training in the field of anesthesia. Moreover, the National Patient Safety Foundation has broadened the study of human factors to all medical specialties. Both groups believe that further study and advances in training can improve patient outcomes and safety.

Reason[5] operationalized error into the following three terms: slips, lapses, and mistakes. A *slip* is defined as an error of execution. It is observable and can simply involve the human action of picking up the wrong syringe or turning the wrong knob on an oxygen flowmeter. A *lapse* is not observable, but involves the inability of a person to correctly recall information from memory, such as the mixture of a lidocaine drip. Finally, a *mistake* is defined as an error in planning rather than an error in execution. Here, a nurse may have planned to actively suction secretions from an endotracheal tube during extubation of a patient. Although the execution was technically correct, the lungs were left devoid of oxygen in the process, which was a mistake in planning.

A common misconception is that errors only happen to lazy incompetent individuals who lack vigilance. On the contrary, errors can happen to any individual despite vigilance, motivation, and dedication. When errors occur, blame should not be placed on the individual; rather, a more enlightened view should be embraced—to understand the breakdown in the system and the resulting harm to a patient. Two compelling themes surface from human factors research: (1) humans are prone to err and (2) most errors are not the result of personal inadequacies or carelessness, but instead are the product of defects in the design of health care environmental systems in which the work occurs. An illustrative case follows.

Sarah, an experienced PACU nurse, was well into her double shift by the time the patient arrived in the unit at 2:00 AM. A 36-year-old woman involved in a motor vehicle crash had just undergone an exploratory laparotomy and splenectomy for intraabdominal bleeding. Thirty minutes after the patient's arrival, an alarm sounded. Sarah noted that the patient's heart rate was 36 beats/min and dropping. Following unit protocol, Sarah quickly reached into the medication cart for atropine and intravenously administered a 0.4-mg dose. Almost instantly, the patient's blood pressure soared to 300 mm systolic on the arterial line monitor and the patient went into cardiac arrest. Despite full resuscitative efforts, the patient did not respond.

Later, as Sarah was cleaning up the bedside stand of all the medications used in the code, she found an empty phenylephrine vial. Immediately, Sarah realized that she had inadvertently given the patient a 10-mg bolus of phenylephrine instead of the intended dose of atropine.

A follow-up root cause investigation discovered that the pharmacy had recently stocked phenylephrine next to atropine in the medication drawer. Both the drugs were manufactured by the same company and came in the same sized vials with the same color snap-off caps. The label for atropine was a light red color, but the phenylephrine label was pink. Instead of placing the blame on Sarah, the suggestion was made that pharmacy immediately tag the vials with a black colored *A* atop the atropine and physically separate the two drugs from one another in the medication cart. The manufacturer was also notified and encouraged to change the labeling system.

Although initially one might question how a nurse could misread or choose not to read the label and give a wrong medication, in retrospect it is easy to see how an experienced nurse could slip while emergently reaching for a medication under conditions of high stress. Such a slip is analogous to a common error among anesthesia providers concerning gas flow meters. At one time, anesthesia gas delivery systems had two similar gas control knobs: one to deliver oxygen and one to deliver nitrous oxide. Slips occurred when anesthesia providers inadvertently turned up the nitrous oxide when they had intended to turn up the oxygen, which resulted in a hypoxic gas mixture being delivered to patients. A human factors approach was chosen to remedy this problem. The oxygen knob was redesigned with deep palpable indentations, whereas the nitrous oxide knob remained smooth. The anesthesia provider then was able to tell by touch alone which knob was in hand. The anesthesia machine was also given a built-in fail-safe mechanism that did not allow the delivery of a hypoxic mixture regardless of how high the nitrous flow was set. This approach to the problem effectively prevented harm to the patient by a hypoxic mixture of gases. Accidents and accident reporting were viewed in these examples as opportunities to design more robust systems to prevent the same type of injury from ever occurring again.

Traditionally, an adverse outcome results in blaming the particular caregiver; however, careful study of the entire system in which the incident occurred usually uncovers multiple factors that contributed to the event.[2] Lack of training, improper equipment maintenance, poor staffing, or an illegible order transcribed incorrectly can individually or jointly contribute to a critical event. In other words, a cascade of events rather than a single event, often results in an adverse outcome. CRM training advocates the systems approach to adverse outcome analysis. The systems approach seeks answers from a macro perspective to discover the contributing factors. A look at policies and administrative decisions that either supported or derailed a critical incident is a radical departure from the traditional "frame and blame" punitive approach used in medicine. This approach should not be interpreted as lessening the responsibility of the person who made an error, but as gaining a better understanding of why the error occurred; only then can the system be adjusted to better

prevent reoccurrence. CRM training strives to make practitioners aware of systemic factors and to work effectively within the context of a large system that might not always support their efforts. The goal of CRM training is to learn from the mistakes of others through an open exchange of information to lessen the contributions of human factors to an adverse event. In this way, students can come to understand the cascade of events that lead to mistakes in a certain situation.

Perianesthesia nurses are at the "sharp end" of the patient encounter; they interface directly with the patient. Many "blunt end" factors, such as the nature of the work, equipment manufacturers, hospital administrations, and other institutional effects, significantly contribute to placing these nurses at that sharp end. When error occurs, it is prudent to examine all causative factors.

CRISIS MANAGEMENT PRINCIPLES

Many approaches, philosophies, and theories of crisis management exist for use in managing complex industries such as health care. One such approach is described by the acronym ERR WATCH, developed by Fletcher[6] to help the practitioner recall the eight essential elements of crisis management (Box 4-1). ERR WATCH also serves as a reminder that the goal of crisis management is the reduction of the element of human error in any given situation. The human factors shaping performance are of prime importance. Limitations exist in a health care provider's ability to quickly and accurately process rapidly changing information during a crisis. When these limitations are understood, many opportunities can be found to improve performance.

The role of PACU nurses is unique in health care delivery. Nurses must not only be familiar with a wide variety of patient conditions and surgical treatments; they must also be educated and prepared to provide care for a multitude of populations, including neonates, small children, adults, and the elderly, all within a single shift. In addition, PACU nurses interact with staff members and physicians from many disciplines and must be able to function with an often unpredictable workload. The following sections discuss these crisis management principles in detail from the perspective of a PACU nurse.

Environment

The perianesthesia period is a potentially tumultuous time for surgical patients; therefore the typical PACU represents a complex and dynamic work environment for nurses. The acuity and diversity of postsurgical patients, dependence on

1. Know Your **Environment**
   - Know equipment function, troubleshooting, and plans for failure.
   - Be aware of staffing levels throughout shift.
2. Use Your **Resources**
   - Be aware of personal limitations.
   - Use texts and references as resources.
   - Plan ahead for probable problems.
3. Frequent **Reevaluation**
   - Evaluate treatments for untoward effects or effectiveness.
   - Gather information from all available sources.
   - Maintain situation awareness.
4. Manage Your **Workload**
   - Prioritize patient needs.
   - Preload and offload tasks.
   - Delegate tasks to others.
5. **Attention** Allocation
   - Resources are limited.
   - Avoid fixation errors.
6. **Teamwork**
   - Communicate changes and new information.
   - Use shared mental models.
7. **Communication**
   - Use closed-loop communication.
   - Avoid blame and criticism of others.
   - Focus on patient needs.
8. Call for **Help**
   - Global check before report.
   - Give a clear concise report to incoming staff.
   - Assign duties as needed.

technology and complex equipment, and inadequate staffing levels contribute to the uncertainty of the environment.

The inherent risk associated with the surgical experience follows patients to the PACU. Each patient brings an underlying medical pathology that might not be recognized until the recovery period. Such pathology can include obstructive sleep apnea, coronary artery disease, and electrolyte imbalances. Perianesthesia nurses are expected to care for patients who have undergone a wide range of surgical procedures that require a similar yet different skill set. PACU nurses must be cognizant of the ill effects of such conditions and be prepared to act on them if necessary.

A multitude of sophisticated monitors and equipment are involved in the care of patients after surgery. Nurses often rely heavily on technical specialists for maintenance and proper functioning of this equipment. Although nurses work with routine equipment on a daily basis, they may need additional training to deal with troubleshooting

and the possibility of catastrophic failure of life-sustaining equipment, such as ventilators, dialysis machines, and intraaortic balloon pumps. Seconds can be critical if the patient is disconnected from any of these life-supporting devices. The nurse's focus remains on the patient while the specialist concentrates on the equipment; however, a cross-over of skills is necessary. Therefore, opportunities for education regarding critical equipment in the environment should be offered to PACU nurses to facilitate an exchange of information and to develop contingency plans for major equipment failures should they occur. Familiarity with such emergency plans is essential and lifesaving.

Unit staffing has a major influence on the PACU nurse's role as a care provider. Open unit layouts are advantageous because nurses are expected to simultaneously monitor and assess multiple patients. Maintenance of an overall awareness of staffing levels throughout a shift enables the nurse to make appropriate assignments and exert some control over the environment. Staffing that appears adequate at one point can quickly become inadequate, unsafe, and inept as staff are called to transport and admit patients, take breaks, or attend meetings. As staffing becomes insufficient, so does the opportunity for assistance should the need arise in an emergency.

Resources

Resources are assets available to PACU nurses that enable them to do their work. The appropriate use of resources allows for safe and effective care for patients after surgery. Resources are often overlooked in an emergency. A nurse's knowledge and skills are indispensable resources while caring for patients in the PACU. However, recognition of personal limitations is also a necessary component of delivery of safe care. An honest self appraisal may reveal multiple factors that influence performance and vigilance.[7] Lack of sleep, boredom, concerns over personal matters, illness, and the influence of medications can adversely affect performance. Because nurses are human, they are not entirely immune to these influences. Knowledge of these factors and the ability to communicate them to coworkers and supervisors can go a long way to overcome their deleterious effects. A request for a lighter assignment may ultimately be safer than an attempt to overcome fatigue after a sleepless night with a sick child. The expectation that every nurse can perform optimally every day is unrealistic.

Critical care texts, drug formularies, and pharmacology manuals provide essential references for many drugs and dosages that are not used routinely. Institutional protocols and procedure guidelines should be kept on the unit for reference as needed. A review of best evidence is prudent when caring for a patient whose condition is atypical. Advanced cardiac life support (ACLS) algorithm cards, for example, are invaluable in the event of an unstable dysrhythmia or cardiac arrest because recall of these detailed protocols is difficult. Many practitioners carry a personal notebook of medications, precalculated drug dosages, and management protocols for quick access if necessary. Given the volume of knowledge necessary to provide the best nursing care, one cannot stay current in all areas without the use of such cognitive resources. Various applications for smart phones, tablets, and other technological devices are available now for health care workers and provide quickly accessible information.

Reevaluation

The critical aspects of an emergency often cause health care providers to lose sight of the proverbial big picture. Thus, the purpose of reevaluation is twofold: to assess the effectiveness of treatment and to provide more comprehensive insight into the problem. For example, a nurse may become involved in initiating a response to a patient in cardiac arrest yet forget to turn the oxygen to 100% on the ventilator. A continuous scan of all monitors and equipment to evaluate change is ideal in order to provide the best care. The risks and benefits of every intervention must be analyzed. Reevaluation helps to draw the focus outward to see whether parameters that were overlooked initially have changed. With baseline data, a better understanding of the trends in these parameters can be realized. The ability to stand back and absorb the situation in its entirety is referred to as *situation awareness* in human factors literature.[8] Situational awareness allows one to grasp the effects of significant changes and to plan instead of merely react to the situation. It is an integral and requisite component for optimal performance and effective decision making in dynamic and complex environments such as the PACU. With continuous reevaluation of the patient, the PACU nurse can report more effectively to incoming help. The PACU nurse is able to detail what has been done and to prioritize subsequent interventions, which helps new team members contribute positively and effectively.

Workload

A typical day in any critical care unit is filled with multiple tasks. Most nurses quickly learn to distribute their workload throughout the shift and to prioritize patient care needs as conditions change.

Experienced nurses frequently use strategies known as *preloading* and *offloading* to balance the demands of patient care. *Preloading* is defined as early preparation for an upcoming procedure. *Offloading* describes the work to be done after care has been rendered. These two strategies can dramatically decrease the workload during busy periods.

An unexpected emergency dramatically and precipitously increases workload. Additional help is essential in completion of the multitude of tasks required during this critical time. As new staff members arrive, they should be assigned a specific task that is appropriate to their education and experience. The charge nurse can page attending physicians and other support personnel to distribute the workload more appropriately to ensure coverage. Registered nurses can administer medications, change ventilator settings, and assist in procedures, whereas other appropriately trained staff can carry blood samples to the laboratory for analysis, obtain blood products from the blood bank, or secure the proper equipment.

Attention Allocation

It is well understood that human beings pay attention to what is most important to them at any given moment in time. Attention is a limited resource; a person can accurately follow only two to three rapidly changing variables at any one time. Multiple direct patient care activities increase the burden on attention. The uncertain nature of a crisis presents a significant opportunity for error, which makes comprehension and analysis of the situation difficult for any one individual. The perianesthesia nurse must be available to make observations, commit to decisions, and continuously evaluate rapidly changing conditions, often for more than one patient.

Fixation on one idea and pauses in thinking are common for health care providers involved in a critical incident. Fixation errors occur in dynamic situations and are often difficult events from which to recover. For example, a PACU nurse may recognize a decrease in oxygen saturation accompanied by elevated peak airway pressures and, with that information, treat the patient for a bronchospasm. While doing so, the nurse may not be receptive to the hypotension, flushing, and rash that signal an allergic reaction. This failure is an example of a *this and only this* fixation error in which one has a reasonable diagnosis in mind and manipulates any additional signs and symptoms to fit that diagnosis. A second common fixation error is labeled *anything but this*, in which treatment is delayed while one seeks additional information in the face of a crisis. The nurse essentially identifies the problem but continues to look for a more manageable diagnosis leading to delayed or improper treatment. The third type of fixation error is called *everything's okay,* in which the health care professional denies a problem in evolution. In this case, a PACU nurse might be witnessing a steady decrease in a patient's oxygen saturation and choose not to respond, telling himself "everything's okay." All health care providers are vulnerable to these types of fixation errors during the time constraints of an evolving emergency. These errors are the result of an overtaxed brain that precludes effective performance given the immense workload.

Teamwork

Nurses in the PACU routinely use teamwork to care for critically ill patients. Flexible assignments, assistance with turning patients, or preparation of medications are just a few ways nurses work together to accomplish their goals.

During the management of a crisis, however, good teamwork is critical. Additional staff members with variable expertise may suddenly join the existing team. Physicians may arrive and begin to order treatments, drugs, and tests. The original PACU team of nurses now becomes multidisciplinary and takes on a new character. New physician residents may be reluctant to take on a leadership role or several may attempt to be the leader simultaneously. Verbal orders may be given but directed at no particular individual. A previously organized environment can rapidly become chaotic and disordered.

Multidisciplinary team training at major health care institutions has shown excellent results from crisis management training. Some team members are trained to acquire effective leadership skills while other team members may be taught to be productive and effective team members. Team members are encouraged to give their input to the leader, to inform leaders of significant changes, to report the administration of drugs and treatments, and to critique problem solving strategies. Information from any source may provide the answer in an ambiguous situation. Recognition that every member of the team has the potential to make valuable contributions is important. The team supports the leader in maintaining good situation awareness and in making the best possible decisions. Ideally, the leader should be willing to consider input from all team members, communicate the diagnosis and plans for treatment, and keep team members informed of progress. By doing so, the team leader keeps the entire team focused on the immediate needs of the patient and further encourages their active role in optimizing the patient's condition.

Communication

Great leadership and teamwork cannot occur without the ability to communicate effectively. The military uses closed-loop communication to ensure that orders are received and understood properly. People must be addressed by name to attract their attention. Once a particular message is stated clearly, look for verbal confirmation that the message was received correctly. "Give some atropine" is better stated as "Bill, give 0.5 mg of atropine IV now." Bill, in turn, should state "I am giving 0.5 mg of atropine IV now." As Bill completes the task, he should inform the leader that it has been done, which verifies that he has successfully completed the task and that he is free to participate in other additional tasks.

High noise levels accompany an emergency situation as many people try to talk at the same time. Speaking in a calm quiet voice does more to attract attention than another shout in the melee. Preceding the statement with the person's name helps to gain attention. Repeating the name may be necessary to divert the person from other activities.

Conflict is common in emotionally charged situations. There have been several published accounts of hostile interactions between health care providers that actually led to violence. To avoid escalation of existing hostility, speak in impersonal terms and avoid making judgments and placing blame on others.

Call for Help

Nurses are accustomed to working together. They rarely have trouble calling for additional help as needed for physical tasks such as getting the code cart, starting additional intravenous lines, or hanging blood products. A second person's opinion, however, may be absolutely critical during the management of a serious situation. Many health care providers believe that they lose credibility with colleagues if they call for assistance in this type of situation. Merit exists in the adage "do what's right for the patient, not what's right for the provider." A call for a second opinion from someone with more expertise is a wise move, not a weak one.

Before help arrives, a global scan of the patient, the equipment, and the monitors is a good practice. This requisite knowledge provides a set of baseline data with which to compare as the treatment progresses and allows the nurse to provide a full report to incoming assistants. When help arrives, incoming staff members should receive a succinct report on what has happened and any treatment that has begun. Information in the report need not include insignificant details, but should convey the information necessary to explicate the situation at hand.

The ERR WATCH principles make sense. Most PACU nurses can use them daily in their practice and have them available when an emergency situation occurs. These principles are universal and can be used to effectively improve performance and positively influence the care given to the postsurgical patient in the complex environment of the recovery room.

SIMULATION IN CRM TRAINING

Simulation is the implementation of artificial representations of complex real-world processes with a sufficient level of fidelity to achieve particular goals.[9] Simulation imitates real phenomena and processes to capture key characteristics and behaviors of real life events. It is an innovative instructional approach that enhances learning and promotes a sense of empowerment on the part of learners by involving them in the decisions that influence their learning. Through simulation, trainees are challenged in novel ways and take more responsibility in their learning. A critical feature of simulation as a learning tool is that learners have the ability to interact with their surroundings experimentally.[9] Using high-fidelity simulated environments, educators and trainers can create models of crisis and chaos where the risk to a real patient is absent.

CRM training for PACU personnel incorporates human patient simulators in high-fidelity critical care environments to simulate rare but life-threatening postanesthesia crises, including inability to ventilate, anaphylactic shock, and cardiac arrest, to name a few. Human patient simulators, sometimes referred to as *mannequins*, are full-body representations of patients that demonstrate physiologic parameters, such as blood pressure, heart rate, airway pressure, oxygen saturation, and central venous and pulmonary pressures. Different models of human patient simulators offer varying degrees of realism, including bleeding, urination, sweating, drooling, pupil constriction and dilation, seizures, chest movement, and peripheral pulses. Standard monitoring equipment is used to display physiologically appropriate measurements of all invasive and noninvasive values. Simulators also have the ability to breathe spontaneously with measurable exhaled carbon dioxide. Furthermore, trainees can assess heart, breath, and bowel sounds. The addition of various props can transform the patient into a full-term parturient, an elderly gentleman, or even a young athlete. Placed within a realistic setting, the human patient simulator becomes lifelike as it converses with trainees via an instructor-speaker microphone.

Human patient simulators come with an accompanying laptop computer and software and are operated by a controller, usually a member of the training team. The controller can steer the human patient simulator to respond to trainee interventions, such as drug and fluid administration, cardiac defibrillation, intubation, and oxygenation. Human patient simulators are highly effective in contributing to the realism necessary to achieve educational objectives.

CRM emphasizes the integration of crisis management principles, including decision making, task management, leadership, communication, situational awareness, and teamwork, in the training of recovery room nurses and team members to manage critical events and crisis situations. Identification and mastering of ideal case management behaviors, including preparation, anticipation, and vigilance, are also a significant goal of CRM training. In addition, factors such as production pressure, problem evolution, and abstract reasoning and their influence on the provider to act efficiently are considered and explored.[10]

CRM training is an experiential teaching approach that brings the daunting characteristics of a perianesthesia crisis to life and ultimately intends to improve efficiency, effectiveness, and safety in the delivery of care to surgical patients. Most CRM training courses have a similar structure that incorporates assigned readings that describe basic principles, a course introduction that details the overall concept, an orientation to the simulated critical care environment, and videotaped critical incident scenarios of which the learner is an active participant performing the duties of a PACU team member under the extreme conditions of a postanesthesia emergency. During a simulated scenario, one learner out of the group is randomly selected to be in the "hot seat" as the team leader while the other members of the group participate in various roles as team members. During a CRM training course, the trainee is able to not only actively apply crisis resource management principles during a crisis but also observe other learners applying these same principles while fulfilling other team member roles.

A video-playback, detailed debriefing session, usually facilitated by course faculty, immediately follows the scenario in an adjacent classroom. *Debriefing* is a discussion among students, guided by faculty, that encourages reflective thought and self review.[11] Debriefing is regarded as an integral part of CRM and occurs in a positive, supportive, nonjudgmental, and nonevaluative environment that allows all participants an opportunity to share their experience, offer comments, and discuss concerns.[11] The primary goal of debriefing is the discussion of the CRM principles as they relate to the outcome. The discussion is focused on essential crisis management principles such as communication, teamwork, and decision making. Trainees are often surprised at their performances as they view the videotape and are able to scrutinize their interaction with other team members. Most importantly, the group examines CRM strategies that can be used to prevent future errors in similar situations. Most participants complete the course feeling better prepared to navigate the complexity inherent in critical events characteristic of the PACU.

Variety of Teaching Goals

Simulation centers provide a safe place for training health care providers. Mistakes made during simulation sessions do not harm actual patients. Procedures can be performed repeatedly until the trainee gains a desired level of confidence and proficiency. New employees can learn the unit's routines or how to admit and care for various types of patients. PACU personnel can work with the actual unit equipment to better understand its operation. Existing staff members could potentially use the simulator to practice rarely performed procedures, learn new skills, or orient to new equipment such as computerized charting. A hands-on opportunity to deliver ACLS protocols is just one example of the potential use of simulation. Personnel can gain experience in the diagnosis and management of rare life-threatening medical crises rarely witnessed in any other setting. Several institutions have developed morbidity and mortality conferences using simulation technology to recreate real cases. Through simulation, many topics can be taught either individually or as part of a more comprehensive critical care course.

For effective management of crises in health care, collaboration of multiple team members, including physicians and nurses, is essential. Simulation provides an opportunity for training health care teams to work collectively and maximize their potential. Studies in aviation and medicine have found that lack of nontechnical skills such as teamwork contributed to most disasters. Until the introduction of full-scale human patient simulators, the training of teams was never formalized. Now, actual teams of nurses, respiratory therapists, physicians, and other health care providers can interact realistically and learn to communicate and

function together as a cohesive unit. This type of training has been performed at various sites and has been found to be effective at improving team performance.[12,13]

SUMMARY

Much of the existing literature on crisis management comes from the field of aviation psychology, air traffic control, and military operations. In an effort to improve quality and safety in health care, formal training in crisis management has been developed and embraced by many disciplines. CRM in health care incorporates concepts such as situation awareness and human error, to ultimately improve provider performance and promote patient safety.

Technical knowledge and skills alone are not adequate for functioning in the complex environment of critical care. Patients today are sicker than ever before. With this increased patient acuity also comes an increasing number of critical events that need prompt and accurate management. Each problem has many possible outcomes that depend largely on the actions or inactions of caregivers. Every patient deserves to have well-trained and knowledgeable care providers who can manage the ordinary events associated with recovery from anesthesia as well as the unexpected ones. CRM training and simulation offer a new approach to help PACU nurses meet these challenges successfully. Like the patients for whom they care, health care professionals are human, and humans are imperfect, which is something that cannot be changed. Through advanced training techniques such as CRM and the use of high-fidelity simulation technologies, perianesthesia nurses can be more prepared for life-threatening emergencies, mitigate the number of preventable mishaps, and better contribute to the overall well-being of the patients for whom they provide care.

REFERENCES

1. Durso FT, et al: En route operational errors and situation awareness, *International Journal of Aviation Psychology*, 8(2):177–194, 1998.
2. Gaba DM, et al: Theory of dynamic decision-making and crisis management. In Gaba DM, et al: *Crisis management in anesthesiology*, New York, 1994, Churchill Livingstone, pp. 5–46.
3. Cooper J, et al: Preventable anesthesia mishaps: a study of human factors, *Quality and Safety in Health Care* 11(3): 277–282, 2002.
4. Cook RI, Woods DD: Human error in medicine. In Bogner MS, editor: *Operating at the sharp end: the complexity of human error*, Hillsdale, NJ, 1994, Lawrence Erlbaum Associates.

5. Reason J: Human error: models and management, *Br Med J* 320(7237):768–770, 2000.

6. Fletcher JL: AANA journal course: update for nurse anesthetists; ERR WATCH: anesthesia crisis resource management from the nurse anesthetist's perspective, *Journal of the American Association of Nurse Anesthetists* 66(6): 595–602, 1998.

7. Whittingham RB: *The blame machine: why human error causes accidents*, Burlington, MA, 2004, Butterworth-Heinemann.

8. Endsley MR, Garland DJ: *Situation awareness analysis and measurement*, Mahwah, NJ, 2000, Lawrence Erlbaum Associates, Inc.

9. Doyle DJ: *Simulation in medical education: focus on anesthesiology,* available at www.med-ed-online.org/f0000053. htm. Accessed May 10, 2011.

10. Gaba DM, et al: Simulation-based training in anesthesia crisis resource management (ACRM): a decade of experience, *Simulation Gaming* 32(2):175–193, 2001.

11. Savoldelli GL, et al: Value of debriefing during simulated crisis management, *Anesthesiology* 105(2):279–285, 2006.

12. Cannon-Bowers JA, Salas E: *Making decisions under stress,* Washington, DC, 2006, American Psychological Association.

13. Weller JM, et al: Evaluation of high fidelity patient simulator assessment of performance of anaesthetists, *Br Journal of Anaesth* 90:43–47, 2003.

5 Infection Prevention and Control in the PACU

Lisa Sturm, MPH, CIC

The increasing prevalence rate of multidrug-resistant organisms combined with the increasing complexity of care and the volume of patients seen in a busy perianesthesia unit underscores the importance of having an infection control program in place.

Patients with a wide range of infectious diseases, some communicable, commonly receive care in the preoperative and postoperative settings. The goal of infection control is prevention of the transmission of pathogenic microorganisms among patients, staff members, and visitors. A multitude of variables needs to be managed for this prevention, ranging from environment, to equipment, to health care worker behaviors and practices.

The following policies and procedures that are based on published guidelines and recommendations can help to minimize the infectious risks present in a perianesthesia care unit. Education, compliance, monitoring, and quality improvement are essential to the success of the infection control efforts.

DEFINITIONS

Adverse Events: Untoward, undesirable, and usually unanticipated events, such as death of a patient, an employee, or a visitor in a health care organization. Incidents such as patient falls or improper administration of medications are also considered adverse events even if there is no permanent effect on the patient.

Airborne Transmission: (Microorganisms that are) carried or transported by the air.

Antibiotic Resistance: The selective pressure of antimicrobial therapy has resulted in the evolution of bacteria that are resistant to certain antibiotics. The resistance patterns of the microbes are constantly changing. These patterns are affected by patterns of antibiotic use, the prevalence of specific microorganisms, the mechanisms of resistance in these organisms, resistance transfer from one organism to another, and the patient population. The risk of infection or colonization with antibiotic-resistant microorganisms is higher among sicker and debilitated patients and in settings of high antimicrobial use and invasive technology (e.g., intensive care unit [ICU]). Infections from antibiotic-resistant organisms are difficult to treat and are often associated with high morbidity rates. These microbes can be spread from patient to patient through transient hand carriage and environmental contamination.

Antimicrobial Prophylaxis: Antibiotics that are given before the surgical incision for prevention of a surgical wound infection.

Artificial Nails: Nails with products affixed to them, such as gel, tips, jewelry, overlays, and wraps.

Attributable Mortality Rate: The death rate (expression of the number of deaths in a population during a specified time frame) that can be linked to a particular cause or source.

Barrier Precautions: The use of garb (e.g., masks, hair coverings, gowns, gloves) for protection to either the health care worker or the patient.

Bloodborne: Microorganisms that are carried or transmitted via the blood or fluids that contain blood.

Bloodborne Pathogens: Pathogenic microorganisms that are present in human blood and can cause disease in humans. These pathogens include, but are not limited to, hepatitis B virus (HBV), hepatitis C virus (HCV), and human immunodeficiency virus (HIV).

Central Line Associated Bloodstream Infection (CLA-BSI): Bacteremia or fungemia that develops in a patient with an intravascular central venous catheter.

Central Venous Catheter: A vascular access device that terminates at or close to the heart or one of the great vessels. An umbilical artery or vein catheter is considered a central line.

Chlorhexidine Gluconate (CHG): An antibacterial agent that is effective against a wide variety of gram-negative and gram-positive organisms and used as a topical antiinfective agent for the skin and mucous membranes.

Clostridium difficile: A bacterium that causes diarrhea and more serious intestinal conditions such as colitis. It is found in the normal gastrointestinal flora in about 3% of healthy adults and in 10% to 30% or more of hospitalized patients. Antibiotic use, even a short course given for prophylaxis or treatment of infections, often changes the normal gastrointestinal flora, which can lead to *C. difficile* overgrowth and toxin production. *C. difficile* accounts for 15% to 25% of all antibiotic-associated diarrhea. *C. difficile* colitis occurs in all ages but is most frequent in middle-aged and older adults or patients with debilitated conditions. *C. difficile* is shed in feces and is spread primarily via the hands of health care personnel who have touched a contaminated surface or item and via direct contact with a contaminated item. Hand hygiene performed with soap and water and thorough disinfection of the environment with diluted bleach reduce the risk of spreading *C. difficile*.

Colonization: Microorganisms that have become established in a habitat in a host but do not cause disease (infection) in this habitat.

Contact (Direct or Indirect): (Microorganisms that are) spread from contaminated hands or objects.

Contact Dermatitis: Inflammation of the skin that results from direct exposure to an irritant.

Contaminated Sharps: Any contaminated object that can penetrate the skin, such as needles, scalpels, broken glass, broken capillary tubes, and exposed ends of dental wires.

Cross Transmission: Horizontal transmission of an organism in the health care setting; patient to patient.

Disinfection: To render free from infection, especially with destruction of harmful microorganisms.

Droplet Transmission: (Microorganisms that are) carried on airborne droplets of saliva or sputum. In general they travel from 0 to 3 feet.

Epidemiology: A branch of medical science that deals with the incidence, distribution, and control of disease in a population.

Exposure Control Plan: A formal document as defined by the Occupational Safety and Health Administration (OSHA) Regulations (Standards, 29 CFR) Bloodborne Pathogens 1910.1030; to exist in any institution with occupational exposure. The document is designed to outline the steps necessary to eliminate or minimize employee exposure.

Extended-Spectrum Beta-Lactamases (ESBL): Beta-lactamase is a type of enzyme responsible for bacterial resistance to beta-lactam antibiotics; among these are penicillins, cephalosporins, carbapenems, and others. In the middle 1980s, new types of beta-lactamase were produced by *Klebsiella* spp. and *Escherichia coli* that could hydrolyze the extended spectrum cephalosporins; these are collectively termed the *extended spectrum beta-lactamases*.

Fecal-Oral: Microorganisms that are spread through ingestion of contaminated feces.

Health Care–Associated Infections: Acquired or occurring in the health care setting.

Health Care Worker Flora: The microorganisms (as bacteria or fungi) that live in or on the bodies of personnel who work in a health care institution.

Hypothermia: Subnormal temperature of the body, defined as temperature less than 36° C.

Immunocompromised: Impairment or weakening of the immune system.

Medical Waste/Regulated Waste: Liquid or semiliquid blood or other potentially infectious materials; contaminated items that release blood or other potentially infectious materials in a liquid or semiliquid state if compressed; items that are caked with dried blood or other potentially infectious materials and are capable of releasing these materials during handling; contaminated sharps; and pathologic and microbiologic wastes that contain blood or other potentially infectious materials.

Microbial Colony Counts: Enumeration via direct count of viable isolated bacterial or fungal cells or spores capable of growth on solid culture media. Each colony (i.e., microbial colony-forming unit) represents the progeny of a single cell in the original inoculum. The method is used routinely by environmental microbiologists for quantification of organisms in air, food, and water; by clinicians for measurement of patient microbial load; and in antimicrobial drug testing.

Moist Body Substances: All body fluids, including blood, body cavity fluids, breast milk, urine, feces, wound or other skin drainage, respiratory and oral secretions, mucous membranes.

Mucous Membranes: Mucous membranes line cavities or canals of the body that open to the outside, including the eyes, ears, mouth, nose, and genitals.

Multidrug Resistant Organisms (MDROs): Microorganisms, predominantly bacteria, that are resistant to one or more classes of antimicrobial agents. Although the names of certain MDROs describe resistance to only one agent (e.g., methicillin-resistant *Staphylococcus aureus* [MRSA], vancomycin-resistant *Enterococcus* [VRE]), these pathogens are frequently resistant to most available antimicrobial agents. These highly resistant organisms deserve special attention in health care facilities. In addition to MRSA and VRE, certain gram-negative bacteria, including those that produce ESBLs and *Klebsiella pneumoniae* carbapenemase–producing organisms are of particular concern.

N95 Respirator: An air-purifying filtering-facepiece respirator that is more than 95% efficient at removing 0.3-μm particles and is not resistant to oil.

Negative-Pressure Isolation Rooms: The difference in air pressure between two areas. A room that is under negative pressure has a lower pressure than adjacent areas, which keeps air from flowing out of the room and into adjacent rooms or areas.

Normothermia: Normal body temperature (i.e., 36° to 38° C).

Nosocomial Infections: Term used historically to denote infections that are acquired or occur in a hospital.

One-Handed "Scoop" Technique: A method of capping a needle if deemed necessary to do so. The needle cap is set on a stable surface and not touched. The needled device then is placed inside the cap with one hand. The cap is then secured into place with the other hand.

Parenteral Exposure: Piercing of mucous membranes or the skin barrier through such events as needle sticks, human bites, cuts, and abrasions.

Pathogenic Microorganisms: An organism of microscopic or ultramicroscopic size that is capable of causing disease.

Personal Protective Equipment (PPE): Specialized clothing or equipment worn by an employee for protection against a hazard. General work clothes (e.g., uniforms, pants, shirts, blouses) not intended to function as protection against a hazard are not considered to be PPE.

Seroconversion Risk: The likelihood of conversion from negative virus status to positive virus status.

Susceptible: Little resistance to a specific infectious disease.

Transient Contamination: A microorganism that exists temporarily on the hands of a health care worker and is not part of the normal flora of the skin.

Vancomycin-Resistant Enterococcus (VRE): A strain of *Enterococcus* species that normally lives in the intestines and sometimes the urinary tract of all people. VRE has learned to resist or survive most antibiotics, including a strong antibiotic called *vancomycin*. VRE is acquired via direct contact (touching) with objects or surfaces that are contaminated with VRE. VRE is not spread through the air. People at risk for VRE infection are those who have chronic illnesses, have undergone recent surgery, have weakened immune systems, or have recently taken certain antibiotics.

Vector: Microorganisms that are spread through insects.

MANAGING THE ENVIRONMENT AND EQUIPMENT

Environment

A safe and clean environment is essential for a reduction in the risk of transmission of microorganisms. Most equipment in a perianesthesia unit that comes into contact with patients is considered to have a low risk of infection transmission, most notably if the equipment is noninvasive and contacts only intact skin. Examples of these items are electrodes, stethoscopes, pulse oximeter devices, blood pressure cuffs, the outside surfaces of equipment (e.g., ventilators, intravenous pumps), and larger surfaces (e.g., tables, wheelchairs, bedside stands, floors, walls). Depending on the item and the nature of the contamination, simple surface cleaning is all that is necessary to ensure safety between uses. Many hospital-grade disinfectants are combined with a cleaning component so that both cleaning and disinfection can be achieved in one step. Disinfection wipes are an appropriate option as well because of their active ingredient. If visible blood or body fluid is present, then a hospital-grade disinfectant approved by the Environmental Protection Agency (e.g., a quaternary ammonium compound, 70% isopropyl, properly diluted bleach, or phenolic) is required per the Occupational Safety and Health Administration (OSHA) Bloodborne Pathogen Standard.[1]

Laundry

The risk of actual disease transmission from soiled linen is negligible, although laundry can harbor large numbers of pathogenic microorganisms. Simple hygienic practices for the processing and storage of linens are recommended for a reduction in the likelihood of transmitting infectious diseases.

Soiled linens should be handled as little as possible and with minimal agitation for prevention of gross microbial contamination of the air and of persons who handle the linens. All soiled linens should be bagged or placed in containers in the care unit; they should never be sorted or rinsed in the location of use. Linens heavily contaminated with blood or other body fluids should be bagged and transported in a manner that prevents leakage.

Commercial laundry facilities often use water temperatures of at least 160° F (71° C) and 50 to 150 ppm of chlorine bleach for removal of significant quantities of microorganisms from grossly contaminated linens. Commercial dry cleaning of fabrics soiled with blood also renders these items free of the risk of pathogen transmission. Last, clean linen should be handled, transported, and stored by methods that ensure its cleanliness.

Furnishings and Equipment

All furnishings in a perianesthesia environment should be evaluated before purchase and assessed for the ability to resist staining and tearing. Furnishing and medical equipment ease of cleaning and ability to withstand harsh disinfections, including 10% diluted bleach, should also be considered. Ease of disassembly for the purposes of cleaning and disinfection should be reviewed. Absorbent upholstery should be avoided if the likelihood of contamination is present. Torn mattress pads and seating should be repaired or replaced promptly for prevention of contamination. All manufacturers' instructions for cleaning and disinfection should be obtained, and the appropriate personnel responsible for this task should be trained initially and regularly thereafter.

Sinks

The number and accessibility of sinks in the perianesthesia care unit is important for increased compliance with hand washing. The *Guidelines for Design and Construction of Hospital and Health Care Facilities,* published and updated periodically by the American Institute of Architects (AIA), should be referenced for current sink allotment recommendations. The guidelines are conceived as minimal construction requirements for hospitals, and the document includes engineering systems, infection control, and safety and architectural guidelines for design and construction. The Joint Commission states that the AIA guidelines should be used during new construction. The current AIA guidelines recommend at least one hand washing station with hands-free or wrist blade–operable controls for every four beds in a postanesthesia care unit (PACU).[2]

Bays and Isolation Rooms

Appropriate space allotment and other design features for patient bays and rooms during new construction and renovation can be obtained from the AIA guidelines reference. Additional local and state stipulations may apply. Provisions should be available for the isolation of infectious patients, but an airborne (respiratory) infection isolation room is not required in a preoperative or postanesthesia care unit. However, each individual setting needs to conduct an infection control risk assessment for the need for an isolation room based on the epidemiology of airborne diseases (e.g., frequency of tuberculosis in the community, medically or surgically treated in the institution).

Traffic Flow

The movement of staff members, patients, visitors, and equipment in the preoperative and PACU setting is an important consideration in the design or renovation of space. Areas in which invasive procedures (e.g., central line insertions) take place should be away from main traffic areas, entrances, and exits to reduce the likelihood of contamination.

GENERAL INFECTION CONTROL PRACTICES

Handwashing

The benefits of hand hygiene in a hospital setting were first recognized by Ignaz Semmelweis in 1847 after the death of his friend from an infection that he contracted after his finger was accidentally punctured with a knife during a postmortem examination. The friend's autopsy showed a pathologic situation similar to that of the women who were dying from puerperal fever in one of the obstetric clinics. Semmelweis immediately proposed a connection between cadaveric contamination and puerperal fever and made a detailed study of the mortality statistics of the obstetric clinic attended by physicians who also performed autopsies with the statistics of the midwives' clinics. The midwives did not participate in autopsies. He concluded that he and the students carried the infecting particles on their hands from the autopsy room to the patients they examined in the clinical setting. Semmelweis concluded that some unknown "cadaveric material" caused childbed fever. He

instituted a policy requiring use of a solution of chlorinated lime for washing hands between autopsy work and the examination of patients and the mortality rate dropped from 12.24% to 2.38%, comparable to the midwives' clinics' rates.[3]

To this day, hand hygiene remains of paramount importance for preventing the spread of disease-causing germs in the perianesthesia setting. Hands should be washed with soap and water for at least 15 to 20 seconds with a hospital-approved liquid or foam soap (bar soap should be avoided). If hands are not visibly soiled, an alcohol-based hand rub can be used. Alcohol-based hand rubs significantly reduce the number of microorganisms on the skin, are fast acting, and cause less skin irritation.[4] They should not be used if the hands are visibly contaminated with blood, body fluids, or soiling. Hand hygiene should be minimally performed before and after patient care, after handling of soiled equipment or linen, after removal of gloves, after use of the restroom, before and after eating, or whenever hands are soiled. Health care personnel should avoid wearing artificial nails and keep natural nails less than one quarter of an inch long if they care for patients at high risk of acquiring infections (e.g., patients in intensive care units or in transplant units).

Adherence to hand hygiene practices has been studied in observational studies of health care workers (HCWs). Compliance rates to follow recommended hand hygiene procedures have been poor, with mean baseline rates of 5% to 81% (overall average, 40%). Perceived barriers to adherence with hand hygiene include skin irritation, inaccessible hand-hygiene supplies, interference with HCW-patient relationships, priority of care (i.e., the patient's needs are given priority over hand hygiene), wearing of gloves, forgetfulness, lack of knowledge of hand hygiene policy, insufficient time for hand hygiene, high workload and understaffing, and the lack of scientific information or education indicating a definite effect of improved hand hygiene on health care–associated infection rates.[5-11]

Frequent and repeated use of hand hygiene products, particularly soaps and other detergents, is a primary cause of chronic irritant contact dermatitis among HCWs.[12] To minimize this condition, HCWs should use hospital-approved hand lotion frequently and regularly on their hands. Small personal-use containers or multiuse pumps that are smaller than 16 ounces (and not refilled) should be used. Lotions that contain petroleum or other oil emollients can affect the integrity of latex gloves; therefore compatibility between the lotion and its possible effects on gloves should be considered at the time of product selection.[1] Last, certain moisturizing products and surfactants have been shown to interfere with the residual activity of chlorhexidine gluconate (CHG), a skin antiseptic in liquid soap. Compatibility between a lotion and its possible effects on the efficacy of certain antiseptic soaps should be considered at the time of product selection.

Personal Protective Equipment

The most common personal protective equipment (PPE) used by HCWs is gloves. The Centers for Disease Control and Prevention (CDC) has recommended that HCWs wear gloves to: (1) reduce the risk of personnel acquiring infections from patients; (2) prevent HCW flora from being transmitted to patients; and (3) reduce transient contamination of the hands of personnel by flora that can be transmitted from one patient to another.[13] OSHA mandates that gloves be worn during all patient care activities that may involve exposure to blood or body fluids that may be contaminated with blood.[1] They should also be worn for direct contact with mucous membranes, nonintact skin, open wounds, or items potentially contaminated with moist body substances. Gloves should also be worn in vascular access procedures. The effectiveness of gloves in prevention of contamination of the hands of HCWs has been confirmed in several clinical studies. Two of these studies, which involved personnel caring for patients with *Clostridium difficile* or vancomycin-resistant *Enterococcus* (VRE), revealed that wearing gloves prevented hand contamination among most personnel who had direct contact with patients.[14-16] Wearing of gloves also prevented personnel from acquiring VRE on their hands when touching contaminated environmental surfaces.[16] Prevention of heavy contamination of the hands is considered important because hand washing or hand antisepsis might not remove all potential pathogens when hands are heavily contaminated.[17,18]

Additional forms of PPE include fluid-resistant gowns, aprons, or other protective clothing. This PPE should be worn to protect clothing and all areas of exposed skin when contact with moist body substances is reasonably anticipated. Gowns shall be used once and discarded after use. Face protection, such as masks and protective eyewear (goggles or glasses with side shields), should be worn to prevent contact of blood or other moist body substances with the mucous membranes of the nose and mouth, which can occur when moist body substances are splashed, sprayed, or splattered. Face shields can be worn in place of protective eyewear and masks.

Standard Precautions

Standard Precautions synthesize the major features of Universal Precautions (Blood and Body Fluid Precaution, designed to reduce the risk of transmission of bloodborne pathogens) and body substance isolation (designed to reduce the risk of transmission of pathogens from moist body substances) and apply to all patients who receive care in hospitals, regardless of diagnosis or presumed infection status. Standard Precautions apply to: (1) blood; (2) all body fluids, secretions, and excretions, except sweat, regardless of whether or not they contain visible blood; (3) nonintact skin; and (4) mucous membranes. Standard Precautions are designed to reduce the risk of transmission of microorganisms from both recognized and unrecognized sources of infection in hospitals.[19]

In addition to the aforementioned use of hand hygiene and PPE, Standard Precautions also encompass the management of patient care equipment. They stipulate that used patient care equipment that is soiled with blood, body fluids, secretions, and excretions should be managed in a manner that prevents skin and mucous membrane exposures, contamination of clothing, and transfer of microorganisms to other patients and environments. Reusable equipment should be cleaned and reprocessed appropriately before use for the care of another patient, and single-use items (or items labeled as disposable) should not be reprocessed and reused and should be discarded properly.

Standard Precautions also encompass the practices of environmental control (e.g., that the hospital has adequate procedures for the routine care, cleaning, and disinfection of environmental surfaces, beds, bedrails, bedside equipment, and other frequently touched surfaces) and ensure that these procedures are followed. Last, Standard Precautions reiterate the importance of the Occupational Health and Bloodborne Pathogens Rule and proper patient placement for prevention of transmission of disease, both of which are discussed later in this chapter.

MANAGEMENT OF THE INFECTED OR CONTAGIOUS PATIENT

The chain of infection is a concept that shows the essential requirements for the perpetuation of a disease-causing microorganism (Fig. 5-1). All infectious diseases are caused by a microorganism (e.g., bacteria, virus, mold, fungi, parasite). For survival, each microorganism sustains itself in a source. The source may be a living host, such as a human or animal, or a nonliving source, such as

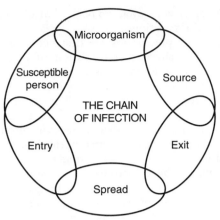

FIG. 5-1 Chain of infection. (Courtesy The Department of Infection Control and Epidemiology at the University of Michigan Hospitals and Health Centers, Ann Arbor, Mich.)

biohazardous waste or a laboratory specimen. To cause disease, the microorganism must have a portal of exit from the source (e.g., respiratory tract, spill) and a method of spread. The six main methods of spread for infectious diseases include airborne, droplet, contact (direct or indirect), bloodborne, vector, and fecal-oral. With its unique method of spread, an organism must find a way to enter its next host. The entry point may be the same as the exit from the source of the infection (such as respiratory route to respiratory route or blood to blood), or it may be different (such as fecal exit to oral entry). The last component to the chain of infection is the susceptible person. A person may be more susceptible because of underlying illness, such as immunocompromise from chemotherapy or AIDS, or because of the risks of an open incision or invasive procedure. Likewise, a person may be less susceptible to the infection as a result of history of vaccination or natural immunity from past exposure or disease.

Communicable Diseases of Concern

Every institution should have a method of identifying patients who pose a public health risk to others, and each perianesthesia unit needs to be aware of the process used for this identification. Certain communicable diseases should be clearly documented in the patient's medical record, and the patient should be placed into appropriate patient precautions or isolation per institutional policy to minimize the infectious risks to others. Infectious diseases that warrant immediate attention include, but are not limited to, bacterial meningitis (or meningitis of unknown infectious etiology), measles (rubeola), mumps, rubella, chickenpox, tuberculosis,

and severe acute respiratory syndrome. Each state in the United States publishes it own reportable disease listing that stipulates reporting requirements. Typically, diseases are reported to the local public health department by the physician or the infection control department. Communication is essential between the patient, health care provider, reporting department in the institution, and public health department to ensure that the chain of infection is broken.

Antibiotic-Resistant Organisms

In addition to the communicable diseases that pose an infectious risk to others, antibiotic-resistant organisms pose a significant threat to others if not properly controlled and managed. Aside from the cross-transmission risks, these organisms also cause an increase in lengths of stay, costs, and mortality rates.[20-25] The most common organisms include methicillin-resistant *Staphylococcus aureus* (MRSA) and VRE. Certain strains of *S. aureus* also have intermediate susceptibility or are resistant to vancomycin (i.e., vancomycin-intermediate *S. aureus* [VISA], vancomycin-resistant *S. aureus* [VRSA]). In addition to the gram-positive organisms are certain gram-negative bacteria, including those that produce extended-spectrum beta-lactamases (ESBLs) and others that are resistant to multiple classes of antibiotics. Examples of resistant gram-negative bacteria include *E. coli*, *Klebsiella pneumoniae*, and *Acinetobacter baumannii*, and organisms such as *Stenotrophomonas maltophilia*.

Because of the differences in the pathogens, the diseases they cause, their routes of transmission, the patients they infect, and the intensity of patient care activities, each institution needs to have tailored infection control strategies. The perianesthesia personnel should be familiar with the epidemiology of the institution's antibiotic-resistant organisms. This information can typically be obtained from the microbiology department or infection control department.

Patients who are vulnerable to colonization and infection include those with severe disease, especially those with compromised host defenses from underlying medical conditions; recent surgery; or indwelling medical devices (e.g., urinary catheters, endotracheal tubes). Hospitalized patients, especially patients in the ICU, tend to have more risk factors than nonhospitalized patients do and have the highest infection rates. Increasing numbers of infections with multidrug-resistant organisms (MDROs) also have been reported to occur outside the ICU.[26]

Ample epidemiologic evidence suggests that MDROs are carried from one person to another via the hands of HCWs. Hands are easily contaminated during the process of care giving or from contact with environmental surfaces in close proximity to the patient. The latter is especially important when patients have diarrhea and the reservoir of the MDRO is the gastrointestinal tract. Studies of poor compliance with hand hygiene policies and glove use indicate a greater likelihood that HCWs will transmit MDROs to other patients. Thus, strategies to increase and monitor adherence to policies are important components of MDRO control programs.[21]

An institutional control program for MDRO includes administrative support, judicious use of antimicrobials, surveillance (routine and enhanced), standard and contact precautions, environmental measures, education, and decolonization.

Isolation and Precautions

The CDC Hospital Infection Control Practices Advisory Committee (HICPAC) has a published guideline that outlines recommendations for isolation precautions in hospitals. Two tiers of HICPAC isolation precautions exist. The first is referred to as *Standard Precautions,* and the second is precautions designed only for the care of specified patients. These additional transmission-based precautions are for patients known or suspected to be infected by epidemiologically important pathogens spread via airborne or droplet transmission or via contact with dry skin or contaminated surfaces.

Standard Precautions

Standard Precautions apply to all patients who receive care in hospitals, regardless of diagnosis or presumed infection status. Standard Precautions apply to: (1) blood; (2) all body fluids, secretions, and excretions except sweat, regardless of whether or not they contain visible blood; (3) nonintact skin; and (4) mucous membranes. Standard Precautions are designed to reduce the risk of transmission of microorganisms from both recognized and unrecognized sources of infection in hospitals. Handwashing is a critical component of Standard Precautions.

Transmission-Based Precautions

Transmission-based precautions are designed for patients who need additional precautions above and beyond Standard Precautions to interrupt transmission of the infectious organism. The three types of transmission-based precautions are airborne precautions, droplet precautions, and contact precautions. These precautions may be combined for diseases that have multiple routes of transmission. When used either singularly or

in combination, they are to be used in addition to Standard Precautions.

Airborne precautions are designed to reduce the risk of airborne transmission of infectious agents. Airborne transmission occurs with dissemination of either airborne droplet nuclei (5 μm or smaller in size of evaporated droplets that may remain suspended in the air for long periods of time) or dust particles that contain the infectious agent. Microorganisms carried in this manner can be dispersed widely by air currents and may become inhaled by or deposited on a susceptible host within the same room or over a longer distance from the source patient, depending on environmental factors; therefore negative-pressure isolation rooms are necessary for these patients. If such a room is not available, the patient should be given a mask to wear and should be segregated away from other patients. Prompt transfer of such patients to negative-pressure isolation rooms should be undertaken to minimize the risk of transmission. During transport, the patient should be masked. Personnel who transport the patient should not be masked. Examples of diseases that require airborne precautions include pulmonary tuberculosis, chickenpox, and disseminated zoster (shingles). Personnel who care for patients in airborne precautions must wear respiratory protection (N95 respirator) when entering the room of a patient with known or suspected infectious pulmonary tuberculosis.[22,23] Susceptible persons should not enter the room of patients known or suspected to have measles (rubeola) or varicella (chickenpox) if other immune caregivers are available. If susceptible persons must enter the room of a patient known or suspected to have measles (rubeola) or varicella, they should wear respiratory protection (N95 respirator).[23] Persons who are immune to measles or varicella need not wear respiratory protection.

Droplet precautions are designed to reduce the risk of droplet transmission of infectious agents. Droplet transmission involves contact of the conjunctivae or the mucous membranes of the nose or mouth of a susceptible person with large-particle droplets (larger than 5 μm) that contain microorganisms generated from an infected person. Droplets are generated from the source person, primarily during coughing, sneezing, or talking, and while performing certain procedures such as suctioning and bronchoscopy. Transmission via large-particle droplets necessitates close contact because droplets do not remain suspended in the air and generally travel only short distances, usually 3 feet or less, through the air. Because droplets do not remain suspended in the air, a negative-pressure room is not needed to prevent droplet transmission. HCWs should wear gowns, gloves, masks, and eye protection when within 3 feet of an infected patient. Because the environment can play a role in harboring contamination, prompt cleaning of visible contamination should be performed. In addition, multiple-patient care items (e.g., blood pressure cuffs, stethoscopes) should be disinfected before use on another patient. Hands can become contaminated through holes in gloves or during removal of PPE and therefore should be promptly washed after patient care and removal of PPE. During patient transportation, patient dispersal of droplets is minimized by the patient wear a mask.

Contact precautions are designed to reduce the risk of transmission of infectious organisms with direct or indirect contact. Direct-contact transmission involves skin-to-skin contact and physical transfer of microorganisms to a susceptible person from an infected or colonized person, such as occurs when personnel turn patients, empty drainage bags, or perform other patient care activities that require physical contact. Indirect-contact transmission involves contact of a susceptible person with a contaminated intermediate object, usually inanimate, in the patient's environment. Examples of diseases that require contact precautions include VRE, MRSA, *C. difficile*, lice, and scabies. Health care workers should wear disposable gowns and gloves when providing direct care to patients in contact precautions. As in droplet precautions, a clean environment is critical to minimize transmission of disease and should be promptly and thoroughly disinfected if contaminated and on patient discharge from the area. Hand-washing is of paramount importance in interrupting the spread of infections from patients in contact precautions and should be practiced diligently. Patients requiring contact precautions can be safely transported in a wheelchair or stretcher without any special requirements. However, a clean barrier (e.g., sheet, gown) should be placed between them and the transport vehicle, which should be disinfected before use with another patient. Health care workers should avoid wearing dirty gowns and gloves during transport to avoid contamination of public spaces.

A synopsis of the types of precautions and the patients who need the precautions is listed in the reference *2007 Guideline for Isolation Precautions: Preventing Transmission of Infectious Agents in Healthcare Settings.*[19] Although prospective identification of all patients who need these enhanced precautions is not possible, certain clinical syndromes and conditions carry a sufficiently high risk to warrant the empiric addition of enhanced precautions while a more definitive diagnosis is pursued. A listing of such conditions and the recommended precautions in addition to Standard Precautions is beyond the scope of this chapter, but can be referred to in the *2007 Guideline for Isolation Precautions.*

Patients who are immunocompromised vary in their susceptibility to health care–associated infections, depending on the severity and duration of immunosuppression. They generally are at increased risk for bacterial, fungal, parasitic, and viral infections from both endogenous (own flora) and exogenous (external) sources. The use of Standard Precautions for all patients and transmission-based precautions for specified patients, as recommended in this guideline, should reduce the acquisition by these patients of institutionally acquired bacteria from other patients and environments.

Prevention of Health Care–Associated Infections

Currently, between 5% and 10% of patients admitted to acute care hospitals acquire one or more infections, and the risks have steadily increased during recent decades. These adverse events affect approximately 2 million patients each year in the United States, result in approximately 90,000 deaths, and add an estimated $4.5 to $5.7 billion per year to the costs of patient care.[24] These infections are referred to as *nosocomial infections* or as *health care–associated infections* (the more recent terminology).

Most health care–associated infections (in descending order of frequency) are caused from urinary tract infections, surgical site infections (SSIs), bloodstream infections, and pneumonia. The perianesthesia nurse can play a major role in preventing all these infections in the surgical population by adhering to time-honored practices such as asepsis and recommended standards of care supported by the literature (often referred to as *evidence-based care*). Published guidelines are available from the CDC on prevention of surgical site infections, intravascular catheter infections, and pneumonia.

One area of surgical patient quality improvement in which perianesthesia nurses can play a significantly active role is the Surgical Care Improvement Project (SCIP), originated by The Centers for Medicare and Medicaid Services (CMS). This project is a national quality partnership of organizations focused on improvement of surgical care with significant reduction in surgical complications. Partners in SCIP believe that a meaningful reduction in surgical complications depends on surgeons, anesthesia providers, nurses, pharmacists, infection control professionals, and hospital executives working together to intensify their commitment to making surgical care improvement a priority.[25] SCIP has identified seven processes or outcome measures related to infection prevention. They are listed in Box 5-1.

The CDC estimates that approximately 500,000 SSIs occur annually in the United States.[26] Patients who have SSIs are up to 60% more likely to spend time in an ICU, are fivefold more likely to be readmitted to the hospital, and have twice the mortality rate compared with patients without an SSI.[27] A targeted process within the SCIP initiative to reduce SSIs is with the appropriate antimicrobial prophylaxis administration process because, despite evidence of effectiveness of antimicrobials to prevent SSIs, previous studies have shown inappropriate timing, selection, and excess duration of administration of antimicrobial prophylaxis. The SCIP measures are: (1) the proportion of patients

who have parenteral antimicrobial prophylaxis initiated within 1 hour before the surgical incision; (2) the proportion of patients who are provided a prophylactic antimicrobial agent that is consistent with currently published guidelines; and (3) the proportion of patients whose prophylactic antimicrobial therapy is discontinued within 24 hours after the end of surgery.[28]

An additional measure gaining momentum in the surgical population because of the SCIP initiative is glucose control. Currently, the measures are limited to specific patient populations undergoing surgery, consistent with evidence-based medicine. The fourth SCIP CMS infection indicator addresses patients for cardiac surgery and the postoperative serum glucose. This recommendation was in part the result of studies such as Latham and colleagues,[29] who concluded that diabetes (odds ratio [OR], 2.76; $p < 0.001$) and postoperative hyperglycemia (OR, 2.02; $p = 0.007$) were independently associated with development of SSIs. Former SCIP CMS infection indicator number 7 has been changed to SCIP indicator number 10. It is based on a study by Kurz and colleagues,[30] who reported SSIs in 18 of 96 patients undergoing colorectal surgery who were hypothermic (19%), but in only 6 of 104 patients who were normothermic (6%; $p = 0.009$).[30]

Another SCIP process targeting SSI reduction is the issue of appropriate hair removal at the surgical site. The *CDC Surgical Site Infection Prevention Guidelines* state that preoperative shaving of the surgical site the night before an operation is associated with a significantly higher SSI risk than either the use of depilatory agents or no hair removal.[31-36] Shaving immediately before the operation compared with shaving within 24 hours before surgery was associated with decreased SSI rates (3.1% versus 7.1%); if shaving was performed more than 24 hours before the operation, the SSI rate exceeded 20%.[33] In addition to when the hair is removed, how it is removed is important as well. In one study, SSI rates were 5.6% in patients who had hair removed with razor shave compared with a 0.6% rate among those who had hair removed with depilatory or who had no hair removed.[33] The increased SSI risk associated with shaving has been attributed to microscopic cuts in the skin that later serve as foci for bacterial multiplication. On the basis of the data, the SCIP recommendation is to avoid shaving surgical sites and to use clippers only if hair removal is necessary immediately before surgery.

The role of the perianesthesia nurse relative to the SCIP initiative varies because of institutional differences in ordering and administration of surgical prophylaxis, glucose control, maintenance of

---

BOX 5-1   **SCIP Process Measures for Prevention of Infection**

SCIP INF 1: Prophylactic antibiotic received within 1 hour before surgical incision.
SCIP INF 2: Prophylactic antibiotic selection for surgical patients.
SCIP INF 3: Prophylactic antibiotics discontinued within 24 hours after surgery end time (48 hours for patients for cardiac surgery).
SCIP INF 4: Patients for cardiac surgery with controlled, 6:00 AM postoperative serum glucose.
SCIP INF 6: Surgery patients with appropriate hair removal.
SCIP INF 9: Urinary catheter removed on postoperative day 1 or 2 with day of surgery being day 0.
SCIP INF 10: Surgery patients for whom either active warming was used intraoperatively for the purpose of maintaining normothermia or who had at least one body temperature equal to or greater than 96.8° F (36° C).

From U.S. Department of Health and Human Services: *Hospital quality initiatives, process of care measures,* available at www.cms.gov/HospitalQualityInits/18_HospitalProcessOfCare-Measures.asp. Accessed September 21, 2011; TMF Health Quality Institute: *SCIP quality indicators,* available at http://hospitals.tmf.org/SCIP/SCIPQualityIndicators/tabid/678/Default.aspx. Accessed September 21, 2011; The Joint Commission: *Specifications manual for national hospital inpatient quality measures,* available at www.jointcommission.org/specifications_manual_for_national_hospital_inpatient_quality_measures/. Accessed September 21, 2011.
INF, Measure related to infection; *SCIP,* Surgical Care Improvement Project.

normothermia, and surgical site hair removal. Nonetheless, active collaboration with the initiative is essential for optimal outcomes.

Another recommendation from the *CDC Surgical Site Infection Prevention Guidelines* relates to a patient's skin hygiene before surgery. A preoperative antiseptic shower or bath decreases skin microbial colony counts. In a study of more than 700 patients who received two preoperative antiseptic showers, chlorhexidine reduced bacterial colony counts ninefold (from 2.83 to 0.3) compared with other products.[37] Although other studies corroborate these findings,[38,39] a Cochrane Review found no added benefit of CHG over other antimicrobial soaps.[40] CHG-containing products need several applications to attain maximal antimicrobial benefit; therefore repeated antiseptic showers are usually indicated.[39] Although preoperative showers reduce the skin's microbial colony counts, they have not definitively been shown to reduce SSI rates.[41] However, from a basic hygiene perspective, a patient's skin should be as clean as possible before surgery. Products are currently available that allow for quick and easy skin cleansing in the perioperative setting. They are CHG based and waterless.

Intravascular devices are regularly inserted into patients in the perianesthesia setting. Care must be taken during insertion and line management to prevent bloodstream infections. The incidence rate of central line–associated bloodstream infection (CLA-BSI) varies considerably by type of catheter, frequency of catheter manipulation, and patient-related factors (e.g., underlying disease, acuity of illness). Peripheral venous catheters are the devices most frequently used for vascular access. Although the incidence rate of local infections or bloodstream infections (BSIs) associated with peripheral venous catheters is usually low, serious infectious complications produce considerable annual morbidity rates because of the frequency with which such catheters are used. However, most serious catheter-related infections are associated with central line venous catheters. A total of 250,000 cases of CLA-BSIs has been estimated to occur annually.[42] The attributable mortality rate is an estimated 12% to 25% for each infection, and the marginal cost to the health care system is $25,000 per episode.[42]

In the perianesthesia setting, the biggest effect on prevention of CLA-BSI is control of the insertion process and adherence to aseptic technique. Best practice recommendations for skin preparation include use of an appropriate antiseptic before catheter insertion and during dressing changes. A 2% chlorhexidine-based preparation is preferred, but tincture of iodine, an iodophor, or 70% alcohol can also be used.[43-46]

The level of barrier precautions needed to prevent infection during insertion of central lines is more stringent then what is required for peripheral venous or arterial catheters. Maximal sterile barrier precautions (e.g., cap, mask, sterile gown, sterile gloves, and large sterile drape) during the insertion of central lines substantially reduces the incidence rate of CLA-BSI compared with Standard Precautions (e.g., sterile gloves, small drapes).[47,48] To further reduce the likelihood of contamination of the line, injection ports should be cleaned with 70% alcohol or an iodophor before the system is accessed, and all stopcocks should be capped when not in use.[49-51]

OCCUPATIONAL HEALTH

The perianesthesia nurse is at risk of occupational exposure to bloodborne pathogens, such as HIV, HBV, and HCV. Seroconversion risk after exposure to HIV is 0.3%, to HBV is 15% to 30% (if unvaccinated), and to HCV is 3% to 10%. Exposure to blood from a patient can occur from parenteral exposure to contaminated sharps (e.g., needle stick injury) or splashes to mucous membranes with blood or body fluids. If a nurse is stuck with a needle or other sharp or gets blood or other potentially infectious materials in the eyes, nose, or mouth or on broken skin, the exposed area should be immediately flooded with water and any wound should be cleaned with soap and water or a skin disinfectant if available. The incident should be reported immediately to the employer, and the nurse should seek medical attention.

The OSHA Bloodborne Pathogen (BBP) Standard outlines the appropriate measures an institution must have in place to control for employee exposures. Each institution is required to have an exposure control plan to be in compliance with the OSHA BBP Standard, which outlines the policies, procedures, and training requirements of the HCWs. Each perianesthesia setting should evaluate its practices and ensure that it has the appropriate safety devices, PPE, and training to minimize risks to the employees who work there.

Recommendations for minimization of exposures include taking care to prevent injuries: with use of needles, scalpels, and other sharp instruments or devices; with handling of sharp instruments after procedures; with cleaning of used instruments; and with disposal of used needles. Used needles should never be recapped or otherwise manipulated with both hands or with any other technique that involves directing the point of a needle toward any part of the body used. Instead, either a one-handed scoop technique or a mechanical device designed for holding the needle sheath should be used. Used needles from disposable syringes should not be removed by hand and should not be bent, broken, or otherwise manipulated by hand. Used disposable syringes and needles, scalpel blades, and other sharp items should be disposed in appropriate puncture-resistant containers that are located as close as practical to the area in which the items were used, and reusable syringes and needles should be placed in a puncture-resistant container for transport to the reprocessing area. Certain states in the United States (currently Michigan and Florida) require sharps waste containing residual medication to be managed in a separate sharps container to prevent pharmaceuticals from entering the routine waste stream.

To minimize exposure to mucous membranes, all procedures that involve blood or other potentially infectious materials shall be performed in such a manner as to minimize splashing, spraying, spattering, and generation of droplets of these substances. PPE should be provided at no cost to employees and should be readily accessible.

Eating, drinking, smoking, applying cosmetics or lip balm, and handling contact lenses are prohibited in work areas with a reasonable likelihood of occupational exposure. Food and drink should not be kept in refrigerators, freezers, shelves, or cabinets or on countertops or bench tops where blood or other potentially infectious materials are present.

Medical waste must be managed properly and in compliance with the OSHA BBP Standard and any state regulations and laws. Regulated waste should be placed in containers that are closable; constructed to contain all contents and prevent leakage of fluids during handling, storage, transport, or shipping; labeled or color-coded per the standard; and closed before removal to prevent spillage or protrusion of contents during handling, storage, transport, or shipping.

The employer must make the HBV vaccination series available to all employees who have occupational exposure and should provide postexposure evaluation and follow-up to all employees who have had an exposure incident.

Perianesthesia nurses should protect themselves against infection from HBV with vaccination with the HBV vaccine, unless contraindicated for medical reasons. With proper administration, the vaccine is approximately 90% (80% to 95%) effective in prevention of infection in susceptible vaccine recipients. Immunity produced by this vaccination possibly will decrease with time and boosters will have to be given to ensure protection.[52] Per OSHA standards, this vaccine must be made available at no cost to the employee and must be accompanied by the necessary training requirements.

Training and training records are an important component in the OSHA BBP Standard. Training records shall include the following information: the dates of the training sessions, the contents or a summary of the training sessions, the names and qualifications of persons who conduct the training, and the names and job titles of all persons who attend the training sessions. Training records shall be maintained for 3 years from the date on which the training occurred.

Twenty-four states, Puerto Rico, and the Virgin Islands have OSHA-approved state plans and have adopted their own standards and enforcement policies. For the most part, these states adopt standards that are identical to the federal OSHA. However, some States have adopted different standards applicable to this topic or may have different enforcement policies.

In 2001, the OSHA BBP Standard was revised to reflect the stipulations of the Needlestick Safety and Prevention Act passed by the U.S. Congress in 2000. This act requires the use of engineering and work practice controls to eliminate or minimize employee exposure to bloodborne pathogens. It requires that the institution perform an annual consideration and implementation of appropriate commercially available and effective safer medical devices designed to eliminate or minimize occupational exposure. It also requires soliciting input from nonmanagerial employees responsible for direct patient care and who are potentially exposed to injuries from contaminated sharps, in the identification, evaluation, and selection of effective engineering and work practice controls and the documentation of the solicitation in the exposure control plan.

In addition to the HBV vaccine, additional vaccines are recommended to ensure that personnel are immune to vaccine-preventable diseases. Optimal use of vaccines can prevent transmission of diseases and eliminate unnecessary work restriction. Prevention of illness through comprehensive personnel immunization programs is far more cost effective than case management and outbreak control. Mandatory immunization programs, which include both newly hired and currently employed persons, are more effective than voluntary programs in ensuring that susceptible persons are vaccinated.[53] National guidelines for immunization of and postexposure prophylaxis for health care personnel are provided by the U.S.

Public Health Service's Advisory Committee on Immunization Practices.[54]

Safe Injection Practices

Per the CDC *One and Only* campaign, since 1999 more than 125,000 U.S. patients have been potentially exposed to a bloodborne pathogen, such as HIV, HBV, or HCV because of an HCW's or facility's unsafe injection practice.[55] A review to quantify the issue in nonhospital settings (e.g., nursing homes, free standing infusion centers, pain clinics) identified 33 outbreaks of HBV or HCV that were epidemiologically linked to lapses in infection control practices, resulting in 448 patients acquiring a bloodborne pathogen infection. Eighteen of these outbreaks were related to syringe re-use or mishandling of medication vials.[56] See Box 5-2 for some basic steps that should be applied to every patient to prevent the transmission of bloodborne pathogens.

BOX 5-2 Steps to Prevent Transmission of a Blood-Borne Pathogen

DO NOT
- Re-use a syringe, even if the needle is changed.
- Administer medication from a syringe to multiple patients, even if the needle is changed in between.
- Combine the leftover contents of single-use vials for later use.
- Use a "community" IV bag of saline for flush syringes for multiple patients.

DO
- Use single-dose vials for parenteral medications whenever possible.
- Use a sterile device to access MDVs and avoid touching the access diaphragm.
- Keep MDVs away from the immediate patient treatment area to prevent inadvertent contamination.
- Always wipe the top of medication vials with 70% isopropyl alcohol before accessing, even if a new vial.
- Discard any vial if the sterility is compromised.
- Do not "double-dip" into MDVs with a used needle and/or syringe. If double-dipping does occur, then discard the MDVs after use on that single patient.
- Use fluid infusion and administration sets (i.e., IV bags, tubings, connections) for one patient only and dispose of them promptly when no longer in use.

IV, Intravenous; *MDV,* multidose vial.

SUMMARY

Providing care in a perianesthesia unit is not without infectious risks for patients and the HCW in the environment. Adherence to published guidelines and institutional policies for minimization of infectious risks is paramount for optimal patient and employee outcomes. Simple tasks such as hand washing can significantly reduce the incidence rate of health care–associated infections and reduce the transmission of disease. Additional measures to ensure a safe and clean environment and equipment further lower the risks. Lastly, the perianesthesia nursing team can play a significant role in the quality improvement process of the surgical patient and can greatly affect outcomes that benefit the patient and the institution.

REFERENCES

1. Occupational Safety and Health Administration: 29CFR Part 1910:1030: *Occupational exposure to bloodborne pathogens: final rule, federal register,* OSHA, Washington, DC, 1991.
2. AIA Facilities Guidelines Institute: *Guidelines for design and construction of healthcare facilities,* Washington, DC, 2010, AIA.
3. Potter P, Semmelweis I, *Emerg Infect Dis* 7:368, 2001, available at http://wwwnc.cdc.gov/eid/content/7/2/pdfs/v7-n2.pdf. Accessed September 20, 2011.
4. Centers for Disease Control and Prevention: Guideline for hand hygiene in health-care settings, *MMWR* 51(RR-16), 2002.
5. Pittet D, et al: Members of the infection control program: compliance with handwashing in a teaching hospital, *Ann Intern Med* 130:26–130, 1999.
6. Larson E, Killien M: Factors influencing handwashing behavior of patient care personnel, *Am J Infect Control* 10:93–99, 1982.
7. Conly JM, et al: Handwashing practices in an intensive care unit: the effects of an educational program and its relationship to infection rates, *Am J Infect Control* 17:330–339, 1989.
8. Dubbert PM, et al: Increasing ICU staff handwashing: effects of education and group feedback, *Infect Control Hosp Epid* 11:91–193, 1990.
9. Larson E, Kretzer EK: Compliance with handwashing and barrier precautions, *J Hosp Infect* 30(suppl):88–106, 1995.
10. Sproat LJ, Inglis TJJ: A multicentre survey of hand hygiene practice in intensive care units, *J Hosp Infect* 26:137–148, 1994.
11. Kretzer EK, Larson EL: Behavioral interventions to improve infection control practices, *Am J Infect Control* 26:245–253, 1998.
12. Tupker RA: Detergents and cleansers. In van der Valk PGM and Maibach HI, editors: *The irritant contact dermatitis syndrome,* New York, 1996, CRC Press.
13. Garner JS, Simmons BP: Guideline for isolation precautions in hospitals, *Infect Control* 4(suppl 4):245–325, 1983.

14. McFarland LV, et al: Nosocomial acquisition of *Clostridium difficile* infection, *N Engl J Med* 320:204–210, 1989.

15. Pittet D, et al: Bacterial contamination of the hands of hospital staff during routine patient care, *Arch Intern Med* 159:821–826, 1999.

16. Tenorio AR, et al: Effectiveness of gloves in the prevention of hand carriage of vancomycin-resistant *Enterococcus* species by health care workers after patient care, *Clin Infect Dis* 32:826–829, 2001.

17. Ehrenkranz NJ, Alfonso BC: Failure of bland soap handwash to prevent hand transfer of patient bacteria to urethral catheters, *Infect Control Hosp Epidemiol* 12:654–662, 1991.

18. Kjrlen H, Andersen BM: Handwashing and disinfection of heavily contaminated hands—effective or ineffective? *J Hosp Infect* 21:61–71, 1992.

19. Siegel JD, et al, and the Healthcare Infection Control Practices Advisory Committee: *2007 Guideline for isolation precautions: preventing transmission of infectious agents in healthcare settings*, available at http://www.cdc. gov/hicpac/2007IP/2007isolationPrecautions.html. Accessed September 12, 2011.

20. Seigel, JD, et al, and the Healthcare Infection Control Practices Advisory Committee: *Management of multidrug resistant organisms in healthcare settings 2006*, available at http://www. cdc.gov/hicpac/pdf/guidelines/MDROGuideline2006.pdf. Accessed September 26, 2011.

21. Institute for Healthcare Improvement: *Reduce healthcare-associated infections*, available at http://www.ihi.org/explore/ HAI/Pages/default.aspx. Accessed March 2007.

22. Centers for Disease Control and Prevention: Guidelines for preventing the transmission of tuberculosis in healthcare facilities, *MMWR* 43(RR-13):1-132, 1994.

23. Department of Health and Human Services, Department of Labor: Respiratory protective devices: final rules and notice, *Federal Register* 60(110):30336–30402, 1995.

24. Burke JP: Infection control—a problem for patient safety, *N Engl J Med* 348:651–656, 2003.

25. MedQIC: *Surgical care improvement project*, available at http://www.jointcommission.org/specifications_manual_ for_national_hospital_inpatient_quality_measures. Accessed September 20, 2011.

26. Wong ES: Surgical site infection. In Mayhall DG, editor: *Hospital epidemiology and infection control*, ed 2, Philadelphia, 1999, Lippincott Williams & Wilkins.

27. Kirkland KB, et al: The impact of surgical site infections in the 1990s – attributable mortality, excess length of hospitalization, and extra costs, *Infect Control Hosp Epidemiol* 20:725–730, 1999.

28. Bratzler DW, Houck PM: Antimicrobial prophylaxis for surgery: an advisory statement from the National Surgical Infection Prevention Project, *Clin Infect Dis* 38:1706–1715, 2004.

29. Latham R, et al: The association of diabetes and glucose control with surgical-site infections among cardiothoracic surgery patients, *Infect Control Hosp Epidemiol* 22(10): 604–606, 2001.

30. Kurz A, et al: Perioperative normothermia to reduce the incidence of surgical-wound infection and shorten hospitalization, *N Engl J Med* 334:1209–1215, 1996.

31. Cruse PJ, Foord R: The epidemiology of wound infection: a 10-year prospective study of 62,939 wounds, *Surg Clin North Am* (60)1:27–40, 1980.

32. Mishriki SF, et al: Factors affecting the incidence of postoperative wound infection, *J Hosp Infect* 16:223–230, 1990.

33. Seropian R, Reynolds BM: Wound infections after preoperative depilatory versus razor preparation, *Am J Surg* 121:251–254, 1971.

34. Hamilton HW, et al: Preoperative hair removal, *Can J Surg* 20:269–271, 1977.

35. Olson MM, et al: Preoperative hair removal with clippers does not increase infection rate in clean surgical wounds, *Surg Gynecol Obstet* 162:181–182, 1986.

36. Mehta G, et al: Computer assisted analysis of wound infection in neurosurgery, *J Hosp Infect* 11:244–252, 1988.

37. Garibaldi RA: Prevention of intraoperative wound contamination with chlorhexidine shower and scrub, *J Hosp Infect* 11(Suppl B):5–9, 1988.

38. Paulson DS: Efficacy evaluation of a 4% chlorhexidine gluconate as a full-body shower wash, *Am J Infect Control* 21(4):205–209, 1993.

39. Hayek LJ, et al: A placebo-controlled trial of the effect of two preoperative baths or showers with chlorhexidine detergent on postoperative baths or showers with chlorhexidine detergent on postoperative wound infection rates, *J Hosp Infect* 10:165–172, 1987.

40. Webster J, Osborne S: Preoperative bathing or showering with skin antiseptics to prevent surgical site infection, *Cochrane Database of Systematic Reviews* 2(CD004985):2006.

41. The European Working Party on Control of Hospital Infections, et al: A comparison of the effects of preoperative whole-body bathing with detergent alone and with detergent containing chlorhexidine gluconate on the frequency of wound infections after clean surgery, *J Hosp Infect* 11:310–320, 1988.

42. Kluger DM, Maki DG: *The relative risk of intravascular device related bloodstream infections in adults* [abstract], Proceeding of the Abstracts of the 39th Interscience Conference on Antimicrobial Agents and Chemotherapy, American Society for Microbiology, 1999, San Francisco.

43. Maki DG, et al: Prospective randomised trial of povidone-iodine, alcohol, and chlorhexidine for prevention of infection associated with central venous and arterial catheters, *Lancet* 338:339–343, 1991.

44. Garland JS, et al: Comparison of 10% povidone-iodine and 0.5% chlorhexidine gluconate for the prevention of peripheral intravenous catheter colonization in neonates: a prospective trial, *Pediatr Infect Dis J* 14:510–516, 1995.

45. Little JR, et al: A randomized trial of povidone-iodine compared with iodine tincture for venipuncture site disinfection: effects on rates of blood culture contamination, *Am J Med* 107:119–125, 1999

46. Mimoz O, et al: Prospective, randomized trial of two antiseptic solutions for prevention of central venous or arterial catheter colonization and infection in intensive care unit patients, *Crit Care Med* 24:1818–1823, 1996.

47. Mermel LA, et al: The pathogenesis and epidemiology of catheter-related infection with pulmonary artery Swan-Ganz catheters: a prospective study utilizing molecular subtyping, *Am J Med* 91(Supp 2):S197–S205, 1991.

48. Raad II, et al: Prevention of central venous catheter-related infections by using maximal sterile barrier precautions

during insertion, *Infect Control Hosp Epidemiol* 15:231–238, 1994.

49. Luebke MA, et al: Comparison of the microbial barrier properties of a needleless and a conventional needle-based intravenous access system, *Am J Infect Control* 26:437–441, 1998.

50. Salzman MB, et al: Use of disinfectants to reduce microbial contamination of hubs of vascular catheters, *J Clin Microbiol* 31:475–479, 1993.

51. Plott RT, et al: Iatrogenic contamination of multidose vials in simulated use: a reassessment of current patient injection technique, *Arch Dermatol* 126:1441–1444, 1990.

52. Occupational Safety and Health Administration: *CPL 2-2 OSHA instruction: subject: hepatitis B risks in the health care system,* Washington, DC, 1983, Office of Occupational Medicine.

53. Bolyard EA, et al: The Hospital Infection Control Practices Advisory Committee: Guideline for infection control in health care personnel, *Am J Infect Control* 26(3):289–354, 1998.

54. Advisory Committee on Immunization Practices (AICP): Immunization of health-care workers: recommendations of the Advisory Committee on Immunization Practices (ACIP) and the Hospital Infection Control Practices Advisory Committee (HICPAC), *MMWR* 46(RR-18): 1–42, 1997.

55. Center for Disease Control and Prevention: *CDC's Role in Safe Injection Practices,* available at http://www.cdc.gov/injectionsafety/. Accessed September 15, 2011.

56. Thompson ND, et al: Nonhospital health care-associated hepatitis B and C virus transmission: United States, 1998-2008, *Ann Intern Med* 150:33-39, 2009.

RESOURCES

Allen G, editor: *Infection prevention in the perioperative setting: zero tolerance for infections, an issue of perioperative nursing clinics.* St. Louis, 2010, Saunders.

Hooper VD, et al.: ASPAN's evidence-based clinical practice guideline for the promotion of perioperative normothermia:Second edition, *J Perianesth Nurs* 25:346–365, 2010.

Block S: *Disinfection, sterilization and preservation,* ed 5, Philadelphia, 2001, Lippincott Williams & Wilkins.

Jensen, PA, et al. Guidelines for preventing the transmission of *Mycobacterium tuberculosis* in health-care settings, *MMWR* 54(RR-17):1–141, 2005.

Needlestick Safety and Prevention Act: public law 106–430, 106th Congress, available at http://www.osha.gov/SLTC/bloodbornepathogens/index.html. Accessed September 12, 2011.

Kaye K: *Infection prevention and control in the hospital, an issue of infectious disease clinics,* St. Louis, 2011, Saunders.

Kerr CM, Savage GT: Managing exposure to tuberculosis in the PACU: CDC guidelines and cost analysis, *J Perianesth Nurs* 11(3):143–146, 1996.

Mangram AJ, et al: Guidelines for the prevention of surgical site infections, *Infect Control Hosp Epidemiol* 20(4):250–278, 1999.

Sullivan EE: The use of contact and airborne precautions in the perianesthesia setting, *J Perianesth Nurs* 17(3):190–192, 2002.

Sullivan EE: Off with her nails, *J Perianesth Nurs* 18(6): 417–418, 2003.

Yokoe DS, et al: A compendium of strategies to prevent health-care-associated infections in acute care hospitals, *Infect Cont and Hosp Epidemiol* 29(Suppl 1): S12–S21, 2008.

6 The Changing Health Care System and Its Implications for the PACU

Xinliang Liu, MBBS, MSc, Carolyn A. Watts, PhD, and
Kenneth R. White, MSN, PhD, RN, MPH, FACHE

The health care system in the United States is one of the nation's largest and most important economic sectors. It consists of all the resources and activities whose primary purpose is to promote, restore, or maintain the health of the American people.[1] Continuous efforts have been made to improve the health care system's ability to produce care that is safe, effective, patient-centered, timely, efficient, and equitable.[2] An emphasis on safety implies that medical care should bring minimal harm to patients. Effectiveness highlights the importance of providing evidence-based services only to those who could benefit. Patient-centeredness emphasizes individualized care and the patients' pivotal role in all clinical decisions. Timeliness underscores the significance of "reducing waits and sometimes harmful delays for both those who receive and those who give care."[2] Efficiency focuses on eliminating waste in the production of medical care, including overuse of medical resources and undue administrative costs. Finally, equity stresses the need for "providing care that does not vary in quality because of personal characteristics such as gender, ethnicity, geographic location, and socioeconomic status."[2] As health technology and the role of government in financing care have increased in the past 10 years, the health care system has played an increasingly important role in people's lives. The rapid development of medical science and technology, changing economic and political environment, and soaring consumer expectations have profoundly changed what health care is and how it can be delivered. It is critical for postanesthesia nurses to understand the nation's health care system.

A health care system is shaped by four functional components: financing, workforce development, service delivery, and regulation.[1] This chapter provides a broad overview of these components, including how the health care system is financed, who provides health care services, what medical services are produced, and role of the government in the health care system. There is also a discussion of the issue of the uninsured population, a summary of the recent health care reform legislation, and an explanation of the implications for the post anesthesia care unit (PACU) and perianesthesia nurses.

HEALTH CARE FINANCING

In the United States, the private sector has a larger role in paying for health care costs than in most developed countries. Public programs are focused on health care for special population subgroups, such as senior citizens, low-income populations, veterans, and active duty and retired military personnel and their dependents. The financial burden of health care is shouldered by three major sponsors in the United States: businesses, households, and governments.[3] Health care costs are billed through private insurance plans, out-of-pocket payments, philanthropic funds, and public programs.

Private Business

Private businesses contribute to approximately one fifth of health care spending, in the form of employer-sponsored health insurance, contribution to Medicare, workers compensation, disability insurance, and worksite health care.[3] Employers are the leading source of health coverage. The majority of employers (69% in 2010) offer health insurance as a fringe benefit to cover their employees as well as their employees' dependents.[4] Federal, state, and local governments, as employers, also make contributions to private health insurance programs to insure public employees. For example, in 2009, the federal government contributed $26.8 billion to the Federal Employees Health Benefits Program to cover more than 8 million federal employees, retirees, and their dependents, including members of the U.S. Congress.[5]

Employer-sponsored health insurance has been designed predominantly through managed care plans of various kinds in recent decades. Managed care plans are lower cost alternatives to conventional indemnity insurance by incorporating a wide range of organizational and financial arrangements to organize, reimburse, and monitor services. The most common type of managed care plans is the preferred provider organization

(PPO). A PPO selectively contracts with hospitals and other providers to form a network and creates financial incentives for members to use network providers. The incentives can include lower deductibles, lower copayment, and coinsurance. The advantage to the PPO is that network providers negotiate lower reimbursement rates in exchange for higher anticipated volume. Another type of managed care plan, the health maintenance organization (HMO), is more restrictive. Members are required to use in-network providers and must be authorized by their primary care physician to see a specialist. HMO plans usually have lower out-of-pocket payments than PPO plans. Point-of-service (POS) plans are hybrids of PPO and HMO plans in which enrollees can choose to pay extra at the point of a particular service to see a non-network provider. Some employers also offer a high-deductible health plan with savings option (HDHP/SO). The annual deductible of a typical HDHP plan can be $2000 or higher for single coverage. Health reimbursement arrangements and health savings accounts are linked with such plans, allowing employees to save for medical expenses on a tax-free basis. In 2010, 58% of covered employees were enrolled in PPOs, followed by HMOs (19%), HDHP/SOs (13%), and POS plans (8%). Approximately 1% were covered by conventional indemnity plans.[4]

Employers and employees both contribute to the cost of employment-based health insurance. Covered employees on average shouldered 19% of the total premium for single coverage and 30% for family coverage in 2009%,[4] approximately $75 monthly for single coverage and $333 monthly for family coverage. Private and public sector employers often vary as to the relative role of health benefits in the total compensation package. From 2000 to 2009, the share of premiums paid by private sector employers dropped from 74.7% to 69.7%. During the same time period, the share paid by the federal government remained at 72% to 73%, whereas state and local governments' contributions increased from 79.2% to 83%.[3]

In addition to premiums, covered employees must also pay deductibles (an amount that must be paid before the health insurance begins to pay), copayments (a set amount paid per visit or service), or coinsurance (a percentage of the cost for services or drugs). In the past few decades, the out-of-pocket liabilities for employees have increased as employers have tried to control the cost of providing health benefits. Some small businesses have ceased to offer health insurance to their employees in the face of soaring health benefit costs.

Not all employers provide health benefits to their employees. Those offering insurance benefits tend to be large firms with well-paid workers.[4] Even if employers offer insurance, employees can choose not to participate if the premium share is too high, the value of the benefits too low, or if the employee has higher value options for coverage elsewhere (e.g., through a spouse). Employer-based insurance coverage is clearly tied to employment. In the economic downturn near the end of the first decade of the twenty-first century, millions of workers lost their jobs and their insurance coverage. Nearly three of five adults who lost a job with health benefits in 2010 became uninsured.[6] Private business health spending decreased 0.5% in 2009, the first decline since 1987, resulting from a 3.2% decrease in employer-sponsored health insurance coverage.[3]

Households

The financial burden of health care on households consists of three parts: health insurance premiums, out-of-pocket payments (deductibles, copayments, and coinsurance), payments for services that are not covered by insurance, and the mandatory Medicare payroll tax for employed individuals. Households contributed to 28% of national health spending in 2009, or 6.2% of personal income.[3] This average, however, conceals the larger burden on low-income families. In 2010, half of adults from families with incomes less than 100% of the federal poverty level (FPL, $22,050 for a family of four) spent 10% or more of their income on health care.[6]

Direct household spending on health care can be strongly influenced by economic conditions. The growth rate of out-of-pocket payments dropped from 3.1% in 2008 to 0.4% in 2009 as consumers postponed medical services during the economic recession.[3]

Governments

Federal and state governments are charged with funding public health-related programs, including Medicare, Medicaid, and the Children's Health Insurance Program (CHIP). The Centers for Medicare and Medicaid Services (CMS) is the federal agency that administers these three programs (Medicaid and CHIP are administered jointly with the states.) The federal government also subsidizes employment-based health insurance through tax laws that allow recipients of employer-based insurance to receive these benefits tax free. This subsidy is estimated to be $177 billion in the year 2011.[7]

Medicare is the nation's largest health insurer. It covers people age 65 or older, those with certain disabilities, and those with end-stage renal disease. The program is organized into four parts. Medicare Part A (Hospital Insurance) pays for inpatient care in hospitals, skilled nursing services, hospice, and home health care. The Part A program is financed primarily through the Federal Insurance Contributions Act tax, which funds Social Security and Medicare. Currently, the Medicare payroll tax is 2.9%, with the worker and the employer each paying 1.45%. Self-employed individuals must pay the entire 2.9% tax.

Medicare Part B (Medical Insurance) covers doctors' services and tests, outpatient care, some home health services, durable medical equipment, and certain preventive services. Part B is financed through premiums paid by enrollees and contributions from general revenues of the U.S. Treasury. Beneficiary premiums are currently set to cover approximately 25% of the per capita cost of Part B. In 2011, the Part B premium is $96.40 for those enrolled before 2010, $110.50 for those enrolled in 2010, and $115.40 for all others. Individuals with yearly incomes higher than $85,000, or couples with income above $170,000, pay premiums that range from $161.50 to $369.10 per month.[8]

Medicare Part C (Medicare Advantage Plan) is an alternative to original Medicare (Part A and Part B). Medicare Advantage Plans are administered by Medicare-approved private insurance companies. Medicare Advantage Plans provide all benefits covered by original Medicare plus some extra coverage, such as vision, hearing, dental, prescription drug coverage, and health and wellness programs at added costs. Medicare pays a fixed monthly fee for each beneficiary to the private insurance companies. Enrollment in Medicare Part C is voluntary; approximately 20% of Medicare beneficiaries sign up for Medicare Advantage Plans.

Medicare Part D (Medicare Prescription Drug Coverage) helps to pay for prescription drugs. People eligible for Medicare participate on a voluntary basis and pay a monthly premium. All prescription drug plans are administered by Medicare-approved private insurance companies. The premium, cost sharing, and drugs covered vary from plan to plan. As of January 2008, more than 25 million Medicare beneficiaries (57%) were enrolled in Part D plans.[9]

Medicaid is a joint federal and state program that provides comprehensive medical and long-term care coverage for individuals with limited income and resources and for those with major disabilities. Although the federal government provides broad guidelines, states have a wide degree of flexibility to design the eligibility criteria and benefit package. For example, California's Medicaid program (Medi-Cal) covered 29% of its total population in 2007, while the Medicaid program in Nevada covered 10% of its population in the same year.[10] Income limits for program eligibility for single adults varied from 17% of the FPL in Arkansas to 215% of the FPL in Minnesota.[11] In general, eligibility rules for children are more generous than for adults in all states. Medicaid plays a key role in ensuring access to care for the low-income population.

CHIP represents another joint effort on the part of federal and state governments. This program provides free or low-cost health insurance coverage to children up to 19 years old in families with incomes exceeding eligibility limits for Medicaid who cannot afford private health insurance. Uninsured children in families with incomes up to $44,100 a year (200% of the FPL for a family of four) are eligible for the CHIP in many states. The program generally covers doctor visits, hospitalizations, prescription drugs, and vision and dental care. Pregnant women and other adults may also be covered by the program. Similar to Medicaid, CHIP is administered by each state under broad federal requirements; therefore eligibility, benefits, premiums, and cost sharing are different from state to state. For the federal fiscal year 2010, a total of 7.7 million children were enrolled in CHIP at some point during the year.[12]

Health care spending by governments amounted to 44% of national health expenditures in 2009, with the federal government accounting for approximately 27% and state and local governments accounting for 16%.[3] Government health care spending is projected to account for more than half of total health care spending by 2012.[13]

The U.S. health care system is the most expensive one in the world. National health spending was $2.5 trillion in total, or $8086 per capita in 2009.[14] The ratio of health spending to the gross domestic product (GDP) reached 17.6%.[14] Health care spending in the United States is significantly higher than in other industrialized countries. For example, France, Switzerland, and Germany devoted 11.2%, 10.7%, and 10.5%, respectively, of their GDP to health care in 2008.[15] The United States spent more than twice as much as relatively rich European countries on health care per capita. Adjusted for purchasing power parity, France spent $3696 per capita on health care in 2008, Germany spent $3737 per capita, and the United Kingdom spent $3129 per capita.[15] National health care expenditures are projected to grow at an average annual rate of 6.1% (1.7 percentage points faster than GDP), climbing to $4.5 trillion, or 19.3% of GDP by 2019.[13]

THE UNINSURED POPULATION

The United States is one of three countries in the Organization for Economic Co-operation and Development (OECD) that do not offer health coverage to all of its citizens (Mexico and Turkey are the other two.) Although the elaborate patchwork of public and private coverage options works well for many of those who have employer-sponsored health benefits or who are eligible for public programs, it has many holes. In 2009, for example, 676,000 elderly people did not qualify for Medicare.[16] Two of every 10 individuals younger than 65 years are not covered by employment-based health insurance, are not eligible for Medicaid or other public programs, and are left uninsured.[16] The resulting uninsured population was 50 million in 2009.[16]

Adults with low and moderate incomes, young adults, and racial or ethnic minority groups, such as Hispanics and blacks, are more likely to be uninsured.[6] Those between 19 and 29 years of age have the highest uninsured rate (28%) of any age group (Fig. 6-1). Noncitizens (legal and undocumented) are approximately

threefold more likely to be uninsured than citizens.[16] Insurance rates vary across states because of differences in average income, employment opportunity, and Medicaid policy at the state level (Fig. 6-2). Massachusetts has an uninsured rate of less than 5%, whereas the rate exceeds 25% in New Mexico, Florida, and Texas.[16]

Having no health insurance negatively affects the financial condition, health-seeking behavior, and health outcomes of the uninsured. Three of five uninsured adults reported having problems paying medical bills or having accrued medical debt, nearly twice the rate of the insured population.[6] Because they have to pay for medical bills out of pocket, the uninsured are inclined to delay or forego needed health care. Two thirds of the adults who were uninsured in 2010 reported experiencing one or more of the following: failing to fill a prescription; skipping a medical test, treatment, or follow-up visit; choosing not to see a doctor when sick; or not seeing a specialist because of cost.[6] Emergency department services are often the only option for the uninsured when medical care is unavoidable. The uninsured are more likely to be in poor health than the insured. Uninsured adults were more than twice as likely to report being in fair or poor health as those with private insurance.[16]

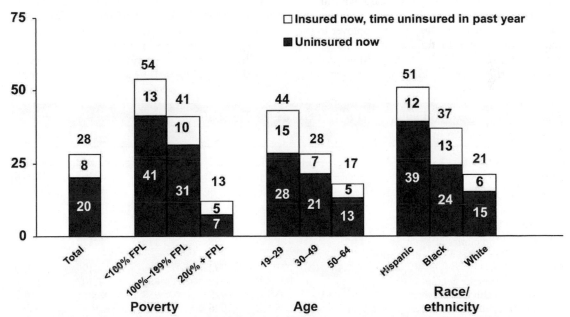

FIG. 6-1 Uninsured rates among adults based on income, age, and race/ethnicity (NOTE: Subgroups may not sum to totals because of rounding). *FPL*, Federal poverty level. (From Collins SR, et al: Help on the horizon: how the recession has left millions of workers without health insurance, and how health reform will bring relief, *The Commonwealth Fund Biennial Health Insurance Survey*, New York, 2011, The Commonwealth Fund.)

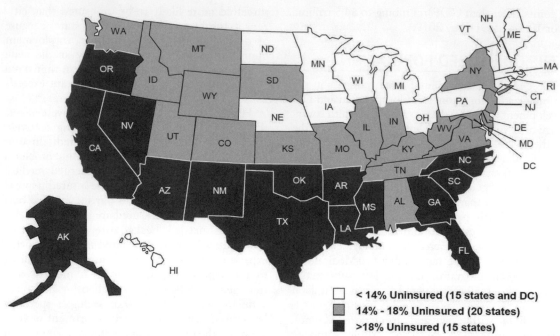

FIG. 6-2 Uninsured rates among nonelderly by state, 2009 to 2010. (From Kaiser Family Foundation: *Kaiser Commission on Medicaid and the Uninsured/Urban Institute analysis of 2010 and 2011 ASEC Supplement to the CPS, two-year pooled data,* available at http://facts.kff.org/chart.aspx?ch=2345. Accessed September 20, 2011.)

HEALTH CARE WORKFORCE

A capable and motivated health care workforce is essential to achieve national health goals. The health care industry is the largest employer in the nation. More than 15 million people worked in this enterprise in 2009 (Table 6-1). Major categories of health care professionals include physicians, dentists, registered nurses, licensed practical nurses (LPNs), pharmacists, health services administrators, and allied health professionals. In addition, millions more work in health-related industries to produce supplies, capital goods, and services for people providing direct patient care.

Physicians are central to the delivery of health care services. They are responsible for the

TABLE 6-1 Persons Employed in Health Service Sites (In Thousands)					
SITE	2005	2006	2007	2008	2009
All employed civilians	141,730	144,427	146,047	145,362	139,877
All health service sites	14,052	14,352	14,687	15,108	15,478
Percent of employed civilians	9.9%	9.9%	10.1%	10.4%	11.1%
Offices and clinics of physicians	1801	1785	1720	1562	1555
Offices and clinics of dentists	792	852	843	774	801
Offices and clinics of chiropractors	163	163	144	139	136
Offices and clinics of optometrists	98	98	114	110	117
Offices and clinics of other health Practitioners	275	292	299	195	220
Outpatient care centers	901	919	881	1,107	1,102
Home health care services	795	928	959	881	967
Other health care services	1045	1096	1334	1647	1747
Hospitals	5719	5712	5955	6241	6265
Nursing care facilities	1848	1807	1689	1779	1869
Residential care facilities, without nursing	615	700	749	673	699

Data from National Center for Health Statistics: *Persons employed in health service sites, by site and sex: United States, selected years 2000–2009,* available at www.cdc.gov/nchs/hus/contents2010.htm#table105. Accessed September 16, 2011.

evaluation, diagnosis, and treatment of patients. Even as insurance companies and health care organizations create incentives to influence the preferences of patients and the practice pattern of physicians, physicians still exert enormous power in controlling and directing the use of medical inputs in the production of health care services. Those wishing to practice allopathic medicine must get a four year undergraduate degree and a doctor of medicine (MD) degree from an accredited medical school, pass a series of the United States Medical Licensing Examination tests offered by the National Board of Medical Examiners, and complete a supervised residency program. Physicians must be licensed by every state in which they practice. Those who wish to further specialize in areas such as cardiology or pediatric surgery must complete a fellowship beyond the residency and typically sit for specialty board examinations to achieve voluntary board certification. Similar requirements exist for practitioners of osteopathic medicine (i.e., doctor of osteopathic medicine).

Physicians can be grouped into generalists and specialists. Generally speaking, physicians trained in general internal medicine, pediatrics, and family medicine are considered to be primary care physicians. Primary care physicians provide services to meet the routine needs of patients, such as health maintenance, initial diagnosis, and continuing treatment of common illness. Physicians who have additional training to practice in a medical specialty are referred to as *specialists*. Typical specialties include anesthesiology, subspecialties of internal medicine, surgical subspecialties, obstetrics and gynecology, dermatology, ophthalmology, and psychiatry.

Physicians can start their own solo practice or join a group practice once they are licensed. The former path has become less popular in recent years because of the capital required to start a private practice, the financial pressure on physician owners, and the burden of marketing and managing the practice. Although most physicians practice in office-based settings, an increasing number of physicians choose to become hospitalists who work full time in a hospital and provide intensive care for hospitalized patients.

Nurses are major caregivers for patients. In addition to supporting care for patients, nurses are the leading force in conducting case management, utilization review, quality assurance, and patient education. Advanced practice nurses (APNs)—clinical nurse specialists, nurse anesthetists, nurse-midwives, and nurse practitioners—assume relatively independent responsibilities for more complicated patient services, for primary care as well as in acute care settings.

Nurses must be licensed by a state's Board of Nursing to practice nursing. The licensure requires graduation from an approved nursing program and the completion of a national examination. Nurses have varying degrees determined by different educational paths. Registered nurses must have a baccalaureate degree in nursing (BSN) offered by a college or university, an associate degree in nursing (ADN) obtained from a community or junior college, or a diploma from an approved hospital nursing program. Licensed practical nurses (LPNs) or licensed vocational nurses (LVNs) must complete a state-approved training program in practical nursing. This program usually takes 1 year. Currently, APNs must have a minimum of a master's degree, with a requirement from the American Association of Colleges of Nursing that the APN have a doctorate of nursing practice (DNP) as a minimum educational level by 2015. The DNP is designed for nurses seeking a terminal degree in nursing practice and offers an alternative to research-focused doctoral programs. The practice doctorate is the graduate degree for advanced nursing practice preparation, including but not limited to the four current APN roles mentioned previously. The majority of nurses work in hospitals. A large proportion of nurses also work in offices of physicians, home health care services, and nursing care facilities. Many nurses have sought careers in other fields such as insurance companies, emergency medical centers, work sites, schools, government agencies, and social assistance agencies.

MAJOR MEDICAL SERVICES

There are three major types of medical services: outpatient services, inpatient services, and long-term care (LTC). Outpatient medical services consist of diagnostic and therapeutic services that do not require an overnight stay in a health care facility. In 2008, there were 956 million visits to physician offices, 110 million visits to hospital outpatient departments, and 124 million visits to hospital emergency departments.[17]

Advances in medical and surgical technology enable increasingly more inpatient services such as surgical procedures, rehabilitative therapies, renal dialysis, and chemotherapy to be performed in outpatient settings. Pressure from payers to reduce medical expenses also promotes the use of ambulatory care settings as alternatives to expensive inpatient care. Currently, as many as 70% of all surgeries are performed in ambulatory settings.[18] Outpatient services can be rendered in physicians' offices, hospital outpatient departments, hospital emergency departments, freestanding ambulatory surgery centers (ASCs), medical laboratories, and hospice facilities and through home health agencies in the patient's home.

Inpatient services refer to medical services received during one or more overnight stays in a health care facility. These services include room and board, physician services, inpatient pharmacy, skilled nursing care, rehabilitation services, and ancillary services. The use of inpatient services per capita has declined over the past 30 years. In 2007, there were 112.4 hospital stays and 540.4 days of inpatient care per 1000 population. In 1980, there were 174.5 stays and 1302.7 days of care per 1000 population.[17] The length of a hospital stay declined sharply after CMS adopted a prospective payment system for reimbursing hospital care in 1983. This system pays a fixed amount for each case in the same diagnosis-related group regardless of the actual days spent in the hospital or services used. The average length of stay in nonfederal short-term hospitals was 4.8 days in 2007 compared with 7.5 days in 1980.[17]

Hospitals are the major source of inpatient services. There were 5815 hospitals in the United States in 2008 (Fig. 6-3). Among them, 5010 were nonfederal, community, short-term hospitals with an average patient stay of less than 30 days.[19] Other types of hospitals serve special population subgroups, including federal hospitals, long-term hospitals, psychiatric hospitals, and hospital units of institutions (e.g., prison hospitals, college infirmaries).

Hospitals can be classified into three main groups by ownership structure: public hospitals, nonprofit hospitals, and for-profit hospitals. Public hospitals are owned by the federal, state, or local government. Federal hospitals serve specific populations, such as Native Americans, veterans, or military personnel and their dependents. State hospitals usually focus on providing mental health services. Public hospitals operated by county, city, and sometimes state governments tend to be community hospitals that are open to the general public. These hospitals usually serve a large proportion of Medicaid and uninsured patients.

Approximately half of the hospitals in the nation are private, nonprofit hospitals. They are owned by local communities or other nongovernmental organizations and operated on a nonprofit basis. Nonprofit hospitals can earn surpluses or accounting profits (i.e., an excess of revenues over expenses), but they may not distribute surpluses to any private shareholder or individual. Nonprofit hospitals receive a tax exemption for federal income tax and are often exempt from local property taxes. They also have access to charitable donations that are tax deductible for donors, and they are tax exempt bond financing.

An increasing number of hospitals are operated as for-profit organizations. These hospitals are typically owned by national or regional health systems; fewer are freestanding facilities. For-profit hospitals operate at a relatively smaller scale. The average number of beds among for-profit hospitals was 121 in 2008 compared with 557 beds for nonprofit hospitals and 131 beds for state and local government hospitals.[19]

With the aging of the population, LTC services delivered to patients with physical or mental disabilities are increasingly important. LTC recipients can be elderly individuals with Alzheimer disease, strokes, complications of diabetes, or visual impairments. Young people with permanent or temporary disabilities may also need LTC. Individuals needing LTC services have varying degrees of difficulty in performing some activities of daily living (ADLs) or instrumental activities of daily living without assistance. *Activities of daily living* refers to basic activities such as bathing, dressing, toileting, eating, and moving from one location to another. Instrumental activities of daily living include more complicated tasks such as preparing food, housekeeping, and handling finances.

In 2009, there were 15,700 nursing homes providing LTC to 1.4 million residents.[17] Nursing homes are the most common providers of LTC.

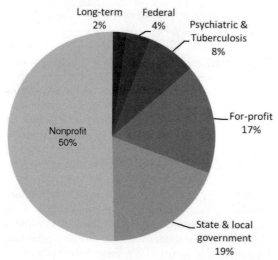

FIG. 6-3 Proportion of hospitals by type of hospital, 2008. (Data from U.S. Census Bureau: *Statistical abstract of the United States: 2011*, available at http://www.census.gov/compendia/statab/cats/health_nutrition/health_care_utilization.html. Accessed July 25, 2011.)

LTC can also be provided by assisted living facilities, home health agencies, or family members and other informal caregivers in various noninstitutional settings. A study by the U.S. Department of Health and Human Services estimated that people who reach age 65 have a 40% chance of entering a nursing home. Among those entering a nursing home, approximately 10% will stay there 5 years or more.[20] Most of the nursing homes are for-profit entities owned by multi-facility chains.

GOVERNMENT'S ROLE IN HEALTH CARE

The government is deeply involved in every aspect of the health care system. Government intervention mainly takes four forms[21]: (1) commodity taxes and subsides (e.g., government at several levels imposes taxes on tobacco to discourage smoking, and the federal government offers tax credits to employers who provide health benefits to their employees); (2) direct provision (the federal government provides medical care to American Indians, veterans, and military personnel and their dependents); (3) transfer programs, such as Medicaid as discussed in the previous section; and (4) regulation (e.g., state licensure of health care professionals.) This section discusses the responsibilities of the federal, state, and local governments with an emphasis on their role as regulators.

Role of the Federal Government

The federal government's duty to protect the health of all Americans and to provide essential human services is executed by the U.S. Department of Health and Human Services. Departmental leadership is provided by the Office of the Secretary, which is directly supported by the Deputy Secretary, Chief of Staff, a number of assistant secretaries, staff offices, and operating divisions (Fig. 6-4). The 11 operating divisions include eight agencies within the U.S. Public Health Service and three human services agencies. In the Public Health Service Division, the National Institutes of Health, the Food and Drug Administration, and the Centers for Disease Control and Prevention are the primary federal agencies that conduct research and establish regulations aimed protecting the health and safety of the U.S. population. CMS is the federal agency that administers Medicare, Medicaid, and CHIP (the last two are administered jointly with states). To achieve better efficiency and improve the overall quality of care, CMS has taken significant steps toward a strategy that links payment to health care providers' performance. For example, after October 1, 2008, CMS ceased to pay for a series of hospital-acquired conditions ("never events") that are deemed as avoidable in most cases through the application of evidence-based guidelines.[22] One of the "never events" is surgical site infection following certain surgical procedures. The CMS payment policy, which is usually adopted by private payers and state governments, imposes financial pressure on health care organizations to redesign the process of care and also requires every health worker to change clinical practices and follow recommended quality guidelines more closely.

Role of State and Local Governments

State governments are responsible for protecting and promoting the health status of their residents. State departments perform a wide variety of services, including health care professional and facility licensing, vital statistics collection, administration of Medicaid, CHIP and other categorical programs, disease surveillance, operation of state mental health hospitals and medical schools, and many others.

Local health departments are frontline agencies for monitoring and protecting the health of the population. Services range from restaurant sanitation inspections, vital statistics collection, disease surveillance, supervision of water and food supplies, and enforcement of local health codes. Local health departments also provide a series of preventive and clinical services, including immunization and vaccination, infectious and noncommunicable disease screening, and treatments for specific diseases. After the terrorist attacks of September 11, 2001, state and local governments have significantly strengthened their capacity for emergency preparedness and response.

2010 HEALTH CARE REFORM

The pressure for health care reform in recent years arose from the severe challenges faced by the health care system. Health spending was consuming a substantial and ever larger share of government, business, and family expenditures. Efforts to control rising costs were largely failing, and the number of uninsured had risen to an unprecedented level. With these facts as backdrop and amid much political wrangling, the Patient Protection and Affordable Care Act (PPACA) and the Health Care and Education Reconciliation Act of 2010, were approved by the U.S. Congress and signed by President Barack Obama in March 2010. These two pieces of legislation aim to overhaul the health care system through expansions of coverage, reform of health insurance market, and delivery system reorganization.[23]

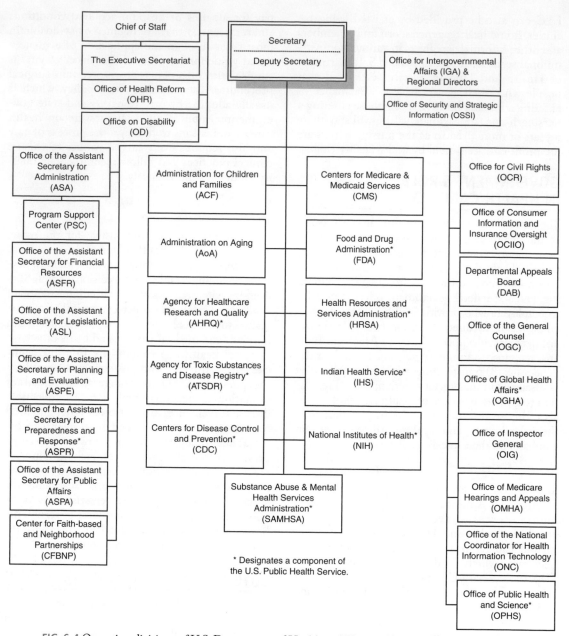

FIG. 6-4 Operating divisions of U.S. Department of Health and Human Services. (From U.S. Department of Health and Human Services: *U.S. Department of Health and Human Services Organizational Chart*, available at www.hhs.gov/about/orgchart/. Accessed September 16, 2011.)

Coverage Expansion

The PPACA expands coverage by requiring most individuals to have qualifying health coverage, subsidizing insurance for individuals and families with income between 133% and 400% of the FPL, encouraging small businesses to offer health benefits to their employees, and expanding Medicaid to individuals and families with income up to 133% of the FPL.

Health Insurance Market Reforms

The legislation creates state-based health insurance exchanges where individuals and small businesses can purchase qualified health insurance products offered by private insurance companies. All plans offered in the exchanges must set premiums based only on age, benefit package, family structure, geographic area, and tobacco use. Before the operation of such exchanges in 2014, a temporary national high-risk pool will be created to provide health coverage to individuals with preexisting conditions. The law requires that group health insurance plans must use no less than 85% (individual and small business insurance no less than 80%) of premium dollars on clinical services, quality, and other nonadministrative costs. The law also extends dependent coverage for children to age 26 and prohibits insurance companies from imposing lifetime maximums on coverage or rescinding coverage after a policy has been written.

Delivery System Reorganization

The PPACA fosters delivery system reorganization by changing Medicare payment rates and rules, and by encouraging innovation through support of pilot projects. Medicare annual market basket updates for inpatient hospital, skilled nursing facility, and other Medicare providers are reduced. Medicare payments to hospitals with excess readmissions or hospital-acquired conditions are reduced. Bonuses will be distributed among health care providers and insurance plans that exhibit higher quality or efficiency. For example, providers organized as accountable care organizations will be able to keep part of the cost savings they achieve for the Medicare program. In addition, the law appropriates funding for pilot programs to develop bundled payments for multiple providers involved in a single episode of care, or to establish a hospital value-based purchasing plan.

Although the legislation has already begun to change the health care system since it was signed into law, its major provisions are not scheduled to become effective until 2014. Given the controversial nature of some of the law's provisions and the numerous efforts underway to modify it, the law's ultimate effect on the U.S. healthcare system is difficult to predict.

IMPLICATIONS FOR THE PACU

PACUs—whether they are located in hospitals, ASCs, or other medical facilities—are strongly influenced by changes in the health care system. For a PACU nurse, effectively managing the intricacies of the health care environment will not only benefit current and future practice, but will also help make the PACU and the health care facility successful.

Working within a Changing Health Care System

Although the managed care movement of the 1990s was dismantled in large part by the providers

and consumer backlash it generated, successful health care organizations of the twenty-first century will operate under many of the principles of managed care. Managed care represented efforts made by market forces to finance and deliver health care in a way that both reduced costs and maintained the quality of care. The concept of managed care originated with prepaid group plans in the post–World War II period. Managed care began to gain momentum during 1970s, when the purchasers of health care (i.e., government and employers) were increasingly frustrated by escalating health care costs. Managed care emerged as a cost-saving alternative to the traditional fee-for-service system. The most important feature of managed care involves closing, in one way or another, the open-ended promises of traditional insurance policies of unlimited volume-based payment for providers and unlimited choice for consumers. Although the rapid growth of managed care in the 1990s encountered a backlash from consumers and providers, the cost control methods in managed care have been widely adopted because the imperative of expenditure control without sacrificing quality did not disappear with the unpopular nomenclature. Approximately 70% of Medicaid recipients and 25% of Medicare beneficiaries receive their benefits through managed care organizations.[24,25] Most of the plans offered by employers are also some form of managed care plan.

The spread of managed care has affected the way that health care is delivered, not only for health care provider organizations but also for the individual nurse at the bedside. It has never been more important for health care professionals to deliver health care services in an increasingly efficient and effective manner, to provide care in the most appropriate and cost-effective settings, to help patients transition from one care setting to another, and to emphasize patient education and preventive services.

Financial Management in the PACU

Historically, surgical services were the most financially profitable area in the hospital. In the era of restricted reimbursement, however, hospitals and ASCs are seeking ways to minimize their costs to increase their profit margins. Therefore, health care professionals must examine the services that are provided to ensure that gains in patient outcomes are worth the costs. For individual nurses in the PACU, understanding the cost structure of postanesthesia care is the first step in delivering cost-effective treatment without compromising quality.

The total cost of care reflects the monetary value of all the resources used to deliver the surgical or medical services. Costs can be broken into two main categories: fixed costs and variable costs.

Fixed Costs

Fixed costs are independent of output. They are considered to be constant in the short-term. Examples of fixed costs in the PACU include monitors, stretchers, intravenous pumps, and the physical plant of the facility itself.[26].

Variable Costs

Variable costs vary with the number of procedures performed or patients treated. These costs are linked directly to the production of services. Dressings, medications, laundry, oxygen and ventilator tubing, and electrocardiographic electrodes are typical variable costs in the PACU. If staff members are paid an hourly wage, the labor cost can be grouped into variable costs as well, because since it is connected to the number of hours worked.

From the perspective of a health care organization, labor costs comprise two parts: direct and indirect labor costs. Direct labor costs represent the amount paid to employees who are directly involved in the production of patient services. Direct labor costs for a PACU are calculated by multiplying the average hourly wage rate of each job class by the number of hours provided in each class and adding the results together.[27] Indirect labor costs are composed of the salaries of those not directly involved in the provision of patient care. Salaries of the nurse manager, unit secretaries, and any other staff who do not provide direct patient care are in this category. This category also contains any portion of staff salaries that are derived from attendance at meetings, in-service education, or other ancillary or support services.

Charges do not accurately reflect the true costs of providing services to a patient. Authors of one study reported that the cost-to-charge ratio for the PACU is 0.54.[26] In other words, the fees charged to patients can be twofold the actual costs. Charges often reflect the market forces of supply and demand and do not necessarily maintain a constant relationship with costs.[26] Charges may also be deliberately set higher to cover costs for other departments that receive no reimbursement, such as medical records and risk management. The actual cost of providing services can be assessed using the microcosting method, in which each input consumed is identified, measured, and valued.[28]

Under pressure from private insurers, government programs, and individual patients to reduce costs and increase efficiency, nurses are increasingly at the forefront of identifying process improvement opportunities that result in cost savings without sacrificing patient care. When nurses develop an understanding of how money flows through an organization, they become among the best advocates for cost-reduction strategies. The individuals at the bedside usually know where money is wasted and how the system can be improved to benefit all parties involved. All they need is to be involved in the decision-making process.

There are many ways that nurses can contribute to the efficiency of patient care. For example, evidence suggests that preexisting pain, anxiety, age, and type of surgery are the four most significant predictive factors for the intensity of postoperative pain.[29] Perianesthesia nurses can identify patients prone to postoperative pain and take proactive actions. As a result, the need for pain medication can be reduced and the costs of the PACU can be lowered. Perianesthesia nurses can also achieve cost savings by ensuring the smooth transition of patients to the community or other care settings. Preprinted instructions are a necessity in patient discharge education. Evidence indicates that patients who receive both verbal and written instructions are more likely to fully understand the care instructions.[30] Perianesthesia nurses must be involved in the creation of these materials and should serve on the patient education committee in their facilities.

Nursing Quality Improvement in the PACU

Quality of care has been a focus for the health care delivery system, especially after the publication of the Institute of Medicine's *Cross the Quality Chasm* report in 2001.[2] In recent years, efforts to control health costs and improve access to care have caused widespread concerns that the quality of care may be compromised.

Nursing staff members are the main source of input in the PACU. By actively participating in quality improvement initiatives, perianesthesia nurses can make a big difference in patient outcomes.

Perianesthesia nurses can begin to set the tone of the patient experience during preoperative teaching. This exchange provides the opportunity for the nurse to explain the postoperative course of care and for the patient to share expectations and concerns. A discussion of what the patient anticipates can help to guide care in the PACU. This type of exchange and follow-through in care costs little and can provide the patient and family with a better PACU experience.

Perianesthesia nurses need to adopt evidence-based practice (EBP) in order to substantially improve the quality of care while at the same time reducing unnecessary services and costs. One commonly used definition of EBP is "the conscientious, explicit, and judicious use of the current best evidence in making decisions about the care of individual patients."[31] An example of EBP is fast-tracking, a process in which patients are moved rapidly through the phases of recovery from anesthesia and are discharged home sooner. A review of published studies concluded that implementation of fast-track recovery pathways in pancreatic surgery is feasible and can achieve shorter hospital stay and reduced costs, with no increase in readmission or perioperative mortality rates.[32] Perianesthesia nurses should pay close attention to quality-related research and update their knowledge frequently to optimize their practice.

To standardize the process of care, various national professional groups, managed care organizations, and government agencies have embarked on the development of clinical practice guidelines. The American Society of PeriAnesthesia Nurses (ASPAN) is responsible for advancing the unique specialty of perianesthesia nursing. Clinical guidelines on normothermia, pain and comfort, postoperative nausea and vomiting, and postoperative discharge nausea and vomiting can be found on the ASPAN web site[33] and should be incorporated into daily practices by PACU nurses.

Cultural Competency in the PACU

The health care system is facing an ever more diverse patient population. In the last three decades, the proportion of the population speaking a language other than English at home has increased as racial and ethnic diversity in the United States have increased.[34] It is estimated that 55 million people spoke a language other than English at home in 2007. Among those for whom English was not the first language, 24.4% spoke English "not well" or "not at all."[34] Communication between patients with limited English proficiency and their providers can be impaired by language barriers, which may lower both patient and provider satisfaction, compromise patient safety, and potentially lead to suboptimal quality of care and health disparities for this population.[35-39] The challenges related to language and culture barriers may be even more prominent in the post–health care reform era because the new legislation will bring in large numbers of previously uninsured people and who are more likely to be from racial or ethnic minority populations.

In this environment, PACUs need to be transformed into culturally competent delivery systems that "acknowledge and incorporate at all levels the importance of culture, assessment of cross-cultural relations, vigilance toward the dynamics that result from cultural differences, expansion of cultural knowledge, and adaptation of services to meet culturally unique needs."[40] Many efforts can be made to improve the ability of postanesthesia nurses to deliver effective and respectful care to patients with cultural or linguistic barriers. These patients should be identified quickly so that care givers can pay special attention to the possible sources of misunderstanding. Special programs, such as translation services, should be made available. Currently, the District of Columbia and 13 states provide Medicaid and CHIP reimbursement for interpreter services.[41] Health care staff members, especially nurses, should be trained to interact effectively with patients from other cultures and languages. PACUs located in communities with large percentages of minorities should employ staff from those populations. Cultural competence strategies should be included in health care facility accreditation and licensure processes.

SUMMARY

The U.S. health care system continues to evolve at a rapid pace. This requires health care organizations and health professionals to constantly make adjustments to the demands of the health care environment. Nurses are perfectly situated to assist with strategies that cut costs while simultaneously improving quality of care. Acquiring the knowledge and skills to deliver health care to an increasingly diverse population is the challenge faced by each perianesthesia nurse. Perianesthesia nursing can make significant contributions to the surgical experience of the patients.

REFERENCES

1. World Health Organization: *The world health report 2000—health systems: improving performance*, Geneva, 2000, World Health Organization.
2. Institute of Medicine: *Crossing the quality chasm: a new health system for the twenty-first century*, Washington DC, 2001, National Academy Press.
3. Centers for Medicare and Medicaid Services: *Health expenditures by sponsors: business, household and government,*

available at https://www.cms.gov/nationalhealthexpend-data/06_nationalhealthaccountsbusinesshousehold government.asp. Accessed February 25, 2011.

4. Kaiser family foundation and health research & educational trust: *2010 Kaiser/Hret employer health benefits survey*, available at http://ehbs.kff.org/pdf/2010/8085.pdf. Accessed May 18, 2011.

5. U.S. Office of Personnel Management: *Federal employees health benefits program handbook*, available at http://www.opm.gov/insure/health/reference/handbook/fehb03.asp#govshare. Accessed May 1, 2011.

6. Collins SR, et al: *Help on the horizon—findings from the commonwealth fund biennial health insurance survey of 2010*, available at http://www.commonwealthfund.org/~/media/Files/Publications/Fund%20Report/2011/Mar/1486_Collins_help_on_the_horizon_2010_biennial_survey_report_FINAL_v2.pdf. Accessed May 18, 2011.

7. Employee Benefit Research Institute: *Tax expenditures and employee benefits: estimates from the FY 2011 budget*, available at http://www.ebri.org/pdf/publications/facts/FS-209_Mar10_Bens-Rev-Loss.pdf. Accessed May 18, 2011.

8. Centers for Medicare & Medicaid Services: *2011 Part B premium amounts for persons with higher income levels*, available at http://questions.medicare.gov/app/answers/detail/a_id/2306/session/L2F2LzEvc2lkL0VRa3J6NnBr. Accessed March 6, 2011.

9. Kaiser Family Foundation: *Prescription drug benefit under Medicare 2008*, available at http://www.kaiseredu.org/Issue-Modules/Prescription-Drug-Benefit-Under-Medicare/Background-Brief.aspx. Accessed March 6, 2011.

10. Kaiser Family Foundation: *Medicaid enrollment as a percent of total population, 2008*, available at http://statehealthfacts.org/comparereport.jsp?rep=54&cat=4&sortc=1&o=a. Accessed May 4, 2011.

11. Kaiser Family Foundation: *Income eligibility limits for working adults at application as a percent of the federal poverty level (FPL) by scope of benefit package*, available at http://statehealthfacts.org/comparereport.jsp?rep=54&cat=4&sortc=1&o=a. Accessed May 12, 2011.

12. Centers for Medicare & Medicaid Services: *FY 2010 number of children ever enrolled year—CHIP by program type*, available at http://www.cms.gov/NationalCHIPPolicy/downloads/FY2010StateCHIPTotalTable_020111_FINAL.pdf. Accessed March 10, 2011.

13. Truffer CJ, et al: Health spending projections through 2019: the recession's impact continues, *Health Affairs* 29(3): 522–529. DOI: 10.1377/hlthaff.2009.1074, 2010.

14. Centers for Medicare & Medicaid Services: *National health expenditures 2009 highlights*, available at http://www.cms.gov/NationalHealthExpendData/downloads/highlights.pdf. Accessed January 28, 2011.

15. Organisation for Economic Co-operation and Development: *Briefing note for OECD Health Data 2010: how does the United States compare*, available at http://www.oecd.org/dataoecd/46/2/38980580.pdf. Accessed January 25, 2011.

16. Kaiser Family Foundation, Kaiser Commission on Medicaid and the Uninsured: *The uninsured: a primer, December 2010*, available at http://www.kff.org/uninsured/upload/7451-06.pdf. Accessed May 18, 2011.

17. National Center for Health Statistics: *Health, United States, 2010: with special feature on death and dying*, Hyattsville, MD, 2011, available at http://www.cdc.gov/nchs/data/hus/hus10.pdf. Accessed May 18, 2011.

18. Medicare Payment Advisory Commission (MedPAC): *Report to the congress: Medicare payment policy. (March 2004), Washington, DC, 2004*, available at http://www.medpac.gov/documents/Mar04_Entire_reportv3.pdf. Accessed April 5, 2011.

19. U.S. Census Bureau: *Statistical abstract of the United States: 2011*, available at http://www.census.gov/compendia/statab/2011edition.html. Accessed May 18, 2011.

20. Centers for Medicare & Medicaid Services: *Long-term care 2009*, available at http://www.medicare.gov/longtermcare/static/home.asp. Accessed March 10, 2011.

21. Folland S, et al: *The economics of health and health care*, ed 6, Upper Saddle River, New Jersey, 2010, Prentice Hall.

22. Centers for Medicare & Medicaid Services: *Hospital-acquired conditions (present on admission indicator)*, available at http://www.cms.gov/HospitalAcqCond/. Accessed July 26, 2011.

23. Kaiser Family Foundation: *Focus on health reform—summary of new health reform law*, available at http://www.kff.org/healthreform/upload/8061.pdf. Accessed March 10, 2011.

24. Centers for Medicare & Medicaid Services: *Medicaid managed care enrollment report, summary statistics as of June 30, 2008*, available at https://www.cms.gov/Medicaid-DataSourcesGenInfo/04_MdManCrEnrllRep.asp. Accessed February 14, 2012.

25. Kaiser Family Foundation: *Medicare advantage 2010. Data spotlight: plan enrollment patterns and trends 2010*, available at http://www.kff.org/medicare/8080.cfm. Accessed May 18, 2011.

26. Macario A, et al: What can the postanesthesia care unit manager do to decrease costs in the postanesthesia care unit? *J Perianesth Nurs* 14:284–93, 1999.

27. Kahl K, Preston B: Identifying the cost of patient care in the postanesthesia care setting, *J Post Anesth Nurs* 3:198–202, 1988.

28. Gold MR, et al: *Cost-effectiveness in health and medicine*, New York, 1996, Oxford University Press.

29. Ip HYV, et al: Predictors of postoperative pain and analgesic consumption: a qualitative systematic review, *Anesthesiology* 111:657–77, 2009.

30. Flacker J, et al: Hospital discharge information and older patients: do they get what they need? *Journal of Hospital Medicine* 2:291–6, 2007.

31. Sackett DL, et al: Evidence based medicine: what it is and what it isn't, *BMJ* 312:71–2, 1996.

32. Ypsilantis E, Praseedom RK: Current status of fast-track recovery pathways in pancreatic surgery, *JOP* 10:646–50, 2009.

33. American Society of PeriAnesthesia Nurses: *Clinical practice guidelines*, available at http://www.aspan.org/ClinicalPractice/ClinicalGuidelines/tabid/3254/Default.aspx. Accessed May 1, 2011.

34. Shin HB, Kominski RA: *Language use in the United States: 2007, American Community Survey Reports, ACS-12*, Washington, DC, 2010, U.S. Census Bureau.

35. Carrasquillo O, et al: Impact of language barriers on patient satisfaction in an emergency department, *J Gen Intern Med* 14:82–7, 1999.

36. Morales LS, et al: Are Latinos less satisfied with communication by health care providers? *J Gen Intern Med* 14:409–17, 1999.

37. Atchison KA, et al: A qualitative report of patient problems and postoperative instructions, *J Oral Maxillofac Surg* 63:449–56, 2005.

38. John-Baptiste A, et al: The effect of English language proficiency on length of stay and in-hospital mortality, *J Gen Intern Med* 19:221–8, 2004.
39. Bard MR, et al: Language barrier leads to the unnecessary intubation of trauma patients, *Am Surg* 70:783–6, 2004.
40. Betancourt JR, et al: Defining cultural competence: a practical framework for addressing racial/ethnic disparities in health and health care, *Public Health Rep* 118:293–30, 2003.
41. National Health Law Program and The Access Project: *Language services action kit: interpreter services in health care settings for people with limited English proficiency*, Washington, DC, 2004, National Health Law Program and The Access Project.

7 Patient Safety and Legal Issues in the PACU

Jacqueline Ross, PhD, RN, CPAN

The current spotlight on patient safety provides nurses with an opportunity and the moral responsibility to call for changes in health care facilities' policies and operations that we know are detrimental to the safety of patients. The challenge is for all nurses to seize this opportunity. (Chapter 20a, p. 5)[1]

Perianesthesia units pose a variety of unique legal and patient safety issues for perianesthesia nurses. Legal issues and patient safety cannot be separated. Patient safety is a paramount concern for nurses, patients, and administrators. (Chapter 4 provides a more comprehensive review of patient safety and adds to the depth of understanding of patient safety concepts in perianesthesia nursing.) The perianesthesia nurse, as a licensed professional nurse, is subject to a set of standards that must be followed to practice nursing. These standards are those that a reasonable and prudent nurse would follow in the state of his or her practice. If the action of a perianesthesia nurse is not reasonable for a perianesthesia nurse and the action causes injury to the patient, a malpractice lawsuit may result. The aim of this chapter is to improve the legal knowledge of perianesthesia nurses and provide some guidance on some potential legal concerns of perianesthesia nurses.

The first section of this chapter includes the ethical values that underlie the formation of laws. This discussion is followed by common legal terminology, along with definitions and some examples. Some of the current approaches to patient safety are discussed. Next, the anatomy of a malpractice claim is explained. From these examples the perianesthesia nurse should have a better understanding of the litigation process with a review of these cases. Finally, the chapter presents some examples of malpractice issues involving nurses practicing in the perianesthesia area including examples of how some cases transpired.

DEFINITIONS

Advance Directive: A written document recognized by state law that provides directions for care of a person in the event that the person is unable to make decisions on treatment choices. Advance directives include do not resuscitate orders, living wills, and durable power of attorney for health care.

Adverse Event: Any injury caused by medical care. Examples include postoperative surgical site infection or a drug reaction. Having an adverse event does not imply a medical error.

Advocacy: Acting on behalf of the patient in an effort to protect that person's rights to make his or her own decisions. Nurses are expected to act as the patient advocate.

Assault: Involves a threat that causes the patient to be in fear of a physical injury. For example, saying "if you do not stay still I will put restraints on you" to a patient could lead to the charge of assault.

Battery: Involves unauthorized touching of a patient's body, for example if a patient has a do not resuscitate order in place but cardiopulmonary resuscitation is performed on the patient. Everyone involved could be charged with battery

Civil Law: A type of law that is concerned with relationships among persons and the protection of a person's rights. Violation of this type of law may cause harm to an individual or property, but no grave threat to society exists.

Confidentiality: A special relationship that exists between the patient and the perianesthesia nurse in which the information discussed is not shared with a third party who is not directly involved in the patient's care. Disclosure of confidential information exposes the perianesthesia nurse to liability for invasion of the patient's privacy and breech of confidentiality malpractice claims.

Consent: A voluntary act on the part of the patient to grant someone a type of care. Implied consent is not expressly written or spoken, but implied when circumstances exist that lead a reasonable person to believe that consent had been given, such as when the failure to act would result in injury (cardiopulmonary resuscitation needed). Expressed consent is either spoken or written and typically involves both.

Contract Law: A law that is concerned with enforcement of an agreement among private individuals.

Contributory Negligence: Used in medical malpractice when it is alleged that the patient's actions or inactions contributed to the injury.

Criminal Law: A type of law that is concerned with relationships between individuals and governments and with acts that threaten society and its order; a crime is an offense against society that violates a law and is defined as a misdemeanor (less serious in nature) or a felony (serious in nature).

Damages: The sum of money a court or jury awards as compensation for a tort action. Damages can be broken down into general damages, which are given for intangible wrongs, such as pain and suffering, disfigurement, interference with ordinary enjoyment of life, and loss of consortium (marital services), that are inherent in the injury itself; special damages, which are the patient's out-of-pocket expenses, such as medical care, lost wages, and rehabilitation costs; and punitive damages, which are the damages sought as punishment for those whose conduct goes beyond normal malpractice.

Defamation: Refers to damage caused to someone's reputation. If the damaging information is written, the defamation is called *libel;* if it is spoken, it is called *slander.*

Defendant: A person who is accused of wrongdoing; in a malpractice claim, the defendant can be a perianesthesia nurse.

Defensive Charting: Extensive documentation that is accurate and factual in the medical record.

Deposition: Out-of-court oral testimony given under oath before a court reporter. The deposition can involve expert witnesses, fact witnesses, defendants, or plaintiffs and can be used to impeach (find inconsistencies or untruths) testimony in trials.

Disruptive, Unprofessional Behavior: Behavior that shows disrespect for others, such as verbal abuse. This behavior impedes the safe delivery of patient care. This behavior is not acceptable and needs to be reported to administrators.

Durable Power of Attorney for Health Care: This advance directive specifies who decides health care decisions for the patient if the patient is incompetent. The patient's condition does not need to be terminal for this advance directive to be in effect. The durable power of attorney for health care must have been signed when the patient was competent, and it applies only to the health care decisions.

Ethics: The distinction between right and wrong based on knowledge, not just opinions. *Ethics* refers to what someone should do or the desired behavior.

Expert Witness: A person with specific knowledge, skills, and experience regarding a specific area, such as perianesthesia nursing, who testifies to the ultimate issue, such as: What was the duty or was the duty violated? Did the violation cause injury? What could the defendant have done to prevent the injury? Did malpractice occur?

Health Insurance: Portability and Accountability Act (HIPAA): This law was enacted to ensure privacy rights and describes how personal health information can be used and how a patient can obtain access to the information.

Human Factor: Safety problems that arise because of the interaction between people, technology, and work environments.

Impaired Nurse: A nurse who is unable to function effectively because of some type of substance abuse, such as alcohol, prescription drugs, and illegal drugs. If you know of an impaired nurse you should report this to your supervisor. Many state boards of nursing have programs in place to assist impaired nurses. Impaired nurses are a threat to patient safety.

Informed Consent: The patient's approval (or that of the patient's legal representative) to a specific care service; informed consent is a legal document. Informed consent can be waived for urgent medical or surgical intervention as long as this exception is so stated in an institutional policy. Types of consents are admission agreement, blood transfusion consent, surgical consent, research consent, and special consent, such as for the use of restraints, client photographs, organ donation, or autopsy. Proceeding without consent can lead to charges of battery or assault. A patient has a right to refuse informed consent. If this occurs make sure to document this. Nurses are only witnessing the signature.

Intentional Tort: Consequences of actions that can be reasonably foreseen, violate duty, or cause injury; in this case, an expert witness is not necessary to bring a case. The actions are closely related to criminal acts in that they involve more intent to do wrong. Types of intentional torts include assault, battery, and false imprisonment.

Interrogatory: The process of discovery of the facts regarding a case through a set of written questions exchanged through the attorneys that represent the parties involved in the case.

Invasion of Privacy: This can entail the disclosure of personal details of a patient, accessing patient's medical records when not involved in the patient's care or using a picture of a patient without their consent.

Jurisdiction: The court's authority to accept or decide cases, which can be based on location or subject matter of the case.

Law: Perianesthesia nurses are governed by civil and criminal law when they are in the role as providers of services, employees of institutions, and private citizens. The types of laws are contract, civil, criminal, and tort. Law mandates behavior and it is written by experts and those in authority (e.g., legislators).

Liability: Proof of liability is described in Box 7-1.

Libel: Libel involves writing something that ruins a patient's reputation.

Living Will: An advance directive that states what the patient wants if they become incompetent and terminal. The living will must have been written when the patient was competent.

Malpractice: Determined if the perianesthesia nurse owed a duty to the client and did not carry out that duty and the client was injured because the nurse failed to perform the duty. The elements of negligence are applied to the determination of malpractice, and usually an expert witness is used to establish standard of care and prove the violation resulted in injury. It involves the conduct of perianesthesia nurses that falls below the professional standard of care.

Minors: A patient who is under the legal age (usually 18 years) as defined by state statute and may not give legal consent; consent must be obtained by a parent or the legal guardian.

Near Miss: An event or a situation that did not lead to a patient injury. An example may be a nurse is about to administer a wrong medication to a patient, but realizes it and does not give the medication. Near misses need to be reported and investigated because they can be used to identify systematic issues.

Negligence: This is a tort that is the failure to provide care that a reasonable person ordinarily would provide in a similar circumstance. The elements that must be established to prove negligence are: (1) an established relationship, (2) the duty established by profession, and (3) a violation of that duty that results in injury.

Nurse Practice Act: A series of statutes that have been enacted by every state legislature to regulate the practice of nursing. In essence, the statutes define the scope of nursing practice and distinguish between nursing practice and medical practice; every professional nurse must review and understand the provisions of the Nurse Practice Act in the state or province in which the nurse works.

Patient's Bill of Rights: A document of client rights that reflects acknowledgement of the client's right to participate in one's own health care, with an emphasis on client autonomy and several laws and standards that pertain to the client's rights.

Plaintiff: The person who files the lawsuit and seeks damages for a perceived wrongdoing; usually the patient or the patient's family.

Post hoc, ergo propter hoc: "After this, therefore because of this"; the theory of the injury has been bypassed as the injury occurred, and that by itself indicates a failure to do what was reasonable and prudent.

Quasi-Intentional Tort: This tort involves more intent than malpractice and includes invasion of privacy and defamation.

Res ipsa loquitur: "The thing speaks for itself." This can be invoked in a medical malpractice case if the case meets the following four criteria or tests: (1) the injury is considered to occur only during failure to exercise ordinary care, skill, or diligence; (2) the injurious actions are under the exclusive control of the practitioner; (3) the patient makes no contribution to the injury; and (4) the reasons for the injury are more attributable to the nurse than to the patient. Allows post hoc reasoning. Some perianesthesia examples of this term would be a burn from improperly used equipment or a foreign body left in a patient from a procedure.

Slander: Stating something that is untrue that ruins the patient's reputation.

Standards of Care: Standards based on various types of evidence as to what is reasonable and prudent behavior for a perianesthesia nurse (health care professional). These standards are usually outlined by the state or province Nurse Practice Acts. Standards are also established through nursing organizations, such as the American Society of PeriAnesthesia Nurses and the American Nurses Association. It is important to note that these standards reflect the minimum care.

Statute: Documented rules for living in a state (state law) or the United States (federal law) that are passed by state legislatures and by Congress.

Statute of Limitation: The time limit that patients have to bring a claim. If the patient fails to meet the statute of limitations, then the case cannot proceed. States differ on the time periods and when the statute starts. The statute can start at the time of the injury, when the patient discovers the injury or when the treatment for the injury stopped.

Tort Law: A civil wrong (not criminal), other than a breach in contract, in which the law allows an injured person to seek damages from the person who caused the injury.

Vicarious Liability: This term indicates that one party is responsible for the actions of another party. This type of liability often occurs with nurses working in a hospital.

ETHICAL VALUES

Ethical values serve as the basis for many of the laws that affect nurses and their practice. These values include: beneficence, nonmaleficence, autonomy, justice, fidelity, and life.[2] Each of these values are discussed briefly, along with some of the laws associated with them (see Chapter 8).

- Beneficence means to "do good." Beneficence reflects the care given by nurses and other health care providers. Health care providers are mandated to provide care for patients. Failure to provide this care often leads to claims of malpractice.[2]
- Nonmaleficence refers to "do no harm." Health care providers may be charged with violating this value through false imprisonment, battery, or assault. Slander and invasion of privacy are other examples.[2]
- Autonomy can also be thought of as freedom. Autonomy includes clinical issues of consent, advance directives, and transplant issues.[2]
- Justice entails fairness. Justice includes the enforcement of antidiscrimination and labor laws.[2]
- Fidelity is accountability on the part of the nurse and promotes truthfulness. Consent issues and confidentiality are incorporated under this value.[2]
- Life entails both the beginning and end of life. Ethics issues involving birth include abortion, stem cell research, and artificial insemination. Issues such as do not resuscitate (DNR), assisted suicide, and quality of life encase some of the values at the end of life.[2]

CURRENT APPROACHES TO PATIENT SAFETY

Medical mistakes often go undetected because health care professionals have too narrowly focused on individual error as the cause of those mistakes. As Lucian Leape notes:

> *Ironically, that unique nature of medical injury, or more precisely our reaction to it, has been the major barrier to reducing medical errors and injury. Shame, guilt,*

and fear prevent many physicians from discussing their mistakes, being honest with patients, and being able to look beyond their individual errors to correct underlying systems failures. They can only try harder. For many lawyers, a sense of just cause, in some cases moral outrage, similarly blinds them to alternatives to tort litigation. Both are misplaced. And both have been manifestly unsuccessful in preventing medical injuries. We have created a monster.[3]

One of the main changes in the approach to patient safety has been a move from the "culture of blame" to a culture of safety. In the past when errors were made the emphasis was on the person making the error, focusing on an individual's inattention, forgetfulness, or carelessness. However, evidence supports the theory that the error is most likely related to problems within the system. One of the main premises with the systems approach is that human beings are fallible and errors are expected. The goal of decreasing medical error is to build defenses into the system. If an error does occur, the emphasis is on why and how the system failed.[4] Administrators should place attention on the conditions in which individuals work, using tasks and teams with a goal to create better systems.

Facilities that focus on the person fail to further investigate possible causes in the error. A person focus includes active failures, such as health care procedural violations and lapses. An active failure occurs at the point of contact and is often referred to as an *error at the sharp end*. These sharp end errors are among the first noticed and often have bad outcomes.[4]

Latent conditions, those conditions that can lay dormant over a long time, refers to the less obvious failures in the system, such as design problems that lead to patient safety issues. These latent conditions are the result of decisions and actions by administrators—those who write policies and design the systems. Latent conditions account for the complexity of the system and how this affects the person at the point of contact. Reason[4] stated there are two kinds of adverse effects arising from latent conditions: error provoking conditions within the local workplace (e.g., poor staffing, fatigue) and long-lasting holes or weaknesses in the defenses (e.g., poor procedures and policies, design and construction deficiencies). Latent conditions can be discovered and corrected before a patient error, leading to a proactive stance. Organizations that strive for this approach are referred to as *high-reliability organizations* (HROs).[5]

HROs are facilities that are consistent in a focus on patient safety and avoidance of errors. The origins of HROs can be traced to the nuclear power and aviation industries. HROs easily identify weak links in patient safety and then strongly and promptly respond to these weaknesses, thus avoiding potential catastrophic errors. Every health care facility differs in its culture, systems issues, and challenges; therefore how health care facilities develop into an HRO will differ. HROs change their cultures to focus on reducing systems failures and have mechanisms in place to respond if a system failure occurs.[5]

HROs function within complex environments that place them at risk for error; for example, hospitals have interdependence among various disciplines from nursing to physicians to support staffs. In addition, within the hospital setting are multiple subcultures. This interdependence continues with the coordination needed to accomplish patient care efficiently and in a safe manner. This coordination also leads to extreme hierarchical differentiation in which roles are defined and differentiated, and decision making often falls to the most knowledgeable in the group. HROs also have high degrees of accountability, and in the health care industry that accountability is primarily to the patient. HROs also require good feedback among its teams and the ability to work under time constraints.[5]

The Agency for Heathcare Research and Quality stresses several important concepts with HROs: resilience, deference to expertise, reluctance to simplify, sensitivity to operations, and preoccupation with failure. Being resilient indicates that the HRO has leaders and staff members who know how to respond to system failure. For an HRO to succeed, listening to the front-line staff, who understand how the processes work, is essential for managers. It is human nature to simplify processes; however, a complex understanding of systematic failures is needed in an HRO. An awareness of the current state of the processes and systems notes risks and aids in the prevention of future errors. HROs also take near misses seriously, using them as a means to further improve systems.[5]

ANATOMY OF A MALPRACTICE CLAIM

Many state laws that govern legal claims for medical malpractice specify that the actions or inactions of nurses and doctors may be the basis for a medical malpractice lawsuit (Box 7-1).[6,7] The legal formula used in most medical malpractice cases is that a nurse, or other health care

BOX 7-1   Elements Needed to Prove Liability

- *Duty:* At the time of injury, a duty existed between the plaintiff and the defendant.
- *Breach of Duty:* The defendant breached duty of care to the plaintiff.
- *Proximate Cause:* The breach of duty was the legal cause of injury to the plaintiff.
- *Damage or Injury:* The plaintiff experienced injury or damages or both and can be compensated by law.

practitioner, must have and use the knowledge, skill, and care ordinarily possessed and used by members of the profession in good standing and that a doctor or nurse is liable if he or she did not have and use them.[8,9] American states are split on whether the standard of care for a health care practitioner should be judged by practitioners in the "same or similar locality" or according to a "national standard" of medical care. A national standard is normally used in cases of medical specialists and nurses.[10,11]

Nurses need to be aware that four elements must be present to prove malpractice: duty, breach of duty, causation, and damages. The first element is duty, which simply means that once you accept responsibility for a patient you owe a duty to act in conformity to the accepted standards of practice. Knowledge of your state's nurse practice act is essential. State boards of nursing differ on what nurses can do within the scope of practice. Often the state practice act is not clear. When in doubt, always double check with the state board of nursing.[12] Accepted standards of practice also include clinical practice guidelines and a facility's policies and procedures. In the past, a community standard of care was accepted. However, most courts now expect adherence to national standards.

If the assumption of duty was established, then there must be a breach of this duty for malpractice. Nurses and other health care professionals can be responsible because of an action or an inaction (omission). This breach of duty of the nurse is measured against what a *reasonably prudent nurse* under the same or similar circumstances would do using objective criteria. The nurse cannot blame fatigue or lack of experience as the cause of the breach.[2] If a nurse thinks he or she is working too many hours or needs more orientation to a unit or new equipment, it is the nurse's duty to report this to the manager. Not following standards of care or policies can be a breach of duty. In addition, expert witnesses can be used to illustrate that a nurse failed to act as a reasonably prudent nurse would in the same situation.

If a breach of duty has been established, then that breach of duty must be related to a damage or causation of the damage. The plaintiff will attempt to show that the injury would not have happened if the health care provider would have acted as a reasonably prudent health care provider would in the same situation. The plaintiff may also attempt to establish causation by stating that if the first injury had not occurred then other injuries would not have resulted.[2]

The final element in a malpractice claim is damage. Damages can be physical, psychological, or monetary.[12] Damages or injury must be present for the fourth element in malpractice to be satisfied—for example, giving the wrong medication to a patient that did not result in injury would not constitute malpractice.[2]

A claim is a demand for financial compensation for an injury that results from medical care. The majority of claims involving nursing issues are handled legally through the facility where the nurse worked during the incident. On rare occasions, hospitals or providers may pay for these claims out of pocket, especially if the damage is small (e.g., lost dentures). However, most claims are reported to the commercial malpractice insurance carrier who then investigates the claim, determines liability issues, and either settles the case out of court, denies liability altogether, or goes to trial. A few claims are dropped by the claimant before trial or are handled via arbitration or mediation.

The first step in a claim involves pleadings that are sent to the defendant. For most nurses, these pleadings will be sent directly to the nurse's place of employment. Legal liability for nurse malpractice generally falls on the responsible nurse or the nurse's employer under the legal doctrine of *respondent superior*. American tort law generally assigns shared responsibility for the nurse's malpractice to the employer, the supervising physician, or both under the doctrine of joint and several liability; therefore both the nurse and the respondent superior codefendants are liable for the full judgment against them, which gives the plaintiff patient the option of suing the nurse, the liability insurance carrier, the nurse's codefendant employer, and any other codefendants (and the liability insurance carriers).[12-14] However, a nurse who has committed malpractice is still primarily liable for damages to the patient plaintiff:

The mere fact that the plaintiff may focus collection efforts against a wealthier [or so-called "deep pockets"] codefendant, such as the nurse's employer, does not eliminate the nurse's liability (or the possibility that the nurse's employer will take some adverse job action, such as discipline or termination, or that the state licensing board will suspend or revoke the nurse's license). A nurse must be satisfied that he or she has [adequate] malpractice insurance, provided by either the self or the employer. In selecting the amount of coverage, the nurse should be aware of any caps or limits on damages that exist under state law.[14]

The pleadings will come in the form of a complaint, which can be specific or generic in terms of allegations, injury, and demands. If a nurse directly receives these pleadings, he or she should take these forms to the facility's legal department. Complaints typically have a time limit to respond. Failure to respond in the allotted time will lead to a judgment against the nurse and will most likely result in no coverage from the malpractice carrier. Once the nurse is aware of the medical malpractice claim, it is important that the case is not discussed with anyone, including peers.[12,13]

When the complaint is received by the malpractice insurer, an attorney will be assigned to monitor the case and provide an answer to the complaint. This answer tends to be direct, short, and often a denial of allegations. It is important to understand that both parties (plaintiff and defendant) can amend their pleadings to the court.[12,13]

The discovery process occurs after the pleadings have started, and this process implies that the parties in the claim will be determining the evidence. The plaintiff may have already, and most likely has, requested all of the medical records. A nurse should never add information to a medical record after receiving a notice of a malpractice claim. This action will result in spoliation of records and implies guilt.[12,13]

Attorneys will most likely send interrogatories to each other, which are written questions that need to be answered by the other party. Each of these questions is examined by the attorney first, because some may be too vague or may be objected to by the attorney. Next, the interrogatory will be sent to the health care provider and written responses will be needed. The attorney will review these responses carefully. When these interrogatories have been reviewed, the health care provider swears to the answers and they become part of the permanent legal record.[12,13]

During discovery, depositions are also taken. Depositions are recorded by a court reporter and answers are given under oath. Nurses should take comfort in the fact that attorneys will take time to prepare them for these depositions. Often attorneys will conduct pre-deposition interviews. Nurses should also be aware that they may be contacted for a deposition, even if they are not a party to the claim.[10-13] Tips for giving a deposition are covered in Box 7-2.

BOX 7-2   Suggested Behaviors When Giving a Deposition

- Look and act like a professional, indicating that you are prepared.
- Be clear, accurate, and concise; do not guess.
- Do not be argumentative with the attorney; this will reflect poorly on you.
- If you are in front of a jury, look at them and the judge when answering questions. (More than 95% of malpractice claims never make it to a jury trial.) Follow the advice of your defense attorney.
- Never give opinions unless asked for them; stick to the facts.
- Speak slowly and in a well-modulated tone of voice.
- Do not allow yourself to be rattled by the opposing attorney.
- If you do not remember a question or do not understand it, ask for it to be repeated or clarified. Do not get caught in the trap of allowing the attorney to use long multipart questions in an effort to confuse you.
- If you have made a statement and later realize it is not correct, do not be afraid to say so, rather than skirt issues or contradict yourself.
- Do not allow yourself to be goaded into an angry or emotional response; remember that you can always ask for a break during a deposition to collect yourself and your thoughts.
- Avoid the use of "always" and "never" and vague comments like "maybe," "I think," or "possibly."
- Only answer the immediate question. Do not provide more information than is asked for by the question.
- After the deposition is completed, you can request a copy to view it for accuracy.
- Be open and honest with your attorney, even if providing some information may be embarrassing. The plaintiff attorney may try to use this information to impede your credibility.
- Do not answer hypothetical questions. If you are directed to do so by the judge, then be sure to state that this is a hypothetical answer and is not based on the case currently being decided.
- Wait until the attorney has finished asking the question. Take a breath and then answer.
- If testifying in front of a jury, try to avoid overuse of medical terms. Attempt to state the facts in terms that are easy to understand.

Both the defense and plaintiff attorneys will use expert witnesses to support their case. In some cases the plaintiff is unable to find an expert witness to support their allegations; the case is often dismissed if this occurs. Medical and nursing expert witnesses rely heavily on their own personal experiences from practice; they may use medical treatises or journals as evidence; they may cite from nursing and medical reference books; and because substantial regional variations exist in the use of many procedures, experts may rely more on anecdotal experiences with little regard for differences in outcome. Some experts comment that the system is not very good, because determining which expert is more believable to the jury generally boils down to a "battle of the experts." Often attorneys on both sides attempt to impeach the qualifications of the expert witness on the other side, questioning qualifications or perhaps attempting to prove that the expert medical witness is unqualified because he or she is not familiar with the practice of nursing in a particular locality or a particular area of expertise. Another factor involved in the credibility of an expert witness is recent clinical experience. Box 7-3 presents ways that perianesthesia nurses can protect themselves against litigation.

When discovery has been completed and the expert witnesses have presented their opinions, the parties will decide how to proceed. Often a settlement offer is made and the parties will negotiate a possible settlement; however, if both sides believe they have a strong case, they will proceed to court. The trial is typically a jury trial and proceeds like a normal jury trial, including a jury verdict. Any jury finding can be appealed.[10,11]

If the case is settled or results in a plaintiff verdict, it is often filed with the National Practitioner Data Bank (NPDB). The NPDB is a central source of information regarding malpractice payments for physicians, nurses, and dentists. The databank became operational on September 1, 1990, and as of 1998 had more than 195,000 reports of malpractice payments, adverse licensure, clinical privileging, professional society membership, Drug Enforcement Agency actions, and Medicare or Medicaid exclusions actions concerning licensed professionals. Approximately 30,000 reports are added each year[15]; however, if the nurse is covered under the hospital policy a claim will not be filed. The NPDB contains only cases that have been settled and does not contain the majority of claims that are dismissed. In addition, the NPDB will also contain information from state boards on disciplinary action and disciplinary action (based on clinical practice) taken by a facility against a health care provider.[2]

BOX 7-3   How to Protect Against Litigation

- Adhere to accepted standard of care.
- Ensure that major aspects of care are met: responsibility, technical competence, and nursing judgment.
- Use appropriate documentation (see Boxes 7-4 and 7-5)
  - Document what you see and do.
  - Do not use judgmental language in documentation.
  - Do not alter the records.
- Avoid medication errors.
  - Violation of the classic five "rights" of medication administration
    - Right drug
    - Right patient
    - Right amount
    - Right route
    - Right time
- Claims based on medication errors are augmented when the perianesthesia nurse:
  - Fails to record the medication administration properly
  - Fails to recognize side effects or contraindications
  - Fails to know patient's allergies
- Recognize and respond to complications.
- Ensure that all equipment functions properly.
- Adequately assess, monitor, and obtain assistance.
- Ensure adequate communication with all members of the health care team.
- Report all incidents or occurrences.
- Do not tolerate disruptive or abusive behavior.
- Demand and provide good, standardized handoffs.
- Properly supervise nursing staff, students, or technicians.
- Know and respect all patient's rights (see Box 7-6).
- Protect a patient's privacy.
- Ensure that informed consent has been given to the patient. If in doubt, have the physician speak with the patient. Remember that, as a nurse, you are just witnessing the patient's signature on the informed consent, but always act as the patient's advocate.
- Follow up on ordered tests.
- Record telephone calls or e-mails, including the time called, the time the call was returned, and what was discussed.
- Include quotes of the patient that may seem important to remember in the future.
- Delegate tasks appropriately to those with verified adequate skill.

In summary, the overarching goal of nursing care is to prevent patient injury. Nurses can work toward this goal by following standards of care and reporting any potential problems to the administration. Because perianesthesia nurses care for multiple patients daily, it is essential that they document their care for easier recollection in the event a claim is filed. Some suggestions for documentation are included in Boxes 7-4 and 7-5.

BOX 7-4   Guidelines for Defensive Charting

- All entries should be accurate and factual.
- Make corrections appropriately and according to agency or hospital policies. *Never* obliterate or destroy any information that is or has been in the chart. This could lead to the charge of fraud or tampering with the records.
- If information exists that should have been charted and was not, the perianesthesia nurse should make a late entry, noting the time the charting actually occurred and the specific time the charting reflects.
- All identified patient problems, nursing actions taken, and patient responses should be noted. Do not describe a patient problem without including the nursing actions taken and the patient response.
- Documentation of why you did not do something that you would routinely do is often as important as documentation of why you did something. An example of this situation is a patient who refuses ambulation; the notation would be, "patient refused to ambulate because of . . ."
- Be as objective as possible in charting.
- Each page of the chart should contain the current date and time.
- Each page of the chart should include the full name and professional designation of every person who makes an entry on that page.
- Follow up with who saw the patient and what measures were initiated, especially in such instances as when the physician visited and calls that were made to the physician for a problem, and record the physician's response, the nursing actions, and the patient's response.
- Ensure that your notes are legible and clearly reflect the information to be documented to assure that the information makes sense and is portrayed accurately.
- Pertinent notes from other providers should also be reviewed to ensure that the medical record shows a coordination of health care team efforts and thoughts.
- Do not use the chart as a means of retaliation against other health care provider.
- Do not add to a document, such as an informed consent, unless the patient initials these additions.
- Do not include anything after the patient signs a document. Get a new document if needed and have the patient sign it as well.

Adapted from Zerwekh J, Garneau AZ: *Nursing today: transition and trends,* ed 7, St. Louis, 2012, Saunders; Hall J: *Law and ethics for clinicians,* Amarillo, Tex, 2002, Jackhal Books.

BOX 7-5   Computer Documentation Guidelines

- Do not ignore any warnings from the computer. These warnings are patient safety reminders.
- Do not allow anyone to have access to your password, even if temporarily.
- Know your hospital policy on late entries and error corrections. Documentation of these types of entries will most likely require a different approach.
- Access information only as needed. Do not access patient records if you are not involved in the care. The consequences of unethical access could lead to criminal and civil proceedings.
- Request in-services for any new implementation of online documentation or new systems.
- Know and follow your institution policy on how to handle patient printouts. Shredding or the elimination of patient identifiers should be included in that policy.

From Brent NJ: *Nurses and the law: a guide to principles and applications,* ed 2, Philadelphia, 2001, Saunders.

SOURCES FOR IDENTIFICATION OF MALPRACTICE IN THE PACU

Because the majority of malpractice claims are dismissed without any settlement, the factors associated with these dismissed claims remain unknown. If claims are settled with health care providers, such as physicians, then this information is reported to the NPDB. Because many claims involving perianesthesia nurses are covered under the facilities' malpractice claims, the information is not captured in the National Practitioners Data Base. As mentioned earlier, many claims are dismissed, and the information related to patient safety is lost; therefore there is a lack of information within the perianesthesia areas in regard to malpractice claims.

A recent analysis of closed malpractice claims involving cases occurring within the PACU was published. This article provided a first snapshot into the malpractice issues and patient safety in the perianesthesia areas, such as ambulatory surgery and PACU.[16]

The most common allegations for claims occurring in the PACU included:
- Improper management of the surgical patient
- Anesthesia related (e.g., damage to teeth)
- Improper anesthesia administration
- Failure to monitor the patient's physiologic status
- Delay in treatment
- Delay in diagnosis
- Wrong medications

Although two of these allegations clearly involved the anesthesia provider (improper anesthesia administration and anesthesia related), many of the other allegations related to the nursing care in the PACU. In fact, 39% of the medical malpractice claims occurring in the PACU had *nursing* listed as the primary responsible party. The top three risk management issues among PACU nurses included clinical judgment (present in 24% of the claims and included failure to monitor the patient and appreciate changes in vital signs), administrative issues (present in 19% of the claims and focused on failure to follow policies and procedures and the need for staff training), and communication issues (present in 19% of the claims and involved communication between providers, as well as poor rapport with another health care provider).[16]

Several of the claims consisted of more than one of these risk management issues, highlighting the complexity of health care. One case included a patient who was recovering from general anesthesia. The PACU nurse recorded that the alarms were on (as were required by policy), but the PACU nurse failed to actually check the alarms and just assumed the alarms were on. None of the alarms, either for the cardiac monitor or the pulse oximeter, were on and the patient experienced respiratory depression, and then had a cardiopulmonary arrest, leading to anoxic brain damage. This is an example of a human factor causing an error in the PACU. The nurse became used to the routine of the monitor alarms being on and failed to check them.

This snapshot included only cases that led to claims handled by one malpractice carrier in the United States; therefore the investigation into malpractice issues in the perianesthesia units remains relatively unknown. This analysis of claims provides insight to PACU nurses on the importance of communication and monitoring of patients.[16] Perianesthesia nurses are an essential player in patient safety.

INDIVIDUAL LIABILITY AND THE STANDARD OF CARE

As stated previously, there is no clear definition of a standard of care for a particular patient during particular circumstances. The standards for evaluation of the delivery of professional nursing services are not normally established by either judge or jury. Instead, the nursing profession itself sets the standards of practice, and the courts enforce these standards in tort suits. This practice requires that both plaintiff and defense attorneys present evidence of the standard of care by use of expert medical witnesses, who are almost always other perianesthesia nurses who practice nursing under

similar circumstances as the defendant nurse. No clear definitions of the standard of care for a particular situation exist.

The development and proliferation of clinical practice guidelines is one of the transforming forces in current medical practice and has aided plaintiff and defense attorneys in developing a more objective case on behalf of their clients. In this area, clinical practice guidelines can be highly useful.[17] As one author states:

> The consistent use of well-developed and medically appropriate practice guidelines has two potentially compelling benefits. First, scientifically reliable guidelines can improve medical practice by reducing the incidence of misdiagnoses and inappropriate treatment decisions . . . Second, if major inroads are made into the process of creating and disseminating guidelines, their use may improve the process of malpractice litigation when the practice of medicine goes awry or when insurance coverage is denied. Clinical practice guidelines are being used by both plaintiff and defense attorneys as evidence of the standard of care in medicine. For this very reason, it may be more useful for practitioners, including nurse anesthetists, to review and implement guidelines rather than to review and analyze published malpractice cases on the same subject![18]

There are several definitions of *clinical practice guidelines*, and the term itself has various synonyms, including clinical pathways, critical pathways, clinical paradigms, practice parameters, treatment protocols, and evidence-based medicine standards. Regardless of the name, the definition includes "systematically developed statements to assist practitioners and patient decisions about appropriate health care for specific clinical conditions."[19] Most guidelines attempt to improve health care providers' decision making by detailing appropriate indications for specific interventions.[20] Recently, authors of one article pointed out the complicated issues that arise with formulation of CPGs and suggest that committees who develop the guidelines allow flexibility, include multiple sources of evidence, and not rely on a small panel to write the guideline. They also maintain that if evidence is sparse, that fact should be openly acknowledged in the guideline.[11] Managed care organizations have embraced practice guidelines in the belief that their use will help control health care costs. A number of health care providers, feeling financial pressure to use such practice guidelines, have rebelled against their use believing that they will lead to a "cookbook" practice of medicine. Although this claim is partly valid, more compelling reasons for health care providers to embrace practice guidelines exist. American health care is subject to too much variation in practice, according to some commentators, and physicians and nurses are inundated with increased research on practice guidelines. Keeping up with all the medical advances worldwide is simply impossible. Accordingly, the advantages of using evidence-based guidelines in medical practice are gaining more widespread approval among health care providers. The Institute of Medicine declared that professional societies can contribute to improvement in patient safety through the promulgation and promotion of practice guidelines and that such guidelines can be written through a more interdisciplinary approach to patient care. Practice guidelines are among the most widely used methods of modification of physician behavior and improvement of patient safety. Significantly, practice guidelines are increasingly cited in court litigation and are used as evidence of a medical standard of care. They can also be raised as an affirmative defense by physicians and nurses in medical malpractice suits to show compliance with accepted medical practice. The American Society of PeriAnesthesia Nurses now has in place two evidence-based clinical practice guidelines. Both of these guidelines were developed using an interdisciplinary approach.[21,22]

Several states have legislated the use of such practice guidelines and provide tort immunity for health care practitioners in exchange for following such guidelines. Finally, because these practice guidelines are widely published on the Internet, failure to access such information is likely to become an important piece of evidence in a malpractice suit, because the failure is evidence that a physician or nurse has failed to stay current in his or her field of practice. With more focus on practice guidelines based on outcomes, it is important that health care practitioners understand the sources of medical malpractice to develop practice guidelines aimed at these patient safety areas.

SUGGESTIONS TO DECREASE LEGAL LIABILITY AND IMPROVE PATIENT SAFETY

Health care providers remain deeply committed to the care and safety of their patients. However, focusing on the blame game—singling out individuals for punishment and retribution and reliance on the court system for compensation to injured patients—has done little to increase patient care overall in American hospitals.[6] The complex nature of the health care industry simply does not lend itself to this process of blaming individuals and allowing the courts to compensate injured patients. Instead, nursing professionals should embrace and encourage a systematic approach to defining quality of patient care and improving patient safety. To this end, the blame game will hopefully give way to developing a root cause analysis of medical errors and near misses and a systematic approach for making patient safety a priority in hospitals.

This is not to say that individual accountability or liability will disappear altogether—it will not. However, a systematic approach to individual liability will result in more focus on detailed credentialing processes, better assessment of professionals within certain job constraints, better licensing techniques, and better continuing educational programs, all geared to keep health care professionals competent and qualified for the particular tasks that they must do. With this new way of ascertaining how medical errors and near misses are made and how they can be avoided, some of the more important patient safety tips include the following:

- Report and investigate all near misses. Everyone can all learn from his or her mistakes, and mistakes that do not cause harm are just as important to understand and investigate as those that do cause harm. Identifying causes of near misses can highlight systems issues that have been overlooked for a long period of time within patient care. Addressing near misses before patient injury is important to improve patient safety and decrease filing of medical malpractice claims.
- Be sure that the hospital has a system to report and investigate all medical errors and near misses by encouraging and rewarding those who report personal mistakes rather than punishing them. Develop a systematic process to question potential medical errors before they happen. Time and again, members of a health care team see problems coming, but they are afraid to question the authority of the person who is about to make a mistake.
- Nurses are sometimes afraid to question physician's orders, but their doubts can often save a patient's life. Develop a policy on questioning authority. Each facility should have a chain of command policy in force, and nurses should not hesitate to use it. Every health care team member has the responsibility for patient outcome.
- Disruptive behavior from any health care provider should not be tolerated. Each health care member is entitled to fair treatment.

- Empower and actively involve your patients in determining their own standard of health care. In an age of patient autonomy and informed consent, patient involvement is acquiring new meaning. Informed consent is no longer a signature on a piece of paper but a process of ongoing communication. The more patients know what to expect from their own treatment protocol, the better they are able to help the nurse do his or her job and improve their own safety during care (Box 7-6).
- Embrace protocols and electronic checklists into practice. Human errors that involve equipment misuse remain a major concern for patients for anesthesia. Studies indicate that indexed electronic checklists are superior to either memorized or nonindexed paper checklists in reducing errors of omission. Airline pilots never fly without them, and neither should nurses.
- Try to avoid workarounds. Workarounds are often started because the system is not working for the end user. For example, a new system of medication delivery is implemented. However, this new system causes twice as much time for the nurse to administer the medication. Nurses then develop workarounds to decrease the time involved. These workarounds provide ample opportunity for medical errors. If you notice workarounds used within in your units, bring it to the attention of management. Again, workarounds tend to indicate a systems issue, which can be fixed if known.[23]
- Remain up-to-date on continuing education. Taking these courses not only improves the nurse's knowledge base, but it provides evidence that the nursing professional is current with the trends in perianesthesia nursing. If a nurse is involved in a lawsuit, lawyers for the plaintiff will likely ask to see his or her continuing education credits.
- Certification makes a difference as it illustrates that the nurse has a basis of knowledge within a specialty. This designation also highlights that the nurse voluntarily sought to advance and validate his or her clinical knowledge.
- Embrace the use of clinical guidelines. Just as checklists and protocols can help to avoid many human mistakes made as the result of doing a repetitive task, clinical guidelines can help to avoid human mistakes made as the result of judgmental error. Guidelines are not a definitive standard of care. However, clinical guidelines help to provide a defense in the medical record. The nurse must justify the reasons for deviating from the clinical guidelines. Untoward risks are part of medical care, but justifying decisions helps in defending medical actions later.
- Know what is covered, excluded, and provided by malpractice insurance. Even with all the previously listed recommendations, errors happen and involvement in a legal claim is often the first time medical professionals learn what insurance they do or do not have. As an employee, a nurse may be covered under a hospital "house" policy. It is important to read and understand that coverage. If job descriptions change dramatically, it is important to get written clarification of coverage from the insurance carrier. All health care professionals should make appointments with their insurance agents to review their medical malpractice policies. Some exclusions may be cause for surprise. Sexual misconduct with a patient is obviously excluded, but often, intentional acts are excluded as well. Know what this means; ask for examples; and know

---

BOX 7-6   Patient Rights When Hospitalized

- Right to considerate and respectful care
- Right to obtain current and understandable material
- Right to be informed about illness, possible treatments, and likely outcome and to discuss this information with the physician
- Right to know the names and roles of the persons who are involved in care
- Right to consent to or refuse a treatment
- Right to have an advance directive
- Right to privacy
- Right to expect that medical records are confidential
- Right to review the medical record and to have information explained
- Right to expect that the hospital will provide necessary health services
- Right to reasonable continuity of care
- Right to know whether the hospital has relationships with outside parties that may influence treatment or care
- Right to consent or refuse to take part in research
- Right to be told of realistic care alternatives when hospital care is no longer appropriate
- Right to know about hospital rules that affect treatment and about changes and payment methods

From Christensen B, Kockrow E: *Foundations of nursing*, ed 4, St. Louis, 2003, Mosby; Paasche-Orlow MK, et al: National survey of patients' bill of rights statutes, *J Gen Intern Med* 24:489–494, 2009.

the coverage dollar amount limitation and tail policy, if any.

Nurses focus on patient safety every day in their practice, but there are some legal considerations which remain. For example, improving patient safety emphasizes the need to report near-misses. To ensure that the reporting of near-misses is not discouraged, the leadership of the organization needs to embrace a culture of safety rather than blame. On the legal side of this reporting is the assurance that this information is safe from discovery and used in manners to improve patient safety. Reporting of near-misses can accentuate system issues before a major injury occurs. This allows the systematic problem to be identified and improved. However, health care workers may not report such events if there is the fear of retaliation or blame. Real leadership is needed, not only on the part of hospital administrators, physicians, and nurse administrators, but bedside nurses as well to incorporate patient safety and the reduction of medical errors as a specific goal. This requires a real change in the way hospitals hire, monitor, and manage their human resources. Also, patients must take responsibility for their own medical care and treatment. It is important that patients are encouraged to speak up if something does not seem right in their care. As Box 7-7 suggests, some methods exist to reduce errors in hospitals and specifically the PACU.

BOX 7-7   Ways to Reduce Errors in Hospitals

- Reduce mental errors by reducing stress and fatigue.
- Expand knowledge and develop programs to minimize inevitable errors by simplifying steps and systems.
- Avoid reliance on memory; simplify tasks and standardize procedures.
- Reduce drug errors of all types by systematizing and using dedicated staff members for use of drug delivery systems.
- Standardize equipment, such as same location in each unit, and identify equipment that is prone to causing errors.
- Training and education: use of simulators and performance certification.
- Use a process-of-care approach, whereby decision making is standardized, and development of error reduction program.
- Improve the structure of the department by having leadership direction that is multidisciplinary with outcome measures and reporting along with use of external benchmarks.
- Be responsive to change and resource allocation.

SUMMARY

The intent of this chapter is to introduce the perianesthesia nurse to the legal components of being a licensed professional nurse. Hopefully the definition section aids in developing an understanding of the legal system and patient safety, and how both affect perianesthesia care. A recent investigation into malpractice issues occurring in the PACU will provide perianesthesia nurses with more insight into potential patient safety issues. Several boxes were presented to help the perianesthesia nurse to understand the importance of defensive charting, patient rights, methods to protect the perianesthesia nurse from litigation, and some ideas on the appropriate actions for giving a deposition.

The perianesthesia nurse should gain a good understanding of the legal process and become more confident when faced with the law. Certainly continuing education, critical thinking, and use of good common sense help in dealing with the legal issues that touch every perianesthesia nurse everyday. In addition, nurses should be involved with activities such as patient safety through simulation and quality and patient safety processes within the institution. Another important element to the legal component to perianesthesia practice is to get involved and visit the hearings conducted by the state board of nursing and the state legislature. With involvement in these legal processes and functions, perianesthesia nurses become more aware of how to protect themselves legally in their practice setting; more importantly, with a better understanding of the legal process, the perianesthesia nurse can influence the direction of many health care issues locally, statewide, and nationally.

REFERENCES

1. Agency for Healthcare Research and Quality: *Patient safety and quality: an evidence-based handbook for nurses,* AHRQ Publication No. 08-0043, Rockville, Md, 2008, available at www.ahrq.gov/qual/nurseshdbk/. Accessed September 13, 2011.
2. Hall J: *Law and ethics for clinicians,* Amarillo, Tex, 2002, Jackhal Books.
3. Leape LL: Foreword: preventing medical accidents: is "systems analysis" the answer? *Am J Law Med* 27:27–37, 2001.
4. Reason J: Human error: models and management, *Br Med J* 320:768, 2000.
5. Agency for Healthcare Research and Quality: *Becoming a high reliability organization: operational advice for hospital leaders,* AHRQ Publication No. 08-0022, Rockville, Md, 2008, available at www.ahrq.gov/qual/hroadvice/. Accessed September 13, 2011.

6. Andrews M: *Nurse's legal handbook*, ed 3, Pennsylvania, 1996, Springhouse.
7. Gic JA: Nursing and the law. In *Legal medicine*, ed 7, St. Louis, 2007, Mosby.
8. William P, Keeton P: *The law of torts*, ed 5, St. Paul, Minn, 1984, West Publishing Co.
9. Pegalis S, Wachsman H: *American law of medical malpractice*, ed 2, Deerfield, Ill, 1992, Clark Boardman Callaghan.
10. Zitter JM: *Standard of care owed to patient by medical specialist as determined by local, "like community," state, national, or other standards* (annotation), 18 A.L.R. 4th 603, 1982.
11. Moffett P, Moore G: The standard of care: legal history and definitions: the bad and good news, *West J of Emerg Med* 12(1):109–112, 2011.
12. Brent N: *Nurses and the law: a guide to principles and applications*, ed 2, St. Louis, 2011, Saunders.
13. Bogart-Brewer J: American Association of Legal Nurse Consultants: *Legal nursing consulting: principles and practice*, Boca Raton, Fla, 1998, CRC Press.
14. Kessler DP, McClellan MB: Do doctors practice defensive medicine? *Q J Econ* 111(2):353–359, 1996.
15. U.S. Department of Health and Human Services: *National practitioner data bank*, available at www.npdb-hipdb.hrsa.gov/. Accessed September 13, 2011.
16. Ross J, Ranum D: Improving patient safety by understanding past experiences in day surgery and PACU, *J Perianesth Nurs* 24(3):144–151, 2009.
17. U.S. Department of Health and Human Services, Agency for Healthcare Research and Quality: *National guidelines clearinghouse*, available at www.guideline.gov/. Accessed September 13, 2011.
18. Finder JM: The future of practice guidelines: should they constitute conclusive evidence of the standard of care? *Health Matrix* 10:67–76, 2000.
19. Field MJ, Lohr KN, editors: *Clinical practice guidelines: directions for a new program*, Washington, DC, 1990, National Academy Press.
20. Sheetz ML: Toward controlled clinical care through clinical practice guidelines: the legal liability for developers and issuers of clinical pathways, *Brooklyn L Rev* 63:1341–1366, 1997.
21. Hooper V, et al: ASPAN's evidence-based clinical practice guideline for the promotion of perioperative normothermia, *J Perianesth Nurs* 24(5):271–287, 2009.
22. Hooper V, et al: ASPAN's evidence-based clinical practice guideline for the prevention and/or treatment of postoperative nausea and vomiting and postdischarge nausea and vomiting in adult patients, *J Perianesth Nurs* 21:230–250, 2006.
23. Odom-Forren J: The normalization of deviance: a threat to patient safety, *J Perianesth Nurs* 26:216–219, 2011.

RESOURCES

Agency for Healthcare Research and Quality: Patient safety network, available at www.psnet.ahrq.gov/default.aspx.
Spath PL, editor: *Error reduction in health care: a systems approach to improving patient safety*, ed 2, San Francisco, Calif, 2011, Jossey-Bass, available at www.psnet.ahrq.gov/resource.aspx?resourceID=21939. Accessed January 2, 2012.

8 Ethics in Perianesthesia Nursing

Alexander Tartaglia, MA, MDiv, DMin, BCC, ACPE Supervisor, Ken Faulkner, MA, MDiv, and Audrey R. Roberson, MS, RN, CPAN, CNS-BC

The concern for ethical practice in the care of patients has a long tradition. Since the times of Hammurabi and Hippocrates, clinicians have identified the need to develop superior technical skills and an understanding of the application of those skills using sound moral judgment. This chapter assists the perianesthesia nurse in developing a framework for understanding ethical obligations to patients, surrogates, and colleagues. Beginning with a definition of ethics, the chapter offers an historic review of landmark cases that contribute to the development of bioethics as a distinct discipline. It describes and outlines the common principles used in the analysis and resolution of ethical concerns.

The chapter proceeds to examine ethical concerns most commonly encountered by perianesthesia professionals, including patient safety, privacy, and informed consent, with particular attention to do not resuscitate orders in the perioperative context. It offers practical guidance to assist clinicians in seeking strategies toward the resolution of ethical dilemmas.

UNDERSTANDING ETHICS

Understanding the nature of ethical reflection requires the establishment of a common language and definition of terms. Foundational questions about the nature of ethics and morality precede movement to particular ethical issues within the moral context of the clinical setting. What do we mean when we use the terms *ethics* and *morality*? What is the nature of a moral dilemma? What is the goal of ethical reflection? How can we know which rules, principles, standards, or guidelines are best for determining appropriate ethical behavior in the resolution of everyday dilemmas?

The terms *ethics* and *morality*, although obviously related, are distinct. *Ethics* is derived from the Greek root *ethos*, meaning "character."[1] *Morality* or *morals* is derived from the Latin word *mores* or *moralis*, meaning "customs, character, or habit."[1]

The ancient terms have a shared meaning. Today, persons engaged in the formal discipline of ethical reflection have a more distinct understanding. Beauchamp and Childress understand ethics as a "generic term for various ways of understanding and examining the moral life" and morality as "norms about right or wrong human conduct that are so widely shared that they form a stable (although usually incomplete) social consensus."[2] Morality informs persons in society as to what behavior or conduct may be considered good or right. Questions of morality include: What is the right thing to do in this circumstance? How should I act in this situation?

Ethics is the formal analysis, study, and reflection on how individuals answer basic questions of moral behavior. As a discipline, ethics is most often associated with the fields of philosophy and theology. As a method of reflection, it asks certain types of questions, such as: How do I determine what is good or bad? How do I justify my actions, and what reasons, rules, principles, standards, or guidelines should direct my decisions? Understood as a formal discipline engaged in the systematic assessment of the morals that exist in the lives of individuals and society, ethics has a twofold task. One task is descriptive in nature, which means that ethics may simply describe in an orderly fashion the values or norms of good or bad behavior that are a part of the social context. The other task is normative, which means that ethics seeks to clarify, justify, and correct those values and norms as they apply in certain circumstances.

The goal of ethical reflection, particularly in health care, has the practical function of assisting individuals or groups in the resolution of moral dilemmas. A dilemma occurs when one is faced with a choice between two or more equally desirable but mutually exclusive options. A moral dilemma is present when a moral obligation exists on both sides of the choice to perform or refrain from performing an action and ethical reasons can be found to support either of the alternatives.[3] The essence of a moral dilemma is conflict. That is, a moral dilemma occurs when an individual or society experiences a conflict between competing values, duties, and obligations in a given situation.

A classic example of a moral dilemma in health care that continues to evade resolution in American society is abortion. Those who support reproductive choice argue on the basis of a woman's right for the freedom to decide what happens to her own body. Supporters of abortion rights give greater weight to the moral status of the mother, as an independent and autonomous agent, than to the developing fetus. Those who oppose abortion argue that the fetus is also a living human with its own independent moral status and, as a human life, deserves equal protection and the same right to a full life as the mother. The conflict is not so much between the mother and the fetus but rather the values and obligations that are owed to each party. Some value the autonomy of the mother more than the fetus. Others value the independent moral status of the developing fetus over the mother's. One cannot equally honor both sets of values or obligations—thus the moral dilemma. A dilemma exists because a reasonable individual can appreciate the need to respect the rights of a woman to make decisions concerning her own body and by association her own destiny and, at the same time, can respect the value of the unborn human life that has the same potential to develop into an equally autonomous individual. As a result, there is a conflict about which obligation should prevail. This simplified version of the abortion debate illustrates the conflict of competing values that are inherent in any moral dilemma.

THE EMERGENCE OF BIOETHICS

Ethical reflection can apply to any arena of life, but in the last few decades, a new term has come to signify ethical reflection in the health care field: *bioethics*, or more precisely, *biomedical ethics*. Bioethics is the application of ethical study and reflection to the life sciences. More recently, the term *clinical ethics* has been used to define ethical reflection in the clinical context of the actual care of patients. Many of the ethical concerns that confront professionals in the perianesthesia context are, by nature, clinical ethics issues.

The emergence of bioethics as a field within health care responds to a series of emerging problems in the second half of the twentieth century. This period represents a time in American history of social foment related to developing individual and civil rights concerns, to the recognition that society has become increasingly pluralistic, and to the rapid development of technologic advances in

medicine. Each of these concurrent historic forces led to novel moral challenges and the need for new ways to address the transformative dilemmas. For many years, medical ethics remained under the purview of physicians, who almost exclusively governed decision making for patients, with discussion or reflection on difficult moral problems encountered in the delivery of care or in medical research kept private. After 1950, a number of noteworthy medical and legal cases emerged in the context of a rapidly changing society, which led to challenges to paternalism and gave rise to bioethics as a new interdisciplinary discipline. David Rothman describes this historic development as one in which physicians slowly became "strangers at the bedside" as other professions more frequently weighed in on the deliberations of medical decision making and recurring ethical dilemmas.

> In the post–World War II period, a social process that had been under way for some time reached its culmination: the doctor turned into a stranger, and the hospital became a strange institution. Doctors became a group apart from their patients and from society as well, encapsulated in a very isolated and isolating universe.[4]

Isolation occurred in part because paternalistic ways of governing health care by physicians began to break down in the face of increasing social challenges. Physicians no longer maintained sole discretion in addressing problems and shaping policy. Individuals from the fields of philosophy, religion, law, journalism, and social sciences began to pay attention to the rumblings of problems in health care and began to organize to address their concerns. A more informed citizenry began to demand a more active voice in decision making and oversight in the delivery of medical care.

PARADIGMATIC CASES

In addition to the larger social movements, the history of the development of bioethics has been fueled by noteworthy medical and legal cases. These cases are significant for leading to profound changes in the way similar medical cases would forever be viewed. These cases reshaped health policy and law and reformed ethical practices in the way other patients in similar circumstances would be treated. The cases led to a different way of perceiving and valuing the moral obligations owed to patients by physicians, researchers, and other health care professionals.

Research with Human Subjects

Among the most sweeping reform in the second half of the twentieth century was in the arena of medical research with human subjects. For much of medicine's history, the improvement of care for patients has been through the trial-and-error method of experimentation. Few therapies, when initially applied, had any guarantee of success, and some were fraught with the risk of further injury or debilitation to the patient. Early medical researchers were practicing physicians whose small-scale experiments were conducted solely for therapeutic benefit. The goal of experimentation was undertaken not as much to benefit future patients as to heal the very individual under the immediate care of the practicing physician.[5] Most research was, at least in its intent, benevolent and humanistic with the Hippocratic ideal of "doing no harm" providing the guiding norm of the experimenter's conduct. Nonetheless, two key events revealed how flagrantly this norm can be ignored when the focus shifts to utilitarian goals other than the safety and welfare of humans.

Nazi Germany will forever be remembered for war crimes committed against the human race. Millions of victims lost their lives not only to the actual military conflict of World War II but also to the mass exterminations of innocent members of "undesirable" ethnic groups and other minorities. The techniques for these exterminations were perfected by Nazi physicians whose gruesome acts were later publicly revealed in the Nuremberg war criminal trials and documented by American observer Dr. Leo Alexander.[6] The trials revealed how physicians and administrators conspired to engage in medical experiments, such as forced sterilizations, poisonings, the infliction of simulated combat injuries, exposure to infections and extreme weather conditions, and ultimately the refinement of euthanasia techniques on those deemed mentally or physically "defective." There were approximately 275,000 victims over a 10-year span of time. After these staggering revelations, an international tribunal of judges developed what is known as the Nuremberg Code, a statement of 10 principles that govern the ethical conduct of medical experimentation with human subjects. At the heart of the code is that the "voluntary consent of the human subject is absolutely essential" and that freedom from coercion, force, duress, or deception be a condition of participation in any form of experimentation. Expanding the moral framework for the conduct of medical research in the Nuremberg Code, the World Medical Association adopted the Helsinki Declaration in 1964.

Unfortunately, the efforts of Nuremberg and Helsinki did not end the problems with human research. Even within the United States, these important principles did not filter into the consciousness or conduct of physician experimenters, which became all too apparent in the infamous research project now known as the Tuskegee Syphilis Study. From 1932 to 1972, the U. S. Public Health Service (USPHS), later known as the Centers for Disease Control and Prevention (CDC), engaged in a research study that involved 400 African American men in Macon County, Alabama. During the course of 40 years, what began as a small time-limited project to improve the treatment of syphilis among poor minorities expanded into a full-blown plan marked by deception and discrimination that yielded no new information about the disease and offered no bona fide treatment for subjects.[7] When the study first began in the early 1930s, the treatment for syphilis consisted of a difficult regimen of arsenic and mercury vaccinations. Although the treatment offered some control, this method proved to be no definitive cure for the illness. The study was initiated with hopes of understanding the disease and finding the definitive cure, but evolved merely into an observation of how the disease progressed through its various stages, culminating in death in many cases.

Participants in the study were led to believe that they were being provided real treatment for what the physician researchers called *bad blood*, a euphemistic term for any kind of blood-related condition. Treatment amounted essentially to various placebos combined with painful nontherapeutic spinal taps. Subjects were induced to participate in the study through the offer of free treatment, meals, and transportation. Free burial insurance was promised on the condition that the research subjects permit an autopsy on their deaths for documentation of the effects of the end stages of the disease. Even after World War II, when the curative antibiotic of penicillin became widely available, subjects of the study were prohibited from receiving it so that researchers might continue to track the disease's effects on the unsuspecting subjects' bodies. The deception and coercion continued until USPHS investigator Peter Buxtun learned of the project from a colleague. Frustrated in his attempts to end the study by working within the USPHS, Buxtun turned to the press, and reporter Jean Heller broke the story in July 1972.[8]

The public and political outcry that followed the revelation of the study culminated in its immediate suspension and Congressional passage of the Federal Research Act of 1974, which created two significant entities.[9] First, the act established what is now known as the Office for Human Research Protections, which mandates that all institutions that receive federal funding for research with human subjects maintain institutional review boards with oversight for the safety and ethical treatment of research subjects. Second, the act established the National Commission for the Protection of Human Subjects of Biomedical and Behavioral Research. The commission, composed of physicians, researchers, attorneys, theologians, and philosophers, was assigned to craft guidelines that would serve as a moral foundation for future human research regulation.[5] By 1979, the commission had arrived at a policy statement known as the *Belmont Report*.[10] The report highlighted three basic ethical principles that guide all medical research involving humans in the United States. The principle of respect for persons requires that participation in research be based on the voluntary informed consent of the subject of the study. The principle of beneficence calls for a comprehensive risk and benefit assessment that weighs the potential harm against the potential benefit to the current subjects or future patients. The principle of justice requires that research subjects be chosen equitably (unlike Tuskegee) and that a fundamental fairness in both benefits gained and risks incurred be shared by research participants. Justice also requires that the more vulnerable members of society, such as children, prisoners, pregnant women, and the mentally challenged, be given added protection in research.

Reforms and regulations that emerged from Tuskegee and the *Belmont Report* now ensure that essential elements be present in every medical or behavioral research study that involves persons. These elements are voluntary participation, informed consent, comprehension by the subject of the nature and purpose of the study, full disclosure of risks and benefits, disclosure of alternatives to participation in research (as in the case of treatment associated with clinical trials), and the option to withdraw from the study without penalty.

More recently, President Barack Obama authorized the Presidential Commission for the Study of Bioethical Issues to conduct a thorough review of domestic and international regulations on human subjects research to determine whether current rules still provide adequate protection. This directive occurs following the new revelations of unethical research in Guatemala from 1946 to 1948 in the U.S. Public Health Services Sexually Transmitted Diseases Inoculation Study.[11]

End-of-Life Cases

Controversial patient care cases involving end-of-life decision making hold a prominent place in the development of the bioethics movement.

Three cases are particularly noteworthy; all involved young women, each of whom was severely incapacitated and unable to participate in decisions regarding life-sustaining therapy. The first landmark case is that of Karen Ann Quinlan.[12] Karen was a 21-year-old woman in New Jersey who, in 1975, suffered a severe anoxic brain injury after an accidental overdose of alcohol and drugs. Karen never regained consciousness and remained dependent on a ventilator for breathing and a feeding tube for nutrition and hydration. Eventually, she was given the diagnosis of a persistent vegetative state (PVS), a neurologic condition characterized by a "complete unawareness of the self and the environment, accompanied by sleep-wake cycles with either complete or partial preservation of the hypothalamic and brainstem autonomic functions."[13] Patients with PVS display "eyes open" unconsciousness and may have gross involuntary movements, but do not respond to external stimuli or engage in any purposeful activity. After some months, Karen's parents came to the realization that their daughter would likely never regain consciousness or the ability to have any meaningful interaction with others. Following what they believed would be her own wishes, they asked physicians to remove the ventilator and allow Karen to die a natural death. Karen's physicians adamantly opposed this idea, believing this to be an act of euthanasia, or worse, murder. Karen's parents then petitioned the courts, and her case eventually came before the New Jersey Supreme Court. The Supreme Court ruled in the parents' favor on the basis that Karen had a fundamental right to privacy and the right not to have treatment continued against her will. The Court wrote that "the State's interest (to preserve life) weakens and the individual's right to privacy grows as the degree of bodily invasion increases and the prognosis grows dim. Ultimately there comes a point at which the individual's rights overcome the State's interest."[12] Physicians slowly weaned Karen from the ventilator while continuing her tube feedings and hydration (Karen's parents never asked for the removal of the tube). Remarkably, Karen lived an additional 10 years before she died in a nursing home in 1986.

A second landmark case is that of Nancy Cruzan, a case sometimes referred to as the first "right to die" case to go before the United States Supreme Court.[14] In 1983, Nancy was a 24-year-old woman who lost control of her vehicle on an icy road late one night in Missouri. She was found lying face down in a ditch after being ejected from her overturned car. Nancy had stopped breathing and had no detectable heartbeat for a brief period of time. Rescue personnel intervened to restore her respiratory and cardiac function. Like Karen Ann Quinlan, Nancy had had an anoxic brain injury that led to the eventual diagnosis of a PVS. Nancy was eventually transferred from an acute care setting to a rehabilitation facility where, despite years of effort, no improvements were seen in her condition. Unlike Karen Ann, Nancy was not dependent on a ventilator but was similarly sustained with a gastrostomy tube for feeding and hydration. Four years after her injury, Nancy's parents asked physicians to remove the feeding tube with the understanding that Nancy would die. They contended that Nancy had remarked about never wanting to be artificially sustained if she could not be "at least halfway normal."[14] Physicians resisted, and Nancy's parents turned to the courts for help. The Supreme Court of Missouri ruled against them with the argument that sufficient evidence of Nancy's true wishes did not exist to justify the withdrawal of life support, particularly in light of the consequence of death. Denial of the Cruzans' wishes on Nancy's behalf led to an appeal to the U.S. Supreme Court and set the stage for one of the most famous medical legal cases in U.S. history.

The U.S. Supreme Court received the case in December 1989 and issued a ruling in June 1990. In somewhat of a split decision, the Court, on Constitutional grounds, affirmed both certain rights and requirements for all parties in determining a course of action in cases like Cruzan's. The Court acknowledged an individual's right to refuse treatment, even such treatment as life-sustaining tube feeding and hydration. Yet the Court went on to say that the state of Missouri could require "clear and convincing evidence" that such refusal was made while that person was still competent. On these grounds, the Cruzan case was remanded to Missouri for further adjudication. The emergence of new evidence that indicated that Nancy would not have wanted life-sustaining treatment in her current condition led to a Missouri lower court permitting the withdrawal of the feeding tube. Nancy died in December 1990.

The Cruzan case, and the memory of the Quinlan case before it, propelled the creation of federal legislation designed for individuals to state their desire to refuse life-sustaining treatment under the conditions set forth by the Supreme Court, even if rendered incompetent and unable to communicate. The Patient Self-Determination Act of 1990 established on a national level the legitimacy of previously written advance directives as valid legal expressions of an individual's desire for no treatment in end-of-life circumstances.[15] These advance directives, often referred to as *living wills* (and in many states including durable power of attorney for health care decisions), in theory meet the "clear and convincing" evidence standard required by the U.S. Supreme Court. Currently, all 50 states recognize and honor some form of written advance directives. However, problems persist in these difficult cases in both the interpretation of generalized written statements and the infrequency of use among the public.[16,17] As the next case shows, the absence of clear communication and understanding among family members over end-of-life wishes in medical care sometimes yields disastrous consequences.

The case of Terri Schiavo is the most recent of the series of tragic end-of-life cases to be pushed onto the national stage.[18,19] Terri was a 26-year-old woman in 1990 when she had a cardiac arrest most likely as a result of an electrolyte imbalance from an ongoing eating disorder. Like Quinlan and Cruzan before her, she had a severe anoxic injury that rendered her a total care patient in a PVS for 15 years, dependent on a percutaneous endoscopic gastrostomy tube for nutrition and hydration. Early on in her care, Terri's husband, Michael, and her parents, Bob and Mary Schindler, were united in efforts to keep Terri alive and restore her to some level of conscious functioning. Within a few years, Michael came to the conclusion that Terri would not make any recovery and sought to remove the feeding tube to allow Terri to die. The Schindlers, deeply religious, vehemently opposed this request. They believed that removal of the tube was an act of murder and that continued aggressive effort could restore Terri to wakefulness. The Schindlers also questioned the diagnosis of PVS; they believed that Terri both recognized and communicated with them in her own limited way.

Fundamental disagreement between Michael and the Schindlers over Terri's fate led to a bitter and international public dispute waged in the courts for more than a decade. The Schindlers petitioned to have Michael removed as Terri's guardian and garnered the support of the Florida state legislature and Governor Jeb Bush, who signed a one-time stay forbidding the removal of the feeding tube pending further legal appeal. On three separate instances, the U.S. Supreme Court refused to hear the case, each time affirming the appropriateness of lower court findings in favor of Michael Schiavo. In the end, Michael's position as Terri's guardian was upheld and the courts allowed the removal of the percutaneous endoscopic gastrostomy tube. Terri died on March 31, 2005, with her husband at her side. After her death, Michael permitted, at the request of the Schindlers, a neuropathologic autopsy that revealed severe atrophy of the brain. The official cause of death by the medical examiner was listed as "complications from anoxic encephalopathy."[20]

The cases of Quinlan, Cruzan, and Schiavo reveal the ongoing struggle that clinicians and families face in making decisions on behalf of patients with incapacitated conditions. The legacy of these cases highlights the continuing difficulties in withdrawing or withholding treatment in the care of patients with life-threatening conditions and little or no hope of recovery. A lack of public consensus has limited the development of social and institutional policy to guide clinicians. Even the closest of kin can sometimes be unclear about what their loved ones would desire in critical cases.[21]

GUIDING PRINCIPLES

With insight gained from history of research with human subjects and difficult end-of-life cases, the bioethics movement developed new ways of valuing and examining ethical dilemmas in patient care. A consensus has emerged on a set of guiding principles to assist health care professionals in the wide variety of clinical situations they may encounter. Tom Beauchamp and James Childress advance the clearest interpretation of these principles emerging over time from the common morality of society and the particular context of the clinical environment. These principles are respect for autonomy, nonmaleficence, beneficence, and justice.[2]

Respect for autonomy refers to the norm of respect for the decision-making capacities of autonomous individuals. Defined as self rule or self governance, *autonomy* means that competent adults have the fundamental right to determine what happens to their bodies and to make choices in treatment options that are consistent with their own beliefs and values.[2] Autonomy is grounded in respect for persons and the inherent dignity and worth of each individual and is reflected in the Code of Ethics of the American Nurses Association.[22] In the clinical setting, the autonomy of the patient is often challenged by the vulnerabilities created by pain, sedative effects, and severe illness as well as the anxiety produced by a lack of understanding of the complexities of the modern health care institution, such as the medical language and jargon used by professionals. The obligation of clinical caregivers is to uphold autonomy by engaging in an ongoing process of informed consent, maintaining privacy and confidentiality, and enhancing, to the greatest degree possible, the mental and emotional capacity of the patient for participating in decision making. In the American context, autonomy is often thought of as the first and most important of the four principles.

Nonmaleficence refers to the obligation of clinicians to prevent harm to patients under their care or to minimize risks of harm to the fullest extent possible. This norm is often linked to the medical framework of the Hippocratic admonition *primum non nocere,* translated to mean "above all, do no harm."[2] The potential for harm to patients in health care can be understood in both broad and narrow terms. Nursing frames this understanding in the ethical obligation to advocate for processes that minimize harm and maximize comfort and support for patients.[22] *Nonmaleficence* refers to the effort made by clinicians to limit physical pain, disability, or even death as a consequence of the treatment process itself. More broadly, the term refers to the duty to alleviate the emotional and spiritual suffering of the patient undergoing the traumatic experience of institutionalization, separation from loved ones, and the inability to make a living among other challenges.

Beneficence is the principle that speaks to the duty of promoting the ultimate welfare of the patient above all other concerns. In common usage, beneficence speaks to acts of mercy, kindness, and charity.[2] As such, beneficence and nonmaleficence may be thought of as two sides of the same coin. Nonmaleficence emphasizes not harming the patient in the effort to do good. Beneficence supports doing good for the patient. Again, the obligation to serve as a patient advocate in a manner that promotes health, well being, and especially safety is a component of sound ethical practice for the nursing professional. In health care, beneficence speaks to the humanitarian values that should underlie decision making and treatments offered to vulnerable persons. It is no accident that the word *hospital* is associated with the term *hospitality*. Beneficence affirms that patients should be treated as valued guests in what can often be a foreboding institutional environment. It also suggests that, although clinicians often are tempted by interests that conflict with the patient's welfare, they should seek to set aside those interests or minimize their effects as much as possible in an effort to maintain professional integrity.

The last and perhaps most elusive principle promoted is the principle of justice. The elusiveness of justice is the result of the wide variety of ways it is defined and understood in society. Within the context of health care, justice is best understood as the obligation of clinicians to distribute fairly the medical benefits, risks, and costs associated with the provision of health care.[2] As such, persons in similar circumstances are to be treated similarly. The challenges to the fairness principle are immeasurable in the modern American health care system. Global challenges are most visible in the debates concerning universal health insurance, equity of access, and financing the health care industry. Clinical challenges to justice are more evident in the struggle to evenly allocate scarce resources, such as organs for transplant and blood products as well as access to care, services, and beds in emergency and critical care areas. Justice for the practicing nurse might be understood again in terms of advocacy, this time in the promotion of equality in the provision of quality care through the use of appropriate standards of practice for all patients.[22]

PERIANESTHESIA ETHICS

Nursing professionals face a complex maze of ethical issues within the perioperative context. The intensity of a fast-pace environment with limited room for error demands not only clinical competence but critical thinking, quick judgment, and clear communication. Vigilance regarding professional functioning and ethical practice is essential for the achievement of positive clinical outcomes within a morally sound arena. Although many issues exist, the ethical issues faced by perianesthesia nurses can be captured within three general categories: (1) informed consent, (2) privacy and confidentiality, and (3) patient safety.

Informed Consent

Informed consent is the process of communication between a patient and physician that results in the authorization or understanding for a specific medical intervention.[23] Informed consent is rooted in respect for persons, patient autonomy, and self determination and formalizes a component of the covenant between the patient and the physician. It is built on the principles of trust and truth telling regarding the use of a particular intervention or treatment to achieve a desired medical outcome.

Despite the clarity of definition for the informed consent process, multiple questions or potential ethical conflicts can arise for nursing staff within the perioperative period. A simple question such as "What were they going to do again?" asked by an anxious patient in the preoperative holding area can set off a series of internal alarms in the mind of a nurse. Does the patient need reassurance or more information? Is it a momentary failure of memory or a lack of adequate understanding of the procedure that prompted the question? Who secured the consent of the patient? How was the request approach conducted? How does the nurse understand the professional and ethical obligations in the face

of a seemingly unsure patient and the pressure of a tight operating room (OR) schedule?

The nurse might begin by seeking verification of a signed written consent form. Whereas the presence of the form might satisfy the technical act of granting consent, it may or may not fulfill the ethical obligation. Informed consent is more than a means of securing a signature. Rather, it is a process of open two-way communication that implies full disclosure and provides detailed information on the nature of a specific procedure. A comprehensive informed consent process not only reviews the diagnosis and purpose of the intervention but also outlines its potential risks and benefits. It includes alternative treatment options, if any, and the risks and benefits of forgoing the treatment procedure. Informed consent assumes that the threshold elements of patient capacity and voluntary nature are met.[24]

Questions may also arise regarding the duration and scope of a signed informed consent. The nurse in the previous scenario may have noticed that the signed consent was properly secured but completed in the surgeon's office nearly 90 days ago. Should the consent still be valid for the patient who is now unsure about the nature of the procedure? What if, inside the OR, the surgeon determines that a change or expansion to the original procedure is indicated? Is the consent still valid? How much latitude is afforded the surgeon? What is the nurse's obligation to confirm that the patient understood the potential surgical outcomes?

Informed consent requires that the process be completed by a clinician able to provide the intervention and in a manner that allows time and space for patients to ask questions, seek clarification, and discuss potential options for care. The content of these discussions should be documented and communicated to members of the interdisciplinary team. An adequate informed consent process is further challenged by potential language barriers, such as complex medical terminology, cultural diversity, and functional limitations among populations with cognitive impairments.[25,26] All these issues underscore the significance of effective communication in the patient-physician relationship and among members of the interdisciplinary team.

What then is the ethical responsibility of the nurse in the holding area who is faced with the patient's question of uncertainty and the surgical team's schedule? To what extent is the nurse's ethical obligation to serve as a patient advocate in support of an informed decision? How might the nurse's obligation be affected for the patient who adds the statement, "At least my surgeon promised to be there for the entire operation," when the nurse knows of that particular surgeon's tendency toward intermittent presence while residents perform most operations? What if the nurse understood from a colleague that the patient's original consent was provided under pressure to comply? Specific questions such as these identify just a few of the immediate moral dilemmas that have implications for clinical practice and patient outcomes.

Resuscitation in the Perioperative Context

A special circumstance of informed consent in the perioperative context is the issue of resuscitation for patients with preexisting "do not resuscitate" (DNR) orders. Cardiopulmonary resuscitation (CPR) is the only medical procedure routinely performed in a hospital without the expressed consent of a patient. Routine management of the patient who is under the influence of anesthesia shares some of the same interventions and characteristics of resuscitation. As such, the practice of routine suspension of DNR orders for patients during anesthesia care in the OR was commonly accepted through the 1980s.

By the mid 1990s, a growing dissatisfaction existed with this practice. The evolution of increased respect for patient autonomy evolved from changes in medical practice and the Patient Self-Determination Act of 1990. Complicating matters was a lack of consistency within organizational policies regarding physicians' obligation to inform patients with existing DNR orders that they would be resuscitated during the perioperative period. Respect for patient autonomy and concern for adequate informed consent procedures challenged old practices and forced the issue onto the agendas of key professional organizations. Emerging from these conversations was support for the practice of required reconsideration. A comprehensive conversation regarding a patient's DNR status during the administration of anesthesia is recommended between the physician and the patient or surrogate, with the result documented and communicated among health care team members. Required reconsideration has since become the predominant recommended approach supported by the American Society of PeriAnesthesia Nurses, the American College of Surgeons, the American Society of Anesthesiologists, the Association of periOperative Registered-Nurses, and the American Association of Nurse Anesthetists.[27-31]

Despite the majority movement toward required reconsideration, a lack of consensus remains on the application of this practice among anesthesiologists, nurse anesthetists, and other perianesthesia nurses.[32,33] Variation among hospital policies that guide the use of CPR for patients with preexisting DNR orders who undergo surgical intervention and anesthesia reflects this diversity of opinion. Currently, three distinct approaches to addressing this issue dominate the landscape. These approaches include: routine or automatic suspension of DNR orders for a defined time period, required reconsideration of the DNR status with a means approach, and required reconsideration of the DNR status with a goals-oriented approach.

A decreasing but still not uncommon practice is the automatic suspension of DNR orders for this category of patients. Complications related to maintenance of a DNR order are well documented in the literature. These complications include: (1) many of the elements of routine care for a patient undergoing general anesthesia are considered resuscitation; (2) failure to exercise resuscitative efforts for this category of patients without certainty of the cause of an arrest is inconsistent with the principles of beneficence and nonmaleficence; (3) failure to suspend DNR orders places the surgeon in an unintended ethical dilemma between patient preferences and surgical outcomes that may be used to evaluate physician practice; and (4) the very ethos of the OR is to sustain life and reluctance is found for practices that might otherwise introduce an avoidable death into that context.

The argument for supporting unrestrained resuscitation is one of clarity for both clinicians and patients or surrogates, but other arguments may also support this position.[34] This position reduces the burden on the provider to differentiate whether the underlying cause of a cardiopulmonary arrest is related to the routine effect of anesthesia rather than the result of the patient's underlying disease process. Unrestrained resuscitation also simplifies the content of conversation between the provider and the patient or surrogate and becomes more a matter of informing the patient or surrogate of hospital policy. Another interpretation is that the practice relieves the patient or surrogate of the burden of a complicated decision in the face of a series of "what if" scenarios that may or may not emerge during surgery.

The minimal ethical obligation in the case of automatic suspension of DNR orders is an intentional and comprehensive conversation between the physician (surgeon or anesthesiologist) and the patient or surrogate before sedation. In the case of automatic suspension of DNR orders, informed consent requires that the physician outlines for the patient the hospital policy, including the duration and context of the suspension. Such clarity minimally offers the patient the opportunity to factor the implications of such a policy into the decision-making process about surgery. Organizational policies that support automatic suspension ideally also incorporate an option for the patient to select another provider, with the recognition that this can have its own complicating factors. In the case of automatic suspension, policies should identify which medical service informs the patient or surrogate. In addition, clear and timely communication should occur with postanesthesia providers regarding the duration of the suspension as the patient progresses through the levels of care from phase I and phase II to extended care.

As previously indicated, patients, surrogates, and clinicians have raised concern regarding the ethical appropriateness of automatic suspensions of DNR orders in the perioperative period, even with the provision of informed discussion. The argument is that such suspension of orders is a violation of a patient's right to self determination and fails adherence to the principle of patient autonomy.[35-44] This position has obvious ethical implications for providers. It requires intentional dialogue with patients or surrogates regarding the options and implications of maintaining or suspending the DNR order during surgery. Organizational policies can mandate such communication and documentation of the conversation, but the ethical challenge to informed consent remains in the details of it. Informed consent in this instance implies that patients or surrogates are offered information about their procedures, including potential risks and benefits, alternative treatment, and the potential implications of foregoing the intervention. Discussion of how resuscitation would be managed in the perioperative period is an essential but complicated discussion. Conversation within this context should be conducted without coercion, in a language that is understandable to patients or surrogates, and with sufficient time to allow questions and concerns to lead to an informed decision.

Clear and consistent communication alone does not readily resolve the complexities of management of a DNR order in the perioperative period.[45] Discussion in the literature on the pragmatics of managing the DNR order in the perioperative period is reflected in two approaches, both supporting the ethical obligation to respect patient autonomy. One position suggests a means or procedure-directed approach that examines routine resuscitative actions and determines which interventions would be offered in the perioperative period. The second position supports an ends-oriented approach that examines the goals of the patient relative to the present procedure. Both options suggest a limited resuscitation approach during the perioperative period, as distinct from

the two extreme options of suspension of DNR orders with unrestrained resuscitative efforts or maintenance of current DNR orders limiting all interventions not immediately associated with routine anesthesia care.

The procedure-directed approach provides a checklist of specific provider interventions.[46] The application of this approach requires consideration of each optional intervention (i.e., those not associated with routine anesthesia care) individually between the patient or surrogate and the surgeon or anesthesia provider.[39] The advantages of procedure-directed orders are the reduction of ambiguity and the consistency of application from one clinician to another throughout intraoperative resuscitation management. The limitations to procedure-directed orders include an expectation that anything but the most likely problems would be anticipated in advance and the lack of flexibility offered the clinician in response to a temporary and readily reversible event.

The goal-oriented approach seeks to incorporate the patient's values as the primary consideration in determination of the extent of resuscitation.[47] Patients offer guidance regarding preferred outcomes but leave specific interventions to the discretion of the provider. Although this approach supports patient autonomy, it also provides a larger role for the provider. The advantage to this approach is that it offers flexibility to the clinician to act in accordance with a broad understanding of patient preferences should an unanticipated event occur in the OR setting.[46] The limiting argument for this position has been that it risks putting unanticipated decision-making power back in the hands of the physician.

Keys to success for either of these approaches are communication and documentation. The complexity of this issue underscores the significant ethical obligations of the perioperative nurse. The obligation to act in the patient's best interest demands that the nurse be knowledgeable and informed, beginning with having a clear understanding of the organization's DNR policy and its specific application to the perianesthesia period.[48] Equally important is that the nurse has knowledge of the DNR status of the patient during that period, including any documentation regarding limited resuscitation and knowledge of the timeframe in the case of temporarily suspended DNR orders.

Privacy and Confidentiality

Maintaining the privacy and confidentiality of patients remains a challenge for health care organizations and clinicians. Privacy and confidentiality are complementary rather than synonymous concepts.[49] *Privacy* suggests that a patient has the right to control general access and distribution of personal information about one's health and implies that boundaries that protect a patient's personal space are respected within a clinical setting. *Confidentiality* relates to the personal trust that intimate information shared by a patient with a clinician is used only for the patient's medical benefit. As such, information is shared with those members of the interdisciplinary team on a need-to-know basis. Information should be shared with third parties only with permission of the patient except in the cases of an identified surrogate for the patient who lacks the decision-making capacity. The ethical responsibility to maintain privacy and confidentiality proceeds from the principle of respect for persons that promotes human dignity and maximized patient control.[50] Such responsibility is particularly critical for the most vulnerable of patients. This responsibility applies to the preoperative setting when marking surgical sites to ensure minimal exposure. It also applies to treatment of patients under the effects of anesthesia by eliminating and addressing derogatory or disrespectful behaviors or communications.[50]

One of the most significant challenges to patient privacy during the perioperative period is the physical setting of the postanesthesia care unit (PACU). More often than not, the PACU is configured as a multipatient care area with only curtains for privacy. Private communications between patients and clinicians are subject to being overheard by other patients or even visitors. Staff members not directly involved in the care of particular patients may encounter neighbors and friends who are recovering from surgery and would have preferred to remain unnoticed. One particular conflict that may emerge stems from the rights of parents who wish to be present when a minor child awakens from surgery. Although sensitivity to the needs of children is shown, the presence of parents in the PACU can compromise the privacy obligated to other patients.

How does the PACU nurse observe multiple patients while ensuring privacy? The typical PACU nurse monitors more than one patient, thus exposing patients to potential violations of personal space in the interest of patient safety. An additional challenge to the nurse can be finding the appropriate way to respond to the physician who performs examinations without properly drawing the curtain or who engages in intimate conversations with patients without proper discretion as to volume and content.

Teaching hospitals carry additional potential dilemmas in maintenance of patient privacy. The parameters of what is ethically permissible or appropriate relative to observation or examination by students or others in training of patients who are anesthetized remains ethically ambiguous. Should examination itself, the type of examination, the number of students observing, the nature and extent of the consent process, or some combination of these factors drive the parameters of ethical appropriateness? Should informed consent include details regarding these parameters? What is the extent of ethical obligation on the perianesthesia nurse to speak up as a patient advocate?

The professional responsibility to maintain confidentiality and privacy is clearly required from the perianesthesia nurse. The exchange of privileged patient information should follow the organization's policies on confidentiality and the code of ethical conduct of the appropriate professional organization, which would include at a minimum the sharing of information on a need-to-know basis and the proper collection of patient data for research purposes.

Patient Safety

The ethical responsibility for all clinicians and health care providers to act in the best interest of patients is no more evident than in the obligation to ensure patient safety. The significance of this obligation on perianesthesia nurses is both organizational and personal. Minimally, this obligation stems from the ethical principle of nonmaleficence. Organizational obligation includes responsibility to ensure that the environment is safe for patients. Critical to patient safety is the requirement that a clinician at any given point in the treatment process has shown appropriate competencies for the level of care being provided. Competency implies possession of the knowledge, skills, attitudes, and behavior to deliver the appropriate level of care on a consistent basis.[51] Clinicians are obligated to know and to function within the standard of care of their professional role and the professional standards of practice within their discipline.[52] This responsibility can be particularly challenging for nurses in the PACU, an environment frequently characterized by overcrowding because of limited intensive care unit beds and staffing shortages and where nurses might be asked to provide care outside the unit's scope of care.[53]

The principle of beneficence speaks to the perianesthesia nurse's responsibility to a wide range of ethical obligations. Ethical dilemmas faced by clinicians can include how to respond to a colleague who appears impaired in some way, what to do regarding the reporting of a medical error, or how to respond to a situation in which a colleague is engaged in deceptive practice or illegal behavior—all situations that affect maintenance of a safe environment and adherence to ethical practice and organizational guidelines. Responsibility extends to the nurse's obligation to follow best practice processes and to take initiative to eliminate errors, such as calling "time out" if guidelines such as those designed to ensure correct site surgery are not followed properly.[54,55]

The transfer of the patient from the OR to the PACU has the potential to introduce a number of ethical dilemmas related to patient safety. One common dilemma faced by the perianesthesia nurse in the PACU setting is the obligation regarding unintended intraoperative awareness. The responsibilities of the nurse in this instance can be multiple. With an interview of the patient who is emerging from the influence of anesthesia to determine whether any recollection of events exists or whether the patient experienced pain during the surgical procedure, the nurse must make an initial assessment. If the finding is affirmative, the nurse must then determine how to communicate the information. Clear documentation of the patient's response and notification of the surgeon and the anesthesia provider are critical. Equally important is communication of the patient's experience to the intensive care unit or floor nurse who will assume care for the patient and who can identify resource personnel who could be available to support the patient who has experienced such trauma. The ethical dilemma becomes more complicated should the perianesthesia nurse discover that a pattern of unintended intraoperative awareness emerges as the result of care by a specific anesthesia provider or surgeon.

The hand-off from the OR to the PACU can be complicated by the pressure of time. What essential information needs to be passed from the OR nurse or the nurse anesthetist to the PACU nurse? How should the transfer of a patient whose condition is marginally stable or the one whose condition is hemodynamically stable but in pain be handled between the nurse anesthetist and the PACU nurse? How could this situation be compromised by a demanding OR schedule that anticipates a speedy return to the OR by the anesthetist? Minimal responsibility in this instance includes documentation of the patient's status on arrival, information on the surgical and anesthesia course, and collaboration in the care of the patient until the PACU nurse accepts responsibilities.[56] The assessment and management of pain in the postoperative period remains a critical ethical obligation and can be a source of tension between the transferring

anesthesia provider and the receiving PACU nurse. This process can be particularly complicated for the pediatric patient or the geriatric patient with cognitive impairment because clinicians may need knowledge and specialized training for such populations.[56] Special care should be taken not to underestimate the level of pain severity and undertreat the patient. The safe transfer of care should be extended again when the patient moves from the PACU to another care setting. Although guidelines for the safe transfer of care have been identified by both the American Society of Peri-Anesthesia Nurses and the American Society of Anesthesiologists, successful patient outcomes in these situations are facilitated with clear and proper communication skills.

A corollary of the ethical principle of respect for persons and the obligation to ensure patient safety is truth telling. The ethical responsibility to tell the truth in medicine exists at both organizational and individual patient levels. Organizationally, the perianesthesia nurse needs to determine the ethical course of action in disclosing potential safety problems under the pressure to move patients efficiently through the system. At an individual patient level, the perianesthesia nurse is challenged to determine the ethical course of action in facilitating disclosure of a medical error, even one seemingly inconsequential.[57]

At one point or another, all health care professionals encounter a case that conflicts with their own personal value system or that creates significant emotional discomfort. Perianesthesia nurses are no different. Nursing professionals should make every effort to anticipate in advance such potential conflicts and reference any organizational personnel policies that address this conflict. Generally speaking, refusal of anticipated conflicts of moral conscious is ethical provided no compromise to patient safety exists.

RESOURCES FOR RESOLVING ETHICAL DILEMMAS

Clear and consistent communication between clinicians and patients and among clinicians continues to be the backbone of good ethical practice. Despite the most diligent practice, ethical dilemmas continue to challenge clinicians. The ethical responsibility for the perianesthesia nurse can become particularly burdensome in the perioperative environment, where issues of power and politics are never far away. Identification of resources to support staff seeking resolution of ethical conflicts can relieve the burden. Managers and supervisors should not be overlooked as resources for assistance. Supervisors should be dependable sources for accessing organizational policies or for support in dealing with colleagues in other disciplines. Staff access to organizational and departmental policies has been enhanced with the use of an institution's Intranet postings. In addition, the code of ethics for nearly all relevant professional nursing organizations is available through Internet web sites. Questions regarding ethical practices related to release of patient information, business practice, or even professional behavior can be referred to ever-expanding corporate compliance programs.

Ethics Committees and Consultation Services

The Standards of The Joint Commission require that hospitals have an identifiable process for the resolution of ethical dilemmas. Subsequently, most hospital-established ethics committees are charged with three functions: the development of policies to address recurrent difficult situations, such as DNR or withdrawal of care orders; education to the organization that addresses issues faced by the organization or its specialty disciplines; and consultation to patients, families, and staff for the mediation of conflicts or exploration of treatment options. Although guidelines to determine the functioning of ethics committees can vary by organization, generally speaking, access to the ethics committee is available to any individual with standing in a case. This access includes patients or surrogates and staff involved in the care of the patient. Consultation services are generally provided by a subcommittee of the membership that possesses some training in clinical ethics. Consultations, whether by the committee as a whole or by subcommittee, serve as nonbinding recommendations that identify the ethically appropriate options of care available to the physician and patient.

Consultation provided by members of the ethics committee can be a critical resource for the perianesthesia nurse who is uncertain about the appropriate ethical course in a given clinical situation. The goal of ethics consultation is the improvement of patient outcomes through a process of reasoned decision making. Consultation typically takes the form of facilitation and dialogue to ensure that the key ethical issues and the essential perspectives of persons with standing in a case are provided adequate voice. The value of ethics consultation is the availability and timely response of a neutral resource to assist staff in the exploration of ethically appropriate alternatives to a situation that lacks consensus. The reality that an ethics consultation, like a medical consultation, is a resource, not a final decision, may disappoint clinicians who seek a quick resolution for a complex situation or an ally to advance a particular position.

Ethics Case Review Methodology

The struggle around ethical dilemmas for most clinicians occurs when a clinical situation creates a conflict of personal values or when the rights of individual patients appear to not be respected. The use of a pragmatic tool to examine a moral problem is a valuable resource for the novice and the experienced clinician. Thoughtful case analysis requires a reasoned methodology ensuring that a reasoned approach is followed and that influential factors are given appropriate consideration. The use of a case-based methodology can facilitate responsible reflection with an objective theoretic framework while attending to the specifics of a particular situation. Detailed case-based approaches are available.[58] In general, the literature points to five common elements for the case review process: assessment and gathering, establishment of ethical questions, identification and analysis of alternatives, selection and implementation, and evaluation.

Assessment and Gathering

The assessment and gathering stage begins with identifying and gathering the medical facts of the case. What is the patient's condition? What treatment options are available? What is the patient's prognosis with and without treatment? What is the patient's capacity to make an informed decision? What are the patient's preferences regarding care alternatives and quality of life factors? For the patient without capacity, were any preferences previously expressed, either verbally or in the form of a written advance directive? If not, what are the preferences expressed by the surrogate? Do any cultural or social factors come into play for the patient or surrogate, such as individual beliefs or values? Identification of potential resources within the organization that could assist in resolving the dilemma is also a key component of assessment and gathering.

Ethical Questions

At this point, identification of the ethical issue or problem should be clarified. What points of conflict are raised by the case? Differentiation of facts and feelings and bracketing of personal agendas are important. Identification of ethical principals relevant to the case becomes the group task.

Identification and Analysis of Alternatives

Difficult ethical situations are often characterized by more than one morally justifiable course of action. Each alternative should be examined within the context of the medical situation and the patient or surrogate preferences and analyzed with attention to institutional issues and third-party interests. Case history, whether prominent in the literature or particular to the organization, also serves as a resource to assist in the consistent treatment of similar ethical situations.

Selection and Implementation

The selection and implementation of a particular course of action is often driven by the medical indications of the case and, when known, the patient or surrogate preferences. In the absence of clear preferences, the *best interest standard* should be factored into the decision. The decision should be defensible by one or more ethical principles. Any treatment alternative selected in an ethically ambiguous situation should be consistent with the goals of a comprehensive plan of care for the patient. Rationale for the selection of an alternative should be communicated to involved parties. At this point, any legal considerations ought to be incorporated before final implementation.

Evaluation

The implementation of any medical decision includes an element of ongoing evaluation. Consideration of the benefit of any intervention and the goals of treatment should be subject to periodic and regular review. Often accomplished through retrospective case review, this consideration includes assessment of desired outcomes and identification of unanticipated complications. On final resolution of a case, final outcomes and any new learning should be communicated to the multiple constituents.

SUMMARY

Clinical ethics continues to develop into a mature field with established acceptance among health care professionals. Codes of professional ethics are the norm for nursing organizations, and there is a growing literature of ethical issues in perianesthesia nursing. Evolving technology and increased emphasis on patient rights presents ever-increasing options for care and considerations for decision making within the medical community. In addressing these issues, the perianesthesia nursing professional has much to contribute. It is crucial to develop the competencies and skills required to be effective clinicians who possess the critical assessment tools necessary to negotiate difficult situations in an environment of culturally diverse values.

REFERENCES

1. *American heritage dictionary of the English language,* ed 3, Boston, 1996, Houghton Mifflin Company.
2. Beauchamp TL, Childress JF: *Principles of biomedical ethics,* ed 6, New York, 2008, Oxford University Press.
3. Fletcher JC, et al: *Clinical ethics: history, content, and resources.* In Fletcher JC, et al, editors: *Introduction to clinical ethics,* ed 2, Hagerstown, Md, 1997, University Publishing Group.
4. Rothman DJ: *Strangers at the bedside: a history of how law and bioethics transformed medical decision making,* New York, 1991, Basic Books.
5. Jonsen AR: *The birth of bioethics,* New York, 1998, Oxford University Press.
6. Alexander L: Medical science under dictatorship, *N Engl J Med* 241:39–47, 1949.
7. Jones JH: *Bad blood,* New York, 1993, The Free Press.
8. Heller J: *Syphilis victims in U.S. study went untreated for 40 years,* NY Times, July 26, 1972.
9. National Research Act of 1974, Pub. L. 93-348.
10. The National Commission for the Protection of Human Subjects of Biomedical and Behavioral Research: *The Belmont report: ethical principles and guidelines for the protection of human subjects of research,* 1979, available at http://www.hhs.gov/ohrp/policy/belmont.html. Accessed on March 16, 2011.
11. Presidential Memorandum: *Review of human subjects protection, released by the White House Office of the Press Secretary,* November 24, 2010.
12. In the matter of Karen Quinlan, an alleged incompetent, 70 NJ 10, 355 A.2d 647, 1976.
13. The Multi-Society Task Force on PVS: Medical aspects of the persistent vegetative state—first of two parts, *N Engl J Med* 330:1499–1508, 1994.
14. Cruzan versus Director, Missouri Department of Health, 497 US 261, 11 S. Ct. 2841, 1990.
15. Patient self determination act of 1990, sections 4206 and 4751 of omnibus reconciliation act of 1990, Pub L No. 101–508 (November 5, 1990).
16. Meisel A, et al: Seven legal barriers to end-of-life care: myths, realities, and grains of truth, *JAMA* 284:2495–2501, 1996.
17. Upadya A, et al: Patient, physician, and family member understanding of living wills, *Am J Respir Crit Care Med* 166:1430–1435, 2002.
18. Gostin LO: Ethics, the Constitution, and the dying process: the case of Theresa Marie Schiavo, *JAMA* 293:2403–2407, 2005.
19. Wolfson J: Erring on the side of Theresa Schiavo: reflections of the special guardian ad litem, *Hastings Center Report* 35(3):16–19, 2005.
20. Thogmartin JR: Medical examiner, district six of the state of Florida: Report of autopsy for Schiavo, Theresa, case #505439, June 13, 2005.
21. Shalowitz D, et al: The accuracy of surrogate decision makers, *Arch Intern Med* 166:493–497, 2006.
22. American Nurses Association: *Code of ethics for nurses,* available at http://nursingworld.org/MainMenuCategories/EthicsStandards/CodeofEthicsforNurses.aspx. Accessed March 17, 2011.

23. American Medical Association: *Informed consent*, available at http://www.ama-assn.org/ama/pub/physician-resources/medical-ethics/about-ethics-group/ethics-resource-center/educational-resources/federation-repository-ethics-documents-online/american-college-physicians/acp-physician-and-patient.page. Accessed January 2, 2012.

24. Boyle RS: *The process of informed consent*. In Fletcher JS, et al, editors: *Fletcher's introduction to clinical ethics*, ed 3, Hagerstown, Md, 2005, University Publishing Group.

25. Galanti GA: Applying cultural competence to perianesthesia nursing, *J Perianesth Nurs* 21(2):97–102, 2006.

26. Sullivan EE: Issues of informed consent in the geriatric population, *J Perianesth Nurs* 19(6):430–432, 2004.

27. American Association of Perianesthesia Nurses: *A position statement on the perianesthesia patient with a do-not-resuscitate advance directive*, available at http://www.aspan.org/Portals/6/docs/ClinicalPractice/PositionStatement/1012/Pos_Stmt_1_DNR.pdf. Accessed March 16, 2011.

28. American College of Surgeons: [ST-19] *Statement on advance directives by patients: "Do not resuscitate" in the operating room*, available at http://www.facs.org/fellows_info/statements/st-19.html. Accessed January 2, 2012.

29. American Society of Anesthesiologists: *Standards, guidelines, statements and other documents*, available at http://www.asahq.org/For-Members/Clinical-Information/Standards-Guidelines-and-Statements.aspx. Accessed March 17, 2011.

30. Association of Operating Room Nurses: *AORN Position Statement on Perioperative Care of Patients with Do-Not-Resuscitate or Allow-Natural-Death Orders*, available at http://www.aorn.org/PracticeResources/AORNPositionStatements/Position_DoNotResuscitate/. Accessed March 17, 2011.

31. American Association of Nurse Anesthetists: *AANA Position Statements, Advisory Opinions, and Considerations*, available at http://www.aana.com/Resources.aspx?id=24804. Accessed March 17, 2011.

32. Fallat ME, Deshpande, JK, and the Section on Surgery, Section on Anesthesia and Pain Medicine, and Committee on Bioethics, American Academy of Pediatrics: Do-not-resuscitate orders for the pediatric patients who require anesthesia and surgery, *Pediatrics* 114(6):1686–1692, 2004.

33. Stack CG, Perring J: Pediatric DNAR orders in the perioperative period, *Pediatric Anesthesia* 19:964–971, 2009.

34. Mohr M: Ethical conflicts during anesthesia "Do not resuscitate" orders in the operating room, *Anesthetist* 46(4):267–274, 1997.

35. Walker RM: DNR in the OR resuscitation as an operative risk, *JAMA* 266(17):2407–2412, 1991.

36. Cohen CB, Cohen PJ: Required reconsideration of "do not resuscitate" orders in the operating room and certain other treatment settings, *Law Med Health Care* 20(4):354–363, 1992.

37. Igoe S, et al: Ethics in the OR: DNR and patient autonomy, *Nurs Manage* 24(9):112A,D,H, 1993.

38. Golanowski M: Do-not-resuscitate: informed consent in the operating room and post anesthesia care unit, *J Post Anesth Nurs* 10(1):9–11, 1995.

39. Craig DB: Do not resuscitate orders in the operating room, *Can J Anaesth* 43(8):840–851, 1996.

40. Lonchyna VA: To resuscitate or not . . . in the operating room: the need for hospital policies for surgeons regarding DNR orders, *Ann Health Law* 6:209–227, 1997.

41. Goldberg S: Do-not-resuscitate orders in the OR—suspend or enforce? *AORN J* 75(2):296–299, 2002.

42. Saver C: Knowing when to stop: DNR in the OR, *OR Manager* 23(11):17–21, 2007.

43. Berlandi JL, Duncan J: Perioperative DNR orders, palliative surgery, and ethics, *Perioperative Nursing Clinics* 3(3):223–232, 2008.

44. Ball KA: Do-not-resuscitate. Orders in surgery: decreasing the confusion, *AORN J* 89(1):140–146, 2009.

45. Ewanchuk M, Brindley PG: Perioperative do not resuscitate orders—doing 'nothing' when 'something' can be done, *Crit Care* 10(4):219, 2006.

46. Guarisco KK: Managing do not resuscitate orders in the perianesthesia period, *J Perianesth Nurs* 19(5):300–307, 2004.

47. Truog RD, et al: DNR in the OR: a goal-directed approach, *Anesthesiology* 90(1):281–295, 1999.

48. Keffer MJ, Keffer HL: The do-not-resuscitate order: moral responsibilities of the perioperative nurse, *AORN J* 59(3):648–650, 1994.

49. DeRenzo EG: Privacy and confidentiality. In Fletcher JS, et al, editors: *Fletcher's introduction to clinical ethics*, ed 3, Hagerstown, Md, 2005, University Publishing Group.

50. Baillie L, Ilott L: Promoting the dignity of patients in perioperative practice, *J Perioper Prac* 20(8):278–82, 2010.

51. Burden N, Saufl N: Why ethical standards? An introduction to the Perianesthesia standards for ethical practice, *J Perianesth Nurs* 16(1):2–5, 2001.

52. Mamaril ME: Standards of perianesthesia nursing practice: advocating patient safety, *J Perianesth Nurs* 18(3):168–172, 2003.

53. Iacono MV: Perianesthesia staffing . . . thinking beyond numbers, *J Perianesth Nurs* 21(5):346–352, 2006.

54. Odom-Forren J: A tragedy unfolds: lessons to learn, *J Perianesth Nurs* 21(5):367–369, 2006.

55. American Association of Perianesthesia Nurses: *A position statement on perianesthesia safety*, available at http://www.aspan.org/Portals/6/docs/ClinicalPractice/PositionStatement/1012/Pos_Stmt_10_Perianes_Safety.pdf. Accessed August 5, 2011.

56. Schroeter K: Pain management: ethical issues for the perianesthesia nurse, *J Perianesth Nurs* 14(6):393–397, 1999.

57. Espin S, et al: Error or "act of God"? A study of patients' and operating room team members' perceptions of error definition, reporting, and disclosure, *Surgery* 139:6–14, 2006.

58. EM Spencer: A case method for consideration of moral problems. In Fletcher JS, et al, editors: *Fletcher's introduction to clinical ethics*, ed 3, Hagerstown, Md, 2005, University Publishing Group.

Evidence-Based Practice and Research

Vallire D. Hooper, PhD, RN, CPAN, FAAN

Perianesthesia nurses are commonly faced with a host of common and uncommon patient scenarios demanding thoughtful, efficient decision making and intervention. The choice of what course of action to take is, in many cases, as important as the action itself. Decisions associated with all aspects of patient care should be evidence based, a process of considerable complexity that involves identifying a clear question or problem, locating sources of information, evaluating the quality and relevance of information, recognizing the contextual elements that may alter the application of that information in a particular setting, and assessing its effect on the patient. The purpose of this chapter is to explore the basic concepts of evidence-based practice (EBP) and their relationship to research as well as to explore the application of EBP in the perianesthesia setting.

DEFINITIONS

Clinical Practice Guideline: Systematically developed statements or guides designed to provide a key link between evidence-based knowledge and health care practice and to offer a mechanism to advance the quality and equity of patient care through the translation of evidence to practice.[1-3]

Evidence-Based Practice: The conscientious and judicious use of current best available evidence in conjunction with clinical expertise and patient values or preference to guide the care given to patients.[1,4-6]

Experimental Design: A study whose purpose is to test cause-and-effect relationships, specifically to examine the effects of an intervention or treatment on selected outcomes. An experimental design always includes an intervention and control group with random assignment to groups.[1,4]

Metaanalysis: A technique for quantitatively integrating the results of multiple similar studies addressing the same research question to produce a single estimate of the effect of the intervention of interest.[4]

Nonexperimental Design: Also called an *observatory* or *exploratory study*, a non-experimental design is a study in which data are collected regarding a phenomena without the introduction of an intervention by the researcher.[1,4]

Prospective Study: Follows patients forward in time, with the use of carefully defined protocols to determine an outcome that is unknown beforehand. This powerful type of research allows the determination of cause-and-effect relationships.[4]

Qualitative Research: The investigation of phenomena using an in-depth and holistic approach, often involving personal interviews and observations.[1,4]

Quantitative Research: The investigation of phenomena involving the use of precise measurement and manipulation of numeric data via statistical analysis.[1,4]

Quasiexperimental Design: A type of design that examines the effect of an intervention on an outcome but lacks one or more characteristics of a true experimental design.[1,4]

Randomized Controlled Clinical Trial: Patients are randomly assigned to a control (receiving the standard treatment or placebo) or intervention group (receiving the new or experimental treatment), and the outcome is measured and compared. Such trials are considered the most reliable and impartial method of determination of treatment effectiveness.[1,4]

Retrospective Study: Looks backward in time, usually with use of medical records or existing databases. This type of study is weaker than a prospective study and permits one to determine only the nature of association between a treatment and outcome.[1,4]

Systematic Review (Integrative Review or Metasynthesis): A rigorous and systematic review of the literature on a like topic involving a clearly defined method for identifying, appraising, and synthesizing the literature and drawing conclusions regarding the question of interest.[1,4]

OVERVIEW OF EVIDENCE-BASED PRACTICE

EBP involves the conscientious and judicious use of the most current and best available evidence along with the clinician's expertise and consideration of the patient's values and preferences to provide patient care.[1,4-6] Evidence-based care has been recognized by the Institute of Medicine as a critical component of safe, quality patient care.[7] Despite the emphasis on evidence-based care and the millions of dollars spent in the development and conduct of research designed to improve patient care,[8] it can take as long as 15 years for this newly discovered knowledge to be translated to clinical practice.[9-11]

Nursing has a long history of applying evidence to practice, dating back to the days of Florence Nightingale; however, little recognized progress was made in the formal EBP movement until the development of the Cochrane Collaboration, established by Archie Cochrane in the early 1970s in the United Kingdom. As this collaboration was evolving, a similar movement was evolving at the McMaster Medical School in Canada. Originally designated as *evidence-based medicine*, the concept has shifted over time to be referred to as *evidence-based practice* and is inclusive of all health care disciplines.[1,4,5]

THE PROCESS OF EVIDENCE-BASED PRACTICE

There are many models to guide the process of EBP. Some of the best known models include the Iowa Model of EBP,[12,13] the Hopkins Model of EBP,[14] the Melnyk/Fineout-Overholt model,[1] and the Rosswurm and Larrabee model.[15,16] Steps common to all EBP models include[1,12,14,15]:
1. Identify the problem or need for change.
2. Refine the question.
3. Locate the evidence.
4. Critically appraise and synthesize the evidence.
5. Design the practice change.
6. Implement the change.
7. Evaluate the outcomes of the practice change.
8. Adjust, integrate, and sustain the change.
9. Disseminate outcomes.

Identify the Problem or Need for Change

The first step in the EBP process is to identify the problem or need for change. Problem identification or "triggers" for change can arise from many sources and can be either knowledge or problem focused.[12] Problem-focused triggers typically arise from clinical problems or data. Perhaps performance improvement data shows an increase in surgical site infection, or clinical observation shows that female laparoscopic patients are having a higher incidence of postoperative nausea and vomiting (PONV) then other patients. Knowledge-focused triggers arise when a nurse or another member of the health care team gains new knowledge about current practice that may show improved patient outcomes. This knowledge may arise from reading journal articles or attending a conference.[12] After the problem is identified, it is important to form a work team that is inclusive of all involved stakeholders. Organizational support, to include commitment of all necessary resources, inclusive of employee time to work on the project, should also be obtained.[12,15]

Refine the Question

One of the most critical components of the EBP process is to form a focused, searchable, answerable clinical question. Successful completion of this task will literally drive the continued evolution of the project. A strong question typically addresses at least four major components (Box 9-1): the patient (or population), intervention, comparison, and outcome (PICO). A fifth component that may be included is time (PICOT).[1]

The patient or population of interest may be further clarified by addressing the age, gender, ethnicity, or disorder (procedure or disease) in the question. Interventions can include elements such as a therapeutic intervention, a diagnostic test, exposure to disease, or a risk behavior. The comparison is the additional intervention that you are considering, such as another medication or nursing intervention, another diagnostic test, or frequently routine therapy or standard of care. The outcome of interest is the result that you are interested in improving or accomplishing. Often, one will evaluate multiple outcomes in an EBP project. The most essential component of an outcome is that it is measurable. Outcomes commonly measured in perianesthesia EBP projects include length of stay in a particular area, pain scores, incidence of PONV or PDNV, and patient satisfaction. Another important outcome measure that should be considered is cost of care.

When the PICO components have been defined, the next step is to organize them into a question. The most common EBP questions are focused on either an intervention, prognosis or prediction, diagnosis or diagnostic test, or etiology.[1] Templates for developing questions using identified PICO components are provided in Box 9-2. Box 9-3 provides an example of the process.

BOX 9-1   PICO Components

P = Patient, population, or disease of interest
I = Intervention of interest
C = Comparison intervention of interest
O = Outcome of interest

From Melnyk BM, Fineout-Overholt E: *Evidence-based practice in nursing and healthcare: a guide to best practice*, ed 2, Philadelphia, 2011, Lippincott Williams & Wilkins.

BOX 9-2   PICO Question Templates

Intervention: In **P**, what is the effect of **I** compared with **C** on **O**?
Prognosis and prediction: In **P**, how does **I** compared with **C** influence or predict **O**?
Diagnosis or diagnostic Test: In **P**, what is the accuracy of **I** compared with **C** in diagnosing **O**?

From Melnyk BM, Fineout-Overholt E: *Evidence-based practice in nursing and healthcare: a guide to best practice*, ed 2, Philadelphia, 2011, Lippincott Williams & Wilkins; Polit DF, Beck CT, editors: *Nursing research: generating and assessing evidence for nursing practice*, Philadelphia, 2008, Lippincott Willims & Wilkins.

BOX 9-3	Sample PICO Components and Question

PICO COMPONENTS
P = Adult PACU patients
I = Acupressure
C = Routine care
O = Incidence of PONV

PICO INTERVENTION QUESTION
In adult PACU patients, what is the effect of acupressure compared with routine care on the incidence of PONV?

RECOMMENDED SEARCH TERMS BASED ON QUESTION
Key search terms: acupressure, PONV
Other possible terms: postoperative, postanesthesia, complications, nausea, vomiting
Search limits: adult

POSSIBLE SEARCH SCENARIO
Step 1 (explode all terms):
• Acupressure
• PONV
• Postoperative complications (MeSH term)
• Nausea
• Vomiting
Step 2:
• Combine postoperative complications and nausea and vomiting
Step 3:
• Combine results from Step 2 and acupressure
Step 4:
• Limit results from Step 3 by adult ages in the search limitations options

PACU, Postanesthesia care unit; *PONV,* postoperative nausea and vomiting.

Locate the Evidence

Key sources of evidence include evidence-based guidelines, evidence-based reviews such as Cochrane Reviews, and original research articles and reviews published in journals. These sources can be located by searching databases and government or specialty practice websites.[17,18] It is always recommended that multiple databases be searched; however, searches of certain databases or other sources may be more productive depending on the type of question posed (Table 9-1).

The process of locating the best evidence is driven by the formulation of a solid question. The PICO components of the question provide the key search terms as well as guides for limiting or narrowing your search. The ideal approach would be to engage the services of a medical librarian who is familiar with EBP searches. The reality, however, is that such resources might not be readily available to the bedside nurse. The first step to embarking on a successful search strategy is to identify the key search terms unique to your particular question. It is often helpful to begin this process by taking the time to make a list of key search words or terms. The most successful searchers are general driven by at least two or three key search concepts.[17] This list should be driven by the PICO components of your question. Using the example question in Box 9-3, key search words would include acupressure and PONV. Other useful search terms may include *postoperative, postanesthesia, nausea, vomiting,* and *complications.* Because PONV can occur in both adult and pediatric populations, it may also be helpful to use the adult population as a search limit.

In most databases, these key search terms will automatically map to medical subject headings, also known as *MeSH terms.*[17] For example, if PONV is not a MeSH term in the database that you are searching, it may automatically map to nausea, vomiting, or postoperative complications. It is recommended that one use the "explode" option for the primary search terms, and then use features such as combining search results using *and* or *or* to further narrow the results. For example, should the search term *PONV* map to a MeSH heading of *postoperative complications,* it may be helpful to fully explode this term, as well as the terms *nausea* and *vomiting.* is the next step is to combine the three terms (i.e., postoperative complications, nausea, vomiting) using *and* to narrow the search to literature specific to PONV. Combine this narrowed search result with the results from the search on the term *acupressure* to capture the literature addressing the use of acupressure for the prevention or treatment of PONV (see Box 9-3). These results may then be narrowed by adult ages using the search limitation options.

If this initial search strategy yields a large number of results that would prohibit a comprehensive review of the references, it may be helpful to further limit the search by levels of evidence. EBP should be guided by the best available evidence. What is considered *best* is guided by the level of the evidence and its relationship to the question of interest. The level of evidence is ranked according to the type of evidence or research design. Numerous evidence hierarchies are available in the literature. All commonly rank systematic reviews, metaanalyses, and high-quality evidence-based clinical practice guidelines as the highest level of evidence, and expert opinion as the lowest level of evidence. A sample evidence hierarchy is provided in Table 9-2.

Table 9-1	Databases and Other Sources for Conducting Literature Searches	
DATABASE OR SOURCE	TYPE OF INFORMATION	ACCESS
Cumulative Index to Nursing and Allied Health Literature (CINAHL)	Excellent database for more nursing focused questions	www.cinahl.com (subscription required)
MEDLINE	Developed by the National Library of Medicine; recognized as the premier source for biomedical literature	www.pubmed.gov
Cochrane Databases	Database of all Cochrane reviews; excellent source for systematic reviews	www.cochrane.org
Joanna Briggs Institute	International source for evidence-based guidelines	www.joannabriggs.edu.au
National Guideline Clearinghouse	Hosted by the Agency for Healthcare Research and Quality; free clearinghouse of clinical practice guidelines	www.guideline.gov
Specialty practice organizations such as ASPAN, ANA, AORN, and SAMBA	Provide evidence-based guidelines or practice recommendations regarding various aspects of anesthesia and perianesthesia care	Access via each organizational web site

Modified from Melnyk BM, Fineout-Overholt E: *Evidence-based practice in nursing and healthcare: a guide to best practice,* ed 2, Philadelphia, 2011, Lippincott Williams & Wilkins; Polit DF, Beck CT, editors: *Nursing research: generating and assessing evidence for nursing practice,* Philadelphia, 2008, Lippincott Williams & Wilkins; Ehrlich-Jones L, et al: Searching the literature for evidence. *Rehabil Nurs* 33:163–169, 2008; Fineout-Overholt E, et al: Teaching EBP: getting to the gold: how to search for the best evidence. *Worldviews Evid Based Nurs* 2:207–211, 2005.

Table 9-2	Evidence Hierarchy
LEVEL	DESCRIPTION
I	Systematic review or metaanalysis of RCTs; evidence-based guidelines based on a systematic review process
II	Evidence from at least one RCT
III	Evidence from at least one quasiexperimental study
IV	Systematic review of descriptive or qualitative studies
V	Evidence from at least one nonexperimental study
VI	Evidence from at least one descriptive or qualitative study
VII	Expert opinion

Modified from Polit DF, Beck CT, editors: *Nursing research: generating and assessing evidence for nursing practice,* Philadelphia, 2008, Lippincott Williams & Wilkins; Newhouse RP, et al: *Johns Hopkins nursing evidence-based practice model and guidelines,* Indianapolis, 2007, Sigma Theta Tau; Fineout-Overholt E, Johnston L: Teaching EBP: asking searchable, answerable clinical questions, *Worldviews Evid Based Nurs* 2:157–160, 2005; Krainovich-Miller B, et al: Evidence-based practice challenge: teaching critical appraisal of systematic reviews and clinical practice guidelines to graduate students, *J Nurs Educ* 48:186–195, 2009; Jones KR: Rating the level, quality, and strength of the research evidence, *J Nurs Care Qual* 25:304–312, 2010.
RCT, Randomized controlled trial.

Critically Appraise and Synthesize the Evidence

The next step in the EBP process is to critically appraise and then synthesize the evidence. A thorough discussion of the specifics guiding the critical appraisal of various research designs is beyond the scope of this chapter. It is helpful to first break out each particular component of an article so that it is possible to easily analyze each section. Questions that can help in organizing an appraisal are outlined in Table 9-3.

Criteria guiding the critical appraisal and ranking of the quality of a piece of evidence are dependent on the type of evidence examined. Table 9-4 provides an overview of specific criteria that should be used to examine certain types of evidence, and Table 9-5 provides some general guidance in judging the overall quality of a specific type of evidence.

It may be helpful to organize this information in tables to better assimilate and synthesize the information.[1,4,15,19] The first step in this process would be to develop evidence tables that include some of the basic evidence components of the article, to include the evidence level and quality ranking (Table 9-6). It may then be helpful to also develop tables summarizing the articles by interventions and specific outcomes of interest. This summary information will then

Table 9-3 Questions to Consider in Appraising Evidence

APPRAISAL QUESTION	APPLICATION TO YOUR EBP QUESTION
What is the research question or purpose of the article?	Does the question or purpose relate to your EBP question?
What is the study design?	
Who or what are the subjects or setting?	Are the subjects or setting similar to that of your EBP question?
What are the predictor (independent) variables?	Are these similar to factors affecting your EBP issue?
What are the outcome (dependent) variables?	Are these the same as the outcomes that you are interested in for your EBP question?
What type of analysis was conducted?	
Are there potential biases?	
What were the results?	Can you apply the results to your EBP question?

From Ehrlich-Jones L, et al: Searching the literature for evidence, *Rehabil Nurs* 33:163–169, 2008.
EBP, Evidence-based practice.

Table 9-4 Evidence-Specific Criteria for Appraising Quality

EVIDENCE TYPE	APPRAISAL CRITERIA
Systematic review	Were the search criteria clearly identified?
	Were clear inclusion or exclusion criteria provided?
	Were all applicable studies identified and included?
	Was a clear process for assessing the quality of the included articles provided?
RCTs	Was a power analysis conducted to establish sample size?
	Were the subjects randomly assigned to groups?
	Were all involved parties blinded to the group (treatment versus control) assignment?
	Were subjects analyzed in the groups to which they were randomly assigned?
Quasiexperimental	All RCT criteria except random assignment to groups
Nonexperimental (descriptive)	Was a power analysis conducted to establish sample size?
	Is the sample representative of the population of interest?
	Are all critical outcomes being measured?
Qualitative	Were the data collection methods adequately described?
	Were negative or discrepant results fully addressed?
	Are the explanations of the results plausible and coherent?

Modified from Melnyk BM, Fineout-Overholt E: *Evidence-based practice in nursing and healthcare: a guide to best practice,* ed 2, Philadelphia, 2011, Lippincott Williams & Wilkins; Polit DF, Beck CT, editors: *Nursing research: generating and assessing evidence for nursing practice,* Philadelphia, 2008, Lippincott Williams & Wilkins; Jones KR: Rating the level, quality, and strength of the research evidence, *J Nurs Care Qual* 25:304–312, 2010.
RCT, Randomized controlled trial.

Table 9-5 Guidelines for Ranking Quality

QUALITY LEVEL	EVIDENCE TYPE	CRITERIA
High	Systematic reviews	Well-defined, reproducible search strategy; consistent results across included studies; criteria-based evaluation of overall strength and quality of included articles; definitive conclusions
	Research	Consistent results based on adequate sample size and control measures; consistent recommendations based on extensive literature review with thoughtful reference to current scientific evidence
	Expert opinion	Expertise clearly evident
Good	Systematic reviews	Reasonably thorough and appropriate search; reasonably consistent results across studies; evaluation of strength and limitations of included studies; fairly definitive conclusions
	Research	Sufficient sample size; some control; reasonably consistent results; fairly definitive results
	Expert opinion	Expertise appears to be credible
Low or major flaws	Systematic reviews	Undefined, poorly defined, or inadequate search strategies; insufficient evidence with inconsistent results; unable to draw conclusions
	Research	Insufficient sample size; numerous confounding variables; inconsistent results; unable to draw conclusions
	Expert Opinion	Expertise not discernable or dubious

From Newhouse RP, et al: *Johns Hopkins nursing evidence-based practice model and guidelines,* Indianapolis, 2007, Sigma Theta Tau.

| | | SAMPLE | | EXCLUSION OR | |
| JOURNAL | RESEARCH | SIZE OR | NO. OF | INCLUSION | POPULATION |
INFORMATION	DESIGN	TYPE	TEMPS	CRITERIA (SIGNIFICANT)	STUDIED
Shinozaki T, Deane R, Perkins FM, 1988; Infrared tympanic thermometer: evaluation of a new clinical thermometer, *Crit Care Med*	Not specified; looks like prospective, descriptive comparative analysis	Not specified	Not specified	Inclusion: body temperature <36° C on admission to SICU	Elective coronary artery bypass surgery patients; all ventilated with heated humidifiers to maintain inspired gas temperature at 34-36° C

Table 9-6   Sample Evidence Table: Temperature Measurement State of Science Code Sheet

Inclusion Criteria: Data based; PA or EA as Gold standard; Tympanic, TA, or Oral comparison; Adult
SICU, Surgical intensive care unit; *PA*, pulmonary artery; *T*, tympanic; *R*, right; *L*, left.

help in interpreting what is and is not supported by the evidence, and thus guide recommended practice changes.

Design and Implement the Practice Change

The next steps of the EBP process are to design and implement the practice change. The results of a critical appraisal and synthesis of the evidence should provide guidance in answering the PICO question, and thus identify the practice change that is indicated. In the case of the sample PICO question in Box 9-3, "In adult PACU patients, what is the effect of acupressure compared with routine care on the incidence of PONV," the evidence search revealed a Cochrane Review that supported the effectiveness of acupressure in reducing the incidence of PONV. Because a Cochrane Review is of the highest level and quality of evidence available, one can be confident that the addition of acupressure should be effective in reducing the incidence of PONV in the adult PACU patient population.

If you have not already done so, one of the first steps in implementing a proposed practice change is to identify and engage all affected staff and stakeholders. From this group, formal implementation teams are built and change leaders or

agents in the targeted implementation unit are identified. Build excitement about the change by identifying the relative advantage of the practice change, both for the practitioner and the patient. Discuss observable benefits. Design an education strategy that incorporates the advantages and benefits of the change and provides an overview of the where's, how's, and why's associated with the proposed change. Listen to staff feedback as the change is previewed and adjust strategies as indicated by staff response and recommendation. Identify possible barriers to implementing the proposed change and develop strategies to help overcome these variables such as technological resources, reminder tools, and documentation resources.[1,15]

When developing the implementation strategy for the practice change, also identify a target unit or patient population in which to first pilot the practice change. Using a targeted implementation plan will facilitate evaluation of outcomes and modification of the practice change or implementation strategy before going with facility-wide implementation. It is also important to collect preliminary outcome data before implementation of the practice change so that clinical outcomes can be compared before and after implementation.[1,15]

SETTING	INVASIVE ROUTE	NONINVASIVE ROUTES	TRAINING/ INTERRATER RELIABILITY/ ACCURACY STANDARD	CONCLUSIONS	LIMITATIONS	EVIDENCE EVALUATION
SICU	PA (American Edwards, connected to American Edwards monitor)	T (1st temperature) R	T, taken on both sides Accuracy: not addressed	PA/T mean difference: 35.0-35.4: 0.3 ± 0.2 35.5-35.9: 0.2 ± 0.3 36.0-36.4: 0.3 ± 0.2 36.5-36.9: 0.4 ± 0.2 37.0-37.4: 0.4 ± 0.2 37.5-37.9: 0.4 ± 0.2 38.0-38.4: 0.4 ± 0.1 38.5-38.9: 0.2 ± 0.2 39.0-39.4: 0.2 ± 0.1 PA/T correlation: $R = 0.98$ L/R ear difference: 0.0 ± 0.1 They conclude that the T is accurate and correlates well to core.	No. of data collectors not specified Training not addressed No. of subjects not specified Technique not specified	Level V; Good

Evaluate the Outcomes of the Change

Outcomes of interest should be measurable and easily identified from the PICO question. The outcome of interest in the sample PICO question (Box 9-3), incidence of PONV, is easily measured. It is also likely that data regarding this issue can be easily abstracted from the medical record to allow for comparison before and after the practice change. Additional measurable outcomes that may also be examined for this question include number and amount of prophylactic or rescue antiemetics given, length of stay in the PACU or phase II setting, patient satisfaction, and overall cost of care. When outcome measures are finalized, a data collection cycle should be established that allows for inclusion of a large enough sample of patients to ensure a true evaluation of the effects of the practice change on targeted patient outcomes.[1,15]

In addition to a quantitatively focused outcome evaluation, it is also important to capture qualitative feedback from the major stakeholders and staff members, as well as patients and family members affected by the practice change, as appropriate. This type of evaluation allows for an opportunity to closely examine process and flow issues that might not be reflected by other outcome measures. This information may indicate the need to refine the implementation strategy before expansion of the practice change across multiple units in the facility.[1,15]

Adjust, Integrate, and Sustain Change

When the proposed practice change has been piloted on a specific unit or target population and the results of that pilot have been analyzed, it is then time to make appropriate adjustments and expand the practice change to other appropriate units or patient populations in the facility. This project expansion requires continued engagement of all stakeholders and affected staff of all affected units. Minor adjustments to the practice change or implementation strategy may be indicated to incorporate needs of a specific unit or patient population. Monitoring of outcome data as well as process and structure issues should also be continued throughout the implementation stage, and then on a periodic basis postimplementation to assure sustainability and incorporation into the practice culture.[15]

Disseminate Outcomes

Outcome dissemination should incorporate numerous internal and external strategies. Daily or at least weekly feedback will be indicated on individual units as the practice change is implemented to allow for celebration of successes and rapid resolution of identified problems. As the practice change is expanded throughout the facility, larger celebrations of success may be indicated to reward good practice and improved patient outcomes. It is also important that the process and outcomes are disseminated outside of the facility via poster and podium presentations as well as journal articles.[1,15] It is only through the sharing of EBP failures and successes that practice can continue to evolve and improve on a national and international level.

RELATIONSHIP OF EVIDENCE-BASED PRACTICE TO BEDSIDE PRACTICE

EBP is the key link between knowledge generation and application of that knowledge to practice. It is the most critical component in improving the safety and quality of patient care,[7] and it should be the standard of practice for all disciplines. EBP is a process that affords the opportunity to explore, implement, and assess interventions that are applied to the patient within the context of all available information. It represents a shift in the culture of health care provision away from exclusive opinion-based, past practice, and precedent decisions toward making health care decisions based on science, research, and evidence, while continuing to incorporate provider expertise and patient preference.

SUMMARY

Today's perianesthesia nurses have an enormous amount of information and experience (personal, collegial, published) from which to draw when providing patient care. Only through the thorough analysis and synthesis of the highest levels and quality of information available, however, can the perianesthesia nurse be assured of providing the highest quality of care available.

REFERENCES

1. Melnyk BM, Fineout-Overholt E: *Evidence-based practice in nursing & healthcare: a guide to best practice,* ed 2, Philadelphia, 2011, Lippincott, Williams, & Wilkins.
2. Larson E: Status of practice guidelines in the United States: CDC guidelines as an example, *Prev Med* 36(5):519–524, 2003.
3. Lia-Hoagberg B, et al: Public health nursing practice guidelines: an evaluation of dissemination and use, *Public Health Nurs* 16(6):397–404, 1999.
4. Polit DF, Beck CT, editors: *Nursing research: generating and assessing evidence for nursing practice,* Philadelphia, 2008, Lippincott, Willims, & Wilkins.
5. Titler MG: The evidence for evidence-based practice implementation. In Hughes RG, editor: *Patient safety and quality: an evidence-based handbook for nurses,* vol 1, Rockville, Md, 2008, AHRQ 113–161.
6. Sackett DL, et al: *Evidence-based medicine: how to practice and teach EBM,* ed 2, Edinburgh, 2000, Churchill Livingstone.
7. Institute of Medicine: *Crossing the quality chasm: a new health system for the 21st century,* Washington, DC, 2001, National Academy Press.
8. Dufault M: Testing a collaborative research utilization model to translate best practices in pain management, *Worldviews on Evidence-Based Nursing,* 1:S26–S32, 2004.
9. Dobbins M, et al: A framework for the dissemination and utilization of research for health-care policy and practice, *The Online Journal of Knowledge Synthesis for Nursing,* 9(7), 2002.
10. Donaldson NE, et al: Outcomes of adoption: measuring evidence uptake by individuals and organizations, *Worldviews on Evidence-Based Nursing,* 1:S41–S51, 2004.
11. Olsen L, et al: *The learning healthcare system: workshop summary (IOM roundtable on evidence-based medicine),* available at http://books.nap.edu/catalog.php?record_id=11903. Accessed April 9, 2009.
12. Cullen L, Adams S: An evidence-based practice model, *J Perianesth Nurs* 25(5):307–310, 2010.
13. Titler M, et al: The Iowa model of evidence-based practice to promote quality care, *Critical Care Nursing Clinics of North America,* 13:497–509, 2001.
14. Newhouse RP, et al: *Johns Hopkins nursing evidence-based practice model and guidelines,* Indianapolis, 2007, Sigma Theta Tau.
15. Larrabee JH: *Nurse to nurse: evidence-based practice,* New York, 2009, McGraw Hill Medical.
16. Rosswurm MA, Larrabee JH: Clinical Scholarship: A model for change to evidence-based practice, *Image: Journal of Nursing Scholarship* 31(4):317–322, 1999.
17. Ehrlich-Jones L, et al: Searching the literature for evidence, *Rehabil Nurs* 33(4):163–169, 2008.
18. Fineout-Overholt E, et al: Teaching EBP: Getting to the gold: how to search for the best evidence, *Worldviews on Evidence-Based Nursing,* 2(4):207–211, 2005.
19. Fineout-Overholt E, et al: Evidence-based practice, step by step: critical appraisal of the evidence: part III, *Am* 110(11):43–51, 2010.
20. Fineout-Overholt E, Johnston L: Teaching EBP: asking searchable, answerable clinical questions, *Worldviews on Evidence-Based Nursing,* 2(3):157–160, 2005.
21. Krainovich-Miller B, et al: Evidence-based practice challenge: teaching critical appraisal of systematic reviews and clinical practice guidelines to graduate students, *Journal of Nursing Education* 48(4):186–195, 2009.
22. Jones KR: Rating the level, quality, and strength of the research evidence, *J Nurs Care Qual* 25(4):304–312, 2010.

10 The Nervous System

Corey R. Peterson, DNP, CRNA

The primary goal of anesthesia, whether general anesthesia, neuraxial anesthesia (spinal and epidural anesthesia), or regional anesthesia, is the alteration of the normal functioning of the nervous system in the body. General anesthesia achieves this primarily by interacting with the central nervous system, whereas regional anesthesia affects the peripheral nervous system. The effects of neuraxial anesthesia bridge both the central nervous system and the peripheral nervous system. Regardless of the type of anesthesia used, patients in the postanesthesia care unit (PACU) will have some alteration in their nervous system functioning. Consequently, the perianesthesia nurse must have an understanding of the basic anatomic and physiologic principles of the nervous system. This chapter provides the perianesthesia nurse with a comprehensive review of both the anatomy and the physiology of the central and peripheral nervous system.

DEFINITIONS

Afferent: Carrying sensory impulses toward the brain.
Autoregulation: An alteration in the diameter of arterioles to maintain a constant perfusion pressure during changes in systemic blood pressure.
Axon: A long, slender projection from the nerve cell body that transmits nerve impulses away from the cell.
Cistern: A reservoir or cavity.
Commissure: White or gray matter that crosses over in the midline and connects one side of the brain or spinal cord with the other side.
Decussate: Refers to crossing of parts from one side of the brain or spinal cord to the other.
Dendrite: Branched projection from the nerve cell body that transmits nerve impulses into the nerve cell.
Dorsal: Posterior.
Efferent: Carrying motor impulses away from the brain.
Glial Cells: Nonneuronal cells that maintain homeostasis for nerve tissue within the central nervous system.

Gray Matter: Central nervous system tissue consisting primarily of nerve cell bodies, glial cells, and capillaries.
Inferior: Beneath; also used to indicate the lower portion of an anatomic part.
Lower Motor Neurons: Neurons of the spine and cranium that directly innervate the muscles (e.g., those found in the anterior horns or anterior roots of the gray matter of the spinal cord).
Myelin: A product of glial cells that forms an insulating layer around axons, allowing faster nerve impulse conduction.
Neuroglia: The supporting structure of nervous tissue that consists of a fine web of tissue composed of neuroglia or glia cells. It performs supportive and nutritive functions for the nerve network but is not directly involved in nerve impulse transmission.
Plexus: A network of nerves.
Postural Reflexes: Reflexes that are basically proprioceptive, concerned with the position of the head in relation to the trunk and with adjustments of the extremities and eyes to the position of the head.
Proprioception: Sensory input from joints, tendons, and muscles that transmit information regarding the position of one body part in relation to another.
Ramus (rami): The primary division of a nerve.
Synapse: A junction between two nerve cells.
Upper Motor Neurons: Neurons in the brain and spinal cord that activate the motor system (e.g., the descending fibers of the pyramidal and extrapyramidal tracts).
Ventral: Anterior.
White Matter: Central nervous system tissue consisting mostly of myelinated axons.

THE NERVOUS SYSTEM

The nervous system can be broadly divided into two components: the central nervous system (CNS) and the peripheral nervous system (PNS). Although these divisions are commonly used, the boundaries between them can be somewhat arbitrary. The flow of sensory information and motor control signals between the two elements of the nervous system is critical for its normal functioning and the health of the individual.

Central Nervous System

The CNS comprises the brain and spinal cord and is exceedingly complex, both anatomically and physiologically. None of the structures in the CNS function in an isolated manner. Neural activity at any level of the CNS always modifies or is modified by influences from other parts of the system, which accounts for the unique nature and extreme complexity of the CNS, much of which remains to be clearly understood.

The Brain

The human brain serves both structurally and functionally as the primary center for control and regulation of all nervous system functions. As such, it is the highest level of control and integration of sensory and motor information in the entire body.

The brain (encephalon) is divided into the following three large areas based on its embryonic development: (1) the forebrain (prosencephalon) contains the telencephalon (cerebrum) with its hemispheres and the diencephalon; (2) the midbrain (mesencephalon) contains the cerebral peduncles, the corpora quadrigemina, and the cerebral aqueduct; and (3) the hindbrain (rhombencephalon) comprises the medulla oblongata, the pons, the cerebellum, and the fourth ventricle.

Forebrain

Telencephalon, Cerebral Cortex

The cerebrum is the largest part of the brain. It fills the entire upper portion of the cranial cavity and consists of billions of neurons that synapse to form a complex network of neural pathways.

The cerebrum consists of two hemispheres interconnected by a large band of neurons known as the *corpus callosum*. Each hemisphere is further subdivided into four lobes that correspond in name to the overlying bones of the cranium. These lobes are the frontal, parietal, temporal, and occipital lobes (Fig. 10-1). Both hemispheres consist of an external cortex of gray matter, the underlying white matter tracts, and the basal ganglia (cerebral nuclei). Each hemisphere also contains a lateral ventricle, which is an elongated cavity concerned with the formation and circulation of cerebrospinal fluid (CSF).

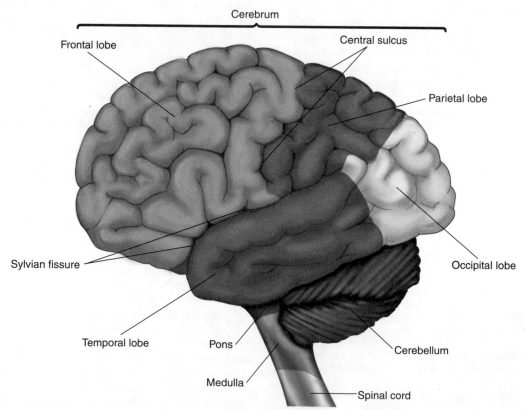

FIG. 10-1 Left lateral view of the brain, showing principal divisions of brain and four major lobes of cerebrum.

The cerebral cortex has an elaborate mantle of gray matter and is the most highly integrated area in the nervous system. It is arranged in a series of folds that dip down into the underlying regions. These folds greatly expand the surface area of the gray matter within the limited confines of the skull. Each fold is known as a *gyrus*. Grooves exist between these gyri. A shallow groove is known as a *sulcus,* whereas a deeper grove is known as a *fissure.*

The cerebral hemispheres are separated from each other from front to back by the longitudinal fissure. The transverse fissure separates the cerebrum from the cerebellum beneath it.

Each hemisphere has three sulci between the lobes. The central sulcus (also known as the *fissure of Rolando*) separates the frontal and parietal lobes. The lateral sulcus (the fissure of Sylvius) lies between the frontal and parietal lobes above and the temporal lobe below. The small parietooccipital sulcus is located between its corresponding lobes (see Fig. 10-1).

The white matter of the cerebrum is situated below the cortex and is composed of three main groups of myelinated nerve fibers arranged in related bundles or tracts. The commissural fibers transmit impulses between the left and right hemispheres. The largest of these fibers is the corpus callosum. The projection fibers are afferent and efferent nerve fibers that transmit impulses between the cortex, lower parts of the brain, and the spinal cord. A notable example is the internal capsule that surrounds most of the basal ganglia and, in part, connects the thalamus and the cerebral cortex. Finally, the association fibers transmit impulses from one part of the cortex to another within the same hemisphere.[1]

Functional Aspects of the Cerebrum

Nearly every portion of the cerebral cortex is connected with underlying structures of the diencephalon, midbrain, and hindbrain, and no areas in the cortex are exclusively motor or exclusively sensory in nature. However, some regions are primarily concerned with the control of motor movement, whereas others are primarily involved in the perception of sensory information. The activities of these areas are integrated by association fibers that compose the remainder of the cerebral cortex. Association fibers play important roles in complex intellectual and emotional processes.

Motor Areas. No single area of motor control exists within the brain because the integration and control of muscle activity depends on the harmonious activities of several areas, including the cerebral cortex, the basal ganglia, and the cerebellum.

Primary Motor Area. The primary motor area of the cerebral cortex is located in the precentral gyrus of the frontal lobe, just in front of the central sulcus, and is concerned mainly with the voluntary initiation of finely controlled movements, such as those of the hands, fingers, lips, tongue, and vocal cords. The amount of area in the primary motor cortex devoted to a particular muscle or muscle group is a reflection of the degree of fine motor control required for the proper functioning of these muscles. For example, the muscles that control speech or the use of the fingers are represented by many more neurons within the primary motor cortex then are the larger muscles of the legs or trunk. This disproportionate representation within the primary motor cortex is a reflection of the relative importance the brain places on the proper control of different muscles.

Axons from the primary motor cortex descend through the internal capsule, midbrain, and the pons to the medulla. These axons are called *pyramidal* because of the shape of the structure they form with the medulla. Within the medulla, most of these axons decussate and continue down into the spinal cord via the lateral corticospinal tracts. Fibers that do not decussate in the medulla descend down the spinal cord via the ventral corticospinal tracts. Most of these fibers eventually decussate at lower levels within the cord. Pyramidal cell axons also connect within the brain with the basal ganglia, the brainstem, and the cerebellum. Generally, these pyramidal motor nerves constitute a direct pathway from the primary motor area to the muscles and are concerned mostly with control of discrete, detailed body movements.

Premotor Area. The premotor area of each hemisphere is located in the cortex immediately in front of the primary motor cortex in the frontal lobe. On the whole, this area is concerned with movement of the opposite side of the body, especially with control and coordination of skilled movements of a complex nature, such as throwing or kicking a ball. In addition to its subcortical connections with the primary motor area, its neurons also have direct connections with the basal ganglia and related nuclei in the brainstem, for example, the reticular formation. Many of the axons from these subcortical centers cross to the opposite side before descending as extrapyramidal tracts in the spinal cord. Collectively, the connections from the premotor area to these related nuclei compose the extrapyramidal system, which coordinates gross skeletal muscle activities that are largely automatic in nature. Examples are postural adjustments, chewing, swallowing, gesticulating during speech, and associated movements that accompany voluntary activities. Certain portions of the extrapyramidal tract also have an inhibitory effect on spontaneous movements initiated by the cerebral cortex and serve to prevent tremors and rigidity. Complete structural and functional separation of the pyramidal and extrapyramidal systems is impossible because they are so closely connected in the harmonious work of executing complex coordinated movements.

Of interest to the PACU nurse is that drugs used during the perioperative period can cause extrapyramidal reactions. More specifically, the neuroleptics, such as the phenothiazines (of which chlorpromazine is the prototypal drug), the butyrophenones, as typified by droperidol (Inapsine) and haloperidol (Haldol), and the antiemetic metoclopramide (Reglan) are known to produce extrapyramidal reactions. The following four types of extrapyramidal reaction exist: drug-induced parkinsonism, akathisia, acute dystonic reactions, and tardive dyskinesia.

Drug-induced parkinsonism, which can occur 1 to 5 days after the administration of the neuroleptic drug, is typified by a generalized slowing of automatic and spontaneous movements (bradykinesia), with a masklike facial expression and a reduction in arm movements. The most noticeable signs of the drug-induced parkinsonism syndrome are rigidity and oscillatory tremor at rest. The treatment is an antiparkinsonian agent, such as levodopa, trihexyphenidyl, and benztropine.

Akathisia, which can occur 5 to 60 days after the administration of a neuroleptic drug, refers to a subjective feeling of restlessness accompanied by a need on the part of the patient to move about and pace back and forth, acute anxiety, and the feeling impending of doom. Treatment requires a reduction in the dosage of the responsible drug and the administration of a benzodiazepine if encountered during the perioperative period.

Acute dystonic reactions may occur after the administration of some psychotropic drugs and are characterized by torsion spasms, such as facial grimacing and torticollis. These reactions are occasionally seen when a phenothiazine is first administered, and they are associated with oculogyric crises. Acute dystonic reactions may be mistaken for hysterical reactions or seizures and can usually be reversed with anticholinergic antiparkinsonian drugs, such as benztropine or trihexyphenidyl.

Tardive dyskinesia is a late-appearing neurologic syndrome that is characterized by stereotypic, involuntary, rapid, and rhythmically repetitive movements, such as continual chewing movements and darting movements of the tongue. Treatment is not always satisfactory because antiparkinsonian drugs sometimes exacerbate tardive dyskinesia. Tardive dyskinesia often persists despite discontinuation of the responsible drug.[2,3]

Two important structural aspects of the premotor area are worth noting for those who care for neurosurgical patients. First, the fibers from both the primary motor and the premotor areas are funneled through the narrow internal capsule as they descend to lower areas of the CNS. This action is significant because the internal capsule is a common site of cerebrovascular accidents that can result in a variety of motor deficits. Second, lesions within one side of the internal capsule result in paralysis of the skeletal muscles on the opposite side of the body because of the crossing of fibers within the medulla.[4]

Motor Speech Area. This area is only one point in the complicated network needed to form spoken and written words. The motor speech area lies at the base of the motor area and slightly in front of it in the inferior frontal gyrus and is also known as the *Broca area.* In right-handed people (most of the population), the language and speech areas are usually located in the left hemisphere. In those who are left-handed, these areas may lie within the right or the left hemisphere.

Prefrontal Area. This area of the frontal lobe lies anterior to the premotor area, has extensive connections with other cortical areas, and is believed to have an important role in complex intellectual activities, such as mathematic and philosophic reasoning; abstract and creative thinking; learning; judgment and volition; and social, moral, and ethical values. The prefrontal area also influences certain autonomic functions of the body with the conduction of impulses directly or indirectly through the thalamus to the hypothalamus, which makes possible certain physiologic responses to feelings such as anger, fear, and lust.

Sensory Areas. Sensory information from one side of the body is received by the somatic sensory area of the opposite hemisphere, which is located in the parietal lobe in the area of the postcentral gyrus. Crude sensations of pain, temperature, and touch can be experienced at the level of the thalamus, but true localization and discrimination of these sensations is a function of the parietal cortex. The activities of the somatic sensory area allow for proprioception, for the recognition of the size, shape, and texture of objects, and for the comparison of stimuli as to intensity and location.

The auditory area lies in the cortex of the superior temporal lobe. Each hemisphere receives impulses from both ears. The visual area is located in the posterior occipital lobe, where extremely complex transformations in the signals conveyed by the optic nerve occur. The right occipital cortex receives impulses from the right half of each eye, and the left occipital cortex receives impulses from the left half of each eye. The olfactory area is believed to be located in the medial temporal lobe, and the gustatory area is located nearby at the base of the postcentral gyrus.

Association Areas. Large areas of the cortex remain for which no discrete function is known. These areas are called *association areas.* They play a major role in the integration of the sensory and motor phases of cortical function by providing complex connections between them.

Limbic System. The principal structural and functional units of the limbic system are the two rings of limbic cortex and a number of related subcortical nuclei, the anterior thalamic nuclei, and portions of the basal nuclei (Fig. 10-2). In general, the limbic system is concerned with a wide variety of autonomic somatosensory and somatomotor responses, especially those involved with emotional states and other behavioral responses. Within the limbic system, the benzodiazepine and opiate receptors have been identified (see Chapters 19, 21, and 22).

The limbic system, which acts in close concert with the hypothalamus, can evoke a variety of autonomic responses, including changes in heart rate, blood pressure, and respiratory rate. This system plays an intimate role in the creation of emotional states, particularly anxiety, fear, and aggression. Stimulation of the limbic system also evokes complex motor responses directly related to feeding behavior. The limbic system has been shown to have major relationships with the reticular formation of the brainstem and is presumed to have a role in the alerting or arousal process. The system is also implicated in the hypothalamic regulation of pituitary activity and may be associated somehow with the memory process for recent events as well. In addition, it is intimately concerned with complex phenomena, such as the control of various biologic rhythms, sexual behavior, and motivation.

Basal Ganglia. A cerebral nucleus is a group of neuron cell bodies within the CNS. Five of these deep-lying masses of gray matter are located within the white matter of each hemisphere and are collectively known as the basal ganglia. These masses are the caudate nucleus, the putamen, the globus pallidus, the substantia nigra, and the subthalamic nucleus. Together, they exert a steadying influence on muscle activity. The basal ganglia are an important part of the extrapyramidal motor

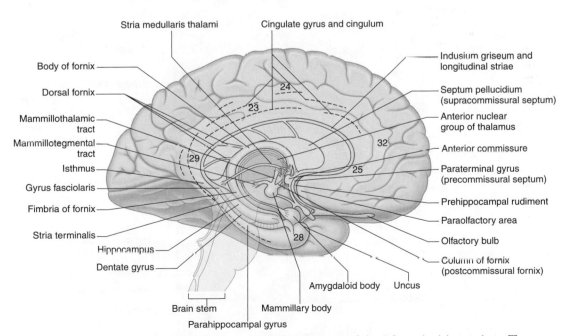

FIG. 10-2 Components of the limbic system. Medial aspect of the left cerebral hemisphere. The approximate locations of some Brodmann areas are indicated. (From Standring S: *Gray's anatomy: the anatomical basis of clinical practice,* ed 40, London, 2009, Churchill Livingstone.)

pathway that connects nuclei with each other, with the cortex, and with the spinal cord. The ganglia also connect with areas in the hindbrain (the red nucleus and the substantia nigra) to assist in the role of smoothing and coordinating muscle movements. Disturbances in these ganglia result in tremor, rigidity, and loss of expressive and walking movements, as seen in Parkinson syndrome.[5]

Diencephalon

The second major division of the forebrain is the diencephalon (Fig. 10-3), which consists of the thalamus and the hypothalamus. The diencephalon also contains the third ventricle and is almost completely covered by the cerebral hemispheres. This portion of the brain has a primary role in sleep, emotion, thermoregulation, autonomic activity, and endocrine control of ongoing behavioral patterns.

The thalamus consists of right and left egg-shaped masses, which compose the greatest bulk of the diencephalon and form the lateral wall of the third ventricle. Each thalamus serves as a relay center for all incoming sensory stimuli, except for taste. These impulses are then grouped and transmitted to the appropriate area of the cerebral cortex. Because of its interconnections with the hypothalamus, the limbic system, and the frontal, temporal, and parietal lobes, this structure is also integrally involved with emotional activities, instinctive responses, and attentive processes.

The hypothalamus is a group of bilateral nuclei that forms the floor and part of the lateral walls of the third ventricle. Extremely complex in function, the hypothalamus has extensive connections with the autonomic nervous system and with other parts of the CNS. It also influences the endocrine system by virtue of direct and

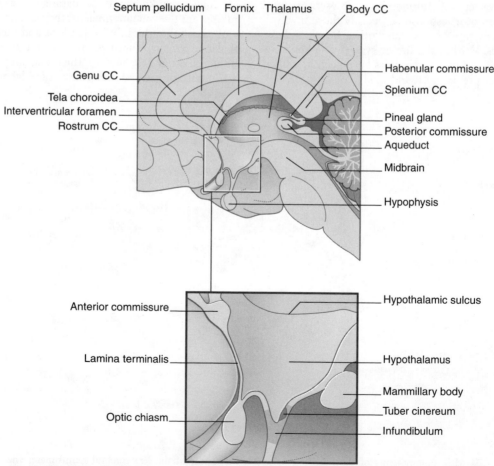

FIG. 10-3 The diencephalon and its boundaries. *CC,* Corpus callosum. (From Fitzgerald MJT, et al: *Clinical neuroanatomy and neuroscience,* ed 6, St. Louis, 2011, Saunders.)

indirect connections with the pituitary gland and the release of its own hormones. In association with these other structures, the hypothalamus participates in the regulation of appetite, water balance, carbohydrate and fat metabolism, growth, sexual maturity, body temperature, pulse rate, blood pressure, sleep, and aspects of emotional behavior. Because of the connection of the hypothalamus with the thalamus and cerebral cortex, emotions can influence visceral responses on certain occasions.[6]

Midbrain

The midbrain, or mesencephalon, is a short narrow segment of nervous tissue that connects the forebrain with the hindbrain. The midbrain is vital as a conduction pathway and as a reflex control center. Passing through the center of the midbrain is the cerebral aqueduct, a narrow canal that serves to connect the third ventricle of the diencephalon with the fourth ventricle of the hindbrain for the circulation of CSF. In addition, cranial nerves III (oculomotor) and IV (trochlear) originate in the ventral aspect of the midbrain.[7]

Hindbrain

The hindbrain, or rhombencephalon, consists of the pons, the medulla oblongata, the cerebellum, and the fourth ventricle (Fig. 10-4).

Pons

The pons is literally the bridge between the midbrain and the medulla oblongata as it lies in front of the fourth ventricle and separates it from the cerebellum. It receives many ascending and descending fibers en route to other points in the CNS. The pons also contains the motor and sensory nuclei of cranial nerves V (trigeminal), VI (abducens), VII (facial), and VIII (acoustic). The roof of the pons contains a portion of the reticular formation, and the lower pons assists in the regulation of respiration.

Medulla Oblongata

The medulla oblongata is an expanded continuation of the spinal cord and is located between the base of the skull, the foramen magnum, and the pons. It is anatomically complex and not usually amenable to surgery. Many of the white fiber tracts between the brain and spinal cord decussate as they pass through the medulla. Centers for many complex reflexes are located in the medulla oblongata and include those for swallowing, vomiting, coughing, and sneezing. The originating nuclei of cranial nerves IX (glossopharyngeal), X (vagus), XI (accessory), and XII (hypoglossal) are found in the medulla oblongata (Table 10-1). Because of these originating nuclei, the medulla has an essential role in the regulation of cardiac, respiratory, and vasomotor reflexes. Injuries to the medulla, such as those that accompany basal skull fracture, often prove fatal.

Cerebellum

The cerebellum overlaps the pons and the medulla oblongata dorsally and is located just below the occipital lobes of the cerebrum. It is separated from the cerebrum by the tentorium, a folded layer of the dura mater. Structurally, the cerebellum comprises two hemispheres with a constricted central portion with a bilayered cortex composed of gray matter. Beneath the gray matter are white fiber tracts that extend like branches of a tree to all parts of the cerebellar cortex. Deep within the white matter are masses of gray matter called the *cerebellar nuclei*. These nuclei connect the cerebellar hemispheres with each other and with areas in the cerebrum, the hindbrain, and the spinal cord.

The cerebellum has no sensory function and does not initiate movement as the cerebrum does. Functionally, it coordinates muscle tone and voluntary movements through important connections via the spinal cord with the proprioceptor nerve fibers in skeletal muscles, tendons, and joints. In addition, the cerebellum is involved in reflexes necessary for the maintenance of equilibrium and posture, through its connections with the vestibular apparatus of the inner ear. The

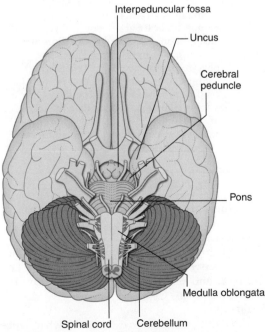

Interpeduncular fossa

Uncus

Cerebral peduncle

Pons

Medulla oblongata

Spinal cord   Cerebellum

FIG. 10-4 Ventral view of the brainstem in situ. (From Fitzgerald MJT, et al: *Clinical neuroanatomy and neuroscience*, ed 6, St. Louis, 2011, Saunders.)

Table 10-1   Cranial Nerves and Their Functions

NUMBER	NAME	TYPE	FUNCTION
I	Olfactory	Sensory	Smell
II	Optic	Sensory	Vision
III	Oculomotor	Mixed: mainly motor	Motion of eye up, in, and down Raising of eyelid Constriction of pupil Accommodation of pupil to distance Proprioceptive impulses
IV	Trochlear	Mixed: mainly motor	Motion of eye down Proprioceptive impulses
V	Trigeminal Ophthalmic branch Maxillary branch Mandibular branch	Mixed	Motor: muscles of mastication Sensory: face, nose, and mouth Proprioceptive impulses from teeth sockets and jaw muscles
VI	Abducens	Mixed: mainly motor	Outward motion of eye; proprioception from eye muscles
VII	Facial	Mixed: mostly motor, some sensory and autonomic	Motor: movement of facial muscles, ear, nose, and neck Sensory: taste and anterior two thirds of tongue Autonomic: secretion of saliva and tears
VIII	Acoustic Cochlear branch Vestibular branch	Sensory	Cochlear: hearing Vestibular: maintenance of equilibrium and posturing of head
IX	Glossopharyngeal	Mixed: motor, sensory, and autonomic	Motor: muscles of swallowing Sensory: taste, posterior third of tongue, and sensation from pharynx Autonomic: impulses to parotid glands and decrease blood pressure and pulse
X	Vagus	Mixed: motor, sensory, and autonomic	Motor, sensory, and autonomic: information to and from larynx, pharynx, trachea, esophagus, heart, and abdominal viscera
XI	Spinal accessory	Mixed: mostly motor	Cranial portion: motor and sensory information to and from voluntary muscles of pharynx, larynx, and palate (swallowing) Spinal portion: motor information to sternocleidomastoid and trapezius muscles May form components of cardiac branches of vagus
XII	Hypoglossal	Mixed: mostly motor	Motor and sensory information to and from tongue muscles Position sense

cerebellum also receives optic and acoustic information, but the specifics of the anatomic pathways involved have not yet been discerned.

Damage to the cerebellum does not result in paralysis or sensory loss. The outcome of damage depends on which portion of the structure is involved. Damage to one part can result in loss of balance, nystagmus, and a reeling gait (cerebellar ataxia). Damage to another area can cause disturbances in the postural reflexes. Posterior lobe disturbances result in changes in voluntary movements, such as discrepancies in force, direction, and range of movements; lack of precision in movements; and, possibly, intention tremors.

Fourth Ventricle

The fourth ventricle is a diamond-shaped space located between the cerebellum posteriorly and the pons and medulla oblongata anteriorly. The ventricle contains CSF.

Brainstem

Authors disagree to some extent as to what structures collectively constitute the brainstem. All agree that it includes the midbrain, the pons, and the medulla oblongata. Some believe that the diencephalon rightly belongs in the group. Whichever grouping is used, all functions of each structure within it may be considered to be basic activities of the brainstem. All the cranial nerves are attached to the brainstem (if the diencephalon is included), with the exception of the olfactory nerve and the spinal portion of the accessory nerve.

Reticular Formation

The reticular formation lies within the brainstem (including the diencephalon). An important function of the reticular formation is its action as an intermediary between the upper and lower motor neurons of the extrapyramidal system. In this way, the reticular formation facilitates or augments reflex activity and voluntary movements. Its motor neurons can be excitatory or inhibitory in action. For example, with inhibition of extensor muscles, it facilitates the action of flexor muscles.

Every pathway that carries information to the brain also contributes afferent fibers to the reticular formation, so that it is kept well informed about conditions of both the outside world and the internal organs. Efferent impulses that leave the reticular formation travel to the cerebral cortex and to the spinal cord. By virtue of its location in and connections with the brainstem and diencephalon, the reticular formation participates integrally in their activities.

Another important function of the reticular formation is the activation and regulation of those brain activities related to attention arousal and consciousness. For this reason, it is often called the *reticular activating system.*

Damage to the reticular formation results in greatly decreased levels of consciousness. When the cerebral cortex is isolated from the reticular activating system by disease or injury of the upper portion of the midbrain, decerebrate posturing occurs. This stereotypical posturing involves the arms and legs being held straight out, the toes being pointed downward, and the head and neck being arched backwards. This abnormal posturing results from the dominant effect of the extensor muscles and a lack of inhibition from opposing motor neurons and flexor muscles. The rigidity is accompanied by a profoundly reduced level of consciousness.

Protection of the Brain

The brain is protected by the cranial bones, the meninges, and the CSF (Figs. 10-5 and 10-6).

Cranial Bones

Eight cranial bones encase the brain and support and protect it from most ordinary bumps and jarring. In the adult, immovable fibrous joints, or sutures, fuse these bones together to form the rigid walls of the box known as the cranium. The base of the cranium is both thicker and stronger than its roof or walls.

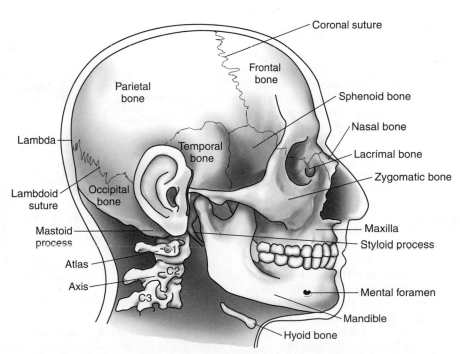

FIG. 10-5 Lateral view of skull, showing relationship of skull and cervical vertebrae to face.

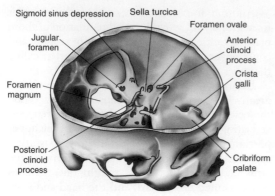

Sigmoid sinus depression   Sella turcica
Jugular foramen   Foramen ovale
                                           Anterior clinoid process
Foramen magnum   Crista galli
Posterior clinoid process   Cribriform palate

FIG. 10-6 Interior of cranial cavity.

The bones of the cranium are the frontal, right and left parietal, occipital, sphenoid, ethmoid, and right and left temporal bones. The frontal bone forms the anterior roof of the skull and the forehead. Within the frontal bone are the frontal sinuses, which communicate with the nasal cavities. The parietal bones form much of the top and sides of the cranium. The occipital bone forms the back and a large portion of the base of the skull. The two temporal bones are complicated and form part of the sides and a part of the base of the skull. Their inner surfaces are not as smooth and regular as the bones previously mentioned. Parts of the temporal bones articulate with the condyles of the lower jaw, and air cells in the mastoid portions of the temporal bones communicate with the middle ear. The sphenoid bone occupies a central portion of the floor of the skull. It alone articulates with each of the other cranial bones. Its middle portion contains the sphenoid sinuses, which open into the nasal cavity. The upper portion of the sphenoid bone has a marked saddlelike depression, the sella turcica, which holds the pituitary gland. The ethmoid bone is light and has a spongy structure. It is located between the orbital cavities and is a cribriform plate that forms the roof of the nasal cavity and part of the base of the cranium. The ethmoid sinuses open into the nasal cavities.

Several features of the cranial bones are particularly noteworthy for the PACU nurse. Among these features is the fact that the air cells in the mastoid portion of the temporal bone may become infected from otitis media or after surgery on the middle or inner ear. This mastoiditis can cause severe complications if it extends through the thin plate of bone that separates it from the cranial meninges. Another point of interest is that surgical access to the pituitary gland is commonly accomplished through the sphenoid bone via the nostrils; one example is transsphenoidal

hypophysectomy. Finally, nasal suctioning is absolutely contraindicated in the patient with cranial surgery because of the danger of perforation of the cribriform plate of the ethmoid bone, which results in leakage of CSF and permits direct access to the brain by infectious organisms.

One main opening is located at the base of the skull and is called the *foramen magnum*. It marks the point at which the brainstem changes structure and becomes identified inferiorly as the spinal cord. Many smaller openings in the skull allow the cranial nerves and some blood vessels to pass through it to and from the face, the jaw, and the neck. The atlas of the vertebral column (C_1) supports the skull and forms a moveable joint with the occipital bone.[7]

Meninges

The meninges (Fig. 10-7) are three fibrous membranes between the skull and the brain and between the vertebral column and the spinal cord. The outer membrane is the dura mater and the inner is the pia mater; between them lies the arachnoid mater.

Dura Mater. The dura mater is a shiny, tough, inelastic membrane that envelops and supports the brain and spinal cord and, by various folds, separates parts of the brain into adjoining compartments. The portion within the skull differs from the dura of the spinal cord in three ways. First, the cranial dura is firmly attached to the skull. The spinal dura has no attachment to the vertebrae. Second, the cranial dura consists of two

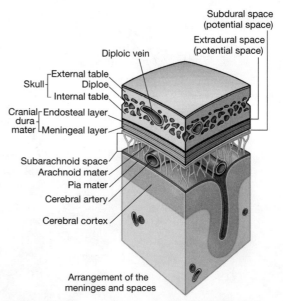

Subdural space (potential space)
Extradural space (potential space)
Diploic vein
External table
Skull — Diploe
Internal table
Cranial dura mater — Endosteal layer
Meningeal layer
Subarachnoid space
Arachnoid mater
Pia mater
Cerebral artery
Cerebral cortex

Arrangement of the meninges and spaces

FIG. 10-7 Arrangement of meninges in the cranial cavity. (From Drake RL, et al: *Gray's anatomy for students*, ed 2, Philadelphia, 2010, Churchill Livingstone.)

layers; it covers the brain (meningeal dura) and lines the interior of the skull bones (periosteal dura). Third, the two layers of the cranial dura are in contact with each other in some places but separate in others where the inner layer dips inward to form the protective partitions between parts of the brain. In addition, the spaces or channels formed by these separations of dural layers are filled with venous blood that is leaving the brain; these spaces are called *cranial venous sinuses* and are an elaborate network unique to the brain (see Fig. 10-7).

There are three major partitioning folds of the meningeal dura. The falx cerebri separates the right and left hemispheres of the cerebrum. The tentorium cerebelli supports and separates the occipital lobes of the cerebrum from the cerebellum. The falx cerebelli separates the two cerebellar hemispheres. The tentorium separates the posterior cranial chamber from the remainder of the cranial cavity and serves as a line of demarcation for describing the site of a surgical procedure or a lesion as either supratentorial or infratentorial.

Encased between the two dural layers are two major groups of venous channels that drain blood from the brain. None of these vascular channels possesses valves, and their walls are extremely thin because of the absence of muscular tissue. The superior-posterior group consists of one paired and four unpaired sinuses. The anterior-inferior group consists of four paired sinuses and one plexus. The sinuses function to drain venous blood into the internal jugular veins, which are the principal vessels responsible for the return of the blood from the brain to the heart (Fig. 10-8).

Arachnoid Mater. The arachnoid is a fine membrane between the dura mater and the pia mater. Between the arachnoid and the dura is the subdural space, a noncommunicating space filled with CSF. The cerebral blood vessels that traverse this space have little supporting structure, which makes them particularly vulnerable to injury at this point.

The arachnoid forms a type of roof over the pia mater, to which it is joined by a network of trabeculae in the subarachnoid space. It does not follow the depressions of the surface architecture. The arachnoid sends small, tuftlike extensions through the meningeal layer of the dura into the cranial venous sinuses. These extensions are called

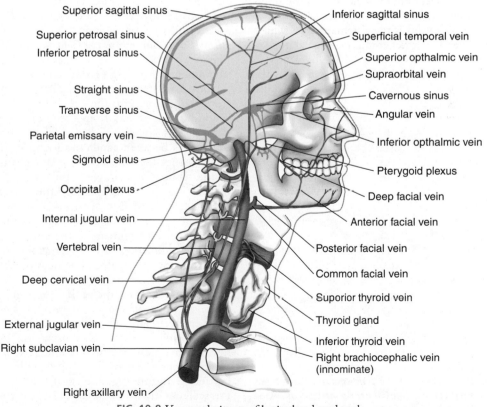

FIG. 10-8 Venous drainage of brain, head, and neck.

the *arachnoid granulations* or *arachnoid villi*. The arachnoid villi serve as a pathway for the return of CSF to the venous blood system. Subarachnoid CSF is most abundant in the grooves between the gyri, particularly at the base of the brain, where the more freely communicating compartments form six subarachnoid cisternae, or reservoirs.

Pia Mater. The inner layer of the meninges, the pia mater, is a fine membrane rich in blood (choroid) plexuses and mesothelial cells. This layer is closely associated with the arachnoid and covers the brain intimately, following the invaginations and convolutions of the brain surface. The veins of the brain lie between threadlike trabeculae in the subarachnoid space. Branches of the cortical arteries in the subarachnoid space are carried with the pia mater and enter the brain substance itself.[5]

Cerebrospinal Fluid System

The CSF is a clear colorless watery fluid with a specific gravity of 1.007. A principal function of this fluid is to act as a cushion for the brain. Because both brain tissue and CSF have essentially the same specific gravity, the brain literally floats within the skull. CSF also serves as a medium for the exchange of nutrients and waste products between the blood stream and the cells of the CNS.

Cerebrospinal fluid is found within the ventricles of the brain, in the cisterns that surround it, and in the subarachnoid spaces of both the brain and the spinal cord (Figs. 10-9 and 10-10). The largest of the cisterns is the cisterna magna, which is located beneath and behind the cerebellum.

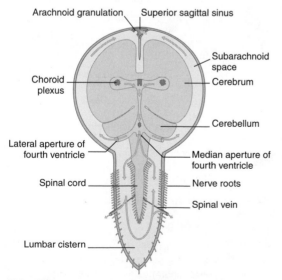

FIG. 10-9 Circulation of cerebrospinal fluid. (From Fitzgerald MJT, et al: *Clinical neuroanatomy and neuroscience*, ed 6, St. Louis, 2011, Saunders.)

Although some CSF is formed by filtration through capillary walls throughout the brain's vascular bed, its primary site of formation is in the choroid plexuses within the ventricles. This formation is achieved with a system of secretion and diffusion. The choroid plexuses are highly vascular, tufted structures composed of many small granular pouches that project into the ventricles of the brain. CSF is formed continuously and is reabsorbed at a rate of approximately 750 mL per day. The net pressure of the CSF is regulated in part by a balance between formation and reabsorption.

The four ventricles of the brain communicate directly with each other. The first and second (lateral) ventricles are elongated cavities that lie within the cerebral hemispheres. The third ventricle is a slitlike cavity beneath and between the two lateral ventricles. The fourth ventricle is a diamond-shaped space between the cerebellum posteriorly and the pons and medulla anteriorly.

The main route of reabsorption of excess CSF is through the arachnoid villi that project from the subarachnoid spaces into the venous sinuses of the brain, particularly those of the superior sagittal sinus. The arachnoid villi provide highly permeable regions that allow free passage of CSF, including protein molecules and some small particulate matter contained within it. The process of osmosis is believed to be mainly responsible for the reabsorption of the fluid.[6]

Blood-Brain Barriers of the Central Nervous System

The amount and rate of diffusion of fluids and dissolved substances across capillary membranes from the plasma into the extracellular fluid surrounding cells differs from tissue to tissue. This difference is largely a function of the structural differences between capillaries found in the different tissues and reflects the physiologic function of the tissue. For example, capillaries within the liver are highly porous, creating little hindrance to the movement of fluid, and dissolve substances such as drugs and proteins between plasma in the extracellular environment of the liver tissue; this reflects the function of the liver as an organ responsible for the synthesis of many substances and the metabolism of many others.

On the other extreme of the spectrum is brain tissue. Brain tissue is highly sensitive to changes in its extracellular environment and the introduction of foreign or unusual substances. To facilitate the maintenance of this uniquely balanced environment, the body has evolved a blood-brain barrier to tightly regulate what may enter the extracellular environment of the brain from the capillaries.

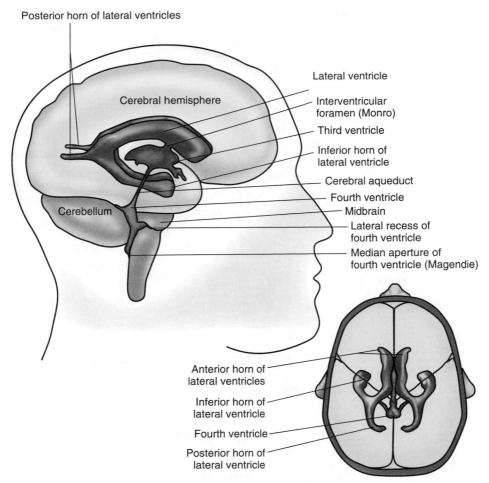

FIG. 10-10 Ventricular system, lateral and superior views.

The site of the blood-brain barrier is not at the surface of the neurons themselves. Rather, it is a series of special adaptations to the capillaries present in the cerebral circulation. These adaptations form a series of physical barriers that act together to prevent the normally rapid transport of substances from the blood to the nervous tissue. These barriers include the tight intercellular junctions between the epithelial cells of the capillaries that appear to effectively reduce permeability. A substantial basement membrane surrounds the capillaries, and an external membrane is provided by the end-feet of the astrocytes between the neurons and the capillaries. This series of physical barriers plays a major role in retarding or preventing the passage of foreign substances into the brain tissue. The integrity of the blood-brain barrier and its ability to control what enters the CNS can break down in areas of the brain that are infected, traumatized, or irradiated or contain tumors.

The speed with which substances penetrate the blood-brain barrier is inversely proportional to their molecular size and directly proportional to their lipid solubility. Only water, carbon dioxide, and oxygen cross the blood-brain barrier rapidly and readily, whereas glucose crosses more slowly and by a facilitated transport mechanism. Water-soluble compounds, electrolytes, and large protein molecules generally cross very slowly or not at all. Most general anesthetics effectively cross the blood-brain barrier because of their high lipid solubility.[8,9]

Arterial Blood Supply to the Brain

The entire arterial blood supply to the brain, with the exception of a small amount that flows in the anterior spinal artery to the medulla, is carried through the neck by four vessels: the two vertebral arteries and the two carotid arteries (Figs. 10-11 and 10-12).

The two vertebral arteries supply the posterior portion of the brain. They ascend in the neck

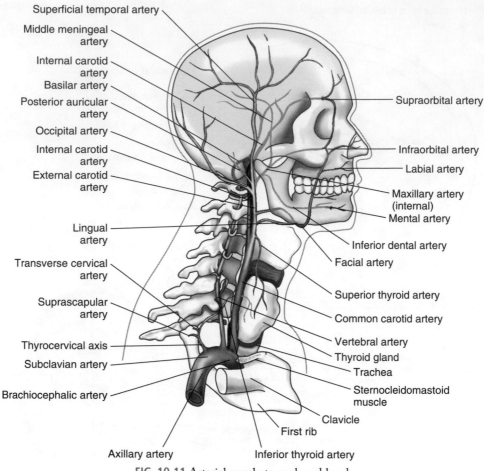

Superficial temporal artery
Middle meningeal artery
Internal carotid artery
Basilar artery
Posterior auricular artery
Occipital artery
Internal carotid artery
External carotid artery
Lingual artery
Transverse cervical artery
Suprascapular artery
Thyrocervical axis
Subclavian artery
Brachiocephalic artery
Axillary artery

Supraorbital artery
Infraorbital artery
Labial artery
Maxillary artery (internal)
Mental artery
Inferior dental artery
Facial artery
Superior thyroid artery
Common carotid artery
Vertebral artery
Thyroid gland
Trachea
Sternocleidomastoid muscle
Clavicle
First rib
Inferior thyroid artery

FIG. 10-11 Arterial supply to neck and head.

through the transverse foramina on each side of the cervical vertebrae, enter the skull through the foramen magnum, and join near the pons to form the basilar artery of the hindbrain. A relatively small volume of the total blood flow to the brain is carried by the vertebral or basilar artery. The circle of Willis, in turn, is formed by the union of the basilar artery and the two internal carotid arteries. Before they join the circle of Willis, these arteries send essential branches to the brainstem, cerebellum, and falx cerebelli.

The circle of Willis is a ring of blood vessels that surrounds the optic chiasm and the pituitary stalk. The circle of Willis gives rise to three pairs of arteries: the anterior, the middle, and the posterior cerebral arteries. Each pair of arteries supplies specific areas of the brain: (1) the anterior cerebral arteries supply approximately half of the frontal and parietal lobes, including much of the corpus callosum; (2) the middle cerebral arteries perfuse most of the lateral surfaces of the hemispheres and send off branches to the

corpus striatum and the internal capsule; and (3) the posterior cerebral arteries supply the occipital lobes and the remaining portions of the temporal lobes that are not supplied by the middle cerebral arteries.[7]

Regulation of Cerebral Blood Flow

The brain has almost no ability to store nutrients. For this reason, it is dependent on a continuous flow of blood to supply the glucose and oxygen required for normal neuronal cell functioning. Even a brief interruption of blood flow, for as short as few seconds, can result in loss of consciousness. The high rate of metabolic demand associated with neuronal cell functioning also requires a relatively large amount of blood flow. In fact, 15% of the total resting cardiac output goes to the brain, which represents approximately 2% of the total body weight.

The body has several mechanisms to ensure the uninterrupted high rate of blood flow required by the brain. As in other tissues in the body, the brain's requirement varies with metabolic activity.

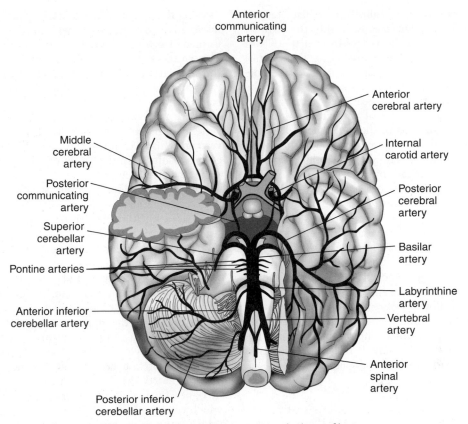

FIG. 10-12 Major arteries as seen on the base of brain.

The more active the brain, the greater the blood supply it requires. Regulation of this blood supply is primarily based upon the concentration of carbon dioxide in the brain tissue. Carbon dioxide is a normal byproduct of neuronal cellular metabolism. The concentration of carbon dioxide in the brain tissue increases as neuronal cellular metabolism increases with an increase in brain activity. This increase in carbon dioxide causes the cerebral vasculature to dilate, increasing blood flow to the brain. The opposite occurs when carbon dioxide concentration declines in the brain. This mechanism is highly sensitive, and even small changes from the normal carbon dioxide levels in the brain can cause significant changes in the volume of cerebral blood flow.

The vessels of the brain will also react to changes in the oxygen concentration of the brain tissue. As the oxygen concentration level falls in the brain, the vasculature will vasodilate to increase cerebral blood flow. An increase in the oxygen level will cause a degree of vasoconstriction. This mechanism is not as sensitive as the one regulated by carbon dioxide. The vasculature changes triggered by alterations in the oxygen concentration do not occur until oxygen levels are significantly increased or decreased from their normal levels.

A third mechanism to maintain blood flow to the brain is called *autoregulation*. Autoregulation ensures a constant cerebral blood flow to the brain despite the normal fluctuations that occur in blood pressure in the body. It achieves this effect by changing the diameter of the vasculature in response to changes in blood pressure. An increase in the blood pressure causes the cerebral vessels to constrict, whereas a decrease in blood pressure causes them to dilate. Autoregulation is effective over the normal range of blood pressures seen in the body, but when blood pressures become very low (a mean arterial pressure [MAP] less than 50 mm Hg) or very high (MAP greater than 150 mm Hg) the mechanism loses its effectiveness and blood flow to the brain becomes pressure dependent. In addition, autoregulation, like the blood-brain barrier, can be lost in cases of trauma, infection, or tumors in the brain.

Intracranial Pressure Dynamics
The bones of the skull form a rigid box that surrounds and contains the brain, CSF, and blood

that is perfusing the brain. Intracranial pressure (ICP) is the pressure created within the skull by the contents; it usually ranges from 4 to 15 mm Hg. Compensatory mechanisms exist that control for minor variations in the changes of the volumes of blood, CSF, and brain tissue within the skull, keeping the ICP nearly constant. If ICP should increase because of an increase in one or more of the contents of the skull, such as a brain tumor or swelling because of a blow to the head, significant injury can result to the brain from lack of blood flow or death owing to herniation of the brain through the base of the skull.

Cerebral Perfusion Pressure

Cerebral perfusion pressure (CPP) is essentially the blood pressure of the brain; it is a reflection of the flow of blood to the brain and usually ranges from 90 to 100 mm Hg. In normal conditions, CPP and resultant blood flow are determined by the difference between the inflow and the outflow pressures. Inflow pressures are represented by the MAP, and in normal conditions the mean outflow pressure is equivalent to the central venous pressure. In situations in which ICP is greater than venous pressure, the following equation applies:

$$CPP = MAP - ICP$$

From this formula, it is obvious that an increase in ICP or a decrease in MAP can compromise CPP and blood flow to the brain. This situation is a common concern for neurosurgical patients during the perioperative period and a critical concern for PACU nurses. Efforts must be simultaneously made to maintain mean arterial pressure while at the same time control the intracranial pressure. Common steps to control intracranial pressure include decreasing brain activity by administering sedative drugs, controlling blood flow to the brain by decreasing carbon dioxide concentration in the brain by hyperventilating the patient, and maintaining a patient in a semi-Fowler's position to optimize venous drainage from the brain. Care must always be taken, though, not to sacrifice mean arterial pressure in an attempt to decrease intracranial pressure, as can happen with the overzealous use of diuretics.[5,10]

Spinal Cord

Protection of the Spinal Cord

Bones of the Spine

The spine is composed of a series of irregular bony vertebrae "stacked" one atop the other to form a strong but flexible column. They are joined by a series of ligaments and intervening cartilages and have two primary functions. Together these structures support the head and trunk. The spine also

protects the spinal cord and its 31 pairs of spinal nerve roots by encasing them in a long canal formed by openings in the center of each vertebra. This vertebral canal extends the entire length of the spine and conforms to the various spinal curvatures and to the variations in size of the spinal cord itself.

There are 7 cervical, 12 thoracic, and 5 lumbar vertebrae. In the adult, the sacrum consists of five vertebrae fused to form one bone. Similarly, the coccyx results from the fusion of four or five rudimentary vertebrae.

Despite variations in their structure, all but two vertebrae share certain anatomic and functional aspects. With the exception of the first and second cervical vertebrae (C1 and C2), all have a solid drum-shaped body that serves as the weight-bearing segment. The posterior segment of the vertebra is called the arch, and each one comprises two pedicles, two laminae, and seven processes (four articular, two transverse, and one spinous). Projecting from the upper part of the body of each vertebra is a pair of short thick pedicles. The concavities above and below the pedicles are the four intervertebral notches. When the vertebrae are articulated, the notches in each adjacent pair of bones form the oval intervertebral foramina, which communicate with the vertebral canal and transmit the spinal nerves and blood vessels.

Arising from the pedicles are two broad plates of bone, the laminae, that meet and fuse at the midline posteriorly to form an arch. Projecting backward and downward from this junction is the spinous process, a knobby projection easily palpated under the skin of the back. Lateral to the laminae, near their junction with the pedicles, are paired articular processes, which facilitate movement of the vertebral column. The two superior processes of each vertebra articulate with the inferior processes of the vertebra immediately above it. The small surfaces where they meet are called *facets*. The transverse processes are located somewhat anterior to the junction of the pedicles and the laminae; they are between the superior and inferior articular processes. These and the spinous processes provide sites for the attachment of muscles and ligaments. The hollow opening formed by the body of the vertebra and the arch is termed the *vertebral foramen*, a protected space through which the spinal cord passes.

Between each of the vertebrae and atop the sacrum is an intervertebral disk composed of compressible tough fibrous cartilage concentrically arranged around a soft pulpy substance called the nucleus pulposus. Each disk acts as a cushionlike shock absorber between the vertebrae. When the intervertebral disk is ruptured, the soft nucleus pulposus can protrude into the vertebral canal, where it can exert pressure on a spinal nerve root and can cause significant, debilitating pain and motor function impairment. This herniated nucleus pulposus may require surgical excision through a laminectomy if the herniation is severe enough.

Many important variations exist among the regional vertebrae. For example, the first cervical vertebra, or atlas, is ring shaped and supports the cranium. It has no body or spinous process and allows for a nodding motion of the head. The second cervical vertebra, or axis, is most striking because of the odontoid process, or dens, that arises perpendicularly to meet with the atlas and allows rotation of the head. The cervical spine as a whole is extremely mobile and is therefore particularly susceptible to acceleration-deceleration and twisting injuries that hyperflex or hyperextend the neck. In addition, the spinal cord is relatively large in this area and therefore sustains damage fairly easily after injury to the cervical spine (Fig. 10-13).

The 12 thoracic vertebrae increase in size as they approach the lumbar area. They are distinctive in that they have facets on their transverse processes and bodies for articulation with the ribs. The thoracic spine is fixed by the ribs, but the lumbar spine is not, which creates a vulnerability that is responsible for an increased incidence rate of fracture or dislocation at T12, L1, and L2. These injuries are typically found in motor vehicle crash victims who were wearing lap seatbelts without shoulder restraints.

The five lumbar vertebrae are large and massive because of their prominent role in weight bearing. They have no transverse foramina. The sacrum, with its five fused vertebrae, is large, triangular, and wedge-shaped. It forms the posterior wall of the pelvis and articulates with L5, the coccyx, and the iliac portions of the hips. The triangular coccyx is formed by four small segments of bone, the most rudimentary part of the vertebral column.[1]

Spinal Meninges

In addition to the bony vertebral column, the spinal cord is covered and protected by the continuous downward projection of the three meninges that perform the same protective function for the brain. The dura mater is the outermost membrane and is a strong but loose and expandable sheath of dense fibrous connective tissue that ends in a sac at the end of the second or third segment of the sacrum and protects the cord and the spinal nerve roots as they leave the cord. The dura does not extend beyond the intervertebral foramina. As noted previously, the spinal dura differs from the cranial dura in that the spinal dura is not attached to the surrounding bone, consists of only one layer, and does not send partitions into the fissures of the cord.

The epidural space is located between the outer surface of the dura and the bones and ligaments of the vertebral canal. It contains a quantity of loose connective tissue, fat, and a plexus of veins. The subdural space is a potential space that lies below the inner surface of the dura and the arachnoid membrane; it contains only a limited amount of CSF.

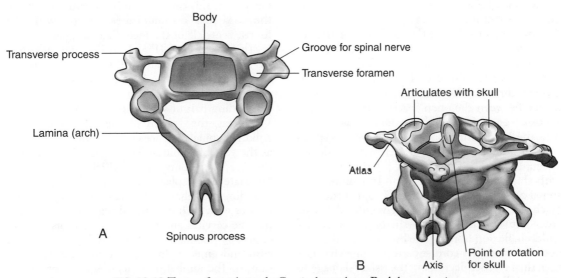

FIG. 10-13 Types of vertebrae. **A,** Cervical vertebrae. **B,** Atlas and axis.

The middle meningeal layer is the arachnoid membrane, which is thin, delicate, and nonvascular; it is continuous with the cranial arachnoid and follows the spinal dura to the end of the dural sac. For the most part, the dura and arachnoid are unconnected, although they are in contact with each other.

The arachnoid is attached to the pia mater by delicate filaments of connective tissue. The considerable space between these two meningeal layers is called the *subarachnoid space*. It is contiguous with that of the cranium and is largest at the lower end of the spinal canal, where it encloses the masses of nerves that form the cauda equina. The spinal subarachnoid space contains an abundant amount of CSF and is capable of expansion to the point of completely filling the entire space included in the dura mater. This subarachnoid space plays a vital role in the regulation of ICP by allowing for the shunting of CSF away from the cranium. When spinal anesthesia is used, the local anesthetic agent is deposited into the subarachnoid space. Because the CSF in the subarachnoid space bathes the spinal nerves as they emerge from the cord, the local anesthetic effectively blocks spinal nerve conduction.

The third and innermost meningeal layer of the spine is the delicate pia mater. Although it is continuous with the cranial pia mater, it is less vascular, thicker, and denser in structure than the pia mater of the brain. The pia mater intimately invests the entire surface of the cord, and, at the point where the cord terminates, it contracts and continues down as a long slender filament (filum terminale) through the center of the bundle of nerves of the cauda equina and anchors the cord at the base of the coccyx.[11]

Lumbar Puncture

The examination of CSF and determination of CSF pressure are frequently of great value in the diagnosis of neurologic and neurosurgical conditions. The collection of CSF is ordinarily accomplished through the insertion of a long spinal needle between the open spaces between L3 and L4 or L4 and L5, through the dura and arachnoid into the subarachnoid space. Because the spinal cord in adults ends at the level of the disk between L1 and L2, danger of injuring the cord with this procedure is minimal. In children, the spinal cord may extend below L3 so that the subarachnoid space is usually safely entered in the areas between L4 and L5. In both adults and children, flexion of the spine by assuming the fetal position raises the cord superiorly somewhat farther, thus further decreasing the risk of damage to the cord. Because the most superior points of the

iliac crests are at the level of the upper border of the spine of L4, they are used as anatomic reference points in selection of the site for lumbar puncture. For a complete description of spinal and epidural anesthesia, see Chapter 25.[12,13]

Structure and Function of the Spinal Cord and the Spinal Nerve Roots

The lowest level of the functional integration of information in the CNS takes place in the spinal cord. Here, information is received in the form of afferent (sensory) nerve impulses from a variety of sensory receptors from the periphery of the body. This information may be processed locally within the cord, but more often is relayed to higher brain centers for additional processing and modification, thus resulting in sophisticated and elaborate motor (efferent) responses. A discussion of the spinal cord primarily involves the consideration of its function as a relay system for both afferent and efferent impulses.

The spinal cord is the elongated slightly ovoid mass of central nervous tissue that occupies the upper two thirds of the vertebral canal. In the adult, it is approximately 45 cm (17 inches) long, although this length varies somewhat among individuals depending on the length of the trunk. The cord is actually an inferior extension of the medulla oblongata and begins at the level of the foramen magnum of the occipital bone.

From that point, the cord continues downward to the upper level of the body of L2, where it narrows to a sharp tip called the *conus medullaris*. From the end of the conus, an extension of the pia mater known as the *filum terminale* continues to the first segment of the coccyx, where it attaches (Fig. 10-14).

The small central canal of the spinal cord contains CSF. This cavity extends the entire length of the cord and communicates directly with the fourth ventricle of the medulla oblongata.

The spinal cord (Fig. 10-15) is composed of 31 horizontal segments of varying lengths. It comprises 8 cervical, 12 thoracic, 5 lumbar, 5 sacral, and 1 coccygeal segment, each with a corresponding pair of spinal nerves attached.

During the growth of the fetus and young child, the spinal cord does not continue to lengthen as the vertebral column lengthens. Consequently, the cord segments, from which spinal nerves originate, are displaced upward from their corresponding vertebrae. This discrepancy becomes greater with each downward segment. For example, the cervical and thoracic nerve roots take an almost horizontal course as they leave the spinal cord and emerge through the intervertebral foramina. The lumbar and sacral nerve roots, however, are extremely long and take an oblique

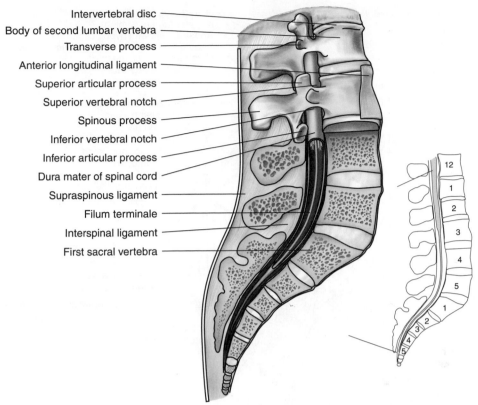

FIG. 10-14 Vertebral column showing structure of vertebrae, filum terminale, and termination of dura mater.

downward course before finally emerging from their appropriate lumbar or sacral intervertebral foramina. The large bundle of nerves lying within the inferior vertebral canal is called the *cauda equina* for its resemblance to a horse's tail (see Fig. 10-15). Several longitudinal grooves divide the spinal cord into regions. The deepest of these grooves is the anterior median fissure. Opposite this, on the posterior surface of the cord, is the posterior median fissure. These fissures divide the cord into symmetric right and left halves that are joined in the central midportion (Fig. 10-16).

Like the brain, the spinal cord comprises areas of gray matter and areas of white matter. Unlike the locations in the brain, the gray matter of the cord is situated deep in its center, whereas the white matter is on the surface. The gray matter of the cord is composed of large masses of nerve cell bodies, along with dendrites of association and efferent neurons and unmyelinated axons, all embedded in a framework of neuroglia cells. The gray matter is also rich in blood vessels. The gray matter has two main functions: (1) synapses within the gray matter relay signals between the periphery and the brain, sometimes via the white matter of the cord; and (2) nuclei in the gray mat-

ter also function as centers for all spinal reflexes and integrate some motor activities within the cord itself, such as the "knee-jerk" stretch reflex.

The white matter of the cord completely invests the gray matter. It consists primarily of long myelinated axons in a network of neuroglia and blood vessels. Its fibers are arranged into bundles called *tracts, columns,* or *pathways* that pass up and down, linking various segments of the cord and connecting the spinal cord with the brain, thus integrating and coordinating sensory and motor functions to or from any level of the CNS.

When viewed in cross section, the gray matter of the cord looks like the letter *H,* two crescent-shaped halves joined together by the gray commissure surrounded by white matter. For descriptive purposes, the four segments of the *H* are called *right* and *left anterior (ventral)* and *posterior (dorsal) horns.* The anterior motor (efferent) neurons lie within the anterior (ventral) gray horns and send fibers through the spinal nerves to the skeletal muscle. The nerve cell bodies that compose the posterior (dorsal) gray horns receive sensory (afferent) signals from the periphery via the spinal nerve roots. The lateral gray horns project from the intermediate portion of the H. The

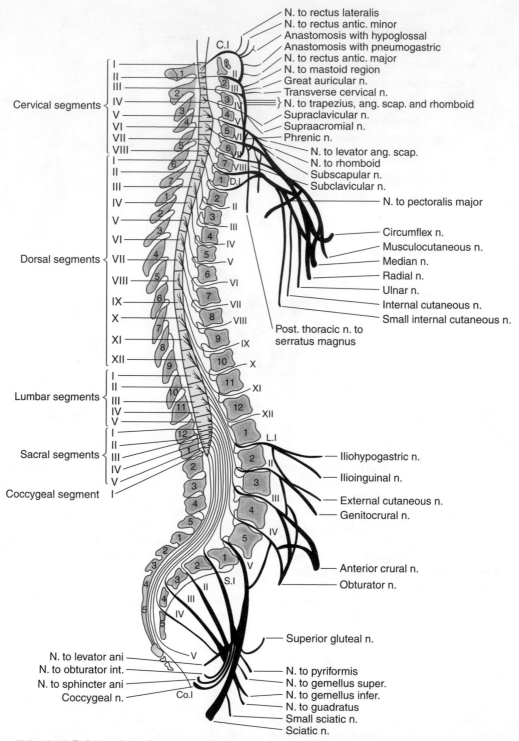

FIG. 10-15 Relationship of segments of spinal cord and their nerve roots to bodies and spinous processes of vertebrae.

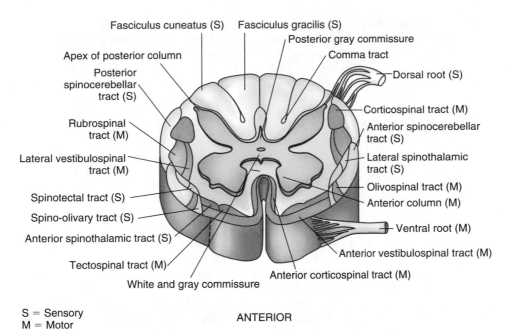

FIG. 10-16 Major ascending and descending tracts of the spinal cord.

nerve cells in these horns (called *preganglionic autonomic neurons*) give rise to fibers that lead to the autonomic nervous system.

The white matter of each half of the cord is divided into the following three columns (or funiculi): ventral, lateral, and dorsal. Each column is subdivided into tracts, which are large bundles of nerve fibers that are arranged in functional groups. The ascending or sensory projection tracts transmit impulses to the brain, and the descending or motor projection tracts transmit impulses away from the brain to various levels of the spinal cord. Some short tracts travel up or down the cord for only a few segments of the cord. These propriospinal (association or intersegmental) tracts connect and integrate separate cord segments of gray matter with one another and consequently have important roles in the completion of various spinal reflexes.

The 31 pairs of spinal nerves are symmetrically arranged. Each nerve contains several types of fibers and arises from the spinal cord by two roots: a posterior (dorsal) and an anterior (ventral) root (Fig. 10-17). The axons that make up the fibers in the anterior roots originate from the cell bodies and dendrites in the anterior and lateral gray horns. The anterior (ventral) root is the motor root, which conveys impulses from the CNS to the skeletal muscles. The posterior (dorsal) root is known as the *sensory root*. Sensory fibers originate in the posterior root ganglia of the spinal nerves.

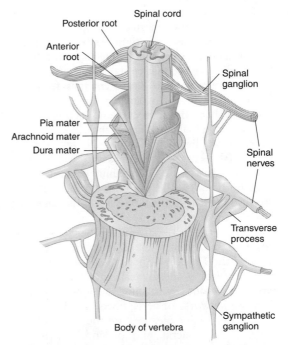

FIG. 10-17 Coverings of the spinal cord. Note how the dura mater extends to cover the spinal nerve roots and nerves. (From Thibodeau GA, Patton KT: *Structure and function of the body*, ed 13, St. Louis, 2008, Mosby.)

PHYSIOLOGIC CONSIDERATIONS IN THE PACU

Each ganglion is an oval enlargement of the root that lies just outside the intervertebral foramen and contains the accumulated cell bodies of the axons that compose the sensory fibers. One branch of the ganglion extends into the posterior gray horn of the cord. The other branch is distributed to both visceral and somatic organs and mediates afferent impulses to the CNS. The cutaneous (skin) area innervated by a single posterior root is called a *dermatome*. Knowledge of dermatome levels is useful clinically in determination of the level of anesthesia after spinal or regional anesthesia (see Chapter 25).[1]

The lateral gray horns of the spinal cord give rise to fibers that lead into the autonomic nervous system, which controls many of the internal (visceral) organs. Sympathetic fibers from the thoracic and lumbar cord segments are distributed throughout the body to the viscera, blood vessels, glands, and smooth muscle. Parasympathetic fibers, present in the middle three sacral nerves, innervate the pelvic and abdominal viscera; therefore the ventral (anterior) root of the spinal nerve is often called the *motor root,* although it is also responsible for the preganglionic output of the autonomic nervous system.

The anterior and posterior roots extend to the intervertebral foramen that correspond to their spinal cord segment of origin. As the roots reach the foramen, the two roots unite to form a single mixed spinal nerve that contains both motor and sensory fibers. As the nerve emerges from the foramen, it gives off a small meningeal branch that turns back through the same foramen to innervate the spinal cord membranes, blood vessels, intervertebral ligaments, and spinal joint surfaces. The spinal nerve then branches into two divisions that are called *rami*. Each ramus contains fibers from both roots. The posterior rami supply the skin and the longitudinal muscles of the back. The larger anterior rami supply the anterior and lateral portions of the trunk and all the structures of the extremities; however, the anterior rami (except those of the 11 thoracic nerves) do not go directly to their destinations. Instead, they are first rearranged without intervening synapses to form intricate networks of nerve fibers called *plexuses*.

The five major plexuses are the cervical, brachial, lumbar, sacral, and pudendal. Peripheral nerves emerge from each plexus and are named according to the region that they supply.

The cervical plexus comprises the first four cervical spinal nerves. The phrenic nerve is the most important branch of the cervical plexus because it supplies motor impulses to the diaphragm. Any injury to the spinal cord above the origin of the phrenic nerve (C4) results in paralysis of the diaphragm and death without mechanical ventilation. Selective anesthesia of the brachial plexuses, which innervate the arms, or pudendal plexuses is often used in regional anesthesia. With the local anesthetic deposited at or near the brachial plexus, the musculocutaneous, median, ulnar, and radial nerves can be anesthetized, thereby allowing painless surgery from the elbow to the fingers. The pudendal nerve, which supplies motor and sensory fibers to the perineum, can be anesthetized with a pudendal plexus block. This type of nerve block is effective in relieving some of the pain of childbirth. Among the nerves given off by the lumbar plexus are the ilioinguinal, genitofemoral, obturator, and femoral nerves. Among those given off by the sacral plexus are the superior and the inferior gluteal nerves.

Anterior rami from the thoracic area do not form a plexus but lead instead to the skin of the thorax and to the intercostal muscles directly. The thoracic and upper lumbar spinal nerves also give rise to white rami (visceral efferent branches), or preganglionic autonomic nerve fibers. Parts of this ramus join the spinal nerves to the sympathetic trunk. The gray ramus is present in all spinal nerves.[14]

Vascular Network of the Spinal Cord

The spinal cord derives its rich arterial blood supply from the vertebral arteries and from a series of spinal arteries that enter the cord at successive levels. Segmentally, the spinal arteries that enter the intervertebral foramina are given off by the intercostal vessels and by the lateral sacral, iliolumbar, inferior thyroid, and vertebral arteries.

The venous supply inside and outside the entire length of the vertebral canal is derived from a series of venous plexuses (Fig. 10-18) that anastomose with each other and end in intervertebral veins. The intervertebral veins leave the cord through the intervertebral foramina with the spinal nerves.

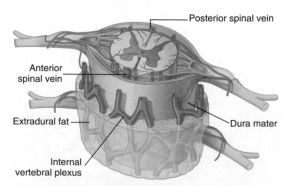

FIG. 10-18 Venous plexuses are veins that drain the spinal cord. (From Drake R, et al: *Gray's anatomy for students,* ed 2, Philadelphia, 2010, Churchill Livingstone.)

Autonomic Nervous System

The autonomic nervous system is composed of the sympathetic and parasympathetic nervous systems. These two divisions of the autonomic nervous system function to regulate and control the visceral functions of the body. In their regulation and control function, they usually work in opposition to each other.

Sympathetic Nervous System

The sympathetic nervous system originates from the thoracolumbar (T1 to L2) segments of the spinal cord. This system is mainly excitatory in physiologic function; however, research indicates that some inhibitory function in the sympathetic nervous system does exist. Because the sympathetic nervous system involves the cardiovascular system and cardiovascular drugs, it is discussed in detail in Chapter 11.

Parasympathetic Nervous System

The parasympathetic nervous system basically functions as an inhibitor of the sympathetic nervous system. It originates in the cranium via cranial nerves III, V, VII, IX, and X. Cranial nerve X, or the vagus nerve, is the most important nerve because it carries about 75% of the parasympathetic nerve impulses. The parasympathetic nervous system also originates in the sacral portion of the spinal cord. Consequently, the parasympathetic nervous system uses the craniosacral outflow tracts.[15] Acetylcholine (ACh) is the main neurotransmitter for the parasympathetic nervous system. The ACh acts on two types of receptors, the muscarinic and nicotinic cholinergic receptors. Because of the pharmacologic implications of the parasympathetic nervous system, it is discussed in detail in Chapters 11 and 23.

SUMMARY

This chapter demonstrates the physiologic concept of regulation and control. The nervous system is highly complex, with both central and peripheral components working in concert. It has electric and chemical neurotransmitters that in many ways functions best in a homeostatic environment. Should the body suffer injury or change in fluid status or temperature, to name a few examples, the nervous system does not function appropriately. Consequently, evaluation of the nervous system by the perianesthesia nurse is an important component of nursing care in the PACU.

REFERENCES

1. Hanson JT: *Netter's clinical anatomy*, ed 2, Philadelphia, 2010, Saunders.
2. Benumof J, Saidman L: *Anesthesia and perioperative complications*, ed 2, St. Louis, 1999, Mosby.
3. Evers A, Maze M: *Anesthetic pharmacology: physiologic principles and clinical practice*, ed 2, Philadelphia, 2011, Churchill Livingstone.
4. Cottrell J, Smith D: *Anesthesia and neurosurgery*, ed 4, St. Louis, 2001, Mosby.
5. Hall J: *Guyton and Hall textbook of medical physiology*, ed 12, St. Louis, 2010, Saunders.
6. Fitzgerald MJT, et al: *Clinical neuroanatomy and neuroscience*, ed 6, St. Louis, 2012, Saunders.
7. Drake R, et al: *Gray's anatomy for students*, ed 2, Philadelphia, 2009, Churchill Livingstone.
8. Brunton L, et al: *Goodman and Gilman's the pharmacological basis of therapeutics*, ed 12, New York, 2010, McGraw-Hill.
9. Stoelting R: *Pharmacology and physiology in anesthetic practice*, ed 4, Philadelphia, 2005, Lippincott Williams & Wilkins.
10. Ganong W: *Review of medical physiology*, ed 23, New York, 2009, McGraw-Hill.
11. Miller R: *Anesthesia*, ed 7, St. Louis, 2009, Saunders.
12. Barash P, et al: *Clinical anesthesia*, ed 6, Philadelphia, 2009, Lippincott Williams & Wilkins.
13. Nagelhout J, Plaus K: *Nurse anesthesia*, ed 4, St. Louis, 2010, Saunders.
14. Miller RD, Pardo M: *Basics of anesthesia*, ed 6, St. Louis, 2011, Saunders.
15. Aitkenhead A, et al: *Textbook of anaesthesia*, ed 5, London, 2007, Churchill Livingstone.

PHYSIOLOGIC CONSIDERATIONS IN THE PACU

11 The Cardiovascular System

Lindsay Cosco, BSN, RN, and Joseph F. Burkard, DNSc, CRNA

The cardiovascular system has a significant impact on the patient recovering from anesthesia. Fortunately, there are many ways available to monitor its status. The cardiovascular system also reflects the status of the patient in the postanesthesia care unit (PACU). More specifically, a return to normal values by the cardiovascular system is a good indicator of the progression of emergence of the patient from anesthesia.[1]

In addition, many drugs used for anesthesia depend on the cardiovascular system to produce their effects. Many of the same drugs also have effects on the cardiovascular system. As a result, the perianesthesia nurse must understand the physiologic principles that relate to the cardiovascular status of the patient in the PACU who has received an anesthetic.

The basic anatomy of certain structures of the cardiovascular system is not covered completely in this chapter because basic nursing texts provide ample material on this subject. However, the clinical correlation between the physiology of the cardiovascular system and perianesthesia nursing care is provided throughout the chapter.[2]

DEFINITIONS

Adrenergic: A term that describes nerve fibers that liberate norepinephrine.
Afterload: The impedance to left ventricular ejection. The afterload is expressed as total peripheral resistance.
Angina Pectoris: Chest pain caused by myocardial ischemia.
Arrhythmia: An abnormal rhythm of the heart, also referred to as *dysrhythmia*.
Arteriosclerosis: Degenerative changes in the arterial walls that result in thickening and loss of elasticity.
Automaticity: The ability of the cardiac pacemaker cells to undergo depolarization spontaneously.
Bathmotropic: Affecting the response of cardiac muscle (or any tissue) to stimuli.
Bigeminy: A premature beat along with a normal heart beat.
Bradycardia: A heart rate of 60 beats/min or less.
Cardiac Arrest: Ventricular standstill.
Cardiac Index: A "corrected" cardiac output used to compare patients with different body sizes. The cardiac index equals the cardiac output divided by the body surface area.

Cardiac Output: The amount of blood pumped to the peripheral circulation per minute.
Cholinergic: Describes nerve fibers that liberate acetylcholine.
Chronotropic: Affecting the rate of the heart.
Conduction: Movement of cardiac impulses through specialized conduction systems of the heart that facilitate coordinated contraction of the heart.
Cor Pulmonale: Pulmonary hypertension as a result of obstruction of the pulmonary circulation that causes right ventricular hypertrophy.
Cyanosis: Bluish discoloration, seen especially on the skin and mucous membranes, as a result of a reduced amount of oxygen in the hemoglobin.
Diastole: The period of relaxation of the heart, especially of the ventricles.
Dromotropic: Affecting the conductivity of a nerve fiber, especially the cardiac nerve fibers.
Ectopic: Located away from a normal position; in the heart, a beat that arises from a focus outside the sinus node.
Ectopic Pacemaker: Focus of ectopic pacemaker shown as premature contractions of the heart that occur between normal beats.
Electrolyte: An ionic substance found in the blood.
Embolism: A blood clot or other substance, such as lipid material, in the blood stream.
Excitability: The ability of cardiac cells to respond to a stimulus with depolarization.
Exsanguinate: To deprive of blood.
Fibrillation: An ineffectual quiver of the atria or ventricles.
Flutter: A condition, usually atrial, in which the atria contract 200 to 400 beats/min.
Heart Block (Complete): A condition that results when conduction is blocked by a lesion at any level in the atrioventricular junction.
Hypertension: Persistently elevated blood pressure.
Hypervolemia: An abnormally large amount of blood in the circulatory system.
Infarction: A necrotic area resulting from an obstruction of a vessel.
Inotropic: Affecting the force of contraction of muscle fibers, especially those of the heart.
Ischemia: Local tissue hypoxia from decreased blood flow.
Leukocytosis: Increased number of white blood cells; a white blood cell count higher than 10,000 per mm^3.
Leukopenia: Decreased number of white blood cells; a white blood cell count lower than 5000 per mm^3.

Murmur: An abnormal heart sound heard during systole, diastole, or both.

Myocardium: The muscular middle layer of the heart between the inner endocardium and the outer epicardium.

Normotensive: With a normal blood pressure.

Occlusion: An obstruction of a blood vessel by a clot or foreign substance.

Pacemaker: The area in which the cardiac rate commences, normally at the sinoatrial node.

Palpitation: A patient's abnormal rate, rhythm, or fluttering of the heart.

Paroxysmal Tachycardia: A period of rapid heart beats that begins and ends abruptly.

Pericarditis: An inflammation of the pericardium.

Peripheral Resistance: Resistance to blood flow in the microcirculation.

Polycythemia: An excessive number of red blood cells, which is reflected in an abnormally high hematocrit level.

Preexcitation Syndrome: When the atrial impulse bypasses the atrioventricular node to produce early excitation of the ventricle.

Preload: The left ventricular end-diastolic volume.

Pulse Deficit: The difference between the apical and radial pulses.

Reentry (Circus Movement): Reexcitation of cardiac tissue by the return of the same cardiac impulse via a circuitous pathway.

Syncope: Fainting, giddiness, and momentary unconsciousness, usually caused by cerebral anoxia.

Systole: The period of contraction of the heart, especially the ventricles.

Thrombosis: The formation of a clot (thrombus) inside a blood vessel or a chamber of the heart.

THE HEART

The Cardiac Cycle

The heart is a four-chambered mass of muscle that pulsates rhythmically and pumps blood into the circulatory system. The chambers of the heart are the atria and the ventricles. The atria, which are pathways for blood into the ventricles, are thin walled, have myocardial muscle, and are divided into the right and left atria by a partition. During each cardiac cycle, approximately 70% of the blood flows from the great veins through the atria and into the ventricles before the atria contract. The other 30% is pumped into the ventricles when the atria contract. On contraction of the right atrium, the pressure in the heart is 4 to 6 mm Hg. The contraction of the left atrium produces a pressure of 6 to 8 mm Hg.[1,2]

Three pressure elevations are produced by the atria, as depicted on the atrial pressure curve. They are termed the *a, c,* and *v waves* (Fig. 11-1). The *a* wave is a result of atrial contraction. The *c* wave is produced by both the bulging of atrioventricular (AV) valves and the pulling of the atrial muscle when the ventricles contract. The *v* wave occurs near the end of the ventricular contraction as the amount of blood in the atria slowly increases and the AV valves close.[1-3]

The ventricles receive blood from the atria and then act as pumps to move blood through the circulatory system. During the initial third of diastole, the AV valves open and blood rushes into the ventricles. This phase is called the *period of rapid filling of the ventricles.* The middle third of diastole is referred to as *diastasis,* during which a small amount of blood moves into the ventricles. During the final third of diastole, the atria contract and the other 30% of the ventricles fills. As the ventricles contract, the AV valves contract and then close, thereby preventing blood from flowing into the ventricles from the atria.[3,4]

As the ventricles begin to contract during systole, the pressure inside the ventricles increases, but no emptying of the ventricles occurs. During this time, called the *period of isometric contraction,* the AV valves are closed. As the right ventricular pressure rises to more than 8 mm Hg and the left ventricular pressure exceeds 80 mm Hg, the valves open to allow the blood to leave the ventricles. This period, termed the *period of ejection,* consumes the first three quarters of systole. The remaining fourth quarter is referred to as *protodiastole,* when almost no blood leaves the ventricles yet the ventricular muscle remains contracted. The ventricles then relax, and the pressure in the large arteries pushes blood back toward the ventricles, which forces the aortic and pulmonary valves to close. This phase is the period of isometric relaxation.

At the end of diastole, each ventricle usually contains approximately 120 mL of blood—the end-diastolic volume. During systole, each ventricle ejects 70 mL of blood, which is the stroke volume. The blood that remains in the ventricle at the end of systole is end-systolic volume and amounts to approximately 50 mL.[3,4]

Cardiac Output

Cardiac output is the amount of blood ejected from the left or right ventricle in 1 minute. In the normal adult with a heart rate of 70 bpm, the cardiac output is approximately 4900 mL. This estimate can be derived with taking the rate of 70 times the stroke volume of 70 mL. User-friendly sophisticated equipment is available to monitor a patient's cardiac output in the PACU. The information derived from serial measurements of the cardiac output can be helpful in assessing the general status of the cardiovascular system and determining the appropriate amount and type of fluid therapy for the patient.[6]

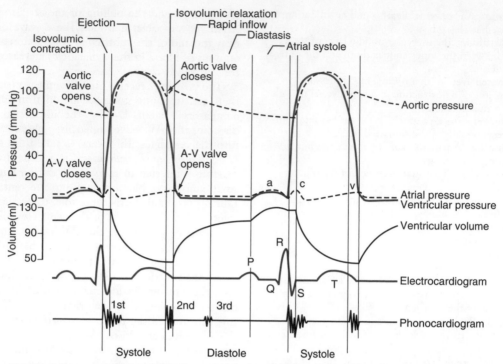

FIG. 11-1 Events of cardiac cycle, showing changes in left atrial pressure, left ventricular pressure, aortic pressure, ventricular volume, electrocardiogram, and phonocardiogram. *A-V,* Atrioventricular. (From Hall J: *Guyton and Hall textbook of medical physiology,* ed 12, Philadelphia, 2011, Saunders.)

The cardiac output is measured with a variety of techniques. Kaplan suggests that the thermodilution method, which uses a pulmonary artery catheter, is the clinical method of choice. For a higher degree of reproducibility, Kaplan recommends a technique of standardization in which the injectate temperature and volume, and the speed of injection, are carefully controlled and duplicated. The most reproducible results have been obtained with injections of 10 mL of cold (1° to 2° C) 5% dextrose in water. It is important to remember that the thermodilution technique measures right-sided cardiac outputs; therefore measurements of cardiac output with the thermodilution technique are usually unreliable for patients with intracardiac shunts.[6,7]

Other methods of calculation of the cardiac output are the Fick and Stewart techniques. The Fick technique involves calculations of the amount of blood needed to carry oxygen taken up from the alveoli per unit of time. This technique is said to be accurate within a 10% margin of error. In the Stewart technique, a known quantity of dye is injected and its concentration is measured after the dye is dispersed per unit of time.[7]

Cardiac output can be influenced by venous return. If the heart receives an extra amount of blood from the veins (↑ preload), the cardiac muscle becomes stretched and the stretched muscle contracts with an increased force to pump the extra blood out of the heart. If the heart receives less blood than normal (↓ preload), according to the Frank-Starling law of the heart, it contracts with less force. This concept is important to the perianesthesia nurse. For example, if a patient is undergoing mechanical ventilation and too much positive end-expiratory pressure is overinflating the lungs, the increased pressure on the inferior vena cava impedes the venous return to the heart, thereby decreasing blood pressure. The blood pressure is derived from the following interacting factors: the force of the heart, the peripheral resistance, the volume of blood, the viscosity of blood, and the elasticity of the arteries. Thus, cardiac output can be seen to play a major role in the maintenance of a normal blood pressure.[6-8]

Arterial Blood Pressure

The arterial blood pressure consists of the systolic and diastolic arterial pressures. The systolic blood pressure is the highest pressure that occurs within an artery during each contraction of the heart. The diastolic blood pressure is the lowest pressure that occurs within an artery during each contraction of the heart. The mean arterial pressure is the average pressure that pushes blood through the systemic circulatory system. Methods of assessing and monitoring the arterial blood pressure in the PACU are discussed in Chapter 27.

Some factors that affect the arterial blood pressure are the vasomotor center, the renal system, vascular resistance, the endocrine system, and chemical regulation. The vasomotor center, located in the pons and the medulla, has the greatest control over the circulation. This center picks up impulses from all over the body and transmits them down the spinal cord and through vasoconstrictor fibers to most vessels of the body. These impulses can be excitatory or inhibitory. One type of pressoreceptor that sends impulses to the vasomotor center is the baroreceptor. The baroreceptors are located in the walls of the major thoracic and neck arteries, in particular, the arch of the aorta. When these vessels are stretched by an increased blood pressure, they send inhibitory impulses to the vasomotor center, which lowers the blood pressure. The aortic and carotid bodies located in the bifurcation of the carotid arteries and along the aortic arch can increase systemic pressure when stimulated by a low partial pressure of oxygen in arterial blood (PaO_2).[9,10]

The renal regulation of arterial pressure occurs through the renin-angiotensin-aldosterone mechanism (see Chapter 13).

The vascular resistance of the systemic vascular system can alter systemic pressure. As the total cross-sectional area of an artery decreases, the systemic vascular resistance increases. Therefore, as the blood flows out of the aorta, a decrease in the arterial pressure in each portion of the systemic circulation is directly proportional to the amount of vascular resistance. This principle is the reason that the arterial pressure in the aorta is much higher than the pressure in the arterioles, which have a small cross-sectional area.

The nervous system, when stimulated with exercise or stress, elevates the arterial pressure via sympathetic vasoconstrictor fibers throughout the body.

Historically, when the radial artery was to be cannulated for direct monitoring of blood pressure and sampling of arterial blood gases in the PACU, a modified Allen test was performed. This test was used for assessing the risk of hand ischemia if occlusion of the cannulated vessel should occur. The modified Allen test is performed with the patient making a tight fist, which partially exsanguinates the hand. The nurse then occludes both the radial and the ulnar arteries with digital pressure. The patient is asked to open the hand, and the compressed radial artery is then released. Blushing of the palm (postischemic hyperemia) should be observed. After approximately 1 minute, the test should be repeated on the same hand with the nurse now releasing the ulnar artery while continuing to compress the radial artery. If the release of pressure over the ulnar artery does not lead to postischemic hyperemia, the contralateral artery should be similarly evaluated. The results of the modified Allen test should be reported as "refill time" for each artery. The modified Allen test at most, is subjective, especially when hand blushing is slow and is rarely done in clinical practice.[11]

Valves of the Heart

The semilunar valves are the aortic and pulmonary valves. They consist of three symmetric valve cusps, which can open to the full diameter of the ring yet provide a perfect seal when closed. During diastole, they prevent backflow from the aorta and pulmonary arteries into the ventricles.

The AV valves are the tricuspid and mitral valves. These valves prevent blood from flowing back into the atria from the ventricles during systole.

Attached to the valves are the chordae tendineae, which are attached to the papillary muscles, which in turn are attached to the endocardium of the ventricles. When the ventricles contract, so do the papillary muscles, thus pulling the valves toward the ventricles to prevent bulging of the valves into the atria (Fig. 11-2).[1,2]

Heart Muscle

The heart muscle comprises three major muscle types: atrial muscle, ventricular muscle, and excitatory and conductive muscle fibers. The atrial

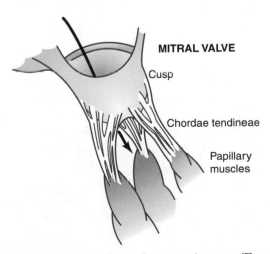

FIG. 11-2 Mitral valve and its attachments. (From Hall J: *Guyton and Hall textbook of medical physiology*, ed 12, Philadelphia, 2011, Saunders.)

and ventricular muscles act much like skeletal muscles. The excitatory and conductive muscles function primarily as an excitatory system for the heart and a transmission system for conducting impulses throughout the heart.

The cardiac muscle fibers are arranged in a latticework; they divide and then rejoin. The constriction of the cardiac muscle fibers facilitates action potential transmission. The muscle is striated, and the myofibrils contain myosin and actin filaments. Cardiac muscle cells are separated by intercalated disks, which are actually the cardiac cell membranes that separate the cardiac muscle cells from one another. The intercalated disks do not hinder conductivity or ionic transport between cardiac muscle cells to any great extent. When the cardiac muscle is stimulated, the action potential spreads to excite all the muscles, which is called a *functional syncytium* (Fig. 11-3). This functional syncytium can be divided into atrial and ventricular syncytia, which are separated by fibrous tissue. However, an impulse can be transmitted throughout the atrial syncytium and then via the AV bundle to the ventricular syncytium. The "all-or-none" principle is in effect: when one atrial muscle fiber is stimulated, all the atrial muscle fibers react if the action potential is met. This principle applies to the entire ventricular syncytium as well.[1,2]

The main properties of cardiac muscle are excitability (bathmotropism), contractility (inotropism), rhythmicity and rate (chronotropism), and conductivity (dromotropism). When cardiac muscle is excited, its action potential is reached and the muscle contracts. Certain chemical factors alter the excitability and contractility of cardiac muscle (Box 11-1).

BOX 11-1   Chemical Factors that Affect Cardiac Muscle Excitability and Contractility

- Causing increase
  - High pH
  - Alkalosis
  - High calcium concentration
- Causing decrease
  - High potassium concentration
  - High lactic acid concentration
  - Acidosis

Conduction of Impulses

The heart has a special system for generating rhythmic impulses. This system for providing rhythmicity and conductivity consists of the sinoatrial (SA) node, the AV node, the AV bundle, and the Purkinje fibers (Fig. 11-4). The SA node is situated at the posterior wall of the right atrium and just below the opening of the superior vena cava. The SA node generates impulses with self excitation, which is produced by the interaction of sodium and potassium ions. The SA node provides a rhythmic excitation approximately 72 times per minute in an adult at rest. The action potential then spreads throughout the atria to the AV node.[1,2]

The AV node is located at the base of the wall between the atria. Its primary function is to delay the transmission of the impulses to the ventricles, which allows time for the atria to empty before the ventricles contract. The impulses then travel

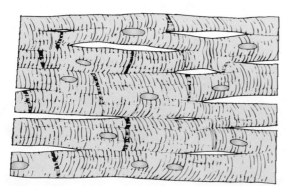

FIG. 11-3 Syncytial nature of cardiac muscle. (From Hall J: *Guyton and Hall textbook of medical physiology*, ed 12, Philadelphia, 2011, Saunders.)

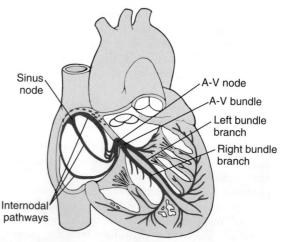

FIG. 11-4 Sinoatrial node and Purkinje's system of the heart. *A-V*, Atrioventricular. (From Hall J: *Guyton and Hall textbook of medical physiology*, ed 12, Philadelphia, 2011, Saunders.)

through the AV bundle, sometimes called the *bundle of His*. The AV node is able to discharge impulses 40 to 60 times per minute if not stimulated by an outside source.

The Purkinje fibers originate at the AV node, form the AV bundle, divide into the right and left bundle branches, and spread downward around the ventricles. The Purkinje fibers can transmit the action potential rapidly, thus allowing immediate transmission of the cardiac impulse throughout the ventricles. The Purkinje fibers are able to discharge impulses between 15 and 40 times per minute if not stimulated by an outside source.

The parasympathetic nerve endings are distributed mostly at the SA and AV nodes, over the atria, and to a lesser extent over the ventricles. If stimulated, they produce a decrease in the rate of rhythm of the SA node and slow the excitability at the AV node. The sympathetic nerves are distributed at the SA and AV nodes and all over the heart, especially the ventricles. Sympathetic stimulation increases the SA node rate of discharge, increases cardiac excitability, and increases the force of contraction.[1,2]

Coronary Circulation

The coronary arteries furnish the heart with its blood supply. The main coronary arteries are on the surface of the heart, but smaller arteries penetrate the heart muscle to provide it with nutrients. The inner surface of the heart derives its nutrition directly from the blood in its chambers.

The coronary arteries originate at two orifices just above the aortic valve. The right coronary artery descends by the right atrium and ventricle and usually terminates as the posterior descending coronary artery. The left coronary artery is usually approximately 1 cm in length and divides into the anterior descending and circumflex arteries. The anterior descending artery usually terminates at the apex of the heart and anastomoses with the posterior descending artery. The anterior descending artery supplies part of the left ventricle, the apex of the heart, and most of the interventricular septum.

The left circumflex artery descends posteriorly and inferiorly down to and terminates in the left marginal artery or communicates with the posterior descending coronary artery. Venous drainage is with superficial and deep circuits. The superficial veins empty into either the coronary sinus or the anterior cardiac veins, both of which drain into the right atrium. The deep veins drain into the thebesian or sinusoidal channels.

The regulation of coronary blood flow is determined primarily with the oxygen tension of the cardiac tissues. The most powerful vasodilator of the coronary circulation is hypoxemia. Other factors that can affect coronary blood flow are carbon dioxide, lactate, pyruvate, and potassium, all of which are released from the cardiac muscle. Coronary artery steal occurs when collateral perfusion of the myocardium is significantly reduced by an increase in blood flow to a portion of the myocardium that is normally perfused. More specifically, drug-induced vasodilatation of normal coronary arterioles can then divert or steal blood flow from potentially ischemic areas of the myocardium perfused by the vessels that have increased resistance (atherosclerotic vessels). Coronary artery steal can occur when arteriolar-vasodilating drugs, such as nitroprusside and isoflurane (Forane), are administered. This situation is especially likely to occur in people who are "stealprone"; they constitute approximately 23% of the patients with coronary artery disease, especially patients who have significant stenosis and occlusions to one or more coronary arteries.[1,2]

Stimulation of the parasympathetic nervous system causes an indirect decrease in coronary blood flow. Direct stimulation is slight because of the sparse amount of parasympathetic nerve fibers to the coronary arteries. The sympathetic nervous system serves to increase coronary blood flow both directly (as a result of the action of acetylcholine and norepinephrine) and indirectly (caused by a change in the activity level of the heart). The coronary arteries have both alpha and beta receptors in their walls (see the section on adrenergic and cholinergic receptors).[12]

Because so much cardiac disease involves the coronary arteries, the anesthetic risk rate increases in patients with cardiac disease. A functional classification of cardiac cases is based on the ability to perform physical activities (Box 11-2). Patients in classes III and IV have a significant risk for surgery and anesthesia and should undergo complete monitoring when they receive care in the PACU.[13]

Effect of Anesthesia on the Heart

Cardiac dysrhythmias are observed in approximately 60% of all patients who undergo anesthesia.[14-15] The inhalation anesthetics, such as isoflurane, sevoflurane, and desflurane, can evoke junctional rhythms or increase ventricular automaticity or both. These anesthetics also slow the rate of SA node discharge and prolong the bundle of His-Purkinje and ventricular conduction times. Along with these changes in rhythm, alterations in the balance of the autonomic nervous system between the parasympathetic and sympathetic systems caused by drugs such as anticholinergics and catecholamines or by light anesthesia can initiate cardiac dysrhythmias. Therefore, in the immediate postoperative

> ### BOX 11-2   Functional Classification of Cardiac Cases
>
> *Class I*: No limitation. Ordinary physical activity does not cause undue fatigue, dyspnea, palpitation, or angina.
>
> *Class II*: Slight limitation of physical activity. Such patients are comfortable at rest. Ordinary physical activity results in fatigue, palpitation, dyspnea, or angina.
>
> *Class III*: Marked limitation of physical activity. Less than ordinary activity leads to symptoms. Patients are comfortable at rest.
>
> *Class IV*: Inability to carry on any physical activity without discomfort. Symptoms of congestive failure or angina are present even at rest. With any physical activity, increased discomfort is experienced.

Modified from Hall J: *Guyton and Hall textbook of medical physiology*, ed 12, Philadelphia, 2010, Saunders.

period, cardiac dysrhythmias are likely because of light anesthesia during emergence or because of the administration of drugs that alter sympathetic activity. Consequently, continuous monitoring of cardiac rate and rhythm is mandated in the PACU.[14,15]

Myocardial Infarction

Acute myocardial infarction is a commonly encountered medical emergency that can occur in the PACU. More than 90% of myocardial infarctions result from disruption of an atherosclerotic plaque with subsequent platelet aggregation and formation of an intracoronary thrombus. The form of myocardial infarction that results depends on the degree of coronary obstruction and associated ischemia. A partially occlusive thrombus is the typical cause of non-ST elevation myocardial infarction. At the other end of the spectrum, if the thrombus completely obstructs the coronary artery, the results are more severe ischemia and a larger amount of necrosis, manifesting as an ST-elevation myocardial infarction.[15,16] The objectives in the management of a patient with an acute myocardial infarction are pain relief, control of complications, salvage of ischemic myocardium, and a return to a productive life. The diagnosis of myocardial infarction is made on the basis of clinical findings, and therapy should be instituted immediately when suspected. (Cardiopulmonary resuscitation is discussed in Chapter 57.) An electrocardiogram performed in the PACU may reveal an injury pattern, but normal electrocardiographic results certainly do not exclude a diagnosis of myocardial infarction.[16]

Physical assessment for a suspected myocardial infarction can include the following subjective findings: (1) pain or pressure, which is usually substernal but may be manifested in the neck, shoulder, jaws, arms, or other areas; (2) nausea; (3) vomiting; (4) diaphoresis; (5) dyspnea; and (6) syncope. The onset of pain can occur with activity but can also occur at rest. The duration may be prolonged, from 30 minutes to several hours. Objective findings can include hypotension, pallor, and anxiety. The blood pressure, pulse, and heart sounds may be normal with an acute myocardial infarction. On auscultation of the chest, the abnormal cardiac findings may include atrial gallop, ventricular gallop, paradoxic second heart sound, friction rub, and abnormal precordial pulsations.[16]

The electrocardiographic pattern can vary by the location and extent of the infarction, but myocardial damage can occur without changes in the electrocardiogram. Some typical features of a transmural infarction are acute ST-segment elevation in leads that reflects the area of injury, abnormal Q waves, and T wave inversion.

Serum Markers of Infarction

Necrosis of myocardial tissue causes disruption of sarcolemma, so that the intracellular macromolecules leak into the bloodstream. Detection of such molecules in the serum, particularly cardiac-specific troponin and creatine kinase MB isoenzyme, serves important diagnostic and prognostic roles.[8-11]

Troponin is a cardiac specific regulatory protein in muscle cells that controls interactions between myosin and actin. Although found in both skeletal and cardiac muscles, the cardiac forms of troponin I and troponin T are structurally unique, and highly specific assays for their detection in the serum have been developed. Cardiac troponin serum levels begin to rise 3 to 4 hours after the onset of chest discomfort, peak between 18 and 36 hours, and then decline slowly, allowing for detection for up to 10 to 14 days after a large infarction.[8-11]

In the absence of trauma, the elevation of CK-MB is highly suggestive of myocardial injury. To facilitate the diagnosis of infarction using this marker, it is common to calculate the ratio of CK-MB to total CK. The ratio is usually greater than 2.5% in the setting of myocardial injury and less than that when CK-MB is from another source. The serum level of CK-MB starts to rise 3 to 8 hours after infarction, peaks at 24 hours, and returns to normal within 48 to 72 hours.[8-11]

Research studies have shown that patients who have had a myocardial infarction within 6 months before surgery have a recurrence rate of 54.5% for a myocardial infarction that could occur during or after the surgical procedure. If the myocardial infarction occurred between 6 months and 2 years before surgery, the rate of recurrence of infarction is between 20% and 25%. Between the second and third years, the incidence rate of reinfarction is approximately 5%. Most studies indicate that 3 years after the original myocardial infarction, the recurrence rate is approximately 1%, which equals the normal rate of myocardial infarction in the general population. Therefore the chance of a patient having an acute myocardial infarction in the PACU can be considered significant. This chance is especially true for patients in the PACU who have had a myocardial infarction within the last 3 years, who have a documented myocardial infarction risk factor (e.g., angina, hypertension, diabetes), or who have some combination of the previous factors.[16-17]

Perianesthesia Nursing Care

The perianesthesia nurse should be constantly alert for complications such as anxiety, arrhythmias, shock, left ventricular failure, and pulmonary and systemic embolisms. Pain and apprehension can be relieved with treatment with morphine sulfate, fentanyl, or hydromorphone (Dilaudid). Oxygen should be administered with nasal prongs because a face mask may increase the patient's apprehension. Continuous cardiac monitoring should be instituted, and the patient should be kept in a quiet area. Drugs such as atropine, lidocaine, digitalis, quinidine, sodium nitroprusside (SNP), phentolamine, and nitroglycerin should be available. A machine for countershock also should be immediately available. Fluid therapy and urine output should be monitored completely for prevention of fluid overload. A pulmonary artery catheter or central venous pressure (CVP) monitor may be used for determining fluid replacement in patients with reduced intravascular volume and hypotension (see the discussion of CVP catheters in the following section). A benign myocardial infarction does not exist; all patients with a diagnosed myocardial infarction need constant competent perianesthesia care.[9,18]

Central Venous Pressure Monitor

The CVP monitor enhances the assessment of venous return and hypovolemia. More specifically, the CVP monitor is used to assess the adequacy of central venous return, blood volume, and right ventricular function. The actual pressure reading obtained from this monitor reflects the pressure in the great veins when blood returns to the heart.

The left ventricular end-diastolic pressure (LVEDP) serves as a good indicator of left ventricular preload. With a patient with a good ejection fraction, the CVP measurement serves as an approximate value for the LVEDP. However, it is important to remember that the CVP has limited value in assessment of left ventricular hemodynamics.

In the immediate postoperative setting, the CVP remains an excellent parameter indicating the adequacy of blood volume. In the hypovolemic state, the CVP is decreased. The administration of appropriate fluids and blood to expand the intravascular space increases the CVP toward the patient's baseline reading. In the clinical setting, no absolute predetermined normal value for a CVP reading exists. The best use of this particular monitoring mode is for serial measurements for assessment of cardiovascular performance. See Chapter 27 for a discussion of the CVP monitor.[4,11,13]

Pulmonary Artery Catheter

The pulmonary artery catheter is used to monitor the central venous, pulmonary artery, and pulmonary capillary wedge pressures. This balloon-tipped catheter with four or five ports is discussed in detail in Chapter 27. Pulmonary artery catheters are used predominantly for cardiothoracic surgical patients and surgical patients with large volume shifts.

In the immediate postoperative period, the pulmonary artery catheter is usually used for patients with clinical shock, compromised ventricular function, and severe cardiac or pulmonary disease. In addition, patients who have had extensive surgical procedures or major cardiovascular surgery can benefit from this monitor. Accurate monitoring of left-sided and right-sided preload along with the rapid determination of cardiac output makes this monitor an excellent parameter for determining mechanical and pharmacologic therapy, with the intended outcome of enhanced cardiac performance and tissue perfusion.[11,13]

CIRCULATORY SYSTEM

Red Blood Cells

The healthy red blood cell (RBC) is in the form of a biconcave disk that can change its shape to move through the microcirculation. The major function of the RBC is the transport of oxygen to the tissue cells; it is also an important factor in carbon dioxide transport. The RBC is responsible for approximately 70% of the buffering power of whole blood in the maintenance of acid-base balance.

RBCs are produced by the bone marrow. The normal rate of production is sufficient to form approximately 1250 mL of new blood per month. This rate is also the normal rate of destruction. The average life span of an RBC is 120 days. The hematocrit value is the percentage of RBCs in the blood. The optimal range in adults is between 30% and 42%. When the hematocrit level is reduced to less than 30%, the oxygen-carrying capacity declines steeply. Moreover, when the hematocrit level rises to greater than 55%, the oxygen-carrying capacity declines because the increase in blood viscosity causes increased work for the heart and decreased cardiac output. The normal amount of hemoglobin in the RBC ranges from 10 to 13.5 g. In fact, the amount and type of hemoglobin determine the oxygen-carrying capacity. Recent evidence indicates that the cutoff value for risk of reduced oxygen-carrying capacity and blood volume is a hemoglobin level of 11 g, a hematocrit of 27%, or both. Transfusion with blood or blood products to raise the level of hemoglobin should be strongly considered for any patient with values lower than the cutoff values.[2]

White Blood Cells

White blood cells (WBCs), or leukocytes, are the body's major defense against infection. The two primary types of circulating leukocytes are polymorphonuclear leukocytes (PMNs) and lymphocytes. The role of the PMNs in combating infection is to migrate to the infectious site in large numbers and phagocytize the invading microbe. The role of the lymphocytes is to mediate immunoglobulin production and act in the delayed hypersensitivity in the type IV reaction (see Chapter 18). Evaluations of the WBC count should focus on the number of PMNs. When the PMN level is less than 1000 per mm³, the incidence rate of infections is increased. Postanesthesia patients with a PMN level of 500 to 100 per mm³ are at great risk of infection.[2]

Some of the major clinical situations that cause a reduction in PMN levels (leukopenia) are viral infections, including human immunodeficiency virus, and cancer chemotherapy.

Blood Platelets

Normal hemostasis requires a proper interaction between blood vessels, platelets, and coagulation proteins. Any dysfunction in any one of the three components has a profound effect on hemostasis. When a tissue injury occurs, the vessel wall undergoes vasoconstriction and activates the extrinsic pathway for coagulation proteins. Platelet adhesion and aggregation occur along with the activation of the intrinsic and extrinsic pathways for the coagulation proteins. The result of this interaction is a hemostatic plug.[2]

Clinical evaluation for proper coagulation focuses on the following four tests: bleeding time (BT), platelet count (PC), prothrombin time (PT), and partial thromboplastin time (PTT). The BT and PC are tests for evaluation of platelet function, and the PT and PTT are tests for evaluation of the coagulation system.

A prolongation of the BT and surgically related hemorrhage seem to be correlated. The normal BT is between 2 and 11 minutes. The test results are considered abnormal when the BT is longer than 12 minutes. The template procedure should be used when the BT is performed because it is more sensitive than older methods. The normal platelet count is between 200,000 and 450,000 per mm³. More specifically, the patient usually tolerates surgery and the postanesthesia phase well in regard to hemostasis with a platelet count of 100,000 per mm³ or higher. Patients with a platelet count of 50,000 to 100,000 per mm³ may have ecchymoses from tissue trauma. If the platelet count is less than 50,000 per mm³, many alterations in bleeding may occur. These patients need constant evaluation and therapy in the postoperative period.[5]

The PTT is a test for evaluation of the intrinsic and common coagulation pathways of the coagulation system. It is most commonly used for monitoring heparin therapy. Normal results are considered to be 25 to 32 seconds, depending on the reagent. Abnormal results are considered to be longer than 35 seconds. The PT is used to examine the extrinsic coagulation system for evaluation of oral anticoagulant therapy. Normal results are based on laboratory control for interpretation. Usually, the control is normal in patients with an appropriately functioning extrinsic coagulation system. When the value is more than 3 seconds greater than the control, the test results are considered to be abnormal. The international normalized ratio (INR) evaluates the extrinsic and common pathway independently of various reagents used in different laboratory setting and in different areas of the world. The normal INR is 1.5 to 2.5. Many institutions report both the PT and INR values.[8] Postoperative bleeding can occur when the patient's preoperative or intraoperative coagulation study results are abnormal. Bleeding tendencies are enhanced by the presence of postoperative hypertension. In addition, when hemostasis is lacking at the suture line or extensive surgical tissue trauma exists, the likelihood of postoperative bleeding is increased. Finally, the use of antibiotics during and after surgery can also increase bleeding tendencies. Therefore the perianesthesia nurse should evaluate the patient's preoperative and intraoperative coagulation study results and examine the surgical incision for bleeding during initial assessment. Certainly, the postoperative trauma patient who has undergone extensive surgical trauma should be constantly monitored for bleeding tendencies, especially if intraoperative antibiotics were administered. If the patient is undergoing anticoagulant therapy, continued monitoring of the anticoagulant activity is mandated. Finally, in the patient with a demonstrated bleeding tendency, maintenance of a normal arterial blood pressure must be ensured. For a complete review of the fluid and electrolyte administration see Chapter 14.[19]

Blood Vessels

The circulatory system can be divided into the systemic and the pulmonary circulation. The systemic or peripheral circulation comprises arteries, arterioles, capillaries, venules, and veins. The walls of the blood vessels, except the capillaries, are composed of three distinct coats: the tunica adventitia, the tunica media, and the tunica intima. The outer layer, the tunica adventitia, consists of white fibrous connective tissue, which gives strength to and limits the distensibility of the vessel. The vasa vasorum, which supplies nourishment to the larger vessels, is in this layer. The middle layer, the tunica media, consists of mostly circularly arranged smooth muscle fibers and yellow elastic fibers. The innermost layer, the tunica intima, is a fine transparent lining that serves to reduce resistance to the flow of blood. The valves of the veins are formed by the foldings of this layer. The capillaries consist of a single layer of squamous epithelial cells, which is a continuation of tunica intima.[2]

The arteries are characterized by elasticity and extensibility. The veins have a poorly developed tunica media and are therefore much less muscular and elastic than arteries.

Microcirculation

Microcirculation is the flow of blood in the finer vessels of the body. It involves the arterioles, capillaries, and venules. The arteries subdivide to the last segment of the arterial system, the arteriole. The arteriole consists of a single layer of smooth muscle in the shape of a tube for conducting blood to the capillaries. As the arterioles approach the capillaries, they lack the coating of smooth muscle and are termed *metarterioles*. At the point at which the capillaries originate from the metarterioles, a smooth muscle fiber (the precapillary sphincter) encircles the capillary. At the other end of the capillary is the venule, which is larger but has a much weaker muscular coat than the arteriole.[2]

The capillaries are usually no more than 4 to 9 mcg in diameter, which is barely large enough for corpuscles to pass through in single file. Blood moves through the capillaries in intermittent flow, caused by the contraction and relaxation of the smooth muscle of the metarterioles and the precapillary sphincter. This motion is termed *vasomotion*. The metarterioles and precapillary sphincter open and close in response to oxygen concentration in the tissues—a form of local autoregulation.

The microcirculation serves three major functions: (1) transcapillary exchange of nutrients and fluids; (2) maintenance of blood pressure and volume flow; and (3) return of blood to the heart and regulation of active blood volume.[2]

ADRENERGIC AND CHOLINERGIC RECEPTORS

The cardiovascular system and the concept of adrenergic and cholinergic receptors are closely related. The perianesthesia nurse must understand the pharmacodynamics of these receptors.[20,21]

Functional Anatomy: The Mediators

Cholinergic is a term used to describe the nerve endings that liberate acetylcholine. The cholinergic neurotransmitter, acetylcholine, is present in all preganglionic parasympathetic fibers, all preganglionic sympathetic fibers, all postganglionic parasympathetic fibers, and all somatic motor neurons. Two exceptions to the general rule are postganglionic sympathetic fibers to the sweat glands and to the vasculature of skeletal muscle. These fibers are considered sympathetic anatomically but cholinergic in terms of their neurotransmitter (i.e., they release acetylcholine as their neurotransmitter).[20,21]

The term *adrenergic* is used to describe nerves that release norepinephrine as their neurotransmitter. Epinephrine may be present in the adrenergic fibers in small quantities, usually representing less than 5% of the total amount of both epinephrine and norepinephrine. The adrenergic fibers are the postganglionic sympathetic fibers, with the exception of the postganglionic sympathetic fibers to the sweat glands and to the efferent fibers to the skeletal muscle (Box 11-3).[20,21]

The adrenal medulla should be considered separately because it is innervated by a preganglionic sympathetic fiber that liberates the neurotransmitter acetylcholine and because the postganglionic portion is the adrenal medulla, which behaves much like a postganglionic sympathetic fiber. The adrenal medulla is therefore stimulated by acetylcholine, which causes the release of both epinephrine and norepinephrine from its chromaffin cells. As opposed to the usual finding of a

---

BOX 11-3   Cholinergic and Adrenergic Nerves

MEDIATOR: ACETYLCHOLINE—CHOLINERGIC NERVES
- Effects
  - All preganglionic parasympathetic fibers
  - All preganglionic sympathetic fibers
  - All postganglionic parasympathetic fibers
  - All somatic motor neurons
  - Postganglionic sympathetic fibers to sweat glands
  - Postganglionic sympathetic vasodilator fibers innervating skeletal muscle vasculature

MEDIATOR: NONEPINEPHRINE—ADRENERGIC NERVES
- Effects
  - All postganglionic sympathetic fibers (except those to sweat glands and efferent fibers to skeletal muscle)

Modified from Nagelhout J, Plaus K: *Nurse anesthesia*, ed 4, St. Louis, 2009, Saunders.

---

preponderance of norepinephrine at the postganglionic nerve fiber terminals, the distribution in the adrenal medulla is 80% epinephrine and 20% norepinephrine. Therefore the neurotransmitter of the adrenal medulla is epinephrine.[2,20,21]

Cholinergic Neurotransmitter: Biochemistry

The neurotransmitter acetylcholine is synthesized from choline and acetate through the enzymatic activity of choline acetylase to form acetylcholine (Box 11-4); it is then stored in vesicles. When acetylcholine is released from a preganglionic fiber, it may then act on the membrane of the preganglionic fiber with a positive feedback mechanism, thus enhancing the release of acetylcholine. The calcium ion facilitates this additional release of acetylcholine. This process is called *excitation-secretion coupling through calcium*.[2,20,21]

Adrenergic Neurotransmitter: Biochemistry

The adrenergic neurotransmitter, epinephrine, begins in the body as phenylalanine, which is hydroxylated to tyrosine, which is again hydroxylated to form L-dopa, an amino acid. This process is probably the weakest step in the biosynthetic chain and may be a possible site of action of an autonomic drug. A soluble enzyme, L-dopa decarboxylase, acts on L-dopa to form dopamine, which in turn is synthesized to norepinephrine. In the adrenal medulla, norepinephrine can be methylated in the cell to form the final product, epinephrine. This reaction is catalyzed by the enzyme phenylethanolamine-N-methyltransferase (see Box 11-4).[20,21]

The storage site of norepinephrine in the adrenergic nerves appears to be in the intracellular granules. Depletion of the total content of norepinephrine through continued nerve stimulation is difficult, but with continuous chronic drug administration, a clinical hypotensive state may be caused by the decreased sympathetic vasomotor tone.

The mechanism of release of norepinephrine from the adrenergic fibers and epinephrine from the adrenal medulla appears to be that of reverse pinocytosis. Pinocytosis is a mechanism by which the membrane engulfs substances in the extracellular fluid. With the influence of the appropriate stimuli, an opening is created through which the soluble contents of a portion of the storage granules are released. The major means of inactivation of norepinephrine is through a mechanism known as *uptake*, in which the released neurotransmitter is recaptured into the neuronal system by the neuron that released it or by neurons adjacent to it and, in some instances, by neurons associated with tissues some distance from the original site of release.

The norepinephrine that is not recaptured is metabolized eventually to vanillylmandelic acid. Epinephrine also undergoes a number of steps in its biodegradation to vanillylmandelic acid. An increase in vanillylmandelic acid concentration in

---

BOX 11-4   Synthesis of Neurotransmitters

CHOLINERGIC

$$\text{Choline} + \text{Acetate} \xrightarrow{\text{Choline acetylase}} \text{Acetycholine}$$

ADRENERGIC

$$\text{Phenylalanine} \longrightarrow \text{Tyrosine} \xrightarrow{\text{Tyrosine hydrolase}} \text{L-dopa} \xrightarrow{\text{L-dopa decarboxylase}}$$

$$\text{Dopamine} \xrightarrow{\text{Dopamine beta oxidase}} \text{Norepinephrine} \xrightarrow{\text{Phenylethanolamine-N-methyltransferase}} \text{Epinephrine}$$

Modified from Nagelhout J, Plaus K: *Nurse anesthesia*, ed 4, St. Louis, 2009, Saunders.

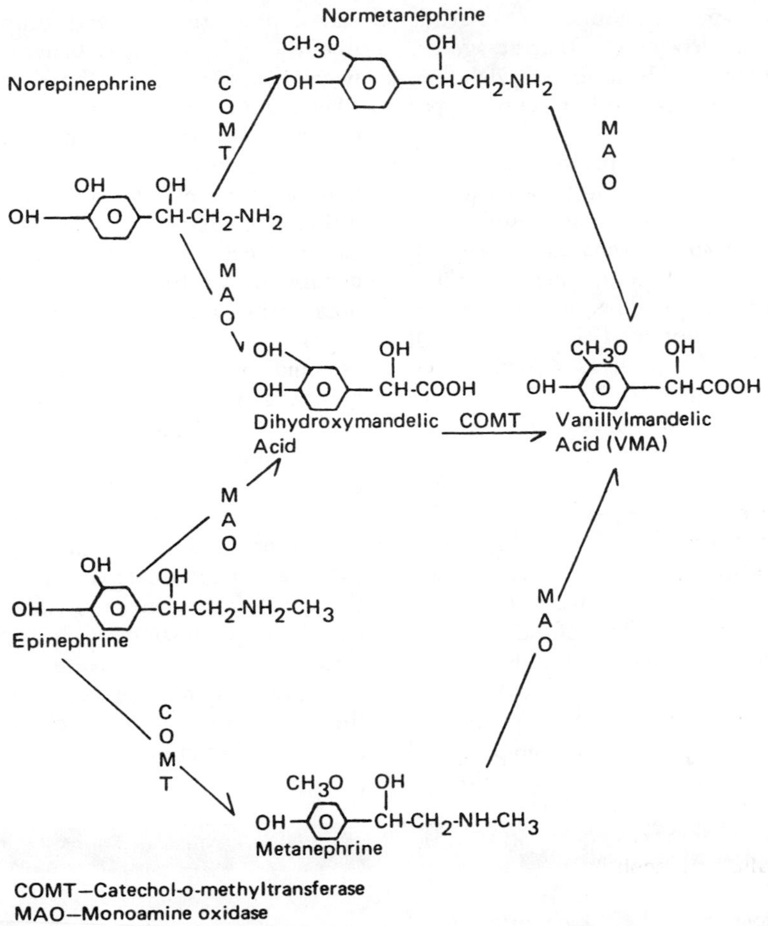

Normetanephrine

Norepinephrine

Dihydroxymandelic Acid — COMT → Vanillylmandelic Acid (VMA)

Epinephrine

Metanephrine

COMT—Catechol-o-methyltransferase
MAO—Monoamine oxidase

FIG. 11-5 Metabolism of epinephrine and norepinephrine. (From Drain CB: Current Concepts on the pharmacodynamics of adrenergic and cholinergic receptors, *AANA J* 44:272, 1976.)

the urine is useful in the diagnosis of conditions such as pheochromocytoma and neuroblastoma (Fig. 11-5).[2,20,21]

When a patient is administered a drug that is a monoamine oxidase inhibitor—such as isocarboxazid (Marplan), pargyline (Eutonyl), phenelzine sulfate (Nardil), or tranylcypromine sulfate (Parnate)—a buildup of epinephrine or norepinephrine can occur and lead to sympathetic hyperactivity. This occurrence is especially likely when substances or drugs such as tyramine or indirect-acting vasopressors, such as ephedrine, are administered.

Cholinergic Receptors

The pharmacologic and physiologic actions of acetylcholine are apparently mediated by its combination with specific cholinergic receptors. The actions of acetylcholine and drugs that mimic acetylcholine are mediated through two types of cholinergic receptors: nicotinic and muscarinic (see Chapter 23).[2,20,21]

When the nicotinic receptors are stimulated, the following responses are observed:
- Stimulation of autonomic ganglia, both parasympathetic and sympathetic.
- Stimulation of the adrenal medulla, which results in the release of both epinephrine and norepinephrine.
- Stimulation of skeletal muscle at the motor endplate.

The muscarinic responses elicited by muscarine and acetylcholine are the following:
- Stimulation or inhibition of smooth muscle in various organs or tissues.
- Stimulation of exocrine glands.
- Slowing of cardiac conduction.
- Decrease in myocardial contractile force.

Nicotinic responses in terms of antagonism can be blocked with drugs such as ganglionic or neuromuscular blocking agents, or both, whereas muscarinic responses are blocked with the class of drugs best typified by atropine.[2,20,21]

PHYSIOLOGIC CONSIDERATIONS IN THE PACU

Muscarine is a specific agonist at muscarinic receptors, whereas nicotine is a specific agonist at nicotinic receptors. However, acetylcholine is capable of stimulating both receptor types (Table 11-1).[2,20,21]

A series of compounds is specific in its ability to combine with acetylcholinesterase and inhibit its activity through competitive inhibition. The prototype compounds in this category are neostigmine (Prostigmin), physostigmine salicylate (Antilirium), pyridostigmine (Regonol, Mestinon), and edrophonium (Tensilon, Enlon).

Belladonna alkaloids such as atropine have adverse effects that are peculiar to the PACU phase of the surgical experience. More specifically, belladonna alkaloids that cross the blood-brain barrier can cause disorientation, violent behavior, or somnolence. Physostigmine salicylate, an anticholinesterase that is capable of penetrating the blood-brain barrier, has been shown to be useful in reversing the adverse effects of belladonna alkaloids on the central nervous system. Physostigmine salicylate is also useful in reversing the disorientation or somnolence caused by drugs such as diazepam, phenothiazines, tricyclic antidepressants, antiparkinsonian drugs, promethazine, and droperidol. Patients in the PACU who may benefit from treatment with physostigmine are those who have received a belladonna alkaloid or neuroleptic type of agent either before or during surgery, who have had disorientation or restlessness or both for more than 30 minutes after anesthesia, and who are difficult to arouse over an appropriate period. Patients with any one of these dysfunctions qualify for treatment and can be given 1-mg increments of physostigmine intravenously at 15-minute intervals until they are conscious and oriented to time, place, and person. After treatment has begun, the perianesthesia nurse should monitor the blood pressure and pulse immediately before and 5 minutes after the administration of physostigmine. In addition, some patients may have side effects from physostigmine, such as nausea, pallor, sweating, and bradycardia. Because glycopyrrolate (Robinul) does not cross the blood-brain barrier, treatment of the side effects of physostigmine is especially helpful. Finally, patients who have undergone treatment with physostigmine probably should remain in the PACU for approximately 1 hour after the administration of the anticholinesterase.[20-23]

Table 11-1	Cholinergic Receptors	
ORGAN STIMULATED BY CHOLINERGIC AGONIST	RESPONSE	TYPE OF CHOLINERGIC RECEPTOR RESPONSE
Heart		
Sinoatrial node	Negative chronotropic effect	Muscarinic
Atria	Decreased contractility and increased conduction velocity	Muscarinic
AV node and conduction system	Decrease in conduction velocity—AV block	Muscarinic
Eye		
Sphincter muscle of iris	Contraction (miosis)	Muscarinic
Lung		
Bronchial muscle	Contraction	Muscarinic
Bronchial glands	Stimulation	Muscarinic
Exocrine Glands		
Salivary glands	Profuse watery secretion	Muscarinic
Lacrimal glands	Secretion	Muscarinic
Nasopharyngeal glands	Secretion	Muscarinic
Adrenal medulla	Catecholamine secretion	Nicotinic
Autonomic ganglia	Ganglion stimulation	Nicotinic Muscarinic
Skeletal Muscle		
Motor endplate	Stimulation	Nicotinic (motor endplate receptor)

Modified from Nagelhout J, Plaus K: *Nurse anesthesia*, ed 4, St. Louis, 2009, Saunders.
AV, Atrioventricular.

Adrenergic Receptors

The stimulation of the sympathetic nervous system can be both inhibitory and excitatory, which has caused considerable confusion. Originally, theories were postulated that this phenomenon handled the release of two different compounds. The variation in the effects of stimulation was later found to be related not to the differences in chemical release but rather to a difference in the receptors' responses to the transmitter.[2]

The adrenergic receptors, which respond to catecholamines, can be subdivided into three main types: dopaminergic, alpha, and beta. The dopaminergic receptors are primarily in the central nervous system and the mesenteric and renal blood vessels. The agonist for these receptors is dopamine. The alpha receptors can be further divided into $alpha_1$ and $alpha_2$ receptors. The postsynaptic $alpha_1$ receptors are excitatory in action, except in the intestine. Stimulation of the $alpha_1$ receptors causes smooth muscle contraction, which results in a vasoconstriction or pressor response. Hence, the $alpha_1$ receptor is activated by the release of norepinephrine, and this released norepinephrine also activates the presynaptic $alpha_2$ receptors to inhibit the further release of norepinephrine. As a result, the $alpha_1$ receptor is activated by the release of norepinephrine, and the released norepinephrine in turn stimulates the $alpha_2$ receptor, thus producing inhibition of the release of norepinephrine and resulting in a negative feedback loop (Fig. 11-6).[24]

The drug clonidine (Catapres) is believed to stimulate the $alpha_2$ receptors, which lower the sympathetic outflow of norepinephrine and ultimately lead to a hypotensive effect. In addition to lowering catecholamine levels, clonidine can reduce the plasma renin activity. This antihypertensive drug enjoys a significant degree of popularity, but it can have a negative effect on the patient in the PACU. More specifically, the clonidine withdrawal syndrome has been reported when the drug has been stopped abruptly. The sequelae of the syndrome resemble pheochromocytoma in that shortly after the withdrawal of the clonidine the patient can have hypertension, tachycardia, and increased blood levels of catecholamines. Treatment of this syndrome usually involves a reinstitution of the clonidine therapy and alpha-adrenergic blocking agents such as phentolamine.[24]

Stimulation of the beta receptor causes vascular smooth muscle relaxation, which then leads to a decrease in blood pressure through a decrease in peripheral resistance. The beta receptor can be divided into two types: $beta_1$ and $beta_2$. $Beta_1$-subtype receptors are found in all cardiac tissue except the coronary vasculature and are responsible

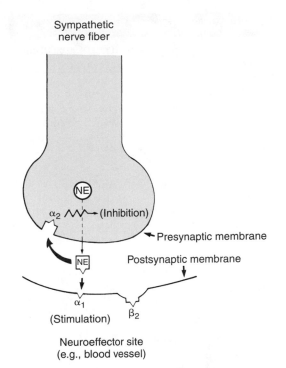

Sympathetic
nerve fiber

NE

$alpha_2$ ⟶ (Inhibition)

← Presynaptic membrane

NE

Postsynaptic membrane

$alpha_1$ $beta_2$
(Stimulation)

Neuroeffector site
(e.g., blood vessel)

FIG. 11-6 Presynaptic and postsynaptic alpha receptors at ending of norepinephrine (NE)-secreting neuron. (From Gardenhire DS: *Rau's respiratory care pharmacology*, ed 7, St. Louis, 2008, Mosby.)

for characteristic effects noted after stimulation of the heart with epinephrine, including the following effects: (1) increase in heart rate; (2) increase in contractile force; (3) increase in conduction velocity; and (4) shortening of the refractory period. $Beta_1$-subtype receptors mediate effects elicited by catecholamines (Table 11-2).[21-24]

The physiology of the beta receptor has many implications for the care of the PACU patient. Once the beta receptor has been activated by first messengers, endogenous catecholamines, or exogenous beta agonists such as isoproterenol, certain biochemical events occur (Fig. 11-7). The enzyme adenylate cyclase, which is located on the plasma membrane, is stimulated with beta-receptor activation. Next, within the cell, adenosine triphosphate is broken down to $3',5'$-adenosine monophosphate (cyclic AMP). The cyclic AMP is then released into the cytoplasm of the cell and acts to modulate cellular activities. Hence, the cyclic AMP is considered to be the second messenger. Cyclic AMP is inactivated to 5-AMP by the enzyme phosphodiesterase.[21-24]

Clinically, isoproterenol or terbutaline can be administered to increase the cyclic AMP levels in the $beta_2$ receptors in the bronchial airways with

Table 11-2	Adrenergic Receptors
RESPONSE	**TYPE OF ADRENERGIC RECEPTOR**
Heart	
Positive inotropic effect	Beta$_1$
Positive chronotropic effect	Beta$_1$
Cardiac arrhythmias	Beta$_1$
Positive dromotropic effect	Beta$_1$
Vascular	
Arterial and arteriolar constriction	Alpha$_1$
Coronary artery constriction	Alpha$_1$
Coronary artery dilatation	Beta$_1$
Arteriolar relaxation	Beta$_2$
Gastrointestinal Tract	
Intestinal relaxation	Alpha$_1$, beta$_1$
Sphincter contraction (usually)	Alpha$_1$
Urinary Bladder	
Bladder relaxation (detrusor)	Beta$_2$
Bladder contraction (trigone and sphincter)	Alpha$_1$
Eye	
Contraction (mydriasis)	Alpha$_1$
Ciliary muscle of iris	Beta$_2$
Metabolic	
Liver glycogenolysis (hyperglycemia)	Alpha$_1$, beta$_2$
Muscle glycogenolysis	Beta$_1$
Lipolysis	Beta$_1$
Oxygen consumption (increases)	Beta$_1$, beta$_2$
Other Smooth Muscle	
Bronchial (relaxation)	Beta$_2$
Spleen (contraction)	Alpha$_1$
Ureter (contraction)	Alpha$_1$
Uterus (contraction)	Alpha$_1$
Uterus (relaxation)— nonpregnant condition	Beta$_2$

Modified from Nagelhout J, Plaus K: *Nurse anesthesia*, ed 4, St. Louis, 2009, Saunders.

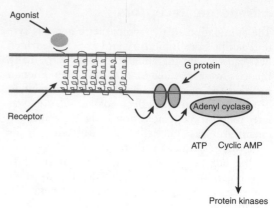

FIG. 11-7 Beta receptors belong to the family of G protein-coupled receptors. The pathway involves binding of an agonist, such as a catecholamine, to an extracellular receptor. *ATP,* Adenosine triphosphate; *cyclic AMP,* 3′,5′-adenosine monophosphate. (From Topol EJ: *Textbook of interventional cardiology,* ed 5, St. Louis, 2008, Saunders.)

the intended result of bronchodilatation. Another way to increase the cyclic AMP levels is inhibition of the action of phosphodiesterase. Caffeine and methylxanthines, such as aminophylline, are inhibitors of the enzyme phosphodiesterase and can be used alone or in combination (for synergistic effects) with the beta agonists to produce the desired bronchodilatation in the patient. It is important to remember that other catecholamine effects are produced by the increase in cyclic AMP levels. Consequently, although aminophylline is considered a bronchodilator, it increases the myocardial contractility and heart rate of the patient, thus mandating that the perianesthesia nurse monitor both respiratory and cardiac function when methylxanthines are administered.

The coronary arteries contain alpha$_1$ and beta$_1$ receptors and therefore also have the ability to vasoconstrict and vasodilate (see Table 11-2). The endogenous catecholamines, norepinephrine and epinephrine, are capable of stimulating both the alpha and the beta receptors.[21-24]

Site of Action of Autonomic Drugs

Methyldopa (Aldomet; the alpha-methylated analogue of L-dopa) is an antihypertensive drug. Methyldopa reduces the sympathetic nerve stimulation through the production of a selective agonist, alpha methylnorepinephrine.[21-24]

Guanethidine has the ability to prevent nerve stimulation and thus inhibit norepinephrine release. Guanethidine interferes with the storage of norepinephrine and, if given chronically, results in a decrease in the amount of norepinephrine stored in adrenergic nerves. Reserpine also shares this latter action with guanethidine. Therefore chronic use of guanethidine and reserpine results in a relative depletion of the norepinephrine content from sympathetic nerves (Table 11-3).

The calcium channel blockers have been found to have considerable value in the treatment of supraventricular tachycardias, angina pectoris, and myocardial infarction. The prototype calcium channel blockers are verapamil (Isoptin), nifedipine (Procardia, Adalat), and diltiazem (Cardizem). All three drugs depress calcium entry into conduction

Table 11-3   Drugs that Interfere with Specific Steps in Process of Chemical (Neurohumoral) Transmission

CHEMICAL TRANSMISSION	ADRENERGIC NERVES	CHOLINERGIC NERVES
Synthesis of mediator	Methyldopa	Hemicholinium
Storage of mediator	Reserpine	—
Release of mediator	Guanethidine	Botulinus toxin
Combination of mediator with its receptor	Phenoxybenzamine (alpha receptor)	Atropine (muscarinic)
	Propranolol (beta receptor)	Nicotine (nicotinic)
Enzymatic destruction of mediator	Pyrogallol (COMT inhibitor)	Physostigmine (cholinesterase inhibitor)
	Tranylcypromine (MAOI)	
Prevention of inactivation of mediator (blocks uptake)	Cocaine	—
Repolarization of postsynaptic membrane (persistent depolarization)	—	Succinylcholine

From Nagelhout J, Plaus K: *Nurse anesthesia*, ed 4, St. Louis, 2009, Saunders.
COMT, Catechol-*O*-methyltransferase; *MAOI,* Monoamine oxidase inhibitor.

tissue and cardiac muscle, which results in a depression of conduction and leads to a reduction of the circus movements. These calcium entry blockers produce hypotension with different mechanisms. Nifedipine, like SNP, decreases the systemic vascular resistance with a compensatory tachycardia, and verapamil and diltiazem lower the cardiac output by exerting a negative dromotropic effect. The effects of the calcium channel blockers can be enhanced with inhalation anesthesia agents such as halothane. Consequently, in the PACU, patients who received an inhalation of anesthetic and are undergoing treatment with a calcium channel blocker may have some hypotension. Therefore the perianesthesia nurse should vigorously monitor the cardiovascular parameters of these patients and report any confirmed hypotension to the attending physician.[20-24]

Dopamine is a naturally occurring biochemical catecholamine precursor of norepinephrine. It exerts a positive inotropic effect and a minimal chronotropic effect on the heart. Therefore, the contractility of the heart is increased without a change in the afterload (total peripheral resistance), which leads to an increase in cardiac output. The increase is in the systolic and pulse pressures, with virtually no effect on the diastolic pressure. Dopamine is not associated with tachyarrhythmias and produces less of an increase in myocardial oxygen consumption than does isoproterenol. Blood flow to peripheral vascular beds may decrease while mesenteric flow increases. One of the major reasons for the increase in the use of dopamine clinically is its dilatation of the renal vasculature. This action is the result of the inotropic effect and decreased peripheral resistance. Therefore the glomerular filtration rate is increased along with the renal blood flow and sodium excretion.[20-24]

Dobutamine (Dobutrex) is synthetically derived from the catecholamine isoproterenol. Consequently, it produces a positive inotropic effect with specificity to the beta$_1$ receptors, thus resulting in an increase in cardiac output with minimal effects on blood pressure, heart rate, and systemic vascular resistance. The drug is usually administered intravenously in a dose range of 2 to 10 mcg/kg/min and is especially useful for patients who are recovering from cardiopulmonary bypass surgery. Dobutamine is sometimes combined with a vasodilator to reduce afterload in an effort to optimize the cardiac output.[20-24]

Hypotension Therapy

Hypotension in the immediate postoperative period is of great concern and deserves the prompt attention of the perianesthesia nurse. When hypotension is detected in the postanesthesia patient, the nurse should first reaffirm the measurements. An incorrectly placed or sized blood pressure cuff or malfunction of the stethoscope can yield incorrect measurements (see Chapter 27). If an arterial catheter transducer system is used, it should be appropriately zeroed and calibrated and the air bubbles removed to ensure that artificially low readings are not observed. In addition, if the patient is hypothermic or receiving alpha-adrenergic agonists such as phenylephrine (Neosynephrine), the patient may have low blood pressures in the radial and brachial arteries, whereas the central blood pressure may be higher. This difference is because of the peripheral vasoconstriction produced by the alpha-adrenergic drugs.[25]

If the hypotension is confirmed, hypovolemia should be considered as a possible cause. The clinical signs of hypotension from hypovolemia include cold, pale, clammy, or diaphoretic skin; rapid, thready pulse; shallow, rapid respirations; disorientation, restlessness, or anxiety; decreased CVP; and oliguria. The nursing assessment of the patient with hypotension should include an inspection of the dressings for excessive bleeding and an evaluation for the clinical signs of hypovolemia. If the patient's circulating blood volume is reduced by more than 15% to 20%, hypotension can ensue. This condition usually happens when the patient has not received appropriate fluid volume replacement during surgery. Other factors in the development of postoperative hypovolemia are ongoing internal or external hemorrhage, sweating, insensible losses, and third-space losses. Third-space losses occur when an exudation of fluid into the tissues occurs (see Chapter 14). Other causes of hypotension include a high alveolar-inflating pressure when a patient is undergoing mechanical ventilation, ventricular dysfunction, myocardial ischemia, and cardiac dysrhythmias. If the hypotension is 30% less than the preoperative baseline blood pressure readings or one or more of the clinical signs of hypovolemia is present, then the attending physician should be notified.[25]

Usual therapy for hypotension in the PACU includes the administration of a high fractional concentration of oxygen, fluid infusion, reversal of residual anesthetic depressant effects, repositioning of the patient to facilitate venous return, reduction in ventilator airway pressures, and administration of vasopressors or anticholinergics or both, such as glycopyrrolate or atropine, as indicated. More specifically, the first line of defense is to return the patient's condition to normovolemia and, in this instance, administer a bolus of crystalloid solution of 300 to 500 mL. The anticholinergics are indicated if sinus bradycardia accompanies the hypotension. The vasopressors exert their effect either directly or indirectly. The direct-acting vasopressor exerts its effect directly on the receptor. Conversely, the pharmacologic action of an indirect vasopressor facilitates the release of norepinephrine from its storage vesicles (primarily the terminal sympathetic nerve fibers), which stimulates the adrenergic receptor to achieve the desired effect. Therefore a direct-acting vasopressor is probably necessary to achieve a response in patients who are depleted of catecholamines by drugs such as reserpine and guanethidine (Table 11-4).[20-25]

Another area of consideration in selection of a vasopressor is the cardiotonic action desired.

Table 11-4 Adrenergic Drugs According to Action

GENERIC NAME	TRADE NAME
Direct-Acting Adrenergic Amines	
Epinephrine	Adrenalin
Norepinephrine	Levophed
Dopamine	Intropin
Dobutamine	Dobutrex
Isoproterenol	Isuprel
Methoxamine	Vasoxyl
Phenylephrine	Neosynephrine
Indirect-Acting Adrenergic Amines	
Metaraminol	Aramine
Mephentermine	Wyamine
Ephedrine	Ephedrine

Metaraminol (Aramine), with its action of norepinephrine release, causes improved cardiac function as a result of its beta-receptor activity. Conversely, phenylephrine and methoxamine (Vasoxyl) possess little or no cardiac effect and exert a pressor action with pure alpha stimulation. The alpha-adrenergic agonists are useful especially for patients who have received a "high" spinal or epidural anesthetic. High levels of regional anesthetics are associated with peripheral vasodilatation and bradycardia because of a sympathetic blockade. Consequently, an alpha-adrenergic agonist produces peripheral vascular vasoconstriction, or a mixed-action alpha and beta drug such as ephedrine can be administered.[20-25]

Drugs that combat hypotension include the cardiac inotropic agents. This class of drugs produces positive inotropic and vasodilating effects and can be considered to be related to digitalis in regard to pharmacologic effects. The major pharmacologic actions of these drugs include increased cardiac output and decreased LVEDP. These drugs are of benefit for the short-term management of congestive heart failure, especially in patients with congestive heart failure who do not have adequate responses to digitalis, diuretics, or vasodilators. Also, the inotropic agents may be valuable in the treatment of cardiogenic shock. This class of drugs can be considered as an alternative to catecholamines for the treatment of low cardiac output in the postoperative period. Drugs in this category include amrinone (Inocor) and milrinone (Primacor). As with other vasopressors, constant monitoring of the patient's vital signs is warranted when inotropic agents are administered.[20-25]

Hypertension Therapy

A hypertensive emergency can occur in the PACU. The patient may arrive in a hypertensive state or become hypertensive during the postanesthesia phase. If the diastolic blood pressure rises to 120 to 140 mm Hg and the patient has a headache, blurred vision, and papilledema along with disorientation, then the physician should be notified immediately.

Before any intervention can be instituted, the cause of the postoperative hypertension must be determined. First, the evaluation should focus on the equipment used to determine the blood pressure; it might not be functioning correctly. For example, the blood pressure cuff may be too narrow; the transducer may not be calibrated correctly; or transducer overshoot may be seen. Next, the evaluation should focus on preexisting diseases. More specifically, the patient may have essential hypertension, and the blood pressure readings may be normal for that patient.

Increased sympathetic nervous system activity causes postoperative hypertension. More specifically, pain, stimulation with an endotracheal tube, bladder distention, and preeclampsia are some of the clinical phenomena that may lead to hypertension. Postoperative pain should be assessed because it can cause a significant degree of hypertension. Pain can be eliminated as a causative factor with determination of whether adequate analgesia exists. If the patient has a significant amount of pain, an analgesic should be administered immediately. In addition, if the hypertension is caused by acute anxiety, the use of sedatives may dramatically reduce the blood pressure. Hypoxemia with hypercarbia from hypoventilation is also a common cause of postoperative hypertension. Therefore, during the evaluation of the patient, the patient's rate and depth of ventilation should be assessed. If the patient has hypoventilation, prompt use of the stir-up regimen is mandated. Another assessment tool in the evaluation of postoperative hypertension is the amount and degree of hypothermia. More specifically, if the patient is shivering, an accompanying increase in blood pressure is seen. Prompt interventions to increase the patient's core temperature to reduce shivering is warranted (see Chapter 53). An assessment of the patient's fluid volume status should be made to determine whether hypervolemia exists because fluid overload can cause postoperative hypertension. In addition, if the patient has acute pulmonary edema caused by hypertensive heart disease, correction of the pulmonary edema usually reduces the blood pressure to acceptable limits. Certainly, whether a hypertensive emergency exists should be determined; if it does, treatment must be started promptly.[20-25]

If pharmacologic antihypertensive therapy is deemed necessary by the physician, the drugs listed in Table 11-5 usually are instituted. For severe postoperative hypertension, SNP is probably the drug of choice. While the SNP is prepared, nifedipine or diltiazem can be given intravenously. Calcium channel blockers decrease blood pressure, cardiac workload, and myocardial oxygen consumption especially in the presence of ischemic heart disease. In addition, the use of nifedipine or diltiazem may preclude the use of a central venous catheter that is required when SNP is given. Once the patient's condition is stabilized, hydralazine (5 to 10 mg) and propranolol (0.2 to 0.5 mg) can be given in repeated intravenous doses to wean the patient off SNP. Propranolol should be titrated to maintain the heart rate at approximately 100 beats/min. Other beta blockers, such as labetalol, metoprolol, and esmolol, can be used intravenously. Esmolol may be the drug of choice because of its short duration of action and rapid onset. The hydralazine can be given as intravenous boluses every 20 to 30 minutes to keep the patient's condition normotensive. Because these drugs are extremely potent and have their own complications, they are discussed briefly in the following sections.[20-25]

Recent research has shown that beta-blockers are able to aid in controlling the sympathetic responses of patients in the perioperative phase of recovery. Controlling sympathetic responses reduces perioperative myocardial ischemia and improves long-term survival in vascular and cardiovascular surgical patients. Research has also shown that the use of alpha-2-agonists such as clonidine and dexmedetomidine in the postanesthesia phase decreases oxygen consumption and improves hemodynamic outcomes.[24]

Dexmedetomidine

Dexmedetomidine is indicated for sedation of patients requiring postoperative mechanical ventilation in the PACU setting. Its indication in the United States was recently expanded to include nonintubated patients requiring sedation for surgery or procedures. Dexmedetomidine is also useful as an adjunct for sedation and general anesthesia in the setting of certain operations and invasive medical procedures, such as colonoscopy. There are no absolute contraindications to the use of dexmedetomidine; its usefulness is limited because the drug cannot be given as a bolus owing to concerns about peripheral alpha-2 receptor stimulation with

Table 11-5   Drugs Used for Treatment of Hypertensive Crisis

DRUG*	ROUTE	INITIAL DOSE	ONSET OF ACTION (MIN)	DURATION OF ACTION	COMMENT
Diazoxide (Hyperstat)	IV	3-5 mg/kg slow bolus	3-5	5-12 hours	
Sodium nitroprusside (Nipride, Nitropress)	IV	0.25-0.5 mcg/kg/min	1-2	<5 min	Titrate dose for desired effect
Nitroglycerin (Tridil, Nitrol IV, Nitrostat IV)	IV	0.25-3 mcg/kg/min	2-5	<5 min	
Phentolamine (Regitine)	IV	5-15 mg bolus; 200-400 mg/L infusion	Immediate	<15 min	Titrate dose for desired effect
Hydralazine (Apresoline)	IV	5-10 mg	15-20	4-6 hours	Given slowly when IV
	IM	10-40 mg	30		
Trimethaphan camsylate (Arfonad)	IV	10-20 mcg/kg/min	1	2-4 min	
Propranolol (Inderal, Ipran)	IV	0.1-0.5 mg slowly, up to 2 mg	10	4-6 hours	May repeat dose
Esmolol (Brevibloc)	IV	50-300 mcg/kg/min	5	20 min	Avoid concentration > 10 mg/mL
Labetalol (Normodyne, Trandate)	IV	0.25 mg/kg	10	4-6 hours	Give slowly
Nifedipine (Procardia, Adalat)	SIV	10 mg	3	7 hours	SIV dose while nitro-glycerin is prepared
	IV	10 mg (slow)	5-10		
Verapamil (Calan, Isoptin)	IV	2.5-5 mg	2-5	4-6 hours	

IV, Intravenous; *IM*, intramuscular; *SIV*, slow intravenous infusion.
*Listed by generic name, with trade name in parentheses.

resulting hypotension. Compared to midazolam, dexmedetomidine was similarly effective for sedation, but shortened the time to extubation. It was associated with less delirium, tachycardia, and hypertension, but more bradycardia. Dexmedetomidine has sedative, analgesic, sympatholytic, and anxiolytic effects that blunt many of the cardiovascular responses in the perioperative period. It reduces the requirements for volatile anesthetics, sedatives, and analgesics without causing significant respiratory depression.[24]

Diazoxide

Diazoxide (Hyperstat) is avidly bound to and inactivated by serum proteins and thus must be given as a rapid intravenous bolus (within 15 seconds) of 3 to 5 mg/kg every 5 minutes. If the desired response is still not obtained after three bolus administrations, the use of SNP should be considered. The major disadvantage of diazoxide as compared with SNP is that diazoxide cannot be titrated in accordance with the patient's response. The onset of action of this drug is within 3 to 5 minutes, and its duration is 5 to 12 hours. Its action is immediate and is achieved through its direct vasodilating effects. Because the drug has more effect on the resistance vessels than the capacitance vessels, it decreases the afterload and has no effect on the preload. Concurrent administration of a loop diuretic, such as furosemide (40 to 80 mg intravenously), is usually advantageous especially if the patient's condition is edematous as a result of either cardiac or renal failure.[22-24]

Clonidine

Clonidine treats high blood pressure by stimulating α_2 receptors in the brain, which decreases cardiac output and peripheral vascular resistance, lowering blood pressure. It has specificity toward the presynaptic α_2 receptors in the vasomotor center in the brainstem. This binding decreases presynaptic calcium levels and inhibits the release of norepinephrine. The net effect is a decrease in sympathetic tone. The antihypertensive effect of clonidine is in fact due to its agonistic effect on the I_1-receptor (imidazoline receptor), which mediates the sympatho-inhibitory actions of imidazoline to lower blood pressure.[22-24]

Sodium Nitroprusside

A compound of unusual chemical structure, SNP (Nipride) is immediately effective in all cases of severe hypertensive crises, including those resistant to diazoxide. Its action is thought to result from the peripheral arteriolar dilatory effect of the drug. Because the drug can lower blood pressure rapidly, careful intravenous administration with constant bedside arterial pressure monitoring is required. The drug is extremely sensitive to light and must be administered through bottles and tubing that are wrapped and protected from the light. Only fresh solutions should be used. Solutions that are more than 4 hours old should be discarded because they may form thiocyanates. Treatment is started with a solution of 250 mL of 5% dextrose in water and 50 mg of SNP (200 mcg/mL) with use of an infusion pump to ensure a precise flow rate. A dose of 1 to 2 mcg/kg/min usually produces a prompt decrease in blood pressure, which returns to control levels within 5 minutes after the drug is stopped. Acute postoperative hypertension can be treated with a one-time single intravenous injection of 50 to 100 mcg of SNP. The onset of action of this drug is 1 or 2 minutes, and its duration of action is 2 to 5 minutes. Because of its unique chemical structure, cyanide is released into the blood stream when the drug is used. The cyanide is quickly converted to thiocyanate by the liver. Thiocyanate toxicity (fatigue, nausea, anorexia, muscle spasms, and disorientation) may result from prolonged use or from high dosages; therefore monitoring of serum thiocyanate levels is advised when the drug is used longer than 24 hours. Toxic symptoms appear with serum thiocyanate levels of 5 to 10 mg/dL, and the compound can be removed rapidly with peritoneal dialysis. As with diazoxide, once blood pressure has been brought to control levels, concomitant use of an oral medication such as guanethidine or methyldopa allows the gradual tapering and discontinuance of SNP.[22-24]

Phentolamine

Phentolamine mesylate (Regitine), an alpha-receptor blocker, is specifically indicated for management of hypertensive crises associated with increased circulating catecholamines. These crises can result from pheochromocytoma or the sudden release of tissue catecholamine stores caused by certain drugs or foods that contain tyramine in patients receiving monoamine oxidase inhibitors (pargyline derivatives, primarily Eutonyl). The antipressor effect of a single intravenous injection is short lived, usually lasting less than 15 minutes; therefore administration of phentolamine with intravenous infusion (200 to 400 g/L) is desirable, along with titration of the dose to achieve the desired pressure level after the blood pressure has been controlled initially with a rapid intravenous dose of 2 to 15 mg. Because the drug blocks only alpha receptors, beta-mediated effects of the circulating catecholamine on the heart must be controlled with the specific beta blocker, propranolol hydrochloride.[22-24]

With rare exceptions, these three drugs (diazoxide, SNP, and phentolamine) can be considered the mainstays of modern therapy in acute hypertensive crises. The other drugs discussed here should be considered second-line drugs. Their primary disadvantages include slower onset of action, rapid development of tachyphylaxis, and marked central nervous system depressant effects. In most instances, the drugs should be used to supplement and initiate long-term control once the acute crisis is resolved with the primary drugs.[22-24]

Hydralazine

Hydralazine (Apresoline) is not effective in hypertensive encephalopathy—complicating acute or chronic glomerulonephropathy; it is used in encephalopathy that has chronic essential hypertension as an underlying cause. Blood pressure is reduced through vasodilatation, which reduces vascular resistance and results in a marked increase in cardiac output and heart rate that can aggravate underlying angina and cardiac failure. The determining factor in this situation is the net change in myocardial oxygen consumption achieved with lowering the elevated afterload; however a decrease in blood pressure produced with hydralazine is not accompanied by a commensurate decrease in renal blood flow; therefore the drug is especially suited for management of hypertensive emergencies associated with renal insufficiency. The initial intravenous dose of 5 to 10 mg should be given. The onset of action of this drug is 15 to 20 minutes, and the duration is 4 to 6 hours. Alternatively, the drug dosage may be increased in 5-mg increments up to 20 mg. The maintenance dose depends on patient response, but is generally 5 to 10 mg intravenously every 4 to 6 hours.[22-24]

Trimethaphan Camsylate

Trimethaphan (Arfonad) is a ganglionic vasodepressor that blocks both the sympathetic and parasympathetic systems at the autonomic ganglia. The effect is primarily orthostatic; therefore large doses must be used to reduce blood pressure in supine patients. The head of the bed should be elevated (reverse Trendelenburg position), if possible, to augment the antipressor action. The dose of this drug is 10 to 20 mcg/kg/min. The onset of action is approximately 1 minute, and the duration of action is 2 to 4 minutes. The 500-mg ampule of trimethaphan is mixed in 250 mL of normal saline solution, which results in a strength of 2 mg/mL. Complications of such ganglionic blockade include atony of the bowel and bladder and paralytic ileus, especially when the drug is used longer than 24 hours. Because of the

commensurate decrease in the glomerular filtration rate when the blood pressure is lowered with the use of this agent, use is not recommended in patients for whom renal insufficiency complicates the hypertensive crisis. The drug's major disadvantage is that it rapidly loses effectiveness after 24 to 72 hours and another agent must be substituted. The drug requires extremely close monitoring by the perianesthesia nurse.[22-24]

Nitroglycerin

Nitroglycerin is a potent vasodilator that produces relaxation of both arterial and venous smooth muscles. The pharmacologic effects of nitroglycerin are mainly on the venous circulation. It produces an increase in venous capacitance, which leads to a reduction in venous return and a decrease in right atrial and pulmonary capillary wedge pressures; therefore the main effect of nitroglycerin is a reduction in the preload. In addition, the myocardial oxygen demand is decreased because of the decrease in myocardial wall tension.[22-24]

Intravenous nitroglycerin may be indicated for treatment of myocardial ischemia, control of hypertension, relief of angina pectoris, and production of vasodilatation for patients with severe congestive heart failure.

When intravenous nitroglycerin is administered in the PACU, an automated infusion pump should be used. The usual dose is between 0.25 and 3 mcg/kg/min. The onset of action for this drug is 2 to 5 minutes, and the duration of action is 3 to 5 minutes. The patient should be continuously monitored for hypotension. Should hypotension occur, an alpha agonist, such as methoxamine, may be used to ensure that the patient's coronary perfusion pressure is maintained. Nitroglycerin migrates into plastic; therefore the perianesthesia nurse should periodically change the plastic tubing on the automated infusion pump and ensure that only glass bottles are used for dilution.[22-24]

Propranolol

Propranolol (Inderal, Ipran) is the prototype beta-blocking drug; consequently, all drugs in this class are compared with propranolol. This drug is known to be nonselective because it blocks both beta$_1$ and beta$_2$ receptors. After administration of this drug, decreased heart rate, contractility, and cardiac output occur. The drug can be administered in single intravenous doses of 0.1 to 0.5 mg, with a maximum dose of approximately 2 mg.[22-24]

Esmolol

Esmolol (Brevibloc) is a cardioselective ultrashort-acting beta-blocking agent with a rapid onset and short duration of action. Because it is cardioselective, esmolol does not appear to affect bronchial or vascular tone at the doses required to reduce the heart rate. This drug has also been shown to blunt the response to endotracheal intubation and can be effective in treatment of postoperative hypertension. In the treatment of postoperative hypertension, a loading dose of 500 mcg/kg should be administered over a 1-minute period. Next, a continuous infusion of 50 to 300 mcg/kg/min should be started. The peak response of esmolol occurs in 5 minutes, with a duration of action of approximately 20 minutes.[22-24]

Labetalol

Labetalol (Normodyne, Trandate) is a drug that possesses antagonist activity at both the alpha and beta receptors. With intravenous administration, it is approximately sevenfold more potent on the beta receptors than on the alpha receptors. More specifically, this drug is an $alpha_1$ antagonist and has antagonist activities on both the $beta_1$ and $beta_2$ receptors. For treatment of postoperative hypertension, a loading dose of 0.25 mg/kg should be administered over a 2-minute period. After this initial dose, intravenous titration to effect should be done at 10-minute intervals to a total of 300 mg. If a continuous infusion is needed, a dose of 2 mg/min can be used.[22-24]

Metoprolol

Metoprolol (Lopressor) is a beta blocker that can be used in patients with reactive and obstructive lung disease because this drug selectively blocks the $beta_1$ effects and consequently blocks the inotropic and chronotropic responses. This selective beta-adrenergic effect is dose related; at high doses, $beta_1$ and $beta_2$ receptors become blocked and airway resistance may increase. For treatment of postoperative hypertension, an intravenous dose of 2 to 5 mg should be used.[22-24]

SUMMARY

The anatomy and physiology of the cardiovascular system has been presented in depth. The electrocardiogram and the electrical activity of the heart were presented, in addition to invasive and noninvasive methods to monitor the cardiovascular system. In addition, myocardial infarction was presented and the various cardiovascular drugs that are currently used were described in detail. One area of medical research is in discovery of new drugs to enhance cardiovascular function. The reader advised to seek the current literature in this area as new methods and drugs continue to be introduced.

REFERENCES

1. Drake R, et al: *Gray's anatomy for students*, ed 2, Philadelphia, 2009, Churchill Livingstone.
2. Hall J: *Guyton and Hall textbook of medical physiology*, ed 12, Philadelphia, 2010, Saunders.
3. Estafanous F, et al: *Cardiac anesthesia: principles and clinical practice*, ed 2, Philadelphia, 2001, Lippincott Williams & Wilkins.
4. Barash P, et al: *Clinical anesthesia*, ed 6, Philadelphia, 2009, Lippincott Williams & Wilkins.
5. Aitkenhead A, et al: *Textbook of anaesthesia*, ed 5, Philadelphia, 2007, Churchill Livingstone.
6. Lake C, et al: *Clinical monitoring: practical applications for anesthesia and critical care*, Philadelphia, 2001, Saunders.
7. Longnecker D, Murphy F: Introduction to anesthesia. In Dripps, et al: Introduction to Anesthesia, ed 9, Philadelphia, 1997, Saunders.
8. Nagelhout J, Plaus K: *Nurse anesthesia*, ed 4, St. Louis, 2009, Saunders.
9. Alspach J: *Core curriculum for critical care nursing*, ed 6, Philadelphia, 2005, Saunders.
10. Atlee J: *Complications in anesthesia*, ed 2, Philadelphia, 2007, Saunders.
11. Smartt S: The pulmonary artery catheter: gold standard or redundant relic, *J Perianesth Nurs* 20(6):373–379, 2005.
12. Gallager C, Issenberg B: *Simulation in anesthesia*, Philadelphia, 2007, Saunders.
13. Ganong W: *Review of medical physiology*, ed 22, New York, 2005, McGraw-Hill Medical.
14. Stoelting R, Miller R: *Basics of anesthesia*, ed 6, Philadelphia, 2011, Churchill Livingstone.
15. Miller R, et al: *Anesthesia*, ed 7, Philadelphia, 2009, Churchill Livingstone.
16. Benumof J, Saidman L: *Anesthesia & perioperative complications*, ed 2, St. Louis, 1999, Mosby.
17. Fisher L: *Benumof's anesthesia and uncommon diseases*, ed 5, Philadelphia, 2007, Saunders.
18. Murray J, Nadel J: *Textbook of respiratory medicine*, ed 2, Philadelphia, 1994, Saunders.
19. Townsend C, et al: *Sabiston textbook of surgery: the biological basis of modern surgical practice*, ed 17, Philadelphia, 2004, Saunders.
20. Stoelting R: *Pharmacology and physiology in anesthetic practice*, ed 4, Philadelphia, 2005, Lippincott Williams & Wilkins.
21. Evers A, Maze M: *Anesthetic pharmacology: physiologic principles and clinical practice*, Philadelphia, 2004, Churchill Livingstone.
22. Kier L, Dowd C: *The chemistry of drugs for nurse anesthetists*, Chicago, 2004, AANA Publishing, Inc.
23. Brunton L, et al: *Goodman and Gilman's the pharmacological basis of therapeutics*, ed 12, New York, 2010, McGraw-Hill Professional.
24. Pandharipande P, Ely EW: Alpha-2 agonists: can they modify the outcomes in postanesthesia care unit, *Current Drug Targets* 6:749–754, 2005.
25. Longnecker D, et al: *Principles and practice of anesthesiology*, ed 2, St. Louis, 1998, Mosby.

PHYSIOLOGIC CONSIDERATIONS IN THE PACU

12 The Respiratory System

Cecil B. Drain, PhD, RN, CRNA, FAAN, FASAHP

Over the last few years, the major feature of inhalational anesthetic agents has been a rapid length of action, which helps to facilitate a rapid emergence from anesthesia. This attribute has, in many ways, made the emergence phase even more critical than in the past. Significant research has been performed on these agents with the result of enhanced patient safety. A major factor of why perianesthesia nursing should always be considered advanced practice nursing in the area of critical care is because of these rapid-acting agents.

The inhalation anesthetic agents depress respiratory function. They also depend largely on the respiratory system for removal during emergence from anesthesia. The other anesthetic agents, such as intravenous agents, also depress respiration. Much of the morbidity and mortality that occurs in the postanesthesia care unit (PACU) can be attributed to an alteration in lung mechanics and a dysfunction in airway dynamics. In fact, 70% to 80% of the morbidity and mortality that occur in the PACU is postulated to be associated with some form of respiratory dysfunction. Consequently, a detailed discussion of the many facets of respiratory anatomy and physiology is presented in this chapter. If the perianesthesia nurse incorporates this information into clinical practice, care of the surgical patient in the immediate postoperative period will be enhanced.

DEFINITIONS

Acidemia: Lower-than-normal blood pH (increased hydrogen ion concentration).

Acidosis: The process that leads to an increase in hydrogen ion concentration in the blood.

Adventitious Sounds: Abnormal noises that may be heard superimposed on a patient's breath sounds.

Alkalemia: Higher-than-normal blood pH (decreased hydrogen ion concentration).

Alkalosis: The process that leads to a decrease in hydrogen ion concentration in the blood.

Apnea: The absence of breathing.

Apneustic Breathing: Prolonged inspiratory efforts interrupted by occasional expirations.

Atelectasis: Collapse of the alveoli.

Bradypnea: Respiratory rate, in the adult, that is less than 8 breaths/min.

Bronchiectasis: Dilatation of the bronchi.

Bronchospasm: Constriction of the bronchial airways caused by an increase in smooth muscle tone in the airways.

Central Sleep Apnea: A cessation of breathing during sleep as a result of transient abolishment of the drive to the respiratory muscles.

Cheyne-Stokes Respirations: Periods of apnea alternating with rhythmic, shallow, and progressively deeper and then shallower respirations that are associated with brain damage, heart or kidney failure, or drug overdose.

Compliance (Lung): A measure of distensibility of the lungs; the amount of change in volume per change in pressure across the lung.

Cyanosis: A sign of poor oxygen transport, characterized by a bluish discoloration of the skin, produced when more than 5 g of hemoglobin per deciliter of arterial blood is in the deoxygenated, or reduced, state.

Dyspnea: A patient's perception of shortness of breath.

Epistaxis: Hemorrhage from the nose.

Hypercapnia: Increased tension of carbon dioxide ($PaCO_2$) in the blood.

Hyperoxemia: Increased tension of oxygen (PaO_2) in the blood.

Hyperpnea: Increased rate of respirations.

Hyperventilation: Overventilation of the alveoli in relation to the amount of carbon dioxide produced by the body.

Hypocapnia: Decreased $PaCO_2$ in the blood.

Hypoventilation: Underventilation of the alveoli in relation to the amount of carbon dioxide produced by the body.

Hypoxemia: Decreased PaO_2 in the blood.

Hypoxia: Inadequate tissue oxygen levels.

Kussmaul Respirations: Rapid, deep respirations associated with diabetic ketoacidosis.

Methemoglobin: Hemoglobin that has the iron atom in the ferric state.

Minute Ventilation ($\dot{V}_E$): The volume of air expired during a period of 1 minute.

Orthopnea: Severe dyspnea that is relieved when the patient elevates the head and chest.

Oxyhemoglobin: Hemoglobin that is fully oxygenated.

Paroxysmal Nocturnal Dyspnea: A sudden onset of severe dyspnea when the patient is lying down.

Partial Pressure: The pressure exerted by each individual gas when mixed in a container with other gases.

Periodic Breathing: A regular waxing and waning of ventilation as a result of fluctuations in central respiratory drive.

Polycythemia: Increased number of red blood cells in the blood.

Rales: Short discontinuous explosive adventitious sounds, usually called *crackles*.

Reduced Hemoglobin: Hemoglobin in the deoxy state (not fully saturated with oxygen).

Respiration: The process by which oxygen and carbon dioxide are exchanged between the outside atmosphere and the cells in the body.

Rhonchi: Continuous musical adventitious sounds.

Sleep Apnea: Repeated absence of breathing during sleep, sometimes hundreds of times during the night and often for 1 minute or longer.

Torr: Units of the Torricelli scale, the classic mercury scale, which is used to express the same value as millimeters of mercury.

Ventilation: The mechanical movement of air in and out of the lungs.

Wheeze: A high-pitched sibilant rhonchus usually produced on expiration.

RESPIRATORY SYSTEM ANATOMY

The Nose

The nose, the first area in which inhaled air is filtered (Fig. 12-1), is lined with ciliated epithelium. Cilia move mucus and particles of foreign matter to the pharynx to be expectorated or swallowed (Fig. 12-2). Other functions of the nose include humidification and warming of the inhaled air and the olfactory function of smell.[1]

Dry gases are often administered during anesthesia. These gases dry the mucous membranes and slow the action of the cilia. The administration of moist gases in the PACU with various humidification and mist therapy devices keeps this physiologic filter system viable. A tracheostomy precludes the functions of the nose, and proper tracheostomy care, including the administration of humidified oxygen, must be instituted.[2]

The blood supply to the nose is provided by the internal and external maxillary arteries, which are derived from the external carotid artery, and by branches of the internal carotid arteries. The venous plexus of the nasal mucosa is drained into the common facial vein, the anterior facial vein, the exterior jugular vein, or the ophthalmic vein. A highly vascular plexus of vessels is located in the mucosa of the anterior nasal septum. This plexus is called the *Kiesselbach plexus* or the *Little area*. In most instances, this area is the source of epistaxis.[3]

Epistaxis can occur in the PACU after trauma to the nasal veins from nasotracheal tubes or to nasal airways during anesthesia. If epistaxis occurs, prompt action should be taken to prevent aspiration of blood into the lungs. The patient should be positioned with the head up and flexed forward toward the chest. Cold compresses applied to the bridge of the nose and neck may be effective in slowing or stopping the bleeding. If the bleeding is profuse, the oral cavity should be suctioned carefully and the attending physician should be notified. A nasal pack or cautery with silver nitrate or electric current may be necessary to stop the bleeding.[4]

The Pharynx

The pharynx originates at the posterior aspect of the nasal cavities and is called the *nasopharynx* until it reaches the soft palate, where it becomes the oropharynx. The oropharynx extends to the level of the hyoid bone, where it becomes the laryngeal pharynx, which extends caudally to below the hyoid bone.[1]

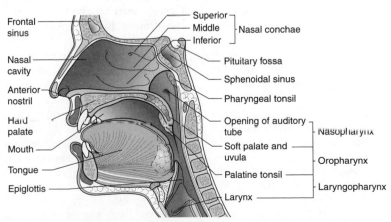

FIG. 12-1 Sagittal section through the nose. (From Watson R: *Anatomy and physiology for nurses*, ed 13, Edinburgh, 2011, Baillière Tindall.)

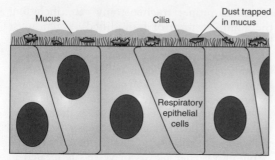

FIG. 12-2 Mucus blanket of nasal airways. Outer (gel-like) layer rests on tips of beating cilia, and inner (water) layer bathes cilia. Particles are trapped on sticky outer blanket and carried posteriorly into nasopharynx by organized beating of cilia. (From Bill RL: *Clinical pharmacology and therapeutics for the veterinary technician,* ed 3, St. Louis, 2006, Mosby.)

The Larynx

The larynx, or voice box (Fig. 12-3), is situated anterior to the third, fourth, and fifth cervical vertebrae in the adult male. It is situated higher in women and children. Nine cartilages held together with ligaments and intertwined with many small muscles constitute the larynx. The thyroid cartilage, the largest, is V-shaped; its protruding prominence is commonly referred to as the *Adam's apple.* The thyroid cartilage is attached to the hyoid bone by the hyothyroid membrane and to the cricoid cartilage. The cricoid cartilage is situated below the thyroid cartilage and anteriorly forms a signet-shaped ring. The signet lies posteriorly as a quadrilateral lamina joined in front by a thin arch. The inner surface of the cricoid cartilage is lined with a mucus membrane. In children younger than 12 years, the cricoid cartilage is the smallest opening to the bronchi of the lungs.

The epiglottis, a cartilage of the larynx, is an important landmark for tracheal intubation that serves to deflect foreign objects away from the trachea. This cartilage is leaf shaped and projects outward above the thyroid cartilage over the entrance to the trachea. The lower portion is attached to the thyroid lamina, and the anterior surface is attached to the hyoid bone and thereby to the base of the tongue. The valleys on either side of the glossoepiglottic fold are termed the *valleculae.*[5]

The arytenoid cartilages are paired and articulate with the lamina of the cricoid through the articular surface on the base of the arytenoid. The anterior angle of the arytenoid cartilage projects forward to form the vocal process. The medial surface of the cartilage is covered by a mucous membrane to form the lateral portion of the rima glottis—that is, the split between the vocal cords. The rima glottis is completed anteriorly by the thyroid cartilage and posteriorly by the cricoid cartilage.

The corniculate cartilages are two small nodules that are located at the apex of the arytenoid. The cuneiform cartilage is a flake of cartilage within the margin of the aryepiglottic folds. It probably serves to stiffen the folds.

The larynx has nine membranes and extrinsic or intrinsic ligaments. Extrinsic ligaments connect the thyroid cartilage and the epiglottis with the hyoid bone and the cricoid cartilage with the trachea. Intrinsic ligaments connect the cartilages of the larynx with each other.

The fissure between the vocal folds, or true cords, is termed the *rima glottidis* or *glottis.* In the adult, this opening between the vocal cords is the narrowest part of the laryngeal cavity. Any obstruction in this area leads to death via suffocation if not relieved promptly. The rima glottidis divides the laryngeal cavity into two main compartments: (1) the upper portion is the vestibule, which extends from the laryngeal outlet to the vocal cords and includes the laryngeal sinus, sometimes called the middle compartment; and (2) the lower compartment, which extends from the vocal cords to the lower border of the cricoid cartilage and thereafter, is contiguous with the trachea.[6]

The muscles of the larynx are also either intrinsic or extrinsic. The intrinsic muscles control the movements of the laryngeal framework. They open the cords on inspiration, close the cords and the laryngeal inlet during swallowing, and alter the tension of the cords during speech. The extrinsic muscles are involved in the movements of the larynx as a whole, such as in swallowing.[4]

The nerve supply to the larynx is from the superior and recurrent laryngeal nerves of the vagus. The superior laryngeal nerve passes deep to both the internal and the external carotid arteries and divides into a small external branch that supplies the cricothyroid muscles that tense the vocal ligaments. The larger internal branch pierces the thyrohyoid membrane to provide sensory fibers to the mucosa of both sides of the epiglottis and the larynx above the cords.[1]

The recurrent laryngeal nerve on the right side exits from the vagus as it crosses the right subclavian artery and ascends to the larynx in the groove between the trachea and esophagus (Fig. 12-4). When the nerve reaches the neck, it assumes the same relationships as on the right. This nerve provides the motor function to the intrinsic muscles of the larynx, with the exception of the cricothyroid, and also provides sensory function to the laryngeal mucosa below the vocal cords.

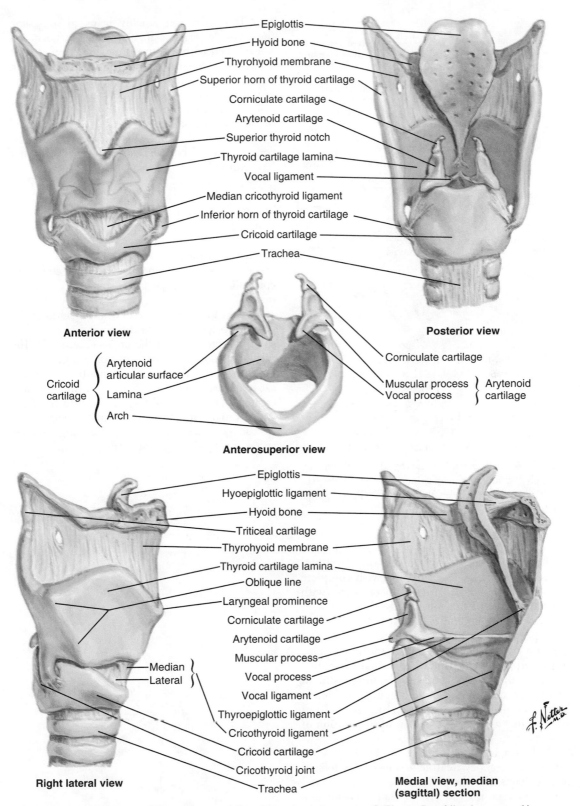

Anterior view

Epiglottis
Hyoid bone
Thyrohyoid membrane
Superior horn of thyroid cartilage
Corniculate cartilage
Arytenoid cartilage
Superior thyroid notch
Thyroid cartilage lamina
Vocal ligament
Median cricothyroid ligament
Inferior horn of thyroid cartilage
Cricoid cartilage
Trachea

Posterior view

Corniculate cartilage
Muscular process } Arytenoid
Vocal process } cartilage

Cricoid
cartilage
Arytenoid
articular surface
Lamina
Arch

Anterosuperior view

Epiglottis
Hyoepiglottic ligament
Hyoid bone
Triticeal cartilage
Thyrohyoid membrane
Thyroid cartilage lamina
Oblique line
Laryngeal prominence
Corniculate cartilage
Arytenoid cartilage
Muscular process
Vocal process
Vocal ligament
Thyroepiglottic ligament
Cricothyroid ligament
Cricoid cartilage
Cricothyroid joint
Trachea

Median }
Lateral }

Right lateral view

**Medial view, median
(sagittal) section**

FIG. 12-3 The larynx. (Netter illustration from www.netterimages.com. © Elsevier Inc. All rights reserved.)

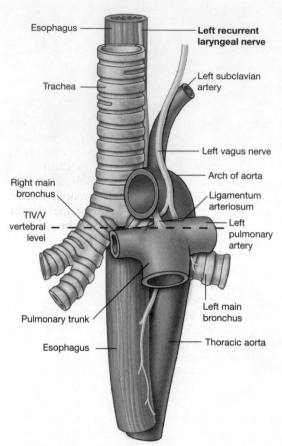

FIG. 12-4 Left recurrent laryngeal nerve passing through the superior mediastinum. (From Drake RL, et al: *Gray's anatomy for students*, ed 2, Philadelphia, 2010, Churchill Livingstone.)

Laryngospasm, a spasm of the laryngeal muscle tissue, may be complete (with complete closure of the vocal cords) or incomplete (with partial closure of the vocal cords). Patients with partial or complete airway obstruction, such as laryngospasm, usually have a paradoxic rocking motion of the chest wall. This motion can be misinterpreted as normal abdominal breathing. As a result, the perianesthesia nurse should always auscultate the patient's lungs to determine the degree of ventilation and should not rely on just a visual assessment of the motion of the chest.

When a laryngospasm occurs in the PACU, prompt emergency treatment is necessary to save the patient's life. The perianesthesia nurse should have someone on the PACU staff summon the anesthesia provider when laryngospasm is suspected. Treatment consists of mask ventilation with sustained moderate pressure on the reservoir bag. This maneuver usually helps to overcome the partial laryngospasm. Complete laryngospasm not relieved with positive pressure within at least 1 minute necessitates more aggressive treatment. Intravenous (0.5 mg/kg) or intramuscular (1 mg/kg) succinylcholine can be administered to relax the smooth muscle of the larynx. Endotracheal intubation may be necessary.[7,8] The nurse must remember that ventilation of the patient's lungs should be continued until complete respiratory functioning has returned.

The Trachea

The trachea is a musculomembranous tube surrounded by 16 to 20 incomplete cartilaginous rings. These C-shaped rings prevent the collapse of the trachea and thereby maintain free passage of air. The trachea is lined with ciliated columnar epithelium, which aids in the removal of foreign material.

The area at the distal end of the trachea at the point of bifurcation into the right and left main stem bronchi is called the *carina* (Fig. 12-5). The carina contains sensitive pressoreceptors, which on stimulation (i.e., with an endotracheal tube) cause the patient to cough and "buck." The angle created at the point of bifurcation into the right and left main stem bronchi is clinically significant to the perianesthesia nurse. This angle varies according to the age and gender of the patient

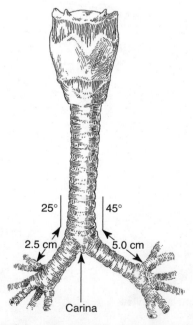

FIG. 12-5 Bifurcation of trachea into main stem bronchi. (From Nagelhout JJ, Plaus KL: *Nurse anesthesia*, ed 4, St. Louis, 2010, Saunders.)

Table 12-1	Variations of Bronchial Bifurcation Angles in Adults and Children	
	RIGHT BRONCHUS (DEGREES)	LEFT BRONCHUS (DEGREES)
Newborn	12-35	30-65
Adult male	20	40
Adult female	19	51

(Table 12-1). The angle at the right main stem bronchus is smaller than the angle at the left main stem bronchus. Foreign material can easily enter the right main stem bronchus at this point. Endotracheal tubes, if advanced too far, usually enter the right main stem bronchus and thereby occlude the left main stem bronchus. As a result, the left lung cannot be ventilated. Signs of this complication include decreased or absent breath sounds in the left side of the chest, tachycardia, and uneven expansion of the chest on inspiration and expiration.[5,9,10]

Bronchi and Lungs

Each primary bronchus supplies a number of lobar bronchi (Fig. 12-6). Humans have an upper, middle, and lower lobe bronchus on the right and only an upper and lower lobe bronchus on the left. Within each pulmonary lobe, a lobar (secondary) bronchus soon divides into tertiary branches that are remarkably constant as to

number and distribution within the lobe. The segment of a lobe aerated by a tertiary bronchus is usually well delineated from adjoining segments by complete planes of connective tissue. These areas of the lung are well defined; therefore pulmonary diseases may be limited to a particular segment or segments of a lobe.

The bronchi bifurcate 22 or 23 times from the main stem bronchus to the terminal bronchi. These bronchi have connective tissue and cartilaginous support. The terminal bronchi branch to the bronchioles with a diameter of 1 mm or smaller and lack cartilaginous support. Bronchioles have thin, highly elastic walls composed of smooth muscle, which is arranged circularly. When the circular smooth muscle is contracted, the bronchiolar lumen is constricted. This circular smooth muscle is innervated by the parasympathetic nervous system (vagus nerve), which causes constriction, and the sympathetic nervous system, which causes dilatation. The patency of the terminal bronchioles therefore is determined by the tonus of the muscle produced by a balance between the two components of the nervous system. Bronchospasm occurs when the smooth muscles constrict or experience spasm, ultimately leading to airway obstruction.

The terminal bronchioles divide into the respiratory bronchioles in which actual gas exchange first occurs. The respiratory bronchioles bifurcate to form alveolar ducts, and these in turn terminate in spherical enclosures called the *alveolar sac*. The sacs enclose a small but variable number of terminal alveoli.[3]

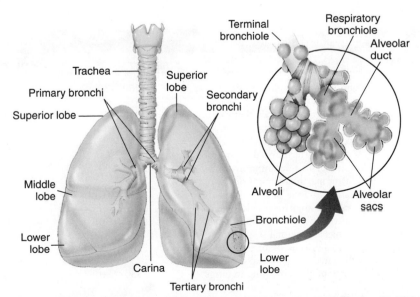

FIG. 12-6 Distribution of bronchi within lungs. Enlarged inset shows detail of alveolus. (From National Association of Emergency Media: *PHTLS prehospital trauma life support* , ed 6, St. Louis, 2007, Mosby.)

The number of alveoli in an average adult's lungs is estimated to be 750 million. The surface area available for gas exchange is approximately 125 m². Alveoli are shaped like soap bubbles in a glass. The interalveolar septum has a supporting latticework composed of elastic collagenous and reticular fibers. The capillaries are incorporated into and supported by the fibrous lattice. The capillary networks in the lungs are the richest in the body.

The lungs receive unoxygenated blood from the left and right pulmonary arteries, which originate from the right ventricle of the heart. The divisions of the pulmonary artery tend to follow the bifurcations of the airway. Typically, two pulmonary veins exit from each lung, and all four veins empty separately into the left atrium. The blood that arrives in the rich pulmonary capillary network from the pulmonary arteries provides for the metabolic needs of the pulmonary parenchyma. Other portions of the lungs, such as the conducting vessels and airways, need their own private circulation. The bronchial arteries, which arise from the aorta, provide the oxygenated blood to the lung tissue. The blood of the bronchial arteries returns to the heart by way of the pulmonary veins.[3]

Each lung is contained in a thin elastic membranous sac called the *visceral pleura*, which is adherent to the external surface of the lung. Another membrane, the parietal pleura, lines the chest wall. These two membranes normally are close to each other. A few milliliters of viscous fluid are secreted between them for lubrication. The visceral pleura continuously absorbs this fluid.

RESPIRATORY SYSTEM PHYSIOLOGY

Lung Volumes and Capacities

Perianesthesia care of the patient is largely based on knowledge of the physiology and pathophysiology of the respiratory system. Dysfunction in lung volumes and capacities that occurs in the patient after surgery is the compelling reason for institution of the stir-up regimen in the PACU. Accordingly, the physiology of the lung volumes and capacities and lung mechanics are described in detail. Table 12-2 provides the definition and normal value for each lung volume and capacity. As shown in Table 12-2 and Fig. 12-7, a lung capacity comprises two or more lung volumes.

Lung Volumes

The tidal volume (V_T) represents the amount of air moved into or out of the lungs during a normal ventilatory excursion. Monitoring of this lung volume is important when the patient is receiving ventilatory support. Because the V_T measurement is highly variable, it is not an extremely helpful parameter in pulmonary function tests. Clinically, the V_T can be estimated at 7 mL/kg. For example, a man who weighs 70 kg has a V_T of approximately 490 mL ($7 \times 70 = 490$).

The expiratory reserve volume (ERV) is the maximal amount of air that can be expired from the resting position after a normal spontaneous expiration. The ERV reflects muscle strength, thoracic mobility, and a balance of forces that

Table 12-2	Lung Volumes and Capacities		
TERMINOLOGY	**DEFINITION**	**HEALTHY MALE* (mL)**	**HEALTHY FEMALE* (mL)**
Tidal volume (V_T)	Volume of air inspired or expired at each breath	660 (230)	550 (160)
Inspiratory reserve volume (IRV)	Maximal volume of air that can be inspired after normal inspiration	2240 (—)	1480 (—)
Expiratory reserve volume (ERV)	Maximal volume of air that can be expired after normal expiration	1240 (412)	730 (300)
Residual volume (RV)	Volume of air remaining in lungs after maximal expiration	2120 (520)	1570 (380)
Vital capacity (VC)	Maximal volume of air that can be expired after maximal inspiration	4130 (750)	2760 (540)
Total lung capacity (TLC)	Total volume of air contained in lungs at maximal inspiration	6230 (830)	4330 (620)
Inspiratory capacity (IC)	Maximal volume of air that can be inspired after normal expiration	2900 (—)	2030 (—)
Functional residual capacity (FRC)	Volume of gas remaining in lungs after normal expiration	3330 (680)	2300 (490)

Adapted from Wylie WB, Churchill-Davidson HC, editors: *A practice of anaesthesia*, ed 4, London, 1978, Lloyd-Luke.
*Data are mean values, with the standard deviation in parentheses.

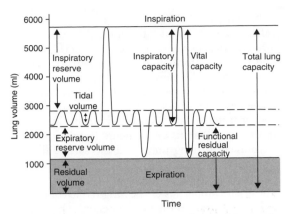

FIG. 12-7 Graphic representation of normal lung volumes and capacities. (From Hall JE: *Guyton and Hall textbook of medical physiology,* ed 12, Philadelphia, 2011, Saunders.)

determine the resting position of the lungs and chest wall after a normal expiration. This lung volume is usually decreased in patients who are morbidly obese (see Chapter 45). This lung volume also is decreased in the immediate postoperative period in patients who have undergone an upper abdominal or thoracic operation.[5,9,10]

The residual volume (RV) is the volume of air that remains in the lungs at the end of a maximal expiration. This lung volume represents the balance of forces of the lung elastic forces and thoracic muscle strength. Patients with skeletal muscle relaxant that was not adequately reversed at the end of the anesthetic period may have an elevated RV because enough muscle strength cannot be generated to force all the air out of the lungs. As the RV increases, more air remains in the lungs so that the air does not participate adequately in gas exchange and becomes dead-space air. As the dead-space volume of air increases, it can impinge on the V_T and hypoxemia can ensue. The importance of the RV is that it allows for continuous gas exchange throughout the entire breathing cycle by providing air to most of the alveoli and it aerates the blood between breaths. Consequently, the RV prevents wide fluctuations in oxygen and carbon dioxide concentrations during inspiration and expiration.[4]

The inspiratory reserve volume (IRV) reflects a balance of the lung elastic forces, muscle strength, and thoracic mobility. The IRV is the maximal volume of air that can be inspired at the end of a normal spontaneous inspiration. Physiologically, the IRV is available to meet increased metabolic demand at a time of excess physical exertion. It assists in moving a larger volume of air into the alveoli through each ventilatory cycle to increase the overall performance and efficiency of the respiratory system.

Lung Capacities

The inspiratory capacity (IC) is the maximal volume of air that can be inspired from the resting expiratory position. The IC is the sum of the V_T and the IRV.

The functional residual capacity (FRC) represents the previously mentioned resting position. The FRC is the volume of air that remains in the lungs at the end of a normal expiration when no respiratory muscle forces are applied. At FRC, the mechanical forces of the lung and thorax are at rest and no air flow is present. Because the FRC is usually reduced in patients who are recovering from anesthesia, this particular lung capacity is of great importance to the perianesthesia nurse when intensive nursing care is rendered. For this reason, breathing maneuvers, such as the sustained maximal inspiration (SMI), are instituted in the PACU to raise the FRC (see the next section on lung mechanics). The FRC represents the sum of the ERV and the RV. A severe increase in the FRC is often associated with pulmonary distention, which is technically a state of hyperinflation of the lung. This state of hyperinflation can be caused by two abnormal conditions: airway obstruction and loss of elasticity. Airway obstruction is exemplified by an episode of acute bronchial asthma; a loss of lung elasticity is usually associated with emphysema. A severe decrease in FRC is associated with pulmonary fibrosis and can be the sequela of postoperative atelectasis.

The vital capacity (VC) is the amount of air that can be expired after the deepest possible inspiration. The VC is the sum of the V_T, the ERV, and the IRV. The VC measures many factors that simultaneously affect ventilation, including activity of respiratory centers, motor nerves, and respiratory muscles, and thoracic maximum, airway and tissue resistance, and lung volume.

The total lung capacity (TLC) is the total amount of air in the lung at a maximal inspiration. The TLC is the sum of the VC and the RV.

Clinical measurements of the TLC, FRC, and RV are difficult because these values include a gas volume that cannot be exhaled; therefore the measurements require sophisticated pulmonary function testing equipment with gas dilution techniques or plethysmography. Measurements of lung volumes and capacities are useful in the evaluation of lung function.[5]

Lung Mechanics
Mechanical Features of the Lungs

Mechanical forces of the respiratory system actually determine the lung volumes and capacities. For an understanding of how these lung volumes and capacities are determined and how they are affected by anesthesia and surgery, the perianesthesia nurse should become familiar with the balance-of-forces concept of the respiratory system (see the section on combined mechanical properties of the lungs and chest wall). The PACU stir-up regimen is designed to increase the postoperative patient's lung volumes and capacities with enhancement of the mechanical forces of the respiratory system.

The lungs and chest wall are viscoelastic structures, one within the other. Because they are elastic, the lungs always want to collapse or recoil to a smaller position. Therefore, as can be seen in the pressure-volume (P-V) curve of the lungs alone (Fig. 12-8), at less than RV the lungs are collapsed and no pressure is transmitted across the lungs (i.e., no transpulmonary pressure). When the lungs are inflated to a volume halfway between RV and TLC, the lungs seek to recoil or collapse back to the resting position equal to or less than RV, which is reflected by an increase in transpulmonary pressure. When the lungs are fully inflated at TLC, a maximal transpulmonary pressure is also exhibited. By analogy, when a balloon is completely deflated, the pressure measured at the mouth of the balloon is zero. When the balloon is partially inflated, the pressure increases as the elastic forces of the balloon try to make the balloon recoil to its resting position. If the balloon is maximally inflated, the elastic recoil of the balloon is greater, as is the pressure measured at the mouth of the balloon.

Pulmonary Hysteresis

Inflation and deflation paths of the P-V curve of the lung are not aligned on top of each other (Fig. 12-9). The path of deformation (inspiration) to TLC is different from the path followed when the force is withdrawn (expiration) from TLC to RV. This phenomenon is known as *pulmonary hysteresis*. The following factors contribute to pulmonary hysteresis: properties of the tissue elements (a minor factor), recruitment of lung units, and the surface tension phenomenon (surfactant).[1]

Elastic Properties of the Lung

The elastic properties of the lung tissue contribute only a small part to the phenomenon of hysteresis.

Recruitment of Lung Units

Recruitment of lung units has an important part in pulmonary hysteresis. For an understanding of recruitment of lung units, the nurse must be familiar with the concept of airway closure. An apex-to-base gradient of alveolar size exists in the lung (Fig. 12-10). This gradient occurs because of the weight of the lung, which tends to pull the lung toward its base. As a result, the pleural pressure is more negative at the apex than at the base of the lung. Ultimately, at low lung volumes, the alveoli at the apex are inflated more than the alveoli at the base. At the base of the lungs, some alveoli are closed to ventilation because the weight of the lungs in that area causes the pleural pressure to become positive. Airways open only when the critical opening pressure is achieved during inflation and the lung units peripheral to them are recruited to participate in volume exchange. This process is called *radial traction* or a *tethering effect*

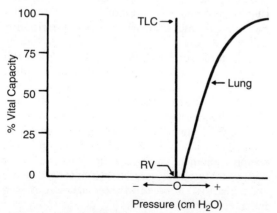

FIG. 12-8 Static deflation pressure-volume curve for lung. Positive pressures represent pressures that tend to decrease lung volume. *TLC*, Total lung capacity; *RV*, residual volume. (From Drain C: Physiology of the respiratory system related to anesthesia, *CRNA* 7: 163–180, 1996.)

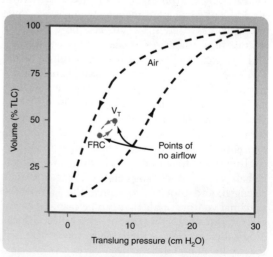

FIG. 12-9 Inflation and deflation paths of pressure-volume curve of lungs. (From Koeppen BM, Stanton BA: *Berne and Levy's physiology*, ed 6 [updated edition], St. Louis, 2010, Mosby.)

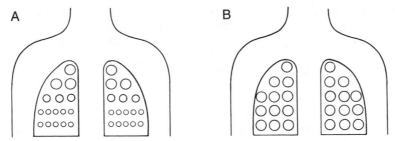

FIG. 12-10 Alveolar size from apex to base of lungs, as subject inhales from residual volume **(A)** to total lung capacity **(B)**.

on airways. An analogy of a nylon stocking can aid in the explanation of this concept. When no traction is applied to the nylon stocking, the holes in the stocking are small. As traction is applied to the stocking from all sides, each nylon filament pulls on the others, which spreads apart all the other filaments; and the holes in the stocking enlarge. Similarly, as one airway opens, it produces radial traction on the next airway and pulls the next airway open; in other words, it recruits airways to open. The volume of air in the alveoli behind the closed airways is termed the *closing volume* (CV). The CV plus the RV is termed the *closing capacity* (CC). The CC normally occurs at less than the FRC.[5]

During the early emergence phase of anesthesia, patients usually have low lung volumes, which can lead to airway closure. Consequently, a postoperative breathing maneuver that has a maximal alveolar inflating pressure, a long alveolar inflating time, and high alveolar inflating volume, such as the SMI or yawn maneuver, should be used to facilitate the maximal recruitment of lung units. With the recruitment of lung units, the FRC could be raised out of the closing volume range and ultimately hypoxemia could be reduced.

Surface Tension Phenomenon

The surface tension phenomenon relates to the action of surfactant on lung tissue. Surfactant is a phospholipid rich in lecithin that is produced by the type II alveolar cells. Surfactant lines the alveolus as a thin surface-active film. This film has a physiologic action of reducing the surface tension of the alveoli and terminal respiratory airways. If the surfactant were not present, the surface tension would be fixed and greater pressure would be needed to keep the alveolus open. As a result, small alveoli would empty into larger ones, atelectasis would regularly occur at low lung volumes, and large expanding pressures would be necessary to reopen collapsed lung units. Surfactant is also an important factor in alveolar inflation because it provides uniformity in the inflation of lung units. In these ways, surfactant helps to impart stability to alveoli in the normal lung. In addition to a

major role in pulmonary hysteresis, surfactant also contributes to lung recoil and reduces the workload of breathing.[8]

Lung Compliance

Several other terms that relate to the P-V curve of the lung deserve attention. One term is *lung compliance* (C_L), which is defined as the change in volume for a given change in pressure or the pressure needed for maintenance of a given volume of inflation. The normal value for C_L is 0.1 L per cm H_2O.

$$C_L = \frac{\Delta V}{\Delta P}$$

where V represents volume and P represents pressure.

Lung compliance is a measurement of the distensibility of the lungs during breathing. According to convention, C_L means the slope on the static deflation portion of the P-V curve over the V_T range; therefore C_L can be said to be the slope of the P-V curve, and it may remain unchanged even if marked changes in lung elastic properties cause a shift of the P-V curve to the left or right. As a result, clinical measurement of lung compliance is done over the V_T range, during deflation. Measurement of the C_L over any other portion of the P-V curve can result in an inaccurate reading as compared with a normal value. Lung elastic recoil (Pst_L) is the pressure exerted by the lung (transpulmonary pressure) because of its tendency to recoil or collapse to a smaller resting state. At low lung volumes, the Pst_L is low; at high lung volumes, the Pst_L is high. This elastic retractive force (i.e., Pst_L) is the result of the overall structural elements of the lung combined with the lung surface tension forces. As mentioned previously, the C_L represents the slope of the P-V curve, and the Pst_L represents the points along the P-V curve. Changes in C_L and Pst_L have dramatic implications in the alteration of lung volumes that occurs in the immediate postoperative period (see the section on postoperative lung volumes).[5]

Equal Pressure Point

The equal pressure point (EPP) has many clinical implications to perianesthesia practice. More specifically, intraoperative and postoperative mechanical ventilations, along with pursed lips and abdominal breathing of the patient with compliant airways, are based on this concept.

The alveoli and airways can be imagined as a balloon in a box (Fig. 12-11). Flow out of the balloon is facilitated by the recoil of the balloon, which forces the air out of the balloon through the neck and out into the atmosphere. The addition of pressure all over the box forces the air out of the balloon at a higher rate of flow. Physiologically, the balloon recoil is analogous to the alveolar recoil pressure. The pressure pushing down on the balloon and its neck corresponds to a positive pleural pressure that is generated on a forced expiratory maneuver. For the air to move out of the alveoli, the alveolar pressure must exceed the pressure at the mouth. The pressure inside the neck of the balloon corresponds to the intraluminal airway pressure. Consequently, the alveolar pressure comprises the recoil pressure of the alveoli and the plural pressure. Also, the pressure to generate air flow decreases down the airway to the mouth (see Fig. 12-11). During a forced expiratory maneuver, the plural pressure pushes down on the alveoli and the airways. If the alveolar recoil pressure is 30 and the plural pressure is 20, the alveolar pressure is 50. The pressure inside the airway (intraluminal pressure) decreases progressively downstream toward the mouth. The EPP occurs when the intraluminal pressure is equal to the plural pressure (20 = 20); from that point, the plural pressure exceeds the intraluminal pressure

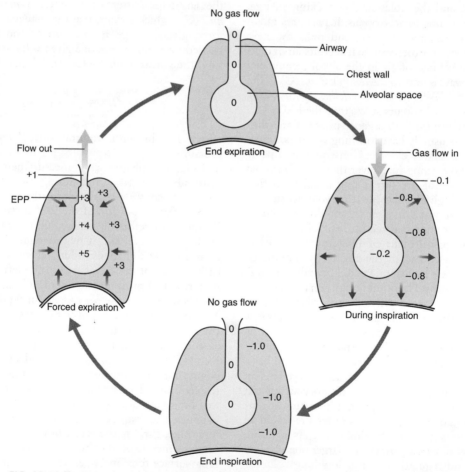

FIG. 12-11 Pressure changes in the chest and lung during inspiration and forced expiration. The pleural pressure around the airways is usually negative (less than atmospheric). During inspiration, the chest wall expands and there is a greater negative pleural pressure, drawing air into the airways. At forced expiration, the pleural pressure may become positive, forcing air out. The equal pressure point (EPP) is where airway pressure equals pleural pressure. (From Naish J: *Medical sciences*, St. Louis, 2009, Saunders.)

and dynamic compression of the airway occurs. Total collapse of the airways from the EPP and the mouth does not normally occur because of the compliance of the airways. Physiologically, the dynamic compression reduces the airways radius and thus results in an increase in flow rates in the compressed area that aids physiologic mechanisms, such as the cough maneuver, to sheer and expel secretions and mucus out of the airways.[5]

In the patient with highly compliant airways (i.e., with chronic obstructive pulmonary disease), the dynamic compression can completely close the airways. The air that is trapped increases the FRC and becomes dead space. The harder the patient tries to expel air, the greater the plural pressure becomes and more dynamic compression occurs; thus a vicious cycle ensues. Interventions to help these patients move air out of the lungs are focused on a reduction of the amount of dynamic compression on the airways. The interventions are to increase the expiratory time and provide physiologic positive end-expiratory pressure (PEEP). Lengthening of the expiratory time aids in reduction of the amount of positive plural pressure on the airways, and physiologic PEEP enhances the airway's intraluminal pressure in the highly compliant airways. In the awake patient with highly compliant airways, abdominal breathing prolongs the expiratory time and pursed-lip breathing provides physiologic PEEP. In the patient who is anesthetized, prolonging the expiratory time (i.e., inspiration:expiration ratio of 1:3) on the ventilator and use of physiologic PEEP (i.e., 5 cm/H_2O) aids in moving air out of the airways.

Pulmonary Time Constant

The pulmonary time constant is similar to the half-life used in assessment of the pharmacokinetic activity of drugs. A time constant represents the amount of time necessary for flow to decrease by a rate equal to half the initial flow. A time constant equals the resistance multiplied by the compliance. Therefore the time necessary to reach each time constant depends on the individual values of resistance and compliance. In normal conditions, the decrease in flow at the first time constant is approximately 37% of the initial flow, or approximately 63% of the total volume added or removed from the lungs. The first time constant represents the time necessary for removing or adding 63% of the total volume of air in the lungs. The decrease in flow rate at the second time constant is approximately 14%, and the percent volume of air added or removed from the lungs is 86%. The decrease in flow at the third time constant is 5%, with a corresponding 95% volume added or removed; therefore the higher the time constant, the more air removed or added to the lungs.[4]

The clinical implications of time constants are extremely important in the perianesthesia care of patients who have received an inhalation anesthetic. Patients who have increased airway resistance or increased C_L, or both, have a prolonged time necessary for filling and emptying of the lungs. The lung units in this situation are referred to as *slow lung units*. The patient with slow lung units usually has chronic obstructive pulmonary disease. Patients with a significant amount of increased secretions also have some slow lung units. Consequently, patients with slow lung units usually have a slow emergence from inhalation anesthesia. Patients with a low C_L, such as patients with pulmonary fibrosis, have fast lung units. As a result, these patients can fill or empty the lungs rather rapidly and have a rapid emergence from inhalation anesthesia.

Mechanical Features of the Chest Wall

Because of its elastic properties, the chest wall always springs out or recoils outward, seeking a larger resting volume. The resting volume of the lungs alone is less than the RV, and the resting volume of the chest wall is approximately 60% of the VC.

The action of the chest wall can be illustrated with the analogy of a wire screen attached around a balloon. The wire screen tends to spring outward so that the screen pulls the balloon open at lower balloon volumes. A measure of the pressure at the mouth of the balloon reflects a negative number. At approximately 60% of the total capacity of the balloon, the screen no longer tends to spring outward. At that point, the addition of air causes the screen to push down on the balloon—a reflection of a positive pressure at the mouth of the balloon. The screen around the balloon can be likened to the chest wall. As shown in Fig. 12-12, at lower lung volumes, the chest wall clearly is inclined to recoil outward, thus creating a negative pressure. At approximately 60% of the VC, the chest wall starts to push down on the lungs, thus creating a positive pressure. The result of the interplay between the chest wall's strong tendency to spring outward and the lung's strong tendency to recoil inward is the subatmospheric pleural pressure.[5]

Pleural pressure can become positive during a cough or other forced expiratory maneuvers. Pneumothorax can occur when the chest wall is opened or when air is injected into the pleural cavity. With this occurrence, the lungs collapse because they naturally recoil to a smaller position; the ribs flare outward because of their natural inclination to recoil outward. Clinically, inspection

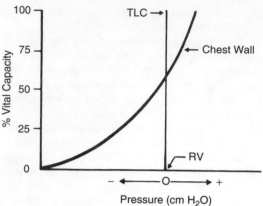

FIG. 12-12 Pressure-volume curve of chest wall during deflation going from TLC to RV. Positive pressures of the chest wall represent pressures that tend to decrease lung size, and negative pressures represent pressures that tend to increase lung volume because of outward recoil tendency of chest wall at approximately 60% of vital capacity or less. *TLC,* Total lung capacity; *RV,* residual volume. (From Drain C: Physiology of the respiratory system related to anesthesia. *CRNA* 7:163–180, 1996.)

of a patient with a pneumothorax may reveal protruding ribs on the affected side.

The two types of pneumothorax are open (simple) and closed (tension). Simple pneumothorax occurs when air flow into the pleural space results in a positive pleural pressure. The lungs collapse because the recoil pressure is not counterbalanced with the negative pleural pressure. Treatment for a pneumothorax can be conservative or more aggressive, depending on the type and amount of pneumothorax. Aggressive treatment consists of the insertion of chest tubes into the pleural space to recreate the negative pleural pressure. This maneuver reestablishes normal ventilatory excursions. In most instances, the air leak between the lung and the pleural space seals after the chest tubes have been removed. If air continues to flow into the intrapleural space but cannot escape, the intrapleural pressure continually increases with each succeeding inspiration. Like a one-way valve, pressure increases and a tension pneumothorax develops. In a brief period, as the intrapleural pressure increases, the affected lung is compressed and puts a great amount of pressure on the mediastinum. Hypoxemia and reduction in cardiac output result, and if treatment is not instituted immediately, the patient may die. Treatment consists of immediate evacuation of the excess air from the intrapleural space with either chest tubes or a large-bore needle. A tension pneumothorax is truly a medical emergency.[2]

Combined Mechanical Properties of the Lungs and Chest Wall

The combined P-V characteristics of the lungs and the chest wall have many implications for the perianesthesia nurse. The combined P-V curve is the algebraic sum of the individual P-V curves of the lungs and chest wall. When no muscle forces are applied to the respiratory system, the FRC is determined by a balance of elastic forces between the lungs and the chest wall (Fig. 12-13). Any pathophysiologic or pharmacologic process that affects the elasticity of either the lungs or the chest wall affects the FRC.

Alterations in the Balance of Pulmonary Forces in the Perianesthesia Patient

During the induction of anesthesia, the shape of the P-V curve of the chest wall is altered. This agent-independent phenomenon is probably the result of loss of chest wall elasticity. Thus the P-V curve of the chest wall of a patient with normal lung function is shifted to the right, the balance of forces occurs sooner, and the FRC decreases (Fig. 12-14). This shift to the right affects the P-V curve of the lung; it also shifts to the right, and secondary changes occur in the lung. More specifically, the changes consist of an increase in lung recoil ($\uparrow Pst_L$) and a decrease in C_L ($\downarrow C_L$). Ultimately, the lung becomes stiffer, and the FRC

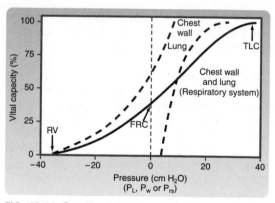

FIG. 12-13 Combined P-V curves of lungs and chest wall. Individual P-V curves of lungs and chest wall are represented with *dashed lines.* They are transposed from static deflation P-V curves of lungs (see Fig. 12-8) and chest wall (see Fig. 12-12). The combined P-V curve is the algebraic sum of deflation curves of the lungs and chest wall. In a combined P-V curve, FRC can be seen to be determined by balance of elastic forces of the lungs and chest wall when no respiratory muscles are applied. *P-V,* Pressure-volume; *TLC,* total lung capacity; *RV,* residual volume; *FRC,* functional residual capacity. (From Koeppen BM, Stanton BA: *Berne and Levy's physiology,* ed 6 [updated edition], St. Louis, 2010, Mosby.)

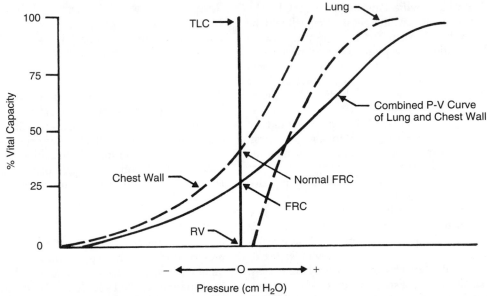

FIG. 12-14 P-V curve representing the lung mechanics of a patient in the immediate postoperative period who has undergone upper abdominal or thoracic surgical procedure. This patient has a loss of chest wall elastic recoil that causes lungs to become less compliant. Consequently, the combined P-V curve shifts to the right, leading to a decline in the FRC because balance of forces occurs at lower lung volumes. *P-V,* Pressure-volume; *FRC,* functional residual capacity; *TLC,* total lung capacity; *RV,* residual volume. (From Drain C: Pathophysiology of the respiratory system related to anesthesia. *CRNA* 7:181–192, 1996.)

decreases and may drop into the closing capacity range. Therefore, during tidal ventilation, some airways are closed to ventilation and ventilation-perfusion mismatching occurs ($\downarrow$ alveolar ventilation/perfusion [$\downarrow V_A/Q_C$]), which ultimately leads to hypoxemia. Research indicates that this phenomenon, coupled with sighless breathing patterns in the PACU, can cause patients to have hypoxemia in the recovery phase of the anesthetic (see the section on postoperative lung volumes).[9]

Pulmonary Circulation

The basic functions of the pulmonary circulation are exchanging gas, providing a reservoir for the left ventricle, furnishing nutrition, and protecting the lungs.

Gas Exchange

The major aspects of gas exchange are discussed in the section on blood gas transport. Because of the implications for perianesthesia nursing care, the concepts of transit time and pulmonary vascular resistance are presented here.

Of the 5 L of blood that flows through the lungs every minute, only 70 to 200 mL are active in gas exchange at any one time. The time a red blood cell (RBC) takes to cross the pulmonary capillary bed is 0.75 seconds, but the RBC takes only 0.25 seconds to become saturated with oxygen—that is, until all the

oxygen-bonding sites on the hemoglobin molecule are occupied. Because the transit time is 0.75 seconds and the saturation time is only 0.25 seconds, the body has a tremendous backup of 0.5 seconds for hemoglobin saturation with oxygen.[5] If the RBCs move across the pulmonary capillary bed at an accelerated pace (decreased transit time), the amount of time available for oxygen to saturate the RBCs is decreased. During stress or exercise, however, the complete saturation of the hemoglobin can still be accomplished because the transit time of a RBC rarely decreases at less than 0.25 seconds.[5]

However, this process is not true for patients with interstitial fibrosis who have a thickened respiratory exchange membrane. These patients may have a normal PaO_2 at rest, but exercise or exertion of surgery increases the cardiac output and decreases the RBC transit time; therefore the hemoglobin does not become completely saturated during its passage through the pulmonary capillary bed. This phenomenon occurs because more time is needed for oxygen to pass through the diseased membrane. For these patients, the lower limit for complete saturation may be 0.5 seconds, not 0.25 seconds. As a result, patients with disorders of the respiratory exchange membrane can have a lower oxygen saturation (SaO_2) on the pulse oximeter with any exertion that could decrease RBC transit time. Clinically, this phenomenon is sometimes called *desaturation on exercise*. Patients in the PACU who are suspected of having this problem should be given low-flow oxygen and be closely monitored for desaturation via a pulse oximeter. Because of the possibility of desaturation, the low-flow oxygen administration should not be discontinued until the patient's condition stabilizes, which could indicate continued administration after the patient is discharged from the PACU. Measures should be started to reduce the extrinsic factors, such as stress, elevated body temperature, and anxiety, which increase the cardiac output.

The pulmonary and systemic circulations have the same pump—the heart. The pulmonary system receives the same cardiac output as the systemic circulation, approximately 5 L/min. The pulmonary circulation, in comparison with the systemic circulation, is a low-pressure system with low resistance to flow, distensible vessels with extremely thin walls, and a small amount of smooth muscle. Many stimuli affect pulmonary vascular resistance. Probably the most potent vasoconstrictor of the lung is alveolar hypoxia. Research indicates that neuroendothelial bodies, which respond to a low PaO_2, may exist close to the pulmonary vascular bed. In addition, the neuroendothelial bodies can liberate prostaglandins or histamine, or both, when alveolar hypoxia is present. Pulmonary vascular resistance does not seem to be affected by the volatile anesthetics such as enflurane and isoflurane. However, nitrous oxide can increase pulmonary vascular resistance, especially in patients with preexisting pulmonary hypertension. Neonates who may or may not have preexisting pulmonary hypertension are prone to developing increased pulmonary vascular resistance when nitrous oxide is administered. If a patient in the PACU is prone to developing increased pulmonary vascular resistance, the effect of nitrous oxide on pulmonary vascular resistance is almost dissipated as a result of the rapid excretion from the lungs of nitrous oxide because of its low blood-gas coefficient.[8]

In the postoperative period, if a patient has atelectasis in some portion of the lungs, the PaO_2 in that particular area of the lungs is reduced. As a result, the neuroendothelial bodies are stimulated to produce increased pulmonary vascular resistance in that area of the lungs. Eventually, the blood is redirected or shunted to areas of the lungs that are adequately ventilated. As a result, the SaO_2 in a patient with atelectasis may indicate hypoxemia (<90%). After 5 to 12 minutes, the SaO_2 may be slightly improved because of the increased pulmonary vascular resistance in the area of atelectasis. Therefore the perianesthesia nurse should continue to use an aggressive stir-up regimen on a patient with atelectasis, even though the patient's SaO_2 values indicate a slight improvement.

Reservoir for the Left Ventricle

In regard to functioning as a reservoir for the left ventricle, the pulmonary veins are considered extensions of the left ventricle.

Nutrition

The pulmonary circulation can be divided into the bronchial circulation and the actual pulmonary circulation. The bronchial circulation carries nutrients and oxygen down to the respiratory bronchioles in the lungs. The bronchial circulation empties its deoxygenated blood via the pulmonary veins to the left heart. The pulmonary circulation carries nutrients to the respiratory bronchioles and the alveoli.[1]

Protection

The role of the lungs in protection is vital for the preservation of the human organism. For example, on the surface of the pulmonary epithelium are invaginations called *caveolae*. Bradykinin and angiotensin I are enzymatically converted on the surface of the caveoli. Ninety percent of the bradykinin is deactivated in the caveoli during each pass through the lungs, and angiotensin I is converted to angiotensin II with angiotensin-converting enzyme in the lungs. In the presence of hypoxia, the conversion of angiotensin I to angiotensin II is inhibited. Also, in the hypoxemic state, less than 12% of the bradykinin is deactivated by the lungs, and in the hypoxemic state the liberated bradykinin then become prostaglandins. Interestingly, the inappropriate levels of prostaglandins as a result of hypoxemia in the chronic state are thought to produce the clubbing of the fingers in patients with long standing chronic hypoxemia. Finally, the pulmonary epithelium also deactivates norepinephrine and serotonin. Serotonin plays an important part in platelet aggregation. Increased levels of serotonin from decreased lung function caused by hypoxia or lung disease lead to a high risk for venous thrombus. The implications for PACU care are that patients who are immobile and hypoxemic ($SaO_2 < 90\%$) should be monitored for pulmonary and systemic thromboemboli.[1]

Water Balance in the Lung

The alveoli stay dry with a combination of pressures and lymph flow (Fig. 12-15). The forces that tend to push fluid out of the pulmonary capillaries are the capillary hydrostatic pressure (P_{cap}) minus the interstitial fluid hydrostatic pressure (P_{is}). The forces that tend to pull fluid into the pulmonary capillaries are the colloid osmotic pressure of the proteins in the plasma of the pulmonary capillaries (π_{pl}) minus the colloid osmotic pressure of the proteins in the interstitial fluid (π_{is}). The Starling equation

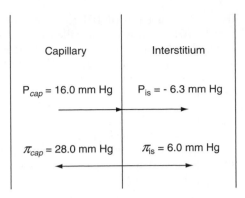

Capillary	Interstitium
P_{cap} = 16.0 mm Hg	P_{is} = - 6.3 mm Hg
π_{cap} = 28.0 mm Hg	π_{is} = 6.0 mm Hg

Systemic - Capillary Membrane

FIG. 12-15 Pressures affecting fluid exchange at the systemic capillaries. Arrows indicate direction of individual pressures causing fluid movement. *Pis*, Interstitial hydrostatic pressure; *Pcap*, capillary hydrostatic pressure; *πis*, interstitial colloid osmotic pressure; *πcap*, plasma colloid osmotic pressure. (From Kacmarek RM, Dimas S: *The essentials of respiratory care*, ed 4, St. Louis, 2005, Mosby.)

describes the movement of fluid across the capillary endothelium:

$$Q_f = K_f (P_{cap} - P_{is}) - \sigma_f(\pi_{pl} - \pi_{is})$$

in which Q_f is the net flow of fluid; K_f is the capillary filtration coefficient, which describes the permeability characteristics of the membrane to fluids; and σ_f is the reflection coefficient, which describes the ability of the membrane to prevent extravasation of solute particles.

Thus, the membrane is permeable to fluid, and in normal circumstances, σ_f is equal to 1.0 in the equation.

With substitution of normal values into the Starling equation:

$$Q_f = K_f[10 \text{ torr} - (-3 \text{ torr})]$$
$$- \sigma_f(25 \text{ torr} - 19 \text{ torr})$$

in which K_f and σ_f are dropped from the equation because they are considered normal and do not affect the outcome of the example; therefore:

$$Q_f = (13 \text{ torr}) - (6 \text{ torr})$$
$$Q_f = +7 \text{ torr}$$

Thus, the pressure favors flow out of the capillaries to the interstitium of the alveolar wall tracts through the interstitial space to the perivascular and peribronchial spaces to facilitate transport of the fluid to the lymph nodes. As a result, a net pressure of 7 torr pushes fluid to the interstitial

space. The lymph flow draining the lungs is approximately 20 mL/h in rate of flow; therefore the lungs depend on a continuous net fluid flux to remain in a consistently "dry" state.[5]

Pulmonary edema, defined as increased total lung water, is associated with dysfunction of any parameter of the Starling equation. Examples of conditions that produce an overwhelming amount of fluid to be drained by the lymphatic system are elevated pulmonary capillary pressure (from left-sided heart failure), decreased capillary colloid osmotic pressure (from hypoproteinemia or overadministration of intravenous solutions), and extravasation of fluid through the pulmonary capillary membrane (from adult respiratory distress syndrome). The earliest form of pulmonary edema is characterized by engorgement of the peribronchial and perivascular spaces and is known as interstitial edema. If interstitial edema is allowed to continue, alveolar pulmonary edema develops.

Pulmonary edema is difficult to assess in the early stages. As the fluid volume increases in the interstitium that surrounds the blood vessels and airways, reflex bronchospasm may occur. A chest radiograph at this time reveals Kerley B lines, which denote fluid in the interstitium. When the lymphatics become completely overwhelmed, fluid enters the alveoli. In the beginning of this pathophysiologic process, fine crackles are heard on auscultation. As pulmonary edema progresses into the alveoli, coarse crackles are heard, especially at the base of the lungs. Because of the direct stimulation of the J receptors in the interstitium, the patient has a tachypneic ventilatory pattern. Initial arterial blood gas values show a low PaO_2 and $PaCO_2$. As the pulmonary edema progresses, the $PaCO_2$ increases because hyperventilation (tachypnea) is not able to counterbalance the rise in the carbon dioxide in the blood. Finally, when the pulmonary edema becomes fulminant, the sputum becomes frothy and blood tinged.[9,11]

Treatment of pulmonary edema is based on the Starling equation. If edema is cardiogenic, the focus of the treatment is a lowering of the hydrostatic pressures within the capillaries. Noncardiogenic pulmonary edema is usually treated with the infusion of albumin to increase the osmotic forces. Diuretics and dialysis also may be used in noncardiogenic edema in an effort to lower the vascular pressures. Positive end-expiratory or continuous positive airway pressure is used with high oxygen concentrations to correct the hypoxemia.

Blood Gas Transport

Respiration is the gas exchange between cellular levels in the body and the external environment. The three phases of respiration are: (1) ventilation, the phase of moving air in and out of the lungs; (2) transportation, which includes diffusion of gases in and out of the blood in both pulmonary and systemic capillaries, reactions of carbon dioxide and oxygen in the blood, and circulation of blood between the lungs and the tissue cells; and (3) gas exchange, in which oxygen is used and carbon dioxide is produced. Blood gas transport is the important link in the carrying of gas to or from the cell.

At sea level, the barometric pressure is 760 torr. Air contains approximately 21% oxygen, which exerts a partial pressure of 159 torr. As described by Dalton's law of partial pressure, the total pressure of a given volume of a gas mixture is equal to the sum of the separate or partial pressures that each gas would exert if that gas alone occupied the entire volume. Therefore the total pressure is equal to the sum of the partial pressures of the major gases in the atmosphere. For example:

$$P_{TOTAL} = PN_2 + PO_2$$

in which P_{TOTAL} is total atmospheric pressure, PN_2 is partial pressure of nitrogen, and PO_2 is partial pressure of oxygen. If the actual numeric quantities then are substituted into the formula[5]:

$$760 \text{ torr} = 601 \text{ torr} + 159 \text{ torr}$$

As expressed in percentages, 100% (total atmospheric pressure) is equal to 79.07% (nitrogen) plus 20.93% (oxygen); therefore nitrogen is 601 torr (0.7907×760), and oxygen is 159 torr (0.2093×760). In the lower airways, water vapor exerts a pressure that can be accounted for with Dalton's law. At the body temperature of 37° C, the water vapor pressure in the lower airways is 47 torr. Because the water vapor pressure affects the partial pressures of both nitrogen and oxygen, it is subtracted from the atmospheric pressure of 760 torr, which results in a pressure of 713 torr (760 torr − 47 torr = 713 torr). For determination of the PO_2 in the lower airways, the percent oxygen (20.93) is multiplied by 713 torr, with a resulting PO_2 of 149.2 torr. The respiratory exchange ratio can be used to understand how the alveolar partial pressure of oxygen is determined. This ratio represents carbon dioxide production divided by oxygen consumption. The normal respiratory exchange ratio is 0.8. Theoretically, then, for every 12 torr of carbon dioxide that is added to the alveolus, 12 torr of oxygen is displaced. Therefore, with no respiratory pathophysiology present, if the $PaCO_2$ is 40 torr, 48 torr of oxygen is removed from the alveolus, in which: $4 \times 10 = 40$ torr (carbon dioxide) and thus $4 \times 12 = 48$ torr (oxygen).

The result is a PaO_2 of 101 torr (149 torr − 48 torr = 101 torr), which is called the *12-10 concept* and is helpful in assessment of arterial blood gas determinations in the PACU (see the section on causes of hypoxemia).

As oxygen diffuses across the pulmonary membrane, the PO_2 is further decreased to 95 torr by a venous admixture. This effect occurs because of vascular shunts that normally redirect 1% or 2% of the total cardiac output either to nonaerated areas in the lungs themselves or directly through the heart, bypassing the lungs.[3]

Oxygen Transport

Oxygen is carried in the blood in combination with hemoglobin or in simple solution. Approximately 98% of oxygen transported from the lungs to the cells is carried in combination with hemoglobin in the RBCs, a reversible chemical combination. The remaining 2% is dissolved in the plasma and in the cytoplasm of the RBCs. The amount of oxygen transported in both forms is directly proportional to the PO_2.

When the blood passes through the lungs, it does not normally become completely saturated with oxygen. Usually, the hemoglobin becomes about 97% saturated. Hemoglobin that is saturated with oxygen is called *oxyhemoglobin*.

Normally, the oxygen content of the arterial blood is 19.8 mL/dL of blood. This total oxygen content in the arterial blood (CaO_2) is equal to the oxygen-carrying capacity of hemoglobin, which is 1.34 times the number of grams of hemoglobin.[3] That number divided by 100 is the oxygen content carried by the hemoglobin. To determine the total amount of oxygen in the blood, the oxygen content that is dissolved in the plasma must be added to the oxygen content of the hemoglobin. The amount of oxygen dissolved in the plasma is determined with multiplication of the PaO_2 by the solubility coefficient for oxygen in plasma, which is 0.003.

Therefore the equation for the total oxygen content in the blood is:

$$CaO_2 = Hb \times 1.34 \times \%Hb \text{ saturation} + (PaO_2 \times 0.003)$$

in which *Hb* is hemoglobin. If the normal values of Hb are 15 g, percent Hb saturation as 97 and PaO_2 as 95 torr are substituted into the equation:

$$CaO_2 = \frac{(15 \times 1.34 \times 97)}{100} + (95 \times .0.003)$$

$$CaO_2 = 19.497 + 0.285$$

$$CaO_2 = 19.782 \text{ mL of oxygen per dL of blood}$$

One must remember that oxygen content is different from oxygen partial pressures. *Content* refers only to the amount of oxygen carried by the blood, not to its partial pressure (PO_2).

In the lungs, venous blood is oxygenated or arterialized. The oxygen bond with hemoglobin is loose and reversible. The bond is also PO_2 dependent—that is, the higher the PaO_2, the greater the oxygen saturation of the hemoglobin. However, the hemoglobin cannot be supersaturated. When all the bonding sites on the hemoglobin molecule are occupied by oxygen, the oxygen is not able to bond to the hemoglobin no matter how much more oxygen is presented to the hemoglobin.

The oxygen-hemoglobin dissociation curve relates the percentage of oxygen saturation of hemoglobin to the PaO_2 value. Note in Fig. 12-16 that the curve is sigmoid in shape with a steep portion between the 10- and 50-torr PaO_2 range, with a leveling off above 70 torr. The flat portion of the curve indicates the capacity to oxygenate most of the hemoglobin despite wide variations in the PO_2 (70 to 98 torr). This flat portion of the curve can be called the *association portion of the curve,* and it corresponds to the external respiration that is taking place in the lungs. The steep portion of the curve indicates the capacity to unload large amounts of oxygen in response to small tissue PO_2 changes. This part of the curve is called the *dissociation portion of the oxygen–hemoglobin dissociation curve.*

As discussed, the normal oxygen content at the association portion of the curve is approximately 19.8 mL of oxygen per deciliter of blood. At the venous dissociation portion of the curve, the content of oxygen is 15.2 mL of oxygen per deciliter of blood. The following formula is used to derive the content of oxygen in the mixed venous blood (CvO_2):

$$CvO_2 = \frac{Hb \times 1.34 \times \%Hb \text{ saturation}}{100} + (PvO_2 \times 0.003)$$

in which PvO_2 is pressure of oxygen in the mixed venous blood.

With substitution of normal values for mixed venous blood of Hb as 15 g, the percent Hb saturation as 75, and PvO_2 as 40 into the formula:

$$CvO_2 = \frac{(15 \times 1.34 \times 75)}{100} + (40 \times 0.003)$$

$$CvO_2 = 15.08 + 0.12$$

$$CvO_2 = 15.20 \text{ mL of oxygen per dL of blood}$$

Therefore, in this example, the net delivery of oxygen to the tissues is 4.6 mL of oxygen per deciliter of blood (19.8 − 15.2 = 4.6).[3]

Factors That Affect Oxygen Transport

The association portion of the oxygen-hemoglobin dissociation curve is not necessarily a fixed line determined solely by the PaO_2. The height and the slope of the curve are dependent on many factors, including pH and temperature. Generally, a decrease in pH (an increase in hydrogen ions) or an increase in body temperature causes a shift of the curve to the right, which leads to a decrease in the height and slope of the curve. Ultimately, less saturation (loading) of the hemoglobin is found for a given PaO_2. As a result, patients who have a low pH or high temperature, or both, probably benefit from a higher fraction of inspired oxygen (FiO_2) than normal for facilitation of an appropriate level of saturation of hemoglobin. However, arterial blood gas determinations should be analyzed before changes in the FiO_2 are made.

At the dissociation portion of the oxygen-hemoglobin dissociation curve, the same is true. This portion is not a fixed line because it also changes position in response to physiologic processes. At the tissue level, metabolically active tissues produce more carbon dioxide and more acid (↓ pH) and have an elevated temperature. These products of metabolism shift the curve to the right. The curve shifts far more in response to physiologic processes in the dissociation portion than in the association part. Metabolically active tissues produce more carbon dioxide and need more oxygen. The effect of carbon dioxide on the curve is closely related to the fact that

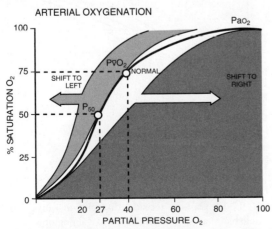

FIG. 12-16 Oxyhemoglobin dissociation curve. (From Frownfelter D, Dean E: *Cardiovascular and pulmonary physical therapy,* ed 4, St. Louis, 2006, Mosby.)

deoxyhemoglobin binds hydrogen ions more actively than does oxyhemoglobin. As a result, at the tissue level, increased carbon dioxide decreases the affinity of hemoglobin for oxygen. The dissociation portion of the curve is shifted to the right and more oxygen is given to the tissue. This effect of carbon dioxide on oxygen transport is called the *Bohr effect*.

2,3-Diphosphoglycerate (2,3-DPG) regulates the release of oxygen to the tissue; it is a glycolytic intermediary metabolite that is more concentrated in the RBCs than anywhere else in the body. High concentrations of 2,3-DPG shift the oxyhemoglobin dissociation curve to the right, which makes oxygen more available to the tissues. Lower concentrations of 2,3-DPG cause a shift of the curve to the left, which ultimately leads to the release of less oxygen to the tissues. The clinical implications of these observations involve the administration of outdated whole blood. Whole blood stored longer than 21 days has low levels of 2,3-DPG. As a result, if outdated blood is administered to a patient, the tissues do not receive an appropriate amount of oxygen because of the shift to the left of the oxygen-hemoglobin dissociation curve.[3]

Pulse Oximetry and the Oxygen Dissociation Curve

Oxygen delivered to the tissues is determined by the cardiac output and the CaO_2. Most of the oxygen is bound to the hemoglobin, and the percentage of the oxygen bound to the hemoglobin is expressed as the SaO_2. The amount of oxygen that is dissolved in simple solution in the arterial blood is the PaO_2. A gradient is set from the lung to the tissues in regard to oxygen delivery and is represented by the oxygen dissociation curve. A normal curve, without any shifts left or right, is determined by the $PaCO_2$, pH, body temperature, and hemoglobin and 2,3-DPG levels. A normal curve is therefore set at values of $PaCO_2$ of 40 torr, pH of 7.4, temperature of 37° C, and hemoglobin of 15 g/dL. With the oxygen dissociation curve (see Fig. 12-16), the PaO_2 can be determined with the SaO_2 reading on the pulse oximeter. For example, an SaO_2 of 90% corresponds to a PaO_2 of 60 torr. With the curve, at an SaO_2 less than 90%, the PaO_2 drops rapidly (the dissociation portion of the curve). Clinically, an SaO_2 of 90% can be considered hypoxemia, and severe hypoxemia occurs when the PaO_2 is less than 40 torr or the SaO_2 is 75%.[10]

Carbon Dioxide Transport

The transport of carbon dioxide begins within each cell in the body. Carbon dioxide is a main byproduct of the energy-supplying mechanisms

of the cell. Approximately 200 mL/min of carbon dioxide is produced within the body at rest. Carbon dioxide is 20-fold more soluble in water than oxygen; therefore it traverses the fluid compartments of the body rapidly. The intracellular partial pressure of carbon dioxide is 46 torr. A 1-torr gradient exists between the cell and the interstitial fluid. Carbon dioxide diffuses out of the cell to the interstitial fluid and has a new partial pressure of 45 torr. When the tissue capillary blood enters the venules, the partial pressure of the carbon dioxide is 45 torr.[10] Carbon dioxide is transported in the blood in three forms: (1) physically dissolved in solution; (2) as carbaminohemoglobin; and (3) as bicarbonate ions.

Carbon Dioxide in Simple Solution

Approximately 12% of the total amount of carbon dioxide transported in the body is physically dissolved in solution.

Carbaminohemoglobin

Approximately 30% of carbon dioxide is transported as carbaminohemoglobin, a chemical combination of carbon dioxide, and hemoglobin that is reversible because the binding point on the hemoglobin is on the amino groups and is a loose bond. This chemical bonding of carbon dioxide with hemoglobin can be graphically described with the use of the carbon dioxide dissociation curve. Two differences are found between the carbon dioxide dissociation curve (Fig. 12-17) and the oxygen-hemoglobin dissociation curve. First, over the normal operating range of blood

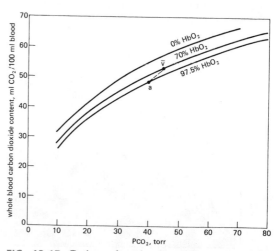

FIG. 12-17 Carbon dioxide dissociation curves for whole blood at 37° C at different oxyhemoglobin saturations. *a*, Arterial point (code: am); $\bar{v}$, mixed venous point. (From Levitzky M: *Pulmonary physiology*, ed 5, New York, 1999, McGraw-Hill.)

the partial pressure of carbon dioxide (PCO$_2$) from 47 torr (venous or PvCO$_2$) to 40 torr (arterial or PaCO$_2$), the slope of the carbon dioxide dissociation curve is nearly linear and not sigmoid like the oxygen-hemoglobin dissociation curve. Second, the total carbon dioxide content is approximately twofold the total oxygen content. Oxygen has a definite effect on carbon dioxide transport. On the upper curve, or venous portion of the carbon dioxide curve, note that the point for the PvCO$_2$ is 47 and the PvO$_2$ is 40. On the lower curve, or arterial carbon dioxide curve, observe the points for the PaCO$_2$ of 40 torr and the PaO$_2$ of 100 torr. Notice how the venous carbon dioxide curve is shifted to the left and is above the arterial curve. This description is the effect of oxygen on carbon dioxide transport, or the Haldane effect. In terms of physiologic significance, the Haldane effect plays a more important role in gas transport than does the Bohr effect. Specifically in the lungs, the binding of oxygen with hemoglobin tends to displace carbon dioxide from the hemoglobin (oxyhemoglobin is more acidic than deoxyhemoglobin). At the tissue level, oxygen is removed from the hemoglobin (as the result of a pressure gradient), which reduces the acidity of the hemoglobin and enables it to bind more carbon dioxide. In fact, because the hemoglobin is in the reduced state (deoxygenated), the hemoglobin can carry 6 volumes percent more carbon dioxide than the amount of carbon dioxide that could be carried by oxyhemoglobin.[4]

Bicarbonate

Sixty-five percent of carbon dioxide is transported as bicarbonate, which is the product of the reaction of carbon dioxide with water. When the carbon dioxide and water join, they form carbonic acid. Almost all the carbonic acid dissociates to bicarbonate and hydrogen ions, as seen in the following equation:

$$CO_2 + H_2O \xrightarrow{\text{Carbonic anhydrase}} H_2CO_3 \rightarrow H^+ + HCO_3$$

This reaction occurs mostly within the RBCs because carbonic anhydrase accelerates the hydration of carbon dioxide to carbonic acid 220 to 300 times faster than if carbon dioxide and water were joined without this enzymatic catalyst.[4]

When the bicarbonate produced in this reaction in the RBCs exceeds the bicarbonate ion level in the plasma, it diffuses out of the cell. The positively charged hydrogen ion tends to remain within the RBC and is buffered by hemoglobin. Chloride, a negatively charged ion that is abundant in the plasma, diffuses into the RBC to maintain electric balance because of ionic imbalance. This movement is called the *chloride shift*. Because of the increase in osmotically active particles within the cell, water from the plasma diffuses into the RBCs. This process explains why the RBCs in the venous side of the circulation are slightly larger than the arterial RBCs (Fig. 12-18).

As the venous blood enters the pulmonary capillaries, the carbon dioxide in simple solution freely diffuses to the alveoli. The carbaminohemoglobin reverses to free the carbon dioxide, which diffuses across the alveoli and is then expired. The hydrogen and the bicarbonate combine to form carbonic acid, which is rapidly broken down by carbonic anhydrase to form carbon dioxide and water. The carbon dioxide then diffuses through the alveoli and is expired.

Not all carbon dioxide is eliminated with pulmonary ventilation. Other buffer systems that remove excess carbon dioxide are acid-base buffers and urinary excretion by the kidneys. The respiratory system can adjust to rapid fluctuations in carbon dioxide, whereas the kidneys may need hours for restoration of a normal carbon dioxide tension.

Acid-Base Relationships

A buffer is a substance that causes a lesser change in hydrogen ion concentration to occur in a solution on addition of an acid or base than would have occurred had the buffer not been present. The buffers can respond in seconds to fluctuations in carbon dioxide tension. Buffers include the carbonic acid–bicarbonate system, the proteinate-protein system, and the hemoglobinate-hemoglobin system.[3]

The pH is a measure of alkalinity or acidity and depends on the concentration of hydrogen ions. Acidic solutions have more hydrogen ions, and alkaline solutions have fewer hydrogen ions.

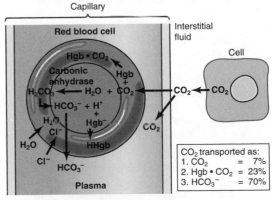

FIG. 12-18 Transport of carbon dioxide in blood. (From Hall JE: *Guyton and Hall Textbook of medical physiology*, ed 12, Philadelphia, 2011, Saunders.)

The pH is described in logarithmic form. Acid solutions have more hydrogen ions and a lower pH, which indicates acidity. If the hydrogen ion concentration is low, then the pH is high and indicates alkalinity. The pH range is from 1 to 14, with 7 as the equilibrium (pK). The normal pH value in extracellular fluid is 7.35 to 7.45, which is slightly alkaline.

The normal bicarbonate level in the extracellular fluid is 24 mEq. Base excess is used to describe alkalosis or acidosis. If a positive base excess number is noted, more base in the extracellular fluid is indicated. If a negative number is reported, the base is being used to neutralize the acid to a point of encroaching on the amount of available base, which is shown with a negative value for the base excess (acidosis).[3]

Respiratory Acid-Base Imbalances

Respiratory acidosis is characterized by a $PaCO_2$ above the normal range of 36 to 44 torr. All other primary processes that tend to cause acidosis are metabolic. Some common causes of carbon dioxide retention and respiratory acidosis are summarized in Box 12-1.

Respiratory alkalosis is characterized by a reduced $PaCO_2$. Hyperventilation frequently causes this disorder. Common causes of excessive carbon dioxide elimination and respiratory alkalosis are summarized in Box 12-2.

BOX 12-1   Common Causes of Carbon Dioxide Retention and Respiratory Acidosis (Hypoventilation)

NORMAL LUNGS
- Anesthesia
- Sedative drugs (overdose)
- Neuromuscular disease
- Poliomyelitis
- Myasthenia gravis
- Guillain-Barré syndrome
- Obesity (pickwickian syndrome)
- Brain damage
- Cardiac arrest
- Pneumothorax
- Pulmonary edema
- Bronchospasm
- Laryngospasm

ABNORMAL LUNGS
- Chronic obstructive pulmonary disease (chronic bronchitis, asthma, and emphysema)
- Diffuse infiltration pulmonary disease (advanced)
- Kyphoscoliosis (severe)

BOX 12-2   Common Causes of Excessive Carbon Dioxide Elimination and Respiratory Alkalosis (Hyperventilation)

NORMAL LUNGS
- Anxiety
- Fever
- Drugs (aspirin)
- Central nervous system lesions
- Endotoxemia

ABNORMAL LUNGS
- Pneumonia
- Diffuse infiltrative pulmonary disease (early)
- Acute bronchial asthma (early)
- Pulmonary vascular disease
- Congestive heart failure (early)

In respiratory alkalosis or acidosis, a linear exchange takes place between the carbon dioxide and bicarbonate concentrations, which is summarized as follows:

- In acute respiratory acidosis, bicarbonate concentration is approximately 1 mEq/L for each 12-torr change in $PaCO_2$.
- In chronic respiratory acidosis, the change in actual bicarbonate concentration is approximately 2 mEq/L for each 12-torr change in $PaCO_2$.
- The change in actual bicarbonate concentration with a chronic change in $PaCO_2$ above the range of 40 torr change is approximately 4 mEq/L for each 12-torr change in $PaCO_2$. This rule holds true for 1 or 2 days after the onset of the disorder because of the slow renal buffer system.

Another rule for determining whether the acid-base disorder is entirely respiratory in origin is that an acute increase in $PaCO_2$ by 12 torr produces a corresponding decrease in pH by 0.07 pH units. In chronic hypercapnia, each increase in $PaCO_2$ by 12 torr results in a corresponding decrease in pH by 0.03 pH units. $PaCO_2$ and pH changes that deviate significantly from these standards suggest that the acid-base disorder is not completely respiratory in origin. For example, if a patient who is recovering from a spinal anesthetic in the PACU has blood gases (room air) of PaO_2 of 92 torr, $PaCO_2$ of 30 torr, and pH of 7.47 compared with preoperative arterial blood gas values (room air) of PaO_2 of 80 torr, $PaCO_2$ of 40 torr, and pH of 7.40, then the rule can be applied. Because the $PaCO_2$ decreased by 12 torr and the pH increased by 0.07 pH units, the patient clearly has respiratory alkalosis and not a metabolic disorder. Moreover, by applying the

12-12 concept, it is likely that this patient probably has acute hyperventilation because the $PaCO_2$ decreased by 12 and thus the PaO_2 should increase by 12, or from 80 to 92 torr.

Metabolic Acid–Base Imbalances

Metabolic acidosis usually results with an increase in nonvolatile acids or a loss of bases from the body. The usual result is a deficit in buffer, base excess, and bicarbonate. Because acidosis stimulates respiration, the $PaCO_2$ usually decreases. The magnitude of the ventilatory response usually differentiates between acute and chronic metabolic acidosis. Some of the common causes of metabolic acidosis are summarized in Box 12-3.

Metabolic alkalosis is produced by an excessive elimination of nonvolatile acids (such as in vomiting, gastric aspiration, and hypokalemic alkalosis) or by an increase in bases (such as in alkali administration or hypochloremic alkalosis caused by some diuretics). A summary of blood gas discrepancies in each condition is provided in Table 12-3.

BOX 12-3 Common Causes of Metabolic Acidosis

- Increased nonvolatile acids
- Diabetes mellitus
- Uremia
- Severe exercise
- Hypoxia
- Shock
- Idiopathic
- Methyl alcohol ingestion (formic acid)
- Aspirin ingestion (salicylic acid)
- Excessive loss of bases (usually $NaCO_3$ from lower gastrointestinal tract)
- Severe diarrhea (e.g., cholera, diarrhea in infants)
- Fistulas (e.g., pancreatic, biliary)

Table 12-3 Summary of Blood Gas Discrepancies in Acidosis and Alkalosis

CONDITION	HCO3−	PCO2	PH
Metabolic acidosis	↓	↓	↓
Respiratory acidosis	↑	↑	↓
Metabolic alkalosis	↑	↑	↑
Respiratory alkalosis	↓	↓	↑

↑, Increased; ↓, decreased.

Matching of Ventilation to Perfusion
Distribution of Ventilation

A gravity dependent gradient of pleural pressure in the upright lung exists at resting lung volumes. The weight of the lung tends to pull the lung tissue toward the base of the lung. As a result, the intrapleural pressure is more negative at the apex of the lung in comparison with the intrapleural pressure at the base and over the V_T range (the alveoli at the apex being more fully inflated compared with the alveoli at the base). Consequently, the alveoli at the base have a greater capacity for volume change during inspiration, whereas the alveoli at the apex are already "stretched," or distended. In a healthy subject who breathes out to RV and then inspires in small steps, the initial inspired air (a small portion) goes to the apex and the base remains completely underventilated. After a certain lung volume is attained, the base of the lung receives almost all the air because of the capacity of the alveoli at the base of the lung for volume change. Therefore, because of the mechanical properties of the lung, the greatest volume change during inspiration from RV to TLC occurs near the base of the lungs.[5]

Distribution of Perfusion

A gravity-dependent gradient for perfusion in the lungs exists; approximately 80% to 90% of blood flow occurs from the middle portion to an area near the base of the lungs. Therefore the blood flow per unit of lung volume increases down the lung from the apex to the base.

Matching

Matching of alveolar ventilation ($\dot{V}_A$) to perfusion ($\dot{Q}_C$) is defined in terms of a certain volume of alveolar gas that is necessary for arterialization of a given volume of mixed venous blood. The normal alveolar ventilation ratio is:

$$\frac{\dot{V}_A}{\dot{Q}_C} = \frac{4000 \text{ mL/min}}{5000 \text{ mL/min}} = 0.8$$

If blood and gas were matched equally throughout the lung, the $\dot{V}_A/\dot{Q}_C$ would be 1. However, in the healthy lung, the matching of ventilation to perfusion is not proportional, which results in varying $\dot{V}_A/\dot{Q}_C$ throughout the lung. More specifically, ventilation at the apex is high as opposed to perfusion, and perfusion is higher than ventilation at the base of the lung. Finally, if all the $\dot{V}_A/\dot{Q}_C$ relationships were added together, the mean ratio would be 0.8.[5]

Causes of Hypoxemia
Hypoventilation

The PaO_2 and $PaCO_2$ are determined with the balance between the addition of oxygen and the removal of carbon dioxide by the alveolar ventilation and the removal of oxygen and the addition of carbon dioxide by the pulmonary capillary blood flow. If the alveolar ventilation is decreased (with no other lung pathologic changes present), the PaO_2 decreases and the $PaCO_2$ increases. In fact, the PaO_2 decreases almost proportionally to the increase in the $PaCO_2$. Recall the calculations made in the 12-12 concept. At any specific inspired oxygen tension, a 12-torr increase in the $PaCO_2$ causes an approximate 12-torr decrease in the arterial oxygen tension. For example, if the normal $PaCO_2$ is equal to 40 torr and the PaO_2 is equal to 95 torr and the patient's alveolar ventilation decreases because of opioids given in the PACU, the $PaCO_2$ increases to 60 torr. The new PaO_2 should be 71 torr (change of 20 torr in the $PaCO_2$, so 12 + 12 = 24 − 95 = 71). Therefore, with assessment of blood gas data and with the 12-10 relationship determined to be present, hypoventilation should be suspected. Note that the 12-10 relationship does not have to be exact, but if the numbers are close to the 12-10 relationship, hypoventilation is the probable cause. An increased FiO_2 value affects the 12-10 relationship. However, most patients in the PACU undergo low-flow oxygen therapy; therefore the FiO_2 is usually between 25% and 50%. Consequently, if the values seem to change proportionally, hypoventilation can still be suspected. Hypoventilation is the most common cause of hypoxemia in the PACU. Nursing interventions should include administration of a higher FiO_2 via low-flow oxygen therapy, stimulation of the patient, use of an aggressive stir-up regimen, and possible pharmacologic reversal of opioids or muscle relaxants.[9]

Ventilation or Perfusion Mismatching

If the 12-10 relationship is not present during the analysis of the arterial blood gases, $\dot{V}_A/\dot{Q}_C$ mismatching is probably the cause. However, it is difficult to determine whether the mismatching problem is the result of increased or decreased $\dot{V}_A/\dot{Q}_C$. As seen in Fig. 12-19 normal $\dot{V}_A/\dot{Q}_C$ exists when appropriate matching of ventilation to perfusion occurs. Decreased $\dot{V}_A/\dot{Q}_C$ occurs when the matching ventilation is reduced in comparison with perfusion of the alveoli, and increased $\dot{V}_A/\dot{Q}_C$ is caused by increased ventilation as compared with perfusion.

Decreased Ventilation to Perfusion

Reduced ventilation, in comparison with perfusion, ($\downarrow \dot{V}_A/\dot{Q}_C$) can be caused by excessive secretions or partial bronchospasm. Intrapulmonary

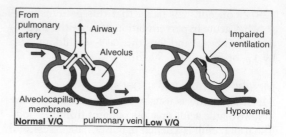
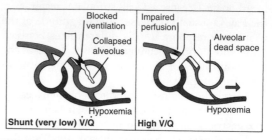

FIG. 12-19 Graphic representation of normal and abnormal matching of ventilation ($\dot{V}_A$) to perfusion ($\dot{Q}_C$). (From Heuther SE, McCance KL: *Understanding pathophysiology*, ed 3, St. Louis, 2004, Mosby.)

shunting results when atelectasis or airway closure occurs. In these situations, oxygen cannot diffuse properly across to the pulmonary capillary blood. In decreased $\dot{V}_A/\dot{Q}_C$, some oxygen diffuses across from the alveoli to the pulmonary capillary blood. Thus, the alveolar-arterial oxygen difference ($PAO_2 - PaO_2$) is slightly reduced. If a large gradient exists in the $PAO_2 - PaO_2$ value, intrapulmonary shunting is probably present. For a patient who is breathing room air, the normal $PAO_2 - PaO_2$ value is between 5 and 15 torr. When a patient is breathing oxygen at a FiO_2 of 0.5 (50%), the $PAO_2 - PaO_2$ value should be approximately 50 torr. A gradient greatly in excess of 50 torr suggests $\dot{V}_A/\dot{Q}_C$ mismatching. The focus of the nursing interventions for improvement of decreased $\dot{V}_A/\dot{Q}_C$ is on airway clearance, reinflation of alveoli, and enhanced patency of the airways. The newly advocated stir-up regimen of turn, cascade cough, and SMI should improve the decreased $\dot{V}_A/\dot{Q}_C$. Percussion or vibration, or both, may also need to be instituted to facilitate secretion clearance. In addition, if partial bronchospasm (expiratory wheeze) is suspected, the attending physician should be consulted about instituting appropriate bronchodilator therapy.

At this point, a clarification of terms used to describe decreased $\dot{V}_A/\dot{Q}_C$ and shunt is in order. Basically, intrapulmonary shunts result in the mixing of venous blood that has not been properly oxygenated into the arterial blood (pulmonary vein). Anatomic shunts, which occur normally, are attributed to the 2% or 3% of the cardiac output that bypasses the lungs. The shunted unoxygenated venous blood comes mainly from the bronchial circulation, which empties into the pulmonary veins, and from the thebesian vessels that drain the myocardium into the left heart. Intrapulmonary shunts occur when mixed venous blood does not become oxygenated when it passes by underventilated, unventilated, or collapsed alveoli. Absolute intrapulmonary shunts, sometimes called *true shunts,* are associated with totally unventilated or collapsed alveoli. Shuntlike intrapulmonary shunts are the areas of low $\dot{V}_A/\dot{Q}_C$ in which blood draining the partially obstructed alveoli has a lower arterial oxygen content than the alveolar capillary units that are well matched. As a result, the presence of anatomic shunts is normal. Abnormal shunts can be classified as physiologic shunts. Physiologic shunts are composed of the anatomic shunts plus intrapulmonary shunts (absolute and shuntlike intrapulmonary shunts).

Increased Ventilation to Perfusion

According to Fig. 12-20, compromise of the circulation to the individual alveolocapillary unit creates an excess of ventilation in comparison with perfusion. If the flow of blood in the pulmonary capillary is partially obstructed, increased $\dot{V}_A/\dot{Q}_C$ results. If the flow of blood is completely obstructed, such as with a pulmonary embolus, only ventilation continues and produces wasted or dead space. Wasted ventilation is the total amount of inspired gas that does not contribute to carbon dioxide removal; it is also known as *physiologic dead space* ($V_Dphysio$). $V_Dphysio$ is that volume of each breath that is inhaled but does not reach functioning terminal respiratory units. $V_Dphysio$

has two components: alveolar and anatomic dead space. Alveolar dead space (V_Dalv), as depicted in Fig. 12-20, is that volume of air contributed by all those terminal respiratory units that are overventilated relative to their perfusion. Anatomic dead space (V_Danat) consists of the volume of air in the conducting airways that does not participate in gas exchange. This category includes all air down to the respiratory bronchioles. The following formula depicts $V_Dphysio$:

$$V_Dphysio = V_Dalv + V_Danat$$

Normally, $V_Dphysio$ consists mainly of V_Danat, with the V_Dalv component being minute, which explains why the normal $V_Dphysio$ volume in milliliters is approximately equal to the weight of a person in pounds. For example, a person who weighs 150 lb has a $V_Dphysio$ of 150 mL. When alveoli become overventilated in comparison with perfused, the V_Dalv increases, which in turn increases the $V_Dphysio$.

The amount of $V_Dphysio$ can be determined with the Bohr equation. Clinically, the Bohr equation is commonly referred to as the V_D/V_T. The ratio of dead space (V_D) to V_T can be used to determine whether the obstruction to pulmonary capillary blood flow is partial ($\dot{V}_A/\dot{Q}_C$) or complete (wasted ventilation). The V_D/V_T can be derived from the following equation:

$$\frac{V_D}{V_T} = \frac{PaCO_2 - P_ECO_2}{P_ECO_2}$$

in which the *PaCO₂* is the arterial carbon dioxide partial pressure and the *P_ECO₂* is the partial pressure of the expired carbon dioxide.

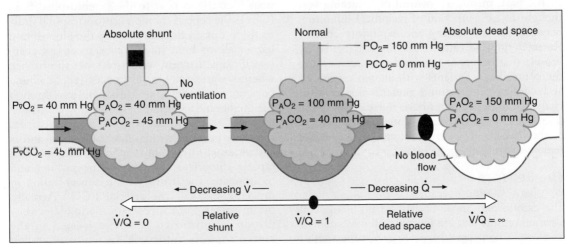

FIG. 12-20 The shunt-dead-space continuum. (From Beachey W: *Respiratory care anatomy and physiology,* ed 2, St. Louis, 2007, Mosby.)

The V_D/V_T ratio is normally 0.3. If the V_D/V_T increases to 0.6, more than half of the V_T is dead space. The minute ventilation (V_E) can double in most patients, but beyond that amount, the effort is too exhausting and a V_D/V_T ratio of more than 0.6 usually mandates that the patient's ventilation be assisted mechanically.

Implications for Perianesthesia Care

In the early postoperative period (including the transport of the patient from the operating room to the PACU), the patient should be considered to have a reduced FRC and hypoventilation and to have some ventilation-perfusion mismatch. All these factors lead to a reduction in arterial oxygenation as reflected by low SaO_2 and PaO_2 values. Hypoxemia can occur during transport to the PACU. Consequently, all patients should receive supplemental oxygenation during transport to the PACU and certainly throughout their stay there. In addition, because these respiratory alterations occur in almost all patients in recovery from anesthesia, pulse oximetry should be used on each patient during transport and in the PACU.

Capnography, however, is a graphic display of instantaneous CO_2 concentration (FCO_2) versus time or expired volume during a respiratory cycle. It provides information about CO_2 production, pulmonary perfusion, alveolar ventilation, and respiratory patterns and is effective in the early detection of adverse respiratory events such as hypoventilation and apnea.[12] Capnography is often used in the PACU on intubated and complex patients, but may also be used with nonintubated complex patients or patients who require sedation.

REGULATION OF BREATHING

In the past, medullary control of breathing was thought to be a function of reciprocal inhibition between the inspiratory and expiratory centers. Research now indicates a more discrete regulatory process that occurs at two levels: the sensors and the controllers.[5] Patients with altered regulation and control of breathing present a significant challenge to the perianesthesia nurse. In addition, anesthesia, surgery, and medications administered in the PACU can have a profound effect on the patient's regulatory processes of breathing.

The Sensors

Peripheral Chemoreceptors

The carotid and aortic bodies are the peripheral chemoreceptors and are located at the bifurcation of the common carotid arteries and at the arch of the aorta, respectively. The carotid and aortic bodies are responsible for the immediate increase in ventilation as a result of lack of oxygen. These peripheral chemoreceptors are composed of highly vascular tissue and glomus cells. The carotid and aortic bodies monitor only the PaO_2, not the CaO_2 of the hemoglobin; therefore the receptors are not stimulated in conditions such as anemia and carbon monoxide and cyanide poisoning.

The carotid bodies are much more important physiologically than are the aortic bodies. The carotid bodies respond, in order of degree of response, to low PaO_2, high $PaCO_2$, and low pH. The carotid bodies respond to a low PaO_2, and the response is augmented by a high $PaCO_2$, a low pH, or both. The physiologic responses to the stimulation of the carotid sinus are hyperpnea, bradycardia, and hypotension. The aortic bodies, however, respond to a low PaO_2 and to a high $PaCO_2$, but not to pH. The results of stimulation of the aortic bodies are hyperpnea, tachycardia, and hypertension.

The carotid and aortic bodies mainly respond to a low PaO_2. This response is commonly called the hypoxic or secondary drive. The impulse activity in these chemoreceptors begins at a PaO_2 of approximately 500 torr. A rapid increase in impulses occurs at a PaO_2 lower than 100 torr. The impulses are greatly increased as the PaO_2 falls to a value less than 60 torr. At less than 30 torr, the impulse activity from the chemoreceptors decreases because of the direct oxygen deficit in the glomus cells. In addition, these peripheral arterial chemoreceptors are stimulated by low arterial blood pressure and increased sympathetic activity.[5]

Central Chemoreceptors

The central chemoreceptors lie near the ventral surface of the medulla. Specifically, these chemosensitive areas are near the choroid plexus (venous blood) and next to the cerebrospinal fluid (CSF). The central chemoreceptors respond indirectly to carbon dioxide because the blood-brain barrier allows lipid-soluble substances (e.g., carbon dioxide, oxygen, water) to cross the barrier, whereas water-soluble substances (e.g., sodium, potassium, hydrogen ion, bicarbonate) pass through the membrane at extremely slow rates. Bicarbonate requires active transport to cross the barrier; therefore carbon dioxide enters the CSF and is hydrated to form carbonic acid. The carbonic acid rapidly dissociates to form hydrogen ion and bicarbonate. The hydrogen ion concentration in the CSF parallels the arterial PCO_2. Actually, the hydrogen ion concentration stimulates ventilation via hydrogen receptors located in the central chemoreceptor area. In summary, carbon dioxide has little direct effect on the stimulation of the receptors in the central chemoreceptor area, but does have a potent indirect effect. This indirect effect is the result of the inability of hydrogen ions to easily cross the blood-brain barrier. For this reason, changes in hydrogen ion concentration in the blood have considerably less effect in stimulating the chemoreceptor area than do changes in carbon dioxide. Consequently, the central chemoreceptor area precisely controls ventilation and therefore the $PaCO_2$. For that reason, the index to the adequacy of ventilation is the $PaCO_2$.

Bicarbonate is the only major buffer in the CSF. The pH of the CSF is a result of the ratio between bicarbonate and carbon dioxide in the CSF. Carbon dioxide is freely diffusible in and out of the CSF via the blood-brain barrier. However, bicarbonate is not freely diffusible and requires active or passive transport to enter or leave the CSF. When an acute increase in the $PaCO_2$ occurs, carbon dioxide enters the CSF and is hydrated, and hydrogen ions and bicarbonate are formed. The hydrogen ion stimulates the chemoreceptors, and the bicarbonate decreases the pH of the CSF. The resultant hyperpnea lowers the blood $PaCO_2$ and thus creates a gradient that favors the diffusion of carbon dioxide out of the CSF. The blood $PaCO_2$ and pH are corrected immediately, but the pH in the CSF requires some time to reestablish a normal carbon dioxide–bicarbonate level because bicarbonate is poorly diffusible. This process is usually not a problem with normal respiratory function. However, for the patient with chronic carbon dioxide retention (chronic hypercapnia) who has hyperventilation to a normal $PaCO_2$ of 40 torr, serious deleterious effects can occur. Patients with a chronically elevated $PaCO_2$ have a higher amount of carbon dioxide and bicarbonate in the CSF, but the ratio is maintained in a chronic situation. In this instance, the patient is breathing at a higher set point. That is, instead of maintenance at 40 torr, the normal $PaCO_2$ for this patient might be maintained at 46 torr and near-normal sensitivity to changes in the $PaCO_2$ may be present. If this patient underwent aggressive ventilation in the PACU with the goal of lowering the $PaCO_2$ to 40 torr, significant negative repercussions could occur. With a lower $PaCO_2$, the carbon dioxide in the CSF diffuses out and the bicarbonate remains because of its inability to diffuse out of the CSF. Thus, an excess of bicarbonate compared with carbon dioxide ($\uparrow$ bicarbonate pool) exists in the CSF and causes the primary stimulus to ventilation to cease. Because the patient's condition is hyperventilation, the $PaCO_2$ decreases and the PAO_2 increases (because of the 12-10 concept). Therefore

the secondary (hypoxic) drive may also become extinguished, and this patient may have no effective drive for ventilation. If patients with chronic hypercapnia are acutely hyperventilated, they must be monitored for apnea once the accelerated ventilation is discontinued. A more appropriate technique is the maintenance of the $PaCO_2$ at the level that is normal for that patient to avoid an apneic situation.[4] Thus, for the patient with chronic carbon dioxide retention who is emerging from anesthesia, an overaggressive stir-up regimen (hyperventilation) should be avoided. The patient should perform the SMI at normal intervals, and the arterial blood gas values should be closely monitored.

In some patients with chronic carbon dioxide retention (chronic hypercapnia), the sensitivity to hydrogen ions via the carbon dioxide may be effectively decreased to the point at which the primary stimulus to ventilation becomes the low PaO_2 at the carotid and aortic bodies. The low PaO_2 becomes an effective stimulus to ventilation, especially when the $PaCO_2$ is elevated. The high $PaCO_2$ augments the response to the low PaO_2 with the peripheral chemoreceptors. For this reason, the patient breathes via the hypoxic drive. Because the carotid bodies are the major peripheral chemoreceptors, patients who use the hypoxic drive may also have bradycardia and hypotension. For that reason, patients with abnormally high preoperative $PaCO_2$ values who have bradycardia and hypotension should be suspected of using the hypoxic drive as the primary drive to ventilation. In the PACU, patients suspected of primary use of this drive should be monitored closely and given oxygen to attain adequate oxygen content (a hemoglobin saturation of between 80% and 90%). The primary goal is to keep the patient oxygenated without extinguishing the main control of ventilation. High-flow techniques that use a Venturi mask that works on the Venturi principle to ensure precise FiO_2 values (i.e., 24% to 50%) can be used with these patients.

Response to Carbon Dioxide

Carbon dioxide is the primary stimulus to ventilation. The carbon dioxide response test is used for assessment of the ventilatory response to carbon dioxide. In this test, the subject inhales carbon dioxide mixtures (with the PaO_2 held constant) so that the inspired $PaCO_2$ gradually increases. Normally the V_E increases linearly as the $PaCO_2$ increases (Fig. 12-21). Some disease states and drugs cause the carbon dioxide response curve to shift to the left or the right. If the curve shifts to the left, the subject is more responsive to carbon dioxide. Factors such as thyroid toxicosis, aggressive personality,

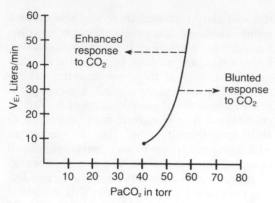

FIG. 12-21 Carbon dioxide response curve. (From Traver G: *Respiratory nursing: the science and the art*, New York, 1982, John Wiley and Sons.)

salicylates, and ketosis shift the curve to the left. A decreased ventilatory response to carbon dioxide occurs when the curve is shifted to the right and is called a *blunted response*. Patients who have a blunted response to carbon dioxide need intensive perianesthesia nursing care. The ventilatory response to an increased concentration of inspired carbon dioxide is blunted by hypothyroidism, mental depression, aging, general anesthetics, barbiturates, and narcotics. Many patients in the PACU either have these conditions or have received these drugs during surgery. This blunted response to carbon dioxide is one of the main justifications for supplemental oxygen administration to all patients who are emerging from anesthesia in the PACU. This response is also the rationale behind the need for critical perianesthesia nursing care that includes frequent assessment and interventions such as the stir-up regimen for prevention of respiratory depression.[1]

Upper Airways Receptors

Receptors that are sensitive to mechanical stimulation and chemical agents and have afferent pathways via the trigeminal and olfactory nerves are located in the nose. Activation of these receptors can cause apnea, bradycardia, and sneezing. When a patient is to undergo nasal intubation, the perianesthesia nurse should monitor for bradycardia and apnea and be prepared for necessary interventions. Atropine or glycopyrrolate (Robinul) may be necessary for the vagolytic effect; succinylcholine may facilitate the intubation. Finally, to provide positive-pressure ventilation, a bag-valve-mask system should be immediately available in case apnea occurs.

Receptors located in the epipharynx are sensitive to mechanical stimulation. Their activation is associated with the sniff or aspiration reflex. Mechanical stimulation of these receptors causes deep inspiration, bronchodilatation, and hypertension. This reflex is a protective reflex that allows material in the epipharynx to be brought down to the pharynx, clearing the nasal airways. In the larynx are irritant receptors that respond to both mechanical and chemical stimulation. Afferent pathways from these receptors travel along the internal branch of the superior laryngeal nerve. Stimulation invokes many responses, including coughing, slow deep breathing, apnea, bronchoconstriction, and hypertension. In addition, the trachea possesses irritant receptors. Stimulation of these receptors can cause responses such as coughing, bronchoconstriction, and hypertension.

During any procedure that involves the intubation of the trachea, the perianesthesia nurse should be prepared to assess the appropriate cardiorespiratory parameters and implement nursing care as necessary.

Lung Receptors

Pulmonary stretch receptors (PSRs) lie within the smooth muscle of the small airways. These receptors are activated by marked distention or deflation (atelectasis) of the lungs. On marked inflation of the lungs, the activation of the PSR leads to a slowing of inspiratory frequency because of an increase in expiratory time. Bronchodilatation and tachycardia also can result from activation of these receptors. The PSRs are thought to be part of the Hering-Breuer reflex. The low threshold for the PSR is present for approximately the first 3 months of life; afterward, the threshold is high throughout adulthood. For the adult, the Hering-Breuer reflex is not important in the control of ventilation except in the anesthetized state. When an adult is administered general anesthesia and ventilation with prolonged maximal lung inflations, a prolonged expiratory time can result because of activation of the PSR.[3]

Of great interest in regard to the pathogenesis of asthma are the irritant receptors that lie between the airway epithelial cells. These receptors respond to chemical irritants (e.g., histamine) and mechanical irritants (e.g., small particles and aerosols) that irritate the pulmonary epithelium. The irritant receptors are mediated by vagal afferent fibers, and on receptor stimulation, bronchoconstriction and hyperpnea occur. The pathogenesis of asthma is suggested to revolve around the sequence of histamine release, which stimulates the irritant receptors and ultimately leads to bronchoconstriction mediated via the vagus nerve.

The J-receptors, or juxtapulmonary capillary–receptors, are located in the wall of the pulmonary capillaries. Like the irritant receptors, the afferent impulses of J-receptors are transmitted to the central nervous system by the vagus nerve. Normal stimuli of the J-receptors include pneumonia, pulmonary congestion, and increased interstitial fluid pressure. Stimulation of these receptors by interstitial or pulmonary edema results in tachypnea, bradycardia, and hypotension.[9] Therefore the nurse should always evaluate the rate of ventilation in the assessment of patients who are at risk for development of pulmonary edema. With the knowledge that interstitial edema usually precedes pulmonary edema and that increased interstitial congestion stimulates the J-receptors, the nurse should consider a rapid shallow breathing pattern to be a danger signal and report it to the attending physician.

Located in the walls of the large systemic arteries, especially in the aortic and carotid sinuses, are stretch receptors called *baroreceptors*. These receptors help to control the systemic blood pressure; they also affect ventilation. When the systemic blood pressure increases, a reflex hypoventilation occurs because of stimulation of the baroreceptors; however, a low systemic blood pressure causes the baroreceptors to produce a reflex hyperventilation. As a result, if a patient in the PACU has a significant amount of hypertension or hypotension, a reflex ventilatory response usually occurs because of the stimulation of the baroreceptors in the large systemic arteries.

The Controllers

The controllers of breathing are located in the central nervous system and comprise two functionally and anatomically separate components. Voluntary breathing is controlled in the cortex of the brain. Automatic breathing is controlled by structures within the brainstem. The spinal cord functions to integrate the output of the brainstem and the cortex. The cortex can override the other controllers of breathing if voluntary control is desired. Examples of voluntary control include voluntary hyperventilation and breath holding.[1,3,5,6]

The Brainstem

Located bilaterally in the upper pons is the pneumotaxic center. This center functions to fine-tune the respiratory pattern with modulating the activity of the apneustic center and regulating the respiratory system's response to stimuli such as hypercarbia, hypoxia, and lung inflation. Near the pontomedullary border is the apneustic center. This center is probably the site of the inspiratory cutoff switch that terminates inspiration. In fact,

apneusis, which consists of prolonged inspirations with occasional expirations, results when the apneustic center has been deactivated. Consequently, the apneustic center is also a fine-tuner of the rhythm of breathing.

Two groups of neurons are located in the medullary center, above the spinal cord: the dorsal respiratory group (DRG) and the ventral respiratory group (VRG). The DRG is composed of inspiratory neurons and is the initial intracranial processing site for many reflexes that affect breathing. It is probably the site of origin of the rhythmic respiratory drive. The DRG sends motor fibers via the phrenic nerve to the diaphragm; it sends inspiratory fibers to the VRG, which is also part of the medullary center. However, the VRG does not send fibers to the DRG; therefore the reciprocal inhibition theory of the regulation of breathing seems unlikely. The VRG is composed of both inspiratory and expiratory cells. The VRG neurons are driven by the cells of the DRG; therefore respiratory rhythmicity and the processing of sensory inputs do not occur initially within the VRG. The major function of the VRG is to project impulses to distant sites and to drive either the spinal respiratory motor neurons (primary intercostal and abdominal) or the auxiliary muscles of breathing innervated by the vagus nerve.

The DRG receives information from almost all the chemoreceptors, the baroreceptors, and the other sensors in the lung. In turn, the DRG generates a breathing rhythm that is fine-tuned by the apneustic center (inspiratory cutoff switch) and the pneumotaxic center. The inspiratory motor impulses are sent to the diaphragm and to the VRG. The VRG then drives spinal respiratory neurons (innervating the intercostal and abdominal muscles) or the auxiliary muscles of respiration innervated by the vagus nerve. Again, the cerebral cortex can override these centers if voluntary control of breathing is desired. In addition, the vagus nerve has a profound effect on many aspects of the control of breathing because the afferent pathways of the vagus nerve from the stretch receptors, J-receptors, and irritant receptors serve to modulate the rhythm of breathing. Therefore any dysfunction that includes transection of the vagi results in irregular breathing patterns, depending on the level of dysfunction (pons or medulla).

Sleep Apnea

The regulation of breathing has been described in detail, and obviously, multiple effects stimulate many levels of receptors to facilitate breathing.

Yet, sleep apnea has become a major health issue and certainly a major concern in the perianesthesia setting. More than 12 million Americans are estimated to have some form of sleep apnea.[13]

Sleep apnea has three forms: obstructive, central, and mixed. Obstructive sleep apnea is caused by an obstruction or blockage of the airway. This obstruction usually occurs in the posterior pharynx, with soft tissue collapse leading to obstruction of the airway. Central sleep apnea is not a single disease entity but includes several disorders in which the definitive event is the withdrawal of effective central drive to the respiratory muscles. The mixed type of sleep apnea is a combination of obstructive and central components. Consequently, sleep apnea can be the result of a variety of pathophysiologic disorders, such as underlying defects in the respiratory controller or neuromuscular systems to include soft tissue collapse.[14,15]

The clinical manifestations of sleep apnea are variable because of the different mechanisms that can produce the syndrome. Fig. 12-22 schematically shows the physiologic responses and clinical features that result from sleep apnea. The risk factors for the development of sleep apnea are presented in Box 12-4, and the presenting symptoms that can be evaluated before surgery at the preoperative interview are presented in Box 12-5.

Management of the patient with sleep apnea begins with a good preoperative screening. Questions that should be asked should include "Do you snore?" and "Do you ever fall asleep easily or sometimes inappropriately?" Other key questions can include "Do you feel tired or groggy when you wake up?," "Do you have headaches in the morning?," "Do you recall waking frequently during the night?," and "Do any of your family members have sleep apnea?"

If obstructive sleep apnea occurs in a patient in the PACU, basic airway care should be given. Certainly sedation is not in the best interest of the patient, as a difficult airway is often present in the PACU. Many times, these patients come to the PACU after a tracheostomy is performed during surgery. Pediatric patients many times have a tonsillectomy and adenoidectomy for treatment of sleep apnea. Airway management should include: avoidance of the supine position, especially in adults; repositioning of the airway; supplemental oxygen; provision for a patent airway; and then application of continuous positive airway pressure via a nose mask, in that order of level of nursing interventions (see Chapter 30). Continuous positive airway pressure has been shown to be effective in patients with central sleep apnea associated with congestive heart failure, and it facilitates a more appropriate emergence from anesthesia or sedation.[15]

POSTOPERATIVE LUNG VOLUMES

Postoperative pulmonary complications are the most common single cause of morbidity and mortality in the postoperative period. The reported incidence rate of postoperative pulmonary complications ranges from 4.5% to 76%.

Patients with Abnormal Pulmonary Function

When patients undergo anesthesia and surgery, certain risk factors predispose them to the development of postoperative pulmonary complications. Patients at the highest risk are those with preexisting pulmonary problems with abnormal pulmonary function before surgery. The other major risk factors associated with postoperative pulmonary complications are chronic cigarette smoking, obesity, and advanced age.

Preexisting Pulmonary Disease

Patients with preexisting pulmonary disease can have clinical or subclinical manifestations of the disease state. Consequently, preoperative pulmonary function tests are valuable when assessing the presence or absence of pulmonary pathophysiology and determining operative risk. Obstructive lung disease (i.e., asthma, emphysema, and chronic bronchitis), the most common category of lung disease, can be assessed with flow-volume measurements. Most pulmonary researchers suggest that a maximal voluntary ventilation that is less than 50% of what is predicted, a maximal expiratory flow rate less than 220 L/min, or a forced expiratory volume in 1 second less than 1.5 L indicates an increased operative risk for pulmonary complications. These flow-volume measurements are valuable predictors of the patient's ability to generate an adequate cough, which is a pulmonary defense mechanism rendered ineffective in the immediate postoperative period by anesthesia and surgery.[9] Consequently, these patients need vigorous informed nursing care in the immediate postoperative period. Priorities of nursing care should include frequent use of the stir-up regimen of turn, cascade cough, and SMI, along with the use of appropriate nursing interventions designed to enhance secretion clearance, which ensures airway patency.

Patients with restrictive lung disease (i.e., pulmonary fibrosis and morbid obesity) represent a

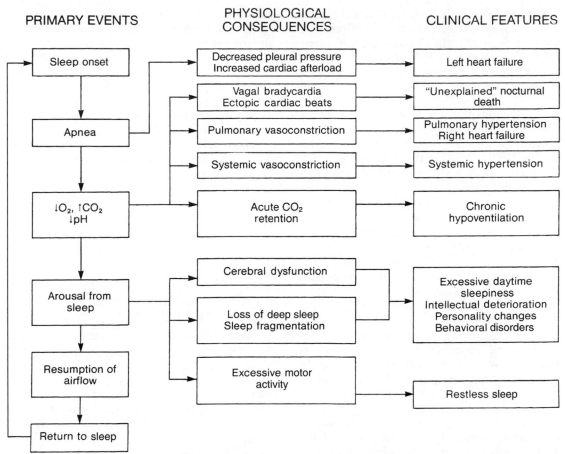

PRIMARY EVENTS   PHYSIOLOGICAL CONSEQUENCES   CLINICAL FEATURES

FIG. 12-22 Schematic of physiologic responses and clinical features that result from sleep apnea. (From Mason RJ, et al: *Murry and Nadel's textbook of respiratory medicine,* ed 4, Philadelphia, 2005, Saunders.)

BOX 12-4   Risk Factors Associated with Sleep Apnea

- Family history of sleep apnea
- Excess weight
- Large neck
- Recessed chin
- Male gender
- Older than 60 years
- Consumption of alcoholic beverages
- History of chronic smoking
- Abnormal structure of the upper airway

From American Sleep Apnea Association: *Sleep apnea,* available at www.sleepapnea.org/learn/sleep-apnea.html. Accessed December 7, 2011.

BOX 12-5   Signs and Symptoms Associated with Sleep Apnea

- Impotence
- Nocturia
- Esophageal reflux
- Depression
- Loud snoring
- Excessive daytime sleepiness
- High blood pressure
- Morning headaches
- Memory problems

From American Sleep Apnea Association: *Sleep apnea,* available at www.sleepapnea.org/learn/sleep-apnea.html. Accessed December 7, 2011.

---

significant risk for postoperative pulmonary complications when pulmonary function test results reveal a VC or a diffusion capacity of less than 50% of predicted values or exercise arterial blood gas values that show slight hypoxemia on exertion. In the PACU, these patients need a vigorous

stir-up regimen with attention to tissue oxygenation via monitoring for hypoxemia. This regimen is needed because, during the surgical experience and in the PACU, physiologic stress can occur. One of the major products of physiologic stress is an increase in cardiovascular parameters, which reduces the transit time of the RBCs across the respiratory gas exchange membrane. Because of the pathologic changes in the respiratory membrane, patients with restrictive lung disease can have desaturation on exertion, such as in the stress reaction.[11]

Cigarette Smoking

Chronic cigarette smoking has been shown to increase the incidence rate of postoperative pulmonary complications. Patients who smoke only 12 cigarettes per day have a sixfold increase in pulmonary morbidity rates in the postoperative period. The incidence rate of pulmonary embolism is higher in the smoker because of increased coagulability produced by chronic cigarette smoking. The ciliated epithelium of the lungs is damaged by chronic cigarette smoking. This damage can cause some blockage of the mucociliary transport system, which finally results in bronchiolar obstruction, infection, and atelectasis. Patients who smoke should be encouraged to stop smoking for at least 2 weeks before surgery to allow the mucociliary transport system to return to a nearly normal level of function. The focus of nursing care for the active chronic cigarette smoker should be similar to the interventions discussed for the patient with obstructive lung disease as the major clinical issue is a thickened pulmonary membrane that inhibits the transport of oxygen to the blood and carbon dioxide crossing over from the blood to the air. This also plays a part in the emergence from anesthesia because patients who are chronic cigarette smokers will have a slow emergence, especially when the anesthesia time exceeds 2 hours.[4]

Obesity

The patient who is markedly overweight has a significant chance of developing postoperative pulmonary complications caused by the altered lung volumes and capacities from the excess adipose tissue. Expansion of the lungs is hindered by an enlarged abdomen, which elevates the diaphragm and adds weight on the chest wall, thereby hindering the outward recoil of the chest wall. This hindrance leads to decreased thoracic wall compliance and ultimately to a reduced FRC. Finally, these complications result in hypoxemia from increased airway closure and $\dot{V}_A/\dot{Q}_C$ abnormalities (see Chapter 45). The goal of nursing interventions in the PACU is the prevention of further airway closure; therefore a vigorous stir-up regimen, including early ambulation, should help prevention of further reduction in the FRC. That measure reduces the

amount of airway closure, alleviates the hypoxemia, and ultimately improves the outcome of the patient.[3,15]

Advanced Age

Patients of advanced age (older than 70 years) have a slightly higher risk of developing postoperative pulmonary complications. A greater decrease in the FRC after surgery in patients of advanced age has been shown. Because the closing volume increases with age, significant airway closure can occur after surgery during tidal ventilation. Although advanced age is not associated with the same degree of risk as the factors previously discussed, it can increase the danger of the other risk factors. However, patients of advanced age should receive a vigorous stir-up regimen in the PACU, if only because of the alterations in lung mechanics.[9]

Physiology of Perianesthesia Pulmonary Nursing Care

Because of the change in the mechanical properties of the lungs and chest wall, patients emerging from anesthesia have decreased lung volumes and capacities (Fig. 12-23). This decrease is especially true of the patient who has undergone a thoracic or upper abdominal surgical procedure.

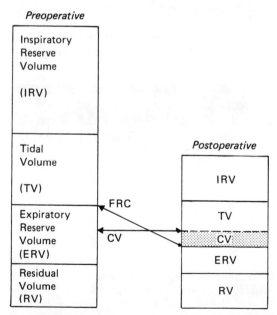

FIG. 12-23 Graphic comparison of preoperative lung volumes to probable lung volumes in immediate postoperative period in patient who has undergone upper abdominal surgical procedure. *FRC*, Functional residual capacity; *CV*, closing volume. (From Drain C: Pathophysiology of the respiratory system related to anesthesia. *CRNA* 7:181–192, 1996.)

In the PACU, a further reduction in lung volumes and capacities may be seen. The major factor that contributes to this reduction in lung volumes in the patient after surgery is a shallow, monotonous, sighless breathing pattern that is caused by general inhalation anesthesia, pain, and opioids. Sighless ventilation can result in an uneven distribution of surfactant and a loss of stability of the small airways and alveoli, which can then lead to alveolar collapse and ultimately to atelectasis. Normally, adults breathe regularly and rhythmically, spontaneously performing a maximal inspiration that is held for approximately 3 seconds at the peak of inspiration. This physiologic process, or SMI, is commonly called a *sigh* or a *yawn*.

In normal lungs, the closing volume is less than the resting lung volume (i.e., the FRC), and airways remain open during tidal breathing. In the immediate postoperative period, patients who have a sighless, monotonous, low-V_T ventilatory pattern usually have a reduced FRC. When the FRC plus V_T is within the closing volume range, the airways that lead to dependent lung zones can be closed effectively throughout tidal breathing (see Fig. 12-23). Inspired gas then is distributed mainly to the upper or nondependent lung zones. Perfusion continues to follow the normal gradient, with higher flows to the dependent areas of the lung.

In the immediate postoperative period, as airway closure occurs, gas is trapped behind closed airways. This sequestered air can become absorbed, and the alveoli then become airless (atelectasis). The atelectasis, as it becomes more widespread, leads to a decrease in ventilation as compared with perfusion (low $\dot{V}_A/\dot{Q}_C$), which results in a widening of the $PAO_2 - PaO_2$ value and ultimately to hypoxemia. In addition, atelectatic areas in the lung provide a culture medium in which pneumonia can develop.

Various investigators have shown a decrease in lung volumes in the postoperative period. Patients who have undergone an upper abdominal surgical procedure have an immediate postoperative decrease in the FRC from hour 1 to hour 2 (Fig. 12-24).[4] The FRC then seems to return to near the baseline value by approximately the fourth postoperative hour. A second subsequent decrease in the FRC is then seen after hour 4, and baseline values are not restored

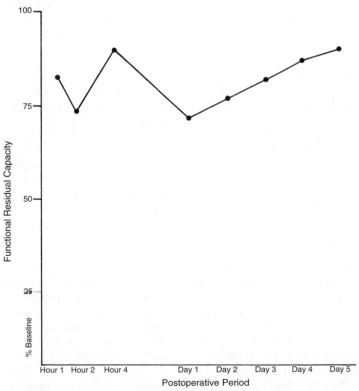

FIG. 12-24 Composite curve of mean values of functional residual capacity in postoperative period. (From Drain C: Anesthesia care of the patient with reactive airways disease, *CRNA* 7:207–212, 1996.)

until 5 days after surgery. A possible explanation of the "peaks and valleys" in the FRC during the postoperative period may be that the first reduction in the FRC is associated with anesthesia and the latter reduction may be from pain. General inhalation anesthesia and pain can dampen the physiologic sigh mechanism. Consequently, all patients who have undergone a surgical procedure, especially those who have incision sites near the thorax or diaphragm, should be strongly encouraged to perform the SMI maneuver both in the PACU and on the surgical unit. The incentive spirometer, a device designed to use positive feedback to encourage the patient to perform the SMI maneuver, can be used by the patient on the surgical unit.

OXYGEN ADMINISTRATION IN THE POSTANESTHESIA CARE UNIT

Administration of oxygen to the patient in the PACU is an important facet in the emergence phase of anesthesia. Oxygen is given to the patient in the PACU primarily because of the blunted or depressed response to carbon dioxide and low lung volumes. Administration of supplemental oxygen during the recovery phase of anesthesia is especially important for the patient who has received a general or spinal anesthetic. The methods of oxygen administration are summarized in Chapter 27.

Perianesthesia Nursing Care

A patent airway must be maintained throughout the administration of oxygen. The patient should be encouraged to cascade cough, perform the SMI, and change positions according to the stir-up regimen discussed in this chapter and in Chapter 27. If a nasal catheter is used, the catheter should be removed every 6 hours for cleansing and reinsertion into the other nostril. In addition, the nasal mucosa should be inspected periodically for dryness when a nasal catheter or prongs are used. Oxygen given in the dry gas form can cause drying and irritation of the mucosa, impair the ciliary action, and thicken secretions; therefore oxygen should always be administered with humidity.

The perianesthesia nurse must receive a report from the anesthesia provider as to the patient's preoperative pulmonary status. Whether the patient has a history of chronic retention of carbon dioxide, as occurs in chronic obstructive pulmonary disease, is especially important to ascertain. As described in this chapter, the patient with carbon dioxide retention who receives oxygen in the PACU should be monitored carefully for any signs of hypoventilation, confusion, or semicomatose condition. If any of these signs appear, the surgeon and anesthesia provider should be notified immediately.

Oxygen Toxicity

When excessive concentrations of inspired oxygen (greater than 60%) are administered to patients for a prolonged period, the eyes, lungs, and central nervous system can be damaged.

Eyes

Premature infants who have a high PaO_2 for longer than 24 hours are at risk for development of retrolental fibroplasia, which is caused by vasoconstriction of the blood vessels of the retina as a result of high oxygen concentrations in the blood. Retrolental fibroplasia presents in an acute form as vascular retinopathy at the developing edge of blood vessels in the premature infant's eye. This presentation is followed by perivascular exudation, tissue hyperplasia, and scar tissue that exerts traction on the retina and leads to retinal detachment and destruction of the infant's vision. Research indicates that the incidence rate of acute retrolental fibroplasia is inversely proportional to birth weight. Most of the clinical research indicates that, to minimize the risk of development of retrolental fibroplasia, the infant's PaO_2 should be maintained between 60 and 90 torr. Perianesthesia nurses should use their best-informed judgment when caring for these infants. As with the adult, the infant who needs a high-inspired oxygen concentration to provide adequate oxygenation should not be denied oxygen because of fear of complications.[6]

Lungs

Concentrations of oxygen greater than 60% damage the lungs within 3 or 4 days. A 120% oxygen concentration administered for 24 to 48 hours also causes pulmonary damage, the signs of which are manifested by type II cell dysfunction in the lung. The type II cells secrete surfactant, and the lack of surfactant in the alveoli leads to alveolar collapse. The hyperoxic environment also stops the ciliary action in the lungs. The early symptoms of this disorder include cough, nasal congestion, sore throat, reduced VC, tracheobronchitis, and substernal discomfort. The early signs of airway irritation may appear when a patient has received 80% to 120% oxygen continuously for 8 hours or longer. The lung appears to indefinitely tolerate oxygen concentrations lower than 40%.[1]

Central Nervous System

Headache is an early indicator of oxygen toxicity. As oxygen toxicity continues to develop, the patient exhibits some confusion. When a patient is receiving a high concentration of oxygen and has these signs and symptoms, the attending physician should be notified. Convulsions usually are not seen in the PACU but can occur when oxygen is delivered in above-normal atmospheric pressure, such as in hyperbaric oxygen chambers.

SUMMARY

The inhalation agents continue to see a significant amount of use in the operating room. They are now time tested and possess excellent qualities that do not have a significant effect on the patient. More specifically, the agents used today are more rapid, do not have a significant effect on the major organ systems, and are easily removed if the patient undergoes appropriate emergence. These factors contribute to the concept of critical care nursing practice in the PACU. This is because of the rapid, maybe even ultrarapid-acting inhalational anesthetic agents that require quick and precise nursing care at the bedside of a patient emerging from anesthesia—advance practice nursing at its best. Nursing research has been conducted in this area, with the PACU patient being used for the clinical trial of breathing methods looking at preoperative and postoperative measurements of the lung volumes and capacities. The research results indicated that the use of the modified stir-up regime or sustained maximal inspiration (SMI), as opposed to the deep-breathing maneuver in emergence of patients during the immediate postoperative period, may be the breathing maneuver of choice. Evidence-based practice suggests that the SMI should be used in the PACU for patients emerging from inhalational anesthesia.

REFERENCES

1. Barrett K, et al: *Ganong's review of medical physiology*, ed 23, New York, 2009, McGraw-Hill Medical.
2. Aitkenhead A, et al: *Textbook of anesthesia*, ed 5, Philadelphia, 2007, Churchill Livingstone.
3. Hall J: *Guyton and Hall textbook of medical physiology*, ed 12, Philadelphia, 2010, Saunders.
4. Nagelhout J, Plaus K: *Nurse anesthesia*, ed 4, St. Louis, 2010, Saunders.
5. Mason R: *Murray and Nadel's textbook of respiratory medicine*, ed 5, Philadelphia, 2011, Saunders.
6. Miller R, et al: *Anesthesia*, ed 7, Philadelphia, 2009, Churchill Livingstone.
7. Brunton L, et al: *Goodman and Gilman's the pharmacological basis of therapeutics*, ed 12, New York, 2010, McGraw-Hill Professional.
8. Stoelting R: *Pharmacology and physiology in anesthetic practice*, ed 4, Philadelphia, 2005, Lippincott Williams & Wilkins.
9. Atlee J: *Complications in anesthesia*, ed 2, Philadelphia, 2007, Saunders.
10. Barash P, et al: *Clinical anesthesia*, ed 6, Philadelphia, 2009, Lippincott Williams & Wilkins.
11. Fisher L: *Anesthesia and uncommon diseases*, ed 5, Philadelphia, 2007, Saunders.
12. Kodali BS: *Why capnography?* available at www.capnography.com/new/index.php?option=com_content&view=article&id=48&Itemid=57. Accessed September 23, 2011.
13. American Sleep Apnea Association, available at www.sleepapnea.org. Accessed on September 14, 2011.
14. Moos D, Cuddeford D: Implications of obstructive sleep apnea syndrome for the perianesthesia nurse, *J Perianesth Nurs* 21(2):103–118, 2006.
15. Passannante A, et al: Anesthetic management of patients with obesity and sleep apnea, *Anesthesiol Clin North Am* 23:479–490, 2005.

RESOURCES

AACN: *Core curriculum for progressive care nursing*, Philadelphia, 2010, Saunders.

Alspach J: *Core curriculum for critical care nursing*, ed 6, Philadelphia, 2005, Saunders.

Bready L, et al: *Decision making in anesthesiology*, ed 4, St. Louis, 2007, Mosby.

Conlay L, et al: *Case files anesthesiology*, New York, 2011, McGraw-Hill Medical.

Drake R, et al: *Gray's anatomy for students*, ed 2, Philadelphia, 2009, Churchill Livingstone.

Deutschman C, Netigan P: *Evidence-based practice of critical care*, Philadelphia, 2010, Saunders.

Dorsch J, Dorsch S: *Understanding anesthesia equipment*, ed 5, Philadelphia, 2007, Lippincott Williams & Wilkins.

Gallager C, Issenberg B: *Simulation in anesthesia*, Philadelphia, 2007, Saunders.

Kaplan J, et al: *Cardiac anesthesia*, New York, 2011, Churchill Livingstone.

Longnecker D, et al: *Anesthesiology*, New York, 2007, McGraw-Hill Medical.

Miller R, Pardo M: *Basics of anesthesia*, ed 6, Philadelphia, 2011, Saunders.

Pasero C, McCaffery M: *Perianesthesia nursing core curriculum: preprocedure, phase I and phase II PACU nursing*, St. Louis, 2011, Mosby.

Schick L, Windle PE: *Perianesthesia nursing core curriculum*, ed 2, Philadelphia, 2010, Saunders.

Shorten G, et al: *Postoperative pain management: an evidence-based guide to practice*, Philadelphia, 2006, Saunders.

Sieber F: *Geriatric anesthesia*, New York, 2006, McGraw-Hill Medical.

Townsend C, et al: *Sabiston's textbook of surgery*, ed 18, Philadelphia, 2008, Saunders.

Vincent J, et al: *Textbook of critical care*, ed 6, Philadelphia, 2011, Saunders.

PHYSIOLOGIC CONSIDERATIONS IN THE PACU

13 The Renal System

Susan J. Fetzer, BA, BSN, MSN, MBA, PhD, CNL

The importance of the renal system in postanesthesia care unit (PACU) care is focused on the ability of the kidneys to metabolize and excrete drugs and to maintain acid-base, electrolyte, and fluid volume balance. The cardiovascular and respiratory systems rely on the ability of the kidneys to maintain homeostasis through physiologic mechanisms. Adequate kidney function is imperative to ensure positive outcomes for the patient recovering from anesthesia in the PACU. When kidney function is impaired, anesthetic drugs cannot be metabolized leading to a prolonged emergence. Impaired kidney function can compromise cardiovascular function when fluids cannot be removed and electrolytes not balanced. With the profound effects that the kidneys have on the patient's recovery, assessment of kidney function is an important consideration in the assessment of the perianesthesia patient. An understanding of renal anatomy and physiology is important to facilitate perianesthesia patient recovery.

DEFINITIONS

Acetonuria: The appearance of acetone in the urine. Acetonuria is present when excessive fats are consumed or when an inadequate amount of carbohydrates is metabolized.

Albuminuria: The presence of protein in the urine, also called *proteinuria*. Albumin is the most common protein found in the urine. This condition usually indicates a malfunction in glomerular filtration.

Anuria: Lack of urine production, less than 50 mL/day.

Azotemia: The presence of nitrogenous products in the blood, usually because of decreased kidney function.

Cystitis: An inflammation of the bladder.

Dysuria: Painful or difficult urination.

Enuresis: Involuntary discharge of urine.

Glomerular Filtration Rate: Volume of fluid filtered through the kidney.

Glycosuria: The presence of glucose in the urine.

Hematuria: The presence of blood in the urine.

Nephritis: Inflammation of the kidney.

Nephrosis: Degeneration of the kidney without the occurrence of inflammation.

Oliguria: A decreased urine formation of less than 500 mL/day or 0.5 mL/kg/h in an adult.

Pyelonephritis: An inflammation of the renal pelvis and calices.

Stricture: An abnormal narrowing; in the urinary tract, a narrowing of the ureter or urethra.

Uremia: The presence of nitrogenous substances in the blood.

Urinary Incontinence: The inability to retain urine in the bladder.

Urinary Retention: Failure to expel urine from the bladder.

ANATOMY OF THE KIDNEYS

The kidneys are two bean-shaped organs in the retroperitoneal spaces at the level of the twelfth thoracic to third lumbar vertebrae. The right kidney is slightly lower than the left. Each kidney weighs approximately 150 g. The notched portion of the kidney is called the *hilum*, which is where the ureter, the renal vein, and the renal artery enter the kidney (Fig. 13-1). The kidney is divided into an outer cortex and an inner medulla.

Blood is supplied to each kidney by a renal artery arising from each side of the abdominal aorta. The rate of blood flow through both kidneys of a man who weighs 70 kg is approximately 1200 mL/min, or approximately 21% of the cardiac output. As the renal artery enters the kidney at the hilum, it divides into the interlobar arteries. Branches from the interlobar arteries divide into afferent arteries that supply the capillaries of the nephrons. The capillaries form the efferent arterioles and divide to form the peritubular capillaries that help to supply the nephron. (Figs. 13-2 and 13-3).

The nephron is the functional unit of the kidney. Together the kidneys contain approximately 2.4 million closely packed nephrons. Each nephron consists of a glomerulus, a proximal convoluted tubule, a loop of Henle, a distal convoluted tubule, and collecting ducts. The blood enters the afferent arteriole and goes into the glomerulus located in the cortex. The glomerulus is a compact network of capillaries encased in a double-layered capsule, the Bowman capsule. Filtered blood flows

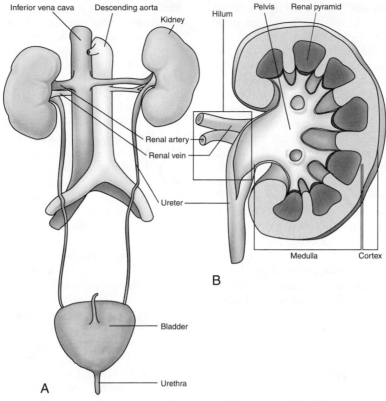

FIG. 13-1 Anatomy of renal and urinary systems. **A,** Urinary system. **B,** Cross section of a kidney.

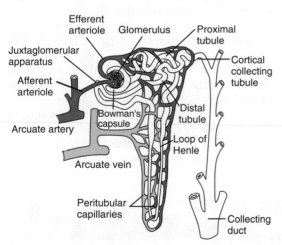

FIG. 13-2 Functional nephron. (From Hall J: *Guyton and Hall textbook of medical physiology*, ed 12, Philadelphia, 2011, Saunders.)

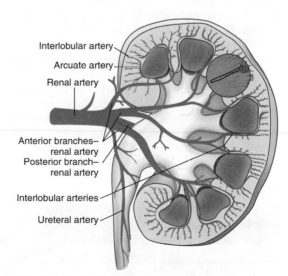

FIG. 13-3 Arterial supply to kidney. Soon after entering the hilum of the kidney, the renal artery divides into several anterior and posterior branches. Branches divide into interlobar arteries, which give off arcuate arteries that course between cortex and medulla.

out of the glomerulus into the efferent arteriole. The portion of the blood that is filtered drains into the proximal convoluted tubule. The renal tubules begin in the Bowman capsule. The pressure gradient, caused by renal artery blood flow, forces fluid to leave the glomerulus and enter the Bowman capsule. The filtrate flows into the proximal convoluted tubule, which is still in the cortex of the kidney, and then into the loop of Henle. The proximal loop of Henle is thick walled, but becomes thin at the distal segment in the medulla of the kidney. The filtrate then flows into the distal convoluted tubule, located in the cortex of the kidney, and passes into the collecting ducts. The collecting ducts traverse the cortex to the medulla, where they merge into the renal pelvis by way of the renal calyces. In the collecting ducts, the filtrate is termed *urine*.

The renal pelvis is a wide, funnel-shaped structure composed of the calyces draining the kidney. The pelvis drains into the ureter, which leads to the bladder.

KIDNEY PHYSIOLOGY

Urine is formed by processes of filtration, reabsorption, and secretion. Filtration occurs as the blood passes through the glomerulus. The force of filtration is a pressure gradient that pushes fluid through the glomerular membrane. Approximately 180 L of water every 24 hours along with other substances is filtered out of plasma by the glomeruli (Table 13-1). Blood cells and heavy particles including proteins are retained in the blood because they are too large to pass through the glomerular epithelium. The presence of red blood cells or protein in the urine usually indicates a pathologic process in the kidney.

Reabsorption occurs in the proximal and distal tubules. Approximately 99% of the water filtered by the glomeruli is reabsorbed. Many substances in the water are reabsorbed with active or passive

transport. Active transport requires energy for movement of the substance across the membrane. Passive transport can be regarded as simple diffusion that does not require energy.

Important constituents of body fluids—substances such as glucose, amino acids, sodium, potassium, calcium, and magnesium—are almost entirely reabsorbed. Certain substances are reabsorbed in limited quantities, such as urea and phosphate, and consequently appear in the urine. In a healthy individual, creatinine is the only filtered substance not reabsorbed and entirely secreted, allowing creatinine to serve as an indicator of glomerular filtration ability. The last process in the formation of urine is secretion. Various substances, including hydrogen and potassium ions, are secreted directly into the tubular fluid through the epithelial cells that line the renal tubules. Secretion plays an important role in promoting the body's acid-base balance.

REGULATION OF KIDNEY FUNCTION

The formation of urine and the reabsorption of substances needed for body function are aided by three physiologic mechanisms: the countercurrent mechanism, autoregulation, and hormonal control.

Countercurrent Mechanism

The countercurrent mechanism is used by the kidneys to concentrate urine. The vasa recta are special capillaries that, with the loop of Henle, form the countercurrent mechanism. Fluids flow in opposite directions between the ascending and descending loops and sections of the vasa recta. The osmolality or weight of particles in solution of the interstitial fluid increases deeper into the medulla. The increase in osmolality results in active transport of particles or solutes into the interstitial fluid. The countercurrent mechanism is useful when the body needs to excrete a large

Table 13-1	Particles Filtered by the Glomerulus, Reabsorbed by the Tubules, and Excreted in the Urine		
PARTICLE	FILTERED (mEq/24 h/170 L)	REABSORBED (mEq/24 h/169 L)	EXCRETED (mEq/24 h/45 L)
Sodium	24,500	24,350	150
Chloride	17,800	17,700	150
Bicarbonate	4900	4900	1
Potassium	700	600	24
Glucose	780	780	0
Urea	870	460	410
Creatinine	12	0	12

amount of waste products yet reabsorb the normal amount of solutes and when the water in the body needs to be conserved, while waste products are eliminated.

Autoregulation

Autoregulation helps to keep the glomerular filtration at a near normal rate, despite fluctuations in arterial pressure. The kidney is able to autoregulate when the mean arterial pressure is between 50 and 150 mm Hg. As arterial pressure increases, the sympathetic innervation to the afferent arterioles causes constriction, thus keeping the glomerular filtration rate constant. When the arterial pressure is low, dilatation of the afferent arterioles serves maintain glomerular filtration. However, sympathetic stimulation can disrupt the autoregulatory process, reducing blood flow despite the mean arterial pressure.

Hormonal Control

Secretion of antidiuretic hormone (ADH) by the posterior pituitary gland is affected by plasma osmolality. When the blood becomes hypertonic, ADH is secreted and water is retained by the kidneys. If the blood is hypotonic, less ADH is formed, causing the kidneys to reabsorb less water and increasing urine formation. ADH acts on the distal tubules and collecting tubules by altering permeability to water.

The juxtaglomerular complex is a group of cells, located just before the glomerulus and in close proximity to the distal tubule, which contain granules of inactive renin. Renin is released in response to reduced arterial blood pressure entering the afferent arteriole of the kidney or a low concentration of sodium in the distal tubule. The released renin acts as an enzyme to convert angiotensinogen to angiotensin I. Angiotensin I is converted to angiotension II by the angiotensin-converting enzyme, which leads to angiotensin II. Angiotensin II stimulates the adrenal cortex to release aldosterone. Aldosterone signals the kidney tubules to increase the reabsorption of sodium and retention of water. Because the renin-angiotensin system causes this reabsorption of water and sodium, it plays a role in the control of arterial blood pressure and is important in the conservation of sodium and control of fluid volume in hypotensive states (Fig. 13-4).

REGULATION OF BODY HOMEOSTASIS

The kidneys play a significant role in regulation of body fluids. The kidneys adjust blood volume and

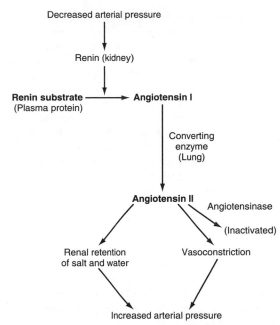

FIG. 13-4 Renin-angiotensin-vasoconstrictor mechanism for arterial pressure control. (From Hall J: *Guyton and Hall textbook of medical physiology*, ed 12, Philadelphia, 2011, Saunders.)

influence extracellular fluid volume, extracellular fluids, electrolytes, and ions. Homeostasis is maintained when the kidneys remove waste products and toxic substances.

The kidneys regulate blood volume through ADH, aldosterone, and the renin-angiotensin mechanism. When the circulating blood volume is excessive, the cardiac output and arterial pressure increases, resulting in greater pressure in the renal artery and the kidney afferent arteriole. Water and sodium are excreted. If the patient is hypovolemic, the kidneys reabsorb fluid to return the blood volume to normal limits.

The extracellular fluid volume is controlled indirectly by the kidneys as blood volume is controlled. The relative ratio of the extracellular fluid volume to blood volume depends on the physical properties of the circulation and of the interstitial spaces, including compliances and dynamics. The kidney maintains the osmolality of the extracellular fluid mainly by regulating the extracellular sodium concentration. Extracellular sodium controls 90% to 95% of the effective osmotic pressure of extracellular fluid. The extracellular concentration of other electrolytes, including potassium, calcium, magnesium, and phosphate ions, is also under renal control.

COMPONENTS OF URINE

The end product of filtration, absorption, and excretion is urine, composed of 95% water and 5% solids. The solids, approximately 60 g/L of urine, are listed in Table 13-2. Urea is derived from the breakdown of amino acids. Uric acid is an end product of purine metabolism, formed from purines ingested as food and from those formed in the body. Creatinine is an end product of creatine, of which 95% is found in muscle tissue. Creatinine is produced during the production of muscle energy.

Creatinine is considered a nonthreshold substance because it is excreted by the kidney in its entirety. High-threshold substances are almost entirely reabsorbed in the kidney. They are an important portion of the blood and are excreted only if they are in an excess concentration. High-threshold substances include glucose, potassium, calcium, and magnesium. Low-threshold substances, such as urea, uric acid, and phosphates, are only minimally reabsorbed by the kidney.

In consideration of the substances found in urine, knowledge of the characteristics of normal urine is useful. Normal urine should be clear and transparent with an amber color, a reflection of urobilin, a byproduct of bilirubin breakdown. Urine is usually acidic because of the excretion of sodium acid phosphate, with a pH of approximately 6. The specific gravity is between 1.003 and 1.025. The volume of urine excreted every 24 hours is approximately 1500 mL.

ACID-BASE BALANCE

The kidneys play a major role in acid-base balance. Although they are the most powerful acid-base regulators, they require several hours to 1 day to return the hydrogen ion concentration to a normal range. In contrast, the respiratory system can react to acid-base imbalances within 1 to 3 minutes.

The pH is an expression of the hydrogen ion concentration in the body fluids. Bicarbonate and carbon dioxide are also factors. The bicarbonate concentration is mainly under renal control, whereas the carbon dioxide is under respiratory control. Approximately 20-fold more bicarbonate than carbon dioxide is in the plasma resulting in a 20:1 ratio. Thus, any change in the 20:1 ratio affects the pH. Any change that affects kidney function affects the bicarbonate portion of the ratio and becomes a metabolic problem. Conversely, any change in the function of the lungs, which affects the carbon dioxide portion of the ratio, is a respiratory problem.

If, for example, a large amount of a bicarbonate solution is rapidly infused into a patient and ventilation does not change (Pco_2 stays constant), the result is a higher value for the bicarbonate and no change in the Pco_2. The net result is a higher pH, which indicates alkalosis, in this case metabolic alkalosis. Conversely, if an acid is infused, the ratio becomes smaller, the pH falls, indicating acidosis, which is termed *metabolic acidosis*.

The kidneys regulate pH by increasing or decreasing the bicarbonate ion concentration in the blood and eliminating hydrogen ions. This regulation is done with a complex series of reactions, which begins with hydrogen ions being secreted into the tubular filtrate. Carbon dioxide, an end product of tubular cell metabolism, combines with water to form carbonic acid (H_2CO_3). The carbonic acid dissociates to form hydrogen and bicarbonate (HCO_3). The hydrogen ion is taken via active transport to the renal tubule and usually exchanges in the tubule with sodium. Via active transport, the sodium moves to the extracellular fluid, where it combines with the bicarbonate that was reabsorbed into the extracellular fluid to form sodium bicarbonate ($NaHCO_3$). In the tubules, the hydrogen ion that was actively transported to the tubule combines with the filtrate bicarbonate to form carbonic acid. The carbonic acid dissociates to form carbon dioxide and water. The carbon dioxide is reabsorbed into the extracellular fluid and eventually excreted by the lungs; the water is excreted as part of the urine.

The kidneys correct alkalosis by decreasing the bicarbonate in the extracellular fluid, which occurs because fewer hydrogen ions enter the tubules because of a low carbon dioxide concentration and because a high bicarbonate concentration exists in the tubules. The bicarbonate cannot be reabsorbed without first combining with the hydrogen; therefore the excess bicarbonate ions

Table 13-2	Principal Constituents of Urine
CONSTITUENTS	**AMOUNT (g/L)**
Organic	
Urea	20-300
Uric acid	0.6-0.75
Creatinine	1.5
Others	2.6
Inorganic	
Sodium chloride	9.0
Potassium chloride	2.5
Sulfuric acid	1.8
Phosphoric acid	1.8
Ammonia	0.5-15
Calcium	0.2
Magnesium	0.2

are lost to the urine as are other positive ions such as sodium and hydrogen. Cellular potassium can exchange with the sodium instead of the cellular hydrogen to conserve the hydrogen, which can help to return the pH to normal limits.

Renal correction of acidosis is achieved by increasing the amount of bicarbonate in the extracellular fluid. An excess of hydrogen ions in comparison with the bicarbonate filtration into the tubules exists. The excess hydrogen ions are secreted into the tubules, where they combine with the phosphate or the ammonia buffer systems. The sodium ions in the tubules move via active transport to the extracellular fluid and combine with the bicarbonate ion to form sodium bicarbonate, which helps correct the acidosis. The urine is acidic because the kidney is excreting excess hydrogen ions.

DIURETIC THERAPY

In the PACU, diuretics are commonly used for blood volume overload (hypervolemia), to reduce intracranial pressure, to maintain kidney function, and to determine the etiology of oliguria. The major side effects of diuretic therapy are related to the contraction of the extracellular fluid volume and alterations in potassium concentrations. Diuretics are categorized according to the site of action on renal tubules and the mechanism altering the secretion of urine. The major categories are osmotic diuretics, thiazide diuretics, potassium-sparing diuretics, loop diuretics, aldosterone antagonists, and carbonic anhydrase inhibitors. Because the use of diuretics is important in the PACU, a brief review of the major categories is provided.

Osmotic Diuretics

Osmotic diuretics are used to evaluate the etiology of oliguria, reduce intracranial pressure, and protection of the kidneys against the development of acute renal failure. Mannitol, the prototype of the osmotic diuretics, is a high-molecular-weight drug given intravenously. The high osmolality draws fluid from the intracellular space and expands the intravascular volume. In the kidneys, the osmotic effect of mannitol on the tubules leads to diuresis. The major concern with mannitol therapy is an increased extracellular fluid volume, which can be of grave consequence in patients with chronic heart failure or impending pulmonary edema. As a result, when administering mannitol the perianesthesia nurse conducts frequent cardiorespiratory assessments and monitors vital signs for indications of vascular overload. Urea is an effective osmotic diuretic; however, this drug has disadvantages that limit its use compared

with mannitol. The major disadvantage of urea is that it causes a significant amount of rebound increase in intracranial pressure and increases the risk of venous thrombosis.

Thiazide Diuretics

Thiazide diuretics are used in the treatment of hypertension, heart failure, and steroid induced edema. One action of thiazides, to increase calcium reabsorption, is beneficial when treating patients with frequent kidney stones. Common thiazide diuretics are chlorothiazide, benzthiazide, and hydrochlorothiazide. Thiazides act on the distal tubule of the loop of Henle to impair the reabsorption of sodium, chloride, and potassium that is excreted with water. Patients receiving long-term thiazide diuretic therapy can have increased urinary losses of water, sodium, chloride, and potassium and some loss of bicarbonate. As a result, these patients are particularly susceptible to hypochloremic hypokalemic metabolic alkalosis.

The most common untoward effect of thiazide diuretics is hypokalemia. Hypokalemia, a reduced serum potassium level, can cause paralytic ileus, severe weakness, hypotension, atrial and ventricular dysrhythmias, and potentiate digitalis toxicity. If treatment for hypokalemia is indicated, intravenous potassium replacement may be given in the PACU.

Potassium-Sparing Diuretics

Potassium sparing diuretics act on the distal convoluted tubule and on aldosterone. The product of their actions is an increased urinary output without potassium loss. The most commonly used potassium-sparing diuretics include triamterene and amiloride A fixed-dose combination of triamterene and hydrochlorothiazide (Dyazide) can also be considered to be in this category of diuretics. The major side effect of potassium sparing diuretics is hyperkalemia, which can occur with excess use or excess potassium supplementation. The symptoms of hyperkalemia include nausea, fatigue, muscular weakness, and cardiac dysrhythmias. For an immediate reduction in the effects of hyperkalemia, calcium gluconate or calcium chloride may be administered. Glucose or insulin in combination with glucose has been used to temporarily reduce dangerous levels of potassium.

A second type of potassium-sparing diuretic is also an aldosterone agonist. Spironolactone acts on the aldosterone receptors in the conducting ducts antagonizing the reabsorption of sodium and chloride by effects of aldosterone. When spironolactone is administered, sodium and chloride reabsorption are increased and potassium excretion is decreased. Because of the decrease in potassium excretion in the conducting ducts, hyperkalemia is a serious side effect of the drug. Spironolactone is indicated for patients with fluid overload from cirrhosis of the liver, nephrotic syndrome, and heart failure. The disadvantage of spironolactone is a slow onset of action and slow metabolism, requiring several days for an effect.

Loop Diuretics

The loop diuretics, including ethacrynic acid, bumetanide, and furosemide, are used primarily in the treatment of pulmonary edema and general edema and in the diagnosis of acute kidney failure. Loop diuretics act on the thick ascending loop of Henle interfering with the concentrating and diluting mechanisms of the kidneys. Major problems with these drugs include deafness (ethacrynic acid), hypokalemia, alkalosis, extracellular fluid volume contraction, and electrolyte imbalance. Because of their potency and ability to act rapidly, loop diuretics are usually the diuretic of choice for the PACU patient. The two major concerns of loop diuretics are hypokalemia and hypovolemia. Serum potassium levels must be monitored closely.

Carbonic Anhydrase Inhibitors

Carbonic anhydrase inhibitors, including acetazolamide (Diamox) act in the proximal renal tubules. The inhibition of the carbonic anhydrase enzyme results in diminished excretion of hydrogen ions and increased excretion of bicarbonate. The net result is a diuresis of alkaline urine. A carbonic anhydrase inhibitor is used to reduce intraocular pressure, which is common in glaucoma and the management of some types of seizures. If this drug is administered to a patient with chronic obstructive pulmonary disease, careful monitoring of the patient's rate of ventilation and $PaCO_2$ level is indicated as excessive bicarbonate is lost in the urine and hypercarbia can occur, which can ultimately lead to central nervous system (CNS) depression. Alkalotic urine is also a risk factor for kidney stones.

EFFECTS OF ANESTHESIA

In patients with normal renal function who receive general inhalation anesthesia, some depression of renal function occurs. All general anesthetics depress renal blood flow, glomerular filtration rate, and urinary flow. Renal function depression is the result of direct and indirect effects of anesthetic agents. Renal blood flow is depressed as a result of renal vasoconstriction or systemic hypotension. Of interest is that the antiemetic and antipsychotic drug droperidol has the smallest effect on renal function. In most instances, the renal depression caused by the anesthetic agents is reversible at the end of the operative procedure.

The stress of surgery and anesthesia trigger a physiologic stress response and release of ADH from the posterior pituitary. When ADH is released, tubular reabsorption of water occurs, which decreases urine volume and increases urine concentration. Other biochemical products of the stress response, namely epinephrine, norepinephrine, and the renin-angiotensin system, also affect the renal system. More specifically, when these amines are liberated, renal blood flow is decreased.

Renal function, as indicated by urine volume and concentration, must be carefully monitored during the emergent phase of the anesthesia. Patients who have undergone major abdominal or thoracic surgery commonly have some diuresis during the immediate postoperative period. However, the stress of surgery may result in fluid volume retention up to 48 hours postoperatively. Monitoring urine volume and concentration is critical in patients after (1) a major surgical procedure; (2) general anesthesia for more than 2 hours; or (3) a significant blood volume replacement during the preoperative or intraoperative phase of the anesthetic experience. Increased abdominal pressure during laparoscopy can compress and compromise the kidneys. Any patient with preoperative indications of compromised renal or cardiovascular function also requires careful monitoring.

EFFECTS OF DRUGS IN PATIENTS WITH COMPROMISED KIDNEY FUNCTION

Kidney disease affects approximately 5% of adults in the United States. Patients with end-stage kidney disease exhibit anemia, body fluid shifts, and alterations in blood albumin and electrolyte levels. Patients may be debilitated and deconditioned. If uremia is present, the CNS may be depressed. When the renal impaired patient exhibits CNS depression, the actions of opioids are intensified and prolonged. Diazepam, which has a 24-hour half-life, is also not a good choice because of its additive effect on the CNS. Drugs that are not metabolized in the body but are typically excreted unchanged by the kidneys are avoided in patients with renal disease. Such drugs include long-acting barbiturates such as barbital and phenobarbital, skeletal muscle relaxants decamethonium and gallamine, and cardiac glycosides digoxin and lanatoside C. Because half the administered dose of the belladonna alkaloids, atropine and hyoscyamine, are excreted unchanged, the dosage of these drugs should be modified by the degree of renal impairment.

In patients with mild to moderate kidney dysfunction, all current inhalation anesthetics can be used in the usual clinical dose range. Because thiopental depends on redistribution for the termination of its action, it may be used in patients with renal impairment. The skeletal muscle relaxants succinylcholine, curare, and pancuronium can be used for patients with compromised kidney function. Vecuronium duration can be prolonged in patients with end-stage kidney disease. Neuroleptanalgesia, a combination of opioid and tranquilizer, when achieved with nitrous oxide and oxygen, is an acceptable technique for the patient with uremia. When droperidol has been administered, which is the prototype neuroleptanalgesic drug, the perianesthesia nurse should monitor the patient for prolonged depressant effects of the drug. More specifically, the tranquilizer component of droperidol has a long half-life; therefore its prolonged effects, coupled with CNS depression from the uremia, may cause the patient to be slow to arouse in the immediate postoperative emergence phase. Consequently, airway patency and cardiovascular parameters are closely monitored. Midazolam, if used as an infusion, can accumulate in patients with compromised kidney function. Propofol is metabolized in the liver and is safe for patients with kidney disease. Nonsteroidal antiinflammatory agents should be avoided because their use can exacerbate renal damage.

ACUTE KIDNEY FAILURE

A sudden decrease in renal function is the hallmark of acute kidney failure. Acute kidney failure will occur in 1 of 100 surgical patients. Patient risk factors include gender (male), age, and diabetes. Additional risk factors include a history of heart failure, hypertension, ascites or preoperative renal insufficiency.[1] Emergency surgery increases the risk of acute kidney failure by 100%, whereas intraperitoneal surgery increases risk by a factor of 3. Acute kidney failure can be due to prerenal, intrarenal, or postrenal causes.

Prerenal refers to system problems preceding blood flow to the kidney, primarily low cardiac output. Low cardiac output can be due to volume depletion, hemorrhage, or myocardial dysfunction. The lack of blood flow to the kidney is the cause of decreased urine output. Ensuring adequate hydration during and after anesthesia along with monitoring blood loss and replacement when indicated can protect renal function.

Intrarenal causes of acute renal failure include acute tubular necrosis. Nephrotoxicity damages the tubular cells of the loop of Henle with changes occurring within hours. Hypotension that results in hypoperfusion to the kidney can also lead to cell death. Patients who have prolonged hypoperfusion because of shock or sepsis and then undergo procedures with contrast dye are at extreme risk. Ensuring that the patient is well hydrated before administering potentially toxic drugs will prevent further damage. The PACU nurse should be aware of any prolonged periods of intraoperative hypotension. Surgical patients who have experienced traumatic injuries can develop rhabdomyolysis. Rhabdomyolysis is caused by the breakdown products of muscle including myoglobin, a large protein molecule. Excessive amounts of myoglobin can clog the glomerulus and the tubules. Additional infusions of isotonic intravenous fluids may be needed during recovery from traumatic muscle damage.

Postrenal failure occurs when urine is blocked from leaving the kidney. Undiagnosed kidney stones or stone movement during percutaneous kidney stone intervention can obstruct the collecting ducts in the kidney pelvis or ureters. Assessment of the free flow of urine may not reveal a blockage until renal failure has occurred.

ASSESSMENT OF KIDNEY FUNCTION

Kidney function is assessed through serum and urine analysis. Because creatinine is a component of urine not reabsorbed back into the tubules it serves as an indicator of glomerular filtration. Every milliliter of glomerular filtrate or urine should contain precisely the same quantity of creatinine as 1 mL of plasma. Serum creatinine is slow to increase when glomerular filtration is impaired and cannot detect the injury in time to intervene effectively; however, serum creatinine is a marker of renal function.

Urine output, usually associated with adequate renal function, is also not a reliable marker of kidney injury. Anuria can be a sign of severe kidney dysfunction, unless the cause is postrenal obstruction. Anuria always requires further assessment. The PACU nurse is more likely to detect persistent oliguria, less than 0.5 mL/kg/h or 25 mL of urine per hour for more than 2 hours. Low urine output can have numerous causes, but constitutes a medical emergency with the surgeon notified immediately.

The urine volume may be abnormally high during emergence from anesthesia. Although intraoperative diuretic administration is a common finding, in conditions creating acute tubular necrosis the increased urine volume represents failure of the tubules to reabsorb the glomerular filtrate. The quality rather than the quantity of the urine provides useful information about the renal state of the patient. Urinalysis can reveal the amount of filtered sodium. Blood in the urine can be caused by postrenal damage.

PREEXISITING KIDNEY FAILURE

More than 26 million people in the United States have chronic kidney disease (CKD). Many have no symptoms, whereas others require dialysis. CKD is defined by the extent of kidney damage and the level of kidney function. Damage for over 3 months with a decreased glomerular filtration rate will classify patients into five stages of CKD. Stage 1 and 2 patients are asymptomatic and are unlikely to be diagnosed until a comorbid condition occurs, such as diabetes or hypertension. Patients with stage 3 CKD experience fatigue, anemia, urine changes, and peripheral edema. Patients with stage 4 CKD have additional symptoms of uremia, anorexia, and numbness and tingling in the extremities. Stage 5 represents progress to a point that the kidneys are no longer able to function at the level needed for daily living and end-stage kidney disease has occurred. Chronic renal failure may last 10 to 20 years before end-stage kidney disease.

Patients with stage 4 or stage 5 kidney disease require creation of an arteriovenous fistula or placement of a temporary vascular shunt to allow hemodialysis. Any patient with CKD can require surgery though their morbidity and mortality risk is substantially increased. In the postoperative period they can be hemodynamically labile. Venous access is difficult because of preexisting vascular disease and the presence of a fistula or shunt. An intravenous catheter is never placed in the same extremity as the fistula or shunt; a blood pressure cuff is never placed above, on, or below the fistula or shunt. Patients with ESRD are scheduled to receive dialysis the day before surgery to optimize volume and electrolyte status. Intravenous fluids are minimized during minor surgery.[2] If extensive surgery is planned, intraoperative dialysis may be required. Patients with ESRD have anemia and coagulation abnormalities because of a lack of erythropoietin and altered platelet function. Bleeding during the PACU stay can be a surgical emergency.

PERIANESTHESIA NURSING CARE

Perianesthesia nursing care centers on recognition and care of the patient at risk for acute kidney failure. The status of the patient's fluid volume should be calculated and evaluated during the admission assessment. Intake includes intravenous fluids and colloidal and blood products. Output includes blood loss, gastrointestinal loss, and urine output. A urine output of less than 0.5 mL/kg/h is not acceptable. The duration of NPO is considered when calculating replacement fluids (125 mL/h NPO). The possibility of third space fluids, particularly during bowel surgery, is considered. When fluid balance is determined, a plan for promoting renal perfusion is discussed with the surgical team. An indwelling urethral catheter may be needed for a patient at risk of kidney failure to monitor moment-to-moment information concerning the volume and quality of urine output. The need for the catheter must be weighed against the risk of a catheter-associated urinary tract infection. For patient safety, urinary catheters must be removed when they are no longer indicated. A bladder scanner should be readily available as a noninvasive assessment of urine production.

If acute kidney failure is apparent, immediate interventions can include larger-than-usual doses of osmotic or loop diuretics. Laboratory analysis for baseline values of serum creatinine, electrolytes, proteinuria, and urine sodium are obtained. Acute kidney failure creates hyperkalemia, which is reflected on the electrocardiogram as high-peaked T waves and depressed S-T segments. The subsequent disappearance of T waves, heart block, and cardiac arrest can occur with increasing levels of potassium.

SUMMARY

A review of the complex anatomy and physiology of the renal system was presented to demonstrate the role the kidney plays in regulating and controlling body systems. Pharmacologic agents administered during the perioperative period must be carefully monitored to avoid kidney damage. Maintaining blood volume and renal perfusion is the key to preserving kidney function. The PACU nurse must be aware of the patient's fluid volume status and carefully monitor the adequacy of urine output. Patients with chronic kidney failure present additional challenges for post anesthesia recovery. Care of the patient requiring genitourinary surgery including renal transplantation is presented in Chapter 41.

REFERENCES

1. Kheterpal S, et al: Development and validation of an acute kidney injury risk index for patients undergoing general surgery: results from a national data set, *Anesthesiology* 110:505–515, 2009.
2. Wagener G, Brentjens T: Anesthetic concerns in patients presenting with renal failure, *Anesthesiol Clin* 28:39–54, 2010.

RESOURCES

Aitkenhead A, et al: *Textbook of anaesthesia,* ed 5, Philadelphia, 2007, Churchill Livingstone.

Atlee J: *Complications in anesthesia,* ed 2, Philadelphia, 2007, Saunders.

Barash P, et al: *Clinical anesthesia,* ed 6, Philadelphia, 2009, Lippincott Williams & Wilkins.

Brunton L, et al: *Goodman and Gilman's the pharmacological basis of therapeutics,* ed 12, New York, 2011, McGraw-Hill.

Miller R, et al, editors: *Miller's anesthesia,* ed 7, Philadelphia, 2010, Churchill Livingstone.

Porth C: *Essentials of pathophysiology,* ed 3, Philadelphia, 2011, Wolters Kluwer.

Stoelting R, Miller R: *Basics of anesthesia,* ed 5, Philadelphia, 2007, Churchill Livingstone.

PHYSIOLOGIC CONSIDERATIONS IN THE PACU

14 Fluid and Electrolytes

Debra Pecka Malina, DNSc, MBA, CRNA

The goal of fluid management in the perioperative period is to maintain adequate intravascular fluid volume, left ventricular filling pressure, cardiac output, systemic blood pressure, and oxygen delivery to tissues. The maintenance of appropriate concentrations of body fluid and electrolytes is essential to normal physiologic function of all body systems. An understanding of basic human physiology in this area along with a brief introduction to the various types and protocols of fluid management of the patient is presented in this chapter.

DEFINITIONS

Anions: Ions that carry a negative charge and migrate to the anode (terminal) in an electric field.
Autologous: Originating within the same person, such as an autotransfusion.
Cations: Ions that carry a positive charge and migrate to the cathode (terminal) in an electric field.
Chvostek Sign: An abnormal spasm of the facial muscles elicited by light taps on the facial nerve that indicates hypocalcemia.
Colloids: Compounds such as red blood cells, albumin, or dextran that, because of size, are retained within a specific fluid compartment and increase the oncotic pressure of that compartment.
Cryoprecipitate: A preparation rich in factor VIII needed to restore normal coagulation in hemophilia. The preparation is collected from fresh human plasma that has been frozen and thawed.
Crystalloids: Balanced electrolyte solutions that are in isotonic solutions of water or dextrose and can move between the intravascular and interstitial compartments.
Edema: Accumulation of fluid in the interstitial spaces.
Hemolysis: A disruption of the integrity of the red cell membrane that causes release of cell contents to include hemoglobin.
Hemostasis: The arrest of bleeding by the interaction of the platelet with the blood vessel wall and the formation of the platelet plug.
Hypercalcemia: Increased plasma concentration of calcium (>5.6 mEq/L).
Hyperkalemia: Greater than 6 mEq/L blood concentration of potassium.
Hypermagnesemia: An increase in the plasma concentration of magnesium (>2.6 mEq/L).

Hypernatremia: An increase in sodium in the plasma of more than 145 mEq/L.
Hypertonic Solutions (Hyperosmotic): Solutions that have an osmolality greater than that of plasma.
Hypocalcemia: Reduced plasma concentration of calcium (<4.4 mEq/L).
Hypokalemia: Less than 3 mEq/L blood concentration of potassium.
Hypomagnesemia: A decrease in the plasma concentration of magnesium (<1.6 mEq/L).
Hyponatremia: A decrease of sodium in the plasma of less than 135 mEq/L.
Hypotonic Solutions (Hypoosmotic): Solutions that have an osmolality less than that of plasma.
Isotonic Solutions: Solutions that have the same osmolality as plasma.
Milliequivalent (mEq): Replaced with the SI units millimole (mmol); mEq/L has been replaced by mmol/L.
Osmolality: A physical property of a solution, one that is dependent on the number of dissolved particles in the solution.
Tetany: A condition characterized by cramps, muscle twitching, sharp flexion of the wrist and ankle joints, and convulsions.
Third Space: Losses of fluid and electrolytes from the extracellular fluid to a nonfunctional space, an acute sequestered space that accompanies surgery.
Trousseau Sign: A test for latent tetany in which carpal spasm is induced with inflation of a sphygmomanometer cuff on the upper arm to a pressure that exceeds systolic blood pressure for 3 minutes.

BODY FLUID BALANCE

Water is the most abundant and essential component of the body. It represents approximately 50% to 60% of adult body weight and 75% to 77% of body weight in infants less than 1 month of age. By approximately 17 years of age, the adult composition is attained; and in a person weighing 154 lb (70 kg), the total body water is approximately 42 L. Because women have higher fat content in their bodies and because fat is essentially free of water, they have a lower water content than men do. Older adults and those with diabetes, hypertension, or obesity also have a lower proportion of water in their bodies.

Body water is the medium within which metabolic reactions take place to facilitate the ionization of electrolytes; it acts as a reagent in many chemical reactions; it transports nutrients to cells and removes waste products; and its high specific heat and heat of vaporization make it especially suitable as a temperature regulator. The total amount of body water remains relatively stable; intake usually slightly exceeds bodily needs and the excess is excreted. Removal or output of water from the body is normally through four types of excretion: through the lungs, gastrointestinal tract, skin, and kidney.

Water intake includes not only the water consumed in beverages but also the fluids obtained from the metabolism of solid foods. The water taken in via beverages and food is referred to as *exogenous water*. Although variance occurs on a day-to-day basis, overall the average adult in a moderate climate with a mixed diet consumes 2500 to 3000 mL daily. Approximately 1000 mL is obtained from beverages and 1500 mL from solid and semisolid foods.

The water formed during metabolism of ingested food is called *endogenous water*. Because metabolism varies with body temperature, the amount of exercise performed, and other factors, the amount of endogenous water available also varies on a daily basis. In a healthy adult who performs a moderate amount of exercise, an average of 300 to 350 mL of endogenous water is available daily. Intake is influenced by the thirst center located in the hypothalamus, which is stimulated by either a decrease in blood pressure or extracellular fluid, or an increase in serum osmolality. If the fluid volume inside the cells decreases, salivary secretion is reduced, thereby causing a dry mouth and the sensation of thirst. In normal circumstances, an individual then drinks and restores the fluid volume (Box 14-1).

Surgical Patient Considerations

The surgical patient experiences even greater fluid losses. Unless the patient is coming to the operating room for a surgical emergency, in most cases adults will be NPO for at least eight hours (Box 14-2). The goal of preoperative fluid therapy is to replace preexisting fluid deficits, normal intraoperative losses (maintenance requirements), and surgical wound losses (third spacing and blood loss).

NPO guidelines are enforced because of the risk of pulmonary aspiration. Over the past few years, fasting times have become more liberal after studies have shown that reduced fasting times lower residual gastric volumes. Furthermore, prolonged fasting can contribute to hypovolemia, hypoglycemia, and patient anxiety. Longer fasting times are generally enforced in patients who are at increased risk for aspiration (Box 14-3).

Lungs

The amount of fluid lost through the lungs varies with the humidity, temperature of inspired air, and the rate and depth of respiration. As a rule, 300 to 400 mL of water is lost daily. This loss of water via the respiratory tract is termed *insensible loss* of water, so named because one is not aware of this loss. The water content of inhaled gases decreases as the ambient temperature decreases. Consequently, the insensible water loss from the lungs is higher in cold environments. Therefore patients with respiratory dysfunction need a greater water intake to offset the increased insensible water loss when they are in cold environments. In addition, an increase in the respiration rate can increase the water loss to as much as 2000 mL, which is significant in patients

---

BOX 14-1   Normal Intake and Output of Water Per Day

INTAKE
Water: 1000 mL
Endogenous water: 1500 mL
Total water intake: 2500 mL

OUTPUT
Insensible loss: 250 mL
Skin: 250 mL
Respiratory tract: 400 mL
Urine: 1500 mL
Feces: 100 mL
Total water output: 2500 mL

BOX 14-2   Summary of Fasting Recommendations

- Clear liquids: 2 hours
- Breast milk: 4 hours
- Infant formula: 6 hours
- Nonhuman milk: 6 hours
- Light meal: 6 hours
  These recommendations apply to healthy patients who are undergoing elective procedures. They are not intended for women in labor.

From American Society of Anesthesiologists Committee on Standards and Practice Parameters: Practice guidelines for preoperative fasting and the use of pharmacologic agents to reduce the risk of pulmonary aspiration: application to healthy patients undergoing elective procedures, *Anesthesiol* 114:495-511, 2011.

BOX 14-3	Patient Conditions at Increased Risk for Aspiration

- Morbid obesity
- Renal failure
- Hepatic dysfunction
- Ascites
- Head injury
- Increased intracranial pressure
- Decreased level of consciousness
- Delayed gastric emptying
- Difficulty swallowing
- Cerebral palsy
- Trauma
- Pain
- Drug overdose
- Difficult airway
- Gastrointestinal obstruction or dysfunction
- Anorexia
- Esophageal disorders
- Diabetes

From Nagelhout J, Plaus K: *Nurse anesthesia*, ed 4, St. Louis, 2010, Saunders; Barash P, et al: *Clinical anesthesia*, ed 6, Philadelphia, 2009, Lippincott Williams & Wilkins.

with chronic obstructive pulmonary disease (see Chapter 48).

Gastrointestinal Tract

The amount of water lost via the feces averages 100 mL per day; however, with vomiting or diarrhea, this loss may be greatly increased. Up to 7000 mL can be lost with diarrhea and 6000 mL with vomiting. The implications to the perianesthesia nurse are great because active vomiting can significantly affect the volume status of the surgical patient. In such cases, fluids should be increased in rate, any ordered antiemetics should be given, and the anesthesia provider should be notified.

Skin

Water lost via the skin can be via insensible (not obvious) or sensible (obvious) loss. There is constant diffusion of moisture from deep body layers to the dry surface where the evaporation occurs. Insensible loss depends largely on environmental humidity. Sensible perspiration refers to loss of water with production of sweat. Sweating is an emergency mechanism for regulation of body temperature when the heat produced by metabolic processes is excessive. The amount of sweat therefore varies with exercise and with body temperature. In a moist atmosphere, sweat may be more visible than in a dry atmosphere, but the

amount of water lost is the same. Despite its role as a protective mechanism, sweating can become a hazard when body water supplies are low because the body continues to lose sweat to maintain its temperature. In the healthy adult who performs moderate exercise in a comfortable environment, approximately 500 mL of water is lost in both sensible and insensible perspiration.

Kidneys

Water loss via the kidneys varies with the supply of body water. The kidneys are able to concentrate the urine, and the specific gravity may approach 1.040 (normal, 1.002 to 1.030); however, if the amount of excess water is great, such as might occur when a large quantity is administered intravenously, the kidneys excrete dilute urine, the specific gravity of which might approach 1.001. In normal conditions, the kidneys excrete approximately 1.5 L per day. In patients who are vomiting or have diarrhea, obviously less water is available, and the kidneys respond promptly by curtailing water loss via urine. The two hormones responsible for control of the volume of urine are antidiuretic hormone from the posterior pituitary and aldosterone from the adrenal cortex. Antidiuretic hormone, by increasing the permeability of the renal distal convoluted tubule and collecting ducts, increases the amount of water reabsorbed and thus decreases the urine volume. Aldosterone increases the renal reabsorption of sodium and of water secondarily. Both hormones are secreted in response to lowered blood volume and serve to control output to balance intake. However, a minimal loss of fluids is obligatory; therefore perioperative monitoring of fluid balance is critical.

Surgical Fluid Loss

Patients undergoing surgery require fluid replacement for that lost through their lungs, gastrointestinal tract, skin, and urine. They also need to have fluid replacement of their NPO deficit, intraoperative fluids lost through blood loss, third space fluid shifts, evaporation through incisions, and tissue manipulation. The amount of replacement is based on the type of fluid used for replacement (i.e., crystalloids, colloids, blood products) and calculations based on a patient's age, sex, and weight.

DISTRIBUTION OF BODY FLUIDS

The fluids in the body can be divided into two compartments along with a potential third compartment or space. The two compartments are normally divided relative to the location of the cell membrane: intracellular (inside the cell) and extracellular (outside the cell). The intracellular fluid (ICF) is estimated to be approximately 40% of the body weight, or approximately 28 L of fluid, and represents approximately two thirds of the total body water. ICF provides a medium for all intracellular activities. The other compartment, the extracellular fluid (ECF), is approximately 20% of the body weight and ranges from 12 to 14 L of fluid. The fluid compartment includes the blood plasma or intravascular fluid, the interstitial fluid (ISF) that bathes the cells, the lymph, the cerebrospinal fluid (CSF), and the transcellular fluids. The transcellular fluids include the synovial fluid, peritoneal fluid, digestive fluids, and fluids of the eye and ear. The lymph, CSF, and the transcellular fluids normally constitute approximately 1% of the body mass. Blood constitutes approximately 4% of the body weight, and the interstitial fluid constitutes 15.7%.[1]

There is a potential third compartment, which is commonly called the *third space*. It is a concept that is defined as a compartment that includes the interstitial spaces that are swollen by local responses to tissue trauma, inflammation, and hormonal influx from the stress of surgery. This third space can occur even when patients have undergone massive surgical procedures and the fluid loss, to include insensible loss, is appropriately replaced. This accumulation of fluid in the third space compartment usually occurs during and immediately after the surgical procedure and is difficult to clinically differentiate from actual blood loss. Clinically, the signs of hypovolemia reflect third space loss and actual fluid loss. The treatment includes infusion of fluids in the range of 3 to 10 mL/kg/h and is usually adequate along with establishment and treatment of the underlying cause (e.g., active bleeding). The third space loss usually resolves in several postoperative days, and the nurse on the unit that receives the patient after the postanesthesia care unit (PACU) should be alert for signs of possible fluid overload as the fluid returns after surgery to the ECF.

Fluid balance involves not only the total amount of body water but also the maintenance of a relatively constant distribution of that water in the different compartments. Circulation of fluid between compartments depends on the relative hydrostatic and osmotic pressures in each compartment. Hydrostatic pressure is the force that pushes fluid from one compartment to the other. If the hydrostatic pressure in the capillaries (blood pressure) exceeds the pressure in the interstitial space, fluid moves from the capillary into the interstitial space. Osmotic pressure is the "pull" of fluids into the compartment; it is

a function of the number of dissolved molecules in the solution and is not influenced by weight or size of the molecule. Electrolytes are the major contributors to the osmotic pressure of the fluids.[2]

The major difference between the two major compartments that make up the extracellular fluid is the much higher protein content in the plasma than in the interstitial fluid. Because capillary membranes are not selectively permeable to small particles, ions and small molecules can exchange rapidly between the plasma and the ISF. However, proteins remain in the plasma because they are too large to cross the capillary barrier. As a result, the electrolyte composition differs slightly from the plasma and the interstitial fluid. The sodium concentration in plasma is slightly greater, whereas the chloride concentration is slightly less than in the interstitial fluid and the sum of the diffusible ions. Thus, the osmotic pressure in the plasma is greater than that of interstitial fluid. The osmotic pressure caused by plasma colloids is called the *colloid osmotic pressure* (COP) or *oncotic pressure*. Protein molecules are responsible for the COP or oncotic pressure. The proteins that exert a COP help to retain the plasma water in the intravascular compartment. Albumin is the major protein in the plasma that contributes to the COP.

The extracellular fluid is regulated carefully by the kidneys to facilitate the cells being bathed in fluid that contains appropriate concentrations of electrolytes to include sodium, potassium, and nutrients. A patient with major abdominal surgery usually excretes large amounts of potassium during the first 48 hours postoperatively and for several days thereafter. As a result, the potassium is usually administered intravenously in the immediate postoperative period. The body has significant stores of potassium; therefore hypokalemia might not be evident for a number of days postoperatively. Potassium levels are generally monitored closely postoperatively, and replacement is administered intravenously when needed. It is important to note that plasma potassium measurements do not exactly predict total body potassium, because potassium is primarily an intracellular ion. From a clinical chemistry point of view, the international standard unit is the millimole (mmol), commonly called the *milliequivalent* (mEq). The clinical implications for the perianesthesia nurse is that patients who undergo major surgery should routinely have potassium levels checked and evaluated before surgery for determining whether they are receiving any non–potassium-sparing diuretics (see Chapter 13).

EDEMA

A delicate balance of pressures keeps fluids passing between compartments (Fig. 14-1). A dynamic equilibrium exists between the plasma and the interstitial fluid because proteins are too large to cross the capillary barrier, which creates a colloid osmotic pressure between the two components. The hydrostatic pressures of the blood and the interstitial fluid tend to oppose each other, which is called the effective filtration pressure. Similarly, the colloid osmotic (or oncotic) pressure is the opposition between the blood and the interstitial fluid. The final common pathway is that these pressures result in a pulling in opposite directions when in appropriate physiologic equilibrium that does not allow fluid to accumulate into the interstitial spaces. Edema then results when either of the two pressures are in dysfunction.

ELECTROLYTES

Electrolytes are any substance in solution that contains free ions that make the substance electrically conductive (e.g., elements, chemicals, minerals). These ions carry an electric charge. The cations are positively charged and include sodium, potassium, calcium, and magnesium. The anions are negatively charged ions and include chloride, bicarbonate, phosphate, sulfate, and ions of inorganic acids such as lactate. Protein also carries a negative charge at physiologic pH. Each of the fluid compartments of the body contains electrolytes. The concentration and specific composition of electrolytes in each compartment vary, and the number of cations in each compartment balances the number of anions to maintain electric neutrality.

The major ions found in the ECF are sodium and chloride. Potassium and phosphate are predominately intracellular ions. The predominance of sodium outside the cell and potassium inside the cell is the result of a cell membrane pump that exchanges sodium and potassium ions. This active transport mechanism requires energy from adenosine triphosphate. Although electrolytes constitute only a small fraction of the body weight, they are essential for facilitation of normal body function. They maintain electroneutrality and chemical conditions in the body fluids, equilibrium between ECF and ICF, and regulation of neuromuscular activity. Monitoring of electrolyte concentrations is usually analyzed before and after surgery, many times requiring blood being drawn in the PACU.

Sodium

Sodium is the major cation in the extracellular fluid. Blood plasma sodium averages 135 to 145 mEq/L and usually does not vary (±5 mEq/L). Variations greater than this can affect many physiologic activities; therefore mechanisms for regulation of sodium concentration are of prime importance in maintenance of balance. Basically, the body regulates sodium with conservation mechanisms when the sodium is low. If body stores of sodium are high, the body excretes sodium via sweat, feces, and, in large part, the kidneys.

The body fluids are maintained in an isotonic state with regulation of the concentration of sodium and its most abundant anion, chloride. Concentration of sodium and chloride in the fluids is maintained primarily with loss or retention of water. Loss of salt is accompanied by loss of water and retention of salt by retention of

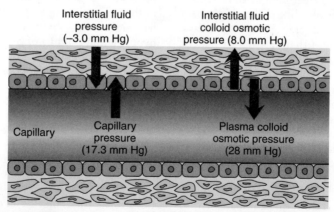

FIG. 14-1 Components of the capillary pressure gradient. Filtration reflects the difference between the combined forces that push fluid out of the capillary (capillary pressure and interstitial fluid colloid osmotic pressure) and those that attempt to hold fluid in the capillary (plasma colloid osmotic pressure and interstitial fluid pressure). (From Copstead LE, Banasik JL: *Pathophysiology*, ed 3, St. Louis, 2005, Saunders.)

water. Water moves into areas where salt is in higher concentration, which is why patients are often placed on a low-salt diet in an effort to reduce fluid overload on the heart and other major organs. However, patients who receive magnesium sulfate can also have impaired fluid excretion.

Of particular interest to the perioperative nurse are patients who have undergone urologic surgery and have been or are currently receiving irrigation fluids in the bladder. These patients are at risk of developing hyponatremia. The most common surgical procedure associated with this complication is a transurethral resection of the prostate. Irrigation fluids typically consist of sorbitol and mannitol or glycine in distilled water. The irrigants are isotonic. The amount of irrigation solution absorbed through the venous sinuses in the bladder averages 10 to 30 mL per minute of resection time. For this reason, the resection time should ideally be limited to 1 hour or less. The absorption of the irrigating fluid results in the fluid entering the vascular system; this can lead to volume overload and ultimately to dilutional hyponatremia.

The resulting lowered serum sodium concentrations can cause serious cardiac and neurologic consequences. Concentrations of sodium at 140 mEq/L are usually associated with the development of cardiac dysrhythmias that can lead to cardiac arrest. Progressive neurologic symptoms include restlessness, confusion, nausea, vomiting, coma, and convulsions.

Hypernatremia is most often caused by a loss of body fluids resulting in excess sodium. Elective surgery should be postponed until sodium levels greater than 150 mEq/L are corrected. Correction of water deficit should take place over 48 hours with hypotonic solutions. Rapid correction can result in seizures, cerebral edema, and coma.[3]

Potassium

Potassium is the most important intracellular cation. Measurement of intracellular potassium is difficult; therefore only extracellular potassium is measured. The normal values are between 3.5 and 5.5 mEq/L. Potassium affects the excitability of nerve and muscle tissue, and is important in the maintenance of cardiac rhythm, deposition of glycogen in liver cells, and transmission and conduction of nerve impulses. It also contributes to cellular energy production. Overall, abnormal potassium concentrations can have serious effects on the contractility of the heart, resulting in dysrhythmias and potential cardiac arrest.

Potassium depletion can be accompanied by changes in plasma potassium concentration. True depletion develops only with a net loss of potassium, whereas a decrease in plasma potassium, hypokalemia, can occur with a shift of potassium from the ECF to the ICF. Decreased intake can cause a mild deficit because the mechanisms for potassium conservation are not as efficient as those for sodium. Severe depletion results from abnormal losses rather than decreased intake. Most common causes of severe potassium loss are usually associated with diuretics (see Chapter 13), vomiting, acute blood loss, gastrointestinal surgery, and nasogastric suctioning. Cardiac arrhythmias, polyuria, confusion, and weakness of skeletal muscle are commonly observed in mild hypokalemia. Hallucinations, diminished reflexes, ST segment depression, widened QRS, flattened T waves, and cardiac arrest result from severe depletion. Oral replacement with potassium chloride is in the range of 60 to 80 mEq/day. Peripheral intravenous (IV) potassium should not exceed 8 mEq/h so as not to irritate veins. Central IV potassium can be infused at 10 to 20 mEq/h. The administration of 0.5 mEq/kg of potassium chloride usually raises the serum potassium concentration by 0.6 mEq/L. If the patient is receiving catecholamine drugs, the increase is approximately 0.1 mEq/L; if the patient is receiving beta-adrenergic antagonists, the serum concentration increases by approximately 0.9 mEq/L. It is important to note that correction of hypomagnesemia may be needed to avoid the increased loss of potassium by the kidneys.

Hyperkalemia is often associated with situations in which cells are injured or destroyed. Examples include chronic and acute renal failure, crush injuries, burn victims, and newborns who receive relatively large transfusions. The administration of succinylcholine, a depolarizing skeletal muscle relaxant, can produce also produce hyperkalemia (discussed in Chapter 23). Accidental lethal doses of supplemental IV potassium have been administered to patients with rapid intravenous infusion in the PACU. Cases have been recorded in which death occurred within 5 minutes of the rapid injection of just 25 mEq of potassium; therefore under no circumstance should potassium chloride be given via IV push.[3]

Calcium

Calcium is one of the major extracellular cations. It is deposited in the bone tissue as crystalline salts composed primarily of calcium and phosphate; the remainder is in the plasma, ISF, and soft tissues. The major fraction of calcium that accounts for its physiologic effects is the ionizable calcium in plasma, of which the normal plasma concentration is maintained between 4.0 and 5.6 mg/dL. The remainder is bound to protein and other substances in nonionizable form, with normal serum calcium levels rending 8.5 to 10.5 mg/dL. Calcium has an important function in neuromuscular transmission, skeletal muscle contraction, blood coagulation, and exocytosis necessary for release of neurotransmitters and autacoids (serotonin, histamine, kinins). In addition, the balance of the appropriate calcium concentration is controlled by the parathyroid hormone, calcitonin, and vitamin D. Calcium also has a reciprocal relationship with phosphate ions.

Hypocalcemia can result from any number of causes; hypoparathyroidism, pancreatitis, renal failure, or decreased serum albumin levels. In hypocalcemia, the nervous system becomes progressively more irritable as the membrane becomes increasingly permeable to sodium. At a certain critical level of calcium, the nerve fibers become so irritable that they begin to fire spontaneously. Impulses pass to skeletal muscles and can cause skeletal muscle spasm, including laryngospasm. Severe tetanic spasms are called *tetany*. Hypocalcemia occurs when the serum calcium concentration is lower than approximately 8 mg/dL. Neuromuscular function becomes increasingly impaired with decreased myocardial contractility, increased central venous pressure, and hypotension. Because of skeletal muscle spasm and potential laryngospasm, when caring for patients with hypocalcemia, the perianesthesia nurse should have appropriate airway equipment readily available for resuscitation.

An increased secretion of parathyroid hormone, most commonly caused by a parathyroid tumor, can cause hypercalcemia. In this situation, nervous system depression results in reduced reflex activity, and depression of muscle contractility results in skeletal muscle weakness, constipation, and loss of appetite. Because some calcium is excreted in the urine, a mild hypercalcemia can induce kidney stones as the calcium combines with phosphate or other anions and precipitates.

Phosphorous

Phosphorous is a major intracellular anion; most of it (85%) is located in the bones. It probably represents the single most important mineral constituent in cellular activity. Normal serum laboratory values range from 3.4 to 4.5 mg/dL for adults and fluctuates with age; it is higher in children. Phosphorous serves many functions, including forming red blood cells (RBCs) and acting as an intermediary in the metabolism of carbohydrates, proteins, and fats (glycolysis). Phosphorous promotes deposition of calcium in the bone and is essential for the delivery of oxygen via the RBCs to body tissues. The small number of phosphorous ions in plasma is important in acid-base balance by way of the phosphate buffer system. Phosphorous is also important in regulation of energy metabolism, in the form of adenosine triphosphate. It is also active in the functions of DNA.

Magnesium

Magnesium is an essential element that is found primarily in muscle and bone. It effects tissue irritability and is a cofactor in various enzyme reactions. Magnesium has a significant effect on cardiac cell membrane ion transport and is essential for activation of many enzyme systems. Magnesium is an essential regulator of calcium within cells and is the natural physiologic antagonist of calcium. In regard to skeletal muscle contraction, the presynaptic release of acetylcholine depends on the actions of magnesium. The current reference values for magnesium range from 1.6 to 2.4 mEq/L.

Hypomagnesemia is frequently overlooked as an electrolyte deficiency. Patients with alcoholism, poor diets or starvation, total parenteral nutrition without supplementation, nasogastric suctioning, or protracted vomiting or diarrhea can have this syndrome. Patients who have undergone cardiopulmonary bypass surgery are susceptible because of the dilutional effects of the pump-priming solutions. Symptoms of acute hypomagnesemia can include Chvostek and Trousseau signs, as with hypocalcemia, stridor, skeletal muscle weakness, seizures, and coma. In the perianesthesia period, ventricular dysrhythmias are usually the most common symptom of hypomagnesemia. Treatment for this syndrome is magnesium 1 to 2 g IV over 15 to 60 minutes or a continuous infusion of magnesium at 0.5 to 1.0 g/h. With severe life-threatening hypomagnesemia, an infusion of magnesium of 10 to 20 mg/kg is usually administered over 10 to 20 minutes.

Hypermagnesemia is a rare clinical phenomenon. The most common cause of hypermagnesemia is the parenteral administration of magnesium as a treatment for pregnancy-induced hypertension. Symptoms of hypermagnesemia include sedation, myocardial depression, relaxed skeletal muscles and, when severe, paralysis of the muscles of ventilation. Treatment of the life-threatening hypermagnesemia is with calcium gluconate (1 g) given intravenously followed by a loop diuretic and increased fluid loading to produce diuresis in an effort to enhance the excretion of the excess magnesium. Monitoring for vasodilation and negative inotropic effects is critical.[2]

PERIOPERATIVE BLOOD AND FLUID REPLACEMENT

Because of many factors (e.g., NPO, insensible fluid loss, surgical stresses of hemostatic function), fluid status, medical and surgical history, and medication regimens should be assessed. If problems with hemostasis are envisioned, coagulation function should be assessed before surgery to ensure appropriate intraoperative and postoperative coagulation. A patient can lose up to 75% of RBC volume if the total blood volume is maintained with the administration of colloid or crystalloid solutions. If the red cells are not replaced, the result is a loss in oxygen-carrying capacity, because RBCs carry approximately 90% of the oxygen in the blood. In the situation of massive transfusions, many complications can arise in the PACU, such as dilutional coagulopathy, acidosis, electrolyte abnormalities, and other long-term consequences as described in Chapter 29.

Assessment of Coagulation

The coagulation function for hemostasis is usually viewed in two separate events. The first event is platelet function, which includes aggregation, adhesion, and release of platelet contents and the coagulation cascade of events, which results in the deposition of a fibrin network to form a clot.

Routine screening tests are commonly performed before surgery and particularly for any patient with a history of bleeding problems. These tests include the platelet count and bleeding time for assessment of platelet function and the prothrombin time (PT) and partial thromboplastin time (PTT) for assessment of the coagulation cascade.

The normal platelet count is 150 to 370 $\times$ 10^9/L. Interestingly, patients with hemostatic stress of a major surgical procedure often begin to have bleeding during the operation when the platelet counts become less than 100 $\times$ 10^9/L. Moreover, certain drugs (e.g., aspirin, clopidogrel, nonsteroidal antiinflammatory drugs, warfarin, some herbal supplements) can also increase surgical bleeding.

Bleeding times are used to measure the primary phase of hemostasis. On the basis of the standardized method, the normal bleeding time is 3 to 10 minutes. This time is elevated in individuals with qualitative platelet abnormalities. A bleeding time greater than 1.5 times the normal is supposed to predict significant hemostatic abnormality. Because of the variability of techniques used with this test, and other more consistent methods, it has fallen out of favor as a reliable measurement.

The PT and the activated partial thromboplastin time (APTT) tests are reliable and accurate. The PT evaluates the extrinsic system of coagulation (requiring a tissue factor to initiate clotting) and is sensitive to defects in fibrinogen and to the clotting factors V, VII, and X. The APTT evaluates the intrinsic system of coagulation (all factors found in the circulation) and is sensitive to defects in fibrinogen, prothrombin, and the factors V, VIII, IX, X, XI, and XII. The PT is evaluated during management of warfarin therapy. The APTT monitors heparin therapy. The normal PT values range between 11 and 13.2 seconds, and the normal APTT range is between 22.5 and 32.2 seconds. The International Normalized Ratio has become a standard test for hemostasis. The range is 0.9 to 1.2 and is a measure of the ratio of the prothrombin time in a specific patient to normal.

Another test, fibrinogen, is also helpful in the prediction of coagulation problems—particularly disseminated intravascular coagulation. The normal value for this test is 195 to 365 mg/dL.[4]

Disseminated intravascular coagulation is an uncontrolled activation of the coagulation system, with consumption of platelets and clotting factors. Diagnosis is based on such factors as the presence of thrombocytopenia, prolongation of the PT and PTT, and increased circulating concentrations of fibrin degradation products in the presence of diffuse hemorrhage. Treatment is focused on removal of the cause, such as hemolytic transfusion reactions, low cardiac output, hypovolemia, and sepsis. The other parameters of treatment include the administration of platelet concentrates and fresh frozen plasma.

CRYSTALLOID AND COLLOID ADMINISTRATION

The use of crystalloid or colloid fluid administration in the PACU is usually based on the purpose of the fluid therapy and replacement in an attempt to maintain the patient's fluid status as normal as possible during and after the surgical procedure. There are many advantages and disadvantages for each type. However, no definitive data seem to support significant differences in outcomes. As a result, the choice of fluid type should be based on the immediate short-term needs of the patient and not on personal preferences and availability of the particular fluid. Some of the factors on which to base the decision are the amount of volume loss, the type of loss amount, and whether the patient has autologous blood available.

Crystalloid fluids are electrolyte solutions dissolved in water or dextrose and water. These electrolytes are impermeable to the cellular membrane, and dextrose crosses cell membranes; however, crystalloids are freely permeable to the vascular membranes. Crystalloid solutions help to determine the total osmotic pressure or osmolality that helps to balance water between the extracellular and the intracellular compartments. Osmolality reflects the number of dissolved particles in solutions. An isotonic solution, such as normal saline, has the same osmolality as plasma, whereas a hypertonic solution has an elevated concentration of particles and a hypotonic solution has fewer dissolved particles than plasma does. Administering hypertonic solutions, such as 3% saline, promotes movement of water from the cells into the plasma and shrinks the brain, whereas hypotonic solutions (e.g., D_5W) expand the brain (Fig. 14-2).

Isotonic crystalloid solutions have a sodium concentration ranging from 130 to 155 mEq/L and an osmolarity of 275 to 310 mOsm/L. The isotonic fluids remain in the extracellular fluid, and the sodium-free solutions are distributed throughout the total body water. Hypertonic crystalloid solutions have a sodium concentration of greater than 150 mEq/L and an osmolarity of greater than 310 mOsm/L.

The normally accepted amount of crystalloid used to replace 1 mL of blood loss is 3 mL of saline or Ringer solution; however, the ratios certainly depend on the circumstances. For example, in patients with major hemorrhage, the ratio can be 1 mL of blood volume replaced with 1 mL of Ringer solution. The ratio can go as high as 10 mL of Ringer to 1 mL of blood volume in the patient with massive trauma who has received large amounts of fluid.

The advantages of crystalloid use are that crystalloids are inexpensive, promote urinary flow, and restore third-space losses. The disadvantages of crystalloid use are that crystalloids can dilute plasma proteins, decrease the colloid pressure, and lead to a filtration from the intravascular to the interstitial compartment, which could result in interstitial pulmonary edema. They have no oxygen carrying capacity. However, crystalloids are an excellent choice for use as maintenance fluids for compensation for insensible losses, as replacement for body fluid deficits, and for special replacements of specific fluids and electrolytes.

Colloids are solutions that contain natural or synthetic molecules that are usually impermeable to the vascular membrane. As a result, they remain predominately in the intravascular space. By doing so, colloids determine the colloid oncotic pressure that helps to balance the water distribution between the intravascular and interstitial spaces. Albumin is the prototype natural colloid and accounts for approximately two thirds of the plasma oncotic pressure. Dextrans 40 and 70, along with hetastarch 6% with an osmolarity of 310 mOsm/L, are the major synthetic colloids in clinical use. The advantages of colloid use are that the solution tends to remain in the intravascular compartment for up to 24 hours, thus causing less peripheral edema and rapidly restoring the circulating volume. In addition, smaller volumes of colloids compared with crystalloids can be used for fluid resuscitation, and the colloids restore the patient volume status sooner and create a sustained increase in plasma volume. Finally, because colloids increase the plasma colloid oncotic pressure, they prevent pulmonary edema. Some of the disadvantages of colloid use include the expense,

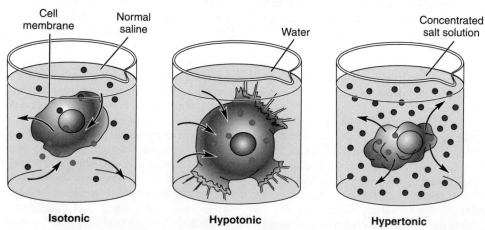

FIG. 14-2 Effects of osmosis—isotonic, hypotonic, and hypertonic solutions. (From Herlihy B: *The human body in health and illness,* ed 4, St. Louis, 2011, Saunders.)

the potential to cause coagulation problems and anaphylactic reactions, and the interference with blood-typing and cross-matching procedures. Although colloids improve the circulating volume, after 24 hours they redistribute into the third space and can exacerbate edema.[5]

Perioperative Replacement for Crystalloid and Colloid Administration

An IV line is usually started before surgery, and maintenance fluids are started to replace the insensible loss from the last intake of oral fluids. Hourly maintenance is generally calculated as the patient's weight in kilograms plus 40 (e.g., 75 kg + 40 = 110 mL/h). During surgery, the insensible loss rate of 2 mL/kg is replaced, along with the maintenance rate. For minimal trauma, 4 mL/kg/h is added. For moderate trauma, 6 mL/kg/h is added, and for severe trauma, 8 to 10 mL/kg/h is added. A colloid solution is often added if the blood loss is greater than 20% of the patient's total blood volume. Total blood volume of an adult male is equal to approximately 5000 mL. PACU monitoring to ensure appropriate fluid support should include vital signs and urine output.

BLOOD COMPONENT THERAPY

Blood is a viscous fluid medium that contains white blood cells (leukocytes), RBCs (erythrocytes), platelets, and plasma. The RBCs are biconcave disks that contain hemoglobin, which transports oxygen and acts as a buffer to help maintain acid-base balance. The membrane of the RBC has antigens, and the plasma contains circulation antibodies. Routine blood typing of blood is performed to identify antigens on the erythrocyte membranes. The ABO and Rh classification systems are two of the common blood group systems. ABO and Rh blood typing is extremely important for preventing incompatibility between donor and recipient. A person with blood type AB+ is termed a *universal recipient* because AB blood has no A or B antibodies in the plasma. Antibodies (Anti-A, Anti-B) are formed whenever membranes lack A or B antigens. These antibodies are capable of causing rapid intravascular destruction of erythrocytes that contain the corresponding antigens. An individual with type O− is termed a *universal donor* because no A or B antigens are present on the RBCs.

During the screening process for compatibility, the ABO and Rh blood typing normally is performed. Next, an antibody screen is performed to detect the presence of the various antibodies in the recipient's and the donor's blood. Only the most common immunogenic allele, the D antigen, is usually addressed. Between 80% and 85% of Caucasians have the D antigen. Individuals lacking this antigen are called Rh negative and usually develop antibodies against the D antigen after exposure to a previous Rh-positive transfusion or pregnancy with an Rh-positive fetus. The last test is the cross match, in which a trial transfusion is simulated.

Donated blood can be stored as whole blood or centrifuged and separated into packed RBCs, leukocytes, platelets, and plasma. Whole blood less than 24 hours old is considered fresh whole blood. Whole blood is used primarily in hemorrhagic shock (massive blood loss > 25% EBV) and contains all blood factors. Platelet activity is less than 5% after 24 hours, and there is reduced content of factors V and VIII. It is not economical for routine use because of blood and blood product shortages. In addition, there is an increased likelihood of allergic transfusion reaction with whole blood. A unit of blood contains 450 mL of blood and 63 mL of anticoagulant. A decrease is seen in RBC adenosine triphosphate and 2,3-diphosphoglycerate levels, which usually resolves with dilution with the patient's blood during transfusion. Blood lactate increases the longer the blood is stored, which can be problematic if multiple blood transfusions are given. Usually sodium bicarbonate is administered to offset the lactate (acid). The patient's potassium also should be monitored because the potassium can be released from the RBC. The patient's pH and PCO_2 are used for evaluation of the need for the sodium bicarbonate. Normal blood storage does not exceed 35 days. RBCs should be administered via a large-gauge needle, and a blood filter and warmer should be used. A standard blood filter removes degenerated platelets, leukocytes, and fibrin accumulation. The standard filter has pores measuring 170 to 230 μm and can be used for up to 2 to 4 units.

The use of autologous blood for transfusions is popular because it reduces the chances for disease transmission and incompatibility and saves the use of banked blood. In this case, the patient donates his or her own blood within 21 to 42 days of operation, depending on the anticoagulant used in the blood storage. The autologous patients are usually given iron supplements and erythropoietin in an effort to keep hemoglobin levels within normal limits.

Another type of autologous blood transfusion is the use of acute isovolemic hemodilution during the operative procedure. In this situation, a portion of the allowable blood loss is collected with a large-bore intravenous cannula. Usually an equal amount of crystalloid is administered to dilute and subsequently reduce the number of RBCs during the operation. Near the end of the operation, the autologous blood is reinfused to provide more RBCs and fresh platelets.

The last type of autologous blood transfusion is the use of intraoperative blood collection systems that collect the blood lost from the operation, which is then reinfused into the patient. Commercial products are available for this collection and collecting. These systems use anticoagulants and provide either washed RBCs or the entire blood products back to the patient. Because of the risk of reinfusion of bacteria or tumor cells, this procedure is not used in patients who are having surgical procedures performed on the bowel or on malignancies.

The role of the perianesthesia nurse in the administration of blood and blood products is critical to the well-being of the patient. The importance of the nurse's checking and rechecking the blood and following all hospital procedures on the appropriate administration of blood or blood products cannot be overstated.

Perioperative Fluid Therapy

Usually, for most healthy patients, blood loss is replaced with crystalloid in which for every 1 mL of blood lost, 3 mL of crystalloid is administered. If a colloid solution is chosen, the blood loss is replaced milliliter for milliliter. That is, for each milliliter of blood loss, 1 mL of colloid solution is administered. If the anemia from blood loss continues, the administration of blood therapy may need to be started.

With the serious consequences of HIV and other blood-borne diseases, the basis for the determination of when to administer blood has been revised. Formerly, if a patient had a hematocrit level of 30 or less or a hemoglobin level of less than 10 g/dL, blood was usually administered. Now, the major factor in the determination of the administration of blood is the hemoglobin. When a patient has a hemoglobin of 7 g/dL or less, blood is usually administered. The formula used in calculation of the approximate allowable loss of blood is that the allowable loss (AL) is equal to the estimated blood volume (EBV) times the preanesthesia hemoglobin ($Hb_{initial}$) minus the target hemoglobin (Hb_{target}), which is divided by the $Hb_{initial}$.

$$AL = \frac{EBV \times Hb_{initial} - Hb_{target}}{Hb_{initial}}$$

For example, for a 70-kg male patient, the estimated blood volume is 5180 mL. For adult men, the total blood volume is equal to 74 mL times the weight in kilograms. In adult women, total blood volume is 70 mL times the weight in kilograms. Our adult male in this example has a hemoglobin level before anesthesia of 13 g/dL. The determination was that the patient should not have the hemoglobin level drop to less than 7 g/dL before blood was administered, and the target hemoglobin value is 7.0 g/dL. Therefore the equation is the following:

$$AL = \frac{5180 \text{ mL} \times 13 \text{ g/dL} - 7 \text{ g/dL}}{13 \text{ g/dL}}$$

Therefore this adult male patient's acceptable blood loss is 2391 mL. The first 2391 mL of blood loss could be replaced with crystalloid or colloids. After that, blood or blood component therapy is usually instituted.[5]

TYPES OF BLOOD COMPONENT THERAPY

Red Blood Cells

RBCs can be described as units derived from a unit of whole blood that has been centrifuged with most of the plasma removed. In addition, RBC units can be diluted with saline solution, but not in normal conditions. This dilution is indicated in older adults, patients with increased oxygen demand, and patients who not have compensation with an increased cardiac output. The RBCs help to restore oxygen transport but do not facilitate blood coagulation. In addition, no medications or other blood products should be added to the RBCs before or during administration. The potential for fluid overload exists during the administration of RBCs, especially in older adults. The perianesthesia nurse should monitor the respiratory status of these patients. Respiratory dysfunction in this situation can include dyspnea and arterial hypoxemia.

Fresh Frozen Plasma

Fresh frozen plasma (FFP) is used for the treatment of bleeding or documented coagulation problems. It should not be used for volume expansion or for replacement of large deficiencies in coagulation factors. FFP is separated from whole blood usually within 8 hours of collection. It can be stored for up to 1 year. It is important to note that various plasma products are available that do not meet the preparation requirements for FFP, including plasma, liquid plasma, thawed plasma, and plasma frozen within 24 hours after phlebotomy.

Platelets

Platelet concentrate is usually suspended in 50 mL of plasma. It is indicated for thrombocytopenia primarily from massive blood transfusion and for thrombocytopathy that is usually drug induced. One unit of platelets usually increases the platelet concentration in the adult by $5000/mm^3$ to $10,000/mm^3$ and in the newborn by $75,000/mm^3$ to $100,000/mm^3$. The platelets are administered via a large-gauge needle with a filter (170 to 220 μm) that is in line.

Cryoprecipitate

Cryoprecipitate is produced with thawing fresh frozen plasma and collecting the precipitate. It can be frozen and stored for up to 1 year. Cryoprecipitate is used for the specific treatment of bleeding associated with deficiencies in fibrinogen, factor XIII, von Willebrand factor, and factor VIII. The cryoprecipitate should be administered within 6 hours after thawing through a standard blood or special component infusion set with an inline 170-μm filter.

Albumin

Albumin is used for acute volume expansion and is considered a colloid. It does not contain any cellular products and is available in 5% or 25% solutions in saline. Albumin is heat treated, which eliminates the possibility of transmitting hepatitis and other diseases.

TRANSFUSION REACTIONS

The appropriate procedures for obtaining the blood sample for type and cross match should be followed. The patient who is receiving the blood should be identified by name and hospital number. Next, the unit of blood should be checked against that patient by checking the name of the patient and hospital number as written on the unit of blood. Two PACU nurses should conduct this identification process.

During the administration of the blood or blood products, the patient should be monitored for acute hemolytic reactions. Although the symptoms of a transfusion reaction may be masked by the depressant effects of the anesthetic, usually an acute hemolytic transfusion reaction is signaled by cardiovascular instability, such as severe hypotension. If a transfusion reaction is suspected, blood should be drawn and sent to the laboratory to have the direct antiglobulin test, which indicates whether a hemolytic transfusion reaction has occurred. This

test is the first test performed by the blood bank (or transfusion medicine) when a transfusion reaction is suspected. Another excellent parameter to monitor is any unexplained bleeding at the operative site. Other signs include pain at the infusion site, anxiety, chills, headache, an increase in temperature, and decreased renal function. If the reaction is an allergic transfusion reaction, the patient has signs of urticaria, stridor, hypotension, and pruritus. A delayed type of hemolytic transfusion reaction may be seen in the PACU. The signs and symptoms include fever and malaise. Laboratory tests that reflect this condition include increased direct bilirubin, decreasing hematocrit, and increased urine urobilinogen levels.

If a hemolytic transfusion reaction is suspected, the PACU nurse should stop the transfusion immediately and attach normal saline solution to the intravenous catheter. The attending physician and the blood bank should be notified, and a specimen of blood should be drawn and sent to the blood bank along with the blood unit and administration set. A specimen of urine should be obtained to send to the laboratory for evaluation for hemoglobin content. Finally, the other units of blood for that patient should be rechecked. See Chapter 29 for further discussion of complications resulting from transfusion of blood products.

VOLUME STATUS ASSESSMENT OF THE PATIENT IN THE POSTANESTHESIA CARE UNIT

Assessment of hypovolemia in the PACU can be difficult because vasoconstriction from events such as surgical stress, intraoperative catecholamine administration, and hypothermia can sometimes compensate for the hypovolemia. Other assessment tools include poor skin perfusion, such as cool, pale, and clammy skin particularly in the feet; oliguria; hypotension; tachycardia; and tachypnea. In addition, the estimated blood loss and the type and amount of replacement fluids recorded on the anesthesia record should be evaluated for excessive blood loss. When these symptoms are seen, the PACU nurse should check the patient for excess bleeding and the IV infusion sites for infiltration. The nurse should also notify the attending physician immediately.

SUMMARY

The objective of this chapter was to provide a broad view of the complex topic of body fluids and electrolytes, and their maintenance and treatment in the perioperative setting. The major electrolytes were presented along with discussion and examples of fluid replacement and fluid loss.

Coagulation is presented in regard to the normal cascade of the various factors and the various laboratory tests that can be used for assessing coagulation from both the intrinsic and extrinsic components. Finally, one of the most important assessment parameters for the perioperative nurse in the PACU is for hypovolemia as a result of blood loss or overall fluid deficit, cardiovascular instability, and electrolyte imbalances.

REFERENCES

1. Hall J: *Guyton and Hall textbook of medical physiology*, ed 12, Philadelphia, 2011, Saunders.
2. Rose B, Post T: *Clinical physiology of acid-base and electrolyte disorders*, ed 5, New York, 2001, McGraw-Hill.
3. Stoelting R, Hillier C: *Pharmacology and physiology in anesthetic practice*, ed 4, Philadelphia, 2005, Lippincott Williams & Wilkins.
4. Brunton L, et al: *Goodman and Gilman's the pharmacological basis of therapeutics*, ed 12, New York, 2011, McGraw-Hill.
5. Nagelhout J, Plaus K: *Nurse anesthesia*, ed 4, St. Louis, 2010, Saunders.

RESOURCES

Aitkenhead A, et al: *Textbook of anaesthesia*, ed 5, Edinburgh, 2007, Churchill Livingstone.
Alspach J: *Core curriculum for critical care nursing*, ed 6, Philadelphia, 2006, Saunders.
Atlee J: *Complications in anesthesia*, ed 2, Philadelphia, 2007, Saunders.
Barrett KE, et al: *Ganong's review of medical physiology*, ed 23, New York, 2010, McGraw-Hill.
Evers A, Maze M: *Anesthetic pharmacology: physiologic principles and clinical practice*, Philadelphia, 2004, Churchill Livingstone.
Fauci AS, et al: *Harrison's principles of internal medicine*, ed 17, New York, 2008, McGraw Hill.
Fleisher LA: *Anesthesia and uncommon diseases*, ed 5, Philadelphia, 2007, Saunders.
Gallager C, Issenberg B: *Simulation in anesthesia*, Philadelphia, 2007, Saunders.
Townsend C, et al: *Sabiston textbook of surgery: the biological basis of modern surgical practice*, ed 18, Philadelphia, 2008, Saunders.
Valchanov K, et al: *Anaesthetic and perioperative complications*, Cambridge, 2011, Cambridge University Press.

The Endocrine System

Andrea Bianco, BSN, MSN, RN, and
Joseph F. Burkard, DNSc, CRNA

Arthur C. Guyton, the great professor of physiology, always began his lecture with, "The essence of physiology is regulation and control."[1] That statement is true for the endocrine system, which is regarded as one of the two physiologic regulating and control systems—the other being the nervous system. Many interrelationships exist between the endocrine and the nervous systems. Dysfunction of the endocrine system is associated with overproduction or underproduction of a single hormone or multiple hormones. This dysfunction may be the primary reason for surgery, or it may coexist in patients who need surgery on other organ systems. To ensure appropriate nursing interventions for the patient with endocrine dysfunction in the postanesthesia care unit (PACU), the perianesthesia nurse must understand the physiology and pathophysiology of the endocrine system.[2,3]

DEFINITIONS

Endocrine Gland: A group of hormone-secreting and hormone-excreting cells.
Gluconeogenesis: The conversion of amino acids into glucose.
Glycogenesis: The deposition of glycogen in the liver.
Hormone: A biochemical substance secreted by a specific endocrine gland and transported in the blood to distant points in the body for regulation of rates of physiologic processes.
Lipolysis: The mobilization of deposited fat.
Releasing Factor: A hormone of unknown chemical structure secreted by the hypothalamus.
Releasing Hormone: A hormone secreted from the hypothalamus.
Stress: A chemical or physical disturbance in the cells or tissues produced by a change either in the external environment or within the body that necessitates a response to counteract the disturbance.
Target Organ: A gland whose activities are regulated by tropic hormones.
Tropic Hormone: A hormone that regulates the blood level of a specific hormone secreted from another endocrine gland.

MEDIATORS OF THE ENDOCRINE SYSTEM: THE HORMONES

A hormone is a biochemical substance synthesized in an endocrine gland and secreted into body fluids for regulation or control of physiologic processes in other cells of the body. Biochemically, hormones are either proteins (or derivatives of proteins or amino acids) or steroids.[1-3]

Protein hormones, such as the releasing hormones, catecholamines, and parathormone, fit the fixed-receptor model of hormone action. In this model, the stimulating hormone, called the *first messenger,* combines with a specific receptor for that hormone on the surface of the target cell. This hormone-receptor combination activates the enzyme adenylate cyclase in the membrane. The portion of the adenylate cyclase that is exposed to the cytoplasm causes the immediate conversion of cytoplasmic adenosine triphosphate into cyclic adenosine monophosphate (AMP). The cyclic AMP then acts as a second messenger and initiates any number of cellular functions.[1-3]

In the mobile receptor model, a steroid hormone, because of its lipid solubility, passes through the cell membrane into the cytoplasm, where it binds with a specific receptor protein. The combined receptor protein-hormone either diffuses or is transported through the nuclear membrane and transfers the steroid hormone to a smaller protein. In the nucleus, the hormone activates specific genes to form the messenger ribonucleic acid (RNA). The messenger RNA then passes out of the nucleus into the cytoplasm, where it promotes the translation process in the ribosomes to form new proteins. Hormones that fit the fixed-receptor model produce an almost instantaneous response on the part of the target organ. In contrast, because of their action on the genes to cause protein synthesis, when the steroid hormones are secreted a characteristic delay in the initiation of hormone response varies from minutes to days.[1-3]

PHYSIOLOGY OF THE ENDOCRINE GLANDS

Pituitary Gland

The pituitary gland rests in the sella turcica of the sphenoid bone at the base of the brain. This gland is divided into anterior and posterior lobes. Because of its glandular nature, the anterior lobe is called the *adenohypophysis;* the posterior lobe is an outgrowth of a part of the nervous system, the hypothalamus, and is called the *neurohypophysis.* The pituitary gland receives its arterial blood supply from two paired systems of vessels: (1) the right and left superior hypophyseal arteries from above and (2) the right and left inferior hypophyseal arteries from below. The anterior lobe receives no arterial blood supply. Instead, its entire blood supply is derived from the hypophyseal portal veins. This rich capillary system facilitates the rapid discharge of releasing hormones that have target cells in the anterior hypophysis.[1-3]

Although the pituitary gland is called the *master gland,* it is actually regulated by other endocrine glands and by the nervous system. The secretion of the hormones of the anterior hypophysis is primarily influenced and controlled by the higher centers in the hypothalamus. Releasing hormones are secreted by the hypothalamic nuclei through the infundibular tract to the portal venous system of the pituitary gland to their respective target cells of the adenohypophysis. Consequently, the hypothalamus brings about fine regulation of the action of the anterior pituitary, and still higher nervous centers apparently further modulate the production of the releasing factors. As a result, the many influences that enter the brain and central nervous system impinge on the anterior pituitary gland either to enhance or to dampen its activity.[1-3]

Hormonal control of the pituitary involves certain feedback systems. For example, corticotropin-releasing hormone stimulates the production and release of adrenocorticotropin (ACTH). The increased concentration of ACTH causes the hypothalamus to decrease its production of corticotropin-releasing hormone, which in turn reduces ACTH production and ultimately reduces the blood level of ACTH. Therefore, when exogenous corticoids are administered chronically, ACTH secretion decreases and the adrenal cortex atrophies. However, the removal of endogenous corticoids with a bilateral adrenalectomy can result in a tumor of the pituitary gland because of the absence of the feedback depression of the corticotropin-releasing hormone.[1-3]

The posterior lobe of the pituitary gland has an abundant nerve supply. Nerve cell bodies in the posterior lobe produce two neurosecretions (antidiuretic hormone and oxytocin), which are stored as granules at the site of the nerve cell bodies. When the hypothalamus detects a need for either neurohypophyseal hormone, nerve impulses are sent to the posterior lobe and the hormone is released by granules into the neighboring capillaries. Consequently, the hormonal function of the posterior lobe is under direct nervous system regulation.[1-3]

Hormones of the Adenohypophysis
Growth Hormone, or Somatotropin

The growth hormone is unique because it stimulates no target gland but acts on all tissues of the body. Its primary functions are maintaining blood glucose levels and regulating skeletal growth. Growth hormone conserves blood glucose by increasing fat metabolism for energy. It enhances the active transport of amino acids into cells, increases the rate of protein synthesis, and promotes cell division. In addition, growth hormone enhances the formation of somatomedin, which acts directly on cartilage and bone to promote growth. The active secretion of growth hormone is regulated in the hypothalamus via growth hormone–releasing hormone. Stimuli such as hypoglycemia, exercise, and trauma cause the hypothalamus to secrete growth hormone–releasing hormone, which is transported to the anterior lobe of the pituitary gland and released into the blood. Secretion of growth hormone can be inhibited by somatostatin, also called *growth hormone–inhibiting hormone,* which is secreted by the hypothalamus and the delta cells of the pancreas.[1-3]

Hyposecretion of the growth hormone before puberty leads to dwarfism, or failure to grow. After puberty, growth hormone hypofunction can result in the condition known as Simmonds' disease. This disease is characterized by premature senility, weakness, emaciation, mental lethargy, and wrinkled dry skin. Giantism is the result of growth hormone hyperfunction before puberty. After puberty, when the epiphyses of the long bones have closed, growth hormone hyperfunction leads to acromegaly. In this disease, the face, hands, and feet become enlarged. Patients with acromegaly are prone to airway obstruction caused by protruding lower jaws and enlarged tongues. Therefore constant vigilance to the respiratory status of these patients is essential in the PACU.[1-3]

Thyroid-Stimulating Hormone, or Thyrotropin

The follicular cells of the thyroid are the target for thyroid-stimulating hormone (TSH). This hormone promotes the growth and secretory activity of the thyroid gland. Production of TSH is regulated in a reciprocal fashion by the blood levels of thyroid hormone and the formation of thyrotropin-releasing hormone in the hypothalamus.[3,4]

Adrenocorticotropin

Adrenocorticotropin promotes glucocorticoid, mineralocorticoid, and androgenic steroid production and secretion by the adrenal cortex. This hormone is released in response to stimuli such as pain, hypoglycemia, hypoxia, bacterial toxins, hyperthermia, hypothermia, and physiologic stress. More specifically, the hypothalamus monitors for these various stressors and on excitation, corticotropin-releasing hormone (CRH) is secreted, which stimulates ACTH secretion from the adenohypophysis. Levels of adrenocortical hormones in the blood regulate secretion of ACTH with a hypothalamic feedback mechanism.[3,4]

Gonadotropic Hormones

Gonadotropic hormones regulate the growth, development, and function of the ovaries and testes. The gonadotropic hormones are the follicle-stimulating hormone and the luteinizing hormone. Secretion of the gonadotropic hormones is stimulated by gonadotropin-releasing hormone; the hormones are secreted by the hypothalamus.[4]

Lactogenic Hormone, or Prolactin

Prolactin stimulates postpartum lactation. Unlike other pituitary hormones, the hypothalamic control of prolactin secretion is predominantly inhibitory.[4]

Melanocyte-Stimulating Hormone

Melanocyte-stimulating hormone exerts its effect on the melanin granules in pigmented skin.

Hormones of the Neurohypophysis
Antidiuretic Hormone, or Vasopressin

During normal activities of daily living, antidiuretic hormone (ADH) is secreted in small amounts into the blood stream for promotion of reabsorption of water by the renal tubules, which leads to a decreased excretion of water by the kidneys. When ADH is secreted in large quantities, vasoconstriction of the smooth muscles occurs and ultimately elevates the blood pressure. The pressor effects of ADH are produced only with large doses that are not in the usual physiologic range. The secretion of ADH is regulated by several feedback loops, one of which involves plasma osmolality. Within the hypothalamus are osmoreceptors, whose function is secretion of ADH when plasma osmolarity is increased. Alternatively, dilution of plasma inhibits ADH secretion. The second feedback loop or major stimulus of ADH secretion is the volume or stretch receptors located in the left atrium. These receptors are activated when the extracellular fluid volume is increased; with this activation, ADH secretion is inhibited. The baroreceptors, which are located in the carotid sinus and aortic arch, are the receptors for the third feedback loop. A decrease in the arterial blood pressure stimulates the baroreceptors, which in turn stimulate a release of ADH. Both the stretch receptors and the baroreceptors transmit neuronal input to the brain via the vagus nerve.[4,5]

Lack of ADH leads to diabetes insipidus. This condition is characterized by the output of a large volume of dilute sugar-free urine.

Oxytocin

Oxytocin produces contraction of uterine muscle at the end of gestation and has a role in milk excretion—that is, in stimulation of the contraction of the surrounding myoepithelial cells of the mammary glands.[4,5]

Pituitary Dysfunction

Hyperfunction rarely involves more than one endocrine gland. Alternatively, hypofunction usually involves more than one endocrine gland, although instances of isolated deficiencies have been reported. A common cause of pituitary hypofunction is compression of glandular cells by the expansion of a functional or nonfunctional tumor. In this situation, an excess of one hormone may coexist with a deficiency of another.[4,5]

Pineal Gland

The pineal gland is situated in the diencephalon just above the roof of the midbrain. This gland is considered an intricate and highly sensitive biologic clock because the secretory activity of the pineal gland is greatest at night. The pineal gland secretes melatonin, which affects the size and secretory activity of the ovaries and other organs. The production and release of melatonin are regulated by the sympathetic nervous system. In fact, the pineal gland is considered a neuroendocrine transducer because it converts nervous system input into a hormonal output.[4,5]

Thyroid Gland

The thyroid gland is located in the anterior middle portion of the neck immediately below the larynx. The gland consists of two lobes that are attached by a strip of tissue called the *isthmus*. Structurally, this gland is composed of tiny sacs called *follicles*. Each follicle is formed by a single layer of epithelial cells that surround a cavity that contains a secretory product known as *colloid*. This colloid fluid consists mainly of a glycoprotein-iodine complex called *thyroglobulin*.[4,5]

On stimulation with TSH, thyroid hormones are produced in the following steps: (1) iodide trapping; (2) oxidation and iodination; (3) storage of the hormones in the colloid as part of the thyroglobulin molecules; and (4) proteolysis, which can be inhibited by iodide, and release of the hormones. The two hormones released from the thyroid gland are triiodothyronine (T_3) and thyroxine (T_4). T_4 represents more than 95% of the circulating thyroid hormone and is considered to be relatively inactive physiologically in comparison with T_3. Consequently, although T_3 has a relatively low concentration, it passes out of the blood stream faster than T_4, has a more rapid action and is probably the major biologically active thyroid hormone. After these hormones are secreted by the thyroid gland, they are transported to all parts of the body by means of plasma proteins, in the form of protein-bound iodinated compounds. As a result, the laboratory test for protein-bound iodine is useful for determining of the amount of circulating thyroid hormone in the blood.[4,5]

T_3 and T_4 regulate the metabolic activities of the body. More specifically, they regulate the rate of cellular oxidation. In addition, they are essential for the normal growth and development of the body. Other metabolic activities that are influenced by T_3 and T_4 are the promotion of protein synthesis and breakdown, increase of glucose absorption and utilization, facilitation of gluconeogenesis, and maintenance of fluid and electrolyte balance. The thyroid hormones are also involved in a feedback mechanism. The concentration of T_3 and T_4 in the blood regulates the secretion of TSH by the anterior pituitary gland. TSH regulates the growth and secretory activity of the thyroid gland.[4,5]

The thyroid gland also secretes thyrocalcitonin, or calcitonin, for maintenance of the proper level of calcium in the blood. More specifically, calcitonin decreases the serum concentration of calcium by counteracting the effects of parathormone and inhibiting the resorption of calcium from the bones.[4,5]

Parathyroid Glands

The parathyroid glands are located on the posterior portion of the thyroid gland. In most instances, one parathyroid gland is present on each of the four poles of the thyroid gland. The parathyroid glands release a polypeptide hormone called *parathormone*. This hormone is the principal regulator of the calcium concentration in the body. Parathormone is released into the circulation by a negative feedback mechanism that depends on the serum concentration of calcium. As a result, a high serum concentration of calcium suppresses the synthesis and release of parathormone and a low serum calcium concentration stimulates the release of the hormone. Normal serum calcium concentrations depend on the regulatory mechanisms, which include parathormone, calcitonin, phosphorus, magnesium, and vitamin D. In fact, the serum calcium concentration is maintained by these regulatory mechanisms within narrow and constant limits. The normal serum calcium level is 9 to 10.3 mg/dL for men and 8.9 to 10.2 mg/dL for women. Serum levels of calcium expressed in milliequivalents per liter are half the value given in milligrams per deciliter.[4,5]

Parathormone influences the rate at which calcium is transported across membranes in the bone, the gastrointestinal tract, and the kidneys. More specifically, calcium release from bone is facilitated by parathormone-induced stimulation of osteoclastic activity. The absorption of calcium by the gastrointestinal tract is enhanced by the parathormone-induced synthesis of vitamin D. Parathormone activates the synthesis of vitamin D and leads to increased tubular reabsorption of calcium and enhanced renal tubular clearance of phosphorus, which results in more calcium entering the circulation.[4,5]

Adrenal Glands

The adrenal glands are located on the apex of each kidney. Each gland consists of an outer portion called the *cortex* and an inner portion called the *medulla*. The medulla is responsible for the secretion of catecholamines (see Chapter 11). The preganglionic fibers of the sympathetic nervous system provide the stimulation that facilitates the liberation of the catecholamines by the medullary cells. The cortex composes the bulk of the adrenal gland and is responsible for the secretion of the steroids. The cortex is divided anatomically and physiologically into three zones: the zona glomerulosa, the zona fasciculata, and the inner zona reticularis. These zones are the sites of secretion of the three major steroid hormones: the mineralocorticoids, the glucocorticoids, and the androgens.[1-5]

The mineralocorticoids are responsible for the maintenance of fluid and electrolyte balance. Aldosterone is, physiologically, the most important mineralocorticoid. The basic action of aldosterone is promotion of the reabsorption of sodium with stimulation of cellular sodium pumps in the target tissue. Overall, aldosterone causes increased tubular reabsorption of sodium and excretion of potassium, which decreases urinary excretion of sodium and chloride and increases urinary secretion of potassium, consequently expanding the extracellular fluid compartment. Aldosterone secretion is increased by ACTH, a depletion in sodium, and an increase in potassium. The secretion of aldosterone is also regulated by the renin-angiotensin system. When the blood supply to the kidneys is low, the juxtaglomerular cells are stimulated to release renin. Renin, which is an enzyme, enters the blood and converts the plasma protein angiotensinogen to angiotensin I. In the lungs and elsewhere, angiotensin I is converted enzymatically to the physiologically active form, angiotensin II. One of the basic actions of angiotensin II is stimulation of the adrenal cortex for secretion of aldosterone. Thus, aldosterone secretion is regulated by the blood pressure and volume; and because it causes retention of sodium and a rise in blood pressure, aldosterone also acts as a feedback mechanism to shut off the further release of renin.[1,4-6]

The glucocorticoids are secreted in the zona fasciculata. Cortisol (hydrocortisone) constitutes approximately 95% of the total glucocorticoid activity, with corticosterone and cortisone constituting the remaining 5%. These hormones function to preserve the carbohydrate reserves of the body with promotion of gluconeogenesis, glycogenesis, lipolysis, and oxidation of fat in the liver. Because they conserve carbohydrates, these hormones serve as functional antagonists to insulin. Finally, these hormones possess an excellent antiinflammatory action. The major regulator of their secretion is ACTH, which is secreted by cells in the anterior pituitary gland.[1,4-6] ACTH is, in turn, modulated by CRH, which is secreted by the hypothalamus. Cortisol serves as a negative feedback mechanism for inhibition of both ACTH and CRH production. Physical and mental stresses stimulate the release of CRH from the hypothalamus. In addition to the catecholamines, cortisol and ACTH are considered to be the major stress hormones.[1,4-7] The androgens, or sex hormones, are actively involved in the preadolescent growth spurt and the appearance of axillary and pubic hair.

Pancreas

Islet of Langerhans cells are scattered throughout the pancreas. The three islet cell types—alpha, beta, and delta—secrete glucagon, insulin, and somatostatin, respectively. Glucagon has several functions that are diametrically opposed to those of insulin. Glucagon is commonly referred to as the *hyperglycemic factor,* and its most important function is to increase the blood glucose level. This increased glucose level in the blood is the result of the effects of glucagon on glucose metabolism—that is, glycogenolysis (in the liver) and increased gluconeogenesis. When the blood glucose concentration decreases to less than 70 mg/dL, the alpha cells secrete glucagon to protect against hypoglycemia. In addition, amino acids enhance the secretion of glucagon. In this instance, the glucagon helps to prevent the hypoglycemia that can result because amino acids stimulate insulin release, which tends to reduce the blood glucose concentration. The secretion of glucagon appears to be inhibited by the release of somatostatin from the delta cells of the pancreas, and because it is a polypeptide, glucagon is rapidly destroyed by proteolytic enzymes.[1,4-7]

Insulin is a protein secreted by the beta cells of the islets of Langerhans in response to elevated levels of blood glucose. Its secretion is inhibited by low blood glucose levels and somatostatin. In addition, insulin secretion can be inhibited by epinephrine, glucocorticoids, and thyroxine. When insulin is secreted by the beta cells, a metabolic state that favors the storage of nutrients is set into action. These physiologic actions include: (1) retention of glucose by the liver; (2) slowing of hepatic glucose release; (3) increase in uptake of glucose by muscle (stored as glycogen) and adipose tissue (stored as triglycerides); (4) translocation of amino acids and neutral fats into muscle and adipose tissue; and (5) retardation of lipolysis and proteolysis. As a result, insulin seems to "open the door" of most of the cell membranes of the body to facilitate the movement of glucose, amino acids, and fatty acids into the cells. Diabetes mellitus, which is a disease that involves the synthesis, storage, and release of insulin, is discussed in detail in Chapter 48.[1,4-7]

Gonads

The hormone testosterone is produced in the interstitial cells of the testes. The synthesis and secretion of this hormone are regulated by luteinizing hormone, which is secreted by the anterior pituitary gland. Testosterone regulates the development and maintenance of the male secondary sexual characteristics and produces some metabolic effects on bone and skeletal muscle. Another action of this hormone is the modulation of male behavior with limbic system stimulation. Estrogen, another gonadal hormone, is secreted by the ovarian follicles in response to the follicle-stimulating hormone and the luteinizing hormone of the anterior pituitary gland and is responsible for the development and maintenance of the secondary sexual characteristics in the female. Estrogen, along with progesterone, which is produced by the cells of the corpus luteum, plays an important role in the menstrual cycle.[1,4-7]

SELECTED SYNDROMES AND DISEASES ASSOCIATED WITH THE ENDOCRINE SYSTEM

Hypoadrenocorticism

A reduction in function of the hormones associated with the pituitary-adrenal axis can develop as a result of: (1) the destruction of the adrenal cortex by degenerative disease, neoplastic growth, or hemorrhage; (2) a deficiency of ACTH; or (3) prolonged administration of corticosteroid drugs. Primary adrenal insufficiency (Addison disease) results from destruction of the adrenal cortex. Although it was previously believed that Addison disease is mainly caused by idiopathic atrophy resulting in an autoimmune dysfunction, new studies suggest that specific targeting of T and B lymphocytes towards steroidogenic organs could also be a likely cause of this disease. Other causes of Addison disease include tuberculosis, histoplasmosis, bilateral hemorrhage from anticoagulation therapy, surgical removal of the adrenal glands, tumor chemotherapy, metastasis to the adrenal glands, and sepsis.[7-14]

A deficiency of ACTH is associated with panhypopituitarism. Patients who have been administered frequent "bursts" of exogenous steroid preparations such as prednisone can have a suppression of output of endogenous corticosteroids because of augmentation of the feedback mechanism to the anterior pituitary gland. Concern about the development of hypoadrenocorticism should be shown in the case of any patient who has received 20 mg of prednisone per day for more than 2 weeks in the preceding 12 months (although author opinions vary on dosage and length of time). The recovery of the normal function of the pituitary-adrenal axis may be as long as 12 months after the discontinuation of steroid therapy. Patients who are even remotely suspected to have hypoadrenocorticism are usually administered steroids before, during, and after surgery.[7-14]

This perioperative steroid coverage is needed because infection, injury, operation, or other stressors activate the pituitary-adrenal axis. If this axis is suppressed (i.e., hypoadrenocorticism), acute adrenal insufficiency (i.e., addisonian crisis) can develop, which is a life-threatening situation that requires prompt action by the PACU nurse. Clinical manifestations of the addisonian crisis include dehydration, nausea, vomiting, muscular weakness, and hypotension, followed by fever, marked flaccidity of the extremities, hyponatremia, hyperkalemia, azotemia, and shock. Therefore the PACU nurse should monitor patients who are even remotely likely to have the addisonian crisis develop. If some of the signs and symptoms appear, the attending physician should be notified immediately. The severely ill patient must be treated while the diagnosis is being confirmed. Dexamethasone 2 to 4 mg is usually administered intravenously along with IV therapy of 5% dextrose in normal saline solution. Dexamethasone is the drug of choice because it does not interfere with the diagnostic tests and yet does provide the needed glucocorticoid. If dexamethasone is not available, administration of a single 100-mg intravenous dose of hydrocortisone is advantageous to obtain both the glucocorticoid and the mineralocorticoid activity. This dose can be followed by 50 to 100 mg of hydrocortisone administered parenterally every 6 hours. During the administration of the treatment, the PACU nurse should continuously monitor the patient's cardiorespiratory status.[7-14]

Syndrome of Inappropriate Antidiuretic Hormone Hypersecretion

The syndrome of inappropriate antidiuretic hormone hypersecretion (SIADH) occurs in the event of continued secretion of ADH in the presence of serum hypoosmolality. More specifically, the feedback loops that regulate ADH secretion and inhibition fail. Usually, both dilution and expansion of the blood volume serve to stimulate a suppression of the release of ADH. However, in SIADH, the feedback loops do not respond appropriately to the osmolar or volume change, and a pathologic positive feedback loop continues, thus resulting in continued production of ADH.[7-14]

When hemorrhage and trauma occur during a surgical procedure, ADH secretion is appropriately elevated. In this situation, SIADH can be induced as a result of overzealous fluid administration. Because of the urinary sodium loss that occurs along with the water retention, the syndrome of acute water intoxication may be seen in the PACU. The symptoms of water intoxication derive from increased brain water, inoperative sodium pump, and hyponatremia. The symptoms begin with headache, muscular weakness, anorexia, nausea, and vomiting and lead to confusion, hostility, disorientation, uncooperativeness, drowsiness, and terminal convulsions or coma. These symptoms usually do not occur if the serum sodium level is higher than 120 mEq/L. Therefore, in patients who have had major vascular surgery, trauma, or hemorrhage, the perianesthesia nurse should assess frequently for the symptoms of SIADH and notify the attending physician if the symptoms become evident. The focus of treatment for SIADH is fluid restriction, diuresis with mannitol or furosemide, and administration of sodium chloride. In addition, the perianesthesia nurse should frequently assess the neurologic signs and cardiorespiratory status of the patient with SIADH and measure and record accurately the intake and output of all fluids.[7-14]

SUMMARY

The hormones secreted by the endocrine system along with the nervous system provide regulation and control of the body. Dysfunction of the production of any one of the hormones can have disastrous effects on the body. Surgery is performed on many of the glands or organs where the secreting endocrine gland is located. Of particular significance to the perianesthesia nurse are the parathyroid glands. One of the adverse outcomes of thyroid surgery is the accidental removal of one or more of the parathyroid glands. This complication is one of many that perianesthesia nurses need to assess when the site of surgery is located near an endocrine gland. The hormone insulin was briefly described, with a more detailed discussion of insulin and diabetes in Chapter 48.[15-18]

REFERENCES

1. Hall J: *Guyton and Hall textbook of medical physiology*, ed 12, Philadelphia, 2011, Saunders.
2. Melmed M, et al: *Williams textbook of endocrinology*, ed 12, Philadelphia, 2011, Saunders.
3. Drake R, et al: *Gray's anatomy for students*, ed 2, Philadelphia, 2009, Churchill Livingstone.
4. Barrett KE, et al: *Ganong's review of medical physiology*, ed 23, New York, 2009, McGraw-Hill Medical.
5. Coursin DB, et al: Endocrine complications in intensive care unit patients, *Semin Anesth Perioperative Med Pain* 21(1):59–74, 2002.
6. Degroot LJ, Jameson L: *Endocrinology*, ed 5, Philadelphia, 2006, Saunders.
7. Aitkenhead A, et al: *Textbook of anaesthesia*, ed 5, Philadelphia, 2007, Churchill Livingstone.
8. Mazzaferri E: *Year book of endocrinology*, St. Louis, 2007, Mosby.
9. Atlee J: *Complications in anesthesia*, ed 2, Philadelphia, 2007, Saunders.
10. Benumof J, Saidman L: *Anesthesia and perioperative complications*, ed 2, St. Louis, 1999, Mosby.
11. Fleisher LA: *Anesthesia and uncommon diseases*, ed 5, Philadelphia, 2007, Saunders.
12. Longnecker D, et al: *Principles and practice of anesthesiology*, ed 2, St. Louis, 1998, Mosby.
13. Miller R, et al: *Miller's anesthesia*, ed 7, Philadelphia, 2009, Churchill Livingstone.
14. Nagelhout J, Plaus K: *Nurse anesthesia*, ed 4, St. Louis, 2010, Saunders.
15. Stoelting R, Miller R: *Basics of anesthesia*, ed 6, Philadelphia, 2011, Churchill Livingstone.
16. Shorten G, et al: *Postoperative pain management: an evidence-based guide to practice*, Philadelphia, 2006, Saunders.
17. Noble K: Thyroid storm, *J Perianesth Nurs* 21(2):119–425, 2006.
18. Townsend CM, et al: *Sabiston textbook of surgery: the biological basis of modern surgical practice*, ed 19, Philadelphia, 2012, Saunders.

PHYSIOLOGIC CONSIDERATIONS IN THE PACU

16 The Hepatobiliary and Gastrointestinal System

Corey R. Peterson, DNP, CRNA

Because a great number of surgical procedures involve the gastrointestinal tract and anesthetic drugs sometimes have a profound influence on this organ system, the perianesthesia nurse in the postanesthesia care unit (PACU) must understand the general functions of the organs of this system. This chapter discusses the overall function of each organ and some of the possible postoperative complications that may involve the gastrointestinal tract. Of specific interest to the perianesthesia nurse is the section on postoperative nausea and vomiting (PONV), which is one of the most common and distressing anesthesia related complications.

DEFINITIONS

Biliary: Pertaining to the gallbladder and bile ducts.
Cholelithiasis: The presence of a common bile duct stone. Also called *chronic cholangitis*.
Diarrhea: Rapid movement of fecal matter through the large intestine.
Enteric System: The gastrointestinal tract.
Gastritis: Inflammation of the gastric mucosa.
Nausea: Conscious recognition of subconscious excitation in an area of the medulla closely related to the vomiting center.
Pancreatitis: Inflammation of the pancreas.
Peptic Ulcer: An excoriated area of the mucosa caused by the digestive action of gastric acid; frequently located in the first few centimeters of the duodenum.
Vomiting: A method for the gastrointestinal tract to rid itself of its contents when almost any part of the upper gastrointestinal tract becomes over irritated, distended, or excitable. The physical act of vomiting results when the muscles of the diaphragm and abdomen contract so that the gastric contents can be expelled.

THE ESOPHAGUS

The esophagus is a pliable muscular tube that extends from the pharynx to the stomach (Fig. 16-1). It is located behind the trachea and in front of the thoracic aorta and traverses the diaphragm to enter the esophagogastric junction, sometimes called the *cardia*. Approximately 5 cm above the junction with the stomach is the lower esophageal sphincter (LES), a circular band of smooth muscle tissue, which functions to prevent the reflux of stomach contents into the esophagus. The normal resting pressure of the LES is approximately 30 torr. This pressure is maintained by stimulation provided by innervation from the vagus nerve. Ordinarily the sphincter remains constricted except during the act of swallowing. Anticholinergic drugs, such as atropine or glycopyrrolate, and pregnancy decrease the resting pressure of the lower esophagus. Drugs that increase the lower esophageal pressure include metoclopramide (Reglan) and antacids. The main function of the esophagus is to conduct ingested material to the stomach.[1,2]

Disorders of the Esophagus

Gastroesophageal reflux disease (GERD) occurs when stomach acid is chronically forced past the LES into the distal portion of the esophagus. Symptoms usually consist of chronic heartburn and substernal pain. Stomach acid refluxes into the esophagus when the pressure in the stomach exceeds the barrier pressure exerted by the LES. This reflux typically occurs because of a weakened LES or an increase in gastric pressure caused by such factors as pregnancy, obesity, or supine positioning. Aside from the distress caused by chronic heartburn, GERD can cause the formation of precancerous cells in the distal esophagus (Barrett's esophagus). In addition, the presence of GERD indicates that the patient has an increased risk of refluxing stomach contents into his or her esophagus and aspirating it in the PACU.

A hiatal hernia occurs when a portion of the upper stomach protrudes or herniates through the diaphragm. Ultimately this causes a stricture or narrowing to form where the diaphragm surrounds the stomach and causes a weakening of the LES. Symptoms of a hiatal hernia include chronic heartburn, pain, and vomiting. Patients with a hiatal hernia need constant observation for active and passive vomiting during the emergent phase of anesthesia. Monitoring patient with a hiatal hernia is especially important if the surgery

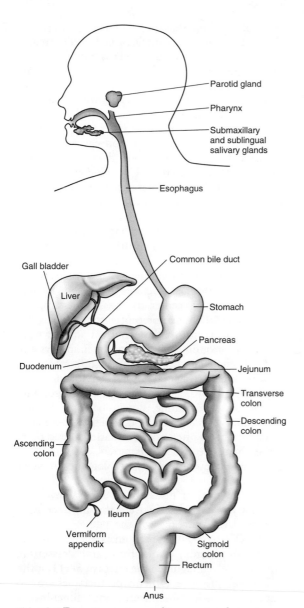

FIG. 16-1 Digestive system and its associated structures.

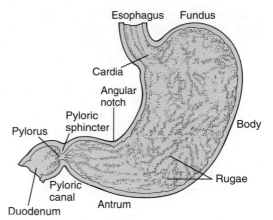

FIG. 16-2 Anatomy of the stomach. (From Hall JE: *Guyton and Hall textbook of medical physiology,* ed 12, Philadelphia, 2010, Saunders.)

extremely acidic. The total gastric secretion on a 24-hour basis is approximately 2 L. This volume normally has a pH of 1 to 3.5. Histamine has a major role in hydrochloric acid production by the parietal cells in the stomach, which is an effect mediated by histamine$_2$ receptors, vagal stimulation, and the hormone gastrin. Activation on any one of these receptors potentiates the response of the other to stimulation. Blockade of the activated receptor produces a reduction in acid response because the potentiating effect of the stimulation is reduced. The third portion of the stomach is the pyloric portion, where a thick viscous mucus and the hormone gastrin are secreted. At the end of the antrum is the pylorus, an opening surrounded by a strong band of sphincter muscle that controls the amount of gastric contents that enter the duodenum.

The vagus nerve (the main nerve for the outflow of the parasympathetic nervous system) provides the nerve supply to the stomach. Stimulation of the vagus causes increased motility of the stomach and the secretion of stomach acid, pepsin, and gastrin. As a result, a vagotomy is sometimes performed during gastric surgery to decrease gastric motility and acid production. This procedure used to be a common surgical treatment for peptic ulcer disease, but is rarely performed now because of great improvements in the medical management of this disorder.

Nervous and hormonal stimulation have profound effects on gastric volume and pH. More specifically, stimulation of the parasympathetic nervous system causes increased gastric secretion, and stimulation of the sympathetic nervous system causes decreased gastric secretion. Consequently, pain and fear, which activate the sympathetic

was performed on an emergency basis when the patient had a full stomach.[3]

THE STOMACH

The stomach can be anatomically divided into the following three sections: the fundus, the body, and the pyloric portion (Fig. 16-2). The fundus is the dome of the stomach, where peptic juice is secreted. The body is the middle portion of the stomach and is lined with parietal cells that secrete hydrochloric acid. The pH of the solution as secreted is approximately 0.8, which is

nervous system, decrease gastric emptying. In addition, the administration of opioids and active labor prolong gastric emptying. Food, depending on the type and amount, passes through the stomach at a variable rate. For example, foods rich in carbohydrates pass through the stomach in a few hours, whereas proteins exit more slowly. The emptying time for fats is the slowest. Fluids, however, pass through the stomach rather rapidly. In fact, 90% of 750 mL of ingested saline solution exits the stomach within 30 minutes. In addition, 150 mL of fluids taken 1 or 2 hours before induction of anesthesia stimulates peristalsis and facilitates gastric emptying. Consequently, the small sips of water taken with the preoperative oral medications may in fact contribute to lower intraoperative and postoperative gastric volumes. It must be emphasized that fasting, regardless of the duration, does not guarantee that the stomach is completely empty of fluids or food.[4,5]

Effect of Pregnancy on Gastric Motility and Secretions

During pregnancy, many alterations occur as a result of the enlarged uterus and altered hormonal state. Because of the enlarged uterus, the stomach and intestine are moved cephalad and the axis of the stomach is shifted to a more horizontal position. The gastric emptying time is increased in women who are at least 34 weeks pregnant. In regard to the gastric volume and pH, no difference between pregnant and nonpregnant states seems to exist. Consequently, pregnant patients who have had nothing by mouth (NPO) for elective surgery do not have any additional risk of aspiration pneumonitis than do nonpregnant patients. However, research findings suggest that pregnant patients who have heartburn may be at greater risk for regurgitation and subsequent development of aspiration pneumonitis. In addition, if intramuscular opioids are given during labor, gastric emptying time is substantially delayed. Epidural anesthesia with local anesthetics does not seem to affect gastric volume or pH; however, if opioids are introduced into the epidural space, a delay in gastric emptying occurs.[6,7]

Postoperative Nausea and Vomiting

Postoperative nausea and vomiting (PONV) continues to be ongoing concern to anesthesia providers and patients, alike. Occurring in as many as one third of all surgical patients and in 80% of high-risk patients PONV is the most commonly occurring postoperative complication. Research shows that surgical patients classify nausea and vomiting as the most undesirable postsurgical complication and identify it as being more undesirable than postoperative pain. In addition to patient dissatisfaction, PONV creates significant health care concerns and increases institutional and individual costs of surgical procedures. Vomiting is associated with wound dehiscence, aspiration, increased intracranial pressure, and increased cardiovascular demand, placing compromised patients at risk for a myocardial infarction. PONV is a common cause of unanticipated hospital admissions, delayed discharge from the PACU, increased demand on provider staffing, and increased material costs. The resulting increased morbidity and mortality, decreased patient satisfaction, and increased health care costs make the prevention and management of PONV a significant priority for health care providers in the surgical setting.

Nausea and vomiting involves a complex interplay between various structures in the body including the vomiting center in the brain stem, the closely associated chemoreceptor trigger zone, the vestibular labyrinth in the ear, vagal afferent neurons in the gastrointestinal tract, the limbic system, and the cerebral cortex. Each of these sites contributes to the triggering of vomiting by releasing single or multiple neurotransmitters, including serotonin, acetylcholine, histamine, dopamine, opioids, and neurokinins. Adding to the complexity, these anatomic structures often possess a variety of receptors for each of the neurotransmitters, each receptor producing its own specific physiologic result when stimulated.

A great deal of research on PONV over the past few years has yielded drugs that have certainly improved the outcomes of the patient in regard to PONV. The 5-HT3 antagonists, such as ondansetron, tropisetron, granisetron, and dolasetron, competitively antagonize the effect of 5-HT at the 5-HT_3 receptor site. Other drug therapies are the antihistamines (promethazine and dimenhydrinate), anticholinergics (scopolamine), neuroleptics (droperidol and triflupromazine), and glucocorticoids, such as dexamethasone. The pathophysiology and pharmacology of PONV is discussed at length in Chapter 29.

With recent research and the advent of new pharmacologic agents, the ability to prevent and efficaciously treat PONV has greatly improved, even for those patients at highest risk for these complications. Under the auspices of the American Society of PeriAnesthesia Nurses, a multidisciplinary panel met to review current literature regarding the prevention and treatment of PONV and formulate a multimodal, multidisciplinary, evidenced-based set of guidelines to guide the practice of those taking care of surgical patients.[8] Chief among these recommendations are that each patient should be assessed for the four evidenced-based risk factors for PONV (female gender, nonsmoker, a history of PONV or motion sickness, and administration of postoperative opioids); pharmacologic interventions should be based on the assessed risk for PONV; multimodal interventions, often consisting of more than one pharmacologic intervention targeting different drug receptors are superior to a single intervention; and rescue therapy should consist of administration of a different class of drug targeted at a different set of receptors than the ones given prophylactically.[8]

The basics of care for vomiting in the PACU setting indicate that the patient should be placed in a head-down position and given oxygen immediately. The purpose of the head-down position is to allow fluid to flow away from the lungs rather than into the lungs. Consequently, the patient should be placed in this position if aspiration is suspected. Fluid should be suctioned rapidly while administration of oxygen continues. If the patient's airway is obstructed by large particles, fingers or forceps should be used to clear the debris and then oxygen should be administered. The physician or anesthesia provider should be notified immediately. Further treatment may include intubation and mechanical ventilation. Steroids and antibiotics may also be administered.

A patient in recovery from a general anesthetic should be assessed for possible passive regurgitation, especially if the patient was not intubated during surgery. Clinical signs include dyspnea, cyanosis of varying degrees, and tachycardia. On auscultation of the lungs, abnormal sounds are usually heard. If the assessment indicates the possibility of this syndrome, oxygen should be administered and the physician notified at once.

The incidence rate for this syndrome is higher in patients who had a full stomach at induction of anesthesia, who underwent intestinal or emergency surgery, or who have a suspected hiatal hernia. The best treatment is prevention. These patients should have a complete return of consciousness before the endotracheal tube is removed. If the endotracheal tube is to be removed in the PACU, the patient should be placed in a lateral position with the head down. Oxygen should be administered, and suction should be available for immediate use before the extubation is performed.[9-12]

THE INTESTINE

The duodenum, which is a part of the small intestine, arises at the pylorus of the stomach and ends at the duodenojejunal junction. The duodenum is divided into the following four segments: superior, descending, transverse, and ascending. The common bile duct and the main pancreatic duct empty into the descending duodenum. The main functions of the stomach and the first portion of the duodenum are to alter the form of food and to supply enzymes for digestion.

The jejunum begins at the descending duodenum at the duodenojejunal angle. It constitutes the first two fifths of the small intestine, and the ileum occupies the distal three fifths of the small intestine. The mesentery, which contains blood vessels, nerves, lymphatics, lymph nodes, and fat, stabilizes the small bowel and prevents it from twisting and constricting its blood supply.

The digestive glands secrete large quantities of water to aid in the digestive process. Between 5 and 10 L of water are estimated to enter the small intestine, and approximately 500 mL leave the ileum and enter the colon. Among the important materials absorbed from the small intestine are sodium, bicarbonate, chloride, calcium, iron, carbohydrates, fats, and amino acids.

Sodium is absorbed by the small intestine at a rate of 25 to 35 g/day. This absorption accounts for approximately 16% of all the sodium in the body. When a patient has extreme diarrhea, sodium can be depleted to a lethal level within a few hours.[13,14]

THE COLON AND RECTUM

At the end of the small intestine is the ileocecal valve, which functions to prevent backflow of fecal material from the colon into the small intestine.

The colon is divided anatomically into the cecum, ascending colon, transverse colon, and descending and sigmoid colon. The functions of the colon are the absorption of water and electrolytes, which occurs principally in the proximal half of the colon, and the storage of fecal material, which occurs in the distal colon. The contents of the cecum are mainly liquid, as compared with the solid material contained in the sigmoid colon. Therefore, if a patient has undergone a colostomy, knowledge of the portion of the colon from which the stoma originates is important for determining whether the excreted fecal material has the normal amount of water content.

Of surgical importance is the appendix, which arises from the cecum at its inferior tip. The appendix represents a special type of intestinal obstruction when it becomes inflamed by hyperplasia of submucosal lymphoid follicles, fecaliths, foreign bodies, or tumors.

The rectum functions entirely as an excretory canal and has no digestive function. It begins anatomically at the distal end of the sigmoid colon and ends at the anus. It is tubular and has two layers. The innermost layer is the lumen of the intestinal tract, and the outermost layer is skeletal muscle of the pelvic floor. The muscle is innervated by the parasympathetic nervous system.[13]

THE ANUS

The anus is the termination of the alimentary canal. It is encircled by striated muscle and innervated by somatic sympathetic and parasympathetic fibers. Because of the parasympathetic innervation of the rectum and anus, parasympathetic stimulation can occur during a rectal examination or surgical procedure. This parasympathetic reflex can also occur when a patient is recovering from a general anesthetic. If a physician deems a rectal examination necessary, the perianesthesia nurse should be prepared to monitor the patient for bradycardia and laryngospasm, which can result from stimulation of the anus and rectum.

THE LIVER

The importance of the liver is generally underestimated. Its proper functioning is critical to almost every other system within the body, and its derangement can compromise normal homeostasis in multiple ways.

The liver is located in the right upper quadrant of the abdomen. It has a dual blood supply that consists of the hepatic artery and the portal vein. The hepatic artery supplies highly oxygenated blood directly from the descending aorta while the portal vein drains blood from the organs of the GI tract. This portal circulation ensures that nutrients, drugs, and other foreign substances absorbed from the GI tract are processed by the liver before they enter the general circulation. The sinusoids, which surround the hepatocytes (liver cells), empty into a venous system that eventually forms the hepatic vein and empties into the inferior vena cava. Approximately 1600 mL of blood per minute flow through the liver; this amount is approximately 30% of the cardiac output. The hepatocytes absorb nutrients from the portal venous blood; store and release proteins, lipids, and carbohydrates; excrete bile salts; synthesize plasma proteins, glucose, cholesterol, and fatty acids; and metabolize exogenous and endogenous compounds.

The liver is the most important storage organ in the body. It absorbs glucose in the form of glycogen, maintains a normal glucose concentration in the body, and stores amino acids, iron, and vitamins. The liver can store up to 400 mL of blood in the sinusoids. If a person loses an appreciable amount of blood, the liver can release stored blood into the circulation to replace what was lost.

The liver performs many vital physiologic functions that have a significant effect on the pharmacologic actions of many of the drugs used in the perioperative period. More specifically, the liver performs biotransformation of drugs with the cytochrome P-450 microsomal enzyme system. Consequently, knowledge of protein synthesis and drug biotransformation is of critical importance to the perianesthesia nurse.

Protein Synthesis

The liver is responsible for the synthesis of most of the proteins found in the plasma. Albumin is the most notable of the plasma proteins synthesized by the liver. Albumin synthesis is regulated by the state of nutrition; therefore a nutritional deficit can result in reduced albumin production. Because many drugs used in anesthesia are protein bound, a reduction in the albumin level can have a significant effect on the pharmacologic action of the drugs. Because the protein-binding sites are reduced, the unbound, pharmacologically active fraction of the drug is increased, which ultimately leads to an increased sensitivity to the drug or a prolonged action. The liver also synthesizes the enzyme pseudocholinesterase (plasma cholinesterase). This protein is the principal enzyme in the metabolism of succinylcholine and the ester-type local anesthetics. Succinylcholine, which is the principal depolarizing skeletal muscle relaxant in use, has an inverse correlation between duration of action and pseudocholinesterase levels. Therefore any patient with suspected liver dysfunction who has received succinylcholine during surgery should be closely monitored for respiratory depression in the immediate postoperative period. Finally, the liver produces a large proportion of the protein substances used in coagulation; therefore patients in liver failure are at risk for coagulopathies.

Drug Biotransformation

The enzymes needed for oxidation and conjugation in the liver are called the *microsomal enzymes*. These enzymes are part of the cytochrome P-450 microsomal system. Exposure to certain drugs, including barbiturates and some anesthetics, can lead to an increase in the amount of microsomal enzymes in the liver. This process is commonly called *enzyme induction.* Enzyme induction increases the rate of drug biotransformation. Patients with severe liver disease may have reduced microsomal activity in the liver. As a result, drugs such as thiopental, diazepam, and meperidine have a prolonged action caused by a decreased rate of drug biotransformation by the microsomal enzymes. Consequently, patients with severe hepatic disease should be closely monitored for respiratory and cardiovascular depression in the PACU phase of the anesthetic experience.[1,5]

THE GALLBLADDER

The gallbladder is a thin-walled, pear-shaped organ attached to the inferior surface of the liver (Fig. 16-3) whose function is to store bile from the liver and release it into the small intestines to aid in the digestion of fats. Anatomically, it is divided into the fundus; the distal tip; the corpus (body), the middle body portion; the infundibulum, a pouch-like structure; and the neck, which leads to the cystic duct. The cystic duct joins the common hepatic duct to form the common bile duct. The common bile duct and the main pancreatic duct of Wirsung usually join at the choledochoduodenal junction, which is a passageway through the duodenal wall. The muscle of the choledochoduodenal junction is the sphincter of Oddi, which regulates the flow of bile into the duodenum. Many common opioid analgesics can produce spasm of the sphincter of Oddi and the duodenum and can increase the pressure in the biliary tree.

Cholelithiasis is a common occurrence in patients with chronic gallbladder disease. As many as 20 million people have some form of cholelithiasis. Gallstones are composed of cholesterol, which is almost insoluble in pure water. The causes of gallstones include an excess of cholesterol in the bile, chronic inflammation of the epithelium, excessive absorption of bile acids from the bile, and excessive absorption of water from the bile. Laparoscopic cholecystectomy is one of the most common abdominal surgeries and offers a clear advancement over the open removal of the gallbladder (see Chapters 40 and 47).[15,16]

THE PANCREAS

The pancreas is situated in the upper abdomen behind the stomach. It is a slender organ that consists of a head, a body, and a tail (Fig. 16-4). Its main duct, through which pass the pancreatic enzymes, runs the entire length of the gland and opens into the duodenum along with the common bile duct. Scattered throughout the pancreas are small clusters of cells called the *islets of Langerhans.* They are responsible for the production and secretion of hormones that they empty directly into the blood stream; therefore the islets of Langerhans are considered an endocrine gland. The following three types of cells are found in the islets of Langerhans: alpha, beta, and delta. The alpha cells are associated with the production of the hormone glucagon, and the beta cells are associated with insulin. The physiologic significance of the delta cells has not been determined.

Insulin is secreted in response to an increase in the concentration of glucose. The secretion of insulin is inhibited when a low concentration of glucose exists. Glucagon is frequently called *hyperglycemic factor,* because it causes hyperglycemia by stimulating the breakdown of liver glycogen with consequent release of glucose into the circulation. It also stimulates gluconeogenesis, which is the formation of glucose from noncarbohydrate sources.

The pancreas excretes juice for digestion of all three major types of food: carbohydrates, fats, and proteins. The pancreatic juice also contains large amounts of bicarbonate ions, which help to neutralize the acidic chyme as it passes into the duodenum from the stomach.

Pancreatitis

Acute pancreatitis is a serious complication of surgery on the biliary tract. It can occur as a result of common duct exploration during gallbladder surgery. Acute postoperative pancreatitis should be suspected with excessive pain, vomiting, fever, tachycardia, persistent ileus, or jaundice. The perianesthesia nurse should be aware of these symptoms, which, if detected, should be reported to the surgeon. Treatment of this disorder may include nasogastric suction,

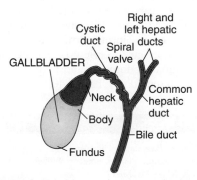

FIG. 16-3 Gallbladder and its extrahepatic ducts. (From Buck CJ: *2012 ICD-9-CM professional edition,* St. Louis, 2012, Saunders.)

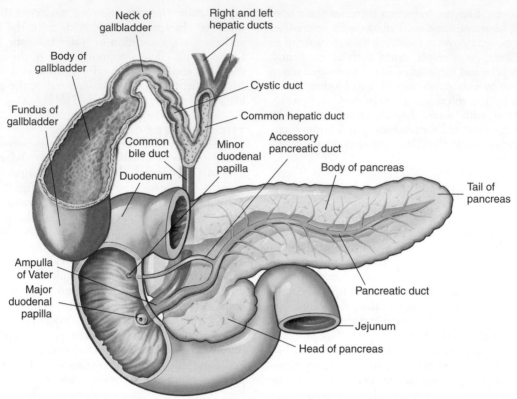

FIG. 16-4 Associated structures of the gallbladder and pancreas. (Modified from Thibodeau GA, Patton KT: *Anatomy and physiology*, ed 7, St. Louis, 2010, Mosby.)

anticholinergic drugs, antibiotics, and replacement of fluids and electrolytes.

THE SPLEEN

The spleen is an oval organ located in the upper left quadrant of the abdominal cavity. Its physiologic functions include the filtering of blood and foreign material, hematopoiesis, and the production of lymphocytes and antibodies in some instances.

The spleen is a highly vascular organ, and approximately 350 L of blood normally flows through it daily. The spleen acts as a reservoir of blood. It can store so many red blood cells that splenic contraction can cause the hematocrit of the systemic blood to increase as much as 3% to 4%.

Normal health is possible after splenectomy because other tissues can assume the functions the spleen normally performs. Splenectomy is usually performed to cure or alleviate hematologic disease or because of its traumatic rupture. Because the spleen is friable and vascular, blood loss from a splenectomy can be high; therefore the perianesthesia nurse must assess the blood loss

and the cardiovascular status of the patient during recovery (see Chapter 40).

SUMMARY

The hepatobiliary and gastrointestinal systems are certainly multidimensional, and the understanding of the anatomy and physiology of these systems is essential to the perianesthesia nurse. The pathophysiologies of selected disorders that pertain to perianesthesia care were presented. Problems such as PONV (see Chapter 29), changes during pregnancy, and drug biotransformation were introduced. A complete overview of the care of the gastrointestinal, abdominal, and anorectal surgical patient is presented in Chapter 40.

REFERENCES

1. Stoelting R: *Pharmacology and physiology in anesthetic practice*, ed 4, Philadelphia, 2006, Lippincott Williams & Wilkins.
2. Evers A, Maze M: *Anesthetic pharmacology: physiologic principles and clinical practice*, ed 2, St. Louis, 2011, Churchill Livingstone.

3. Hines RL, Marschall KE: *Stoelting's anesthesia and co-existing disease*, ed 5, Philadelphia, 2008, Elsevier.

4. Barash P, et al: *Clinical anesthesia*, ed 6, Philadelphia, 2009, Lippincott Williams & Wilkins.

5. Hall J: *Guyton and Hall textbook of medical physiology*, ed 12, Philadelphia, 2011, Saunders.

6. Miller R, et al: *Miller's anesthesia*, ed 7, Philadelphia, 2009, Churchill Livingstone.

7. Stoelting R, Miller R: *Basics of anesthesia*, ed 6, St. Louis, 2011, Churchill Livingstone.

8. American Society of PeriAnesthesia Nurses: ASPAN'S evidence-based clinical practice guideline for the prevention and/or management of PONV/PDNV, *J Perianesth Nurs* 21(4), 230-250, 2006.

9. Brunton L, et al: *Goodman and Gilman's the pharmacological basis of therapeutics*, ed 12, New York, 2010, McGraw-Hill Professional.

10. Hornby PJ: Central neurocircuitry associated with emesis, *Am J Med* 111 (Suppl 8A): 106S-112S, 2001.

11. Murphy M, et al: Identification of risk factors for postoperative nausea and vomiting in the perianesthesia adult patient, *J Perianesth Nurs* 21(6):377–384, 2006.

12. Odom-Forren J, et al: Evidence-based interventions for post discharge nausea and vomiting: a review of the literature, *J Perianesth Nurs* 21(6):411–430, 2006.

13. Drake R, et al: *Gray's anatomy for students*, ed 2, St. Louis, 2009, Churchill Livingstone.

14. Nagelhout J, Plaus K: *Nurse anesthesia*, ed 4, St. Louis, 2009, Saunders.

15. Hansen JT: *Netter's clinical anatomy*, ed 2, Philadelphia, 2010, Saunders.

16. Townsend CM, et al: *Sabiston textbook of surgery: the biological basis of modern surgical practice*, ed 19, Philadelphia, 2012, Saunders.

PHYSIOLOGIC CONSIDERATIONS IN THE PACU

The Integumentary System

Debra Pecka Malina, DNSc, MBA, CRNA

The integumentary system consists of the hair, nails, and skin and performs many functions that influence the perianesthesia nursing interventions in the postanesthesia care unit (PACU). Although the skin has many functions, the most important is to act as a barrier between the internal and external environments. In addition, skin plays an important role in body temperature and fluid regulation, excretion, secretion, vitamin D production, sensation, appearance, and many other functions. The integumentary system is the body's largest organ and first line of defense against many communicable diseases and mechanisms of injury that could cause permanent harm.

In the hospital setting, patients are at risk for many unwanted infections caused by pathogens and normal flora that are present in the environment. The intent of this chapter is to provide the reader with the anatomy and physiology of the integumentary system. It will provide background information to assist the perianesthesia nurse in understanding infection control and aseptic technique. There will be an overview of the patient with acquired thermal injury. Greater understanding of the integumentary system will facilitate the perianesthesia nurse in providing the needed vital care to the patient with a compromised first line of defense.

DEFINITIONS

Desquamation: The process by which dead cells are shed at a fairly constant rate.
Dermis: Corium, or the second layer of the skin.
Epidermis: Multilayered outer covering of the skin.
Frostbite: Trauma caused by the crystallization of tissue fluids in the skin or subcutaneous tissue.
Integumentary System: Skin and cutaneous tissue.

INTEGUMENTARY SYSTEM ANATOMY

The skin, or integument, provides a boundary between the internal and external environments of the body. With aging, the skin becomes thinner with less elasticity and diminished collagen. There is less inflammatory response and integumentary

immunity protection with aging. Skin generally accounts for about 15% of the total body weight. The skin is divided into two major layers: the epidermis and the dermis, which includes the hypodermis (Fig. 17-1). Depending on location, skin varies in number of layers and thickness. The soles of the feet and palms of the hands have the thickest skin (approximately 1.5 mm) and have five layers. Eyelids have the thinnest skin (approximately 0.10 mm) and have four layers.

Epidermis

The outermost layer of the skin is called the *stratum corneum*. It is composed of dead keratinocytes that are continually sloughing as new ones replace them. In addition to dead cells, the corneum also contains keratin, surface lipids, and dirt. The epidermis does not have any blood vessels.

Dead cells are shed at a fairly constant rate with a process called *desquamation*. The epidermis also has keratinizing and glandular appendages. Keratinizing appendages develop into hair and nails; glandular appendages include the sweat, scent, and sebaceous glands. The pigment that determines skin color (i.e., melanin) is also found in the epidermis in structures called *melanosomes*. Manufactured by melanocytes, melanosomes are transported to the keratinocytes and surround them. When skin is exposed to the sun or ultraviolet radiation, the quantity of melanosomes increases, causing a change in skin color.

The innermost layer of epidermis is the stratum basale/germinativum, which contains squamous cells, and is the site of origin for squamous cell carcinoma. Squamous cell cancer is more aggressive than basal cell carcinoma, and often invades surrounding tissues and lymph glands. It is often found on surfaces of the skin which have the most exposure to the sun.

The cells of the lowest, or basal, layer of the epidermis are constantly dividing and producing epidermal cells. Basal cell cancer develops from this layer. It tends to be slow growing, is the most common skin cancer (8 out of 10 cases are basal cell cancer), and has a high rate of recurrence. It is usually found in areas of the body with the most sun exposure.

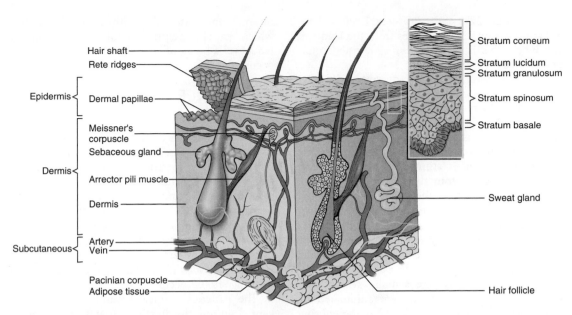

FIG. 17-1 Layers of epidermis. (From Monahan FD, et al: *Medical-surgical nursing health and illness perspectives*, ed 8, St. Louis, 2007, Mosby.)

The granular layer, or stratum granulosum, contains three or four layers of cells. It is composed of cells called *keratinocytes*, which undergo a maturation process called *keratinization*. This process produces lipid granules that form waterproof structures and helps in preventing fluid loss and evaporation through the skin into the environment.

Dermis

The dermis, or corium, lies below the epidermis and consists of collagen, elastic, and reticular fibers. It also contains blood vessels, nerves, lymphatics, and smooth muscle.

Hypodermis

The hypodermis functions as a shock absorber and heat insulator. Located under the dermis, it comprises fat, smooth muscle, and adipocytes. These cells store and accumulate necessary fats. The hypodermis acts as a site of energy production, and insulation. This area of the body stores fat in characteristic locations: hips on women, abdomen in men.[2]

INTEGUMENTARY FUNCTIONS

The skin has many important functions, the most important of which is to act as a barrier between the internal and external environments. In addition, the skin has an important role in body temperature and fluid regulation, excretion, secretion, vitamin D production, sensation, appearance, and many other functions that have yet to be determined.

Thermoregulation

Skin, subcutaneous tissue, and fat in the subcutaneous tissue provide heat insulation for the body. Heat is lost from the body to the surroundings by radiation, conduction, convection, and evaporation (Fig. 17-2). Radiation of heat from the body accounts for approximately 60% of the total heat loss. In this mechanism, heat is lost in the form of infrared heat waves. Conduction of heat to objects represents approximately 3% of the total heat loss, whereas conduction of heat to the air represents approximately 15% of the total heat loss. When water is carried away from the skin by air currents, convection of heat occurs. Evaporation constitutes

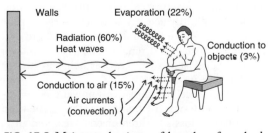

FIG. 17-2 Major mechanisms of heat loss from body. (From Hall JE: *Guyton and Hall textbook of medical physiology*, ed 12, St. Louis, 2011, Saunders.)

approximately 22% of the heat loss. Even without sweating, water still evaporates from the skin and the lungs; this is called *insensible loss* and totals approximately 600 mL/day.

The skin regulates body temperature by conserving heat in a cold environment. Sweating can lower the body temperature in hot environments. The sweat glands are innervated by the sympathetic and parasympathetic nervous systems. When the anterior hypothalamus, in the preoptic area of the brain, is stimulated by excess heat, impulses are sent from this area by way of the autonomic pathways to the spinal cord. From the spinal cord through the sympathetic outflow tracts, the impulses go to the skin all over the body. The sweat glands are innervated by sympathetic nerve fibers. However, in these specific fibers, the neurotransmitter is acetylcholine. Consequently, these fibers are actually sympathetic cholinergic nerve fibers and are stimulated by epinephrine or norepinephrine. Norepinephrine is a catecholamine that is a hormone and neurotransmitter that assists with the fight-or-flight response. It is responsible for cutaneous vasoconstriction and has been associated with the pain of fibromyalgia.[3]

The sweat gland consists of two portions: a deep subdermal coiled portion that secretes the sweat and a duct portion that conducts the sweat to the skin. Sweat has a pH of 3.8 to 6.5 and contains sodium, chloride, potassium, calcium, lactic acid, and urea; therefore sweating is an act of excretion and secretion.

Protection

The skin protects the body from injurious physical, chemical, electric, thermal, or biologic stimuli. Of particular importance to the perianesthesia nurse is the presence of bacteria on the skin that can cause infection when a patient's skin barrier is broken. Normal florae of the skin include *Staphylococcus, Streptococcus,* and *Corynebacterium* organisms. Diphtheroids are also widely distributed on the skin, especially in moist areas. The normal pH of the skin is 4 to 6.5, resulting from production of lactic acid and residues of amino acids. This slightly acid environment serves a protective mechanism by inhibiting bacterial growth. Diabetic, cardiac, and renal patients tend to have more alkaline skin surfaces, thus being at higher risk for skin infections.[4]

When intact, the skin stops unwanted organisms from entering the body and at the same time prevents the loss of water, electrolytes, and proteins to the external environment. When the skin is broken (e.g., surgical incision, ulceration, abrasion, rash, venipuncture), the barrier between the internal and external environments is broken, which is why aseptic technique is important whenever a break of the skin is anticipated or has occurred.

IMPORTANCE OF ASEPTIC TECHNIQUE

Because all skin has disease-causing organisms on its surface, skin can never be sterile. Precautions should be taken to reduce the number of pathogenic organisms that may be introduced into a wound. Good hand washing technique is the most important activity in the prevention of disease transmission. Hands should be washed using traditional hand washing techniques, or using one of the new sanitizing gels before caring for any patient. When hands are visibly soiled, traditional washing should occur.[5]

The patient's surgical wound site should be kept clean, and the dressings should remain sterile, dry, and intact. If any question arises about sterility because of excess bleeding, fluid, or physical contamination, the dressing should be changed per protocol. Special precautions to reduce the introduction of opportunistic organisms should be taken with patients who are prone to infection. This group includes patients who are obese, anemic, or debilitated; those with vascular insufficiency, chronic obstructive pulmonary disease, and diabetes mellitus; and those with an immune deficiency, including patients who are undergoing chemotherapy or chronic steroid therapy or who have acquired immunodeficiency syndrome. Aseptic technique in wound care for these patients should include isolation techniques, such as the wearing a surgical mask and using sterile gloves and drapes.

Standard Precautions in the Postanesthesia Care Unit

The Centers for Disease Control and Prevention developed a guideline for preventing transmission of infectious agents in health care settings.[6] This document is discussed in Chapter 5 with more complete information on the standard precautions in the PACU.

Sterile Technique for Intravenous Therapy

Establishment of an intravenous infusion should be accomplished via sterile technique. The site chosen for venipuncture and cannula (needle) placement should be prepared using aseptic technique according to institutional policies and guidelines. There are many good quality prepackaged IV prep kits. In general though, all IV preparation includes thorough cleaning of the site with alcohol or Betadine-based preparation solutions, the use of sterile angiocatheters, supplies, and an occlusive dressing over the cannulated site. After the intravenous administration route is established, the cannula should be securely anchored to prevent irritating back-and-forth motion and to avoid potential transport of cutaneous bacteria into the puncture wound.

Burn Injuries

A burn, no matter how small, represents a total body assault. The postoperative care of the patient with burn injury can be most challenging to the perianesthesia nurse. These patients usually have a complex array of physiologic complications, from deranged fluid and electrolyte balance to respiratory complications. These patients are also routinely suffering from psychologic problems related to pain, disfigurement, anxiety, and potential permanent lifestyle changes. With their first line of defense against external assaults disrupted, temperature regulation of the burn patient is compromised. It is difficult to maintain normothermia in these patients; the perioperative nurse must take care to prevent burn patients from experiencing hypothermia or hyperthermia. Infection is the most common complication of a burn injury. Meticulous, aseptic skin care is of primary importance. Nursing care of the patient with a burn injury is complex; the reader should refer to Chapter 55 for a discussion of specific pathophysiologic processes, assessment, and nursing interventions for the patient with a burn injury in the PACU.

The four main types of burn injuries include radiation, chemical, electrical, and thermal. A thermal injury can result from extreme cold or heat. Cold (frostbite) and burns are the causes of thermal injury. The most common type of burn injury is the thermal burn caused by excessive heat most commonly from fire, steam, and flammable or hot liquids. Metabolic disturbances and problems in maintenance of thermal control can be challenging. In hospitalized burn patients, mortality can range as high as 25%.

The terms *partial thickness, deep,* and *full thickness* are commonly used in the classification of burn injuries. The terms *first degree, second degree, third degree,* and sometimes *fourth degree* are based on the degree of destruction, depth, and surface appearance of the burn wound (Fig. 17-3). Ambroise Paré, a French surgeon from the 1500s, developed the burn classification system that is still in use today.

Caustic agents, which can be either acid or base, produce chemical burns. Without immediate,

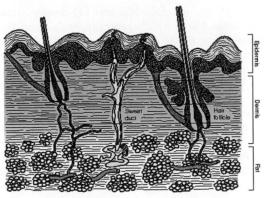

FIG. 17-3 Cross section of skin depicting levels contained in split-thickness and full-thickness skin grafts. (From Townsend T, et al: *The biological basis of modern surgical practice,* ed 18, Philadelphia, 2008, Saunders.)

aggressive treatment, these agents can continue to cause further destruction of fascia, fat, muscle, and bone. Electrical burns, which result from direct contact with electric voltage, are deceiving in appearance. Although only the entrance and exit wounds may be visible, massive damage is often sustained as the high-energy sources follow conductive muscle and nerves. This damage may involve cardiac as well as skeletal structures. Arrhythmias, often fatal, can occur. Damage may necessitate amputation of extremities. Thermal injury often occurs in addition to the electric burn from the heat of arcing currents or ignited clothing.

Superficial or first-degree burns damage only the outer layer of skin (epidermis). Partial thickness or second-degree burns injure the outer layer and the layer underneath. Full-thickness or third-degree burns cause severe injury or destruction to the deepest layer of skin, tissues, hair follicles, and sweat glands. A fourth degree burn involves bone, muscle, and often organs. Full-thickness burns are often the least painful, because nerve endings have been destroyed, causing the absence of sensation.

A partial-thickness burn heals without grafting. Grafting is required when part of the skin has been damaged or destroyed, but enough epithelial cells remain in the skin to provide new epidermis. The partial-thickness burn can also be referred to as a *first-degree* or *second-degree burn.* Partial-thickness burns can be divided into three categories: (1) superficial burns, in which partial skin loss is seen but no dermal death and therefore no slough; (2) intermediate partial-thickness burn, typically characterized by healing from the level of the hair follicles; and (3) deep partial-thickness burn, which typically heals from the level of the sweat ducts. A deep dermal burn is a partial-thickness burn that can heal without grafting. However, if the burn is complicated by infection or mechanical trauma, it is likely to be converted into a full-thickness burn. Full-thickness, or third-degree, burns cause destruction of all the skin. No viable epithelial elements are present, and destruction of the subcutaneous tissue, muscles, and bones may be seen. The wound must be grafted because the skin will not regenerate.[7]

The effects of burns ranges from redness and a burning sensation to edema, blisters, excruciating pain, debilitating and devastating scarring, shock, and death. Burn patients often require frequent, numerous surgeries to remove dead tissue (debridement), release scarring, and apply split thickness skin grafts or one of the many other applications now available: artificial skin, cultured skin autografts, or collagen-based allograft membranes.[8] As a result, the perianesthesia nurse may see these patients repeatedly in the preoperative and PACU areas.

SUMMARY

It is important for the perianesthesia nurse to have an understanding of the anatomy and physiology of the integumentary system in order to appropriately care for patients who are at risk because of disturbances in this system. The importance of following aseptic technique and universal precautions cannot be understated. With all the possible infectious agents and opportunistic organisms seen in the surgical arena, the perianesthesia nurse needs an understanding of the basics of the integumentary system as presented here. For a more comprehensive description of PACU infection control, see Chapter 5 for aseptic technique; and for care of the patient with burn injury, see Chapter 55.

REFERENCES

1. Drake R, et al: *Gray's anatomy for students*, Philadelphia, 2005, Churchill Livingstone.
2. Marks JG, Miller J: *Lookingbill and Marks principles of dermatology*, ed 4, St. Louis, 2006, Saunders.
3. Blumenfeld H, Taylor LA: The role of serotonin norepinephrine reuptake inhibitors in the treatment of fibromyalgia: a guide for the physician assistant, *The Internet Journal of Academic Physician Assistants*, 4(2): 2009, available at http://www.ispub.com/journal/the_internet_journal_of_academic_physician_assistants/volume_4_number_2_7/article_printable/the_role_of_serotonin_norepinephrine_reuptake_inhibitors_in_the_treatment_of_fibromyalgia_a_guide_for_the_physician_assistant.html. Accessed January 14, 2012.
4. Graham-Brown R, Bourke J: *Mosby's color atlas and text of dermatology*, ed 2, St. Louis, 2007, Mosby.
5. Center for Disease Control and Prevention: *Handwashing: clean hands save lives*, available at http://www.cdc.gov/handwashing. Accessed January 14, 2012.
6. Siegel JD, et al, and the Healthcare Infection Control Practices Advisory Committee: *2007 Guideline for isolation precautions: preventing transmission of infectious agents in healthcare settings*, available at http://www.cdc.gov/hicpac/2007IP/2007isolationPrecautions.html. Accessed January 14, 2012.
7. Nagelhout J, Plaus K: *Handbook of nurse anesthesia*, ed 4, St. Louis, 2010, Saunders.
8. ECRI Institute: *Skin substitutes for treatment of burns*, Plymouth Meeting, PA, 2009, ECRI Institute.

RESOURCES

Aitkenhead A, et al: *Textbook of anesthesia*, ed 5, Philadelphia, 2007, Churchill Livingstone.
Atlee J: *Complications in anesthesia*, ed 2, Philadelphia, 2007, Saunders.
Barash P, et al: *Clinical anesthesia*, ed 6, Philadelphia, 2009, Lippincott Williams & Wilkins.
Fisher L: *Benumof's anesthesia and uncommon diseases*, ed 5, Philadelphia, 2007, Saunders.
Hall J: *Guyton and Hall textbook of medical physiology*, ed 12, Philadelphia, 2011, Saunders.
Monahan FD, et al: *Medical-surgical nursing health and illness perspectives*, ed 8, St. Louis, 2007, Mosby.
Walls R, et al: *Rosen's emergency medicine: concepts and clinical practice*, St. Louis, 2009, Mosby.

18 The Immune System

Zohn Centimole, MS, CRNA

During the past three decades, a virtual explosion of information about the immune system has occurred. Diseases once believed to be based in other physiologic systems are now found, as a result of medical research, to have origins in the immune system. Through this improved understanding, the immune system is better viewed as a constellation of responses to a foreign invasion. These responses summarily result in the ability of the body to resist the effects of most toxins and organisms that may cause it damage. Today, in the postanesthesia care unit (PACU), perianesthesia nurses must treat patients with immunosuppression, hypersensitivity type reactions, or patients who have immune diseases, such as acquired immunodeficiency syndrome (AIDS). An informed appreciation of the physiology and pathophysiology of the immune system is essential for the appropriate perianesthesia care of the surgical patient.

DEFINITIONS

Acquired Immunity: The ability of the human body to develop an extremely powerful specific immunity against most invading agents.

Active Acquired Immunity: Immunity that develops when a person comes into direct contact with a pathogen either by contracting the disease produced by the pathogen or by vaccination against the disease.

Antibody: A globulin molecule with the potential to attack agents that are foreign to the host.

Antigen: A protein, large polysaccharide, or large lipoprotein complex that stimulates the process of acquired immunity.

B Lymphocytes or Bursa-Dependent Cells: Immunocompetent lymphocytes that are named for the preprocessing that occurs in the bursa of Fabricius of birds and is responsible for humoral immunity.

Cellular or Cell-Mediated Immunity: A type of acquired immunity that uses sensitized lymphocytes as the primary defense.

Clone: A group of cells that originate from a single parent cell.

Humoral Immunity: A type of acquired immunity that uses antibodies as the primary defense.

Immunity: The ability of the human body to resist almost all types of organisms or toxins that can damage tissues and organs.

Immunodeficiency Disease: Immunosuppression that results from a deficiency of a single humoral antibody group or from a combined deficiency of both T cell and B cell systems.

Immunosuppression: A state of nonresponsiveness of the immune system to antigenic challenge.

Innate Immunity: General processes in the human body, other than those of acquired immunity, that are responsible for protection against organisms and toxins.

Lymphopenia: Decreased function of the lymphoid organs.

Passive Acquired Immunity: Immunity that results when a person receives immune cells or immune serum produced by someone else.

Phagocytosis: The envelopment and digestion of bacteria or other foreign substances.

Sensitized Lymphocytes: Lymphocytes that are made competent by processing to facilitate immunologic activity, such as attachment to and destruction of a foreign agent.

Stem Cells: Unspecialized cells that give rise to specific specialized cells such as T and B lymphocytes.

T Lymphocytes: Sensitized lymphocytes that are responsible for cellular immunity.

PHYSICAL AND CHEMICAL BARRIERS

The body's first line of immunologic defense is the mechanical barrier provided by the epithelial surface. Some parts of the epithelium have extensions from their surface, such as the cilia and the mucus in the respiratory system. These extensions provide an additional physical barrier to the entrance of foreign substances and an efficient removal system. Hydrochloric acid, which is thought to have bactericidal action, is secreted in the stomach. As an additional defense, the skin produces chemicals that inactivate bacteria. The surfaces of the boundary tissues also have specific defenses in the form of secretory antibodies. Consequently, surgical incisions, intravenous cannulation, and many other invasive procedures can cause major breaks in the first line of defense. Therefore the perianesthesia nurse should use good aseptic or sterile technique to prevent an overwhelming bacterial invasion through the boundary tissues.

INNATE IMMUNITY

Innate or nonspecific immunity is the body's second line of immunologic defense against foreign material. In this type of immunity, activation occurs during each exposure to an invading substance. The primary function of the innate immune system is discriminating self from nonself; however, the mechanisms of innate immunity cannot identify the specific invader.

Phagocytosis is the primary mechanism of innate immunity. The cells in the body that carry out the phagocytic functions of innate immunity are monocytes, which are macrophages, and neutrophils (polymorphonuclear leukocytes), which are microphages. The overall immunologic functions of phagocytes are to localize the antigen and to destroy, inactivate, or process it for handling by other components of the immune system. Antigens are usually a protein with a molecular weight of at least 10,000 daltons. The process of phagocytosis can be enhanced with the combination of an antigen and a plasma protein called opsonin, a substance associated with the immune system. Finally, phagocytosis gives transitory protection to the body so that it is not overwhelmed by foreign materials before the immune system (acquired immunity) is activated.

ACQUIRED IMMUNITY

Acquired or adaptive immunity is the body's third line of immunologic defense. Acquired immunity is mediated by the capability of specific antibodies or sensitized lymphocytes to recognize and to react to antigens from the offending agent. Two closely allied types of acquired immune mechanisms occur in the body: humoral immunity and cellular (cell-mediated) immunity.

Humoral Immunity

Humoral immunity is conferred by circulating antibodies that are found in the globulin fraction of blood proteins; therefore these antibodies are called *immunoglobulins* (Ig). Production of the immunoglobulin begins with the lymphocytic stem cells in the bone marrow. These stem cells, which are incapable of forming antibodies, make pre–B lymphocytes that are taken up by the lymph nodes and processed in the as yet unidentified "bursa-equivalent" tissue. These processed B lymphocytes are then released into the blood, where they become entrapped in the lymphoid tissue. On stimulation with an antigen, the B lymphocyte specific for that antigen enlarges, divides, and differentiates into plasma cells that have specificity for that antigen. The plasma cells then produce and secrete an antibody or sensitized lymphocyte.

During the first exposure to the antigen, lymphocytes from one specific type of lymphoid tissue form clones. The clones are responsive only to the antigen responsible for initial development. On the second stimulation by the same antigen, the clones proliferate rapidly, thus leading to the formation of a large amount of antibody. Some cells in this clone mature to form plasma cells, whereas other cells of the clone become B lymphocyte memory cells.

When the immune system responds to the first presentation of the antigen, the immune system remembers the antigen by means of the B lymphocyte memory cell. The immune system can remember the antigen for years. In other words, on the first stimulation by an antigen, the plasma cells produce antibodies (immunoglobulins) as the primary response. The primary response is usually evident approximately 4 to 10 days after the initial exposure to the antigen.

On the second stimulation by the same antigen, a second response occurs. This secondary response, in which a massive amount of antibody specific to the antigen is produced within 1 or 2 days, lasts for months. The secondary response is more rapid, stronger, and more persistent than the primary response because of the memory cells and clones that are produced by the initial exposure to the antigen. If the T lymphocytes are activated by the same antigen, the T lymphocyte helper cells enhance the response of the B lymphocytes; therefore, because of this cooperative effort, the total number of lymphocytes in the lymphoid tissue increases markedly. On second exposure to an antigen, the same plasma cell can produce the particular antibody needed and can convert from one type of antibody secretion to another as needed. When the specific antibodies from the plasma cells are no longer needed, further production of the antibodies is suppressed by the antibodies themselves or by T lymphocyte suppressor cells (Fig. 18-1).

Immunoglobulins, or antibodies, once secreted by the plasma cells, protect the body against invading agents with the following three mechanisms of action: (1) attacking the antigen; (2) activating the complement system, which results in cell lysis; and (3) activating the immediate hypersensitivity reaction, which localizes the invader and may negate its virulence. More specifically, antibodies can inactivate the invading antigen with precipitation, agglutination, neutralization, or complement fixation. Precipitation occurs when an insoluble antibody forms a complex with a soluble antigen, such as tetanus toxin, and the

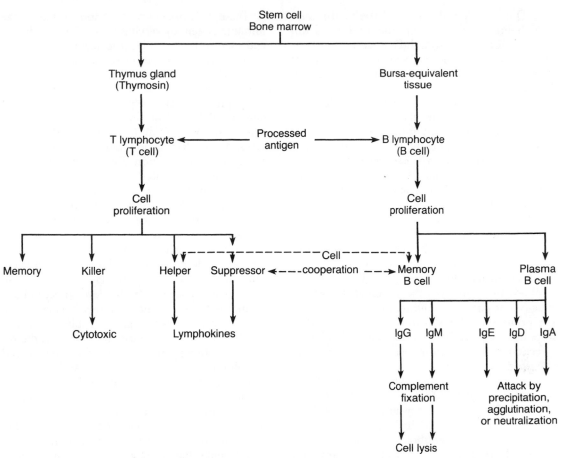

FIG. 18-1 Schematic overview of humoral and cellular immunologic pathways and resulting effector substances or mechanisms of activity.

resulting antigen-antibody complex becomes insoluble and precipitates. When antigens are bound together and react with an antibody, agglutinated aggregates occur. Neutralization is achieved when antibodies cover the toxic sites of an antigenic agent or when antibodies counteract toxins released by bacteria. Rarely are the potent antibodies able to attack a cell membrane directly and cause lysis. However, one of the powerful effects of the binding of the antigen-antibody complex is the activation of complement, which serves to amplify this interaction. More specifically, when IgG or IgM binds to an antigen, the complement system is activated and a cascade system of nine different enzyme precursors (C1 through C9) reacts sequentially. The final result of the activation of the complement system is puncture of the antigen's cell membrane (cell lysis) and rupture of its cellular agents.

The immunoglobulins are large proteins (molecular weights from 150,000 to 900,000 daltons) with specific structural arrangements of polypeptide chains with specific amino acid sequences. The immunoglobulins are divided into five primary classes on the basis of structural arrangements: IgA, IgD, IgE, IgG, and IgM. Each of the immunoglobulins are described as follows.

IgA is a small molecule that constitutes approximately 15% of the total immunoglobulins and is present in most body secretions. Secretory IgA is effective against viruses and some bacteria that invade the mucous membranes. Secretory immunity is also mediated by IgA. The secretory antibodies are found on the mucosal surfaces of the oral cavity (saliva), the lungs (sputum), and the intestinal and urogenital tracts and in mammary secretions. This secretory IgA differs from other antibodies in that it has a protein molecule, called a *secretory piece*, attached to it. IgA activates the complement system through a particular sequence of events called the *properdin pathway*. The complement system is complex cascade of activations of more than 20 proteins that result in the improved ability of phagocytes' cell killing.

IgD constitutes about 1% of the total immunoglobulins. The exact function of IgD is unknown. Similar to IgA, IgD is situated in the upper respiratory mucosa and works to activate B lymphocytes. IgD has been described as "an ancestral surveillance system at the interface between immunity and inflammation."[1] IgD has also been suggested for relationships in antibody activity directed toward insulin, penicillin, milk proteins, diphtheria toxoid, thyroid antigens, and the products of abnormal tissue growth.

IgE is present in minute quantities (approximately 0.002% of total serum immunoglobulins) and is associated with type I immediate hypersensitivity reaction.

IgG is the smallest antibody by size, but constitutes approximately 75% of the total plasma antibodies. The complement system is activated when an antigen binds to IgG. IgG is the only antibody that can cross the placental barrier and thus confer passive immunity to the fetus. IgG is the primary antibody involved in the secondary response. It is active against many bloodborne infectious agents such as bacteria, viruses, parasites, and some fungi.

IgM is the largest antibody by size; it constitutes approximately 10% of plasma antibody. IgM is found almost exclusively in body serums because of its large size and inability to cross membranes; it is the first antibody that responds to an antigen. IgM is involved in the primary antibody response, effectively marking antigens for phagocytic destruction. In addition, IgM is effective in the activation of the complement system.

Cellular Immunity

Cellular immunity is the second type of specific immunity; it uses T lymphocytes and macrophages. Some specific functions of the cellular immunity system are protection against most viruses, slow-acting bacteria, and fungal infections; mediation of cutaneous delayed hypersensitivity reactions; rejection of foreign grafts; and immunologic surveillance.

The T lymphocytes, like the B lymphocytes, originate from primitive stem cells and go through stages of maturation (see Fig. 18-1). When the immature lymphocyte leaves the bone marrow, it migrates to the thymus gland, where it is acted on by the hormone thymosin. The T lymphocyte then becomes mature and immunocompetent. The origin of the name *T lymphocyte* is derived from this thymus-dependent maturation. These mature T lymphocytes can circulate in the blood and lymph, or they may come to rest in the inner cortex of the lymph nodes, where they may form subgroups of T lymphocytes.

These T lymphocytes function overall in the immune system by serving in regulatory, effector, and cytotoxic capacities. The regulatory T lymphocytes are the helper or suppressor T lymphocytes. These lymphocytes amplify or suppress responses of other T lymphocytes or responses of B lymphocytes. The helper T lymphocytes produce a soluble factor that is necessary, in some instances, for antibody formation by B lymphocytes. This helper action is most important for IgE and IgG production. The underproduction of helper cells is associated with AIDS. The suppressor T lymphocytes appear to regulate or suppress the activity of B lymphocytes in the production of antibodies. Evidence indicates that the suppressor T lymphocytes can become pathologically active against helper T lymphocytes and other aspects of cellular immunity. For this reason, these suppressor T lymphocytes may have a role in immune tolerance and in the development of autoimmune disease, such as myasthenia gravis. Effector T lymphocytes are probably responsible for the delayed hypersensitivity reactions, the rejection of foreign tissue grafts and tumors, and the elimination of virus-infected cells. Effector T lymphocytes have antigen receptors on their surfaces that are significant in the initiation of cellular immunity. When an antigen enters the body, it undergoes processing by the phagocytes. The antigen then travels to the regional lymph node, which drains the area of antigen invasion. In this lymph node, the T lymphocyte recognizes the antigen, binds to the antigen, and proliferates. The T lymphocyte becomes sensitized when it comes into contact with the antigen. In addition, memory T lymphocytes result from this interaction. On a second exposure to the antigen, a more intense, efficient, and rapid cellular immunity results. This contact also results in the release of lymphokines by the T lymphocyte. Some of the lymphokines are: (1) chemotactic factor, which recruits phagocytes into the area; (2) migration inhibitory factor, which prevents the migration of phagocytes away from the area; (3) transfer factor, which induces noncommitted T lymphocytes to form T lymphocytes of the same antigen-specific clone as the original cells; (4) lymphotoxin, which is a nonspecific cellular toxin; and (5) interferon, which inhibits the replication of viruses.

The direct cellular cytotoxicity that is mediated by cellular immunity involves cytotoxic lymphocytes, or killer cells, and macrophages. The role of these cytotoxic T lymphocytes is not well established; however, they are believed to be involved in nonspecific killing of viruses, rejection of allografts, and immune surveillance of malignant diseases.

HYPERSENSITIVITY REACTIONS

The immune system serves mainly as protection from harmful substances; however, in some instances, the activation of the immune system can cause deleterious effects, which is *termed allergic response* or *hypersensitivity reaction*. This response represents a magnified or inappropriate reaction by the host to an antigenic substance; it can result in immunologic disease. Hypersensitivity reactions are divided into four major categories: type I, type II, type III, and type IV hypersensitivity reactions (Table 18-1).

Type I Hypersensitivity Reaction (Anaphylactic, Immediate)

Type I hypersensitivity reaction occurs in persons who were previously sensitized to a specific antigen. The antibodies formed against that antigen are of the IgE classification. The term *reagins* is used to describe these IgE antibodies. Reaginic antibodies bind to mast cells in tissues that surround the blood vessels and to blood basophils. When the previously sensitized host is reexposed to the same antigen, the antigen reacts with the reaginic antibody that is attached to the cell and an immediate swelling, and then rupture of the basophil or mast cell results in a release of chemical mediators into the local environment. These chemical mediators include: (1) histamine, which causes local vasodilatation and increased permeability of the capillaries; (2) slow-reacting substance of anaphylaxis, which causes prolonged contraction of some smooth muscle, such as that of the bronchi; (3) chemotactic factor, which draws neutrophils and macrophages into the area of the antigen-antibody reaction;

and (4) lysosomal enzymes, which elicit a local inflammatory reaction. These chemical mediators act on the "shock organs," such as the mucosa, skin, bronchi, and heart. The resulting clinical manifestations of the type I reaction include urticaria, allergic rhinitis, allergic asthma, and, in severe cases, systemic anaphylaxis.

Type II Hypersensitivity Reaction (Cytotoxic)

In the type II hypersensitivity reaction, the antigen and the antibody complex react, thereby injuring the cell membrane or a surface tissue with direct destruction by antibody of cellular elements. The antibodies involved in the type II reaction are either IgG or IgM, and the reaction is enhanced by complement. Hemolytic anemia is an example of a type II reaction that affects the red blood cells (RBCs). For example, when penicillin is absorbed on the RBC membrane, the interaction of antipenicillin antibody, penicillin, and complement causes a reaction that results in the lysis of RBCs.

Type III Hypersensitivity Reaction (Arthus)

The type III hypersensitivity reaction involves the formation of immune complexes of antigen and antibody (IgG or IgM). These immune complexes precipitate in and around small vessels and damage the target tissue by activating complement over several hours. Also involved in this process is an inflammatory reaction that is initiated by the gathering of inflammatory cells and the release of vasoactive amines from platelets. As this process continues, polymorphonuclear leukocytes phagocytize the immune complexes and cause inflammation

PHYSIOLOGIC CONSIDERATIONS IN THE PACU

Table 18-1	Categories of Hypersensitivity Reactions			
TYPE	**MECHANISM**	**OUTCOME**	**REACTION TIME**	**EXAMPLES**
I (Anaphylactic)	Antigen-IgE reaction at surface of mast cells and basophils	Release of mediators	Immediate	Asthma, hay fever, systemic anaphylaxis
II (Cytotoxic)	Binding of IgM or IgG with antigens on surface of cell; enhanced by complement fixation	Cell lysis and tissue damage	Variable	Hemolytic anemia, Goodpasture disease
III (Arthus)	Microprecipitation of immune complex formed by antigen and IgM or IgG; enhanced by complement fixation	Tissue damage and release of vasoactive substances	4-18 hours	Serum sickness, farmer's lung, allergic alveolitis, glomerulonephritis, SLE
IV (Delayed)	Direct interaction of antigen with sensitized T lymphocytes	Release of mediators and tissue damage	24-48 hours	Contact dermatitis, tuberculosis

Ig, Immunoglobulin; *SLE,* systemic lupus erythematosus.

and necrosis of the blood vessels and surrounding tissue because of the release of lysosomal enzymes. Serum sickness and systemic lupus erythematosus are clinical examples of type III hypersensitivity reactions.

Type IV Hypersensitivity Reaction (Delayed or Cell-Mediated)

Type IV hypersensitivity reaction is the only hypersensitivity reaction that does not involve antibodies. In the type IV reaction, the exposure to an antigen and the subsequent binding of the antigen with antigen-specific reactive T lymphocytes initiate the production of lymphokines from the T lymphocytes, with tissue damage as the end result. The antigen responsible for the type IV reaction can be bacterial, fungal, protozoan, or viral. Contact dermatitis, allograft rejection, and delayed response in tuberculin skin tests are examples of delayed hypersensitivity reactions.

LATEX ALLERGY

The prevalence rate of confirmed allergic reactions among health care workers ranges from 5% to 10%. Similarly, recent studies indicate that 8% to 12% of the health care population becomes sensitized to latex. Since the 1980s when universal precautions were instituted to prevent the spread of human immunodeficiency virus, hepatitis viruses, and other infectious agents, health care workers have routinely worn latex gloves as a protective barrier. In addition, the Occupational Safety and Health Administration instructed health care workers to wear protective material as a barrier. A great demand then occurred for surgical gloves. As a result, the accounts of the amount of latex proteins found in surgical gloves varied.

Many products contain latex; at home, these products include rubber bands, some carpets, earphones, and mouse pads. In the hospital setting, tourniquets, pressure cuff tubing, and urinary catheters often contain latex. In the perianesthesia area, possible routes of exposure include contact with mucosa, direct contact of particles with an open surgical wound, and aerosolized particles that are bound to the powder in the latex article. Interestingly, these particles can stay suspended for up to 5 hours.

The degree of reactions to latex varies; irritant contact dermatitis is basically a nonallergic reaction. Symptoms such as dry, itchy, or irritated areas that may be red and cracked usually occur within the first 6 to 24 hours after exposure. The reaction can be caused by exposure to powders added to the gloves, repeated hand washing and drying, or the use of cleaners and sanitizers. Because this reaction

is not a true allergy, it usually clears after the irritant is removed.

Allergic contact dermatitis is also a nonallergic reaction. Symptoms, which usually occur within 24 to 48 hours, include erythema, vesicles, papules, pruritus, blisters, and crusting of the area that touched the latex. This type of response is caused by the chemical additives that are used in the manufacture of latex and are usually thiurams or carbamates.

Of major concern is the type I immediate hypersensitivity, which is the IgE-mediated response. This response usually occurs within minutes of exposure to the latex; however, it can occur within a few hours in some cases. A mild reaction is characterized by skin redness, urticaria, and itching. Severe reactions can produce acute rhinorrhea, sneezing, angioedema, bronchospasm, and anaphylactic shock.[2]

Many organizations are investigating latex allergies, and the American Society of Anesthesiologists has a document that can be found on the Internet (http://ecommerce.asahq.org/publicationsAndServices/latexallergy.pdf). Also, the American Association of Nurse Anesthetists has an excellent web site on latex allergies (http://www.anesthesiapatientsafety.com/patients/latex/fact_sheet.asp). Another expert guideline for management of latex allergies and safe latex use is from the American College of Allergy, Asthma, and Immunology (http://www.acaai.org/allergist/allergies/Types/latex-allergy/Pages/latex-allergies-safe-use.aspx).

The best treatment for a latex allergic response is avoidance. Patients who are at risk for an allergic reaction caused by latex are listed in Box 18-1. Health care personnel with known sensitivity should carry their own nonlatex gloves, usually made of vinyl or neoprene. They also should use nonlatex tourniquets and latex-free or glass syringes and should use stopcocks to inject drugs. Intravenous line tubing should have no latex ports, or if the latex ports exist, they should be taped. Box 18-2 summarizes the various recommendations for patients with known latex allergic reactions or a risk of reactions.

If a reaction to latex develops in the patient in the PACU, the first intervention is removal of the patient from ongoing exposure to the latex. The reactions can vary from mild respiratory reactions that can be treated on a symptomatic level to hives, which can occur immediately to several hours after exposure, and to a type I hypersensitivity anaphylactic reaction.

Treatment for the type I reaction should consist of first carefully looking for the latex allergen, such as rubber drains in the wound, inadvertent

---

BOX 18-1 Patients Who Should Be Strongly Considered at Risk for an Allergic Reaction to Latex

A complete medical history is the most reliable screening examination for prediction of a reaction to latex.

- History of atopic immunologic reactions
- History of contact dermatitis
- History of documented immunologic reactions of unknown etiology during a medical or surgical procedure
- History of allergies to food products, including fruits, nuts, bananas, avocados, celery, figs, chestnuts, and papayas
- Neural tube defects, including spina bifida, myelomeningocele/meningocele, and lipomyelomeningocele
- Multiple operations in the past
- Repeated bladder catheterizations

---

use of latex gloves, latex that contains urinary draining tubes, or intravenous tubing. In addition, remove all latex from the patient bedside; change gloves, discontinue antibiotics and blood administration, maintain the airway, administer 100% oxygen, intubate the trachea if necessary, and maintain intravascular volume support. Once the

diagnosis of type I IgE-mediated anaphylaxis has been confirmed, epinephrine should be administered intravenously in doses of 0.1 mg/kg and titrated to effect. These small doses stabilize the patient's condition and avoid ventricular tachycardia and malignant arrhythmias.

The increasing recognition of latex allergy and accurate testing that is available has led to a decrease in the number of latex allergic persons. Advances in the understanding of these processes should allow this trend to continue.[2] In the meantime, many health care facilities have become latex free environments to protect both employees and patients.

IMMUNOSUPPRESSION

With the advent of organ transplantation, patients often arrive in the PACU in an immunosuppressed state. Consequently, the perianesthesia nurse must have a basic knowledge of the forms of immunosuppression and the appropriate nursing care measures that can be implemented for the patient with immunosuppression.

Forms of Immunosuppression

The unresponsive state of the immune system may be caused by a natural tolerance to self-antigens, to a pathologic state, or to induced immunosuppression. Researchers are attempting to understand

---

BOX 18-2 Summary of the Recommendations for Perianesthesia Care of Patients with Known or Risk of Latex Allergic Reactions

PREOPERATIVE AND INTRAOPERATIVE CARE

- Remove all latex products from the operating room.
- Use a latex-free reservoir bag on the anesthesia machine, oral airways, endotracheal tubes, and laryngeal mask airways.
- Use a latex-free breathing circuit with plastic mask and bag.
- Anesthesia ventilator must have a latex-free bellows.
- Place all monitoring devices, cords, and tubes (oximeter, blood pressure cuffs, electrocardiograph wires) in stockinet and secure with tape to prevent direct skin contact.
- Cover all rubber injection ports on intravenous bags with tape and label them "Do not inject fluid through ports."
- Use intravenous tubing without latex ports or cover with tape.
- Use nonlatex gloves.
- Use nonlatex tourniquets.
- Draw medication directly from opened multidose vials.

- Draw up medications immediately before the beginning of the case.
- Use latex-free or glass syringes.
- Use stopcocks to inject drugs.

POSTANESTHESIA PHASE OF CARE

- Place a sign on the door and flag the chart of the patient to alert personnel to the hypersensitivity.
- Ensure that the patient recovers in a private area.
- Use good handwashing techniques.
- Use only latex-free syringes and gloves.
- Use ampules or remove stoppers from vials before use.
- Cover injection ports on minibags and use latex-free tubings.
- Remain alert for signs and symptoms (hypotension, tachycardia, and bronchospasm) of a latex allergy response and have appropriate emergency drugs and equipment available.

immunosuppression by artificially manipulating the immune system to produce a natural tolerance to self-antigens. Pathologic states such as lymphoma and leukemia are examples of the second form of immunosuppression, in which the immune system becomes unresponsive because of the pathologic changes in the immunocompetent cells. Induced immunosuppression can be accomplished with the administration of an antigen, antisera, or antibody; hormones and cytotoxic drugs; radiation; or surgery. For the most part, induced immunosuppression is used for tissue and organ transplants.

For patients with allergies, the administration of low-dose antigen provides relief in some instances from the antigen-antibody reaction. This desensitizing process produces antibodies that block the interaction between the antigen and the antibody-producing cells. Another method of providing tolerance to self-antigens is with the administration of antisera or antibody in an attempt to coat the antigenic sites. The object is to prevent immunocompetent cells from combining with the antigen. This method of immunosuppression is 100% effective in the prevention of Rh factor sensitization and ultimately erythroblastosis fetalis. Corticosteroids produce immunosuppression by reducing the amount of T and B lymphocytes that circulate in the blood, by blocking lymphokine release, and by decreasing the number of monocytes. Cytotoxic drugs are used in the treatment of cancer and autoimmune diseases. The most popular drugs are azathioprine and cyclophosphamide. These drugs suppress immune system function by killing unstimulated lymphocytes. X irradiation suppresses most of the immunocompetent cells with the induction of a profound lymphopenia. Surgical removal of the thymus gland, spleen, or lymph nodes may alter the immune response with the removal of tissue needed for the maturation of both the cellular and the humoral immune systems.

Perianesthesia Care of the Patient with Immunosuppression

The major responsibilities of the perianesthesia nurse who cares for the patient with immunosuppression are prevention of infection and early diagnosis and treatment of infection. Opinions differ regarding the placement of the patient who is nonleukopenic in protective isolation. However, if the peripheral leukocyte count is less than 2000 cells/mm^3, the patient probably will benefit from protective isolation. Before the patient is admitted to the PACU, sources of cross contamination should be eliminated. Blood pressure cuffs and other equipment that are to be used directly on the patient should be cleaned and disinfected with appropriate solutions. Aseptic technique should be followed at all times. In addition, needle puncture sites and surgical wounds should be cleaned and dressed with appropriate cleaners and ointments. If urinary catheters are used, open skin should be monitored closely for the beginning signs of infection. Patients with immunosuppression might not show the classic symptoms of infection. The temperature of the patient with immunosuppression should be closely monitored, and if it rises above 38° C, the attending physician should be notified immediately. Rectal thermometers should be avoided because they can cause mucosal injury and contamination.

Anesthetics and Immune Function

The invasive procedures involved in an anesthesia practice compromise many of the physical barriers described previously. Tracheal intubation, venous access devices, central neuraxial access, and mucous membrane contact are all vectors of infection. The inflammatory side effects of surgical procedures provide an ample breeding ground for the newly introduced flora.

Anesthetic agents themselves have long been associated with immune dysfunction. Over two decades ago, Nakagawara and colleagues demonstrated that inflammatory precursors were inhibited when exposed to inhalation anesthetics.[3] Macrophage phagocytotic ability is also reduced by the common inhalation anesthetic isoflurane.[4] Similarly, monocyte, neutrophil, and macrophages are inhibited by intravenous propofol in a dose dependent fashion.[5] Proper universal precautionsand careful caution against contamination of the described vectors, are crucial for positive patient outcomes.

SUMMARY

The physiology of the immune system has been presented. This area of medical physiology has been enhanced in its degree of research and treatment with the onset of AIDS and the organ transplant surgeries that depend on drugs and such for suppression of the immune system. Many new pathophysiologic processes will be discovered in the near future that are related directly to the immune system.

REFERENCES

1. Chen K, Cerutti A: The function and regulation of immunoglobulin D, *Current Opinion in Immunology* 23(3):345–352, 2011.
2. Shah D, Chowdhury MMU: Rubber allergy, *Clin in Dermatology* 29:278-286, 2011.
3. Nakagawara M, et al: Inhibition of superoxide production and Ca2+ mobilization in human neutrophils by halothane, enflurane, and isoflurane, *Anesthesiology* 64:4–12, 1986.
4. Kotani N, et al: Intraoperative modulation of alveolar macrophage function during isoflurane and propofol anesthesia, *Anesthesiology* 89:1125–32, 1998.
5. Mikawa K, et al: Propofol inhibits human neutrophil functions, *Anesthesia & Analgesia* 87:695–700, 1998.

RESOURCES

American Association of Nurse Anesthetists: *Talking points about latex allergies*, available at http://www.anesthesiapatientsafety.com/patients/latex/talking_points.asp. Accessed June 2, 2011.
American Society of Anesthesiologists: *Natural rubber latex allergy: considerations for anesthesiologists*, available at http://ecommerce.asahq.org/publicationsAndServices/latexallergy.pdf. Accessed June 2, 2011.
Atlee J: *Complications in anesthesia*, ed 2, St. Louis, 2007, Saunders.

Brunton L, et al: *Goodman and Gilman's the pharmacological basis of therapeutics*, ed 12, New York, 2011, McGraw-Hill.
Fleisher L: *Anesthesia and uncommon diseases*, ed 5, St. Louis, 2007, Saunders.
Gorringe-Moore R: Immunology and the lung. In Traver G, editors: *Respiratory nursing: the science and the art*, New York, 1982, John Wiley & Sons.
Groenwald S: Physiology of the immune system, *Heart Lung* 9(4):645–650, 1980.
Hall J: *Guyton and Hall textbook of medical physiology*, ed 12, Philadelphia, 2011, Saunders.
Jocius M: Immunohematology and transfusion reaction, *AANA J* 50(1):42–48, 1982.
Murray J: *The normal lung*, ed 2, Philadelphia, 1986, Saunders.
Paskawicz J, Chatwani A: Latex allergy: a concern for anesthesia personnel, *Am J Anesth* 28:435–441, 2001.
Rana A, Luskin A: Immunosuppression, autoimmunity, and hypersensitivity, *Heart Lung* 9(4):651–657, 1980.
Spindler J, et al: Intramuscular ketorolac and morphine in the treatment of moderate to severe pain after major surgery, *Pharmacotherapy* 10:51S–58S, 1990.
Sussman G, Gold, M: *Guidelines for the management of latex allergies and safe latex use in health care facilities*, Arlington Heights, IL, 2010, American College of Allergy, available at http://www.acaai.org/allergist/allergies/Types/latex-allergy/Pages/latex-allergies-safe-use.aspx. Accessed June 2, 2011.
Trevor AJ, et al: *Basic and clinical pharmacology*, ed 11, New York, 2009, McGraw Hill.

PHYSIOLOGIC CONSIDERATIONS IN THE PACU

19 Basic Principles of Pharmacology

John J. Nagelhout, PhD, CRNA, FAAN

A thorough understanding of the pharmacology of the drugs used in perianesthesia care is necessary to ensure the best outcomes in surgical patients. Anesthesia care continues to evolve, and the judicious use of a number of selective, potent drugs in various combinations represents the cornerstone of current practice. Consequently, a comprehensive review of the principles and concepts of pharmacology is presented in this chapter. The specific actions and uses of drugs related to perianesthesia care are discussed in the physiology chapters in Section II, as are the concepts of anesthetic agents in the chapters in Section III. The pharmacology of individual drugs can be best understood in relation to the physiologic functions they affect and their common clinical applications.

A significant portion of this chapter is dedicated to an overview of drug interactions, because modern anesthesia care requires balancing the administration of multiple drugs throughout the perianesthesia period. These drugs include anesthesia-related agents, the patient's existing medications, including herbal agents, and other over-the-counter preparations.[1] Clinically, at least 10% of the patients for perianesthesia are taking some form of herbal preparation.[2] Consequently, knowledge of the principles of pharmacology becomes a meaningful and useful tool in the delivery of nursing care to the patient in the postanesthesia care unit (PACU).

DEFINITIONS

Additive Effect: Occurs when a second drug with properties similar to the first is added to produce an effect equal to the algebraic sum of the effects of the two individual drugs. Shorthand often used is $1 + 1 = 2$.

Agonists: Drugs such as dopamine that attach and activate specific receptors.

Antagonists: Drugs such as naloxone (Narcan) that attach to a specific receptor and do not activate the receptor, but prevent an agonist or body chemical such as a neurotransmitter from stimulating the receptor.

Competitive Antagonist: When the concentration of the antagonist is higher than the agonist concentration resulting in reversal or antagonism of the agonist. Examples include naloxone (Narcan) reversing fentanyl or flumazenil (Romazicon) reversing midazolam (Versed). Shorthand often used is $1 + 1 = 0$.

Cross Tolerance: Tolerance to a drug because of an existing tolerance to a similar drug. An example of cross tolerance is a patient who has developed a tolerance to morphine due to repeated administration will also require higher doses of all other opioids as well.

Efficacy of a Drug: Refers to the maximum effect that can be produced by a drug.

Hyperreactivity: An abnormal reaction to an unusually low dose of a drug. For example, patients with Addison disease, myxedema, or dystrophia myotonica have hyperreactivity to unusually low doses of barbiturates.

Hypersensitivity (Anaphylaxis): A drug-induced antigen-antibody reaction. The particular hypersensitivity reaction can be either an immediate (anaphylactic) or a delayed reaction. Hypersensitivity reactions can occur with succinylcholine, antibiotics, and many other drugs that are administered in the PACU (see Chapter 18).

Hyporeactivity: An indication that a person needs excessively large doses of a drug to obtain a therapeutic or desired effect.

Idiosyncrasy: An adverse drug reaction that occurs in a small number of persons and has no correlation to dosage or of type of therapy. Postoperative liver dysfunction following halothane administration is an example.

Pharmacodynamics: The study of the mechanisms of action of drugs and other biochemical and physiologic effects on the body.

Pharmacokinetics: The study of the movement of drugs throughout the body, including the processes of absorption, distribution, biotransformation or metabolism, and excretion.

Potency of a Drug: The dose necessary of a particular drug to produce a specific effect that is designated as the *effective dose* (ED). When that effect is achieved in a particular percentage of patients, it is quantified as ED50 for 50% of the patients and ED95 for 95% of the patients who show an effect to the drug.

Potentiation: The enhancement of the action of one drug by a second drug that has no detectable action of its own. Shorthand commonly used is $1 + 0 = 3$.

Receptors: The portion on or in a cell, usually a protein complex, at which attachment of drugs leads to a physiologic response. The receptors are selective in that they recognize and bind only to specific pharmacologic or physiologic agents.

Synergistic Effect: Addition of a second drug to a drug with properties similar to the first that results in an effect greater than the algebraic sum of the effects of the two individual drugs. Shorthand often used is $1 + 1 = 3$.

Tachyphylaxis: An acute drug tolerance—for example, succinylcholine administered by intravenous drip. Over time, a higher drip rate is needed to achieve the necessary response.

Tolerance: A type of hyporeactivity that is acquired during chronic exposure to a drug in which unusually large doses are needed to reach a desired effect. A prime example is a person who has become dependent on opioids and needs larger than normal doses to elicit the desired therapeutic response.

DRUG RESPONSES

Drugs are given via a chosen route of administration at a specific dose with the expectation of a desired response. Many factors affect the time of onset, the efficacy, and the duration of action of a particular drug. The perianesthesia nurse must be aware of the basic principles of drug actions within a biologic system. A review of the basic concepts of drug responses is presented, with particular emphasis on the patient in the PACU.

Pharmacokinetic Actions

Pharmacokinetics is the pharmacology subspecialty that studies the absorption, distribution, metabolism, and elimination of a drug in the body. Consequently, pharmacokinetics can be viewed as what the body does to a drug after it is administered.

Systemic Absorption by Various Routes of Administration

Oral Route of Administration

When a drug is administered orally, it is absorbed in the small intestine, which has a large surface area. A drug must be lipid soluble to cross the gastrointestinal lining. After such absorption, the drug passes to the liver by way of the portal veins before it can enter the systemic circulation. The liver extracts and metabolizes some of the drug in a process termed the *first-pass hepatic effect*. The drugs that are particularly subject to this effect are agents such as propranolol, metoprolol, verapamil, chlorpromazine, and morphine; therefore these drugs are administered in much higher doses orally than intravenously.[3]

Oral administration of drugs in the PACU has some distinct disadvantages. For example, nausea and vomiting can occur and reduce the amount of the drug available for absorption by the small intestine. In addition, the absorption process can be affected, because the gastric volume and pH are altered either by preoperative drugs or anesthesia and surgery.

Sublingual Route of Administration

The sublingual route of administration has several important advantages over the oral route, because the sublingual route bypasses the first-pass hepatic effect. This route can be particularly favorable in the PACU for drugs such as nitroglycerin. A nitroglycerin tablet be placed sublingually in an intubated as well as a cooperative awake patient.[4]

Subcutaneous and Intramuscular Routes of Administration

These routes of administration require simple diffusion from the site of injection into the systemic circulation and are dependent on blood flow to the injection site. Consequently, these administration routes can result in variations in absorption particularly in the PACU when patients are hypothermic and hypotensive and usually have some peripheral vasoconstriction. Subcutaneous absorption is slow and is reserved for drugs such as insulin or hormones, for which a slow, continuous absorption is advantageous. Intramuscular injections produce a more rapid action and are a common practice in the PACU. In addition, if a patient with a hypothermic condition in the PACU is administered a drug either subcutaneously or intramuscularly, absorption can be delayed. However, when the patient undergoes rewarming, a significant amount of the drug can be rapidly liberated from the injection site, thus causing a large concentration of the drug in the systemic circulation and an exaggerated effect.[3]

Intravenous Route of Administration

This route of administration facilitates the delivery of a desired concentration of a drug in a rapid and precise fashion by single bolus injection or continuous infusion. In the PACU, because patients have an intravenous line, it is the most popular means of drug administration.

Aerosolized Medications to the Respiratory Tract

The aerosolized route of administration facilitates direct delivery from inhaled aerosols to a targeted organ, which reduces the systematic drug exposure and side effects. Many aerosol delivery devices can be used for administration of bronchoactive inhaled aerosols. The most commonly used method of administration in the PACU is the aerosolized nebulizer, in which a specific amount of drug is administered in a solution of normal saline and is nebulized with a ventilator or oxygen delivery devices. Other devices for delivery of the drug either orally or nasally via inhalation are the metered dose inhaler (MDI) with or without a holding chamber or spacer device, the small volume nebulizer (SVN), and the dry powder inhaler (DPI). The MDI, SVN, and the DPI devices deliver approximately the same percentage of the drug to the target organ, the lungs, with the MDI increasing the patient flow rates better than the SVN and the DPI.[4]

Drug Distribution

A drug's distribution in the body is envisioned as entering various defined compartments. A compartment represents a theoretic space. A mathematic model can be used to describe the pharmacokinetics of the disposition of a drug. A two-compartment model is usually used in depiction of a central compartment and a peripheral compartment. The central compartment includes plasma and blood cells and highly perfused tissues such as the heart, lungs, brain, liver, and kidneys. The peripheral compartment represents all other fluids and tissues in the body. With this two-compartment model, a drug can be introduced into the central compartment, move into the peripheral compartment, and then return to the central compartment where removal from the body occurs. The two-compartment model is constructed with the serum concentration versus time and is called the *plasma concentration curve*. From this curve, the distribution and elimination half-times and other kinetic parameters of the drug can be calculated. A drug like propofol will rapidly distribute into the brain when given intravenously, causing a rapid onset of sedation. It also quickly redistributes from the tissues into the blood, resulting in a short duration of action.[5]

Metabolism and Elimination

The major mechanisms for elimination of a drug from the body are hepatic and renal clearance. The half-life ($t_{1/2}$) of a drug is the time at which 50% of the total amount of the drug has been eliminated from the body. The elimination half-life ($t_{1/2\beta}$) is the time that the plasma concentration is at 50% of the elimination phase; the $t_{1/2\beta}$ is directly proportional to the volume distribution of the drug and inversely proportional to the drug clearance. Consequently, when the $t_{1/2\beta}$ for a particular drug is known, a large initial dose called a *loading dose* of a drug can be given to achieve a therapeutic concentration. The drug can then be given via infusion or in multiple doses at calculated intervals, based on the $t_{1/2\beta}$, for a steady-state plasma concentration. In addition, the time necessary for elimination of a particular dose of a drug can be predicted with the $t_{1/2\beta}$. Usually, 95% of the drug can be eliminated in five half-lives.[6]

Removal of Drugs from the Systemic Circulation

Drugs are principally cleared from the systemic circulation via the hepatic, biliary, and renal systems. The hepatic system has a high blood flow and can extract many lipid-soluble drugs from the systemic circulation. In the liver, drugs undergo biotransformation and for the most part become pharmacologically inactive. Enzyme induction or a decrease in protein binding enhances the hepatic clearance of some drugs (see Chapter 16). After they have been metabolized in the liver, drugs can be transported to the biliary system or the kidney for excretion. Some drugs, such as the glucuronides, are actively transported to the bile and excreted in an inactive form.[6]

The kidneys secrete many water-soluble drugs in their unchanged form or as hepatic metabolites. Renal excretion of drugs depends on the following major physiologic processes that occur in the kidneys: glomerular filtration, active tubular secretion, and passive tubular reabsorption. Appropriate renal function is needed for facilitation of many of the drugs administered in the perioperative period. Consequently, concern about renal function should merit creatinine clearance or serum creatinine level tests, because these laboratory tests correlate well with renal drug elimination.[6]

Effects of Physiologic Dysfunction on Pharmacokinetic Action

Renal Disease

Kidney disease reduces the effectiveness of drug clearance and results in a prolongation in the action of the drugs that rely on the kidneys for their removal. In renal drug clearance, the laboratory test of creatinine clearance, for measurement of glomerular filtration (see Chapter 13), can be used for prediction of the degree of a drug's renal clearance. In patients who are anephric or in patients with severe kidney disease, the elimination clearance is decreased and the $t_{1/2}B$ is increased, thus prolonging the effects of the drugs, especially with repeated administrations.[7]

Hepatic Disease

Patients with hepatic diseases such as cirrhosis may have difficulty clearing some anesthetic drugs from the body. Liver function testing is unreliable for predicting the level of impairment in hepatic clearance of drugs. Any patient with documented liver disease should be considered at risk for decreased clearance of drugs. Therefore, in patients with documented hepatic disease, all drugs administered in the PACU should be titrated to desired effect for an appropriate pharmacologic outcome.[8]

Cardiovascular Disease

Cardiovascular diseases that cause a reduction in tissue perfusion have a significant effect on drug distribution and clearance. For example, when lidocaine is administered to patients with congestive heart failure, the dose should be reduced by half because of changes in volume distribution and clearance. Patients who have undergone cardiopulmonary bypass surgery can have a hemodilution of drugs. Patients with cardiac disease should have their medications given at lower doses over longer dosing interval with careful monitoring.[9] Drugs used in the PACU are listed in Table 19-1.

DRUG-DRUG INTERACTIONS

When a patient simultaneously receives two or more drugs, the drugs might interact to cause a different action than expected including an adverse outcome. Patients are often given drugs other than the ones associated with anesthesia and surgery. As a result, the potential for a drug-drug interaction is present in these patients (Table 19-2). These interactions are divided into two broad categories: pharmacokinetic and pharmacodynamic.

Pharmacokinetic Interactions

Interactions of two or more drugs that produce alterations in absorption, distribution, metabolism, or excretion are known as *pharmacokinetic interactions*. Therefore, when one drug alters any pharmacokinetic parameter of another, with a resultant alteration in the concentration of the drug at the receptor site, a pharmacokinetic interaction has taken place. In other words, the absorption, distribution, or elimination of the drug concentration at the receptor site is changed, which results in an altered pharmacologic response.

Absorption

The absorption of one drug can be enhanced or inhibited by another drug. With the addition of epinephrine to solutions of local anesthetics, the absorption of the anesthetic is prolonged through the vasoconstrictive action of epinephrine. The local vasoconstriction produced by epinephrine delays the systemic absorption of the local anesthetic, and the effect of the local anesthetic ultimately is prolonged. When a patient has been administered a preoperative aluminum-containing antacid and then is administered tetracycline in the late postoperative period, absorption of the tetracycline is reduced.[10]

Distribution

Pharmaceutical incompatibility is one type of pharmacokinetic distribution interaction. This situation occurs, for example, when one drug reacts chemically with another. In this situation, when one drug (e.g., aspirin) displaces another drug (e.g., phenytoin) from plasma protein-binding sites, the blood concentration of the free drug is increased, which can result in altered blood levels.[10]

Biotransformation

When patients are administered enzyme-inducing agents, such as barbiturates and the antibiotic rifampin, the activity of the enzyme systems of the liver is increased. This increase results in a more rapid metabolism and excretion of drugs that are metabolized by a particular liver enzyme system. For example, if a barbiturate is administered to a patient who is receiving a stabilized dose of the anticoagulant warfarin, the warfarin blood level may be reduced, which can result in a lowered prothrombin time. If this situation occurs (stabilization with an anticoagulant and administration of an enzyme-inducing agent) and the barbiturate is discontinued, the nurse must monitor the patient for the potentially more serious problem of excessive anticoagulation and hemorrhage.

The drug cimetidine (Tagamet) is sometimes administered before surgery for a reduction in the amount of gastric secretion and for a possible increase in the gastric pH. Cimetidine is a potent inhibitor of drug metabolism and can slow the elimination of antipyrine, warfarin, diazepam, and propranolol. This effect results in an increased drug concentration and enhanced pharmacologic effect of the latter drugs.[11]

Excretion

The pharmacokinetic parameters of concern in excretion relate to one drug facilitating or hindering the excretion of another. An example occurs when probenecid is administered together with penicillin. The outcome of this interaction is that the pharmacologic actions of penicillin are

Text continues on page 246

Table 19-1   Drugs Used in the Postanesthesia Care Unit: Perianesthesia Drug List

DRUG	ROUTE	ONSET	PEAK	DURATION OF ACTION	CLASSIFICATION
Adenosine (Adenocard)	IV	<20 sec	20-30 sec	1 min	Antiarrhythmic
Acetaminophen (Ofirmev)	IV	15 min	30 min	6 hours	Nonopioid analgesic, antipyretic
Acetaminophen (Acephen, Feverall)	Rectal (suppository)	30 min	1 hour	6 hours	Nonopioid analgesic, antipyretic
Albuterol (Proventil, Ventolin)	INH	<5 min	30 min-2 hours	3-6 hours	Bronchodilator
Alfentanil (Alfenta)	IV	1-2 min	1-2 min	10-60 min	Opioid agonist
	Epidural	5-15 min	30 min	30-60 min	
Aminocaproic acid (Amicar)	IV	1-2 hours	—	8-12 hours	Hemostatic agent
Aminophylline	IV	1-2 min	30-60 min	4-10 hours	Bronchodilator
	PO	<30 min	1-5 hours	4-8 hours	
Aprepitant (Emend)	IV	30	2 hours	24 hours	Antiemetic
Atenolol (Tenormin)	IV	5 min	5 min	12-24 hours	β-Blocker
	PO	30-60 min	2-4 hours	24 hours	
Atracurium (Tracrium)	IV	2-5 min	3-5 min	20-35 min	NMB
Atropine	IV, cardiac	30-60 sec	1-2 min	15-30 min	Anticholinergic
	IV, dry	30-60 min	60-90 min	4 hours	
	IO	1-2 min	5-10 min	1-2 hours	
	ETT	10-20 sec	1-2 min	30-45 minutes	
	IM	5-40 min	20-60 min	2-4 hours	
	INH	3-5 min	15-90 min	3-6 hours	
Bumetanide (Bumex)	IV	1-5 min	15-30 min	4 hours	Loop diuretic
Bupivacaine (Marcaine)	Epidural	4-7 min	30-45 min	2-7 hours	Local anesthetic
	Infiltration	2-10 min	30-45 min	3-7 hours	
	Spinal	<1 min	15 min	2-4 hours	
Butorphanol (Stadol)	IV	1-2 min	5-10 min	3-4 hours	Analgesic (agonist-antagonist combination)
	IM	10-15 min	30-60 min	3-4 hours	
Captopril (Capoten)	PO	<15 min	1-2 hours	2-6 hours	ACE inhibitor
Clevidipine (Cleviprex)	IV	1-2 min	5-10 min	15 min	Calcium channel blocker
Chloroprocaine (Nesacaine)	Epidural	6-12 min	10-20 min	30-60 min	Local anesthetic; not to be used for spinal anesthesia
Cimetidine (Tagamet)	IV	30-45 min	60-90 min	4-5 hours	Histamine receptor antagonist
	PO	15-45 min	1-2 hours	2-4 hours	
Cisatracurium (Nimbex)	IV	1-4 min	2-7 min	22-65 min	Nondepolarizing NMB
Clonidine (Catapres, Dixarit)	PO	30-60 min	2-4 hours	6-8 hours	Antihypertensive
	IV	30-60 min	2-4 hours	6-10 hours	
	Epidural	<15 min	3-4 hours		
Cocaine HCl	Topical	<1 min	2-5 min	30-120 min	Topical anesthetic; vasoconstrictor
	PO	30-60 min	—	2-4 hours	
	IM	20-60 min	—	2-3 hours	Opioid agonist
Cyclosporine (Sandimmune)	PO	1-6 hours	8-12 hours	1-4 days	Immunosuppressant

Table 19-1   Drugs Used in the Postanesthesia Care Unit: Perianesthesia Drug List—cont'd

DRUG	ROUTE	ONSET	PEAK	DURATION OF ACTION	CLASSIFICATION
Dantrolene (Dantrium)	IV	<5 min	60 min	3 hours	Skeletal muscle relaxant; for treatment of malignant hyperthermia
	PO	1-2 hours	4-6 hours	8-12 hours	
Desflurane (Suprane)	INH	1-2 min	—	Emergence in 8-9 min	Inhalational anesthetic agent
Desmopressin (DDAVP)	IV	30 min	1.5-3 hours	8-20 hours	Synthetic vasopressin analogue
	Intranasal	<60 min	1-5 hours	8-20 hours	
Dexmedetomidine (Precedex)	IV	1-3 min	5-10 min	Effects last 3-5 min after discontinuance of IV infusion	α_{2b}-Receptor agonist sedative agent
Dexamethasone	IV	<8 hours	12-24 hours	36-54 hours	Long-acting corticosteroid
(Decadron)	IM	<8 hours	1-2 hours	72 hours	
(Respihaler)	INH	<20 min	2-4 hours	12 hours	
(Turbinaire)	Intranasal	<15 min	—	12-24 hours	
Diazepam (Valium)	IV	1-5 min	4-8 min	15-60 min	Benzodiazepine
	IM	15-30 min	—	3-6 hours	
	PO	30-60 min	1-2 hours	3-6 hours	
Digoxin (Lanoxin)	IV	5-30 min	1-5 hours	3-4 days	Inotropic agent
	IM	30 min	4-6 hours	3-4 days	
	PO	30 min to 2 hours	6-8 hours	3-4 days	
Diltiazem (Cardizem)	IV	1-3 min	2-7 min	1-3 hours	Calcium channel blocker
	PO	30 min	2-3 hours	4-6 hours	
	PO, extended	1-3 hours	4-11 hours	18-24 hours	
Diphenhydramine (Benadryl)	IV	<3 min	1-2 hours	3-6 hours	Antihistamine
	PO	1 hour	1-2 hours	4-6 hours	
Dobutamine	IV	2 min	1-10 min	5-10 min	Vasopressor (adrenergic agonist)
Dolasetron (Anzemet)	IV	5-15 min	30-60 min	8-12 hours	Antiemetic
Dopamine (Intropin)	IV	2-4 min	5 min	<10 min	Catecholamine
Doxapram (Dopram)	IV	20-40 sec	1-2 min	5-12 min	Respiratory and cerebral stimulant
Droperidol (Inapsine)	IV, IM	3-10 min	30 min	8-16 hours	Tranquilizer, antiemetic
Edrophonium (Enlon, Tensilon)	IV	30-60 sec	1-5 min	5-20 min	Anticholinesterase
	IM	2-10 min	5-10 min	10-40 min	
Enalapril (Vasotec)	PO	1 hour	4-6 hours	12-24 hours	ACE inhibitor
Enalaprilat (Vasotec IV)	IV	10-15 min	1-4 hours	6 hours	ACE inhibitor
Enoxaparin (LMWheparin)	Subcut	20-60 min	3-5 hours	12 hours	Anticoagulant
Ephedrine	IV	<30 sec	2-5 min	10-60 min	Sympathomimetic
	IM	1-3 min	<10 min	30-60 min	

Continued

Table 19-1   Drugs Used in the Postanesthesia Care Unit: Perianesthesia Drug List—cont'd

DRUG	ROUTE	ONSET	PEAK	DURATION OF ACTION	CLASSIFICATION
Epinephrine (Adrenalin)	IV	<30 sec	2-3 min	5-10 min	Catecholamine
	ETT	15-30 sec	15-25 min	—	
	INH	1 min	1-5 min	1-3 hours	
	Subcut	5-15 min	20 min	—	
Esmolol (Brevibloc)	IV	1-2 min	5-6 min	10-20 min	Cardioselective blocker
Ethacrynic acid (Edecrin)	IV	5-15 min	30 min	2 hours	Loop diuretic
Etidocaine (Duranest)	Infiltration	3-5 min	5-15 min	2-3 hours	Local anesthetic
	Epidural	5-15 min	15-20 min	3-5 hours	
Etomidate (Amidate)	IV	30-60 sec	1 min	5-14 min	Nonbarbiturate hypnotic
Famotidine (Pepcid)	IV	<30 min	30 min	8-12 hours	H_2 antagonist
	PO	20-45 min	1-3 hours	8-12 hours	
Fenoldopam (Corlopam)	IV (continuous infusion)	5 min	15 min	Rapidly metabolized after discontinued	Antihypertensive
Fentanyl (Sublimaze)	IV	<30 sec	3-7 min	30-60 min	Opioid agonist
	Epidural, spinal	4-10 min	<30 min	3-8 hours	
	IM	<8 min	20-30 min	1-2 hours	
	Transdermal	12-18 hours	1-3 days	3 days	
Flumazenil (Romazicon)	IV	1-2 min	6-10 min	45-90 min	Benzodiazepine-receptor antagonist
Furosemide (Lasix)	IV	2-5 min	20-30 min	2 hours	Loop diuretic
	PO	30-60 min	1-2 hours	4-8 hours	
Glucagon	IV, IM	5 min	2-20 min	10-30 min	Antihypoglycemic
Glipizide (Glucotrol)	PO	60-90 min	2-3 hours	10-24 hours	Hypoglycemic
Glycopyrrolate (Robinul)	IV	1-3 min	3-5 min	2-3 hours	Anticholinergic
	IM	15-30 min	30-45 min	2-7 hours	
Granisetron (Kytril)	IV	2-4 min	5-8 min	24 hours	Serotonin receptor antagonist
Haloperidol (Haldol)	IV	5-30 min	1 hour	6-8 hours	Long-acting tranquilizer
Heparin (Liquaemin, Pan heparin)	IV	Immediate	Dose-dependent	Dose-dependent	Anticoagulant
	Subcut	20-30 min	2-4 hours	12-16 hours	
Hetastarch (Hespan)	IV	15-30 min	1 hour	24-48 hours	Plasma expander
Hyaluronidase (Wydase)	Subcut	Immediate	—	30-60 min	Enzyme to increase absorption
Hydralazine (Apresoline)	IV	5-20 min	10-60 min	2-4 hours	Direct-acting arterial vasodilator
	IM	10-30 min	30-80 min	2-8 hours	
	PO	30-120 min	2 hours	2-8 hours	
Hydrocortisone sodium succinate (Solu-Cortef)	IV, IM	5 min	—	30-36 hours	Corticosteroid
Hydromorphone (Dilaudid)	IV	<60 sec	5-20 min	2-4 hours	Opioid (mixed)
	IM, PO	15-30 min	30-60 min	4-6 hours	
Ibutilide fumarate (Covert)	IV	Immediate	10 min	10-30 min	Antiarrhythmic
Insulin, Lente	Subcut	1-4 hours	7-15 hours	18-26 hours	Antidiabetic agent
Insulin, NPH	Subcut	1-2 hours	4-12 hours	18-26 hours	
Insulin, Regular	Subcut	30-60 min	1-5 hours	5-8 hours	

Table 19-1   Drugs Used in the Postanesthesia Care Unit: Perianesthesia Drug List—cont'd

DRUG	ROUTE	ONSET	PEAK	DURATION OF ACTION	CLASSIFICATION
Insulin, Semilente	Subcut	1-3 hours	4-10 hours	12-16 hours	
Insulin, Ultralente	Subcut	4-8 hours	14-24 hours	28-36 hours	
Insulin, NPH 70/Regular 30	Subcut	30 min	2-12 hours	24 hours	
Ipratropium (Atrovent, Itrop)	INH	15-30 min	1-2 hours	4-5 hours	Cholinergic blocker for reactive airways disease
Isoflurane (Forane)	INH	1-2 min	—	15 min after discontinued	Inhalational general anesthetic
Isoproterenol (Isuprel)	IV	Immediate	1 min	1-5 min	Sympathomimetic
Ketamine (Ketalar)	IV	30-60 sec	1 min	5-15 min	Dissociative anesthetic
	IM	3-4 min	5-8 min	12-25 min	
Ketorolac (Toradol)	IV	<1 min	30 min	4-6 hours	Nonsteroidal antiinflammatory
	IM	<10 min	45-60 min	4-6 hours	
	PO	30-60 min	1-3 hours	3-7 hours	
Labetalol (Normo-dyne, Trandate)	IV	1-3 min	5-15 min	15 min to 2 hours	Adrenergic antagonist
	PO	20-40 min	1-4 hours	4-12 hours	
Lansoprazole (Prevacid)	PO	1 hour	2 hours	>24 hours	Proton pump inhibitor
Lidocaine (Xylocaine)	IV	45-90 sec	1-2 min	10-20 min	Local anesthetic
	Epidural	5-15 min	20-30 min	60-120 min	
	Infiltration	<60 sec	20-30 min	30-120 min	
	Spinal	<60 sec	<10 min	60-90 min	
Lorazepam (Ativan)	IV	1-5 min	20-40 min	4-6 hours	Benzodiazepine
	PO	20-30 min	2 hours	10-20 hours	
Magnesium sulfate	IV	Immediate	2-3 min	30 min	Anticonvulsant
Mannitol (Osmitrol)	IV, diuresis	15-60 min	1-3 hours	3-8 hours	Osmotic diuretic
	Epidural	<15 min	60 min	3-8 hours	
	IV, IOP	30-60 min	1-2 hours	4-6 hours	
Meperidine (Demerol)	IV	1-3 min	5-20 min	2-4 hours	Synthetic opioid agonist
	IM	5-10 min	30-50 min	2-4 hours	
	PO	10-45 min	60 min	2-4 hours	
Mepivacaine (Carbocaine)	Epidural	5-15 min	15-45 min	3-5 hours	Local anesthetic
	Infiltration	3-5 min	15-45 min	45-90 min	
Metaproterenol (Metaprel)	INH	<60 sec	60 min	1-4 min	Bronchodilator
Methadone (Dolophine)	IV	1-3 min	15 min	6 hours	Synthetic opioid
	IM	3-60 min	30-60 min	6 hours	
	PO	30-60 min	45 min	6 hours	
Methohexital (Brevital)	IV	<30 sec	30-120 sec	5-10 min	Ultra–short-acting barbiturate
	Rectal	5-7 min	5-10 min	45-90 min	
Methylene blue (Urolene Blue)	IV	<1 min	<1 hour	Varies	Antidote for methemoglobinemia
Methylergonovine (Methergine)	IV	Immediate	5-10 min	45 min	Oxytocic
	IM	2-5 min	30 min	3 hours	

Continued

Table 19-1   Drugs Used in the Postanesthesia Care Unit: Perianesthesia Drug List—cont'd

DRUG	ROUTE	ONSET	PEAK	DURATION OF ACTION	CLASSIFICATION
Metoclopramide (Reglan)	IV	1-3 min	30-60 min	1-2 hours	Dopamine-receptor antagonist-antiemetic
	IM	10-15 min	30-60 min	1-2 hours	
	PO	30-60 min	1-2 hours	1-2 hours	
Metoprolol (Toprol)	IV	<5 min	20 min	5-8 hours	β-Blocker
	PO	<15 min	90 min	12-19 hours	
Midazolam (Versed)	IV	1-5 min	2-5 min	15-90 min	Benzodiazepine
	IM	10-15 min	30-60 min	1-3 hours	
	PO	10-15 min	30-60 min	2-6 hours	
Milrinone (Primacor)	IV	2 min	15 min	2 hours	Inotropic agent
Morphine	IV	<1 min	20 min	2-7 hours	Opioid agonist
Morphine (Duramorph)	Epidural	60 min	90 min	6-18 hours	Opioid agonist
	IM	1-5 min	30-60 min	3-7 hours	
	PO	15-60 min	30-60 min	3-7 hours	
	PO, extended	60-90 min	1-4 hours	6-12 hours	
	Spinal	<60 min	1-2 hours	12-24 hours	
Nalmefene HCl (Revex)	IV	2 min	5 min	4-6 hours	Opioid antagonist
	IV	2-3 min	15-30 min	3-6 hours	
	IM	15 min	30-60 min	3-6 hours	
Naloxone (Narcan)	IV	1-2 min	5-15 min	1-4 hours	Opioid antagonist
	IM	2-5 min	5-15 min	1-4 hours	
Naltrexone (ReVia, Trexan)	PO	5 min	1 hour	24-72 hours	Opioid antagonist
Neostigmine (Prostigmin)	IV	<3 min	7 min	45-60 min	Anticholinesterase
Nicardipine (Cardene)	IV	1 min	15 min	3 hours	Calcium channel blocker
	PO	<30 min	30-60 min	3 hours	
Nifedipine (Procardia)	PO	15-20 min	30-120 min	4-12 hours	Calcium channel blocker
	PO, extended	20-30 min	6 hours	24 hours	
	SL	5 min	20-45 min	4-12 hours	
Nitroglycerin	IV	1-2 min	1-5 min	3-5 min	Peripheral vasodilator
	Ointment	20-60 min	3-6 hours	—	
	SL	1-3 min	30-60 min	—	
	Transdermal	40-60 min	18-24 hours	—	
Nitroprusside (Nipride, Nitropress)	IV	30-60 sec	—	1-10 min	Peripheral vasodilator
Nitrous oxide (N_2O)	INH	1-5 min	—	5-10 min after discontinued	General inhalation anesthetic
Nizatidine (Axid)	PO	30-60 min	30 min-3 hours	8-12 hours	H_2-receptor antagonist
Norepinephrine (Levophed)	IV	<60 sec	1-2 min	2-10 min	Catecholamine
Omeprazole (Prilosec)	PO	1 hour	2 hours	72 hours	Proton pump inhibitor
Ondansetron (Zofran)	IV	<30 min	1-1.5 hours	12-24 hours	Serotonin (5-HT₃) receptor antagonist 5-HT₃
Oxazepam (Serax)	PO	30 min	2 hours	8-12 hours	Benzodiazepine
Oxytocin (Pitocin)	IV	<30 sec	20-40 min	60 min	Oxytocic
	IM	3-5 min	40 min	2-3 hours	
Palonosetron (Aloxi)	IV	5-15 min	2-4 hours	24-72 hours	Antiemetic

Table 19-1   Drugs Used in the Postanesthesia Care Unit: Perianesthesia Drug List—cont'd

DRUG	ROUTE	ONSET	PEAK	DURATION OF ACTION	CLASSIFICATION
Pancuronium (Pavulon)	IV	1-3 min	3-5 min	40-90 min	Nondepolarizing skeletal muscle relaxant
Phentolamine (Regitine)	IV	1-2 min	—	10-15 min	Alpha-adrenergic blocker
	IM	5-20 min	—	30-45 min	
Pentobarbital (Nembutal)	IV	Immediate	1-2 min	15 min	Barbiturate
Phenylephrine (Neo-Synephrine)	IV	<30 sec	1 min	15-20 min	Alpha-adrenergic agonist
Ointment	Ointment	30 min- 4 hours	—	—	
Phenytoin (Dilantin)	IV	3-5 min	1-2 hours	22 hours	Anticonvulsant
Physostigmine (Antilirium)	IV	3-8 min	5-10 min	30 min- 5 hours	Anticholinesterase
Prilocaine (Citanest)	Subcut	1-2 min	<30 min	30 min- 1.5 hours	Local anesthetic
	Epidural	5-15 min	<30 min	1-3 hours	
Procainamide (Pronestyl)	IV	Immediate	5-15 min	2.5-5 hours	Antiarrhythmic
Procaine (Novocain)	Subcut	2-5 min	<30 min	15-30 min	Local anesthetic
	Spinal	2-5 min	<30 min	30 min- 1.5 hours	
	Epidural	5-25 min	<30 min	30 min- 1.5 hours	
Prochlorperazine (Compazine)	IV	3-5 min	15-30 min	3-4 hours	Antiemetic, antipsychotic
	IM	10-20 min	15-30 min	3-4 hours	
	PO	30-40 min	2-4 hours	3-4 hours	
	Rectal	60 min	3-4 hours	—	
Promethazine (Phenergan)	IV	3-5 min	1-2 hours	2-8 hours	Phenothiazine, H_1-receptor antagonist
	IM	20 min	1-2 hours	2-8 hours	
Propofol (Diprivan)	IV	30-60 sec	1 min	5-20 min	Nonbarbiturate anesthesia induction agent
Propanolol (Inderal)	IV	<2 min	1 min	1-6 hours	Alpha-adrenergic receptor antagonist
	PO	30 min	60-90 min	8-12 hours	
Protamine sulfate	IV	30-60 sec	<5 min	2 hours	Heparin antagonist
Ranitidine (Zantac)	IV	<15 min	1-2 hours	6-8 hours	H_2-receptor antagonist
	PO	<30 min	2-3 hours	8-12 hours	
Remifentanil (Ultiva)	IV	1-5 min	—	Opiate effect ceases 18 min after discontinued	Opioid
Ritodrine HCl (Yutopar)	IV	Immediate	—	3-6 hours	α_2-Adrenergic agonist; tocolytic agent
Rocuronium (Zemuron)	IV	45-90 sec	1-3 min	30-120 min	Nondepolarizing NMB agent
Ropivacaine HCl (Naropin)	Subcut	1-5 min	—	2-6 hours	Amide local anesthetic
	Epidural	5-13 min	—	3-5 hours	
Salmeterol (Serevent)	INH	10-20 min	30 min	12 hours	α_2-Adrenergic agonist

Continued

CONCEPTS IN ANESTHETIC AGENTS

Table 19-1	Drugs Used in the Postanesthesia Care Unit: Perianesthesia Drug List—cont'd				
DRUG	**ROUTE**	**ONSET**	**PEAK**	**DURATION OF ACTION**	**CLASSIFICATION**
Scopolamine (Transderm-Scop)	IV	Immediate	—	30-60 min	Anticholinergic
	IM	30 min	—	4-6 hours	
	Transdermal	4 hours	—	72 hours	
Sodium citrate (Bicitra)	PO	2-10 min	60 min	60-90 min	Nonparticulate neutralizing buffer
Somatostatin (Zecnil)	IV	5-10 min	45 min	1 hour	Synthetic somatostatin
Sotalol HCl (Betapace)	PO	1 hour	2.5-4 hours	4-6 hours	Antiarrhythmic
Sodium bicarbonate	IV	2-10 min	10-30 min	30-60 min	Neutralizing buffer
Sodium citrate	PO	<60 sec	3-4 min	2 hours	Neutralizing buffer
Sodium nitroprusside	IV	30-60 sec	1-2 min	1-10 min	Antihypertensive
Succinylcholine (Anectine, Quelicin)	IV	30-60 sec	1 min	4-6 min	Depolarizing skeletal muscle relaxant
	IM	2-3 min	10-30 min	—	
Sufentanil (Sufenta)	IV	1-3 min	3-5 min	20-45 min	Opioid agonist
	Epidural, spinal	4-10 min	<30 min	2-4 hours	
Terbutaline (Brethine)	INH	5-30 min	1-2 hours	3-4 hours	α_2-Adrenergic agonist
	PO	30 min	2-3 hours	4-8 hours	
	Subcut	15 min	30-60 min	1.5-4 hours	
Tetracaine (Pontocaine)	Spinal	<10 min	15-60 min	1.25-3 hours	Local anesthetic
Thiopental (Pentothal)	IV	30-60 sec	20-40 sec	5-15 min	Ultra–short-acting barbiturate
Torsemide (Demadex, Presaril)	IV	10 min	1-2 hours	6-8 hours	Loop diuretic
Vancomycin (Vancocin)	IV	15-30 min	4-6 hours	8-12 hours	Antimicrobial agent
Vasopressin (Pitressin)	IV	15-30 min	30-60 min	2-8 hours	Antidiuretic hormone
Vecuronium (Norcuron)	IV	2-3 min	3-5 min	25-40 min	Nondepolarizing NMB agent
Verapamil (Isoptin)	IV	2-5 min	<10 min	30-60 min	Calcium channel blocker
	PO	30 min	1-2 hours	3-7 hours	
Vitamin K (Aquamephyton)	IM, IV, Subcut	1-3 hours	—	6-48 hours	Water-soluble vitamin
Warfarin (Coumadin)	PO	Up to 5-7 days	—	2-5 days after therapeutic dose reached	Anticoagulant

Adapted from Nagelhout J, Plaus K: *Handbook of nurse anesthesia*, ed 4, St. Louis, 2010, Saunders; *2007 Mosby drug consult*, St. Louis, 2007, Mosby.

IV, Intravenous; *INH*, inhalation; *PO*, by mouth; *NMB*, nondepolarizing neuromuscular blocker; *IO*, intraosseous; *ET*, endotracheal tube; *IM*, intramuscular; *ACE*, angiotensin-converting enzyme; *DDAVP*, 1-deamino-8-D-arginine vasopressin; *Subcut*, subcutaneous; *NPH*, neutral protamine Hagedorn; *IOP*, intraocular pressure; *SL*, sublingual.

prolonged because probenecid delays the excretion of penicillin. This effect can be considered a desirable drug-drug interaction.[10]

Pharmacodynamic Interactions

Pharmacodynamic interactions occur when one drug alters the pharmacologic effects of another drug. For example, when a patient is treated with an antibiotic such as an aminoglycoside or polymyxin and receives a skeletal muscle relaxant such as rocuronium, a prolonged neuromuscular blockage can result. Another example is a patient who receives thiazide diuretic therapy and has resultant hypokalemia. If the patient is administered digitalis, digitalis toxicity can result.[12]

Table 19-2 Drug-Drug or Drug-Induced Interactions in Postanesthesia Care Unit

DRUG	INTERACTIONS	RESULT	MECHANISM
Antihypertensive Drugs			
Propranolol	Inhalation anesthetics	Bradycardia, hypotension	Additive effect
	Lidocaine	Enhanced negative inotropic effect	Propranolol reduces liver blood flow and lidocaine clearance
Lidocaine	Nondepolarizing muscle relaxants	Increased duration of neuromuscular blockade	Synergistic effect
Digitalis	Succinylcholine	Arrhythmias	Direct effect or caused by hyperkalemia that can be induced by succinylcholine
Quinidine	Digitalis (digoxin)	Can produce digitalis intoxication	Decreases digitalis clearance and increases concentration of digitalis
Propranolol	Heparin	Myocardial depression	Heparin increases free fatty acids, which displace propranolol from plasma protein binding sites, leading to increased free propranolol
Quinidine	Myasthenia gravis plus skeletal muscle relaxants	Postoperative respiratory depression	Blockade of acetylcholine receptors at neuromuscular postsynaptic membrane
Digitalis	Thiazide diuretics	Increased potassium excretion by kidneys	Combined effect of two drugs on kidneys promotes potassium excretion
Antibiotics			
Neomycin Streptomycin Dihydrostreptomycin Polymyxin A Polymyxin B Colistin Viomycin Paromomycin Kanamycin Lincomycin Gentamicin Tetracycline	Nondepolarizing skeletal muscle relaxants	Potentiates nondepolarizing muscle relaxants, respiratory depression	Neuromuscular blockade caused by reduction in amplitude of end-plate potential
Opioids			
Morphine Meperidine Fentanyl Sufentanil Remifentanil	Inhalation anesthetics	Potentiation, respiratory, and cardiovascular depression	Depressant effects of inhalation anesthetics and opioids are additive
Meperidine	Enovid	Birth control pill potentiates meperidine	Excess female sex hormones with oral contraceptive therapy, which may slow metabolism of meperidine
Meperidine	Norinyl MAOI	MAOI interacts with meperidine metabolite	Type I: Seizures Type II: Hypotension

Continued

Table 19-2	Drug-Drug or Drug-Induced Interactions in Postanesthesia Care Unit—cont'd		
DRUG	INTERACTIONS	RESULT	MECHANISM
Sympathomimetic Amines			
Epinephrine	Inhalation anesthetics	Cardiac arrhythmias	Anesthetic agents may sensitize myocardium to endogenous and exogenous catecholamines
Electrolytes			
Increased extracellular potassium	Skeletal muscle relaxants	Increased resistance to depolarization and greater sensitivity to nondepolarizing muscle relaxants	Acute increase in extracellular potassium increases end-plate transmembrane potential, thus causing hyperpolarization
Decreased extracellular potassium	Skeletal muscle relaxants	Increased effects of depolarizing muscle relaxants and increased resistance to nondepolarizing muscle relaxants	Acute decrease in extracellular potassium lowers resting end-plate transmembrane potential
Increased calcium levels	Nondepolarizing skeletal muscle relaxants	Decreased response	Calcium increases quantal release of acetylcholine and enhances excitation-contraction coupling mechanism
Magnesium ions	Muscle relaxants	Potentiation	Magnesium ions cause partial muscle relaxation by blocking release of acetylcholine
Calcium chloride	Digitalis	Additive effect on heart	High concentrations of calcium inhibit positive inotropic actions of digitalis and potentiate digitalis toxicity
Miscellaneous			
Furosemide Thiazide Ethacrynic acid	Nondepolarizing skeletal muscle relaxants	Intensified neuromuscular block	Electrolyte imbalance (hypokalemia)
Procaine Lidocaine	Nondepolarizing and depolarizing skeletal muscle relaxants	Enhanced neuromuscular blockade	Decreased end-plate potential
Lithium	Nondepolarizing and depolarizing skeletal muscle relaxants	Potentiated neuromuscular blockade	Lithium ions are substituted for sodium ions at presynaptic level
Chlorpromazine	Nondepolarizing skeletal muscle relaxants	Enhanced neuromuscular blockade	Potentiation of neuromuscular blockade
All inhalation anesthetics	Nondepolarizing skeletal muscle relaxants	Augment block in dose-dependent manner	Central nervous system depression or presynaptic inhibition of acetylcholine
Insulin	Corticosteroids, oral contraceptives, loop and thiazide diuretics	Reduction in effects	Insulin antagonizes effects
Hydrocortisone Dexamethasone Prednisolone	Phenobarbital	Decreased effects of the steroids	Increased metabolism

MAOI, Monoamine oxidase inhibitor.

DRUG-DRUG INTERACTIONS AND THE PACU

Antibiotics

Aminoglycoside and polymyxin antibiotics have been reported to interact with some anesthetic agents and with skeletal muscle relaxants. Streptomycin and the other aminoglycoside antibiotics gentamicin, tobramycin, amikacin, neomycin, kanamycin, and paromomycin can produce a partial neuromuscular blockade by inhibiting the release of acetylcholine from the presynaptic membrane and by altering calcium mobility in muscles. When a nondepolarizing skeletal muscle relaxant such as rocuronium is administered to a patient who receives an aminoglycoside antibiotic, the neuromuscular blockade is intensified and pharmacologic reversal is difficult.[9]

Opioids

Probably the most significant and dangerous drug-drug interaction that can occur in the perianesthesia period is the interaction between meperidine (Demerol) and monoamine oxidase inhibitors (MAOIs). The presumed physiologic dysfunction is that the MAOI decelerates the breakdown of meperidine because of N-demethylase inhibition by the MAOI. The result of the interaction between these two drugs is either a type I response that includes seizures, agitation, rigidity, and hyperpyrexia or a type II response that is depressive in nature and characterized by hypotension, respiratory depression, and coma.

Every perianesthesia nurse has probably observed the drug-drug interaction between opioids administered in the PACU and the inhalation anesthetic agents administered in the operating room. If the anesthetic agent has not been completely eliminated and the patient is administered an opioid, an additive effect between the two drugs occurs. The outcome of this interaction is usually respiratory depression resulting from the combined depressant effects.

If the two drugs have interacted in this way, an opioid antagonist, such as naloxone (Narcan), can be administered to reverse the respiratory depression produced by the opioid. However, naloxone does not reverse respiratory depression produced by inhalation anesthetic agents such as sevoflurane, desflurane, or isoflurane.[13]

Steroids

The use of exogenous steroids administered to a patient with steroid dependency is not actually an interaction of two drugs that alters one of the pharmacokinetic parameters, however the problems that can result will be discussed.

Patients with adrenocortical insufficiency cannot withstand the stress of anesthesia and surgery. For example, if a patient with chronic obstructive pulmonary disease has been treated with long-term steroids, there is usually some degree of adrenocortical insufficiency. As a result, the patient may react to surgery and anesthesia with hypotension, respiratory depression, or delayed recovery. To prevent a hypotensive crisis during the perioperative period, these patients are usually given a maintenance dosage of corticosteroids before, during, and after the surgical procedure.

If these symptoms appear in a patient in the PACU who did not receive this steroid coverage, the preferred treatment is hydrocortisone (see Chapter 15).[14] Major drug groups and intended outcomes in respiratory care are listed in Table 19-3.

SPECIAL CONSIDERATIONS IN PHARMACOLOGY ASSOCIATED WITH PERIANESTHESIA CARE

Sedative Drugs for PACU Patients

Patients in the PACU sometimes need sedation for a variety of reasons, most commonly fear, pain, loss of control, confusion, noise, lights, and alarms. These stimuli can cause a stress response that is experienced by some patients in the PACU; sedative drugs are sometimes used to prevent the adverse physiologic effects of stress, such as increased oxygen consumption, tachycardia, hypertension, and exacerbated hyperglycemia. The drugs that are most commonly used for sedation in the PACU are listed in Box 19-1. The institution of drugs to promote sedation is a difficult task in the PACU because the patient may have residual effects of the intraoperative anesthetic agents still active in the body. A bedside sedation scoring system is helpful in determining the degree of sedation and predicting when concerns about oversedation should be realized. Although many sedation scoring systems are available, the Ramsay Sedation Scoring System appears to be appropriate for assessing drug-induced sedation. The Ramsay Scale consists of six scoring levels. The first three levels (Table 19-4) are usually administered while the patient is awake, and levels 4 through 6 are assessed during varying degrees of sleep. Because oversedation is associated with increased risk of edema, thromboemboli, gastric regurgitation, and aspiration, to name a few, patients in the

Table 19-3	Major Drug Groups and Intended Outcome in Respiratory Care	
DRUG GROUP	**INTENDED PHYSIOLOGIC RESPONSE**	**GENERIC AGENT (TRADE NAME)**
Adrenergic agents	Alpha-adrenergic stimulation produces bronchial relaxation to reduce airway resistance and improve flow rates in patients with obstructive lung disease	Epinephrine, isoproterenol (Isuprel), isoetharine (Bronkosol), terbutaline (Brethine), metaproterenol (Metaprel), albuterol (Ventolin), pirbuterol (Maxair), bitolterol (Tornalate), salmeterol (Serevent), procaterol (Mescalcin)
	Alpha-adrenergic stimulation produces bronchial relaxation, peripheral vascular vasoconstriction, and nasal decongestion	Ephedrine, phenylephrine (Neo-Synephrine)
Anticholinergic agents	Relaxation of cholinergic (vagal)-induced bronchoconstriction to improve flow rates in patients with obstructive lung disease	Ipratropium (Atrovent)
Mucoactive agents	Modification of properties of respiratory tract mucus to facilitate clearance of secretions	Acetylcystine (Mucomist), dornase alfa (Pulmozyme)
Corticosteroids	Reduce inflammation in respiratory tract	Dexamethasone (Decadron), beclomethasone (Vanceril), triamcinolone (Kenalog), flunisolide (Aerobid), fluticasone (Flonase/Flovent), budesonide (Rhinocort)
Antiasthmatic agents	Inhibits chemical mediators of inflammation to help prevent onset of asthma attack	Cromolyn (Intal), nedocromil (Tilade), zafirlukast (Accolate), zileuton (Zyflo), montelukast (Singulair)
Antiinfective agents	Inhibits or stops specific infective agents, such as *Pneumocystis carinii* (pentamidine) or respiratory syncytial virus (ribavirin), or for management of *Pseudomonas aeruginosa* in cystic fibrosis (tobramycin)	Pentamidine, ribavirin (Rebetron), tobramycin (TOBI)
Exogenous surfactants	Enhances lung compliance by reducing surface tension; approved for direct intra-tracheal instillation	Colfosceril (Exosurf), beractant (Survanta)

Adapted from Rau J: Recent developments in respiratory care pharmacology, *J Perianesth Nurs* 13:362, 1998.

BOX 19-1	Drugs Commonly Used in the Postanesthesia Care Unit for Sedation

- Dexmedetomidine
- Fentanyl
- Lorazepam
- Midazolam
- Haloperidol
- Propofol

PACU should have Ramsay Sedation levels in the range of 3 or less.[15,16]

Herbal Medicines

During the past few years, the use of herbal products has greatly increased, and many patients receiving care in the PACU are taking one or more of these preparations. Research into the effect of herbal medications during the perioperative period is lacking, particularly in the area of the effect on postoperative outcomes. In response, the American Society of Anesthesiologists has issued a statement cautioning patients who take herbal products to refrain from those medications at least 2 weeks before surgery.[17] Because of the possible negative perianesthesia outcome caused by herbal products, a brief overview of the more popular herbal products is presented in Table 19-5.

Drugs Used in the Postanesthesia Care Unit

Because of all the possible drugs used in the PACU, Table 19-1 presents most of the drugs that can be used in the perianesthesia care of the surgical patient.

SUMMARY

The intent of this chapter is to provide the perianesthesia nurse with a review of the drugs that are currently used in the perianesthesia period.

Table 19-4   Ramsay Sedation Scoring System

RAMSAY SCORE	CLINICAL PARAMETERS FOR BEDSIDE ASSESSMENT OF SEDATION	GLOBAL DEGREE OF SEDATION
1	Anxious, restless, perhaps agitated	
2	Cooperative and oriented	Varying degrees of awake state
3	Easily arousable, responds appropriately	
4	Brisk response to light glabellar tap or loud auditory stimulus	
5	Sluggish response to glabellar tap or auditory stimulus	Varying degrees of asleep state
6	Asleep, does not respond to previous stimuli	

From Prielipp R, Young C: Current drugs for sedation of critically ill patients, *Semin Anesthesia Perioperative Med Pain* 20: 85-94, 2001.

Table 19-5   Herbal Drugs and Possible Interactions with Anesthesia

HERB	ACTIONS	KEY COMPONENT	UNTOWARD EFFECTS
Aristolochia	Aphrodisiac and anticonvulsant	Aristolochic acid	Nephrotoxic and cardiogenic
Ephedra	Weight loss, stimulant, ergogenic	Ephedrine	Adrenergic stimulant; hypertension, bronchodilatation, diuresis, tachycardia
Feverfew	Temperature reduction, migraine prophylaxis, treatment of rheumatoid arthritis	Parthenolide	Risk of bleeding, insomnia, anxiety; should be discontinued 1 week before surgery
Garlic	Reduction in blood pressure, decrease in total cholesterol	Allicin	Risk of postoperative bleeding; should be discontinued 1 week before surgery
Ginger	Decreases platelet aggregation, antiemetic, motion sickness	Oleoresins	Risk of postoperative bleeding; should be discontinued 1 week before surgery
Ginkgo	Improved cognitive function, chronic venous insufficiency, decreases RBC aggregation, memory loss	Ginkgo biloba extract	Significant risk of postoperative bleeding; should be discontinued 1 week before surgery
Ginseng	Stress reduction, increased physical performance, improved cardiovascular function, anticancer properties, antioxidant	Ginsenosides	Insomnia, irritability, and mania; interactions with digoxin, warfarin, and lithium; should be discontinued 1 week before surgery
Golden seal	Laxative, antiinflammatory, antiemetic	Berberine, hydrastine	Seizures, respiratory depression, hypertension, electrolyte imbalance
Kava	Anxiolytic, analgesic, muscle relaxant, anticonvulsant, local anesthetic properties	Kavapyrones	MAOI, platelet aggregation inhibition, potentiate anesthetics; should be discontinued 1 week before surgery
St. John's Wort	Antidepressant, sedative, hypnotic	Hypericin, pseudohypericin	Should not be administered with other antidepressants; potential to interact with amphetamines and adrenergic stimulants; prolongs effects of anesthesia because antidepressants may be used in perioperative period; should be discontinued 1 week before surgery.
Valerian	Sedative, muscle relaxant	Valerianic acid	Potentiates sedatives, including anesthetics

RBC, Red blood cell; *MAOI*, monoamine oxidase inhibitor.

An overview of the pharmacodynamics and pharmacokinetics was presented, and the common drugs were presented in table form along with the drug-drug interactions and an overview of the drugs used in sedation. Finally, because many people take some form of herbal drugs, a brief overview is present on this area of pharmacology.

REFERENCES

1. Lee A, et al: Incidence and risk of adverse perioperative events among surgical patients taking traditional Chinese herbal medicines, *Anesthesiology* 105:454–61, 2006.
2. Moss J, Yuan C: Herbal medicines and perioperative care, *Anesthesiology* 105:441–2, 2006.
3. Bardal SK, et al: *Applied pharmacology*, St. Louis, 2011, Saunders.
4. Chisholm-Burns MA, et al: *Pharmacotherapy: principles and practice*, ed 2, New York, 2010, McGraw-Hill.
5. Katzung BG, et al: *Basic and clinical pharmacology*, ed 11, New York, 2009, McGraw Hill.
6. Brunton L: *Goodman & Gilman's the pharmacological basis of therapeutics*, ed 12, New York, 2011, McGraw-Hill.
7. Rang HP, et al: *Rang and Dale's pharmacology*, ed 6, London, 2007, Churchill Livingstone.
8. Hall JE: *Guyton and Hall textbook of medical physiology*, ed 12, Philadelphia, 2011, Saunders.
9. Nagelhout J, Plaus K: *Nurse anesthesia*, ed 4, St. Louis, 2010, Saunders.
10. Dipiro JT, et al: *Pharmacotherapy: a pathophysiologic approach*, ed 7, New York, 2008, McGraw-Hill.
11. Miller RD, et al: *Miller's anesthesia*, ed 7, Philadelphia, 2009, Churchill Livingstone.
12. Barasch PG, et al: *Clinical anesthesia*, ed 6, Philadelphia, 2009, Lippincott Williams & Wilkins.
13. Longnecker DE, et al: *Anesthesiology*, New York, 2008, McGraw-Hill.
14. Elisha S: *Case studies in nurse anesthesia*, Sudbury, Mass, 2011, Jones and Bartlett.
15. Atlee JL: *Complications in anesthesia*, ed 2, Philadelphia, 2007, Saunders.
16. Fleisher LA: *Anesthesia and uncommon diseases*, ed 5, Philadelphia, 2006, Saunders.
17. Kaye AD, et al: Perioperative anesthesia clinical considerations of alternative medicines, *Anesthesiol Clin North America* 22(1):125–39, 2004.

20 Inhalation Anesthesia

Cecil B. Drain, PhD, RN, CRNA, FAAN, FASAHP

The inhalation anesthetic agents have undergone a significant transition over the last three decades. Inhalation agents used in the past possessed many positive attributes to include postoperative analgesia and sedation. The emergence from the inhalation anesthetic was slow and not without its difficulties. Research on the inhalational anesthetic agents has been positive and productive, leading to the use of rapid-acting agents. Patients emerge from anesthesia in minutes instead of hours. As a result, patients can be discharged rapidly from perianesthesia care and ultimately the health care facility. It is important to understand the many physiologic and pharmacologic effects of all the anesthetic agents, both used presently and in the past.

The inhalation anesthetic agents in use today have survived the many examinations of research, and clinically they have been shown to add significant safety factors and improved outcomes for perianesthesia patients. Research continues in this area; for example, xenon is under evaluation as an inhalation anesthetic agent.[1] Other volatile agents are undergoing evaluation, all in an effort to find the inhalational agent that best represents all the facets of anesthesia, such as muscle relaxation, sedation, analgesia, amnesia, with minimal effects on the major organ systems of the body.

To anticipate a patient's reaction on emergence from an inhalation anesthetic in the postanesthesia care unit (PACU), the perianesthesia nurse should have a thorough understanding of the pharmacologic concepts of inhalation anesthesia. It is difficult to predict the exact nature of each patient's emergence from inhalation anesthesia because of the complexity of these agents, coupled with drug interactions and the various levels of physical health. An understanding of some general principles prepares the perianesthesia nurse for the most commonly expected outcomes.

DEFINITIONS

Adjustable Positive-Pressure Relief (APR) Valve: Used for release of excessive gas on the circle system of an anesthesia machine.

Amnesia: A component of anesthesia in which the patient is unable to recall the events that occurred during the administration of the inhalational anesthetic.

Analgesia: A component of anesthesia in which the patient is unable to experience pain.

CO_2 Absorption Canisters: Located in a circle system on an anesthesia machine that clears rebreathed gas that contains carbon dioxide by passing through a canister containing a chemical carbon dioxide absorbent.

Delirium: A portion of a stage of anesthesia in which the patient has a transient disturbance during a loss of consciousness accompanied by a change in cognition that has a fluctuating course.

Diffusion Hypoxia: Sometimes referred to as the *Fink phenomenon;* refers to the rapid exit of nitrous oxide and thus partial reduction of the percentage of oxygen that can be inhaled during the immediate (first 4 to 5 minutes) emergence phase of recovery from anesthesia. Supplemental oxygen and the use of the modified stir-up regime negate this effect of nitrous oxide on emergence.

Effective Dose (ED): The dose of a drug necessary to produce a certain effect in a certain percentage of patients. For example, the ED_{50} is the term for when a drug produces a particular effect in 50% of patients.

Hypnosis: A component of anesthesia in which the patient becomes unconscious.

Inhalation Anesthesia: Anesthetic substances, in either volatile or gaseous form, that are inhaled via an anesthesia machine.

Lacrimation: Tears from the lacrimal glands on the medial side of the tissue surrounding the eyes.

Minimal Alveolar Concentration (MAC): A measure of potency of inhalation anesthetic agents; occurs when the equilibrium end-tidal anesthetic concentrations, expressed as a fraction of 1 atm, prevent movement in response to surgical skin incision in 50% of human subjects.

Muscle Relaxation: A component of anesthesia in which the patient has reduced tension of the skeletal muscle.

Nociception: A component of anesthesia in which the patient is unable to sense pain.

Scavenger System: Used to reduce exposure to escaping gases from the anesthesia machine; a waste gas suction tube (scavenger) is connected to the adjustable positive-pressure relief valve and anesthesia ventilator relief valve, and the gases are then vented to the outside atmosphere via an operating room suction system.

Solubility Coefficient: The ratio of the concentration of an anesthetic in blood or other tissue to that in a gas phase when the two are in equilibrium.

Sympatholysis: A component of anesthesia in which the patient is blocked from having an autonomic response to nociceptive (painful) stimuli.

Vaporizer: A device on the anesthesia machine that converts liquid anesthetics into metered amounts of vapor that are added to the fresh gas mixture to produce a known concentration of the vaporized form of the inhalational anesthetic agent.

BASIC CONCEPTS

Evolution of the Signs and Stages of Anesthesia

The five components of anesthesia are hypnosis, analgesia, muscle relaxation, sympatholysis, and amnesia. In the past, when diethyl ether was the primary general anesthetic, assessment of anesthetic depth with the signs and stages of anesthesia was simple; the patient could be monitored by assessing the pupils, respiratory activity, muscle tone, and various reflexes. The ether signs and stages were devised to provide a means of assessing the depth of anesthesia. The first three stages were described by Plomley in 1847; 1 year later, John Snow added a fourth stage: overdose.[2] During

World War I, Guedel more accurately defined and described the signs and stages of anesthesia. A graphic representation of these signs and stages is provided in Fig. 20-1.

With the advent of modern anesthesia, which includes the addition of fluorinated inhalation anesthetic agents, muscle relaxants, and various pharmacologic adjuncts, the usual predictable signs and stages as described by Guedel were abolished. Currently in the PACU, many of these pharmacologic adjuncts have an affect on predicting the depth of anesthesia. The classic signs and stages provide some help in the assessment and care of the patient after surgery. Many times in modern anesthesia practice, these signs and stages provide a basic language for describing the level of anesthesia during and after surgery. Consequently, a brief description, including the incorporation of some of the pharmacology of the modern anesthetics, is given.

Stage I begins with the initiation of anesthesia and ends with the loss of consciousness. It is commonly called the *stage of analgesia*. This stage has been described as the lightest level of anesthesia and represents sensory and mental depression. Stage I is the level of anesthesia used with nitrous oxide. Patients are able to open their eyes on command, breathe normally, maintain protective reflexes, and tolerate mild painful stimuli.

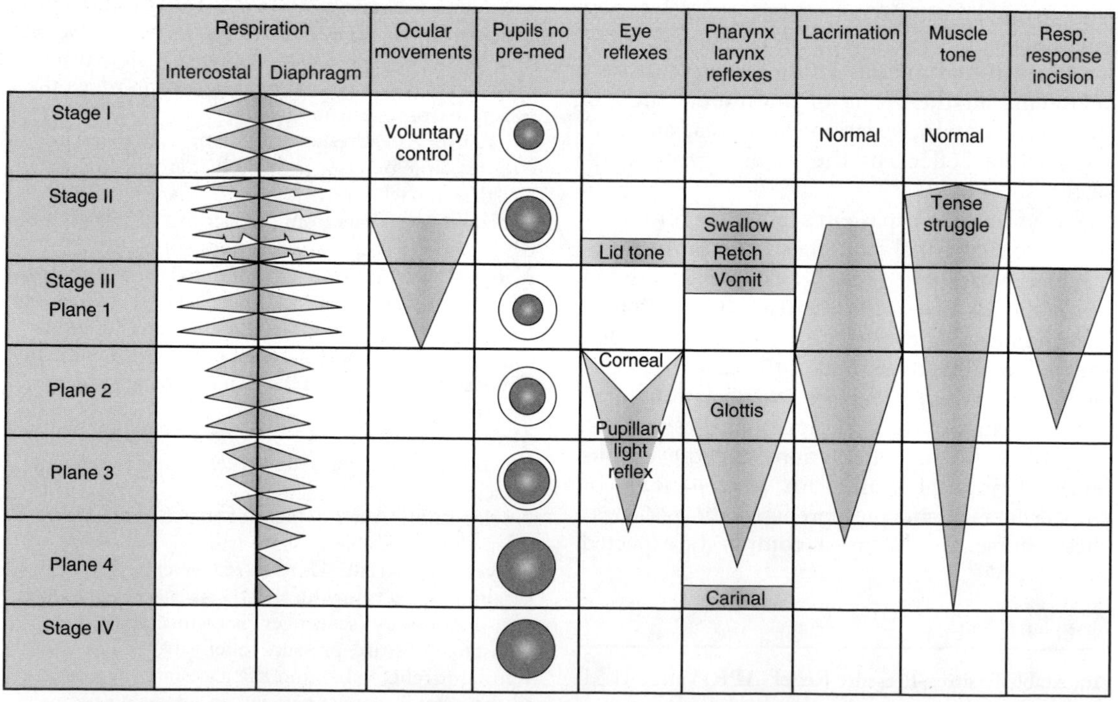

FIG. 20-1 Signs and reflex reactions of stages of anesthesia. (Adapted from Gillespie NA: Signs of anesthesia, *Anesth Analg* 22:275, 1943.)

Stage II starts with the loss of consciousness and ends with the onset of a regular pattern of breathing and the disappearance of the lid reflex; this is also called the *stage of delirium*. This stage is characterized by excitement, and so many untoward responses such as vomiting, laryngospasm, and even cardiac arrest can take place during this stage. With the use of anesthetic agents that act much more rapidly than ether, this stage is passed rather quickly. In addition, the induction of anesthesia is usually facilitated with short-acting barbiturates that expedite a short duration of stage II.

Stage III is the stage of surgical anesthesia. With ether anesthesia, this stage is defined as lasting from the onset of a regular pattern of breathing to the cessation of respiration. At this stage of anesthesia, response to surgical incision is absent. The modern concept of minimal alveolar concentration (MAC) is predicated in part with the signs and stages of surgical anesthesia. MAC is exceeded by a factor of 1.3 in stage III because most patients do not respond to surgical incision at this level of anesthesia. Patients who receive 1.3 MAC anesthesia[3] have a depression in all elements of nervous system function—that is, sensory depression, loss of recall, reflex depression, and some skeletal muscle relaxation. From this point, with the modern anesthetics, increased MAC results in further respiratory, cardiovascular, and central nervous system (CNS) depression. The difficulty is that each of the newer agents affects the clinical signs, such as blood pressure, differently. Consequently, monitoring of the level of anesthesia depends on the particular properties of each agent.

Most surgical procedures in which ether anesthesia was used were performed at this stage of anesthesia, which is divided into four planes.[4] Plane 1 is entered when the lid reflex is abolished and respiration becomes regular. During this plane, the vomiting reflex is gradually abolished. The nurse working in the PACU must know that swallowing, retching, and vomiting reflexes tend to disappear in that order during induction and reappear in the same order during emergence from anesthesia.

Plane 2 lasts from the time the eyeballs cease to move and become concentrically fixed to the beginning of a decrease of activity of the intercostal muscles, or thoracic respiration. The reflex of laryngospasm disappears during this plane. Plane 3 is entered when intercostal activity begins to decrease. Complete intercostal paralysis occurs in lower plane 3, and respiration is produced solely by the diaphragm. Plane 4 lasts from the time of paralysis of the intercostal muscles to the cessation of spontaneous respiration.

Tracheal tug often appears in association with deep anesthesia and intercostal paralysis. This effect represents an unopposed action of the diaphragm, which displaces the hilum of the lung and thereby increases traction on the trachea.

Stage IV lasts from the time of cessation of respiration to failure of the circulatory system. This level of anesthesia is called the *stage of overdose*.

When ether was used as the sole inhalation agent, these signs and stages were seen in reverse order on emergence from the anesthetic. No one clinical sign can be considered a reliable indicator of anesthetic depth by itself. All clinical signs must be viewed in the context of the patient's status along with the particular characteristics of the individual anesthetic agent used.

Some of the more reliable indicators of depth of anesthesia for the more modern inhalation anesthetics include changes in breathing pattern, eye movement, lacrimation, and muscle tone. Because the ventilation is under autonomic control, it is the most sensitive indicator of depth of anesthesia. In the PACU, a patient who uses diaphragmatic ventilation without the intercostal muscles should be considered to be in surgical anesthesia. As the ventilatory pattern returns to a more normal rate, rhythm, and pattern, the patient can be considered to be in light anesthesia and about to have total emergence. Eye movement as opposed to pupillary size is a good indicator of anesthetic depth. Light anesthesia is present with eye movement. Deeper anesthesia is present when the eyes are close together in a cross-eyed position. Lacrimation does not occur during surgical anesthesia when a patient receives desflurane (Suprane), isoflurane (Forane), or sevoflurane (Ultane). Conversely, if a patient received one of those drugs and has tearing, light anesthesia can be considered to be present. As the depth of anesthesia is increased, the amount of muscle tone decreases. Therefore, if a patient in the PACU lacks muscle tone, especially in the jaw and abdomen, the patient should be considered to be in a surgical depth of anesthesia. With the assessment of the degree of muscle tone, the perianesthesia nurse must critically assess the degree of reversal of skeletal muscle relaxants (see Chapter 23) before determining the depth of anesthesia with the criterion of muscle tone. Finally, because the determinants of anesthesia depth have such a high degree of variability, all possible assessment tools should be incorporated into the care of the patient in the PACU. The bottom line is constant vigilance of the patient's physiologic parameters during emergence from anesthesia and the institution of appropriate nursing interventions based on an ongoing assessment.

Pharmacokinetics of Inhalation Anesthetics

The pharmacokinetics of inhalation anesthetics involve uptake, distribution, metabolism, and elimination. Basically, this involves a series of partial pressure gradients starting in the anesthesia machine to the patient's brain for induction, and vice versa for emergence. The object of anesthesia is a constant and optimal partial pressure in the brain. The key to attainment of anesthesia is the alveolar partial pressure (PA) in equilibrium with the arterial partial pressure (Pa) and brain partial pressure (Pbr) of the inhaled anesthetic.[4] The partial pressure of an inhalation anesthetic in the brain is used to determine the depth of anesthesia. The more potent the anesthetic, the lower the partial pressure of the agent needed to produce a certain depth of anesthesia.

Movement of Inhalation Anesthetic from Anesthesia Machine to Alveoli

The determinants of the PA are the inspired partial pressure of the inhalation anesthetic, the characteristics of the anesthesia machine's delivery system, and the patient's alveolar ventilation. The inhaled partial pressure (PI) is the concentration of the inhalation anesthetic that is delivered from the anesthesia machine. The effect of the PI on the rate of increase in the PA is called the *concentration effect*. The higher the inhaled concentration, the more rapid the induction of anesthesia. The anesthesia machine's delivery system has an effect on the depth of anesthesia and the speed of induction and emergence. For example, the rate of uptake of an anesthetic agent administered via inhalation can be reduced with the diffusion of the anesthetic agent into the rubber tubing of the anesthesia machine, the small losses of anesthetic agent from the body via diffusion

across skin and mucous membranes, and, to a lesser extent, the metabolism of the agents by the body.

Alveolar ventilation plays the primary role in delivery of the anesthetic gas. It is determined in large part by the minute ventilation ($\dot{V}_E$). If the $\dot{V}_E$ is high, the anesthetic concentration increases quickly in the alveoli, as does the concentration in the arterial blood. This concept is important to understand because the reverse also is true. In the emergence phase of anesthesia, a good $\dot{V}_E$ is important to ensure elimination of the anesthetic agent.

Movement of Inhalation Anesthetic from Alveoli to Arterial Blood

The movement of the inhalation anesthetic agent from the alveoli to the arterial blood depends on the blood-gas partition coefficient and the cardiac output. The rate at which the anesthetic is taken up by the blood and tissues is governed in part by the solubility of the agent in blood. This is expressed as the *blood-gas partition coefficient*, or the *Oswald solubility coefficient*, and is defined as the ratio of the concentration of an anesthetic in blood to that in a gas phase when the two are in equilibrium (Table 20-1). This concept is difficult to understand because the more soluble the anesthetic agent is, the slower the agent is in producing anesthesia. This effect is because the blood serves as a reservoir and a large volume of the agent must be introduced to attain an equilibrium between the blood partial pressure and the partial pressure in the lungs.

The blood conveys the anesthetic agent to the tissues. Consequently, a normal cardiac output is needed for facilitation of the movement of the inhalation anesthetic through the tissues to the brain. The partial pressure increases most rapidly in the tissues with the highest rates of blood flow. Of interest is the great variation in blood perfusion of certain tissues in the body.

Table 20-1 **Properties of Inhalant Anesthetic Agents**				
	PARTITION COEFFICIENT			
ALVEOLAR AGENT	**BLOOD-GAS**	**OIL-GAS**	**BLOOD-BRAIN**	**MINIMAL CONCENTRATION (% IN OXYGEN)**
Isoflurane (Forane)	0.97	93.7	1.6	1.15
Desflurane (Suprane)	0.42	20.7	1.3	6.58
Sevoflurane (Ultane)	0.69	53.4	1.7	1.71
Nitrous oxide	0.47	1.4	1.1	104.0

The body tissue compartments can be divided into the following major groups:
- The vessel-rich group, which consists of the heart, brain, kidneys, hepatoportal system, and endocrine glands
- The intermediate group of perfused tissues, which consists of muscle and skin
- The fat group, which includes marrow and adipose tissue
- The vessel-poor group, which has the poorest circulation per unit volume and comprises tendons, ligaments, connective tissue, teeth, bone, and other avascular tissue

The vessel-rich group of tissues receives 75% of the cardiac output; thus, the brain becomes saturated rapidly with an anesthetic agent administered via inhalation. On termination of the anesthetic, the reverse takes place, and the agent is rapidly removed from the brain.

The tissue tensions of the inhaled anesthetic increase and approach the arterial blood tension and ultimately the PA. One of the tissue groups that affects both the induction and the emergence from anesthesia is the fat group. The oil-gas partition coefficient best exemplifies the process involved with the affinity of anesthesia agents to adipose tissue and ultimately the emergence from anesthesia. The oil-gas partition coefficient is defined as the ratio of the concentration of the anesthetic agent in oil (adipose tissue) to that in a gaseous phase when the two are in equilibrium (see Table 20-1). The oil-gas partition coefficients seem to parallel anesthetic requirements. In fact, it is possible to calculate the MAC by knowing the oil-gas partition coefficient. With the constant of 150, the calculated MAC for an anesthetic with an oil-gas partition coefficient of 100 is 1.5%.

Because some anesthetic agents are highly fat soluble, they tend to be readily absorbed by the adipose tissue. This characteristic affects uptake of the anesthetic agent, but of more importance is the prolonged recovery phase that usually ensues with a high oil-gas partition coefficient, such as in the case of halothane. Because adipose tissue is poorly perfused by blood, the adipose tissue releases the agent slowly to the blood at the termination of the anesthesia. Redistribution then takes place; some of the agent is eliminated by the lungs, which are vessel rich, and some is distributed to the brain. The recovery period becomes significantly extended when the administration time of the anesthetic agent is prolonged to allow for complete saturation of the adipose tissue.

Halothane (Fluothane) was the classic inhalation anesthetic from the 1960s to the 1990s.

Inclusion of halothane in the discussion is helpful because all the inhalation anesthetic agents currently in use have almost the same partition coefficients. Halothane has an oil-gas partition coefficient that is approximately twice that of isoflurane, desflurane, or sevoflurane; therefore, with use of halothane as the marker, the newer inhalation agents are twice as fast during induction and emergence as before. All three of the inhalational anesthetics currently in use are used in a variety of settings, and all possess a blood-gas partition coefficient less than 1 (see Table 20-1).

Movement of Inhalation Anesthetic from Arterial Blood to the Brain

The transfer of the inhalation anesthetic from the arterial blood to the brain depends on the blood-brain partition coefficient of the agent and the cerebral blood flow. The blood-brain partition coefficient for most of the inhalation anesthetics is between 1.3 and 2 (see Table 20-1). The concentration gradient during induction of anesthesia is as follows:

$$PA > Pa > Pbr$$

During maintenance of surgical anesthesia, the brain tissue becomes saturated with the anesthetic agent and the brain tissue is in equilibrium with the alveolar and arterial concentration. Consequently:

$$PA = Pa = Pbr$$

Emergence of Inhalation Anesthesia

When the administration of the anesthetic is terminated, a reverse gradient takes place. In this instance, the PA is almost zero because only oxygen is administered during the emergence phase. The gradient that develops is as follows:

$$PA < Pa < Pbr$$

This gradient favors the removal of the anesthetic agent from the brain tissue. The partial pressure in the tissues declines first and is followed by that in the arterial blood. The agent returns to the lungs and is then eliminated into the atmosphere. The factors that affect the rate of elimination of the agent are the same ones that determine how rapidly an anesthetic agent takes a patient to surgical anesthesia. If a short procedure is performed (less than 1 hour), complete equilibrium among PA, Pa, and Pbr might not have occurred, and the recovery from anesthesia is more rapid. The reverse is true; during long procedures in which equilibrium occurs, a prolonged emergence may be anticipated.

Potency of Inhalation Anesthetic Agents

Potency is determined by factors such as absorption, distribution, metabolism, excretion, and affinity for a receptor. The potency of the anesthetic agent refers to its ability to take the patient through all the stages of anesthesia to respiratory and circulatory arrest without the occurrence of hypoxia or the use of preanesthetic medication. Certainly, circulatory and respiratory arrests are not desired outcomes of the use of anesthetic agents; these features are used merely to describe the potency of anesthetic agents that are used clinically. For example, isoflurane is 100% potent compared with nitrous oxide, which is 15% potent. Isoflurane, when administered with oxygen to meet the patient's metabolic needs and when given without premedication, takes the patient to circulatory and respiratory arrest, whereas nitrous oxide administered with oxygen takes the patient only to the first portion of surgical anesthesia and no further. Therefore, clinically speaking, potency of a drug makes little difference as long as the drug that is to be administered has an effective dose for a particular patient, which is why the concept of ED was developed. The ED is the dose of a drug necessary to produce certain effects in a certain percentage of patients. For example, an ED_{50} means that a drug produces a particular effect in 50% of the patients.[4]

Another method of determination of potency is with the use of the MAC. The MAC is found with determining the alveolar concentration (at 1 atm) needed for prevention of gross muscular movement in response to painful stimuli in 50% of anesthetized patients. The lower the MAC value, the more anesthetic potency of the inhalation anesthetic. Consequently, the MAC defines the therapeutic effect of inhalational anesthetics as the prevention of movement in response to surgical stimulation.[4]

The potency of an inhalation anesthetic agent with the MAC as the tool of assessment varies with the patient's age, state of health, clinical conditions, and concurrent use of other drugs (with depressant effects). The factors that modify the MAC are presented in Box 20-1. MAC awake is the anesthetic dose at which a patient responds to commands; it is also the dose of anesthetic at which most patients lose consciousness and recall. MAC awake usually corresponds with stage I of anesthesia. Another term used with MAC is *MAC-Block Adrenergic Response,* which is the MAC needed to block the adrenergic and cardiovascular responses to incision; it corresponds to stage III, plane III anesthesia.

BOX 20-1   Factors That Modify Minimum Alveolar Concentration

Factors that increase MAC
- Young age
- Hyperthermia
- CNS stimulation
- Physostigmine
- Alcohol dependency

Factors that decrease MAC
- Elderly age
- Hypothermia
- Acute alcohol ingestion
- CNS depressants
  - Benzodiazepines
  - Barbiturates
  - Propofol
- Tranquilizers
- Opioids
- Pregnancy
- Alpha 2–adrenergic agonists
  - Clonidine
  - Dexmedetomidine

Modified from Longnecker D, et al: *Anesthesiology,* New York, 2007, McGraw Hill Medical.
MAC, Minimum alveolar concentration; *CNS,* central nervous system.

TECHNIQUES OF ADMINISTRATION

The inhalation anesthetics are usually administered by means of an anesthesia machine (Fig. 20-2). The anesthesia machine is essentially a breathing circuit that conveys the agent and oxygen to the patient. It consists of a mask, corrugated tubing, an absorber for removal of expired carbon dioxide, a reservoir bag, unidirectional valves, adjustable positive-pressure relief (APR) valve, and vaporizers (Fig. 20-3).[5]

Circle Systems

A variety of techniques can be used to deliver gaseous agents with the anesthesia machine by adding or removing certain features. The most common technique used is the semiclosed circle method, in which some rebreathing of expired gases occurs by opening the APR valve to vent some of the gas to the atmosphere. The closed circle method is used when low gas flows are desired. In this technique, the APR valve is completely closed and complete rebreathing of expired gases occurs. A carbon dioxide absorber is used in both the semiclosed and the closed techniques.

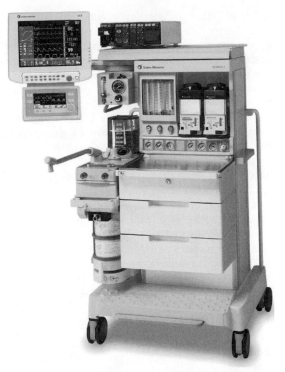

FIG. 20-2 Anesthesia machine apparatus. (Used with permission from Datex-Ohmeda, Madison, Wis.)

INHALATION AGENTS

Inhalation anesthetic substances can be divided into the following two groups: volatile and gaseous. Volatile anesthetic agents are chemicals in the liquid state at room temperature that have a boiling point above 20° C. Ethyl chloride, which has a boiling point of 12° C, is also included in this class of anesthetic agents. The volatile inhalation anesthetic agents are divided into two major categories: the halogenated hydrocarbons and the ethers. Examples of the halogenated hydrocarbons are isoflurane, desflurane, and sevoflurane; diethyl ether is an example of the ethers. The gaseous anesthetic agents, such as nitrous oxide, are in the gaseous state at room temperature. The anesthetic agents currently in use have evolved from the traditional inhalation anesthetics that are not in use today: cyclopropane, chloroform, and diethyl ether.

Modern Inhalation Anesthetics
Isoflurane (Forane)

Isoflurane, an analogue of enflurane, is also a halogenated methyl ethyl ether; it produces a dose-related depression of the CNS.[6] In contrast with enflurane, this anesthetic agent does not produce convulsive electroencephalographic abnormalities.

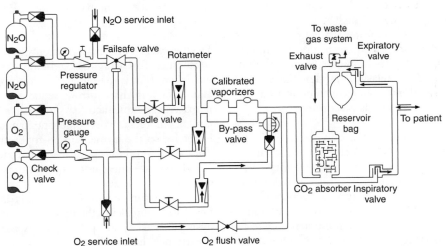

FIG. 20-3 Anesthesia machine circuit. Oxygen and nitrous oxide enter the machine from cylinders or from hospital service supply. Pressure regulators reduce cylinder pressure to approximately 3 kg/cm². Check valves to prevent transfilling of cylinders or gas flow from cylinders to service line. Fail-safe valve prevents flow of nitrous oxide if oxygen supply fails. Needle valves in flowmeters control flows to rotameters. Calibrated vaporizers provide preselected concentration of volatile anesthetics. Gases are delivered to the circle absorber, where unidirectional valves ensure flow from patient through the carbon dioxide absorber. Excess gas is vented through exhaust valve into waste gas scavenger system. Reservoir bag compensates for variations in respiratory demand. (Adapted from Dripps RD, et al: *Introduction to anesthesia: the principles of safe practice*, ed 7, Philadelphia, 1988, Saunders.)

Isoflurane reduces the systemic arterial blood pressure and total peripheral resistance; however, during isoflurane anesthesia, the heart rate is usually increased and the cardiac output usually remains within normal limits. This agent produces respiratory depression and skeletal muscular relaxation in a dose-related fashion, because isoflurane markedly potentiates the actions of the nondepolarizing muscle relaxants. Of interest to the perianesthesia nurse is the fact that isoflurane does not sensitize the myocardium to catecholamines to the same extent as halothane does. Thus, the chance of dysrhythmias is reduced when the patient has received isoflurane anesthesia.

The recovery phase is rapid because of isoflurane's low blood-gas partition coefficient of 0.97.[3,6] The patient awakens promptly and is lucid within 15 to 30 minutes after termination of the anesthetic. However, clinical observation indicates that if the anesthesia time with isoflurane is longer than 45 to 60 minutes, the patient will probably have a slower emergence phase than expected, given that the drug has such a low blood-gas partition coefficient.

The lung volumes and capacities, as measured with the Wright respirometer, return to normal in less than 30 minutes along with the ability to raise the head, protrude the tongue, cough on command, and converse clearly. The blood pressure and pulse remain stable. Shivering is seen in 2% of patients, and nausea and vomiting occur only occasionally.

Isoflurane possesses some excellent qualities: a lack of sensitization of the heart to catecholamines, cardiovascular stability, limited biodegradation, good neuromuscular relaxation, and no CNS excitatory effects. Isoflurane isa major component in the practice of most anesthesia practitioners.

Sevoflurane (Ultane)

Sevoflurane is a 100% potent inhalation anesthetic agent that has a blood-gas solubility coefficient of 0.69,[6] which is near nitrous oxide and thus makes it an extremely rapid-acting agent. Consequently, patients emerge from sevoflurane anesthesia in a matter of minutes when they have received this drug as the sole agent. One must remember that a rapid recovery from an inhalation anesthetic usually mandates the need for analgesic drugs in the immediate postoperative period.[7]

The drug is not irritating to the respiratory tract, and the degree of patient acceptance is high. Sevoflurane can be used in place of halothane for the induction of anesthesia in children[8]; it tends to decrease the blood pressure by decreasing the systemic vascular resistance.

Like all other inhalation agents, this drug is a respiratory depressant and blunts the ventilatory response to an increased $PaCO_2$. This drug undergoes some metabolism at approximately the same degree as does enflurane. The metabolites of sevoflurane include fluoride and hexafluoroisopropanol. On the basis of a number of studies, no evidence of toxicity has been shown in regard to the biodegradation of this agent, probably because of sevoflurane's rapid ventilatory excretion, in which the metabolic byproducts do not seem to be significantly detrimental to the patient.

Like the other ethers, sevoflurane does not sensitize the heart to catecholamines and hence does not predispose to arrhythmias. This inhalation agent reduces cerebrovascular resistance and can increase intracranial pressure in a dose-related manner. In regard to its effect on skeletal muscle function, it enhances the action of the skeletal muscle relaxants. However, because of the drug's rapid elimination, this characteristic does not have a significant effect on the care of a patient in the PACU who has received sevoflurane during surgery.

Sevoflurane possesses many outstanding qualities. It has great precision and control over anesthetic depth, it does not depress kidney or liver function, it has little effect on heart rate, and, most of all, it is extremely rapid, which speeds up the emergence of the patient in the PACU.

Desflurane (Suprane)

Desflurane is a fluorinated ether that is similar to isoflurane. This drug has a blood-gas partition coefficient that is the same as cyclopropane (0.42) and even less than nitrous oxide, which makes it extremely rapid acting.[6] As with sevoflurane, patient emergence is extremely rapid and analgesia is needed in the immediate postoperative period. This drug produces a dose-related decrease in blood pressure and cardiac output that is slightly greater than the depression seen with equivalent doses of isoflurane. Because this drug is an ether-type inhalation agent, the incidence rate of cardiac dysrhythmias when epinephrine is administered is extremely low.

The pungency of desflurane irritates the respiratory tract and causes coughing, breathholding, and laryngospasm. Consequently, the drug is not recommended as an inhalation induction agent, especially in the pediatric age group. This drug depresses respiration in the same fashion as does sevoflurane and thus blunts the response to an increased $PaCO_2$. Desflurane produces a dose-related reduction in cerebrovascular resistance. Desflurane also enhances the neuromuscular blockade produced by skeletal muscle relaxants. However, like sevoflurane, this action is not of consequence for the patient in the PACU because of its extremely rapid ventilatory excretion during emergence.[8] Finally, as opposed to sevoflurane, this drug resists biodegradation and is almost totally eliminated by the respiratory system and therefore does not have a negative effect on the kidney or liver.

Desflurane represents a new era in inhalation anesthesia in regard to its effects on the care of the patient in the PACU. More specifically, because of the low solubility of desflurane, rapid emergence will become common, and a more rapid release from the PACU and a shorter length of stay in the hospital may be possible.

Nitrous Oxide

Nitrous oxide is the only inorganic gas used as an anesthetic agent. It is marketed in blue steel cylinders as a colorless liquid at a pressure of 30 atm. As the pressure is released, nitrous oxide returns to the gaseous state. It is readily soluble in water and heavier than air. Nitrous oxide was probably the first anesthetic agent to be used extensively. The fact that it is still used indicates that, when used properly, it is a valuable and safe anesthetic agent.

Nitrous oxide supports combustion—that is, if a burning match is put into a jar that contains nitrous oxide, it will continue to burn. However, this agent is not explosive. Although the nitrous oxide molecule contains oxygen, that oxygen is unavailable for respiration because nitrous oxide does not decompose in the body.

Nitrous oxide is a 15% potent agent; therefore the maximum depth of anesthesia that can be produced while the patient's metabolic need for oxygen is supplied is the middle of plane 1 of stage III anesthesia. This agent has no side effects unless hypoxia is present. It is nontoxic and nonirritating; however, nitrous oxide can cause postoperative nausea and vomiting, particularly in the ambulatory surgical setting when the procedure lasts for 1 hour, and probably for 2 hours or more.[9] Nitrous oxide is a rapid-acting agent in part because of its blood-gas partition coefficient of 0.47.[6] This agent does not combine with hemoglobin but is carried in physical solution in the blood. It is excreted mostly unchanged by the lungs, although a small fraction is excreted through the skin. It does not sensitize the heart to epinephrine, and it provides a fair amount of analgesia. Even in subanesthetic concentrations, nitrous oxide has an analgesic effect in humans, and 20% concentrations of the gas have been claimed to be as effective as 15 mg

of morphine sulfate. If this agent were more potent, it would probably be considered an almost perfect anesthetic.

In current anesthesia practice, nitrous oxide serves an important role because it is administered alone and in combination with various agents. Recently, the balanced technique of anesthesia has been favored because of the number of negative factors associated with some of the more potent volatile inhalation anesthetics. The balanced technique consists of the administration of opioids that may or may not be in combination with a tranquilizer, a muscle relaxant, nitrous oxide, oxygen, and barbiturates.[3] All the elements of anesthesia or nervous system depression are met: sensory block (analgesia), motor block (muscle relaxation), reflex block, and mental block (narcosis). When nitrous oxide is administered with a potent volatile inhalation anesthetic such as desflurane, it acts as a carrier and provides an additional analgesic effect. The second gas effect occurs because of nitrous oxide's rapid uptake, after which the potent volatile agent takes the patient to the desired surgical plane. The reverse takes place at termination of the anesthetic.

The solubilities of nitrogen and nitrous oxide differ greatly. Nitrous oxide is 30-fold more soluble than nitrogen. An enclosed gas-filled space in the body expands if gas within it is more soluble than the gas respired. For this reason, any enclosed gas-filled cavity in the body expands because of the slow exchange of nitrogen from the cavity for the rapid exchange of large volumes of nitrous oxide from the blood, which is why the use of nitrous oxide is not recommended in surgical procedures for intestinal obstruction or pneumothorax. Nitrous oxide has been shown to dislodge a tympanoplasty graft because of the expansion of the air pocket in the middle ear. Consequently, in surgical procedures that involve the middle ear, the administration of nitrous oxide is usually avoided. Of interest to the perianesthesia nurse is the possible role of nitrous oxide in altering the pressures in the middle ear; nitrous oxide has been suggested to cause nausea and vomiting from the resulting increased pressure in that area.

Diffusion hypoxia after nitrous oxide anesthesia is another area of concern for the perianesthesia nurse. This effect is sometimes called the *Fink phenomenon*. It occurs when not enough nitrous oxide is removed from the lungs at the end of the surgical procedure. Normally, 100% oxygen is administered at the end of the procedure for removal of the nitrous oxide, which is called *nitrous oxide washout*. Diffusion hypoxia is directly related to the dilution of alveolar gas by the rapid diffusion of the nitrous oxide out of the blood. This outpouring of nitrous oxide into the alveoli occurs during the first 1 to 5 minutes after the nitrous oxide has been discontinued. In addition, the rapid movement into the alveoli can cause a dilutional effect of the $PACO_2$ and ultimately a reduction in the stimulus to breathe. Therefore administration of oxygen via mask to all patients who are admitted to the PACU is highly advisable. This maneuver forestalls the development of severe hypoxia if some unpredicted airway problem occurs. Another measure for avoiding this complication is the provision of adequate verbal and physical stimulation to the patient to promote good ventilatory effort. This approach should include encouraging the patient to sigh every 5 minutes to ensure adequate removal of the anesthetic gases.

ASSESSMENT OF THE EFFECTS OF INHALATION AGENTS IN THE PERIANESTHESIA CARE UNIT

In assessment of the patient's degree of emergence from inhalation anesthesia, the nurse must understand the pharmacologic effects of each anesthetic agent and of the preoperative medications used. In addition, the rate of recovery from inhalation anesthesia is predictable based on the solubility of the anesthetic agent, alveolar ventilation, and duration of the anesthetic. Each anesthetic agent is essentially a depressant drug. Certain volatile agents, such as sevoflurane, desflurane, and isoflurane, possess a high degree of myocardial and respiratory depressant properties. One parameter for monitoring of the emergence phase with administration of these agents is the vital signs. Preanesthetic baseline vital sign readings are reliable postoperative indicators of the patient's cardiorespiratory status and can be used in the assessment of the patient's stage of recovery. When this assessment is made, however, all other factors of the patient's condition must also be considered.[10] Total assessment of the patient recovering from anesthesia is discussed in Chapter 27. Most inhalation anesthetics cause some degree of depression of the respiratory system. Consequently, the $PaCO_2$ increases in a dose-related manner, frequency increases, and tidal volume is reduced. Because of the respiratory depression that all patients have after anesthesia and surgery, the perianesthesia nurse must use the stir-up regimen that encourages the patient to perform the sustained maximal inspiration maneuver (see Chapter 27).

To understand the emergence phase of inhalation anesthesia, the nurse also needs a basic understanding of blood-gas and oil-gas partition coefficients. Anesthetic agents are usually administered in combinations, often with nitrous oxide as the carrier gas. The combination of agents usually consists of a 100% potent agent, a carrier agent, and oxygen to meet the metabolic needs of the patient. The agent with the highest blood-gas partition coefficient takes the longest time to be removed from the body. Therefore, if a isoflurane–nitrous oxide–oxygen combination is administered to a patient, the isoflurane, which has the highest blood-gas partition coefficient, is eliminated the most slowly.

Along with the factors attributed to the blood-gas partition coefficient, those attributed to the oil-gas partition coefficient should be considered in an evaluation of length of time of emergence from the anesthetic. When the intraoperative phase is of long duration, an agent with a high oil-gas partition coefficient redistributes into the adipose tissue. As mentioned previously, because the vascular supply to adipose tissue is sparse, the release of the agent to the blood is slow and the emergence is prolonged. Both coefficients must be kept in mind in prediction of the length of the emergence phase from an inhalation anesthetic agent. Isoflurane, for example, has the low blood-gas partition coefficient of 0.97, and a rapid recovery from its administration would be expected. However, isoflurane has a high oil-gas partition coefficient of 93.7; therefore, when it is administered for longer than 2 hours, the adipose tissue is saturated and emergence from the anesthetic agent is prolonged. Nitrous oxide, desflurane, and isoflurane have low blood-gas and oil-gas partition coefficients.[7]

Inhalation agents, because of their depressant effect on the hypothalamus, disrupt the regulation of body temperature that may be manifested by either a reduction or an elevation, depending on the environmental temperature.[10] In the recovery phase, the emerging patient should be monitored for hypothermia or hyperthermia. Serious heat loss can occur in newborns and create difficulties in the reestablishment of adequate ventilatory effort after surgery. Body temperature should be monitored in patients who were febrile before surgery and who received atropine before or during the operative procedure. Agents such as isoflurane that have a direct vasodilatory effect on vascular smooth muscle can cause a temperature drop of 1° C in esophageal temperature. Shivering and tremors have been reported during the postoperative period after isoflurane anesthesia, although these phenomena have mostly been associated with a generalized loss of muscle tone during surgery and anesthesia.

Water and electrolyte balance is affected by inhalation anesthesia.[1] Pituitary and adrenocortical systems appear to be affected in such a way that water and sodium retention and potassium loss occur after anesthesia. This balance is also affected in part by the stress of surgical trauma. Decreased glomerular filtration, increased tubular reabsorption, and varying degrees of oliguria exist in the recovery phase because of renal vasoconstriction. If renal blood flow is not impaired, glomerular function quickly returns to normal after the operation. The increased tubular reabsorption of water usually persists for 36 to 48 hours, but may continue for several days in elderly patients.

SUMMARY

Perianesthesia practice has been changed dramatically over the last few decades. PACU nursing care has also dramatically changed, reflecting the major changes in the pharmacologic actions of the inhalational anesthetic agents. To appreciate the present day practice in the PACU, a good understanding of the evolution of these agents will enhance the present day practice of perianesthesia nursing.

The inhalation anesthetic agents have moved from the first anesthetic discovered in 1846, ether, to derivatives of ether (methoxyflurane); to Penthrane, which was introduced in the early 1960s; to halothane (Fluothane), which was a halogenated hydrocarbon type drug introduced in the late 1960s; and to the current inhalational drugs described in this chapter. The anesthetic agents available for the anesthesia practitioner has in some ways become simplified, and the current selection of agents offers many advantages to the older drugs. For the perianesthesia nurse, this movement in the use of inhalational anesthetic agents has been positive. Previously, the patient would emerge rather slowly. With the current inhalation agents, patients wake up rather quickly. With the advent of these faster acting agents, the perianesthesia nurse is now confronted with new or more profound nursing care issues, such as pain, confusion, and awareness during anesthesia. Consequently, Chapter 31 has been devoted to pain and its physiology, and Chapters 28 and 29 are devoted to the nursing interventions for the sequelae of confusion and awareness with anesthesia.

The administration of inhalation agents has also become more simplified, and gone is the equipment used during the ether to Penthrane days. However, for the assessment of potency, the MAC is still used; and because many practitioners still use the signs and stages first described by Guedel, a description is included in this chapter. In addition, the prediction of emergence of the patient recovering from an inhalational anesthetic can be aided with a firm knowledge of the movement of the anesthetic through the various vascular groups along with the various partition coefficients. Finally, an overview of the assessment of a patient recovering from inhalational anesthesia is provided with a detailed discussion presented in Chapter 27.

Inhalation anesthetic agents used in modern practice have become more simplified, but that is not to be taken out of context. These highly rapid-acting agents have in fact justified the fact that advance practice critical care nursing is the level of care provided in the PACU. These rapid-acting agents require nurses in the PACU to possess a strong knowledge base and the ability to rapidly react to critical situations that can and do occur in the PACU.

REFERENCES

1. Jordan B, Wright E: Xenon as an anesthetic agent, *AANA J* 78(5):387–392, 2010.
2. Longnecker D, Murphy F: *Dripps/Eckenhoff/Vandam introduction to anesthesia*, ed 9, Philadelphia, 1997, Saunders.
3. Stoelting R: *Pharmacology and physiology in anesthetic practice*, ed 4, Philadelphia, 2005, Lippincott Williams & Wilkins.
4. Miller R, Pardo M: *Basics of anesthesia*, ed 6, Philadelphia, 2011, Saunders.
5. Dorsch J, Dorsch S: *Understanding anesthesia equipment*, ed 5, Philadelphia, 2007, Lippincott Williams & Wilkins.
6. Brunton L, et al: *Goodman and Gilman's the pharmacological basis of therapeutics*, ed 12, New York, 2010, McGraw-Hill Professional.
7. Pasero C, McCaffery M: *Pain assessment and pharmacologic management*, St. Louis, 2011, Mosby.
8. Jones R: Desflurane and sevoflurane: inhalation anesthetics for this decade? *Br J Anaesth* 65:527–536, 1990.
9. Stancer-Smiley B, Paradise N: Does the duration of N$_2$O administration affect postoperative nausea and vomiting? *Nurse Anesth* 2(1):13–20, 1991.
10. Nagelhout J, Plaus K: *Nurse anesthesia*, ed 4, St. Louis, 2010, Saunders.

RESOURCES

American Association of Critical-Care Nurses: *Core curriculum for progressive care nursing*, Philadelphia, 2010, Saunders.
Aitkenhead A, et al: *Textbook of anesthesia*, ed 5, Philadelphia, 2007, Churchill Livingstone.
Alspach J: *Core curriculum for critical care nursing*, ed 6, Philadelphia, 2005, Saunders.
Atlee J: *Complications in anesthesia*, ed 2, Philadelphia, 2007, Saunders.
Barash P, et al: *Clinical anesthesia*, ed 6, Philadelphia, 2009, Lippincott Williams & Wilkins.

CONCEPTS IN ANESTHETIC AGENTS

Barrett K, et al: *Ganong's review of medical physiology*, ed 23, New York, 2009, McGraw-Hill Medical.

Bready L, et al: *Decision making in anesthesiology*, ed 4, St. Louis, 2007, Mosby.

Brunton L, et al: *Goodman and Gilman's the pharmacological basis of therapeutics*, ed 12, New York, 2010, McGraw-Hill Professional.

Conlay L, et al: *Case files anesthesiology*, New York, 2011, McGraw Hill Medical.

Davis P, et al: *Smith's anesthesia for infants and children*, ed 8, St. Louis, 2011, Mosby.

Drake R, et al: *Gray's anatomy for students*, ed 2, Philadelphia, 2009, Churchill Livingstone.

Deutschman C, Netigan P: *Evidence-based practice of critical care*, Philadelphia, 2010, Saunders.

Dorsch J, Dorsch S: *Understanding anesthesia equipment*, ed 5, Philadelphia, 2007, Lippincott Williams & Wilkins.

Fisher L: *Anesthesia and uncommon diseases*, ed 5, Philadelphia, 2007, Saunders.

Gallager C, Issenberg B: *Simulation in anesthesia*, Philadelphia, 2007, Saunders.

Hall J: *Guyton and Hall textbook of medical physiology*, ed 12, Philadelphia, 2011, Saunders.

Hines R, Marschall K: *Handbook for Stoelting's anesthesia and co-existing disease*, ed 3, Philadelphia, 2009, Saunders.

Hines R, Marschall K: *Stoelting's anesthesia and co-existing disease*, ed 5, Philadelphia, 2008, Saunders.

Kaplan J, et al: *Cardiac anesthesia*, New York, 2011, Churchill Livingstone.

Kier L, Dowd C: *The chemistry of drugs for nurse anesthetists*, Chicago, 2004, AANA Publishing, Inc.

Kulli J, Koch C: Does anesthesia cause loss of consciousness? *Trends Neurosci* 14(1):6–10, 1991.

Longnecker D, et al: *Anesthesiology*, New York, 2007, McGraw Hill Medical.

Miller R, et al: *Miller's anesthesia*, ed 7, New York, 2010, Churchill Livingstone.

Miller R, Pardo M: *Basics of anesthesia*, ed 6, Philadelphia, 2011, Saunders.

Moos D, Cuddeford D: Implications of obstructive sleep apnea syndrome for the perianesthesia nurse, *J Perianesth Nurs*, 21(2):103-118, 2006.

Mason R: *Murray and Nadel's textbook of respiratory medicine*, ed 5, Philadelphia, 2011, Saunders.

Nagelhout J, Plaus K: *Nurse anesthesia*, ed 4, St. Louis, 2010, Saunders.

Passannante A, et al: Anesthestic management of patients with obesity and sleep apnea, *Anesthesiol Clin North Am* 23:479–490, 2005.

Sandberg W, et al: *The MGH textbook of anesthetic equipment*, New York, 2011, Churchill Livingstone.

Schick L, Windle PE: *Perianesthesia nursing core curriculum: preprocedure, phase I and phase II PACU nursing*, ed 2, Philadelphia, 2010, Saunders.

Shorten G, et al: *Postoperative pain management: an evidence-based guide to practice*, Philadelphia, 2006, Saunders.

Sieber F: *Geriatric anesthesia*, New York, 2006, McGraw-Hill Medical.

Shorten G, et al: *Postoperative pain management: an evidence-based guide to practice*, Philadelphia, 2006, Saunders.

Stoelting R: *Pharmacology and physiology in anesthetic practice*, ed 4, Philadelphia, 2005, Lippincott Williams & Wilkins.

Townsend C, et al: *Sabiston's textbook of surgery*, ed 18, Philadelphia, 2008, Saunders.

Vincent J, et al: *Textbook of critical care*, ed 6, Philadelphia, 2011, Saunders.

White P: *Perioperative drug manual*, ed 2, Philadelphia, 2005, Saunders.

21 Nonopioid Intravenous Anesthetics

Cecil B. Drain, PhD, RN, CRNA, FAAN, FASAHP

Intravenous anesthetics are grouped by primary pharmacologic action into nonopioid and opioid intravenous agents. The nonopioid agents are further grouped into the barbiturates, nonbarbiturates, and sedatives. These drugs can be injected in a rapid intravenous fashion for induction of anesthesia, or they can be used via continuous infusion pump for maintenance of anesthesia. Many of the nonopioid intravenous anesthetic drugs have stood the test of time. In fact, they are now being used more frequently in the postanesthesia care unit (PACU) because the less serious side effects than the opioid agents. Intravenous anesthetics have a wide range of use in the perioperative period. In current anesthesia practice, the use of intravenous drugs is commonplace. The time-tested use of the inhalation anesthetic agents has demonstrated that the agents possess some definite disadvantages. Because of the biotransformation hazards that have been reported with the halogenated inhalation anesthetics, other techniques have been sought for general anesthesia. Because of their safety factors coupled with ease of use, the nonopioid intravenous anesthetic agents have certainly found their place in the practice of anesthesia for enhancement of patient outcomes.

DEFINITIONS

Agonist: A drug that has a specific receptor affinity that produces a predictable response.
Antagonist: A drug that has the ability to block the effects of an agonist drug at the receptor site.
Anterograde Amnesia: The inability to recall events that occur after the onset of amnesia.
Antianalgesic: Administration of a drug that partially blocks the analgesic effects of other drugs that produce analgesia.
Antiemetic: A drug that prevents or alleviates nausea and vomiting.
Cardiostimulatory: Stimulation of the cardiovascular system.
Dissociative: Anesthesia that is characterized by analgesia and amnesia without loss of respiratory function.
Esterases: A chemical group that breaks down certain enzymes.

Extrapyramidal: Effects of the structures outside the cerebrospinal pyramidal tracts of the brain that are associated with movement of the body.
Gamma-Aminobutyric Acid (GABA): An amino acid that functions as an inhibitory neurotransmitter in the brain and spinal cord.
Hypertriglyceridemia: Type I hyperlipoproteinemia.
Neuroleptanalgesia: A state of profound tranquilization with little or no depressant effect on the cortical centers.
Parenterally: Treatment other than through the digestive system.
Resedation: Sedation that recurs after clinical signs indicate that the sedation has ceased.
Sedatives: Substances that have a calming effect.
Sympatholytic: Antiadrenergic effects.
Sympathomimetic: A pharmacologic agent that mimics the effects of stimulation of the sympathetic nervous system.
Thrombophlebitis: Inflammation of a vein accompanied by the formation of a clot.
Torsades de Pointes (TdP): Potentially fatal heart arrhythmia.
Vagotonic: Augmenting the parasympathetic activity by stimulating the vagus nerve.

MECHANISM OF ACTION OF THE NONOPIOID INTRAVENOUS ANESTHETICS

The nonopioid drugs appear to interact with gamma-aminobutyric acid (GABA) in the brain. GABA is an inhibitory neurotransmitter, and activation of the GABA receptors by GABA on the postsynaptic membrane causes inhibition of the postsynaptic neuron. The barbiturates appear to bind to the GABA postsynaptic receptor, with the net result of hyperpolarization of the postsynaptic neuron and inhibition of neuronal activity and ultimately loss of consciousness. Conversely, etomidate (Amidate), which is a nonbarbiturate induction agent, probably antagonizes the muscarinic receptors in the central nervous system (CNS) and acts as an agonist to the opioid receptors.[1] The resultant action of these drugs is a loss of wakefulness.

Sedatives, such as the benzodiazepines, bind to specific receptors in the limbic system. These benzodiazepine receptors use GABA as part of the neurotransmitter system. After the benzodiazepines have bound to the receptor, the action of GABA is enhanced, which leads to the hyperpolarized state and ultimately to inhibition of neuronal activity.[2] The drug flumazenil is a specific benzodiazepine receptor antagonist. Consequently, after the administration of a benzodiazepine agonist, flumazenil can be administered. The pharmacologic actions on the benzodiazepine receptor are reversed, and neuronal activity resumes.

BARBITURATES

Intravenous anesthesia began with barbiturate anesthesia. The long-acting barbiturates were introduced clinically in 1927, but Tovell and Lundy did not begin to use thiopental in clinical anesthesia practice until 1934. Since then, barbiturate anesthesia had great popularity until the late 1990s; with the advent of propofol, thiopental is used in approximately 5% of the general anesthetics today.

Thiopental

Because of its historical significance, thiopental sodium (Pentothal) will be discussed in length. Today, this drug is rarely available in most hospitals and is used in rare instances. Probably the most profound explanation of why thiopental is not used is because of the excellent drug actions of propofol (Diprivan). Thiopental is most commonly injected intravenously to induce or sustain surgical anesthesia. It is usually used in conjunction with a potent inhalation anesthetic and nitrous oxide–oxygen combinations. The main reason for the use of other anesthetic agents with thiopental is that thiopental is a poor analgesic. For surgical procedures that are short and require minimal analgesia, thiopental and nitrous oxide–oxygen combinations can be used. This technique is commonly called the *pent-nitrous technique*. Thiopental is also used: (1) for maintenance of light sleep during regional analgesia; (2) for control of convulsions; and (3) for rapidly quieting a patient who is too lightly anesthetized during a surgical procedure.

The mode of action of thiopental involves a phenomenon of redistribution. Thiopental has the ability to penetrate all tissues of the body without delay. Because the brain, as part of the vessel-rich group, is highly perfused, it receives approximately 10% of the administered intravenous dose within 40 seconds after injection. The patient usually becomes unconscious at this time. The thiopental then redistributes to relatively poorly perfused areas of the body. In the brain, the level of thiopental decreases to half its peak in 5 minutes and to one tenth in 30 minutes. Recovery of consciousness usually occurs during this period. Recovery can be prolonged if the induction dose was excessive or if circulatory depression occurs to slow the redistribution phenomenon. Thiopental is metabolized in the body at a rate of 10% to 15% per hour.

Thiopental is a respiratory depressant.[3] The chief effect is on the medullary and pontine respiratory centers. This depressant effect depends on the amount of thiopental administered, the rate at which it is injected, and the amount and type of premedication given to the patient. The response to carbon dioxide is depressed at all levels of anesthesia and is abolished at deep levels of thiopental anesthesia; therefore apnea can be an adverse outcome of high-dose thiopental.

Myocardial contractility is depressed and vascular resistance is increased after injection of thiopental. The result is that blood pressure is hardly affected, although it may be transiently reduced when the drug is first administered (when the vessel-rich group is highly saturated).

In addition to being nonexplosive, thiopental has the advantages of: (1) rapid and pleasant induction; (2) reduction of postanesthetic excitement and vomiting; (3) quiet respiration; (4) absence of salivation; and (5) speedy recovery after small doses. The disadvantages of the drug are adverse respiratory actions, including apnea, coughing, laryngospasm, and bronchospasm. Extravenous injection can result in tissue necrosis because of its highly alkaline pH (10.5 to 11).

Perianesthesia Care

Because thiopental can have an antianalgesic effect at low concentrations, some patients who have pain may be irrational, hyperactive, and restless during the initial recovery phase. The patient may exhibit some shivering related to lowered body temperature, which can result from a cold operating suite. Of concern to the perianesthesia nurse is the patient admitted with cold, clammy, and cyanotic skin. This effect occasionally occurs with thiopental and is caused, in part, by the peripheral vasoconstrictive action of the drug.

If the anesthesia time exceeds 1 hour or if the total dose of thiopental exceeds 1 g, patients may have a delayed awakening time because of the redistribution of thiopental. This phenomenon is particularly common in obese patients because the drug is highly fat soluble. At present, no antagonist exists for the barbiturates; therefore airway management and monitoring of cardiovascular status are important.

Methohexital

Methohexital is an ultra–short-acting barbiturate intravenous anesthetic agent. It is usually indicated for short procedures in which rapid complete recovery of the patient is needed. Like thiopental, methohexital is rarely administered, primarily because of the excellent drug actions of propofol (Diprivan). Methohexital is approximately threefold more potent as thiopental, and the recovery time from anesthesia is extremely rapid (4 to 7 minutes) because the drug is redistributed from the CNS to the muscle and fat tissues, and a significant portion of the drug is metabolized in the liver.[1] Consequently, the clearance of methohexital is approximately fourfold faster than that of thiopental. Methohexital causes about the same degree of cardiovascular and respiratory depression as does thiopental. This drug can cause coughing and hiccups and, after injection, excitatory phenomena may appear, such as tremor and involuntary muscle movements.

NONBARBITURATES

Propofol

Propofol (Diprivan) is a rapid-acting nonbarbiturate induction agent. It is administered intravenously as a 1% solution and is the most popular intravenous anesthetic in use. The dose for induction is 2 to 2.5 mg/kg.[4] The dose should be reduced in elderly patients and in patients with cardiac disease or hypovolemia. In addition, propofol in combination with midazolam acts synergistically. In fact, the dose of propofol can be reduced by 50% when it is administered in combination with midazolam. When propofol is used as the sole induction agent, it is usually administered over 15 seconds and produces unconsciousness within approximately 30 seconds. Emergence from this drug is more rapid than emergence from thiopental or methohexital, because propofol has a half-life of 2 to 9 minutes[5]; therefore the duration of anesthesia after a single induction dose is 3 to 8 minutes, depending on the dose of the propofol. A major advantage of this drug is its ability to allow the patient a rapid return to consciousness with minimal residual CNS effects. Moreover, the drug's low incidence rate of nausea and vomiting is of particular importance to perianesthesia nursing care. In fact, propofol may possess antiemetic properties.

Propofol decreases the cerebral perfusion pressure, cerebral blood flow, and intracranial pressure. It produces a reduction in the blood pressure similar in magnitude to or greater than thiopental in comparable doses. The decrease in blood pressure is also accompanied by a reduction in cardiac output or systemic vascular resistance. This reduction in blood pressure is more pronounced in elderly patients and in patients with compromised left-ventricular function. As opposed to the reduction in blood pressure, the pulse usually remains unchanged after the administration of propofol because of a sympatholytic or vagotonic effect of the drug. As a result, bradycardia can be assessed after injection of propofol in some patients. In this instance, an anticholinergic drug such as atropine or glycopyrrolate (Robinul) can be administered to reverse the bradycardia.

Propofol has a profound depressant effect on both the rate and depth of ventilation. In fact, after the induction dose is administered, apnea normally occurs. The incidence rate of apnea is greater after propofol than after thiopental and may approach 100%. Consequently, if propofol is administered in the PACU, the perianesthesia nurse should be prepared to support the patient's ventilation and, if necessary, intubate the patient[6] (see Chapter 30).

Clinically, this drug is useful for intravenous induction of anesthesia, especially for outpatient surgery.[7] The drug is also an excellent choice for procedures that require a short period of unconsciousness, such as cardioversion and electroconvulsive therapy. In addition, propofol can be used for sedation during local standby procedures. This drug does not interfere with or alter the effects of succinylcholine because it has such a rapid plasma clearance. Propofol can be used during surgery in a continuous intravenous infusion, and the patients still emerge from anesthesia in a rapid fashion without any CNS depression. This drug can be used in the PACU as a continuous infusion, and the level of sedation can be adjusted by titration to effect.[6] The typical infusion rates for sedation with propofol are between 25 and 100 mcg/kg/min.

With administration within 12 hours of intravenous sedation, propofol is characterized by a more rapid recovery from its sedative effects than midazolam. When propofol is discontinued, extubation can be performed in a short time; propofol is cleared rapidly because of redistribution to fatty tissue and hepatic metabolism to inactive metabolites.

Long-term or high-dose infusions can result in hypertriglyceridemia, which is usually associated with elevated levels of pancreatic enzymes and possibly with pancreatitis. After long infusions, plasma concentrations of propofol gradually increase unless the infusion rate is decreased over time. Current data seem to indicate that the recovery from propofol is less rapid after 12 hours of intravenous sedation. Propofol is contraindicated in patients who are sensitive to soybean oil, egg lecithin, or glycerol and is not recommended for PACU or intensive care unit (ICU) administration in children because of the possibility of emergence agitation.[8]

Perianesthesia Care

When a patient has received propofol for induction or even via continuous infusion, the perianesthesia nursing care should be based mainly on the other drugs that were used during surgery, because propofol is so rapid and has no cumulative effects; its effects are normally dissipated within 8 to 10 minutes. Consequently, the patient usually arrives in the PACU awake and in pain; therefore analgesics should be titrated to effect. Titration is recommended in the immediate postoperative period because propofol and opioid analgesics can have a synergistic effect.

Propofol is a major component used in modern clinical anesthesia practice. It offers many advantages and few disadvantages. More specifically, propofol has one major advantage over all the other intravenous induction agents: early awakening. It can be used in the PACU if indicated. The major concern for the perianesthesia care of the patient who has received this drug is the level of postoperative pain. The nursing assessment and appropriate interventions for pain are the most important aspects of care of the patient who has received this drug.[6]

Etomidate

Etomidate (Amidate), which is a derivative of imidazole, is a short-acting intravenous hypnotic that was synthesized in the 1960s by the laboratories of Janssen Pharmaceutica (Beerse, Belgium). It is not related chemically to the commonly used hypnotic agents. This drug is a mere hypnotic and does not possess any analgesic actions. Etomidate is safe for administration to patients because it has a high therapeutic index. Metabolism of this drug is accomplished by hydrolysis in the liver and by plasma esterases, with the final metabolite being pharmacologically inactive. The cardiovascular effects of etomidate are minimal; when the drug is injected in therapeutic doses, only a small blood pressure decrease and a slight heart rate increase may be observed. Etomidate causes a minimal reduction in the cardiac index and the peripheral resistance. This drug does not seem to produce arrhythmias, which is why etomidate is used in place of propofol as an induction agent for patients with cardiac dysfunction. Respiratory effects include a dose-related reduction in the tidal volume and respiratory frequency, which can lead to apnea.[1] Laryngospasm, cough, and hiccups can occur during injection of this drug; however, the severity of these clinical phenomena can be reduced with an opiate premedication.

Although this drug causes some pain at the site of injection, it does not appear to cause a release of histamine. Spontaneous involuntary movements and tremor have been observed after the injection of etomidate. These involuntary movements can be reduced with an opiate premedication. Etomidate reduces both intracranial and intraocular pressure and therefore is considered safe for use in patients with intracranial pathologic conditions. This short-acting hypnotic is particularly well suited for the induction of neuroleptanalgesia and inhalation anesthesia. The induction dose ranges from 0.2 to 0.3 mg/kg, which produces sleep in 20 to 45 seconds after injection; the patient wakes within 7 to 15 minutes after induction.

Research has shown that etomidate inhibits steroid synthesis and that patients who receive etomidate via continuous infusion have marked adrenocortical suppression for as long as 4 days.[1] Even when etomidate is administered as a single dose, adrenal function is suppressed for 5 to 8 hours. Consequently, after the administration of etomidate, a decrease is seen in cortisol, 17-alpha-hydroxyprogesterone, aldosterone, and corticosterone levels. Therefore etomidate is administered only to selected patients and is no longer administered via continuous intravenous infusion.[1,5]

SEDATIVES

Benzodiazepines

The benzodiazepines, which are sedatives, have enhanced the anesthetic outcomes of the surgical patient. They depress the limbic system without causing cortical depression. More specifically, they interact with the inhibitory neurotransmitter GABA and thus result in reduced orientation (hypnotic effect), retrograde amnesia, anxiolysis, and relaxing of the skeletal muscle.[1,2] Opiates and barbiturates enhance the hypnotic action of the benzodiazepines.

Midazolam

Midazolam has become a popular drug in anesthesia practice and in the perianesthesia care of surgical patients. Midazolam can be used for premedication, cardioversion, endoscopic procedures, and induction of anesthesia and as an intraoperative adjunct for inhalation anesthesia. It also is an excellent agent for sedation during regional anesthetic techniques. The principal action of midazolam is on the benzodiazepine receptors in the CNS, particularly on the limbic system, which results in a reduction in anxiety and profound anterograde amnesia. This drug also has excellent hypnotic, anticonvulsant, and muscle-relaxant properties.

The water-soluble midazolam may offer some advantages over diazepam. It causes depression of the CNS by inducing sedation, drowsiness, and finally sleep with increasing doses. Midazolam is three to four times as potent as diazepam, has a shorter duration of action, and has a lesser incidence rate of injection pain and postinjection phlebitis and thrombosis. More specifically, this drug has a rapid onset of action, a peak in action between 10 and 30 minutes, and a duration of action between 1 and 4 hours. Midazolam administered at a dose of 0.2 mg/kg produces a decrease in blood pressure, an increase in heart rate, and a reduction in systemic vascular resistance. Midazolam should be used with caution in patients with myocardial ischemia and in those with chronic obstructive pulmonary disease.[9] Postoperative patients who have a substantial amount of hypovolemia should not receive midazolam. In addition, midazolam does not affect intracranial pressure.[4,10] Consequently, this drug can be used safely in neurosurgical patients in addition to patients with intracranial pathophysiology.

This drug can be administered in the PACU[11]; therefore the postanesthesia nurse must monitor the patient for respiratory depression after injection because midazolam causes a dose-dependent respiratory depression. Given that every patient in the PACU has received a plethora of depressant drugs during surgery, midazolam can be potentiated easily when administered in the PACU. Because of this potentiation factor, any dose of midazolam administered in the PACU should be considered effective enough to cause profound respiratory depression. Therefore, oxygen and resuscitative equipment must be immediately available, and a person skilled in maintaining a patent airway and supporting ventilation should be present. Extra care also should be observed in patients with limited pulmonary reserve and in the elderly and debilitated with reduction of the dosage of midazolam by 25% to 30%.

Midazolam can be given via continuous infusion for patients who need sustained sedation.[7] However, midazolam has a pH-dependent diazepine ring; at physiologic pH, the ring can close, causing CNS penetration. In addition, its metabolites are partially active, all of which make midazolam not the drug of choice for long-term sedation. Midazolam is sometimes used in the treatment of critically ill patients who are agitated. The guidelines for use can be found in Box 21-1.

Diazepam

Diazepam (Valium) is still a popular drug in anesthesia practice. Because of its ability to allay apprehension, diazepam is indicated for use as a premedicant, as an adjunct to intravenous anesthesia, and as an induction agent. Recovery is usually not prolonged when diazepam is used for the induction of anesthesia. Diazepam can be used as the sole anesthetic agent for short diagnostic and surgical procedures and can be used as sedation to make local anesthesia more acceptable to the patient.

The principal action of diazepam is the depression of limbic system function. Important actions of diazepam are the production of anterograde amnesia for as long as 48 hours after surgery, reduction of anxiety, and provision of minimal cardiovascular depressant effects.[1] Clinical doses of diazepam cause a slight degree of respiratory depression; when it is combined with an opiate, the chance of respiratory depression, including apnea, is greatly increased.

Diazepam may possess some muscle-relaxant properties. Diazepam has been reported to be antagonistic to depolarizing neuromuscular blocking agents, such as succinylcholine, and the action of the nondepolarizing neuromuscular blocking agents (e.g., vecuronium) are reported to be potentiated.

BOX 21-1   Guidelines for the Use of Midazolam for the Treatment of Agitation in the Postanesthesia Care Unit and Critical Care Setting

- Indications: For patients with respiratory or cardiac dysfunction; promotes anxiolysis and amnesia
- Onset of action: 1 to 5 minutes
- Peak of action: 2 to 5 minutes
- Duration of action: 15 to 90 minutes
- Doses:
  - Load: 1 to 4 mg IV over 2 to 3 minutes
  - Maximal load: 5 mg in 1 hour (without intubation) 10 mg in 1 hour (with intubation)
  - Maintenance load: 1 to 5 mg/h (IV push)
- Intravenous infusions: 1 to 50 mg/h; no oral form available
- Tapering: Decrease infusion rate by 10% to 25% of maintenance rate every 24 hours; should be discontinued by day 4

IV, Intravenous.

Diazepam has been used clinically for psychomotor and petit mal seizures because of its anticonvulsant actions.[2,12]

Because many patients who undergo cardioversion are debilitated, diazepam can be used as sedation for this procedure. Increments of 2.5 to 5 mg can be given at 30-second intervals until the speech of the patient is slurred or light sleep occurs. At the time of electric discharge, the patient may have brief muscle contraction and slight arousal. When this technique is used, a significant number of the patients have complete amnesia regarding the event. Diazepam can also be used to provide anesthesia in endoscopic and dental procedures and to control behavior on emergence from ketamine.[7] Finally, this drug also has strong anticonvulsant activity and can stop generalized seizure activity.

Intramuscularly administered diazepam can be painful to the patient, and absorption is often poor. When diazepam is administered intravenously, thrombophlebitis often occurs. With intravenous administration of diazepam, the drug should be injected slowly, directly into a large vein. The drug should not be mixed with other drugs or diluted. The onset of action of diazepam administered intravenously is immediate, and the duration of action varies from 20 minutes to 1 hour. With intramuscular administration, its onset of action is approximately 10 minutes, and the duration of action may be as long as 4 hours. Adverse reactions to diazepam include hiccups, nausea, phlebitis at the site of injection, and occasional acute hyperexcited states.

Lorazepam

Lorazepam (Ativan), a long-acting benzodiazepine, is used as a premedication in current clinical anesthesia practice and as a long-acting slow-onset benzodiazepine for sedation in the PACU and ICU. This drug has actions similar to those of diazepam, but has a slow onset of action from 20 to 40 minutes; the pharmacologic activity can last as long as 24 hours.[9] Lorazepam produces profound anterograde amnesia, tranquilization, and a reduction of anxiety, and the drug provides good cardiovascular and respiratory stability. Therapeutic plasma concentrations are achieved in approximately 3 hours when the drug is given orally. The drug is well absorbed via the intramuscular route; however, the patient has a significant amount of pain during the injection of the drug. Lorazepam can also be injected intravenously, and the patient may have some burning on injection. Because of its slow onset and long duration, lorazepam is mainly used as a preanesthetic medication. If this drug has been administered in the preoperative period, the effects of lorazepam may last well into the postoperative period because of its prolonged action. If an opioid is administered in the PACU to a patient who received lorazepam before surgery, the nurse should monitor for increased opioid sedation and respiratory depression because of the potentiation of the opioid by lorazepam.

Caution should be taken with use of lorazepam in the PACU for sedation. Lorazepam does not have any active metabolites. This long-acting but slow-onset benzodiazepine is often delivered via intermittent boluses, but also can be administered as a continuous infusion. Peak effects are not observed for 30 minutes. However, the solvent for lorazepam contains polyethylene glycol 400 and propylene glycol, both of which have been implicated in the development of lactic acidosis, acute tubular necrosis, and hyperosmolar coma when lorazepam is used in prolonged high-dose infusions.[12] The toxic threshold for this effect has not been defined; therefore high-dose infusions should be avoided, and monitoring for these side effects should be initiated.

Lorazepam is sometimes used in the treatment of critically ill patients who are agitated. The guidelines for use can be found in Box 21-2.

Benzodiazepine Antagonists
Flumazenil

Flumazenil (Romazicon), a benzodiazepine antagonist, antagonizes or reverses the effects of benzodiazepine-induced sedation at the benzodiazepine receptors. Consequently, it reverses the

---

BOX 21-2   Guidelines for the Use of Lorazepam for the Treatment of Agitation in the Postanesthesia Care Unit and Critical Care Setting

- Indications: For patients with respiratory or cardiac dysfunction; promotes anxiolysis and amnesia
- Onset of action: 1 to 5 minutes
- Peak of action: 20 to 40 minutes
- Duration of action: 4 to 6 hours
- Doses:
  - Load: 1 to 2 mg IV over 1 to 2 minutes
  - Maximal load: 4 mg in 1 hour (without intubation)
    6 mg in 1 hour (with intubation)
  - Maintenance load: 1 to 3 mg every 1 to 2 hours (IV push)
  - Intravenous infusions: 1 to 5 mg/h
- Precautions: Paradoxic effects can occur
  - Not dialyzed
  - Tapering: Decrease infusion rate by 10% to 25% of maintenance rate every 24 hours

CNS effects of benzodiazepines, such as the sedation produced by diazepam and midazolam. This drug also reverses the other effects produced by benzodiazepine agonists, including anxiolytic, muscle-relaxant, ataxic, and anticonvulsant actions. However, flumazenil may not be effective in the treatment for benzodiazepine-induced hypoventilation or respiratory failure. This drug is specific for the benzodiazepines and, more specifically, their receptors. Consequently, this drug does not reverse the effects of barbiturates, opiates, and ethanol. Flumazenil should be used with great caution in patients who have a history of epilepsy or chronic benzodiazepine use, because reversal with flumazenil in these patients can result in seizures. The incidence rate of postoperative nausea and vomiting is increased after flumazenil has been administered.

The usual reversal dose for flumazenil is 0.4 mg administered intravenously in 0.1-mg increments. Flumazenil should be administered slowly to avoid the adverse consequences of abrupt wakening. A maximum dose for this drug is 1 mg. The onset of action is usually within 5 minutes, with a duration of action between 1 and 2 hours. Flumazenil has a shorter duration of action than most of the benzodiazepines, and consequently the risk of resedation can occur after the initial reversal dose was administered. This risk is especially true when high doses of benzodiazepines were previously administered. Therefore, after the administration of flumazenil, the patient should be monitored for resedation and other residual effects of benzodiazepines in the PACU and on the receiving unit. If signs of resedation develop, flumazenil should be given at 20-minute intervals as needed to reverse the sedation. In this situation, no more than 1 mg should be given at any one time, and no more than 3 mg should be given within a 1-hour period.[5] This drug should prove to be a valuable asset in the care of the patient who has received an excessive dose of a benzodiazepine, such as midazolam or diazepam. Consequently, flumazenil is useful during surgery, after surgery, and in the ICU.[6]

Physostigmine
Physostigmine (Antilirium) is an anticholinesterase that crosses the blood-brain barrier. Its action is inhibition of the enzyme acetylcholinesterase, which results in an increase in the availability of acetylcholine at the receptors that are affected by the benzodiazepines in the CNS. The preponderance of acetylcholine counteracts the negative effects of glycine and GABA. Consequently, this drug provides a nonspecific reversal of the CNS side effects of the benzodiazepines, scopolamine, and ketamine. The dosage is 0.5 to 1 mg, and it should be administered slowly to prevent untoward cholinergic side effects.[1] Because this drug is a nonspecific agent, a number of vagally mediated cholinergic side effects can occur after its administration. These effects include nausea, vomiting, salivation, bradycardia, bronchospasm, and seizures. Because of its nonspecific properties, physostigmine is rarely used for the reversal of the untoward effects of the benzodiazepines.

Butyrophenones
The butyrophenones are a class of sedatives that produce a state of profound calm and immobility in which the patient appears to be pain-free and dissociated from the surroundings. They are a potent inhibitor of the chemoreceptor trigger zone–mediated nausea and vomiting. These drugs have some profound side effects, but seem to be useful in anesthesia and postanesthesia care of the surgical patient. The two major butyrophenones used in clinical practice are haloperidol and droperidol.

Haloperidol
Haloperidol (Haldol) is a butyrophenone tranquilizer that has limited use in anesthesia practice because of its long duration of action and its high incidence rate of extrapyramidal reactions[4]; however, it has been found to be an excellent antiemetic. The drug is not approved for intravenous use and is usually administered intramuscularly at a dose of 2 to 5 mg. It is used in the treatment of psychoses and as an antiemetic. Haloperidol is sometimes used in the treatment of critically ill patients who are agitated. The guidelines for use can be found in Box 21-3.

Droperidol
Droperidol (Inapsine) can be used alone or in combination with fentanyl (Sublimaze) as part of a neuroleptanalgesic technique. Droperidol is rarely used during surgery for the purposes of being a component of anesthesia, but it is administered in small doses for its antiemetic effect after surgery. It produces a state of calm, disinclination to move, and disconnection from surroundings. The drug has an alpha-adrenergic blocking effect, which offers some protection against the vasoconstrictive components of shock; it leads to good peripheral perfusion; and it unmasks hypovolemia. More specifically, when a patient has compensation for a borderline hypovolemic state with activation of the alpha-vasoconstriction mechanisms, vital signs are normal. When a drug such as droperidol is administered to this patient, by virtue of droperidol's alpha-blocking properties, the signs of hypovolemia appear; therefore the patient's hypovolemia is "unmasked." Droperidol

---

BOX 21-3   Guidelines for the Use of Haloperidol for the Treatment of Agitation in the Postanesthesia Care Unit and Critical Care Setting

- Indications: For patients with respiratory or cardiac dysfunction; promotes anxiolysis and amnesia
- Onset of action: 5 to 30 minutes
- Peak of action: 1 hour
- Duration of action: 6 to 8 hours
- Doses:
  - Load: 2.5 to 5 mg IV over 1 to 2 minutes
  - Maximal load: 20 mg in 1 hour (with and without intubation)
  - Maintenance load: When condition is controlled by loading dose, can decrease dose by 50% or by increasing dosing interval
- Precautions: Precipitates with heparin
  - Decreases epinephrine and dopamine activity
  - Contraindicated in Parkinson's disease
  - Not dialyzed

---

also protects against epinephrine-induced arrhythmias and has an antiemetic effect. In fact, because of its excellent antiemetic properties, droperidol is sometimes administered toward the end of the surgical procedure or in the PACU to reduce the risk of vomiting and aspiration in anxious patients. The antiemetic dose of droperidol is between 1 and 2.5 mg and can be given intravenously. Because of its alpha-blocking properties, this drug can be administered in the PACU on a short-term basis to reduce the afterload.

Droperidol is similar to chlorpromazine (Thorazine) in its CNS effects; however, its mechanism of action is different. Droperidol is more selective than chlorpromazine because it provides more tranquility with less sedation and has less effect on the autonomic nervous system. Droperidol has been classified as a neuroleptic and has some adverse effects that should be assessed throughout the PACU phase. Droperidol may cause hypotension because of its alpha-adrenergic blocking effect and peripheral vasodilatation. It may cause extrapyramidal excitation, such as twitchiness, oculogyric seizures, stiff neck muscles, trembling hands, restlessness, and occasionally, psychologic disturbances (e.g., hallucinations). These excitation can be reversed with atropine or antiparkinsonian drugs such as benztropine mesylate (Cogentin) and trihexyphenidyl hydrochloride (Artane).[2] Clinically, patients who have received droperidol have reported the dichotomy of appearing outwardly calm while feeling terrified

inside and unable to express how they feel. As a result, the perianesthesia nurse should provide emotional support to all patients who have received droperidol.

Droperidol is known to potentiate the action of barbiturates and opioids. It has a high therapeutic margin of safety with a rapid onset of 10 minutes, and its activity is lessened in 2 to 4 hours, although some effects last as long as 10 to 12 hours.

Droperidol is the prototype neuroleptic drug. A neuroleptic drug is one that reduces motor activity, lessens anxiety, and produces a state of indifference in which the person can still respond appropriately to commands. Neuroleptanalgesia is a state of profound tranquilization with little or no depressant effect on the cortical centers; therefore neuroleptanalgesia is achieved with the combination of a neuroleptic such as droperidol and a potent opioid analgesic such as fentanyl. A step further is neuroleptanesthesia, the combination of a neuroleptanalgesic (droperidol plus fentanyl), a skeletal muscle relaxant, and nitrous oxide and oxygen. The main objective in the development of neuroleptanesthesia is to provide, for all types of operations, a technique that does not depress the metabolic, circulatory, or central nervous systems as severely as do the inhalation anesthetics when used alone. Droperidol is rarely used as the neuroleptic component; other sedatives are used in its place, such as midazolam and fentanyl.

The U.S. Food and Drug Administration (FDA) strengthened the warnings and precautions in the labeling for droperidol because the drug was associated with fatal cardiac arrhythmias. More specifically, research has shown QT prolongations that indicate delayed recharging of the heart between beats within minutes after injection of droperidol at the upper end of the labeled dose range. Prolonged QT is dangerous because it can cause a potentially fatal heart arrhythmia known as *torsades de pointes*. The new warning is intended to facilitate the focus on the potential for cardiac arrhythmias during administration and to urge the practitioner to consider the use of alternative medications in patients at high risk for cardiac arrhythmias.

Perianesthesia Care

In the immediate postoperative period, the awakening from neuroleptanesthesia is usually rapid, extremely smooth, and uneventful. A striking feature is the extension of analgesia well into the postoperative period. It is difficult to explain the mechanism of such a prolonged pain-relieving effect with a drug such as fentanyl, in which the onset is so rapid and the duration of action is so short.

Nursing personnel in the PACU should constantly assess the patient for signs of respiratory depression when droperidol is used, even in small doses for its antiemetic properties. Opioids should be titrated to effect in patients who have received low-dose droperidol. If droperidol was used as the neuroleptic component of the anesthetic, the dose of opioid agonists is recommended to be reduced to as little as one fourth to one third the usual dose because of the additive potentiating effects of droperidol.

The patient should be encouraged to cough and perform the sustained maximal inspiration (SMI) maneuver in the PACU (see Chapters 12 and 28). Patients who have received even low-dose droperidol can drift back to sleep unless they are encouraged to move about the surroundings. The perianesthesia nurse will find that, because the analgesia extends into the postoperative period, the patient who has received droperidol is more willing to cough and perform the SMI maneuver. The perianesthesia nurse should use verbal stimulation with these patients because, if ordered, the patient will be able to take a deep breath; otherwise, respiration may remain slow and shallow, or the patient may even become apneic. Consequently the perianesthesia nurse must remain with the patient, provide verbal stimulation, and actively monitor for any signs of respiratory depression.

The perianesthesia nurse should monitor for extrapyramidal symptoms; although rare, these symptoms have been detected as long as 24 hours after a single administration of droperidol. Most of the reported extrapyramidal reactions occurred in children younger than 12 years of age. Because of the length of action of droperidol, the perianesthesia nurse is recommended to provide information about the drug to the nursing personnel on the surgical units via hospital in-service education programs, even when the drug is given in small doses as an antiemetic.

NONSTEROIDAL ANTINFLAMMATORY DRUGS

Ketorolac

Ketorolac (Toradol) is an analgesic that is classified as a nonsteroidal antiinflammatory drug (NSAID). Its mode of action is inhibition of the prostaglandin synthetase enzyme; therefore ketorolac has analgesic, antiinflammatory, and antipyretic actions. An intramuscular dose of 30 mg of this drug is equal to approximately 12 mg of morphine or 100 mg of meperidine in degree of postoperative pain relief. This drug can be administered via either the intravenous or intramuscular route (see Table 19-1). When it is used with supplemental opioids, ketorolac is an excellent postoperative analgesia. For acute postoperative pain, an initial loading dose of 30 mg can be administered intramuscularly. Ketorolac can be administered every 6 hours thereafter at a dose of 15 mg. The duration of analgesia, but not the peak analgesic effect, is increased when the dose is increased beyond its recommended dose range of 15 to 60 mg. Ketorolac should be given at a lower dose range for patients with renal disease, for the elderly (older than 70 years) and for patients who weigh less than 50 kg. Because this drug is an NSAID and not an opioid, its lack of effect on psychomotor activities and on the respiratory system makes it an ideal analgesic for outpatient surgery.

Clinically, for the advantage of the peak effects of ketorolac, the drug is sometimes administered intramuscularly approximately 1 hour before the end of the surgical procedure. In this instance, the patient usually emerges from anesthesia in an analgesic state that lasts well into the immediate postoperative period. For an effective analgesic plan in the PACU, the postanesthesia nurse must determine whether ketorolac was given during surgery to avoid analgesic overmedication.

Indomethacin

Indomethacin is another NSAID that may be useful in the relief of moderate to severe postoperative pain. Its featured drug action is to reduce the amount of substance P, a neuropeptide that causes pain, fever, and inflammation.

This drug has been shown to reduce postoperative pain in the PACU and in particular, patients recovering from a cholecystectomy when used as a rectal suppository.[13] It is hoped that more research will be conducted in the PACU to determine the effectiveness of pain reduction using NSAIDs such as indomethacin.

Nonopioid Medications

OFIRMEV (acetaminophen) is the first intravenous formulation of acetaminophen in the United States. It is indicated for the management of mild to moderate pain, management of moderate to severe pain with adjunctive opioid analgesics, and reduction of fever. It is for use with patients who are adults or children age 2 years or older. This new drug has become an important component of a multimodal approach to postoperative pain management.[14]

OFIRMEV is administered over a 15-minute period. The onset of analgesia occurs within 5 to 10 minutes of intravenous administration, with the peak analgesic effect within 1-hour a duration of 4 to 6 hours. It should be used with caution in patients who have hepatic impairment; however, it has not been shown to affect platelet function or increase surgical bleeding, which means it can be used during the perioperative period. Acetaminophen can potentiate the anticoagulant effects of warfarin; it does not cause the gastric irritation that has been attributed to NSAIDs.[14] Intravenous acetaminophen may decrease the consumption of opioids by postoperative patients. OFIRMEV will become part of a multimodal approach to pain management that will affect patient comfort and satisfaction and lead to increased patient safety with fewer required opioid rescues.[14]

Other Sedative Medications

Dexmedetomidine

Dexmedetomidine (Precedex) is a newer alpha-2 agonist, like clonidine, that is a novel sedative with analgesic properties that controls stress, anxiety, and pain and does not cause respiratory depression. Like clonidine, its mechanism of action is as an agonist of alpha-2 receptors in certain parts of the brain. Consequently, this drug facilitates patient comfort, compliance, and comprehension by providing sedation along with the ability to rouse the patient.

Dexmedetomidine is sevenfold more selective for the alpha receptors and has a shorter duration of action and is considered a full agonist for the alpha-2 receptors. Consequently, it is an excellent drug to decrease the amounts of inhalation anesthetics and opioids. It is also an effective drug in attenuating the cardiostimulatory and postanesthetic delirium effects of ketamine. Dexmedetomidine increases the range of temperatures that do not trigger the thermoregulatory defenses; therefore it is likely to produce some perioperative hypothermia and to be an effective treatment for postoperative shivering.

With stimulation of the alpha-2 receptors, dexmedetomidine decreases the systolic blood pressure; the systemic vascular resistance is little affected, and the cardiac output, which is initially decreased, returns toward predrug levels. The homeostatic cardiovascular reflexes are maintained, and the problems of orthostatic hypotension are avoided.

In the PACU, if dexmedetomidine is administered via intravenous infusion, the nurse should monitor the patient for significant episodes of bradycardia and hypotension. If intervention is necessary, decreasing or stopping the dexmedetomidine infusion and increasing the rate of intravenous fluid administration along with elevation of the lower extremities may be all that is

Table 21-1	Ramsay Level of Sedation Scale
CLINICAL SCORE	LEVEL OF SEDATION ACHIEVED
6	Asleep, no response
5	Asleep, sluggish response to light glabellar tap or loud auditory stimulus
4	Asleep, but with brisk response to light glabellar tap or loud auditory stimulus
3	Patient responds to commands
2	Patient cooperative, oriented, and tranquil
1	Patient anxious, agitated, or restless

needed; if the hypotension continues, vasopressor agents may be necessary (see Chapter 11). If the bradycardia continues, the PACU nurse may need to intervene by obtaining a physician order for an anticholinergic such as atropine or glycopyrrolate. A dexmedetomidine infusion is not recommended to last more than 24 hours. Because dexmedetomidine resembles the alpha-2 adrenergic agent clonidine, abrupt withdrawal of the drug can result in symptoms associated with abrupt stoppage of clonidine. Consequently, when dexmedetomidine is discontinued, symptoms that include nervousness, agitation, headaches, and a rapid rise in blood pressure should be monitored and reported to the anesthesia provider immediately.

Dexmedetomidine is usually administered with a controlled infusion device. The drug should be titrated to the desired clinical effect, which is usually less than 3 on the Ramsey Sedation Scale (Table 21-1). Generally, a loading infusion of 1 mcg/kg over 10 minutes followed by a maintenance infusion of 0.2 to 0.6 mcg/kg/h, and the rate of the maintenance infusion can be adjusted to achieve the desired level of sedation.

DISSOCIATIVE ANESTHETICS

Ketamine

Traditionally, general anesthetic agents achieved control of pain with depression of the CNS. Ketamine is an anesthetic agent that has been introduced has a totally different mode of action. It selectively blocks pain conduction and perception, leaving those parts of the CNS that do not participate in pain transmission and perception free from the depressant effects of the drug. Ketamine is a dissociative drug because patients whose conditions are totally analgesic usually do not appear to be asleep or anesthetized, but rather disassociated from the surroundings. The drug is nonbarbiturate and nonopioid. It is administered parenterally and has a short duration. Early laboratory studies with ketamine suggested that most of the drug's activity is centered in the frontal lobe of the cerebral cortex.

The clinical characteristics of ketamine consist of a state of profound analgesia combined with a state of unconsciousness. The patient usually has marked horizontal and vertical nystagmus. The eyes are usually open and shortly become centered and appear in a fixed gaze. The pupils are moderately dilated and react to light. Respiratory function is usually unimpaired, except after rapid intravenous injection, when it may become depressed for a short time. Ketamine is sympathomimetic in action and is beneficial to patients with asthma because of its bronchodilating effect. When patients receive ketamine, the pharyngeal and laryngeal reflexes remain intact. The tongue usually does not become relaxed, and the airway usually remains unobstructed. Ketamine accelerates the heart rate moderately and increases both the systolic and the diastolic pressure for several minutes, after which the pulse and blood pressure return to preinjection levels. Finally, ketamine increases cerebral blood flow and, consequently, intracranial pressure. Therefore this drug definitely is contraindicated in patients who are at risk for increased intracranial pressure.[15]

Ketamine can be administered intramuscularly or intravenously. The intramuscular dose 6.5 to 13 mg/kg, and the anesthesia lasts from 20 to 40 minutes. The intravenous dose is usually 1 to 4 mg/kg, with anesthesia lasting 6 to 10 minutes. Complete recovery from ketamine varies according to the duration of surgery and the amount of ketamine used throughout the procedure. When a single dose of intravenous ketamine is used, recovery time is usually rapid and does not exceed 30 minutes. When supplemental intravenous doses need to be administered, more particularly when supplemental intramuscular doses are necessary, recovery is often markedly prolonged, sometimes as long as 3 hours.

Perianesthesia Care

When patients emerge from ketamine anesthesia, they may go through a phase of vivid dreaming, with or without psychomotor activity manifested by confusion, irrational behavior, and hallucinations. The perianesthesia nurse should be aware that such psychic aberrations are usually transient and appear to be preventable by avoiding early verbal or tactile stimulation of the patient, which helps to prevent fear and anxiety reactions. Short-acting barbiturates administered intravenously can effectively control the psychic responses sometimes seen after the administration of ketamine. Pediatric patients seem to be less prone to these psychic disturbances. Results of a study revealed that droperidol may be effective in eliminating some of the adverse psychic emergence phenomena of ketamine. Other sedatives such as diazepam have also been found effective in suppression of these phenomena. In addition, the drug dexmedetomidine (Precedex) can help suppress this adverse phenomena. When a patient is admitted to the PACU, the nurse should be aware of any sedatives or whether dexmedetomidine has been administered to the patient.

On arrival in the PACU, the patient should be secluded from auditory, visual, and tactile stimuli and be observed for any signs of respiratory depression. Mechanical airway obstruction, particularly when caused by marked salivation, accounts for most of the instances of respiratory insufficiency after ketamine anesthesia. When the patient does not have adequate respiratory exchange, oxygen should be administered via mask until it is restored. Other important signs to watch for are persistent blood pressure elevation, tachycardia, bradycardia, dreaming, delirium, hallucinations, euphoria, and increased muscle tone. All PACU personnel must know that attempts to rouse patients while they are still unable to see, hear, and orient themselves may set off a chain of anxiety reactions that may ultimately lead to severe psychomotor responses and even more irrational behavior. Should the patient have this augmented psychomotor behavior, dexmedetomidine (Precedex) or one of the benzodiazepine sedation drugs can be administered to facilitate a reduction in the aberrant behavior.

The widespread use of ketamine requires an entirely different approach to perianesthesia nursing care. It should also be noted that ketamine coupled with a small dose of a benzodiazepine may be continued in a low-dose intravenous for sedation and pain relief in the PACU. Certainly, the agent has some deficiencies, but commonly overlooked is the fact that it is one of the safest anesthetics. Its safety justifies its important place in the drugs used by the anesthesiologist. Ketamine appears to be an excellent anesthetic for pediatric patients, as the sole agent for short procedures, for induction of anesthesia in patients at extremely poor risk, and for patients with burns that necessitate surgical treatment. Certain adult orthopedic and diagnostic procedures have also been found suitable for the use of ketamine anesthesia. Ketamine continues to be popular for certain types of anesthetic procedures. Because ketamine is a dissociative agent, its actions should be well

CONCEPTS IN ANESTHETIC AGENTS

understood by the PACU staff to ensure effective informed care of the patient.

SUMMARY

The nonopioid agents are gaining popularity because they are becoming more opioid-like without the side effects. In addition, the induction agents have changed from thiopental to propofol in a short time. The same can be said for the benzodiazepines in the perioperative patient; midazolam is preferred to diazepam. In both cases, the newer drugs offer distinct advantages during surgery and, more importantly, after surgery in the PACU. Finally, the drug ketamine has continued over the years to serve as an excellent anesthetic for specific situations. In addition, the PACU stay for the patient who has received ketamine has improved significantly because of the many adjunct drugs that can be used to prevent the psychic aberrations associated with that drug in the PACU. If fact, because ketamine has demonstrated many positive effects on the relief of postanesthesia pain, it is an agent that can be used in a low-dose intravenous infusion in the PACU with minimal side effects. In an effort to reduce the length of stay of the patient and to provide appropriate post anesthesia pain relief, the nonopioid pharmacologic agents are becoming an important component of intraoperative and postanesthesia care.

REFERENCES

1. Brunton L, et al: *Goodman and Gilman's the pharmacological basis of therapeutics*, ed 12, New York, 2010, McGraw-Hill Professional.
2. Stoelting R: *Pharmacology and physiology in anesthetic practice*, ed 4, Philadelphia, 2005, Lippincott Williams & Wilkins.
3. Aitkenhead A, et al: *Textbook of anesthesia*, ed 5, Philadelphia, 2007, Churchill Livingstone.
4. Miller R, Pardo M: *Basics of anesthesia*, ed 6, Philadelphia, 2011, Saunders.
5. Nagelhout J, Plaus K: *Nurse anesthesia*, ed 4, St. Louis, 2010, Saunders.
6. Schick L, Windle PE: *Perianesthesia nursing core curriculum: preprocedure, phase I and phase II PACU nursing*, ed 2, Philadelphia, 2010, Saunders.
7. Blouin R, Gross J: Ventilation and conscious sedation, *Semin Anesth* 15(4):335–342, 1996.
8. Key K, et al: Use of propofol and emergence agitation in children: a literature review, *AANA J* 78(6):468-473, 2010.
9. Barash P, et al: *Clinical anesthesia*, ed 6, Philadelphia, 2009, Lippincott Williams & Wilkins.
10. Fisher L: *Anesthesia and uncommon diseases*, ed 5, Philadelphia, 2007, Saunders.
11. Shorten G, et al: *Postoperative pain management: an evidence-based guide to practice*, Philadelphia, 2006, Saunders.
12. Borchardt M: Review of the clinical pharmacology and use of the benzodiazepines, *J Perianesth Nurs* 14(2):65–72, 1999.
13. Babar M, et al: Effect of preoperative rectal indomethacin on postoperative pain reduction after open cholecystectomy, *J Perianesth Nurs* 25(1):7–10, 2010.
14. Groudine S, Fossum S: Use of intravenous acetaminophen in the treatment of postoperative pain, *J Perianesth Nurs* 26(2):74–80, 2011.
15. Rakic A, Golembiewski J: Low-dose ketamine infusion for postoperative pain management, *J Perianesth Nurs* 24(4):254–257, 2009.

RESOURCES

American Association of Critical-Care Nurses: *Core curriculum for progressive care nursing*, Philadelphia, 2010, Saunders.
Aitkenhead A, et al: *Textbook of anesthesia*, ed 5, Philadelphia, 2007, Churchill Livingstone.
Alspach J: *Core curriculum for critical care nursing*, ed 6, Philadelphia, 2005, Saunders.
Atlee J: *Complications in anesthesia*, ed 2, Philadelphia, 2007, Saunders.
Barash P, et al: *Clinical anesthesia*, ed 6, Philadelphia, 2009, Lippincott Williams & Wilkins.
Barrett K, et al: *Ganong's review of medical physiology*, ed 23, New York, 2009, McGraw-Hill Medical.
Bready L, et al: *Decision making in anesthesiology*, ed 4, St. Louis, 2007, Mosby.
Brunton L, et al: *Goodman and Gilman's the pharmacological basis of therapeutics*, ed 12, New York, 2010, McGraw-Hill Professional.
Conlay L, et al: *Case files anesthesiology*, New York, 2011, McGraw-Hill Medical.
Davis P, et al: *Smith's anesthesia for infants and children*, ed 8, St. Louis, 2011, Mosby.
Drake R, et al: *Gray's anatomy for students*, ed 2, Philadelphia, 2009, Churchill Livingstone.
Deutschman C, Netigan P: *Evidence-based practice of critical care*, Philadelphia, 2010, Saunders.
Fisher L: *Anesthesia and uncommon diseases*, ed 5, Philadelphia, 2007, Saunders.
Gallager C, Issenberg B: *Simulation in anesthesia*, Philadelphia, 2007, Saunders.
Hall J: *Guyton and Hall textbook of medical physiology*, ed 12, Philadelphia, 2011, Saunders.
Hines R, Marschall K: *Handbook for Stoelting's anesthesia and co-existing disease*, ed 3, Philadelphia, 2009, Saunders.
Hines R, Marschall K: *Stoelting's anesthesia and co-existing disease*, ed 6, Philadelphia, 2012, Saunders.
Kaplan J, et al: *Cardiac anesthesia*, New York, 2011, Churchill Livingstone.
Kier L, Dowd C: *The chemistry of drugs for nurse anesthetists*, Chicago, 2004, AANA Publishing.
Kulli J, Koch C: Does anesthesia cause loss of consciousness? *Trends Neurosci* 14(1):6–10, 1991.
Longnecker D, et al: *Anesthesiology*, New York, 2007, McGraw-Hill Medical.
Miller R, et al: *Miller's anesthesia*, ed 7, Philadelphia, 2009, Churchill Livingstone.
Miller R, Pardo M: *Basics of anesthesia*, ed 6, Philadelphia, 2011, Saunders.

Mason R: *Murray and Nadel's textbook of respiratory medicine,* ed 5, Philadelphia, 2011, Saunders.

Nagelhout J, Plaus K: *Nurse anesthesia,* ed 4, St. Louis, 2010, Saunders.

Pasero C, McCaffery M: *Pain assessment and pharmacologic management,* St. Louis, 2011, Mosby.

Pasero C, McCaffery M: Orthopaedic postoperative pain management, *J Perianesth Nurs* 22(3):160–174, 2007.

Prielipp R, Young C: Current drugs for sedation of critically ill patients, *Semin Anesthesia Perioperative Med Pain* 20(2): 85–94, 2001.

Reves J, et al: Midazolam: pharmacology and uses, *Anesthesiology* 62:310–324, 1985.

Sandberg W, et al: *The MGH textbook of anesthetic equipment,* New York, 2011, Churchill Livingstone.

Schreiber J, et al: Prevention of succinylcholine-induced fasciculation and myalgia, *Anesthesiology* 103:877-884, 2005.

Sieber F: *Geriatric anesthesia,* New York, 2006, McGraw-Hill Medical.

Stoelting R: *Pharmacology and physiology in anesthetic practice,* ed 4, Philadelphia, 2005, Lippincott Williams & Wilkins.

Townsend CM, et al: *Sabiston textbook of surgery: the biological basis of modern surgical practice,* ed 19, Philadelphia, 2012, Saunders.

Vincent J, et al: *Textbook of critical care,* ed 6, Philadelphia, 2011, Saunders.

White P: *Perioperative drug manual,* ed 2, Philadelphia, 2005, Saunders.

CONCEPTS IN ANESTHETIC AGENTS

22 Opioid Intravenous Anesthetics

Cecil B. Drain, PhD, RN, CRNA, FAAN, FASAHP

Opioid intravenous anesthetics constitute a major portion of the clinical anesthesia process. These drugs enhance the effectiveness of the inhalation anesthetics. More specifically, the opioids meet much of the analgesic portion of the anesthesia process. The addition of the opioids to the drugs used for general anesthesia can reduce the concentration of the inhalation anesthetic; as a result, a safer anesthetic can be administered to the patient. Because opioids are used to manage acute and chronic pain and are administered for general inhalation anesthesia, sedation, and pain relief during regional anesthesia, the implications for the postanesthesia nursing care of the surgical patient are profound.

The immediate postanesthesia phase is when the patient is most vulnerable to complications (see Chapter 29).[1] Many drugs that have residual anesthetic effects well into the postanesthesia period are used in modern anesthesia care. These agents include the potent inhaled agents, muscle relaxants, benzodiazepines, and opioids. Respiratory depression is the most common adverse event in the postanesthesia care unit (PACU); therefore the use and understanding of the various opioid agents optimize patient outcomes. In addition, the reduction of pain in the PACU is one of the primary focuses of care in the perianesthesia phase. In addition to assessing pain, the perianesthesia nurse must take into the evaluation of pain the preoperative, intraoperative, and postanesthesia phase of the surgical patient. Because all pain-reducing drugs must be taken into account during the pain assessment in the PACU, the mixed action or agonist-antagonist combination drugs are presented in this chapter. With a detailed description of the major opioids used in the perianesthesia period provided, the PACU nurse will be able to make excellent informed decisions in regard to the anticipated outcome of the patient of pain reduction and comfort.

DEFINITIONS

Agonist: A drug with a specific cellular or receptor affinity that produces a predictable response.
Antagonist: A drug that exerts an opposite action to that of another or competes for the same receptor site or sites.

Breakthrough Pain: A transient increase in the intensity of pain from a baseline pain level that is no greater than moderate.
Dysphoria: A disorder of affect that is characterized by depression and anguish.
Endogenous: Originating inside the body.
Endorphins: These opioid peptides are produced in the body and are composed of many amino acid (protein) substances that attach to opioid receptors in the central nervous system and the peripheral nervous system for reduction of pain.
Exogenous: Originating outside the body.
Fixed Chest Syndrome: Rigidity of the diaphragmatic and intercostal muscles.
Mydriasis: Dilation of the pupil of the eye.
Opiate Receptor: Receptors that are transmembrane proteins that bind to endogenous opioid neuropeptides and exogenous morphine and similar compounds. They are designated mu, kappa, and delta subtypes of the opiate receptor.
Opioid: A drug that contains opium or a derivative of opium along with semisynthetic or synthetic drugs that have opium-like properties.
Piloerection: Erection of the hairs of the skin.
Spasmolytic: Stoppage of muscle group contractions.

CONCEPT OF OPIOIDS AND OPIOID RECEPTORS

Opioids are the substances, either natural or synthetic, that are administered into the body (exogenous) and bind to specific receptors to produce a morphine-like or opioid agonist effect. The endogenous opioids are the endorphins. The endorphins, which are produced in the body, attach to the opioid receptors in the central nervous system (CNS) to activate the body's pain modulating system. The term *opioid* is used because of the multitude of synthetic drugs with morphine-like actions; with the advent of receptor physiology, *opioid* has replaced the term *narcotic,* which is derived from the Greek word for "stupor" and usually refers to both the production of the morphine-like effects and the physical dependence.[2]

The naturally occurring alkaloids of opium are divided into two classes: phenanthrene and benzylisoquinoline. The principal phenanthrene series of drugs includes morphine, codeine, and thebaine. Papaverine and noscapine, which lack opioid activity, represent the benzylisoquinoline alkaloids of opium.[3]

The synthetic opioids have been produced with the modification of the chemical structure of the phenanthrene class of drugs. Drugs such as fentanyl (Sublimaze) and meperidine (Demerol) are examples of synthetic opioids.[2,4]

The identification of specific opioid receptors has enhanced the understanding of the agonist and antagonist actions of this category of drugs. The opioid receptors are located in the CNS, principally in the brain stem and spinal cord. These receptors have been determined by the pharmacologic effect they produce when stimulated by a specific agonist along with how the effect is blocked by a specific antagonist. The three major categories of opioid receptors are the mu (μ), delta (δ), and kappa (κ).[4,5]

The mu receptors are mainly responsible for the production of supraspinal analgesia effects with stimulation. These receptors are further divided into mu-1 and mu-2 types. Activation of the mu-1 receptors results in analgesia; when the mu-2 receptors are stimulated, hypoventilation, bradycardia, physical dependence, euphoria, and ileus can result. The mu receptors are activated by morphine, fentanyl, and meperidine. The drug that is specific to the mu-1 receptor is meptazinol, which is supraspinal in regard to analgesia; the mu-2 receptor analgesia occurs at the spinal level. Other characteristics of the mu-1 and mu-2 receptors are summarized in Table 22-1. Stimulation of the kappa receptors results in spinal analgesia, dysphoria, hallucinations, hypertonia, tachycardia, tachypnea, mydriasis, sedation, and miosis, with little effect on ventilation. The drugs that possess both opioid agonist and antagonist activities, such as nalbuphine (Nubain), have their principal action on the kappa opioid receptors. The delta opioid receptors, when stimulated, serve to modulate the activity of the mu receptors and cause depression and urinary retention. The drug naloxone (Narcan) attaches to all the opioid receptors and thus serves as an antagonist to all the opioid agonists (see Table 22-1).[2,4]

CONCEPTS IN ANESTHETIC AGENTS

Table 22-1 Characteristics of Various Opioid Receptors

EFFECTS	MU RECEPTOR		KAPPA RECEPTOR	DELTA RECEPTOR
	MU-1	MU-2		
Analgesia	Supraspinal	Spinal	Supraspinal, spinal	Supraspinal, spinal; modulates mu-receptor activity
Cardiovascular effects	Bradycardia	Bradycardia		
Respiratory effects		Depression	Possible depression	Depression
Central nervous system effects	Euphoria; sedation; prolactin release; hypothermia; catalepsy; indifference to environmental stimulus	Euphoria; dopamine turnover; possible growth hormone release	Sedation; dysphoria; psychotomimetic reactions (hallucinations, delirium)	
Pupil	Miosis	Miosis	Miosis	
Gastrointestinal effects		Inhibition of peristalsis; nausea, vomiting		
Genitourinary effects	Urinary retention	Urinary retention	Diuresis (inhibition of vasopressin release)	Urinary retention
Pruritus		Yes		Yes
Physical dependence	Low abuse potential	Yes	Low abuse potential	Yes

From Nagelhout J, Plaus K: *Nurse anesthesia*, ed 4, St. Louis, 2010, Saunders.
Other opioid subtypes exist in animals, such as kappa-1, kappa-2, and kappa-3. Mu-1 and mu-2 agonists have not been developed for human use.

Opioids

Opioids, or narcotics, are used often in anesthesia practice. They are usually used in the nitrous-opioid (balanced) techniques, which involve the use of an opioid, nitrous oxide, and oxygen, with or without a muscle relaxant, and propofol for induction.

The effects of opioids generally last well into the PACU phase, and every perianesthesia nurse should have a good knowledge of the pharmacologic actions of each opioid that is administered to the patient in the perioperative phase of the surgical experience.

The administration of opioids in the perioperative period is not without the concern of overdose. The major signs of overdose with opioids are miosis, hypoventilation, and coma. If the patient becomes severely hypoxemic, mydriasis can occur. Airway obstruction is a strong possibility because the skeletal muscles become flaccid. Hypotension and seizures can also occur. The treatment for an opioid overdose is mechanical ventilation and the slow titration of naloxone. Consideration must always be given to the fact that some patients who become overdosed with an opioid may indeed be already physically dependent. Naloxone can precipitate an acute withdrawal syndrome.[2]

Meperidine Hydrochloride

Meperidine (Demerol) was discovered in 1939 by Eisleb and Schauman. Because it is chemically similar to atropine, it was originally introduced as an antispasmodic agent and was not used as an opioid anesthetic agent until 1947. The main action of this drug is similar to morphine; it stimulates the subcortical mu receptors, which results in an analgesic effect. Meperidine is approximately one tenth as potent as morphine and has a duration of action of 2 to 4 hours. The onset of analgesia is prompt (10 minutes) after subcutaneous or intramuscular administration. All pain, especially visceral, gastrointestinal, and urinary tract, is satisfactorily relieved. This drug causes less biliary tract spasm than morphine; however, in comparison with codeine, meperidine causes greater biliary tract spasm. It produces some sleepiness but causes little euphoria or amnesia. Meperidine increases the sensitivity of the labyrinthine apparatus of the ear, which explains the dizziness, nausea, and vomiting that sometimes occur in ambulatory patients.[2,4]

This opioid may slow the rate of respiration, but the rate generally returns to normal within 15 minutes after intravenous injection. The tidal volume is not changed appreciably. In equivalent analgesic doses, meperidine depresses respiration to a greater extent than does morphine. Some authors have noted that meperidine can release histamine from the tissues. Occasionally, urticarial wheals form over the veins where meperidine has been injected. The usual treatment is discontinuation of the use of meperidine and, if the reaction is severe, administration of diphenhydramine (Benadryl). Diphenhydramine further sedates the patient, however, and should be administered only if truly warranted.

Meperidine in therapeutic doses does not cause any significant untoward effects on the cardiovascular system. When this drug is administered intravenously, it usually causes a transient increase in heart rate. With intramuscular administration, no significant change in heart rate is observed. One of the major concerns with this drug is orthostatic hypotension, probably caused by meperidine's interference with the compensatory sympathetic nervous system reflex. After administration of meperidine, a patient should be repositioned slowly in a "staged" approach to avoid any possibility of hypotension.

Meperidine is generally metabolized in the liver; less than 5% is excreted unchanged by the kidneys. However, because of a toxic metabolite of meperidine, patients who are administered this drug may have seizures.[2] Meperidine is partially metabolized to normeperidine which has some analgesic effects, but more importantly, lowers the seizure threshold and can induce CNS excitability. Meperidine probably should not be administered to elderly patients because renal dysfunction may occur and less tolerance to normeperidine.

Because of its spasmolytic effect, meperidine is the drug of choice for biliary duct, distal colon, and rectal surgery. It offers the advantages of little interference with the physiologic compensatory mechanisms, low toxicity, smooth and rapid recovery, prolonged postoperative analgesia, excellent cardiac stability in patients at poor risk, and ease of detoxification and excretion.[2,4,5] Meperidine is used most often with procedures now, and not typically for long-term pain management because of the effects of normeperidine over time.

Morphine

Morphine, one of the oldest known drugs, has only recently been used as an opioid intravenous anesthetic agent. Alkaloid morphine is from the phenanthrene class of opium. The exact mechanism of action of morphine is unknown. In humans, it produces analgesia, drowsiness, changes in mood, and mental clouding. The analgesic effect can become profound before the other effects are severe and can persist after many of the side effects have almost disappeared. With direct effect on the respiratory center, morphine depresses respiratory rate, tidal volume, and minute volume. Maximal respiratory depression occurs within 7 minutes after intravenous injection of the drug and 30 minutes after intramuscular administration. After therapeutic doses of morphine, the sensitivity of the respiratory center begins to return to normal in 2 or 3 hours, but the minute volume does not return to preinjection level until 4 or 5 hours have passed.

The greatest advantage of morphine is the remarkable cardiovascular stability that accompanies its use. It has no major effect on blood pressure, heart rate, or heart rhythm—even in toxic doses, when hypoxia is avoided. Morphine does, however, decrease the capacity of the cardiovascular system to adjust to gravitational shifts. This effect is important to remember because orthostatic hypotension and syncope may easily occur in a patient whose care necessitates a position change. This phenomenon is primarily the result of the peripheral vasodilator effect of morphine. Therefore a position change for a patient who has received morphine should be accomplished slowly, with constant monitoring of the patient's vital signs.

Morphine can cause nausea and vomiting, especially in ambulatory patients, because of direct stimulation of the chemoreceptor trigger zone. The emetic effect of morphine can be counteracted with opioid antagonists and phenothiazine derivatives such as prochlorperazine (Compazine), dexmedetomidine (Precedex), or the 5-HT$_3$ receptor antagonist ondansetron (Zofran). Histamine release has been noted with morphine, and morphine also causes profound constriction of the pupils, stimulation of the visceral smooth muscles, and spasm of the sphincter of Oddi.[5-7]

Morphine is detoxified by conjugation with glucuronic acid. Ninety percent is excreted by the kidneys, and 7% to 10% is excreted in the feces via the bile.[2]

Morphine is used in the balanced, or nitrous-opioid, technique with nitrous oxide, oxygen, and a muscle relaxant. This technique is useful for cardiovascular surgery and other types of surgery in which cardiovascular stability is necessary. The patient may arrive in the PACU still narcotized from morphine with an endotracheal tube in place. Mechanical ventilation for 24 to 48 hours is usually warranted. Morphine may or may not be supplemented during the time of ventilation. This type of recovery procedure facilitates a pain free state and maximum ventilation of the patient during the critical phase of recovery. Morphine can also be used to provide basal narcosis when regional anesthesia is used.

In the PACU, morphine is an excellent drug for the control of postoperative pain. When given intravenously, this drug has a peak analgesic effect in approximately 20 minutes, with a duration of approximately 2 hours. With intramuscular administration, the onset of action is approximately 15 minutes, with a peak effect attained in 45 to 90 minutes and a duration of action of approximately 4 hours.

Methadone

Methadone was introduced in the late 1930s in Germany and in the 1940s in the United States. The drug was originally introduced to help treat chronic pain, opioid abstinence syndromes, and heroin addiction. It has seen a resurgence in popularity for clinical use in the PACU for pain relief.

Methadone undergoes slow metabolism and is high in lipid solubility, which makes it longer lasting that morphine-based drugs, with a duration of action up to 24 hours that allows for less frequent dosing. It is a good drug for treating chronic pain, especially in patients who are thought to have a propensity for drug dependence. Methadone can be administered orally and intravenously; when administered intravenously at a dose of 20 mg, methadone produces postoperative analgesia that lasts more than 24 hours.

The actions of this synthetic opioid agonist resemble morphine; side effects include depression of ventilation, miosis, constipation, and biliary tract spasm. Clinically, the sedative and euphoric actions of methadone appear to be less than those produced by morphine.[5]

Hydromorphone

Hydromorphone (Dilaudid), which is a derivative of morphine, was developed in Germany in the 1920s and released to the mass market in the late 1920s. The drug has a renewed popularity for the PACU and can be administered intravenously, intramuscularly, rectally, or orally. The drug profile in regard to its analgesia and side effects is similar to morphine. Hydromorphone is recommended for patients in renal failure because of its virtual lack of active metabolites after its breakdown in the liver. It has a high solubility and a rapid onset of action and appears to have less troublesome side effects and dependence liability profile as compared with morphine. Because of its high lipid solubility, hydromorphone can be administered via epidural or spinal for a wide area of anesthesia as compared with duramophine.[2]

Hydromorphone, like all opioids, is a CNS depressant and has actions and side effects similar to morphine. Its depressant effects can be enhanced with beta-blockers and alcohol. The duration of action of this drug is approximately 2 hours, with a peak action in approximately 30 minutes with intravenous administration.

Fentanyl

Janssen and colleagues[8] introduced a series of highly potent meperidine derivatives that were found to render the patient free of pain without affecting certain areas in the CNS. Fentanyl (Sublimaze) appeared to be of special interest. In regard to analgesic properties, fentanyl is approximately 80- to 125-fold more potent as morphine and has a rapid onset of action of 5 to 6 minutes and a peak effect within 5 to 15 minutes. The analgesia lasts 20 to 40 minutes when administered intravenously. Via the intramuscular route, the onset of action is 7 to 15 minutes; the analgesia usually lasts 1 to 2 hours. When fentanyl is administered as a single bolus, 75% of the drug undergoes first-pass pulmonary uptake. That is, the lungs serve as a large storage site and this non-respiratory function of the lung (see Chapter 12) limits the amount of fentanyl that actually reaches the systemic circulation. If the patient receives multiple doses of fentanyl via single injections or infusion, the first-pass pulmonary uptake mechanism becomes saturated and the patient has a prolonged emergence because of increased duration of the drug. Consequently, during the admission of the patient to the PACU, the postanesthesia nurse must determine the frequency and amount of intraoperative fentanyl administration. Patients who have received a significant amount of fentanyl via infusion or via titration should be continuously monitored for persistent or recurrent respiratory depression. In addition, fentanyl has been implicated in what is called a *delayed-onset respiratory depression*. In some patients, a secondary peak of the drug concentration in the plasma occurs approximately 45 minutes after the apparent recovery from the drug. This syndrome can occur when some of the fentanyl becomes sequestered in the gastric fluid and then can become recycled into the plasma in approximately 45 minutes. Therefore, in the PACU, all patients who have received fentanyl should be continuously monitored for respiratory depression for at least 1 hour from the time of admission to the unit.[2]

Fentanyl can be administered during surgery at three different dose ranges, depending on the type of surgery and the desired effect. For example, the low-dose range of 2 to 20 mcg/kg attenuates moderately stressful stimuli. The moderate dose range is 20 to 50 mcg/kg and strongly obtunds the stress response. The megadose range of as much as 150 mcg/kg blocks the stress response

and is particularly valuable when protection of the myocardium is critical.[4]

Fentanyl shares with most other opioids a profound respiratory depressant effect, even to the point of apnea. Rapid intravenous injection can provoke bronchial constriction and resistance to ventilation caused by rigidity of the diaphragmatic and intercostal muscles. This is commonly called the *fixed chest syndrome*, which can occur when any potent opioid analgesic is administered too rapidly via the intravenous route. Should this syndrome occur, intravenous subclinical administration of succinylcholine (15 to 25 mg) relieves the rigidity of the chest wall muscles. When succinylcholine is administered for this purpose, the perianesthesia nurse should be prepared to ventilate the patient's lungs until the skeletal muscle relaxant properties of succinylcholine subside.

Fentanyl, unlike most opioids, has little or no hypotensive effects and usually does not cause nausea and vomiting. Because of its vagotonic effect, it may cause bradycardia, which can be relieved with atropine or glycopyrrolate. Fentanyl can be reversed with the opioid antagonist naloxone, which also reverses analgesia. Should fentanyl be reversed with naloxone in the PACU, the perianesthesia nurse should continue to monitor the patient for the possible return of respiratory depression, because the duration of the respiratory depression produced by the fentanyl may be longer than the duration of action of naloxone.

Fentanyl can be used alone in a nitrous-opioid technique. It also is used in the PACU in the form of a low-dose intravenous drip for pain relief; however, fentanyl is usually given slowly intravenously in the PACU for breakthrough pain (see Table 22-2 for helpful calculation of milligram to microgram dosage information).

Table 22-2	Example of Conversion of Dosage Calculations from Milligrams to Micrograms	
MILLIGRAMS	MICROGRAMS	MILLILITERS OF FENTANYL
0.025	25	0.5
0.05	50	1.0
0.10	100	2.0
0.15	150	3.0
0.20	200	4.0
0.25	250	4.5
0.50	500	10.0
1.00	1000	20.0

Sufentanil

Sufentanil is an analogue of fentanyl and is approximately fivefold to sevenfold more potent as fentanyl. Anesthesia with sufentanil can be induced more rapidly, with basically the same technique as that used for fentanyl, without an increase in the incidence rate of chest wall rigidity. However, sufentanil can produce chest wall rigidity; therefore if it is administered in the PACU, equipment for administration of oxygen with positive pressure and the skeletal muscle relaxant succinylcholine should be on hand. The incidence rate of hypertension with sufentanil is lower than with comparable doses of fentanyl. Bradycardia is infrequently seen in patients who receive sufentanil, and when high-dose sufentanil is used in combination with nitrous oxide-oxygen, the mean arterial pressure and cardiac output may be decreased. The recovery time from sufentanil from the time of injection is about the same as with fentanyl, because sufentanil is rapidly eliminated from tissue storage sites; consequently, the duration of action of sufentanil is about the same as with fentanyl. In addition, the incidence rates of postoperative hypertension, the need for vasoactive agents, and the requirements for postoperative analgesics are generally reduced in patients who are administered moderate or high doses of sufentanil in comparison with patients given inhalation agents. Of particular interest to the perianesthesia nurse is that sufentanil has an additive effect that is seen in patients who receive barbiturates, tranquilizers, other opioids, general anesthetics, or other CNS depressants. This effect is especially true of benzodiazepines because they can potentiate a profound hypotensive action. Therefore, when sufentanil is combined with any of these drugs, particular attention should be paid to any signs of decreased respiratory drive, increased airway resistance, or hypotension. Immediate countermeasures include maintenance of a patent airway with proper positioning of the patient, placement of an oral airway or endotracheal tube, and administration of oxygen. If indicated, naloxone should be used as a specific antidote for management of the respiratory depression. The duration of respiratory depression after overdose with sufentanil may be longer than the duration of action of the naloxone. Consequently, the patient should be constantly observed for the recurrence of respiratory depression, even after the initial successful treatment with naloxone. Hypotension can be treated with reversal with naloxone; however, fluids and vasopressors may be indicated (see Chapter 11).[4]

Alfentanil

Alfentanil is another analogue of fentanyl that is approximately one tenth as potent and has approximately one third the duration of action of fentanyl. The onset of action of this drug occurs in 1 or 2 minutes, and the duration of action is 20 to 30 minutes. Alfentanil appears to have significant advantages over currently available opioid anesthetics. For example, it has no cumulative drug effects, and once the infusion of alfentanil is terminated, the emergence time is predictable. Alfentanil, like fentanyl, produces minimal hemodynamic effects and offers a high therapeutic index. In fact, the therapeutic index for alfentanil is higher than those of fentanyl and other opioids. A therapeutic index is the ratio of the lethal dose to the effective dose; the higher the therapeutic index, the farther the lethal dose from the dose used for the desired effect. More specifically, the therapeutic index of fentanyl is 270, which means that it is approximately four times safer than morphine. The therapeutic index of alfentanil is approximately 2.5 times more favorable than that of fentanyl.[9-11]

Alfentanil, in addition to its place in the operating room, may also have important uses in the PACU. Its rapid onset and brief duration of action make it advantageous for the immediate pain relief needs of PACU patients. As previously stated, the drug has approximately one third the potency of fentanyl, but its onset of action is at least three times faster; its duration is one third that of fentanyl, and it has a high therapeutic index, which makes alfentanil well suited for pain relief in the immediate postoperative period. The drug produces few cardiovascular effects and thus should be of great value in preventing dangerous reflexes, such as tachycardia during intubation. Clinical observation indicates that the recovery time for this drug is extremely rapid. Therefore patients who receive this drug during surgery most likely have pain early in the immediate postoperative period, and the appropriate analgesic should be administered.

Remifentanil

Remifentanil is a selective mu opioid agonist that has an analgesic potency almost equal to fentanyl and twentyfold more potent than alfentanil. This drug has some excellent pharmacologic properties in that it is brief in action, titratable, and noncumulative; it lacks histamine release; and it has a rapid recovery after the discontinuation of the drug. The onset of this drug is within 1 minute. When the drug is discontinued, it is metabolized quickly; its effects disappear within 4 minutes. The remifentanil anesthetic technique is excellent for suppression of the stress response and allows for excellent depression of neurologic responses. In regard to the immediate postanesthesia period, remifentanil is better than most intravenous opioid drugs in regard to residual effects because it has a rapid recovery and less risk of postoperative respiratory depression.

This drug should probably not be used in the PACU; however, if the drug is administered in the PACU, it should be administered only by an anesthesia provider who is experienced in the administration of the drug. Some of the adverse effects of the drug may accompany its administration.[1,12,13]

Remifentanil is given via intravenous infusion with an infusion pump and should never be administered via intravenous bolus. The drug can produce the fixed chest syndrome and can also cause nausea and vomiting, respiratory depression, and mild-to-moderate depression of the heart rate and blood pressure.

Partial Agonist-Antagonist Drugs

The partial agonist-antagonist drugs represent a category of drugs that have a primary opioid effect by using the competitive antagonist properties on the mu opioid receptor and an agonist at the kappa and sigma receptors, all leading to providing analgesia. This category of drugs has a low addiction potential, providing mild to moderate pain relief.

Pentazocine

Pentazocine (Fortral, Talwin), an opioid agonist and antagonist analgesic, was first synthesized in 1959. The drug has significant activity and a low addiction potential. It is approximately one third as potent as morphine when given intramuscularly. Its advantage over morphine is that it can be given orally. Pentazocine can be used before and after surgery for the relief of pain from abdominal, cardiac, genitourinary, orthopedic, neurologic, and gynecologic surgery. The observed side effects of this drug include sedation, dizziness, nausea, and vomiting, but these occur infrequently.

Studies of the relative potency of this drug indicate that 30 mg of pentazocine is analgesically equivalent to 10 mg of morphine and 75 mg of meperidine. Pentazocine has been established to relieve severe pain and is approximately twofold to fourfold less potent than morphine when administered parenterally.[2,4,14-16]

Pentazocine can be used in the nitrous-opioid technique. The respiratory depression produced by pentazocine is potentiated when general anesthetics are used concomitantly. Pentazocine produces an increase in systolic blood pressure and

does not appear to have depressant effects on cardiac output. The drug should be used with caution in patients with renal or hepatic impairment. Pentazocine depresses the respiratory system in a manner comparable with morphine in equivalent analgesic doses. Tolerance to the analgesic effect of the drug does not appear to develop as it does with other opioids. Because pentazocine is an opioid antagonist at the mu receptors, administration of this drug to a patient who depends on opiates can induce abrupt withdrawal symptoms.

The onset of analgesic activity of pentazocine is approximately 2 or 3 minutes when it is given intravenously and 15 to 20 minutes when given intramuscularly. The duration of action is approximately 3 hours. When given orally, the drug is approximately one third as potent as when it is given intramuscularly.[2,13]

Butorphanol

Butorphanol is a synthetic analgesic that is chemically related to the nalorphine-cyclazocine series with both opioid and antagonist properties. More specifically, it serves as an agonist at the kappa and sigma opioid receptors. In regard to its analgesic potency, it is approximately fivefold more potent than morphine, thirtyfold more potent than meperidine, and twentyfold more potent than pentazocine. Butorphanol can produce sedation, nausea, and respiratory depression. The respiratory depression is plateaulike in that 2 mg of butorphanol depresses respiration to a degree equal to 10 mg of morphine. The magnitude of respiratory depression with butorphanol is not appreciably increased at doses of 4 mg. The duration of the respiratory depression is dose related and is reversible with naloxone. Intravenous administration of butorphanol can produce increased pulmonary artery pressure, pulmonary wedge pressure, left-ventricular end-diastolic pressure, systemic arterial pressure, and pulmonary vascular resistance. Consequently, this drug increases the workload of the heart, especially in the pulmonary circuit. Because of its antagonist properties, butorphanol is not recommended for patients who are physically dependent on opioids, because butorphanol can precipitate withdrawal symptoms in those patients. See Table 22-3 for an overview of the clinical pharmacology of butorphanol.[4]

Nalbuphine

Nalbuphine (Nubain) is a potent analgesic with opioid agonist and antagonist actions. It is chemically related to oxymorphone and naloxone. This drug is an antagonist at the mu receptors, a partial agonist at the kappa receptors, and an agonist at

Table 22-3	Comparison of Five Analgesics that Use Morphine as Drug with Primary Opioid Effects				
	MORPHINE	**MEPERIDINE**	**PENTAZOCINE**	**BUTORPHANOL**	**NALBUPHINE**
Indication	Moderate to severe pain	Moderate to severe pain	Moderate to severe pain	Moderate to severe pain	Moderate to severe pain
Recommended IM dose (mg)	10	50-100	30	2	10
Recommended IV dose (mg)	4-10	25-50	30	1	10
Time for onset of analgesia	Rapid IV, 30 min IM	Rapid IV, 30 min IM	Rapid IV, 20 min IM	Rapid IV, 30 min IM	Rapid IV, 15 min IM
Duration of analgesia (h)	4	2-4	3-4	3-4	3-6
Respiratory depression	High	High	Occurs, but less than with morphine	Occurs, but less than with morphine	Occurs, but less than with morphine
Cardiovascular effect	Decreases cardiac workload	Decreases cardiac workload	Increases cardiac workload	Increases cardiac workload	Good cardiac stability
Abuse syndrome	High	High	Occurs; induces withdrawal syndrome	Occurs; induces withdrawal syndrome	Occurs; induces withdrawal syndrome

IM, Intramuscular; *IV*, intravenous.

the sigma receptors. Nalbuphine is as potent as morphine and approximately threefold more potent as pentazocine on a milligram basis. At a dose of 10 mg/kg, nalbuphine causes the same degree of respiratory depression as does 10 mg of morphine. At higher doses, nalbuphine exhibits the same plateau effect as butorphanol (i.e., respiratory depression is not increased appreciably with higher doses). The respiratory depression produced by nalbuphine can be reversed with naloxone. Nalbuphine does not appear to increase the workload of the heart or to decrease cardiovascular stability. This drug has a lower abuse potential than does morphine; however, if it is given to a patient who is physically dependent on opioids, withdrawal symptoms may appear. Signs of withdrawal include abdominal cramps, nausea and vomiting, lacrimation, rhinorrhea, anxiety, restlessness, elevation of temperature, and piloerection. If these symptoms appear after the injection of nalbuphine, the administration of small amounts of morphine can relieve the objective effects of the syndrome. See Table 22-3 for an overview of the clinical pharmacology of nalbuphine.[4]

Opioid Antagonists

Opioid antagonists are used to reverse opioid-induced respiratory depression. An opioid antagonist, such as naloxone (Narcan), is a drug that completely antagonizes the effect of an opioid.

Naloxone

Naloxone (Narcan), a pure antagonist, reverses the depressant effects of opioids. More specifically, this drug antagonizes the opioid effects at the mu, kappa, and sigma receptors. This drug also reverses the analgesic effect of the opioid, which is important in assessing the patient's respiratory effort. Naloxone should be titrated according to the patient's response. Usually, 0.1 to 0.2 mg given slowly intravenously should be adequate for reversal. The onset of action of naloxone is 1 or 2 minutes. If after 3 to 5 minutes inadequate reversal has been achieved, naloxone administration may be repeated until reversal is complete. If the patient shows no sign of reversal, assessment of other pharmacologic agents administered is indicated. Drugs such as halothane, barbiturates, and muscle relaxants are not reversed with naloxone.

The duration of action of naloxone is 1 to 4 hours, depending on the route and amount of drug used. If long-acting opioids were used, the patient must be monitored for respiratory embarrassment after the administration of naloxone because the depressant activity of the opioid may return. If this phenomenon occurs, supplemental doses of naloxone can be used. The intramuscular route of administration has been shown to produce a longer lasting effect.

An excessive dose of naloxone can increase blood pressure, a finding that may be seen as a response to pain. Too rapid reversal can induce nausea, vomiting, diaphoresis, and tachycardia. During the reversal procedure, the vital signs should be monitored; naloxone should be used with caution in patients with cardiac irritability.[4,5]

Naloxone does not produce respiratory depression as do other opioid antagonists. It also does not produce any significant side effects or pupillary constriction. Naloxone reverses natural or synthetic opioids and the opioid-antagonist analgesic pentazocine. Because reversal may precipitate an acute withdrawal syndrome, naloxone should be administered with great caution in patients who are physically dependent on opioids.

Nalmefene

Nalmefene (Revex) is similar in chemical structure to naloxone and is considered a long-acting opioid antagonist. It has a rather rapid onset of 2 to 5 minutes, with a duration of action of approximately 8 hours. Nalmefene, when given at the usual dose range, produces the same clinical effects as naloxone.

In the PACU, the dose of this drug for reversal of respiratory depression is 0.1 to 0.5 mcg/kg slowly titrated intravenously at 2- to 5-minute intervals. This drug should be titrated slowly with observation for a return of respiratory effort. When the patient has a return of the appropriate rate and volume of breathing, titration should be stopped and a constant vigilance of the rate and volume of respiration should be continued throughout the PACU stay. This drug should not be administered in a dose of more than 1.6 mcg because this does not elicit additional effects. As with naloxone, nalmefene should not be administered to a patient with opioid dependency. Both drugs should always be titrated slowly to all patients in case a patient is opioid dependent. If the PACU nurse is titrating these drugs and signs of acute opioid withdrawal are seen, titration should stop immediately.

Naltrexone

Naltrexone (Revia) is a pure mu and kappa, and to a lesser extent delta, opioid receptor antagonist; therefore its actions are similar to naloxone. This drug can produce sustained opioid antagonist activity for as long as 24 hours, with a peak action in 8 to 12 hours. This drug can only be administered orally and is used in opioid detoxification because it can facilitate withdrawal; once the patient has undergone complete detoxification, naltrexone can prevent relapses to opioids by blocking the euphoric effects of the opioid. In addition, note that naltrexone is used to treat alcohol dependence;

therefore the same can be said in regard to titrating the drug slowly because it can also cause acute alcohol withdrawal.

SELECTED METHODS OF OPIOID ADMINISTRATION

Intrathecal and Epidural Routes of Administration

For management of acute and chronic pain, the opioids can be administered via the subarachnoid or epidural space. The technique is called the *neuraxial administration of opioids*. This concept of pain relief is based on the fact that opioid receptors exist in the substantia gelatinosa on the dorsal horn of the spinal cord. More specifically, mu, kappa, and delta opioid receptors are located in the substantia gelatinosa. The pain relieved with the administration of neuraxial opioids is usually of the visceral as opposed to the somatic type. When the opioid is administered via the epidural space, it crosses the epidural space to the opioid receptors in the spinal cord. Consequently, the dose of the opioid, when administered into the epidural space, is usually 10 times the dose of the opioid if it were administered via the subarachnoid space.

When 0.1 to 0.2 mg of preservative-free morphine (Duramorph) is administered into the subarachnoid space (intrathecal), the maximum concentration is reached in 5 to 10 minutes, with a duration of 80 to 200 minutes. When 5 mg of morphine is administered into the epidural space in the lumbar region, analgesia can last for as long as 24 hours. The patient should obtain pain relief in 30 to 60 minutes after injection. If appropriate pain relief is not achieved, incremental doses of 1 to 2 mg can be administered. The maximum dose in a 24-hour period is 10 mg.[5]

After spinal surgery, epidural morphine administered with the continuous epidural technique has advantages and disadvantages. Its advantage is a profound degree of pain relief, especially for the first 12 to 18 postoperative hours. However, disadvantages are related to displacement of the epidural catheter and the length of action of the epidural morphine. If the epidural catheter becomes displaced and the morphine has been injected, only partial pain relief ensues. Because of the possibility of profound respiratory depression, opioids must be administered cautiously. In fact, a nonopioid drug such as ketorolac may be especially useful in this circumstance. Depending on the anticipated amount and length of pain, a patient-controlled analgesia (PCA) device can be started in the patient for an immediate result of pain resolution. In addition, the postanesthesia nurse can have a profound effect on reducing the pain threshold by repositioning and reassuring the patient. The new technology of apnea monitors or end-tidal carbon dioxide monitors can be useful in detecting hypoventilation or apnea that can be created by the opioid in this technique. Therefore the use of either monitor on patients who are receiving epidural morphine certainly aids the postanesthesia nurse in monitoring for respiratory dysfunction.[4]

Other opioids that can be administered epidurally are fentanyl and sufentanil.[14] These drugs offer some advantages over morphine; they are more suited for continuous infusion techniques because of their rapid onset and short duration of action. Because they have such a rapid clearance from the cerebrospinal fluid, less chance exists for these drugs to spread toward the head (rostral spread). Rostral spread, which is associated more with morphine, has been shown to produce side effects such as nausea, pruritus, and the previously discussed delayed respiratory depression syndrome. Naloxone reverses this side effect; however, the analgesic effect also is reversed. In this instance, nalbuphine administration should be considered to reverse the respiratory depression and preserve some of the analgesia.

Patient-Controlled Analgesia

For the reduction of pain, the intramuscular injection of opioids and nonopioids has long been the standard route of administration used by nursing personnel. This method of administration has the advantage of simplicity and no requirement for specialized equipment. Its disadvantages include variable uptake, pain on injection, and patient dissatisfaction with the level of pain relief. Patient dissatisfaction is based on the cyclic effect of pain. If a level of analgesia were produced, the adverse effects of pain could be controlled. Intravenous administration offers some advantages over the intramuscular approach. The administration of an opioid via the intravenous route offers the patient an immediate reduction in pain. However, this reduction is only temporary because no appropriate blood level of the opioid has been established.

For an appropriate level of analgesia, a loading dose, followed by titration to effect, based on the pharmacokinetics of the opioid drug is used during surgery. The maintenance of an appropriate blood level of the opioid to achieve and maintain a level of analgesia is the goal of this technique. The blood level of the drug is called the *minimum effective analgesic concentration*

(MEAC). Research has shown that the MEAC varies among individuals. Through the use of technology, the principles of this intraoperative technique have been continued into the immediate postoperative period. Intravenous PCA is the method of choice for patients who need continued analgesia. The peaks and valleys of analgesia can be avoided without the patient becoming totally dependent on the nurse's response for pain relief. PCA allows the patient more control of the situation by allowing the patient to seek out a particular level of analgesia—the MEAC.[4,5,14]

In the PACU, the patient is administered a loading dose of the intravenous opioid to achieve the MEAC and then a PCA infusion pump is set up for the patient. The PCA pump is programmed for the administration of a particular opioid based on the patient's analgesic needs and the pharmacokinetics of the drug to be administered. The parameters to be programmed are the bolus dose, the lockout interval, and the low-dose continuous basal infusion rate. Consequently, with a "push of a button" on the PCA pump, the patient can attain immediate analgesia and receive the benefits of controlled pain relief with low-dose continuous infusion of the opioid.

The amount of the self-dose bolus should be low to avoid an acute increase in blood levels of the drug above the MEAC because, along with the concern about overdose, blood levels above the MEAC have no analgesic value. The lockout interval, or delay, is the setting used to block the use of the self-dose bolus button for a period of time. During this time, the PCA pump does not deliver the drug, even when the patient pushes the button. The lockout interval is usually short, so that the patient can self-administer small incremental doses to maintain the MEAC, but the interval should be long enough to prevent overdosage. The basal infusion rate is usually set at a rate necessary to provide analgesia when the patient is resting. See Table 22-4 for a suggested protocol for drug administration in PCA.

Patient-Controlled Epidural Analgesia

The concept of PCA has been adapted to epidural analgesia or PCEA. In this instance, the PCA infusion pump can be attached to the epidural catheter. The opioid drugs that can be used in this technique are fentanyl and sufentanil. They can be used with great success for analgesia after cesarean section. The basal infusion rate keeps the patient analgesic and comfortable. The patient can self-administer a bolus

Table 22-4	Protocol for Opioid Administration in Intravenous PCA			
	LOADING DOSE		**INTERVAL DOSE**	
DRUG	**ADULT**	**BY WEIGHT**	**ADULT**	**BY WEIGHT**
Morphine	0.5-4 mg every 10 min (total, 6-16 mg)	0.05 mg/kg (total, 0.05-0.2 mg/kg)	0.5-2 mg	10-20 mcg/kg
Meperidine (Demerol)	12.5-25 mg every 10 min (total, 50-125 mg)	0.5-1.5 mg/kg	5-10 mg	0.1-0.2 mg/kg
Fentanyl (Sublimaze)	25-50 mcg every 5 min (total, 50-300 mcg)	0.05-2.0 mcg/kg (total, 0.5-4 mcg/kg)	10-30 mcg	0.25-0.5 mcg/kg

Adapted from Nagelhout J, Plaus K: *Nurse anesthesia,* ed 4, St. Louis, 2010, Saunders.
PCA, Patient-controlled analgesia. Basal rate or interval dose rate is optional because demand-only mode of PCA is often prescribed. Lockout intervals range generally between 6 and 12 minutes.

of the opioid if the analgesia provided with the basal infusion rate is not sufficient. In addition, the bolus opioid facilitates additional analgesia needed for turning and early ambulation. A suggested protocol for both fentanyl and sufentanil is provided in Tables 22-5 and 22-6.

Table 22-5	Protocol for Administration of Fentanyl* via PCEA System for Patients After Cesarean Section		
		SURGICAL	
	PACU	**UNIT**	**FOR PAIN**
Bolus (mcg)	100	—	50-100
Dose (mcg)	40	40	50-60
Lockout (min)	10	10	10
Basal rate (mcg/h)	60	60	60-80
Limit (mcg/h)	260	260	310-380

Adapted from Pasero C, McCaffery M: *Pain assessment and pharmacologic management*, St. Louis, 2011, Mosby.
PCEA, Patient-controlled epidural analgesia.
*Mix fentanyl in 20-mcg/mL solution.

Table 22-6	Protocol for Administration of Sufentanil via PCEA System for Patients After Cesarean Section		
		SURGICAL	
	PACU	**UNIT**	**FOR PAIN**
Bolus (mcg)	30	—	20
Dose (mcg)	8	4	8
Lockout (min)	10	10	10
Basal rate (mcg/h)	6	6	6
Limit (mcg/h)	46	26	26

Adapted from Miller R, Pardo M: *Basics of anesthesia*, ed 6, Philadelphia, 2011, Saunders.
PCEA, Patient-controlled epidural analgesia; *PACU,* postanesthesia care unit.

Because of the possibility of rostral spread, an apnea monitor is suggested for use on patients who are receiving patient-controlled epidural analgesia.[4,5,14] (See Chapter 31.)

Monitoring the Patient Receiving Opioids in the PACU

In addition to routine monitoring for the patient receiving opioids in the PACU, the respiratory rate should be monitored for not only the rate but also the trend. For example, if the respiratory rate decreases from 18 to 16 to 12 in a 45-minute interval, strong suspicion exists that excessive opioid effect has occurred and the modified stir-up regime should be instituted.

Along with monitoring of respiratory rate and depth, peripheral pulse oximetry and, if necessary, detection of expired carbon dioxide or arterial blood gas monitoring can be used. The nervous system clinical indicators of significant opioid action should also be monitored and include observation for excess sedation, lethargy, apathy, dysphoria, nausea, vomiting, pruritus (especially facial), miosis, and cough suppression.[4,14]

If the patient is determined to have opioid-induced respiratory depression, prophylactic supplemental oxygen should be administered and the modified stir-up regime should be instituted. If the patient is difficult to arouse, the airway should be supported and manually assisted ventilation with bag and mask may be needed. Should the patient have excessive secretions or vomitus, a person skilled in airway management should be summoned because tracheal intubation may be necessary. Pharmacologic treatment should include the use of naloxone. For the adult, treatment should start with lower doses such as 0.1 mg and titrate to effect to lessen the adverse cardiovascular effects that can occur when the opioid is completely reversed with high-dose naloxone.

OPIATE DETOXIFICATION IN THE PACU

Many methods of opioid detoxification have been developed since problems with addiction have occurred. The most common methods of opioid detoxification are methadone withdrawal, clonidine withdrawal, clonidine–naltrexone withdrawal, and anesthesia-assisted rapid opiate detoxification (AAROD).[4]

The technique of AAROD is in its experimental stages but has advantages over the other methods of detoxification, in that it is rapid and less costly than the other forms of treatment. In this method, the patient is admitted to the psychiatric unit of the hospital to ensure nothing-by-mouth status and a premedication is usually administered. The patient is usually administered multiple preprocedural oral medications, including clonidine (Catapres) to suppress the withdrawal symptoms, ondansetron (Zofran) to prevent nausea and vomiting, and metoclopramide (Reglan) to decrease gastric acidity. The patient is admitted to the PACU the next morning, and the procedure is initiated. Monitoring of this patient usually includes a continuous cardiac monitor, pulse oximeter, and a noninvasive blood pressure monitor. Oxygen is usually administered by nasal cannula, and emergency resuscitation equipment, including intubation equipment and cardiac arrest cart, is immediately available. Before the initiation of the procedure, midazolam and ondansetron may be given; and depending on the patient, droperidol (Inapsine) in small doses may be given as opposed to midazolam and ondansetron. Next, light sedation is produced with a propofol infusion, and the patient is given intravenous naloxone. The patient has withdrawal signs and symptoms that usually include mydriasis, piloerection, and a mild increase in heart rate and blood pressure. After approximately 45 minutes, the propofol is discontinued and routine postanesthesia nursing care is provided. Emotional support and reassurance certainly are important to ensure an appropriate outcome. Once the patient's condition is stabilized, a report should be given to the receiving nurse on the psychiatric unit, and the patient is discharged from the PACU and transported to the psychiatric unit.

SUMMARY

The use of the "balanced" anesthesia method of administration is becoming the method of choice in the intraoperative care of the surgical patient. This technique has a primary focus using opioids throughout or at the end of the procedure in an effort to provide postoperative pain relief. An excellent working knowledge of the pharmacology of opioids is critical in the administration of perianesthesia care for the surgical patient. Opioids possess excellent qualities for pain relief; however, with incorrect administration or the absence of appropriate monitoring, drastic negative outcomes can occur. With the advent of newer opioids, working with the anesthesia care team is important for prevention of adverse outcomes.

The pure opioid agonists were presented as were the mixed action agonist-antagonists. Appropriate reversal drugs were also presented with the methods of administration of these drugs in the PACU.

REFERENCES

1. Atlee J: *Complications in anesthesia*, ed 2, Philadelphia, 2007, Saunders.
2. Brunton L, et al: *Goodman and Gilman's the pharmacological basis of therapeutics*, ed 12, New York, 2010, McGraw-Hill Professional.
3. Hines R, Marschall K: *Stoelting's anesthesia and co-existing disease*, ed 5, Philadelphia, 2008, Saunders.
4. Nagelhout J, Plaus K: *Nurse anesthesia*, ed 4, St. Louis, 2010, Saunders.
5. Stoelting R: *Pharmacology and physiology in anesthetic practice*, ed 4, Philadelphia, 2005, Lippincott Williams & Wilkins.
6. Shorten G, et al: *Postoperative pain management: an evidence-based guide to practice*, Philadelphia, 2006, Saunders.
7. Stancer-Smiley B, Paradise N: Does the duration of N$_2$O administration affect postoperative nausea and vomiting? *Nurse Anesth* 2(1):13–20, 1991.
8. Stanley TH: The history and development of the fentanyl series, *J Pain Symptom Manage* 7(3):S3–7, 1992.
9. Aitkenhead A, et al: *Textbook of anesthesia*, ed 5, Philadelphia, 2007, Churchill Livingstone.
10. Barash P, et al: *Clinical anesthesia*, ed 6, Philadelphia, 2009, Lippincott Williams & Wilkins.
11. Fisher L: *Anesthesia and uncommon diseases*, ed 5, Philadelphia, 2007, Saunders.
12. Blouin R, Gross J: Ventilation and conscious sedation, *Semin Anesth* 15(4):335–342, 1996.
13. Miller R, et al: *Miller's anesthesia*, ed 7, New York, 2010, Churchill Livingstone.
14. Pasero C, McCaffery M: *Pain assessment and pharmacologic management*, St. Louis, 2011, Mosby.
15. Pasero C, McCaffery M: Orthopaedic postoperative pain management, *J Perianesth Nurs* 22(3):160–174, 2007.
16. Shorten G, et al: *Postoperative pain management: an evidence-based guide to practice*, Philadelphia, 2006, Saunders.

RESOURCES

American Association of Critical-Care Nurses: *Core curriculum for progressive care nursing*, Philadelphia, 2010, Saunders.
Alspach J: *Core curriculum for critical care nursing*, ed 6, Philadelphia, 2005, Saunders.

CONCEPTS IN ANESTHETIC AGENTS

Babar M, et al: Effect of preoperative rectal indomethacin on postoperative pain reduction after open cholecystectomy, *J Perianesth Nurs*, 25(1):7–10, 2010.

Barrett K, et al: *Ganong's review of medical physiology*, ed 23, New York, 2009, McGraw-Hill Medical.

Borchardt M: Review of the clinical pharmacology and use of the benzodiazepines, *J Perianesth Nurs* 14(2):65–72, 1999.

Bready L, et al: *Decision making in anesthesiology*, ed 4, St. Louis, 2007, Mosby.

Conlay L, et al: *Case files anesthesiology*, New York, 2011, McGraw-Hill Medical.

Davis P, et al: *Smith's anesthesia for infants and children*, ed 8, St. Louis, 2011, Mosby.

Deutschman C, Netigan P: *Evidence-based practice of critical care*, Philadelphia, 2010, Saunders.

Dorsch J, Dorsch S: *Understanding anesthesia equipment*, ed 5, Philadelphia, 2007, Lippincott Williams & Wilkins.

Drake R, et al: *Gray's anatomy for students*, ed 2, Philadelphia, 2009, Churchill Livingstone.

Gallager C, Issenberg B: *Simulation in anesthesia*, Philadelphia, 2007, Saunders.

Hall J: *Guyton and Hall textbook of medical physiology*, ed 12, Philadelphia, 2011, Saunders.

Hines R, Marschall K: *Handbook for Stoelting's anesthesia and co-existing disease*, ed 3, Philadelphia, 2009, Saunders.

Jones R: Desflurane and sevoflurane: inhalation anesthetics for this decade? *Br J Anaesth* 65:527–536, 1990.

Kaplan J, et al: *Cardiac anesthesia*, New York, 2011, Churchill Livingstone.

Katoh T, et al: Blood concentration of sevoflurane and isoflurane on recovery from anesthesia, *Br J Anaesth* 69:259–262, 1992.

Key K, et al: Use of propofol and emergence agitation in children: A literature review, *AANA J* 78(6):468–473, 2010.

Kier L, Dowd C: *The chemistry of drugs for nurse anesthetists*, Chicago, 2004, AANA Publishing, Inc.

Kulli J, Koch C: Does anesthesia cause loss of consciousness? *Trends Neurosci* 14(1):6–10, 1991.

Longnecker D, et al: *Anesthesiology*, New York, 2007, McGraw-Hill Medical.

Mason R: *Murray and Nadel's textbook of respiratory medicine*, ed 5, Philadelphia, 2011, Saunders.

Miller R, Pardo M: *Basics of anesthesia*, ed 6, Philadelphia, 2011, Saunders.

Moos D, Cuddeford D: Implications of obstructive sleep apnea syndrome for the perianesthesia nurse, *J Perianesth Nurs* 21(2):103–118, 2006.

Prielipp R, Young C: Current drugs for sedation of critically ill patients, *Semin Anesthesia Perioperative Med Pain* 20(2): 85–94, 2001.

Passannante A, et al: Anesthetic management of patients with obesity and sleep apnea, *Anesthesiol Clin North Am* 23:479–490, 2005.

Rakic A, Golembiewski J: Low-dose ketamine infusion for postoperative pain management, *J Perianesth Nurs* 24(4): 254–257, 2009.

Redai I, et al: Are volatile anesthetics cardioprotective agents? *Semin Anesthesia Perioperative Med Pain* 20(2):95–100, 2001.

Reves J, et al: Midazolam: pharmacology and uses, *Anesthesiology* 62:310–324, 1985.

Sebel P, Larson J: Propofol: a new intravenous anesthetic, *Anesthesiology* 71:260–277, 1989.

Short T, Chui P: Propofol and midazolam act synergistically in combination, *Br J Anaesth* 67:539–545, 1991.

Sandberg W, et al: *The MGH textbook of anesthetic equipment*, New York, 2011, Churchill Livingstone.

Schick L, Windle PE: *Perianesthesia nursing core curriculum: pre-procedure, phase I and phase II PACU nursing*, ed 2, Philadelphia, 2010, Saunders.

Shepherd M: Multidisciplinary approach to developing guidelines for use of anesthetic agents in an intensive care unit, *Anesthesia Today* 6(1):15–18, 1995.

Sieber F: *Geriatric anesthesia*, New York, 2006, McGraw-Hill Medical.

Vincent J, et al: *Textbook of critical care*, ed 6, Philadelphia, 2011, Saunders.

White P: *Perioperative drug manual*, ed 2, Philadelphia, 2005, Saunders.

23 Neuromuscular Blocking Agents

Cecil B. Drain, PhD, RN, CRNA, FAAN, FASAHP

Neuromuscular blocking drugs, or muscle relaxants, have been used in clinical anesthesia since the early 1940s. Significant advances have been made in understanding the physiology of neuromuscular transmission and the pharmacology of muscle relaxants and have contributed greatly to clinical anesthesia as it is currently practiced. Interestingly, muscle relaxants have taken the same path as the inhalational anesthetic agents—rapid onset and a short duration of action. Muscle relaxants are not used exclusively in the field of anesthesia; in postanesthesia care units (PACUs), intensive care units, and emergency department settings, these drugs may be needed to enhance patient care. Muscle relaxants are used: (1) for facilitation of endotracheal intubation; (2) for procedures that necessitate muscle relaxation, such as intraperitoneal and thoracic surgery; (3) in ophthalmic surgery for relaxation of the extraocular muscles; (4) for termination of laryngospasm and elimination of chest wall rigidity, which can occur after rapid intravenous injection of a potent opioid; and (5) for facilitation of mechanical ventilation with production of total paralysis of the respiratory muscles.

DEFINITIONS

Action Potential: The passage of an electric impulse at any point on the nerve fiber where the inside becomes positive and the outside becomes negative; also referred to as *action current*.

Anticholinesterase: A drug that inhibits or inactivates the action of acetylcholinesterase.

Antimuscarinic (Anticholinergic): A drug that blocks the effects of acetylcholine receptors and results in the inhibition of the transmission of parasympathetic nerve impulses.

Clinical Duration: In reference to the use of neuromuscular blocking agents, the time from the administration of the drug to 25% recovery of the train-of-four twitch response.

Defasciculation: A result of the administration of a subclinical dose of a nondepolarizing skeletal muscle relaxant for prevention of the skeletal muscle twitches that occur after the administration of the depolarizing skeletal muscle relaxant succinylcholine.

Depolarizing Skeletal Muscle Relaxant: A skeletal muscle relaxant that after administration produces skeletal muscle twitches by stimulating the nicotinic receptors on the neuromuscular end plate and remaining on

the end plate for 3 to 5 minutes, which leads to muscle paralysis. Skeletal muscle function returns as the pseudocholinesterase metabolizes the succinylcholine, usually between 3 and 5 minutes.

End Plate Potential (EPP): One action potential at the myoneural junction.

Excitation-Contraction (E-C) Coupling: The entire process of muscle contraction, starting with the electric and then the chemical stimulus to the process of the release of calcium in the sarcoplasmic reticulum, which causes the muscle fibers (actin and myosin) to slide and thus contract.

Extraocular Muscles: The six sets of muscles that control the movement of the eyeball.

Fasciculations: Skeletal muscle twitches.

Muscarinic: Subset receptors of the parasympathetic nervous system.

Myopathy: An abnormal condition of skeletal muscle characterized by muscle weakness and wasting.

Neurohumoral Transmission: Combined electric and chemical transmission of an impulse.

Nicotinic: Subset of the parasympathetic nervous system.

Nondepolarizing Agents: Drugs that cause paralysis of skeletal muscle by blocking neural muscular transmission at the myoneural junction.

Onset Time: In reference to the use of neuromuscular blocking agents, the time from the administration of the drug to maximum effect.

Pseudocholinesterase: An enzyme that acts like cholinesterase and metabolizes acetylcholine.

Recovery Index: In reference to the use of neuromuscular blocking agents, the time from the train-of-four twitch index of 25% to 75% recovery of the twitch response.

Total Duration of Action: In reference to the use of neuromuscular blocking agents, the time from drug administration to 90% recovery of the train-of-four twitch response.

Train-of-Four Ratio: A term used in reference to neuromuscular blocking agents in which a comparison is made between the fourth twitch of the train-of-four with the first twitch; when the fourth twitch is 90% of the first twitch, recovery from the neuromuscular blocking agent is indicated.

PHYSIOLOGY OF NEUROMUSCULAR TRANSMISSION

Because of the frequent and routine intraoperative and postoperative use of drugs that alter neuromuscular function, a review of the anatomy and physiology of the neuromuscular system is important, with an emphasis on the chemical changes that occur at the receptor sites. Activation of skeletal muscle is both an electric and a biochemical event. The term *conduction* refers to the passage of an impulse along an axon to a muscle fiber. Transmission applies to passage of a neurotransmitter substance across a synaptic cleft (neuromuscular junction). The combined electric and chemical event is called *neurohumoral transmission.*[1]

As the fine terminal branch of a motor neuron approaches the muscle fiber, it loses its myelin sheath and forms an expanded terminal that lies close to a specialized area of muscle membrane called the end plate (Fig. 23-1). Between the end of the muscle fiber and the end plate is the synaptic cleft, or neuromuscular junction. This space between the nerve and muscle fibers is approximately 20 nm wide. Acetylcholine is the biochemical neurotransmitter involved in the initiation of muscle contraction. Acetylcholine or cholinergic receptors are classified as nicotinic and muscarinic, respectively. The acetylcholine receptors are stimulated by acetylcholine. Anticholinesterase drugs such as neostigmine (Prostigmin), edrophonium chloride (Tensilon, Enlon), and pyridostigmine (Regonol) produce an increase in acetylcholine at the acetylcholine receptor. Therefore the pharmacologic effects of the anticholinesterase drugs are on both the nicotinic and muscarinic receptors. The nicotinic receptors

are further classified as either N_1 or N_2 receptors. The N_1 receptors are located at the presynaptic cleft and influence the release of acetylcholine. The N_2 receptors are situated on the postsynaptic cleft in the neuromuscular junction and, when occupied by acetylcholine, open their channels to allow the flow of ions down the cell membrane, thus resulting in the skeletal muscle contraction. The nondepolarizing neuromuscular blocking agents such as pancuronium (Pavulon) produce a block of the N_2 receptor and thus cause an inability of the channel to conduct ions, which results in skeletal muscle paralysis. Extrajunctional nicotinic receptors are located throughout the skeletal muscles. Their activity is normally suppressed by normal neural activity. However, when a patient has prolonged sepsis, inactivity, denervation, or burn trauma in the skeletal muscles, a proliferation of these extrajunctional nicotinic receptors results. As a result, these patients usually have an exaggerated hyperkalemic response when succinylcholine is administered.[1]

The muscarinic receptors are also subdivided into M_1 and M_2 receptors. M_1 receptors are located in the autonomic ganglia and the central nervous system, and M_2 receptors are located in the heart and salivary glands. Atropine and glycopyrrolate (Robinul) block both the M_1 and the M_2 receptors.[2]

Acetylcholine is formed in the body of the nerve cell and the cytoplasm of the nerve terminal and is stored in the small membrane-enclosed vesicles for subsequent release. A quantum is the amount of acetylcholine stored in each vesicle and represents approximately 10,000 molecules of acetylcholine. The presynaptic membrane contains discrete areas of specialization that are thought to be sites of release of the transmitter. These presynaptic active zones lie directly opposite the N_2 cholinergic receptors, which are located on the postsynaptic membrane. This alignment ensures that the acetylcholine diffuses directly to the N_2 receptors on the postsynaptic membrane quickly and in a high concentration. The N_2 receptor, which responds to the neurotransmitter acetylcholine, is a glycoprotein that is an integral part of the postsynaptic membrane of the neuromuscular junction (see Fig. 23-1). New evidence indicates that a positive feedback mechanism also exists at the neuromuscular junction. Acetylcholine has a presynaptic action; therefore acetylcholine receptors are located on the presynaptic membrane. This positive feedback mechanism enhances the mobilization and release of acetylcholine. Finally, the enzyme that hydrolyzes acetylcholine is acetylcholinesterase, which is located in the neuromuscular junction.[3]

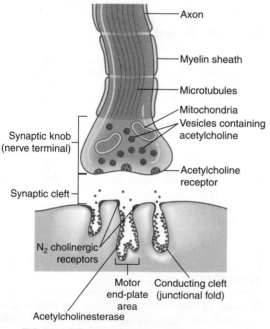

Axon

Myelin sheath

Microtubules

Mitochondria

Vesicles containing acetylcholine

Synaptic knob (nerve terminal)

Acetylcholine receptor

Synaptic cleft

N_2 cholinergic receptors

Motor end-plate area

Conducting cleft (junctional fold)

Acetylcholinesterase

FIG. 23-1 Myoneural junction at resting state.

The initiation of skeletal muscle contraction occurs as a result of applying a threshold stimulus. An action potential that travels down the axon causes depolarization of the presynaptic membrane. As a result of this depolarization, the membrane permeability for calcium ions is increased and the calcium enters, or influxes, into the presynaptic membrane. Calcium acts to unite the vesicle to the presynaptic membrane and causes the rupture of that coalesced membrane, thus releasing acetylcholine into the fluid of the synaptic cleft (Fig. 23-2).

The acetylcholine molecules released from the nerve terminal into the synaptic cleft are subject to two main processes: (1) attachment to N_2 cholinergic receptors located on the postsynaptic membrane, which leads to an opening of calcium channels that results in the movement of sodium into the region and generates an end plate potential (EPP); and (2) attachment of acetylcholine to the presynaptic nicotinic receptor, which enhances the release of more acetylcholine. When enough EPPs are generated, an action potential is propagated and spreads throughout the muscle and causes a change in the ionic permeability of the muscle sarcolemma. This process results in the release of calcium from the sarcoplasmic reticulum with a resultant increase in free calcium concentration in the muscle fiber. The process of excitation-contraction (E-C) coupling then takes place within that skeletal muscle cell. The physiologic outcome of E-C coupling is the contraction of the skeletal muscle. The increased concentration of calcium in the muscle fiber leads to an interaction between troponin-tropomyosin and actin. This interaction causes the active sites on actin to be exposed and interact with myosin and slide together, thus resulting in muscle contraction. This sliding of actin and myosin is sometimes called the *ratchet effect*.[3] The contraction of the muscle fibers is terminated when calcium is pumped back into the sarcoplasmic reticulum of the muscle fibers. The calcium is stored in the sarcoplasmic reticulum for use when another action potential is generated.

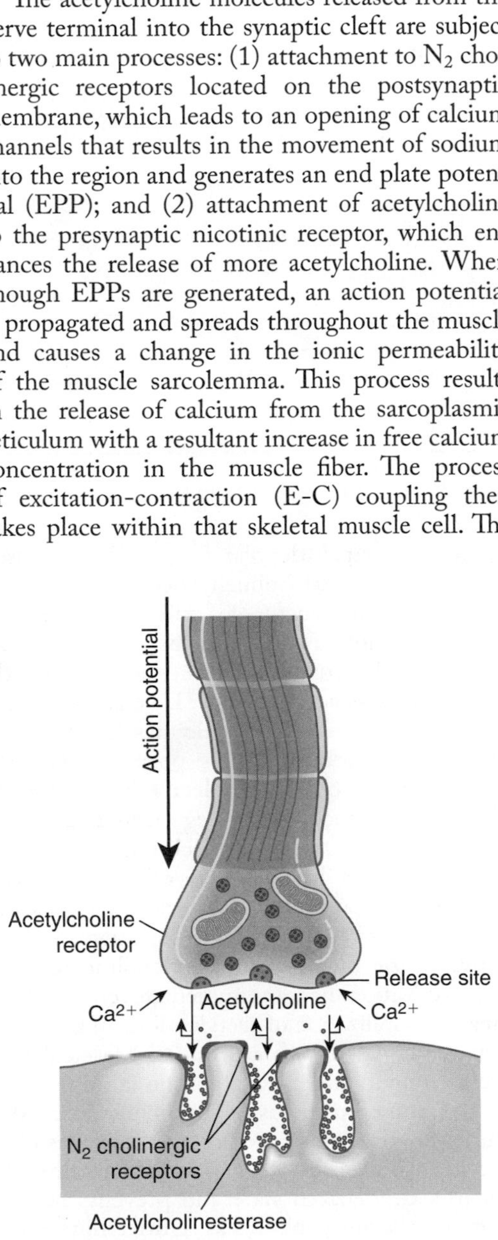

Regulation and control of skeletal muscle contraction are also based on the enzymatic breakdown of acetylcholine. As previously discussed, the stimulus must be strong enough to release enough acetylcholine to bind to the postsynaptic N_2 cholinergic receptor. This process of competition between the postsynaptic N_2 receptor and acetylcholinesterase allows for some degree of regulation of the excitation process and for the recovery of the muscle cell membrane. The molecules of acetylcholine either diffuse in a random fashion to the N_2 receptor or are destroyed by acetylcholinesterase. As the concentration gradient begins to decrease because of the destruction of acetylcholine by acetylcholinesterase, the N_2 receptor gives up its acetylcholine, which is then destroyed, and the skeletal muscle relaxes. A small portion of the acetylcholine can escape the acetylcholinesterase in the synaptic cleft and migrate into the extracellular fluid and from there into the plasma. Acetylcholine within the plasma is then destroyed by plasma acetylcholinesterase, or pseudocholinesterase, which is produced in the liver.[1]

PHARMACOLOGIC OVERVIEW OF THE SKELETAL MUSCLE RELAXANTS

With the anatomy and physiology of neuromuscular transmission as background, the principal pharmacologic actions of the nondepolarizing and depolarizing skeletal muscle relaxants are discussed. Table 23-1 presents a pharmacologic overview of the commonly used skeletal muscle relaxants.

The prototypical nondepolarizing skeletal muscle relaxants are pancuronium and vecuronium (Norcuron). Pancuronium is an inhibitor of acetylcholine, is chemically viewed as two acetylcholine-like fragments, and has a bulky inflexible nucleus. This drug attaches to the N_2 cholinergic receptors on the postsynaptic membrane and prevents depolarization. The skeletal muscle relaxant vecuronium has a chemical structure that is similar

FIG. 23-2 Myoneural junction when threshold stimulus is applied.

Table 23-1	Pharmacologic Overview of Commonly Used Neuromuscular Blocking Drugs				
	PANCURONIUM (PAVULON)	VECURONIUM BROMIDE (NORCURON)	ATRACURIUM BESYLATE (TRACRIUM)	CISATRACURIUM BESYLATE (NIMBEX)	ROCURONIUM BROMIDE (ZEMURON)
Nondepolarizing	Yes	Yes	Yes	Yes	Yes
Depolarizing	No	No	No	No	No
Intubation dose (IV mg/kg)	0.06-0.1	0.08-0.1	0.4-0.5	0.1-0.2	0.1
Intubation time (injection to relaxation; min)	4	2.5-3	2-2.5	2.8-3.4	1-2
Muscle relaxation dose (IV mg/kg)	0.04-0.08	0.05-0.06	0.2-0.5	2.5	0.6-1.0
Recovery time (min)	84-114	30-60	30-45	55-75	30-90
Reversible	Yes	Yes	Yes	Yes	Yes
Time to reversal (after initial dose; min)	40-60	25-30 (for 0.1 mg/kg), 40-80 (for 0.2 mg/kg)	20-35	10-15	5-10
Cumulative effects	Yes	Slight	No	No	No
Fasciculations and muscle soreness	No	No	No	No	No
Risk of histamine release	Slight to none	No	Minimal	No	No
Cardiovascular effects	Slight increase in pulse and increase in BP	None	Few	None	None

IV, Intravenous; *BP*, blood pressure.

to a monoquaternary compound. The principal pharmacologic action of this drug is to block the postsynaptic N_2 cholinergic receptor; in this way, it stops acetylcholine from binding to the receptor, which results in a competitive neuromuscular blockade. The nondepolarizing skeletal muscle relaxants also block the presynaptic cholinergic receptor and thus result in binding of the acetylcholine and thereby prevent activation of the positive feedback mechanism.[4]

The pharmacologic actions of the nondepolarizing skeletal muscle relaxants can be reversed with anticholinesterase drugs such as neostigmine. In effect, these drugs increase the quantum of acetylcholine at the postsynaptic membrane by preventing destruction of the acetylcholine by acetylcholinesterase. This process promotes a more effective competition by the released acetylcholine with the nondepolarizing skeletal muscle relaxant that is occupying the N_2 receptor. Because of the increased availability and mobilization of the acetylcholine, the concentration gradients favor acetylcholine and remove the nondepolarizing agents from the N_2 receptor, with the resultant return to normal contraction of the skeletal muscle.

The principal depolarizing skeletal muscle relaxant is succinylcholine (Anectine, Sucostrin). The molecular structure of this drug resembles two acetylcholine molecules back to back. Because of this structure, succinylcholine has the same effects as acetylcholine. Like acetylcholine, the succinylcholine molecule has a quaternary ammonium portion that is positively charged. This positively charged molecule is attracted by electrostatic action to the negatively charged N_2 receptor. When the succinylcholine attaches to the receptor, a brief period of depolarization occurs that is manifested by transient muscular fasciculations. Succinylcholine also attaches to and activates the presynaptic acetylcholine receptor. This activation has an immediate effect of increased mobilization of acetylcholine in the motor nerve terminals, which explains why fasciculations are commonly observed after the administration of an intravenous bolus of succinylcholine. After the depolarization of the N_2 receptor takes place, succinylcholine promotes and maintains the receptor in a depolarized state and prevents repolarization. Succinylcholine has a brief duration of action because of its rapid hydrolysis of the succinylcholine by the enzyme pseudocholinesterase, which is contained in the liver and plasma. The actions of succinylcholine cannot be pharmacologically reversed.[5]

NONDEPOLARIZING NEUROMUSCULAR BLOCKING AGENTS

Long-Acting Nondepolarizing Skeletal Muscle Relaxants
Pancuronium Bromide

Pancuronium bromide (Pavulon) was introduced into clinical anesthesia in 1972. This drug has shown value (particularly in terms of its safety, cardiovascular stability, and skeletal muscle relaxant properties) and is receiving widespread clinical use.

Chemically, pancuronium bromide is a biquaternary aminosteroid and is related to the androgens; however, it has no hormonal activities. Pancuronium is reversible with an anticholinesterase agent, such as neostigmine, that is administered in combination with an anticholinergic such as glycopyrrolate or atropine. This particular skeletal muscle relaxant has been shown clinically to be extremely difficult to reverse pharmacologically within the first 20 to 30 minutes after injection. In the PACU, if a skeletal muscle relaxant is needed for a short duration, another reversible skeletal muscle relaxant, such as vecuronium or atracurium, should be chosen. Approximately 30 to 40 minutes after injection, pancuronium is easily reversed with the combination of an anticholinesterase and anticholinergic drug preparation. Pancuronium is best suited for surgical procedures that last more than 1 hour; it is well suited for patients who need complete muscle relaxation with continuous mechanical ventilation. The dose for adults is approximately 0.08 to 0.1 mg/kg body weight. Relaxation lasts 60 to 85 minutes. If relaxation is necessary past this initial period, subsequent doses should be decreased to 0.02 to 0.04 mg/kg body weight.

Pancuronium bromide does not produce ganglionic blockade, but it does block the M_2 cholinergic receptors in the heart. Consequently, when pancuronium bromide is administered, a slight 10% to 15% increase in heart rate is observed.[6] Pancuronium activates the sympathetic nervous system by promoting the release of norepinephrine and blocking its uptake at the adrenergic nerve endings. After administration of this drug, a modest increase in mean arterial pressure and cardiac output is produced. Although isolated cases of histamine release have been reported, pancuronium can probably be used in patients who have a marginal allergy history. Pancuronium

bromide is compatible with anesthetic agents used clinically and is safe for use in most patients when a nondepolarizing skeletal muscle relaxant is indicated. However, pancuronium bromide is not indicated when a nondepolarizing muscle relaxant is to be used with caution. In addition, pancuronium should not be used in patients who are undergoing chronic digitalis therapy because cardiac dysrhythmias have been reported. Finally, myocardial ischemia has been reported in patients with coronary artery disease when pancuronium is used. This ischemia is probably associated with the cardiac acceleration properties of the drug.

Pancuronium bromide should be avoided in patients with a history of myasthenia gravis. It is contraindicated in patients with true renal disease because a major portion of the drug is excreted unchanged in the urine. This agent is contraindicated in patients known to be hypersensitive to it or to the bromide ion.

Intermediate-Acting Nondepolarizing Skeletal Muscle Relaxants
Vecuronium Bromide

Vecuronium (Norcuron) is a nondepolarizing skeletal muscle relaxant with a more rapid onset of action and a shorter duration of action than pancuronium. Actually, vecuronium is pancuronium without the quaternary methyl group in the steroid nucleus. Because of this structural difference, vecuronium has no effect on heart rate, arterial pressure, autonomic ganglia, or the alpha and beta adrenal receptors. The potency of vecuronium is equal to or slightly greater than that of pancuronium. Vecuronium has little or no cumulative effect. Although a portion of vecuronium is metabolized, most of the drug is excreted unchanged in the urine and bile. However, the neuromuscular blockade produced by vecuronium is not prolonged by renal failure. The duration of neuromuscular blockade produced by vecuronium is increased in patients with impaired hepatic function. Of clinical interest is that vecuronium, like atracurium, is less influenced by general inhalation anesthetics than is pancuronium.[7] The pharmacologic action of this drug is easily reversed with the combination of an anticholinesterase and an anticholinergic drug.

The onset of action of vecuronium is between 2.5 and 3 minutes, with the normal dose of 0.08 mg/kg intravenously. Because of the rapid onset of action, vecuronium can be used for rapid-sequence intubation. In this instance, a doubling of the dose of vecuronium to 0.2 mg/kg can be used to achieve intubation conditions within 45 seconds to 2 minutes. Another method for use of vecuronium for intubation is the priming technique. The object of this technique is to administer a small priming dose of vecuronium several minutes before the intubation dose is given to shorten the onset of neuromuscular blockade. The usual priming dose is 0.015 mg/kg; after 3 minutes, an intubation dose of 0.1 mg/kg is administered. The onset of neuromuscular blockade should be between 70 and 90 seconds. The main drawback of this technique is the potential development of symptoms of partial neuromuscular blockade. Sensations reported are heavy eyelids, blurred vision, and difficulty in swallowing. Therefore, if this technique is used in the PACU, the nurse should warn patients of the possible symptoms, and ventilatory support should always be available.

Because of concerns about the priming technique, the timing technique was developed. In the timing technique, which is used mainly in the operating room, the patient is given vecuronium before sodium pentothal. Consequently, the induction of anesthesia is specifically timed to the onset of clinical muscular weakness. In this technique, the patient is given 0.1 to 0.2 mg/kg of vecuronium intravenously. At the onset of weakness, as determined with the peripheral nerve simulator, a 1.0- to 2.5-mg/kg bolus dose of propofol is given. Intubating conditions occur within 1 minute.[4]

Vecuronium is primarily used for intraoperative skeletal muscle relaxation and facilitation of mechanical ventilation in the critical care setting. Long-term infusions of this drug in the critical care situation can result in a prolonged recovery and an inability to pharmacologically reverse vecuronium, because the metabolites are still in active form. If corticosteroid therapy is being used for patients with multiorgan failure, this prolonged effect can be exacerbated.

The dose is 0.05 to 0.2 mg/kg for skeletal muscle paralysis, and the onset is 1 to 3 minutes, with a duration between 30 and 90 minutes. Prolonged skeletal muscle relaxing effects can be prolonged with patients with hepatic disease. No significant cardiac effects for this drug have been reported.

Atracurium Besylate

Atracurium (Tracrium) is a nondepolarizing skeletal muscle relaxant that offers an advantage over other skeletal muscle relaxants in that it does not depend on renal or hepatic mechanisms for its elimination. In fact, this quaternary ammonium compound breaks down in the absence of plasma enzymes through what is called *Hofmann elimination* and, to a lesser extent, through ester hydrolysis. Hofmann elimination is a nonbiologic method of degradation that occurs at a physiologic temperature and pH.

Atracurium is less potent than pancuronium and has a rapid onset of 1 to 3 minutes and a duration of action of 30 to 45 minutes. For endotracheal intubation in the PACU setting, 0.3 to 0.5 mg/kg of atracurium should provide adequate skeletal muscle relaxation for intubation in about 2.5 minutes. For maintenance of mechanical ventilation in the PACU setting, an infusion rate of 10 mcg/kg/min of atracurium may be used. When the infusion has been discontinued, spontaneous ventilation by the patient occurs in approximately 30 minutes.[1] The effects can be reversed with a combination of anticholinesterase and antimuscarinic in 12 to 15 minutes after the discontinuation of the atracurium infusion.

Atracurium has many distinct advantages, such as its neuromuscular blockade not being prolonged by renal failure or impaired hepatic function; it has little or no cumulative effect and is not influenced significantly by the specific general inhalation anesthetic dose or concentration. Finally, this drug has little or no cardiovascular effect and is easily antagonized with the combination of an anticholinesterase and an anticholinergic.

Cisatracurium Besylate

Cisatracurium (Nimbex) is a stereoisomer of atracurium that is approximately threefold more potent as atracurium, but with fewer side effects; it is degraded by the same metabolic pathway as atracurium (i.e., the Hofmann elimination mechanism).

The average adult intubation dose of cisatracurium is 0.2 mg/kg and has an onset of approximately 90 seconds, a peak in 3 to 5 minutes, and a duration of action of 40 to 50 minutes. A supplemental dose of 0.03 mg/kg provides an additional 20 minutes of skeletal muscle relaxation. For maintenance of a stable state of skeletal muscle relaxation in the PACU, cisatracurium can be administered via infusion at a rate of 1 to 2 mcg/kg/min.[8]

This drug has all the assets of atracurium plus a great advantage over atracurium of less histamine release. It does not have any particular effect on the cardiovascular system, and because it undergoes an organ-independent clearance, it can be used in patients with hepatic or renal failure without a noticeable change in duration of action. It is well suited for many patients who undergo intermediate to long surgical procedures.

Short-Acting Nondepolarizing Skeletal Muscle Relaxants
Rocuronium Bromide

Rocuronium (Zemuron) is a nondepolarizing skeletal muscle relaxant with a chemical structure related to vecuronium. It has a rapid onset (1 to

1.5 minutes) and a short duration of action of 30 to 120 minutes, depending on the total dose of the drug. The onset and duration of action are not altered in obese patients when the dose is based on the actual body weight. In patients who are older than 65 years, the duration of action is slightly prolonged. In pediatrics, the onset and duration is slightly faster.

Because rocuronium has such rapid effects and short duration of action, spontaneous recovery from neuromuscular blockade is possible. However, if a patient arrives to the PACU with spontaneous ventilation after rocuronium administration during surgery that was not reversed with anticholinesterase and an anticholinergic, the patient still should be monitored in the PACU for neuromuscular function with the use of a peripheral nerve stimulator (PNS). In addition to use of the PNS, the patient should be evaluated for adequate clinical evidence of an adequate return of neuromuscular function with evaluation of the 5-second head lift, adequate phonation, ventilation, and upper airway maintenance.[1]

Rocuronium can be used in patients with renal failure and has a low potential for histamine release. Although rare, its actions are prolonged in patients with cirrhosis of the liver. The muscle relaxant actions of rocuronium are potentiated by the inhalation anesthetics, which makes a prediction of a total recovery from neuromuscular blockade variable. Because rocuronium produces minimal cardiovascular effects, it does not have significant histamine-releasing effects.

Rocuronium can be used as an agent of choice for nondepolarizing rapid sequence intubation in the PACU when appropriate intubation doses are used because it has such a fast onset and short duration of action and therefore is useful in intraoperative and postoperative periods. At a dose of 0.6 to 1.0 mg/kg, rocuronium provides excellent intubating conditions in 60 to 90 seconds for both children and adults. Therefore, before the intubation is attempted, the patient should undergo ventilation with 100% oxygen until appropriate paralysis of the skeletal muscle occurs to facilitate the intubation. The maintenance dose for rocuronium for adults is between 0.1 and 0.2 mg/kg and for children is 0.08 to 0.12 mg/kg intravenously. If rocuronium is to be used for continuous infusion, the initial rate is 0.01 to 0.012 mg/kg/min; at the desired level of neuromuscular blockade, the infusion of this drug can be individualized according to the patient's twitch response as monitored with the use of the PNS. The research indicates that infusion rates can range from 0.004 to 0.016 mg/kg/min. In assessment of the maintenance dosing of rocuronium, it

should be administered at 25% of control T1, which is three twitches of the train-of-four. The infusion solutions for rocuronium can be prepared in solutions of 5% glucose and water or lactated Ringer solution. When the infusion is completed, the unused portions of the infusion solutions should be discarded.[4]

Reversal of Nondepolarizing Neuromuscular Blocking Agents

For restoration of neuromuscular transmission, the antagonist must displace the competitive neuromuscular blocking agent from the nicotinic receptor sites and open the way for depolarization of the postjunctional membrane. The antagonist is an antiacetylcholinesterase that blocks the enzymatic action of acetylcholinesterase located in the postsynaptic clefts so that acetylcholine is not hydrolyzed. The result is a buildup of acetylcholine at the end plate at the N_2 cholinergic receptor. The accumulated acetylcholine displaces the competitive neuromuscular blocking agent, which diffuses back into the plasma and thus reestablishes neuromuscular transmission.

Neostigmine and pyridostigmine are usually the anticholinesterase drugs of choice because of their long duration of action and reliability as compared with edrophonium chloride. However, research has shown that edrophonium chloride is an effective reversal agent of neuromuscular blockades produced by vecuronium and atracurium. Atropine or glycopyrrolate, both antimuscarinic (anticholinergic) drugs, can be administered immediately before or in conjunction with the anticholinesterase for minimization of the muscarinic effects of the anticholinesterase drug. The muscarinic effects include bradycardia, salivation, miosis, and hyperperistalsis. These effects are produced at lower concentrations of the anticholinesterase-type drug when administered (acetylcholine nicotinic effects are at the autonomic ganglia and the neuromuscular junction). Consequently, when an anticholinesterase drug is administered for reversal of the nondepolarizing neuromuscular blocking agent at the N_2 receptor, an antimuscarinic drug is also given for prevention of the adverse muscarinic cholinergic effects associated with the high dose of anticholinesterase. Generally, 2.5 mg of neostigmine is the maximum dose necessary for reversal; however, the suggested limit is 5 mg. The method is administration of 0.4 mg atropine or 0.2 mg glycopyrrolate intravenously over a 1-minute period, observation for an increase in pulse rate, and then administration of 0.5 mg neostigmine intravenously and monitoring for the reversal. This procedure can be repeated until reversal has been achieved or until the limit of neostigmine that can be given is reached. If edrophonium chloride is indicated for reversal, the dose is 0.5 mg/kg with 0.007 mg/kg of atropine.

Neostigmine should be administered cautiously. Cardiac monitoring is essential, especially in elderly or debilitated patients and in patients with cardiac disease. Atrioventricular dissociation and other dysrhythmias can be initiated by the anticholinesterases.[7]

Pyridostigmine is an analogue of neostigmine. It facilitates the transmission of impulses across the myoneural junction by inhibiting the destruction of acetylcholine by acetylcholinesterase. Clinical data indicate a lower incidence rate of muscarinic side effects with this drug than with neostigmine. Like neostigmine, pyridostigmine should be administered with caution in patients with bronchial asthma or cardiac problems. Signs of overdose are related to muscarinic and nicotinic receptor stimulation (Box 23-1). The muscarinic side effects are blocked with atropine or glycopyrrolate. Nicotinic responses can be blocked with drugs such as ganglionic or neuromuscular blocking agents. The recommended dose for reversal is 0.15 mg/kg of intravenous pyridostigmine, in combination with 0.007 mg/kg of intravenous atropine. Full recovery occurs within 15 minutes in most patients; in other patients, 30 minutes or more may be necessary.

Another parasympatholytic agent, glycopyrrolate, has been substituted for atropine in the reversal technique. Its advantages over atropine are a longer duration of action and a lower incidence rate of arrhythmias; it causes small slow changes in the heart rate, and it does not cross the blood-brain barrier. The usual reversal dose is 1 mg of neostigmine and 0.2 mg of glycopyrrolate

in a 2-mL mixture. This dose can be repeated if reversal is inadequate.[1]

Sugammadex (Bridion) is a selective skeletal muscle relaxant binding agent that is effective in reversing the steroidal neuromuscular blocking drugs such as rocuronium, vecuronium, and pancuronium. Essentially, the mode of action of this drug is to form a tight bond with the steroidal neuromuscular blocking agents. The drug has minimal side effects and no anticholinesterase or anticholinergic drugs are required in the reversal using sugammadex. The dose for this drug is 2 to 4 mg/kg with a return to a full train-of-four approximately 3 minutes after injection. This drug appears to have significant clinical benefits compared with anticholinesterase and anticholinergic drugs for reversal.[9,10] The drug is approved for use in Europe and is under consideration but not yet approved for use by the U.S. Food and Drug Administration.

DEPOLARIZING NEUROMUSCULAR BLOCKING AGENTS

Succinylcholine

Succinylcholine (Anectine, Quelicin, Sucostrin) represents a valuable pharmacologic advance in modern anesthesia and in critical care, areas in which resuscitation is required. This agent is usually included as one of the drugs available for emergencies, especially with endotracheal intubation. Outside the operating room, succinylcholine is used for electroshock therapy, for relief of profound laryngospasm, for control of convulsions from tetanus, for management of ventilation of the flail chest, and during reduction of fractures or dislocations.

Although succinylcholine is widely used in the United States, it has side effects and complications that can be avoided with a basic understanding of the pharmacology of the drug.

Succinylcholine acts at the N_2 postsynaptic cholinergic receptor by causing a persistent depolarization of the end plate. It also acts on the presynaptic cholinergic receptor by causing an initial increase in acetylcholine at the motor end plate. This reaction is why patients who receive succinylcholine have fasciculations with initial administration. Succinylcholine is a synthetic quaternary ammonium compound with a chemical structure that closely resembles that of acetylcholine. The typical intravenous dose of succinylcholine to produce flaccid paralysis is 0.5 to 1.5 mg/kg; onset is 30 to 60 seconds with a duration of 5 to 10 minutes.[1] The drug is hydrolyzed rapidly by plasma pseudocholinesterase, an enzyme produced

---

BOX 23-1	Observable Responses to Stimulation of Receptors

NICOTINIC
- Stimulation of autonomic ganglia: both sympathetic and parasympathetic
- Stimulation of adrenal medulla, resulting in the release of both epinephrine and norepinephrine
- Stimulation of skeletal muscles at the motor end plate

MUSCARINIC
- Stimulation or inhibition of smooth muscle in various organs or tissues
- Stimulation of exocrine glands (i.e., salivary and sweat glands)
- Slowing of cardiac conduction
- Decrease in myocardial contractile force

by the liver, to succinylmonocholine and choline. Succinylmonocholine is further hydrolyzed by pseudocholinesterase and true cholinesterase, which are found in the erythrocyte, to succinic acid and choline (Box 23-2).

Advantages and Uses

Succinylcholine has certain advantages that, in most instances, justify its clinical use. Its rapid onset of action, coupled with its short duration of action, has made this drug valuable when: (1) rapid intubation is necessary; (2) laryngospasm is irreversible with positive pressure; (3) the skeletal muscles are rigid and prevent good ventilatory excursion; (4) procedures require a short duration of skeletal muscle relaxation, such as reduction of dislocations and fractures; and (5) electroconvulsive therapy is used to decrease the negative effects of seizures. Continued use over a 30-year period has shown succinylcholine to produce complications that can, in most instances, be prevented if the basic pharmacodynamics of the drug are understood.

In emergencies, succinylcholine remains the major muscle relaxant for facilitation of endotracheal intubation. Succinylcholine is contraindicated in children and adolescent patients except when used for emergency tracheal intubation or in instances in which immediate securing of the airway is necessary.

When this drug is used for a rapid-sequence intubation, the succinylcholine-induced fasciculations and the associated increase in gastric pressure should be reduced or eliminated with an intravenous injection of a small amount (3 mg per 70 kg of body weight) of vecuronium. This defasciculating dose of vecuronium should be administered 1 or 2 minutes before the intravenous bolus injection of succinylcholine of 1.5 mg/kg.

Untoward Reactions

Because hydrolysis of succinylcholine depends on enzymatic activity, an understanding is important of the atypical responses that may occur. Pseudocholinesterase activity in the plasma may be increased or decreased. Cases with increased activity are congenital and occur rarely. Patients with atypical pseudocholinesterase are resistant to succinylcholine and do not relax well. The

reductions in pseudocholinesterase activity may be acquired or congenital. Acquired deficiencies are more important to understand because they are more common. They occur with liver disease, severe anemia, malnutrition, prolonged pyrexia, pregnancy, and recent renal dialysis. Drugs such as quinidine and propranolol (Inderal) inhibit pseudocholinesterase, as do echothiophate iodide eye drops (Phospholine). Patients with low pseudocholinesterase activity have a prolonged response to these drugs.

Atypical pseudocholinesterase occurs alone in approximately 1 in 2800 people; this atypical form is inherited.[6] Patients with genetically induced deficiencies of pseudocholinesterase have been seen to remain apneic for as long as 48 hours after a usual dose of succinylcholine. These patients need mechanical ventilation and constant nursing care. Patients with documented pseudocholinesterase deficiency should be advised to wear a Medic Alert bracelet. If anesthesia is necessary, these patients should be administered nondepolarizing skeletal muscle relaxants, such as pancuronium, vecuronium, and rocuronium, because these drugs can usually be reversed.

Disadvantages and Side Effects

Succinylcholine can be administered via single injection or continuous infusion. The single-injection method is used when neuromuscular relaxation is needed for a short time, such as facilitation of endotracheal intubation. The usual intubation dosage of succinylcholine is 1 mg/kg intravenously. During the first intravenous injection, cardiovascular status usually remains normal. If the injection must be repeated, the patient may have profound bradycardia and various arrhythmias; therefore monitoring of the patient's cardiovascular status with succinylcholine administration is important, especially if the dose is repeated.

Because children and adolescent patients are more likely than adults to have undiagnosed myopathies, a nondepolarizing skeletal muscle relaxant such as rocuronium (Zimuron) should be used for routine procedures in the PACU. More specifically, except when used for emergency tracheal intubation or in the instance in which immediate securing of the airway is necessary,

---

BOX 23-2   Succinylcholine Metabolism

Succinylcholine $\xrightarrow{\text{Pseudocholinesterase}}$ Succinylmonocholine and choline

Succinylmonocholine $\xrightarrow{\text{True and pseudocholinesterase}}$ Succinic acid and choline

succinylcholine is contraindicated in children and adolescent patients because a patient with a myopathy in this age group who is administered succinylcholine can have acute fulminating destruction of skeletal muscle (rhabdomyolysis) that results in hyperkalemia and cardiac arrest.

If succinylcholine must be administered to an adolescent or child, the patient must be monitored completely because the patient is especially prone to bradycardia, even on the initial injection of succinylcholine. This complication can be easily overcome with prior administration of glycopyrrolate or atropine sulfate, either alone or mixed with succinylcholine. This method appears to be the safest way of administering intravenous succinylcholine in this age group.

A disadvantage of the single-injection method with succinylcholine is that it causes fasciculations of the muscles. These "mini" contractions are a result of the initial depolarization of the skeletal muscle from the positive feedback mechanism of initial stimulation of the presynaptic acetylcholine receptor. These contractions frequently lead to muscle pain, which is usually noted by the patient the day after surgery. This effect is particularly true in patients who are ambulatory soon after surgery. In ambulatory patients, muscle pains (myalgia) occur in 60% to 70% of cases. The incidence rate decreases to 10% in those patients confined to bed.[11] Symptoms include pain in the neck, back, and abdomen; pain when blinking the eyes; pain when smiling; and generalized pain when ambulatory. These objective symptoms are usually noticed first by the nurse in the PACU. Skeletal muscle pain around the neck area is sometimes described to the perianesthesia nurse as a sore throat caused by the endotracheal tube; in fact, the pain is caused by the myalgia from the succinylcholine. The pain usually does not require analgesics and subsides in 1 or 2 days. The fasciculations can be prevented by administering a nondepolarizing neuromuscular blocking drug at a pretreatment dose of between 5% and 10% of its normal intubation 2 to 4 minutes before the injection of succinylcholine. If a pretreatment nondepolarizing drug was administered, the dose of succinylcholine should be increased by about 70%.

When succinylcholine is administered to patients in the presence of extensive burns, severe trauma, severe abdominal infections, tetanus, neuromuscular disease, or neurologic lesions such as paraplegia and quadriplegia, a release of potassium from the damaged muscle and nerve cells can result. The common denominator appears to be either massive tissue destruction or central nervous system injury with muscle wasting. This pathophysiologic process results when denervated muscle is stimulated by succinylcholine because of the extrajunctional nicotinic receptors proliferated during the skeletal muscle destruction. After activation of the nicotinic receptor by succinylcholine, response is enhanced in the ionic channels, with a resultant increase in the release of potassium into the circulation. Elevation of the serum potassium level has been reported as high as 10 to 15 mEq/L. The result of this potassium elevation is cardiac dysrhythmias and cardiac arrest. The peak time for this reaction is 7 to 10 days after the injury. However, the critical period for these reactions is 1 to 180 days after trauma. Consequently, succinylcholine is contraindicated in patients who have injuries of major multiple traumas, extensive denervation of skeletal muscle, or upper motor neuron injury.[12]

Succinylcholine has been implicated as one of the trigger agents of malignant hyperthermia. Chapter 53 contains a complete description of the pathophysiology and treatment of malignant hyperthermia.

In pediatric and adult patients anesthetized with halothane combined with succinylcholine as the muscle relaxant, an unusual incidence of plasma myoglobin has occurred. Myoglobin is an intracellular muscle protein and therefore should not be released into the plasma. If myoglobin is found in the plasma, it can only mean that the muscle membrane has been injured.

Succinylcholine can be administered in a drip infusion during a procedure that requires skeletal muscle relaxation for a longer period than a single injection can provide. It is usually administered in a 0.1% to 0.2% solution. If the infusion is administered for a prolonged period, the type of block can gradually change from a depolarizing block to a characteristic nondepolarizing block. The change is always from depolarization to nondepolarization, never in the reverse direction. This type of block is called a *dual* or *phase II block*.[4] The exact time relationship and the mechanism of action are still uncertain. Treatment is via mechanical ventilation and careful monitoring of the patient until the dual block disappears.

Succinylcholine increases intraocular pressure by approximately 7.5 mm Hg in both children and adults, in part because of the contraction of the extraocular muscles. When administered before succinylcholine to prevent contraction of the extraocular muscles, a nondepolarizing neuromuscular blocking drug does not completely extinguish the increase in intraocular pressure. Therefore, even if succinylcholine is used with a neuromuscular blocking drug, it is contraindicated in patients in whom an increase in intraocular pressure would be detrimental.

Factors that Influence the Neuromuscular Blocking Agents

Fluid Balance

Patients who are dehydrated are reported to be extremely sensitive to skeletal muscle relaxants. This finding is probably true because: (1) dehydration decreases neuromuscular excitability; (2) the contracted extracellular fluid compartment permits an increase in the plasma concentration of the relaxant and thus intensifies the relaxant action; and (3) renal function is slowed and the elimination time of the relaxant and its metabolites is prolonged.

Sodium

A deficit of sodium may prolong the neuromuscular block. Experimental evidence indicates that a sodium deficiency itself can result in a partial neuromuscular block.

Potassium

Potassium deficiency appears to increase the blocking action of pancuronium and other nondepolarizing neuromuscular blocking agents. Alternatively, depolarizing neuromuscular blocking agents are required in larger amounts when potassium deficiency exists. Depolarization is prevented to some extent because a potassium deficiency appears to stabilize the muscle end plate. Potassium depletion can occur from decreased intake or excessive loss, such as in chronic pyelonephritis, primary aldosteronism, chlorothiazide therapy, and chronic diarrhea.

Magnesium

An increase in magnesium concentration causes a flaccid paralysis clinically similar to that caused by a nondepolarizing neuromuscular blocking agent. The principal action of magnesium is that it can enter the nerve terminal and replace or decrease the amount of calcium that enters, which stabilizes the postsynaptic membrane. Ultimately, depression of the release of acetylcholine occurs and reduces the EPP, which causes a partial neuromuscular block. Consequently, magnesium enhances a neuromuscular block produced by a nondepolarizing agent and, to a lesser extent, potentiates the block produced by succinylcholine.

Calcium

A deficiency in calcium prolongs the effects of nondepolarizing neuromuscular blocking agents by reducing the amount of acetylcholine released and by inhibiting neuromuscular transmission. The depolarizing neuromuscular blocking agents are also potentiated because a low calcium level aids depolarization. Conversely, the administration of calcium chloride solution in calcium deficiency states antagonizes the nondepolarizing effects of agents such as pancuronium. Calcium chloride has a pronounced antagonism to the respiratory depressant effects of succinylcholine.

pH and Carbon Dioxide

The neuromuscular blocking effect of pancuronium is intensified in acidosis and in states of elevated carbon dioxide tension. With drugs such as rocuronium and succinylcholine, the neuromuscular blocking action is diminished. Alkalosis by itself decreases the effects of pancuronium. Hyperventilation has been thought to augment the abdominal muscle relaxation produced by pancuronium. One explanation of this phenomenon is that changes in pH or plasma concentrations of pancuronium reflect a change in binding to the receptor substance.

Catecholamines

Epinephrine and ephedrine have a type of reversal effect on skeletal muscle. Clinically, an antagonism to pancuronium has been shown. This effect is caused by an increase in acetylcholine release, the inhibition of acetylcholinesterase, a decreased excitability of muscle fibers, and the release of potassium with administration of epinephrine and ephedrine.

Mycins

Several antibiotics have a nondepolarizing neuromuscular blocking property because the aminoglycoside antibiotics potentiate the neuromuscular blockade by inhibiting the presynaptic release of acetylcholine. The resulting clinical difficulties are related to a combination of factors, including large doses of antibiotics, parenteral administration into body cavities that represent a large surface area for absorption, and concomitant use of a neuromuscular blocking agent. Neomycin and streptomycin have been implicated the most frequently (Box 23-3).

Cardiac Antidysrhythmic Drugs

When administered intravenously, lidocaine potentiates a preexisting neuromuscular blockade that occurs because lidocaine stabilizes the postsynaptic membrane and depresses the skeletal muscle fibers. Quinidine interferes with the presynaptic release of acetylcholine at the neuromuscular junction. Consequently, it intensifies the neuromuscular blockade of both depolarizing and nondepolarizing skeletal muscle blocking agents. Finally, calcium channel blocking agents inhibit

> **BOX 23-3**   Neuromuscular Blocking Properties of Various Antibiotics
>
> **ANTIBIOTICS THAT INCREASE THE ACTION OF THE NONDEPOLARIZING AGENTS**
> - Dihydrostreptomycin
> - Neomycin
> - Streptomycin
> - Kanamycin
> - Gentamicin
> - Polymyxin A
> - Polymyxin B
> - Lincomycin
> - Colistin
> - Tetracycline
>
> **ANTIBIOTICS THAT INCREASE THE ACTION OF SUCCINYLCHOLINE**
> - Neomycin
> - Streptomycin
> - Kanamycin
> - Polymyxin B
> - Colistin
>
> **ANTIBIOTICS THAT DO NOT EXERT ANY NEUROMUSCULAR BLOCKING ACTIVITY**
> - Penicillin
> - Chloramphenicol
> - Cephalosporins

the calcium entry, with a resultant reduction in acetylcholine release followed by a reduction in neuromuscular function.

Temperature

Hypothermia antagonizes the action of pancuronium and potentiates the action of succinylcholine. During the recovery phase of an anesthetic, when a neuromuscular blocking agent has been administered, young infants should be specifically monitored for return of skeletal muscle tone. This rule is especially in effect when a nondepolarizing relaxant is administered to infants, who are prone to have some hypothermia because of their immature heat-regulating systems.

Inhalation Anesthetics

The inhalation anesthetics produce a dose-dependent enhancement of the neuromuscular blockade of the nondepolarizing neuromuscular blocking agents. More specifically, this blockade is most pronounced when a patient has received isoflurane. Nitrous oxide only produces minimal potentiation of nondepolarizing neuromuscular blocking agents. This potentiation of the neuromuscular blockade by the inhalation anesthetics results from depression of

the central nervous system and ultimately reduces skeletal muscle tone. Consequently, patients in the PACU who have received nondepolarizing neuromuscular blocking agents during surgery and have not completely emerged from the inhalation anesthetic should be closely monitored with a peripheral nerve stimulator for a reduction in skeletal muscle function. In addition, an aggressive stir-up regimen should be instituted for these patients.

ASSESSMENT OF NEUROMUSCULAR BLOCKADE

In a study conducted in the 1940s, injection with D-tubocurarine (a nondepolarizing skeletal muscle relaxant) first caused motor weakness and then total muscle flaccidity. The small rapidly moving muscles, such as those of the fingers, toes, eyes, and ears, are involved before the long muscles of the limbs, neck, and trunk. The intercostal muscles and finally the diaphragm become paralyzed, and respiration ceases.

The perianesthesia nurse should know the order of the return of muscle function after a patient has received a nondepolarizing muscle relaxant. The recovery of skeletal muscle function is usually in reverse order to that of paralysis; therefore the diaphragm is ordinarily first to regain function. The order of appearance of paralysis after injection with a nondepolarizing neuromuscular blocking agent can be assessed electromyographically as follows:

1. Small-sized muscle groups: oculomotor muscles, muscles of the eyelids; muscles of the mouth and face; small extensor muscles of the fingers, followed by the flexor muscles of the fingers
2. Medium-sized muscle groups: muscles of the tongue and pharynx; muscles of mastication; extensor muscles of the limb, followed by flexor muscles of the limbs
3. Large-sized muscle groups: neck muscles, shoulder muscles, abdominal muscles, dorsal muscle mass
4. Special muscle groups: intercostal muscles, larynx, diaphragm

The order of paralysis is essentially the same after injection with a depolarizing neuromuscular agent, except that the flexor muscles are paralyzed before the extensor muscles. Patients who arrive in the PACU must be evaluated for residual effects from a neuromuscular blocking agent that was administered during surgery. In most instances, the action of the nondepolarizing neuromuscular blocking agent is pharmacologically reversed at the end of the operation before the patient is admitted to the PACU; however, any patient who has received a neuromuscular blocking agent should be closely watched for signs of residual drug action. The goal of the assessment of the recovery from nondepolarizing neuromuscular blocking agents with the train-of-four is a ratio of more than 75%. The residual actions of the depolarizing muscle relaxants are similar to those of the nonpolarizing muscle relaxants, and the same nonrespiratory parameters and respiratory variables can be used in evaluation of the neuromuscular blockade. The evoked (electric stimulation) responses differ between the depolarizing and nondepolarizing neuromuscular blocking agents.

The PNS (Fig. 23-3) can be used in the PACU for assessment of the type and degree of

a neuromuscular blockade. This electric device can be used to stimulate the ulnar nerve at the wrist or elbow, and, on stimulation of the ulnar nerve, the nurse can observe the contraction of the fingers. Fig. 23-4 graphically shows the train-of-four test. The assessment of the depth of neuromuscular blockade with electric stimulation is useful when more than 70% of the N_2 receptors are blocked by a skeletal muscle relaxant. However, in most instances, if the patient has a normal tidal volume, vital capacity, and maximal inspiratory force and can lift the head for 5 seconds, the use of the PNS is not warranted. If identification of the type of neuromuscular blockade used (depolarizing or nondepolarizing) is needed, or if some of the aforementioned parameters are marginal, the train-of-four or sustained tetanus with the PNS can be used to provide the objective data for assessment.

Although the mechanisms that produce the nondepolarizing block differ from the depolarizing block, the diagnostic criteria with a PNS for assessment of a nondepolarizing and phase II dual block are basically the same. The hallmark of a nondepolarizing neuromuscular blockade is an inability to sustain contraction in response to a tetanic stimulus and posttetanic potentiation. A tetanic stimulus is the usual 50 Hz of current for 5 seconds (sustained tetanus) produced by a PNS. Posttetanic facilitation is a twitch after the response to tetanic stimuli higher than the twitch immediately before tetanus. If a patient has a partial nondepolarizing neuromuscular block, an unsustained contraction called *fade* is seen after the initial tetanic stimulus (Fig. 23-5). Fade is caused by the decreased mobilization of acetylcholine in the nerve terminal, because the presynaptic acetylcholine receptor is blocked by the nondepolarizing muscle relaxant. The responses to electric stimulation result from the interaction of acetylcholine released and the number of N_2 cholinergic receptors occupied by the relaxant. In patients with a partial nondepolarizing neuromuscular block, the first three single electric stimuli are of enough intensity to produce a twitch, but the twitch produced is not of the same magnitude as a twitch produced in a subject who has not received a nondepolarizing skeletal muscle relaxant (see Fig. 23-5). The three electric stimuli cause the normal quantum of acetylcholine to be released at the synaptic cleft; however, in this instance, the reduction in twitch magnitude is the result of the number of acetylcholine receptors being occupied by the

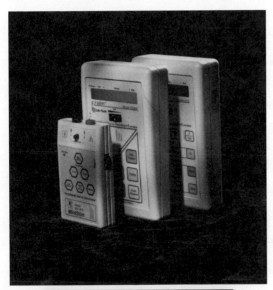

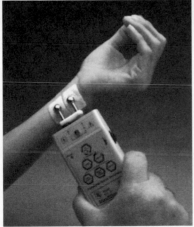

FIG. 23-3 Peripheral nerve stimulator. (Courtesy Life-Tech, Stafford, Tex.)

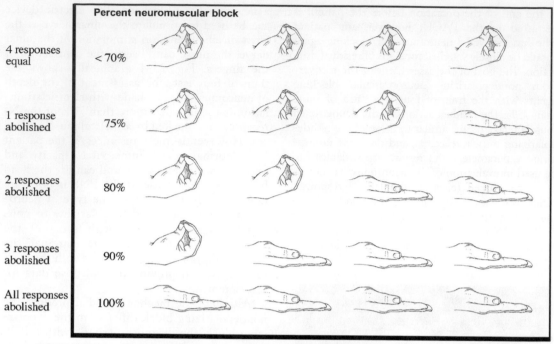

FIG. 23-4 Train-of-four suppression. (From Nagelhout J, Plaus K: *Nurse anesthesia*, ed 4, St. Louis, 2010, Saunders.)

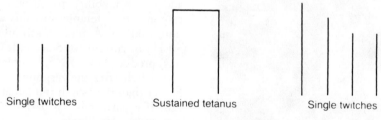

Without nondepolarizing neuromuscular blockade

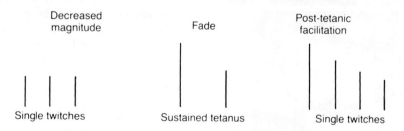

With nondepolarizing neuromuscular blockade

FIG. 23-5 Magnitude of posttetanic facilitation without and with nondepolarizing neuromuscular blockade. (Adapted from Donati F: Monitoring neuromuscular blockade. In Saidman L, Smith NT, editors: *Monitoring in anesthesia*, ed 3, Woburn, Mass, 1993, Butterworth-Heinemann.)

nondepolarizing relaxant. Consequently, if the patient has had a complete nondepolarizing neuromuscular block in which all the N_2 cholinergic receptors were occupied, no twitch is elicited from the three electric stimuli.

In a healthy subject, when a tetanic stimulus is applied for 5 seconds, the quantum of acetylcholine that is released decreases during the stimulus period. In addition, only a fraction of nicotinic cholinergic receptors are activated at any one time to trigger an action potential. The excess in nicotinic cholinergic receptors is the safety margin of neuromuscular transmission. Consequently, in the healthy subject who receives a tetanic stimulus, the magnitude of the twitch response is maintained because of the large nicotinic cholinergic receptor pool; however, if 75% of the nicotinic receptors are occupied by a nondepolarizing neuromuscular relaxant, for example, the twitch response is not maintained and fade (unsustained contraction) occurs because the usual margin of safety of excess acetylcholine receptors has been abolished. Between the termination of a tetanic stimulus and the first single-twitch stimulus, a buildup of acetylcholine occurs in the presynaptic knob. Thus, after sustained tetanus, when the first electric stimulus is administered, the height of the first twitch is greater than the pretetanic twitches. These large posttetanic twitches (posttetanic facilitation) return to the pretetanic height as the acetylcholine mobilization also returns to the pretetanic level. Finally, more than 70% of the nicotinic cholinergic receptors must be occupied before this tetanic stimulation test is sensitive enough for detection of neuromuscular blockade.

The major drawback to the delivery of a 50-Hz tetanic stimulus to an awakened patient in the PACU is pain and general discomfort. For the patient who is awake and reactive, the train-of-four stimulation is better for assessment of the degree of neuromuscular blockade caused by nondepolarizing skeletal muscle relaxants. In this test, the ulnar nerve is used, and four supramaximal electrical stimuli—2 Hz, 0.05 seconds apart—are administered with a PNS. This test, which produces minimal discomfort to the awakened patient, is sensitive only when more than 70% of the nicotinic cholinergic receptors are occupied. The index of neuromuscular blockade in this test is the ratio of the fourth to the first twitch amplitude. More specifically, when the fourth response is abolished, a 75% block exists (Fig. 23-6). When the third and second responses to stimulation are abolished, the respective reductions in neuromuscular blockade are 80% and 90%. Finally, when all four twitch responses are absent, a 100%, or complete, block exists.

The depolarizing neuromuscular blockade is characterized by an absence of posttetanic potentiation, a decreased response to a single impulse, a decreased amplitude (but sustained response to a tetanic stimulus), and, if present, a train-of-four ratio between the first and fourth stimulus that is greater than 70%.[12] Refer to Table 23-2 for a complete overview of the commonly used monitoring

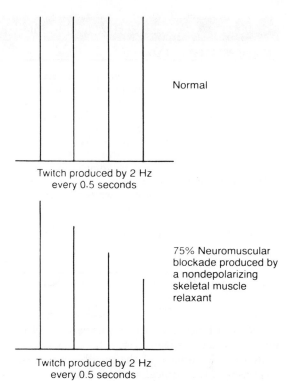

FIG. 23-6 Diagrammatic illustration of train-of-four in normal response and 75% neuromuscular blockade produced by nondepolarizing skeletal muscle relaxant.

tests and Table 23-3 for some key points related to the neuromuscular reversal.

SPECIAL PROBLEMS IN THE POSTANESTHESIA CARE UNIT

A prolonged response to succinylcholine sometimes occurs because a patient does not possess the proper blood level of pseudocholinesterase. Other causes of a prolonged response include: (1) overdose; (2) temperature changes; (3) acid-base imbalance; (4) carcinoma; (5) antitumor agents; (6) antibiotics; (7) myasthenia gravis; and (8) liver disease.

If a patient who arrives in the PACU is apneic, controlled respiration must be initiated and maintained as long as necessary. Careful monitoring of vital signs and evaluation of renal function are important. The neuromuscular block can be identified with the PNS. If electrical stimulation results in vigorous contractions, the apnea is unlikely to be the result of residual neuromuscular block. Consideration must then be given to other agents that may have caused the apneic state. The response of patients with neuromuscular disorders to muscle relaxants may

Table 23-2	Neuromuscular Monitoring Methods	
MONITORING TEST	**DEFINITION**	**COMMENTS**
Single twitch	Single supramaximal electric stimulus ranging from 0.1-1 Hz	Requires baseline before drug administration; generally used as qualitative rather than quantitative assessment
Train-of-four	Series of four twitches at 2 Hz every half second for 2 sec	Reflects blockade from 70% to 100%; useful during onset, maintenance, and emergence
Tetanus	Generally consists of rapid delivery of 30-, 50-, or 100-Hz stimulus for 5 sec	Should be used sparingly for deep block assessment; painful
Posttetanic count	50-Hz tetanus for 5 sec, 3-sec pause, then single twitches of 1 Hz	Used only when train-of-four or double-burst stimulation response is absent; count less than eight indicates deep block, and prolonged recovery is likely
Double-burst stimulation	Two short bursts of 50-Hz tetanus separated by 0.75 sec	Similar to train-of-four; useful during onset, maintenance, and emergence; may be easier for detection of fade than with train of four; tactile evaluation

From Nagelhout J, Plaus K: *Nurse anesthesia*, ed 4, St. Louis, 2010, Saunders.

include resistance, increased response, hyperkalemia, and even cardiac arrest. Table 23-4 is presented as a summary of the possible untoward responses in the clinical setting.

Dual or Phase II Block

Various terms are used to describe the different types of blocks that succinylcholine is able to produce. The phase I block is synonymous with the depolarizing block the drug ordinarily produces. It is characterized by a dose-dependent reduction in a single twitch without fade after a well-sustained tetanus and no posttetanic facilitation when the PNS is used.

Phase II block is also known as a *dual block, desensitization,* or *open channel block.* This block is caused by a conformational change in the presynaptic and postsynaptic cholinergic receptors. This anatomic change results in desensitization to the stimulation of acetylcholine because of the prolonged depolarization at the motor end plate. The characteristics of this block as shown with the PNS are fade in response to tetanic stimuli, posttetanic potentiation, and antagonism with drugs such as neostigmine. The same clinical features are seen when vecuronium is used; however, this similarity does not mean that the two blocks are the same, because good evidence suggests that the vecuronium and succinylcholine phase II blocks differ in several respects. Some clinicians believe that the phase II block produced by succinylcholine can be reversed with anticholinesterases, such as edrophonium, which has a shorter duration of action than neostigmine. Edrophonium is used in this situation because it either reverses or potentiates the block. If potentiation occurs, it is

of a shorter duration than if neostigmine were used. Most experts believe that routine reversal to antagonize the dual block is unwarranted. Ventilation of the patient with a wait for return of the normal neuromuscular transmission is more advisable. See Box 23-4 for a summary of the differentiating characteristics of a depolarizing (phase I) block and a nondepolarizing (phase II) block.

Residual Paralysis

Residual paralysis is the reappearance after surgery of the pharmacologic actions of a nondepolarizing skeletal muscle relaxant that was administered during surgery.[11] Other terms that are associated with this are *compromised ventilation, partial reversal,* or *reduced train-of-four.* This complication arises when renal insufficiency exists. The interesting facet of this complication is that even when a nondepolarizing skeletal muscle relaxant is reversed sufficiently at the end of the anesthetic, residual paralysis may still occur for as long as 8 hours. This reappearance may be partly caused by the fading of the effect of the neostigmine.

Symptoms of residual paralysis include clinical evidence showing a reduction of the return of neuromuscular function with evaluation of the 5-second head lift, adequate phonation, ventilation, and upper airway maintenance along with a poor twitch response with the PNS.

If symptoms appear, the required level of the reversal agent (neostigmine) must be maintained until that portion of the nondepolarizing skeletal muscle relaxant has been eliminated so that symptoms do not reappear. If residual

Table 23-3   Key Points Related to Tests of Neuromuscular Transmission and Reversal

TEST	ACCEPTABLE CLINICAL RESULT TO SUGGEST NORMAL FUNCTION	APPROXIMATE PERCENTAGE OF RECEPTORS OCCUPIED WHEN RESPONSE RETURNS TO NORMAL VALUE	COMMENTS, ADVANTAGES, AND DISADVANTAGES
Tidal volume	At least 5 mL/kg	80	Necessary, but insensitive as indicator of neuromuscular function
Single twitch strength	Qualitatively as strong as baseline	75-80	Uncomfortable; need to know twitch strength before relaxant administration; insensitive as indicator of recovery but useful as gauge of deep neuromuscular blockade
Train-of-four	No palpable fade	70-75	Uncomfortable, but more sensitive as indicator of recovery than single twitch; used as gauge of depth of block with counting number of responses perceptible
Sustained tetanus at 50 Hz for 5 sec	At least 20 mL/kg	70	Very uncomfortable, but reliable indicator of adequate recovery
Vital capacity	At least 20 mL/kg	70	Requires patient cooperation, but is goal for achievement of full clinical recovery
Double-burst stimulation	No palpable fade	60-70	Uncomfortable, but more sensitive than TOF as indicator of peripheral function; no perceptible fade indicates TOF of at least recovery of 60%
Inspiratory force	At least −40 cm H_2O	50	Difficult to perform with endotracheal intubation, but reliable gauge of normal diaphragmatic function
Head lift	Must be performed unaided with patient supine and sustained for 5 sec	50	Requires patient cooperation, but remains standard test of normal clinical function
Hand grip	Sustained at level qualitatively similar to preinduction	50	Sustained strong grip, although also requires patient cooperation; is another good gauge of normal function
Sustained bite	Sustained jaw clench on tongue blade	50	Very reliable with patient cooperation; corresponds with TOF of 85%

Modified from Miller R, et al: *Miller's anesthesia*, ed 7, New York, 2010, Churchill Livingstone; Nagelhout J, Plaus K: *Nurse anesthesia*, ed 4, St. Louis, 2010, Saunders.
TOF, Train-of-four.

CONCEPTS IN ANESTHETIC AGENTS

paralysis occurs, the postoperative use of morphine and similar opioids should be avoided because these agents enhance a residual neuromuscular block sufficiently to make it clinically significant. Finally, because the patient becomes extremely fearful, constant verbal reassurance by the PACU nurse helps to reduce stress and anxiety.

Bradycardia

Another problem that occurs in the PACU is the appearance of bradycardia when a patient has received an atropine-neostigmine combination at the end of the anesthetic. The bradycardia is usually the result of the longer duration of action of neostigmine compared with that of atropine.[12] The treatment for this problem is glycopyrrolate.

Table 23-4	Summary of Response of Patients with Neuromuscular Disorders to Muscle Relaxants		
DISORDER	PATHOPHYSIOLOGY	RESPONSE TO NONDEPOLARIZING MUSCLE RELAXANT	RESPONSE TO DEPOLARIZING MUSCLE RELAXANT
Hemiplegia	Sequelae of CVA; caused by upper motor neuron in cerebral motor cortex	Resistance	Hyperkalemia can occur as early as 1 week and as late as 6 months after stroke
Parkinson disease	Extrapyramidal disorder	Normal	Hyperkalemia may occur
Multiple sclerosis	Demyelinating disorder of CNS	Normal	Hyperkalemia may occur
Diffuse intracranial lesions	No focal neurologic deficits or muscular denervation or paralysis (i.e., ruptured cerebral aneurysm)	Normal	Hyperkalemia and possible cardiac arrest
Tetanus	Acute infectious disease of CNS caused by endotoxin released by *Clostridium tetani*	Normal	Hyperkalemia and possible cardiac arrest
Paraplegia and quadriplegia	Traumatic or pathologic transection of spinal cord and interruption of pyramidal tracts	Increased response	Hyperkalemia as early as 3 weeks and as late as 85 days after spinal cord injury
Amyotrophic lateral sclerosis	Degenerative disease of motor ganglia in anterior horn of spinal cord and of spinal pyramidal tracts	Increased response	No reports of hyperkalemia in ALS; however, myotonia-like contracture may occur in patients with ALS; avoid succinylcholine in patients with significant muscular denervation
Muscular denervation	Result of traumatic peripheral nerve damage; muscles undergo atrophy	Normal response	Muscular contracture and hyperkalemia
Myasthenia gravis	Postsynaptic reduction in number of ACh receptors caused by autoimmune disease	Increased response and prolongation of effects	Resistance and early appearance of phase II (dual) block
Myasthenic syndrome	Differs clinically and electromyographically from myasthenia gravis; associated with small cell carcinoma of lung and results in presynaptic lesion at neuromuscular junction	Exaggerated response	Exaggerated response
Myotonia	Lesion in muscle fiber distal to neuromuscular junction; common symptom is delayed relaxation of skeletal muscles after voluntary contractions	Increased and prolonged; some report normal response	Unpredictable; many reports of increased rigidity
Muscular dystrophy	Disorder of muscle fiber proper that may be caused by neurogenic disorder	Normal to prolonged response; ocular muscular dystrophy has very high sensitivity to D-tubocurarine	Unpredictable; best to avoid use of succinylcholine

CVA, Cerebrovascular accident; *CNS,* central nervous system; *ALS,* amyotrophic lateral sclerosis; *ACh,* acetylcholine.

BOX 23-4 Summary of the Differentiating Characteristics of Phase I and Phase II Blocks

DEPOLARIZING (PHASE I) BLOCK
- Muscle fasciculation preceding the onset of neuromuscular blockade
- Sustained response to titanic stimulation
- Absence of posttetanic potentiation, stimulation, or facilitation
- Lack of fade to train-of-four or double-burst stimulation
- Block antagonized by prior administration of nondepolarizer as pretreatment (approximately 20% more succinylcholine necessary)
- Block potentiated by anticholinesterase drugs

NONDEPOLARIZING (PHASE II) BLOCK
- Absence of muscle fasciculation
- Appearance of tetanic fade and posttetanic potentiation, stimulation, or facilitation
- Train-of-four and double-burst fade
- Reversal with anticholinesterase drugs
- In rare cases, may be produced by an overdose and desensitization with succinylcholine at doses more than 6 mg/kg

From Nagelhout J, Plaus K: *Nurse anesthesia,* ed 4, St. Louis, 2010, Saunders.

Glycopyrrolate should not be administered, however, until other causes of bradycardia are eliminated, such as pain, hypoventilation, and a full bladder.

SUMMARY

The neuromuscular blocking agents used in modern perianesthesia practice produce excellent results with fewer disadvantages compared with the drugs presented in the previous edition of this book. It is remarkable how the art and science of anesthesia has narrowed down the number of agents to be used in clinical practice to the most popular and those that possess excellent advantages over the neuromuscular agents used in the past. An overview of the process of excitation-contraction coupling was presented as were the current drugs in use. An in-depth approach was used in the discussion of the pharmacologic reversal of the nondepolarizing neuromuscular agents and in a discussion of the various methods of monitoring a patient who has received a skeletal muscle relaxant during surgery. Finally, an overview of the PACU nursing care was presented (an in-depth discussion on this topic can be found in Chapter 28).

Neuromuscular blocking agents are useful agents in the operating room for facilitation of the optimum surgical field for the physician to use life-saving skills effectively. In the PACU, neuromuscular blocking agents can be used for life-saving situations and facilitation of mechanical ventilation. In the PACU, these agents should only be administered by a practitioner skilled in airway management. For patients in the PACU who require mechanical ventilation and need neuromuscular blocking agents to enhance ventilatory care, the PACU nurse should be acutely aware that, besides the skillful use of the neuromuscular blocking agent, the patient also needs appropriate sedation and verbal support during that most fearful time of care.

REFERENCES

1. Stoelting R: *Pharmacology and physiology in anesthetic practice,* ed 4, Philadelphia, 2005, Lippincott Williams & Wilkins.
2. Barrett K, et al: *Ganong's review of medical physiology,* ed 23, New York, 2009, McGraw-Hill Medical.
3. Hall J: *Guyton and Hall textbook of medical physiology,* ed 12, Philadelphia, 2011, Saunders.
4. Nagelhout J, Plaus K: *Nurse anesthesia,* ed 4, St. Louis, 2010, Saunders.
5. Longnecker D, et al: *Anesthesiology,* New York, 2007, McGraw-Hill Medical.
6. Miller R, Pardo M: *Basics of anesthesia,* ed 6, Philadelphia, 2011, Saunders.
7. Barash P, et al: *Clinical anesthesia,* ed 6, Philadelphia, 2009, Lippincott Williams & Wilkins.
8. Aitkenhead A, et al: *Textbook of anesthesia,* ed 5, Philadelphia, 2007, Churchill Livingstone.
9. Kopman A: Sugammadex: A revolutionary approach to neuromuscular antagonism, *Anesthesiology* 104:631–633, 2006.
10. Naguib M: Sugammadex: another milestone in clinical neuromuscular pharmacology, *Anesth Analg* 104(3):575–581, 2007.
11. Atlee J: *Complications in anesthesia,* ed 2, Philadelphia, 2007, Saunders.
12. Fisher L: *Anesthesia and uncommon diseases,* ed 5, Philadelphia, 2007, Saunders.

RESOURCES

American Association of Critical-Care Nurses: *Core curriculum for progressive care nursing,* Philadelphia, 2010, Saunders.
Alspach J: *Core curriculum for critical care nursing,* ed 6, Philadelphia, 2005, Saunders.
Ball C: Unraveling the mystery of malignant hyperthermia, *Anaesth Intensive Care* 35(Suppl 1):26–31, 2007.
Bready L, et al: *Decision making in anesthesiology,* ed 4, St. Louis, 2007, Mosby.

Brunton L, et al: *Goodman and Gilman's the pharmacological basis of therapeutics*, ed 12, New York, 2010, McGraw-Hill Professional.

Conlay L, et al: *Case files anesthesiology*, New York, 2011, McGraw-Hill Medical.

Cope T, Hunter J: Selecting neuromuscular-blocking drugs for elderly patients, *Drugs Aging* 20(2):125–140, 2003.

Davis P, et al: *Smith's anesthesia for infants and children*, ed 8, St. Louis, 2011, Mosby.

Drake R, et al: *Gray's anatomy for students*, ed 2, Philadelphia, 2009, Churchill Livingstone.

Deutschman C, Netigan P: *Evidence-based practice of critical care*, Philadelphia, 2010, Saunders.

Dorsch J, Dorsch S: *Understanding anesthesia equipment*, ed 5, Philadelphia, 2007, Lippincott Williams & Wilkins.

Gallager C, Issenberg B: *Simulation in anesthesia*, Philadelphia, 2007, Saunders.

Hines R, Marschall K: *Handbook for Stoelting's anesthesia and co-existing disease*, ed 3, Philadelphia, 2013, Saunders.

Kaplan J, et al: *Cardiac anesthesia*, New York, 2011, Churchill Livingstone.

Kervin W, et al: Residual neuromuscular blockade in the immediate postoperative period, *J Perianesth Nurs* 17:152–158, 2002.

Kier L, Dowd C: *The chemistry of drugs for nurse anesthetists*, Chicago, 2004, AANA Publishing, Inc.

Pasero C, McCaffery M: *Pain assessment and pharmacologic management*, St. Louis, 2011, Mosby.

Schick L, Windle PE: *Perianesthesia nursing core curriculum: preprocedure, phase I and phase II PACU nursing*, ed 2, St. Louis, 2010, Saunders.

Schreiber J, et al: Prevention of succinylcholine-induced fasciculation and myalgia, *Anesthesiology* 1037:877–884, 2005.

Shorten G, et al: *Postoperative pain management: an evidence-based guide to practice*, Philadelphia, 2006, Saunders.

Sieber F: *Geriatric anesthesia*, New York, 2006, McGraw-Hill Medical.

Vincent J, et al: *Textbook of critical care*, ed 6, Philadelphia, 2011, Saunders.

24 Local Anesthetics

Daniel D. Moos, MS, EdD, CRNA

Local anesthetics are used to render a portion of the body insensate to painful stimuli through reversible nerve conduction blockade. Erythroxylon coca, the source of cocaine, was used in antiquity. In 1855, cocaine was isolated from the coca bean and rapidly found a place in modern medicine. In 1884, Carl Koller demonstrated its ability to anesthetize the eye, and William Halsted used cocaine for infiltration and nerve blocks. Cocaine had two major problems: toxicity and physical dependence. The first ester local anesthetic suitable for injection, procaine, was introduced in 1905. In 1948, Lofgren introduced the first clinically useful amide local anesthetic.[1,2] The use of local anesthetics for anesthesia and/or postoperative analgesia continues evolve. Advances in pharmacology and technology have increased the use of local anesthetics. Perianesthesia nurses should understand the basic physiology of nerve conduction, pharmacology of local anesthetics, and identification and treatment of complications that may arise from their use.

DEFINITIONS

Conduction Block Anesthesia: Local anesthetic injected in the immediate vicinity of a major nerve plexus (brachial plexus, lumbar plexus, and neuraxial anesthesia).

Field Block Anesthesia: Local anesthetic injected, in a fanlike manner, into tissue surrounding an incision or puncture site.

Infiltration Anesthesia: Local anesthetic injected at an incision or puncture site.

Intravenous Anesthesia: Lidocaine is injected into the vein of an exsanguinated extremity with an inflated tourniquet.

Neuraxial Blockade: A generic term that encompasses both spinal and epidural anesthesia.

Peripheral Nerve Block: Local anesthetic deposited in the immediate vicinity of an individual nerve to produce anesthesia.

Topical Anesthesia: Local anesthetic applied to skin or mucous membranes (pharyngeal cavity or urethra). Systemic absorption from the mucous membranes is rapid. Excessive dosing can lead to toxicity.[3-5]

NERVE PHYSIOLOGY AND CONDUCTION

Neurons convey information to and from the central nervous system (CNS). Sensory information is transmitted from the periphery by afferent neurons to the CNS. Motor impulses are transmitted by efferent neurons from the CNS to the periphery. Individual neurons contain a cell body, dendrites, and axons. Dendrites are multiple extensions of the cell body that transmit information toward the cell body. An axon is a single extension that transmits information away from the cell body. Axons are enveloped in a cell membrane known as the axolemma. Endoneurium is the connective tissue that envelops individual nerve fibers. Several nerve fibers form fascicles and are in turn covered with perineurium. Several fascicles covered with perineurium are bundled together and covered by connective tissue to form the epineurium that encompasses the entire nerve (Fig. 24-1).[4-7]

Neurons contain positive and negative charges. At a resting state, the inside of the cell is more negative than the more positive extracellular charge. Within the neuron there are potassium (K+) ions, which have positive charges (cations), and proteins, which have negative charges (anions). The negatively charged proteins are impermeable to the walls of the cell, whereas the positively charged K+ ions are small enough to diffuse through small openings. Because negative ions attract positive ions, there is an accumulation of K+ within the neuron. The ratio of intracellular K+ to extracellular K+ is approximately 30:1. Extracellularly, sodium (Na+) is found in abundance. The ratio of extracellular Na+ to intracellular Na+ is approximately 10:1. Sodium ions are less permeable to the cell membrane and gain access through passive diffusion. Sodium specific channels are closed at this time, so the amount of Na+ that reaches the cell is low. In addition, the NA+/K+ pump actively maintains the gradient between extracellular Na+ and intracellular potassium. For every three Na+ ions that are removed from inside the cell, two K+ ions are

311

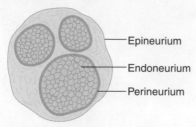

FIG. 24-1 Transverse section of a peripheral nerve. (From Miller RD, et al: *Miller's anesthesia,* ed 7, Philadelphia, 2009, Churchill Livingstone.)

replaced (Fig. 24-2). The net difference between the intracellular K+ (negative) and extracellular Na+ (positive) results in a resting membrane potential of −70 to −90 millivolts.[4,7,8]

Depolarization results in an intracellular change from negative to positive. This occurs because Na+ specific channels are opened (or activated), allowing Na+ to enter the cell. As Na+ enters the cell, additional Na+ channels are opened, resulting in a positive feedback loop. Potassium-specific channels are opened, allowing K+ to move out of the cell and into the extracellular space. When membrane potential becomes reversed, to approximately +35 millivolts, the movement of Na+ into the cell and K+ out of the cell stops (Na+ channels become inactivated) and the Na+/K+ pump restores the membrane potential back to a resting state (Na+ channels are at a resting state; Fig. 24-3).[4,7,8]

An action potential at a singular point will cause additional areas to also depolarize; this is

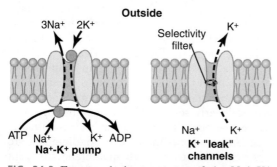

FIG. 24-2 Functional characteristics of the Na⁺-K⁺ pump and of the K⁺ "leak" channels. The K⁺ leak channels also leak Na⁺ ions into the cell slightly, but are much more permeable to K⁺. *ADP,* Adenoside diphosphate; *ATP,* adenosine triphosphate. (From Hall JE: *Guyton and Hall textbook of medical physiology,* ed 12, Philadelphia, 2011, Saunders.)

called *propagation*. Action potentials must reach threshold to continue propagation (all or none response). In unmyelinated nerves, action potentials are propagated along Na+ and K+ gates located in close proximity, and the conduction rate is slow (0.1 to 2.0 m/sec; Fig. 24-4). Myelinated nerves are, in effect, insulated. Ions cannot move through the myelin. Nodes of Ranvier represent an interruption in the myelin. It is here that action potentials can stimulate depolarization and propagation of an impulse. Because the nodes of Ranvier are spaced farther apart, saltatory conduction occurs, resulting in a faster conduction rate (3-120 m/sec; Fig. 24-5).[4,7,8]

Local anesthetics work at the level of the Na+ channel to prevent action potentials from being potentiated and not by altering resting or threshold potential. Local anesthetic molecules are stereospecific and bind within the Na+ channel or near its opening. Local anesthetic molecules have a greater affinity for receptors during their open or inactive state. When local anesthetic molecules bind with the Na+ channel, it prevents a conformational change and the influx of Na+, and depolarization slows. Eventually the minimum blocking concentration of the local anesthetic prevents an action potential from being achieved, and electrical conduction is blocked (Fig. 24-6).[4,7,9]

NERVE FIBER TYPE AND LOCAL ANESTHETIC EFFECTS

Peripheral nerves are divided into three classifications based on diameter, myelination, and conduction velocity. A and B peripheral nerves are myelinated, whereas C fibers are not. A fibers have the fastest conduction velocities, followed by B and C fibers. A fibers are further divided into alpha (α), beta (β), gamma (γ), and delta (δ) fibers. A-α fibers have the fastest conduction velocities and are motor neurons (efferent). A-β fibers are slower than A-α fibers but similar to A-γ fibers in conduction velocity, and are sensory (afferent) neurons that detect touch, pressure, and proprioception. A-γ fibers have a similar conduction speed to A-β fibers and are motor neurons (efferent) to muscle spindles and responsible for reflexes. A-δ fibers have the slowest conduction velocity of the A fibers, are sensory (efferent) for sharp pain (also known as *fast pain* such as an incision or pin prick) and temperature. B fibers have a slower conduction velocity than the A fibers and are preganglionic sympathetic neurons (efferent). C fibers are unmyelinated, have the slowest conduction velocity, and are postganglionic sympathetic neurons (efferent). C fibers transmit slow

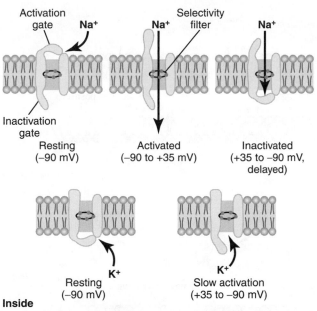

FIG. 24-3 Characteristics of the voltage-gated sodium *(top)* and potassium *(bottom)* channels. (From Hall JE: *Guyton and Hall textbook of medical physiology,* ed 12, Philadelphia, 2011, Saunders.)

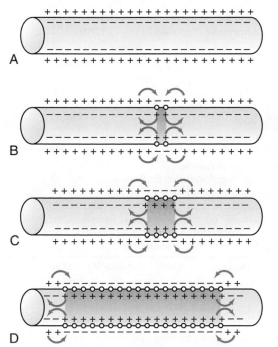

FIG. 24-4 Propagation of action potentials in both directions along a conductive fiber. **A,** A normal, resting nerve fiber. **B,** A nerve fiber that suddenly develops increased permeability to sodium in its midportion. **C** and **D,** Sodium channels in these new areas immediately open, and the explosive action potential spreads. (From Hall JE: *Guyton and Hall textbook of medical physiology,* ed 12, Philadelphia, 2011, Saunders.)

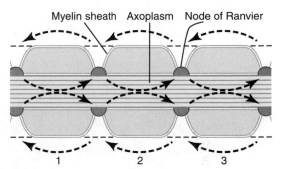

FIG. 24-5 Saltatory conduction along a myelinated axon. Flow of electrical current from node to node is illustrated by the arrows. (From Hall JE: *Guyton and Hall textbook of medical physiology,* ed 12, Philadelphia, 2011, Saunders.)

pain (generalized ache or burning sensation) and temperature (Table 24-1).[3,4,7,9]

Classification of peripheral nerves is important in determining the sequence of local anesthetic blockade. B fibers are the most sensitive. Dilation of cutaneous blood vessels is often the first sign of local anesthetic onset. C fibers and A-δ are next in sensitivity, resulting in the inability to feel cool sensations such as an alcohol wipe. Next in sensitivity are the A-γ, A-β, and A-α fibers, which result in the loss of sensation, pressure, proprioception, and finally motor paralysis. Local anesthetic

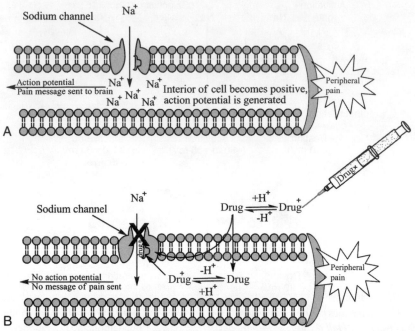

FIG. 24-6 Mechanisms of action for local anesthetics. **A,** Diagram of the axon of a sensory nerve cell transmitting the *pain* message to the CNS via depolarization of the nerve cell. **B,** Local anesthetic drugs, in their ionized form, bind to the sodium channel and prevent sodium from entering the nerve cell. The action potential is thus blocked, and the message of pain is not sent to the brain. (From Friel CJ, et al: Local anesthetic use in perioperative areas, *Perioperative Nurs Clin* 5:203–214, 2010.)

Table 24-1	Classification of Nerve Fibers	
FIBER TYPE	**MYELIN**	**FUNCTION**
A-α	+++	Motor (efferent: to skeletal muscle)
A-β	++	Touch, pressure, proprioception (afferent: from skin)
A-γ	++	Motor (efferent: to muscle spindles)
A-δ	++	Pain (sharp, fast) and temperature (efferent: from skin)
B	+	Preganglionic sympathetic (efferent: to vascular smooth muscle)
C	None	Pain (dull, slow) and temperature (afferent from skin); postganglionic sympathetic (efferent: to vascular smooth muscle)

From Schick L, Windle PE, editors: *Perianesthesia nursing core curriculum: preprocedure, phase I and phase II PACU nursing,* ed 2, St. Louis, 2010, Saunders.

concentration must be adequate to block nerve fibers. It takes twice the concentration of local anesthetic to block motor fibers as it does to block sensory and sympathetic fibers require the least. The order of blockade onset is B fibers > C fibers = A-δ fibers > A-γ fibers > A-β fibers > A-α fibers. Recovery from local anesthetic is the opposite (Box 24-1).[3,4,7,9]

LOCAL ANESTHETIC PHARMACOLOGY

Chemistry and Stereoisomerism

A local anesthetic molecule contains a lipophilic group, an intermediate bond, and a hydrophilic group. The lipophilic (attracted to fat) portion of

BOX 24-1   **Sequence of Nerve Blockade**

- Motor paralysis
- Loss of proprioception (awareness of body or extremity position)
- Pressure sense abolished
- Tactile sense lost
- Slow and fast pain
- Temperature discrimination lost
- Sensation of warmth by patient
- Block of cold temperature fibers
- Vasomotor block dilation of skin vessels and increased cutaneous flow

the molecule is aromatic, usually an unsaturated benzene ring. Classification is dependent on the intermediate bond, which is either an ester (–CO–) or an amide (–HNC–). The hydrophilic (attracted to water) group is generally a tertiary amine and proton acceptor (Fig. 24-7).[4,10,11] The lipophilic and hydrophilic portions of the

molecular structure are crucial to its ability to cross tissue barriers and reach their site of action. The intermediate bond determines the type of local anesthetic, affecting metabolism and potential for allergic reactions.[4] Commonly administered amides and esters are noted in Box 24-2.

Most local anesthetics are stereoisomers. Optical isomers (enantiomers) are mirror images of each other with the same chemical formula, but structurally cannot be superimposed on one another. Most medications are racemic mixtures containing more than one isomer. Because drug receptors are stereospecific and stereoselective, administering a medication that contains stereoisomers means that the clinician is administering more than one medication. Each enantiomer may exhibit differences in absorption, distribution, potency, toxicity, and therapeutic action (Fig. 24-8). Advances in pharmacology have allowed the development of two pure S-enantiomers: ropivacaine and levobupivacaine. Both exhibit advances in safety because they are less toxic than racemic preparations,[9,11,12] although they are still capable of causing toxicity.[13]

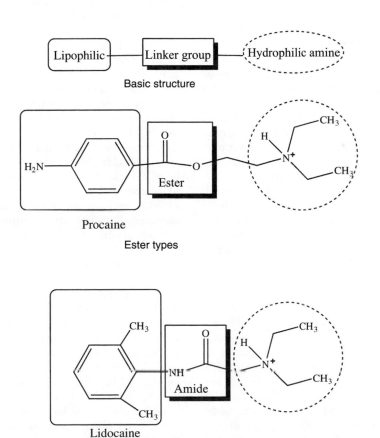

FIG. 24-7 Chemical structure of local anesthetics. (From Friel CJ, et al: Local anesthetic use in perioperative areas, *Perioperative Nurs Clin* 5:203–214, 2010.)

Amides	Esters
Bupivacaine	Benzocaine
Etidocaine	Chloroprocaine
Levobupivacaine	Cocaine
Lidocaine	Procaine
Mepivacaine	Tetracaine
Prilocaine	
Ropivacaine	

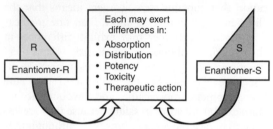

FIG. 24-8 Optical isomers (enantiomers). (Courtesy Daniel Moos.)

Pharmacodynamics

Pharmacodynamics is the study of a medication's effect on the body.[5] Local anesthetics are weak bases and exist as charged (ionized, water soluble) and uncharged (non-ionized, lipid soluble) particles. For local anesthetics to reach their site of action—the nerve fiber—they must transverse biologic barriers. Ionized local anesthetics do not pass through the cell membrane easily; however, non-ionized local anesthetics cross the barrier of the cell membrane, gaining access to the sodium channel. Non-ionized local anesthetics do not readily bind with $Na+$ channels; however, ionized local anesthetics will bind easily. The ratio of ionized to non-ionized local anesthetic is pH dependent. The pH at which a basic medication contains a 50% concentration of ionized and 50% non-ionized local anesthetic is known as *pKa*. Injectable local anesthetics vary in pKa from 7.6 to 9.0. The closer the local anesthetics pKa is to physiologic pH, the faster the onset (chloroprocaine is an exception). Confounding this is commercial preparation of local anesthetics. To stabilize local anesthetics, manufacturers prepare them as a hydrochloride salt with a pH of 6 to 7. If the local anesthetic contains epinephrine, it must placed in an even more acidic environment (pH of 4 to 5), resulting in less non-ionized local anesthetic to cross tissue and thus a slower onset. The same holds true when local anesthetic is injected into infected (acidotic tissue).[4,7,9,11,13]

Potency and duration of action of a local anesthetic is closely correlated to lipid solubility. In general, the more lipid soluble the local anesthetic, the more potent it is and the longer its duration of action. Potent local anesthetics bind with proteins and neural tissue readily, lending to their longer duration of action and toxicity potential. Bupivacaine, levobupivacaine, ropivacaine, etidocaine, and tetracaine are the most potent. Lidocaine, mepivacaine, and prilocaine are moderate, whereas procaine and chloroprocaine are the least potent.[4,7,9,14]

Pharmacokinetics

Pharmacokinetics is the study of a medication's absorption, distribution, metabolism, and excretion.[5] Absorption of local anesthetics is dependent on site of injection, dose, vasoconstrictor, pharmacologic profile, and individual physiologic factors.[3,4,11] Vascularity of tissue has a direct effect on systemic absorption (increases uptake and may lead to toxicity). Absorption of local anesthetic from highest to lowest is as follows: intravenous, tracheal, intercostal, caudal, epidural, brachial plexus, sciatic, and subcutaneous.[3,11,14] Total dose is closely related. The greater the dose, the greater the systemic absorption.[7] Attention to the total dose is important to avoid toxicity. Epinephrine can be added to decrease systemic absorption and prolong duration of action through local vasoconstriction. Norepinephrine and phenylephrine can be added but are less efficacious. The ability of epinephrine to decrease systemic absorption varies by local anesthetic and injection site. The addition of epinephrine for peripheral nerve blocks and epidurals increases duration of action and decreases blood levels by 10% to 30% for lidocaine, mepivacaine, and bupivacaine, but does not alter duration or blood levels for ropivacaine and levobupivacaine. Attention should be placed on the total dose of epinephrine to avoid deleterious effects.[4,7,9] All local anesthetics, with the exception of cocaine and ropivacaine, cause a degree of vasodilatation. Vasodilatation results in increased blood flow to the area of injection and absorption. Lidocaine results in greater local vasodilation than mepivacaine and prilocaine, whereas bupivacaine, levobupivacaine, and etidocaine produce the same degree of vasodilatation.[4] Local anesthetics also vary in protein binding. Local anesthetics that are highly protein bound are absorbed less readily. Protein binding varies from 6% for procaine, which is the least, to greater than 97% for levobupivacaine. Least to greatest protein bound is as follows: procaine < prilocaine < lidocaine < tetracaine < mepivacaine < ropivacaine = etidocaine < bupivacaine

< levobupivacaine.[3,4,9] A final factor in determining the absorption rate of local anesthetics are individual physiological conditions. Extremes of age are a factor because newborns have immature hepatic function, and the elderly have decreased hepatic enzyme function and blood flow resulting in increased in blood concentrations. During pregnancy, doses of local anesthetic should be decreased by one third because of hyperdynamic circulation and hormonal changes that can result in toxicity. Renal, hepatic, and cardiovascular disease can affect local anesthetic pharmacokinetics.[4,7,14,15]

Uptake of local anesthetics results in their distribution to various tissues. The initial rapid disappearance phase (α) includes uptake into highly perfused tissue (brain, lung, liver, kidney, and heart). The lungs act as a large reservoir and decrease initial blood concentrations. The slow phase of disappearance (β) includes distribution to the gut and muscle. Muscle provides a large reservoir for local anesthetics.[4,7,14] During pregnancy, amide local anesthetic molecules can be transferred across the placenta and accumulate in an acidotic environment; this is known as *ion trapping*.[3,9]

Metabolism depends on classification: amide or ester. Amides are metabolized primarily in the liver through cytochrome P-450 system. Extremes of age and disease processes that affect liver perfusion and enzyme activity alter hepatic elimination of amides. Individual amides exhibit different clearance rates (prilocaine > etidocaine > lidocaine > mepivacaine > bupivacaine> ropivacaine). Esters undergo rapid hydrolysis in the blood, which limits toxicity. Plasma cholinesterase is the primary enzyme responsible.[4,9] Caution should be used in patients with a acquired or genetic pseudocholinesterase deficiency, which can decrease metabolism and lead to potentially toxic blood concentrations.[4,16] Metabolism of some ester local anesthetics results in the production of p-aminobenzoic acid (PABA), a known allergen. It is this byproduct of metabolism that makes ester local anesthetics more likely than amides to result in an allergic reaction.[4,14]

Maximum Doses

Maximum doses are general guidelines derived from animal studies in an attempt to identify median effective and toxic doses. Health care providers should take into account the site of injection, the addition or absence of epinephrine, and individual medical conditions such as age, renal, hepatic, cardiac disease, and pregnancy.[15] Refer to Table 24-2 for maximum doses of local anesthetics.

INDIVIDUAL LOCAL ANESTHETICS

Table 24-2 contains a summary of local anesthetic information.

Additional Local Anesthetics

Etidocaine (Duranest) is a long-duration, slow-onset amide local anesthetic introduced in 1972. It can be used for infiltration, peripheral nerve block, and epidural anesthesia. Maximum dose is 300 mg plain and 400 mg with epinephrine. Etidocaine does not enjoy widespread use because it produces a profound and long motor block.[2,3] Prilocaine (Citanest) is a moderate-duration, slow-onset amide local anesthetic introduced in 1960. It can be used for infiltration, intravenous regional block, peripheral nerve block, and epidural anesthesia. The limiting factor is its metabolism to O-toluidine, which can cause methemoglobinemia (see Complications). Prilocaine is not used in the United States, with the exception of eutectic mixture of local anesthetics (EMLA) cream.[3,7,11] Benzocaine is an ester local anesthetic that exists as a weak acid. Because it is non-ionized, it is used only as a topical local anesthetic. Onset is rapid, duration is short, and the maximum dose is 200 to 300 mg. Benzocaine is the most commonly implicated local anesthetic in methemoglobinemia. When using benzocaine, it is important that the manufacturer's recommendations are strictly followed and patients are monitored for this complication.[9,14] EMLA cream is a mixture of 2.5% prilocaine and 2.5% lidocaine that can be applied topically to decrease the discomfort associated with venipuncture, and it is particularly useful when starting intravenous lines on children. Dosing is based on patient weight and surface area, and manufacturer dosing recommendations require strict adherence. Application should occur on intact skin because absorption may be rapid with breaks in the integument. Onset is slow, and depth of penetration is limited. EMLA should not be used in infants younger than 3 months, infants 3 to 12 months old receiving additional medications that may predispose them to methemoglobinemia (i.e., nitrates, dapsone, sulphonamides, benzocaine), and children who may be predisposed to hereditary or congenital methemoglobinemia.[11,25-27]

COMPLICATIONS

Vigilant monitoring for and recognition of allergic reactions, methemoglobinemia, and local anesthetic toxicity are essential to the institution of life saving interventions (Table 24-3).

Table 24-2   Local Anesthetic Agents: Esters and Amides

LOCAL ANESTHETIC	USES AND DOSES	ONSET AND DURATION	DISCUSSION
Esters			
Procaine (Novacaine)	*Topical:* 10%-20% *Infiltration:* 0.25%-0.5% *Nerve block:* 1%-2% *Maximum dose:* 5-6 mg/kg plain (400 mg); 8.5 mg/kg with epinephrine (600 mg)	*Onset:* Slow for infiltration and nerve block; fast for spinal block *Duration:* 30 min plain; 60 min with epinephrine	Introduced in 1905 Limitations include short duration, low potency, and poor stability Undergoes rapid hydrolysis to PABA; less than 50% excreted unchanged in the urine Not commonly used for surgical anesthesia in the operating room
Chloroprocaine (Nesacaine)	*Infiltration:* 1% *Nerve block:* 1%-2% *Epidural block:* 2%-3% *Maximum dose:* 11 mg/kg plain (800 mg); 15 mg/kg with epinephrine (1000 mg)	*Onset:* Fast (6-12 min) *Duration:* 30 min plain; 60 min with epinephrine	Not topically active Short-duration ester manufactured in preservative-free and preservative-containing solution (sodium bisulfate and methylparaben) Not administered for spinals due to the risk of neurotoxicity Preservative-free solutions should be used for epidurals Twelvefold more potent than procaine One of the safest local anesthetics in regard to systemic toxicity Hydrolyzed to inactive metabolites and excreted in the urine
Cocaine	*Topical:* 4%-20% *Maximum dose:* 3 mg/kg	*Onset:* Fast *Duration:* 10-55 min	Moderate duration ester Vasoconstrictor and used topically only Inhibits reuptake of norepinephrine and dopamine; may cause constriction of coronary arteries Limitations include toxicity, sympathetic stimulation, and abuse potential Partially metabolized in the liver and by ester hydrolysis
Tetracaine (Pontocaine)	*Topical:* 0.5%-1% *Infiltration:* 0.1%-0.25% *Maximum dose:* 1.5 mg/kg plain (100 mg); 2.5 mg/kg with epinephrine (200 mg)	*Onset:* Slow *Duration:* (Topical) 55 min; (Spinal) 1-1.5 hours plain; (Spinal) 2-3 hours with epinephrine	Potent, long-acting ester developed in 1930 May be used topically Most commonly used for spinal anesthesia Cerebral spinal fluid does not contain pseudocholinesterase enzymes and must be absorbed systemically to be metabolized Metabolized slower than other esters
Amides			
Lidocaine (Xylocaine)	*Topical:* 2%-4% *Nerve block:* 1%-2% *Epidural:* 1%-2% *IRVA:* 0.5% *Maximum dose:* 4.5 mg/kg plain (300 mg) for other blocks; 7 mg/kg with epinephrine (500 mg); (Topical) 3 mg/kg (less due to rapid absorption); (IRVA) 250 mg	*Onset:* Fast; (Topical) 2-4 min *Duration:* 1-2 hours plain; 2-6 hours with epinephrine for nerve block and infiltration; 1-1.5 hours for spinal or epidural anesthesia	Moderate duration amide introduced in 1948 One of the most common and versatile local anesthetics in current use; rapid onset, intense analgesia, good penetration, and stable Not commonly used for spinal anesthesia due to risk of transient neurological symptoms Metabolized by oxidative dealkylation in the liver; liver disease may reduce elimination and place the patient at risk for toxicity

Compiled from references 2-4, 7, 9, 14, 17-24.
IRVA, Intravenous regional anesthesia.

Table 24-2   Local Anesthetic Agents: Esters and Amides—cont'd

LOCAL ANESTHETIC	USES AND DOSES	ONSET AND DURATION	DISCUSSION
Mepivacaine (Carbocaine)	*Infiltration:* 0.5%-1% *Nerve block:* 1%-2% *Maximum dose:* 4.5 mg/kg plain (300 mg); 7 mg/kg with epinephrine (500 mg)	*Onset:* Fast *Duration:* 45-90 min plain; 2-6 hours with epinephrine	Moderate duration amide introduced in 1957 Similar to lidocaine except slightly longer duration, less toxicity, and less localized vasodilation
Ropivacaine (Naropin)	*Epidural:* 0.1%-0.2% (analgesia); higher concentrations for anesthesia *Nerve block:* 0.5%-1% *Maximum dose:* 200 mg	*Onset:* Fast *Duration:* 2-6 hours	Rapid-onset, long-duration amide local anesthetic that exhibits many advantages over bupivacaine; introduced in 1996 A single enantiomer with a lower risk of toxicity than bupivacaine, which makes it a primary choice for peripheral nerve blocks and epidurals Less motor blockade at lower doses than bupivacaine making it an ideal agent for epidural analgesia Clearance is higher and elimination half-life is shorter than for bupivacaine Metabolized by cytochrome P-450 system in the liver; less than 1% is excreted unchanged Unique in its ability to cause localized vasoconstriction, which eliminates the need to add epinephrine
Bupivacaine (Sensorcaine; Marcaine)	*Infiltration:* 0.1%-0.25% *Nerve block:* 0.25%-0.5% *Spinal:* 0.5%-0.75% *Epidural:* 0.125% for analgesia; higher concentrations for anesthesia *Maximum dose:* 2.5 mg/kg plain (175 mg); 3 mg/kg with epinephrine (225 mg)	*Onset:* Slow *Duration:* 2-4 hours plain; 3-7 hours with epinephrine	Potent, long-duration local anesthetic introduced in 1973; widely used but limited by reports of cardiotoxicity Produces profound sensory analgesia with minimal motor blockade at low doses Development of less toxic, potent long acting amides has reduced its use for peripheral nerve blocks and epidurals Commonly used for spinal anesthesia Primarily metabolized in the liver
Levobupivacaine (Chirocaine)	Concentrations used are similar to bupivacaine *Maximum dose:* 2.5 mg/kg plain; 3.2 mg/kg with epinephrine (150 mg)	*Onset:* Slow *Duration:* 4-11 hours	Long duration S-enantiomer of bupivacaine; because it is a pure isomer, it exhibits less toxicity than bupivacaine Exhibits many of the same characteristics of bupivacaine in regard to potency, onset, and duration

CONCEPTS IN ANESTHETIC AGENTS

Table 24-3	Local Anesthetic Complications*		
	ALLERGIC REACTION	**METHEMOGLOBINEMIA**	**LOCAL ANESTHETIC TOXICITY**
Signs and symptoms	Hypotension, tachycardia, dysrhythmias, cardiovascular collapse, shock, broncho-spasm, cyanosis, dyspnea, hypoxia, angioedema, urticaria, and pruritus	Cyanosis, chocolate colored blood, headache, weakness, dizziness, tachycardia, dyspnea, pulse oximetry reading of 80%-85%, seizures, coma, dysrhythmias, and heart failure	Central nervous system: Dizziness, drowsiness, tinnitus, circumoral numbness, confusion, dysphoria, agitation, loss of consciousness, seizures Cardiovascular: Bradycardia, asystole, hypotension, tachycardia, ventricular fibrillation, ventricular tachycardia, wide complex arrhythmias, ST changes, chest pain, hypertension, ventricular ectopy
Basic Care	Airway Breathing Circulation	Airway Breathing Circulation	Airway Breathing Circulation
Treatment	Large-bore needles to administer crystalloids and colloids Epinephrine titrated to effect; starting dose 50-100 mcg and titrate to effect Diphenhydramine, 1-2 mg/kg IV; usual dose, 25-50 mg; maximum dose, 100 mg Bronchodilators for continued bronchoconstriction Glucocorticoids should be considered Monitor for rebound symptoms in a critical care setting	Cooximetry for diagnosis of methemoglobin levels Methylene blue, 1-2 mg/kg over 5 min; may be repeated every hour up to a maximum of 7 mg/kg Monitor patient for up to 24 hours for reoccurrence in a critical care setting	Seizures treated with benzodiazepines ACLS: Consideration to the potentially counter-productive effects of epinephrine, lidocaine, phenytoin, beta blockers, and calcium channel blockers in this setting 20% lipid emulsion in a dose of 1.5 mL/kg rapid bolus; infusion of 0.25 mL/kg/min Up to two additional boluses may be administered Infusion can be increased to 0.5 mL/kg/min for continued hypotension (maximum dose in first 30 min of lipid resuscita-tion is 10 mL/kg) Make preparations for cardiopulmonary bypass Patients whose conditions are stabilized should be monitored in a critical care setting for reoccur-rence

Compiled from references 4, 14, 33-36, 38-40, 43-47.
*Treatment for adult patients.
IV, Intravenous; *ACLS,* advanced cardiac life support.

Allergic Reactions

True allergic reactions to local anesthetics are rare.[28-30] Allergy to ester local anesthetics are more common than amides because they are me-tabolized to PABA, a known allergen.[4,14] Allergic reactions may be related to preservatives added to local anesthetics. Methylparaben, propylpara-ben, and sulfites are added to a number of con-sumer goods, including local anesthetics, to enhance shelf life. Prior exposure to methylpara-ben or propylparaben is likely, and there is a known cross-reactivity between PABA and these preservatives. In addition, sulfites are known to cause allergic reactions.[10,31] Sulfonamides are similar to PABA. Patients reporting allergic reactions to sulfonamides should not be exposed to ester- or paraben-containing local anesthetics.[31] Allergic reactions are more likely to occur related to exposure to substances such as skin preps, latex, or other medications administered in close proximity.[32] Additional patient-reported allergic reactions may be related to prior experiences resulting in anxiety or rapid systemic absorption (e.g., dental procedures). Anxiety can lead to vasovagal reactions during injection, and rapid systemic absorption of epinephrine containing local anesthetics can lead to palpitations, shortness of breath, syncope, and toxicity.[31]

Allergic reactions can be divided into four types based on the causative agent and immune systems response (see Chapter 18). Of immediate concern are anaphylactic reactions. Anaphylaxis is a type I reaction that results in the release of a number of substances, including histamine and leukotrienes, through mast cell and basophil activation. Clinical signs and symptoms include hypotension, tachycardia, dysrhythmias, cardiovascular collapse, shock, bronchospasm, cyanosis, dyspnea, hypoxia, angioedema, urticaria, and pruritus. Immediate treatment is required to reduce mortality and morbidity.[33-35]

In the event of anaphylaxis, the health care provider should stop the administration of the offending agent; administer 100% oxygen and assist with respiration if the patient is apneic or hypoventilating; and initiate CPR for patients in cardiac arrest. Large-bore intravenous lines should be used to administer intravenous crystalloid fluids or colloids as needed. Large volumes are required because of increased vascular permeability and significant hypotension.

Hemodynamics should be supported by vasopressors. Epinephrine is the first medication of choice because it helps to restore vascular tone, support blood pressure, and reverse bronchoconstriction. Initial bolus doses of 50 to 100 mcg in adult patients are administered and subsequently tailored to patient response. Antihistamines (e.g., diphenhydramine, 1 to 2 mg/kg intravenously; usual dose is 25 to 50 mg, with a maximum dose of 100 mg), bronchodilators, and glucocorticoids are considered and administered as needed. When the reaction has been controlled, the patient is closely monitored for a rebound of symptoms.[34,35]

Methemoglobinemia

Methemoglobinemia can be caused by benzocaine (most common), prilocaine, lidocaine, and tetracaine.[36,37] Some institutions have discontinued the use of benzocaine, and others have suggested that it not be used.[36,38] Methemoglobin is a form of hemoglobin that is unable to carry oxygen. When an agent such as benzocaine is administered, ferrous iron ($Fe+3$) is oxidized to ferric iron ($Fe+2$) either directly or during metabolism. Signs and symptoms include: cyanosis, chocolate-colored blood, headache, weakness, dizziness, tachycardia, dyspnea, seizures, coma, dysrhythmias, and heart failure. Pulse oximetry readings range from 80% to 85% regardless of the severity. The gold standard in diagnosis is cooximetry, available with arterial blood gas analysis. Supportive treatment includes supplemental oxygen and hemodynamic support. Definitive treatment is methylene blue. The dose for adults is 1 to 2 mg/kg over 5 minutes; this can be repeated once every hour up to a maximum of 7 mg/kg. For newborns, the dose should be reduced to 0.5 mg/kg IV. Methylene blue should not be used in patients with a history of glucose-6-phosphate dehydrogenase (G6PD) deficiency; ascorbic acid should be used instead. Patients are monitored for 24 hours for possible recurrence.[36,38-40] When benzocaine is administered, manufacturers' guidelines should be followed and minimal amounts should be delivered. Contraindications include patients with cardiopulmonary disease (e.g., smokers, asthma, bronchitis, emphysema, heart disease), extremes of age (elderly and infants), and patients with known G6PD deficiency, hemoglobin M disease, NADH-MHb reductase deficiency, or pyruvate-kinase deficiency.[38]

Local Anesthetic Toxicity

Local anesthetic (LA) toxicity occurrence has been estimated at 4 per 10,000 epidurals and 7.5 to 20 per 10,0000 peripheral nerve blocks.[41] Toxicity is due to high plasma concentrations affecting neurologic and cardiovascular systems. Toxicity may be due to inadvertent intravascular injection.[9] A test dose before injecting local anesthetics help to confirm that the needle–catheter is outside a vessel; it contains 3 mL of 2% lidocaine with 1:200,000 (15 mcg) concentration of epinephrine. If positive, the heart rate and systolic blood pressure will increase by at least 20 beats/min and 15 mm Hg. Test doses might not be reliable in the presence of beta blockers, advanced age, and general anesthesia.[41] Excessive dosing is a common cause and combining local anesthetics are cumulative and do not lessen the risk.[14] Systemic absorption can result in toxicity and is related to total dose, vascularity of injection site, vasoconstrictor use, and individual local anesthetic used.[9]

Classic signs and symptoms are described as progressive as blood concentrations of local anesthetics increase. CNS symptoms progress from circumoral or tongue numbness and tinnitus up to seizures and coma (Fig. 24-9).[4] The most common CNS symptoms are seizures; followed by dizziness, drowsiness, tinnitus, circumoral numbness, confusion, dysphoria, agitation, and loss of counciousness.[42] Threshold for CNS toxicity is lower for potent local anesthetics (bupivacaine, tetracaine, and etidocaine) and in patients experiencing hypercarbia or metabolic acidosis.[4] Higher blood concentrations lead to cardiovascular symptoms.[4,14] Bradycardia and asystole are the most common manifestations, followed by hypotension, tachycardia, ventricular fibrillation or ventricular tachycardia, wide complex arrhythmias, ST changes, pain dyspnea, hypertension, and ventricular ectopy.[4,14,42] Blood concentrations resulting in cardiovascular toxicity are generally three times the amount that result in seizures. Hypoxia, hypercarbia, acidosis, cardiovascular disease, and pregnancy are predisposing factors that increase the risk for cardiovascular toxicity.[3,4,14,42]

The most common regional anesthetic techniques that result in LA toxicity are epidural, axillary, and interscalene blocks. Toxicity occurs more frequently in females, and age plays a role with 45% of the patients younger than 16 or older than 60 years. Most signs and symptoms of LA toxicity occur within 5 minutes, but up to 25% may occur later. Patients receiving local anesthetic infusions through epidural or peripheral nerve catheters may exhibit signs and symptoms of toxicity hours to days later. Signs and symptoms of LA toxicity can occur in any order, including CNS, CNS and cardiovascular symptoms occurring at the same time, or cardiovascular toxicity occurring without CNS symptoms. This highlights the importance of vigilance regarding changes in the patient's condition that indicate toxicity is occurring.[42]

Initial treatment of LA toxicity should focus on airway, breathing, and circulation. The patient should have a patent airway and 100% oxygen administered. Seizure activity should be controlled with a benzodiazepine. Propofol should not be used if cardiovascular depression is occurring or impending. CPR and ACLS should be instituted. In patients with LA toxicity, epinephrine may increase dysrhythmias; lidocaine will add to the toxicity; and phenytoin, beta blockers, and calcium channel blockers may contribute to cardiovascular depression.[43-46]

Cardiovascular collapse is the most serious and difficult complication to treat. Bupivacaine, etidocaine, and tetracaine are the most cardiotoxic. Treatment for local anesthetic toxicity has recently been standardized.[46,47] Lipid emulsion therapy is a crucial component for successful resuscitation and is theorized to create an additional compartment for local anesthetic molecules to bind, reducing the amount of molecules that bind within the cardiovascular system.

Complications of lipid emulsion therapy in this setting have not been reported.[43-46] Current recommendations include an initial bolus of 20% lipid emulsion in a dose of 1.5 mL/kg rapidly over 1 minute, followed by a continuous infusion at 0.25 mL/kg/min. If cardiovascular collapse continues, up to two additional boluses can be administered. If the patient remains hypotensive, the infusion can be increased to 0.5 mL/kg/min. Lipid infusion should continue for a minimum of 10 minutes after the patient has been stabilized. The maximum dose administered in the initial 30 minutes is 10 mL/kg. Preparation should be made for cardiopulmonary bypass. After stabilization, the patient should be monitored in an intensive care setting for potential recurrence of signs and symptoms of toxicity.[43-46]

The perianesthesia nurse is crucial in assisting the anesthesia provider in monitoring the patient during the placement of a regional anesthetic. If epinephrine-containing solutions or a test dose with epinephrine are administered, close monitoring of changes in heart rate and blood pressure should occur. Maintaining verbal contact with the patient is essential to assess the patient for changes in level of consciousness or initial CNS signs and symptoms that accompany toxicity. Continuous monitoring of the patient's electrocardiogram and blood pressure should occur to detect changes in rhythm or hypotension. A high level of suspicion for LA toxicity should be maintained during block placement and for up to 30 minutes thereafter.[4,42,46]

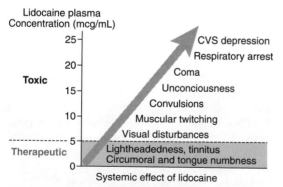

FIG. 24-9 Toxicity progression of lidocaine. (From Nagelhout J, Plaus K, editors: *Nurse anesthesia*, ed 4, St. Louis, 2010, Saunders.)

SUMMARY

Perianesthesia nurses have an important role in the treatment of acute pain. Several modes of analgesia are combined to bring comfort to the patient recovering from surgery.[48] Local anesthetics continue to be an important pharmacologic mainstay, and their use appears to be increasing as a result of advances in their administration. It is imperative that perianesthesia nurses understand the physiology of nerve conduction, pharmacology of local anesthetics, and identification and treatment of potential complications related to their administration.

REFERENCES

1. Morgan GE, et al: The practice of anesthesiology. In Morgan GE, et al, editors: *Clinical anesthesiology*, ed 4, New York, 2006, McGraw-Hill.
2. Ruetsch YA, et al: From cocaine to ropivacaine: the history of local anesthetic drugs, *Curr Top Med Chem* 1:175–182, 2001.
3. Brown C: Anesthetic agents and adjuncts. In Schick L, Windle PE, editors: *Perianesthesia nursing core curriculum: preprocedure, phase I and phase II PACU nursing*, ed 2, St. Louis, 2010, Saunders.
4. Nagelhout J: Local anesthetics. In Nagelhout J, Plaus K, editors: *Nurse anesthesia*, ed 4, St. Louis, 2010, Saunders.
5. Venes D, editor: *Tabor's cyclopedic medical dictionary*, ed 21, Philadelphia, 2009, F.A. Davis Company.
6. Hadzic A, Vloka JD: Essential regional anesthesia anatomy. In Hazic A, Vloka JD, editors: *Peripheral nerve blocks: principles and practice*, New York, 2004, McGraw-Hill.
7. Berde CB, Strichartz GR: Local anesthetics. In Miller RD, editor: *Miller's anesthesia*, ed 7, Philadelphia, 2010, Churchill Livingstone.
8. Hall JE: Membrane potentials and action potentials. In Hall JE: *Guyton and Hall textbook of medical physiology*, ed 12, Philadelphia, 2011, Saunders.
9. Stoelting RK, Hillier SC: Local anesthetics. In Stoelting RK, Hillier SC, editors: *Pharmacology & physiology in anesthetic practice*, ed 4, Philadelphia, 2006, Lippincott Williams & Wilkins.
10. Friel CJ, et al: Local anesthetics use in perioperative areas, *Perioperative Nursing Clinics* 5:203–214, 2010.
11. Drasner K: Local anesthetics. In Stoelting RK, Miller RD, editors: *Basics of anesthesia*, ed 5, Philadelphia, 2007, Churchill Livingstone.
12. Joyce JA: A pathway toward safer anesthesia: stereochemical advances, *AANA J* 70:63–67, 2002.
13. Zink W, Graf BM: The toxicity of local anesthetics: the place of ropivacaine and levobupivacaine, *Curr Opin Anaesthesiol* 21:645–650, 2008.
14. Morgan GE, et al: Local anesthetics. In Morgan GE, et al, editors: *Clinical anesthesiology*, ed 4, New York, 2006, McGraw-Hill.
15. Rosenberg PH, et al: Maximum recommended doses of local anesthetics: a multifactorial concept, *Reg Anesth Pain Med* 29:564–575, 2004.
16. Soliday FK, et al: Pseudocholinesterase deficiency: a comprehensive review of genetic, acquired, and drug influences, *AANA J* 78:313–320, 2010.
17. Novacain (procaine hydrochloride injection, solution) (package insert), Lake Forest, Ill; Hospira, Inc; 2005.
18. Nesacaine (chloroprocaine hydrochloride injection) (product monograph), Mississauga, Ontario; AstraZeneca; 2006.
19. Lidocaine hydrochloride injection (package insert), Shirley, NY; American Regent, Inc; 2003.
20. Carbocaine (mepivacaine hydrochloride injection) (package insert), Lake Forest, Ill; Hospira, Inc; 2009.
21. Allegri M, et al: Efficacy of drugs in regional anesthesia: a review, *Eur J Pain* 3:41–48, 2009.
22. Naropin (ropivacaine hydrochloride monohydrate injection solution) (package insert), Schaumburg, Ill; APP Pharmaceutical, LLC; 2009.
23. Marcaine (bupivacaine hydrochloride injection, solution) (package insert), Lake Forest, Ill; Hospira, Inc; 2004.
24. Chirocaine (levobupivacaine injection) (package insert), Stamford, Conn; Purdue Pharma L.P.; 2000.
25. Couper RTL: Methaemoglobinaemia secondary to topical lignocaine/prilocaine in a circumcised neonate, *J Paediatr Child Health* 4:206–207, 2000.
26. Pesatura KA, Matthews M: Topical anesthesia use in children, *US Pharm* 34:HS-4–HS-7, 2009.
27. EMLA Patch (transdermal therapeutic system) (package insert), Wilmington, Del; AstraZeneca; 2004.
28. Balestrieri PJ, Ferguson JE: Management of a parturient with a history of local anesthetic allergy, *Anesth Analg* 96:1489–1490, 2003.
29. Morais-Almeida M, et al: Allergy to local anesthetics of the amide group with tolerance to procaine, *Allergy* 58:827–828, 2003.
30. Caron AB: Allergy to multiple local anesthetics, *Allergy Asthma Proc* 28:600–601, 2007.
31. Finucane BT: Allergies to local anesthetics-the real truth, *Can J Anaesth* 50:869–874, 2003.
32. Harboe T, et al: Suspected allergy to local anesthetics: follow up in 135 cases, *Acta Anaesthesiol Scand* 54:536–542, 2010.
33. Nitti JT, Nitti GL: Anesthetic complications. In Morgan GE, et al, editors: *Clinical anesthesiology*, ed 4, New York, 2006, McGraw-Hill.
34. O'Donnel MP: The immune system and anesthesia. In Nagelhout J, Plaus K, editors: *Nurse anesthesia*, ed 4, St. Louis, 2010, Saunders.
35. Stevenson J: Trauma care. In Schick L, Windle PE, editors: *Perianesthesia nursing core curriculum: preprocedure, phase I and phase II PACU nursing*, ed 2, St. Louis, 2010, Saunders.
36. Guay J: Methemoglobinemia related to local anesthetics: a summary of 242 episodes, *Anesth Analg* 108:837–845, 2009.
37. Golembiewski J: Local anesthetics, *J Perianesth Nurs* 22:285–288, 2007.
38. Food and Drug Administration: *FDA Public Health Advisory: Benzocaine sprays marketed under different names including Hurricane, Topex, and Cetacaine*, available at http://www.fda.gov/cder/drug/advisory/benzocaine.htm. Accessed September 23, 2010.
39. El-Husseini A, Basin P: Is threshold for treatment of methemoglobinemia the same for all? A case report and literature review, *Am J Emerg Med* 28:748, 2010.

CONCEPTS IN ANESTHETIC AGENTS

40. Moos DD, Cuddeford JD: Methemoglobinemia and benzocaine, *Gastroenterol Nurs* 30:342–345, 2007.
41. Mulroy MF: Systemic toxicity and cardiotoxicity from local anesthetics: incidence and preventative measures, *Reg Anesth Pain Med* 27:556–561, 2002.
42. DiGregorio G, et al: Clinical presentation of local anesthetic systemic toxicity: a review of published cases 1979-2009, *Reg Anesth Pain Med* 35:179–185, 2010.
43. Clark MK: Lipid emulsion as rescue for local anesthetic-related cardiotoxicity, *J Perianesth Nurs* 23:111–117, 2008.
44. Manavi MV: Lipid infusion as a treatment for local anesthetic toxicity, *AANA J* 78:69–78, 2010.
45. Winberg G: *Lipid Rescue-Practice Advisory*, available at http://lipidrescue.org. Accessed July 13, 2010.
46. Neal JM, et al: ASRA practice advisory on local anesthetic systemic toxicity, *Reg Anesth Pain Med* 35:152–161, 2010.
47. Corcoran W, et al: Local anesthetic-induced cardiac toxicity: a survey of contemporary practice strategies among academic anesthesiology departments, *Anesth Analg* 103:1322–1326, 2006.
48. Krenzischek DA, et al: Pharmacology for acute pain: implications for practice, *J Perianesth Nurs* 23:S28–S42, 2008.

Regional Anesthesia

Daniel D. Moos, MS, EdD, CRNA

Regional anesthesia provides several benefits over general anesthesia. It reduces the number of medications required to induce and maintain general anesthesia, avoids insertion of an airway device, and decreases mortality and morbidity. Specifically it has been found that regional anesthesia decreases the incidence of deep vein thrombosis, pulmonary embolism, transfusion, pneumonia, respiratory depression, myocardial infarction, and renal failure while preserving immune function that may decrease the incidence of infection. In addition, regional anesthesia may have a positive effect on postoperative cognitive function and enhance the return of gastrointestinal mobility.[1] Risks include transient or permanent nerve trauma, local anesthetic toxicity, and technique specific complications.[2] Considerations include patient selection, surgeon preference, and surgical procedure. Regional anesthetic techniques should increase as technological advances improve block placement, research supports its benefits, and pharmacologic advances improve the safety of local anesthetics.

DEFINITIONS

Analgesia: Medications administered to reduce or relieve painful stimuli.[3]

Anesthesia: Medications administered to render the entire or portion of the body insensible to painful stimuli.[3]

Alpha-Adrenergic Vasopressors: Medications resulting in peripheral vascular constriction to increase blood pressure. Phenylephrine, a pure alpha agonist with a fast onset and duration of 5 to 20 minutes, is most commonly administered. Phenylephrine can cause reflex bradycardia secondary to baroreceptor stimulation. Norepinephrine is less commonly administered and in low doses has primarily an alpha agonist effect (see Chapter 11).[4]

Combined Spinal Epidural Technique: Combines the administration of a spinal anesthetic with the placement of an epidural catheter. An epidural needle is placed into the epidural space. A spinal needle is then passed through the epidural needle and medication is injected into the subarachnoid space for spinal anesthesia. The spinal needle is withdrawn and an epidural catheter is placed. The epidural catheter can be used to prolong the duration of anesthesia or to administer postoperative analgesia.[5]

Dermatome Level: Spinal nerve roots innervate skin in horizontal 1- to 2-inch bands. Each dermatome corresponds to a specific spinal nerve root. Knowledge of dermatome levels allows the perianesthesia nurse to assess the level of neuraxial blockade. Assessment of dermatome levels can be accomplished with a small pin, wet cotton ball, or alcohol wipe.[6]

Ephedrine: A vasopressor that has direct effects on alpha and beta receptors. It indirectly stimulates the release of catecholamines. Onset is fast, with a duration of action of 1 to 1.5 hours.[4]

Epidural Block: Placement of local anesthetic in the epidural space that results in blockade of the spinal nerves as they exit the subarachnoid space. An epidural can be used as a sole anesthetic, with general anesthesia, or postoperative analgesia. It can be placed in the thoracic or lumbar epidural space.[6]

High Spinal Block: Excessive spread of local anesthetic within the subarachnoid space which leads to apnea, loss of consciousness, and hypotension.[7]

Neuraxial Blockade: Generic term applied to spinal, epidural, or caudal anesthetics.[6]

Palsy: Traumatic injury to a peripheral nerve that results in a loss of motor and normal sensory function.[3]

Paralysis: Traumatic injury to a central nervous system nerves resulting in the loss of motor function and normal sensory function.[3]

Postdural Puncture Headache (Spinal Headache): Headache characterized by an increased intensity of symptoms when in an upright position and a decrease or absence when in supine; caused by a leak of cerebral spinal fluid after the dura has been transversed with a needle.[7]

Tuffier's Line: Landmark used to identify appropriate levels for administration of neuraxial blockade. A line drawn across the iliac crests will generally cross the interspace of L3-L4.[5]

NEURAXIAL ANESTHESIA AND ANALGESIA

Anatomy of the Spine

The vertebral column provides support and attachment to the skull, thorax, and pelvis. It is composed of 33 vertebrae (7 cervical, 12 thoracic, 5 lumbar, 5 sacral, and 4 coccygeal). Each thoracic vertebra articulates to a corresponding rib. Individual vertebra consists of a pedicle, transverse body, superior articular process, inferior articular process, and spinous process. Individual vertebral bodies have an intervertebral disk connecting them while two superior and inferior articular processes articulate above and below each vertebra. Pedicles are notched superiorly and inferiorly; this allows a space for individual spinal nerves to exit from the spinal cord. The anatomy of the bony spine affects the administration of neuraxial blocks. The spinous process and lamina of a vertebra create the posterior boundary of the spinal canal. Angulation of the spinous process affects needle orientation during insertion. In the lumbar area, spinous processes are almost horizontal with flexion. In the thoracic area they are angled in a caudad fashion with flexion. A second factor is the size of the interlaminar spaces. The larger the interlaminar space the easier the access. Generally the lumbar interlaminar spaces are larger than those in the thoracic region.[5,8,9]

Ligaments of the vertebral column are responsible for maintaining shape of the column, providing support, and protection of the spinal cord. Vertebral bodies and disks are connected by the anterior and posterior longitudinal ligament on the anterior side of the vertebral column and the supraspinous ligament, intraspinous ligament, and ligamentum flavum on the posterior side (Fig. 25-1). When a midline spinal puncture is made, the needle traverses these three ligaments.[5,8,9]

The spinal cord is a continuation of the medulla oblongata, occupying the upper two thirds of the vertebral canal. It is approximately 18 inches long and ends at the lower border of L1 in most adults. The spinal cord ends in the conus medullaris and cauda equina. Nerve roots are not fixed, as the spinal cord is, making it difficult to cause trauma to nerve roots; this makes it safe to place a spinal needle below L2 in the adult patient. The lower portion of the spinal cord becomes the filum terminale, which connects to the bone of the coccyx and holds the spinal cord in place.[8-10] The spinal cord is encased by three membranes: dura, arachnoid, and pia mater. The outermost membrane, dura mater, consists of two layers. Between the dura and the ligamentum flavum is the epidural space, a potential space filled with loose fatty tissue and blood vessels. Local anesthetics are injected in this space for epidural anesthesia. The arachnoid layer consists of a thin membranous sheath. The innermost layer is called the *pia mater* and is separated from the arachnoid mater by a subarachnoid space filled with cerebrospinal fluid (CSF). The subarachnoid space is where local anesthetics are deposited for spinal anesthesia (Fig. 25-2). The total CSF volume in the adult is approximately 100 to 150 mL, with 25 to 35 mL of the volume residing within the subarachnoid space. CSF, continually produced by the choroid plexuses, is reabsorbed into the blood through the arachnoid villi, granulation, and to a small extent through epidural veins. The specific gravity of CSF, which ranges between 1.004 and 1.009, affects the spread of local anesthetic solution depending on its baricity. A hyperbaric medication will move toward dependent areas because it is heavier than CSF, whereas a hypobaric solution will do the opposite. Isobaric medications stay within the general area of injection.[5,8,9]

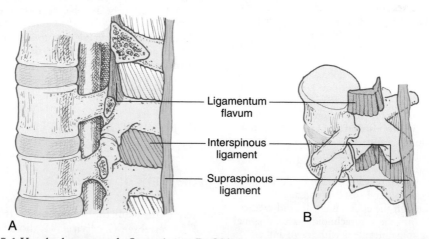

Ligamentum flavum

Interspinous ligament

Supraspinous ligament

A   B

FIG. 25-1 Vertebral anatomy. **A,** Sagittal view. **B,** Oblique view of the lumbar vertebrae showing the ligamentum flavum thickening in the caudad extent of the intervertebral space and in the midline. (From Miller RD, et al: *Miller's anesthesia*, ed 7, Philadelphia, 2009, Churchill Livingstone.)

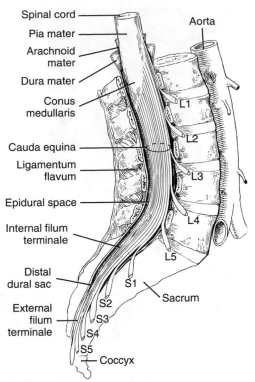

Spinal cord
Pia mater
Arachnoid mater
Dura mater
Conus medullaris
Cauda equina
Ligamentum flavum
Epidural space
Internal filum terminale
Distal dural sac
External filum terminale

Aorta
L1
L2
L3
L4
L5
S1
S2
S3
S4
S5
Sacrum
Coccyx

FIG. 25-2 Extension of the spinal cord to the second lumbar vertebra. (From Nagelhout J, Plaus K, editors: *Nurse anesthesia*, ed 4, St. Louis, 2010, Saunders.)

Thirty-one pairs of spinal nerves travel from the spinal cord and exit at their respective intervertebral foramina (C1-S5). There are 8 cervical, 12 thoracic, 5 lumbar, 5 sacral, and 1 coccygeal pair of spinal nerves. These nerves are blocked by the local anesthetic medication to produce anesthesia or analgesia. Spinal nerve roots vary in size and can be divided into dorsal roots (primarily sensory) and anterior roots (primarily motor).[5,8,9]

Spinal Versus Epidural Blocks

Spinal and epidural blocks are neuraxial blocks. Both block spinal nerve roots, the site of administration differs as does the mechanism of action (Table 25-1). A spinal anesthetic blocks spinal nerve roots as they pass through the CSF, resulting in blockade of sensory, motor, and autonomic impulse transmission whereas epidural anesthesia and analgesia blocks spinal nerve roots outside the subarachnoid space. Epidurals require a large dose of local anesthetic to allow for diffusion through anatomic barriers, such as the dura, and spreads horizontally and vertically within the epidural space. The epidural space is vascular, and there is a risk of local anesthetic toxicity (see Chapter 24). Spinal anesthesia is accomplished by administering a small dose of local anesthetic within the subarachnoid space. Spinal anesthesia is a single injection through a needle and reduces the time for administration but does not allow for repeated dosing. Epidural anesthesia is administered through a catheter that is placed through a needle, may require more time to place, may be dosed again, and used for postoperative analgesia. Spinal anesthesia is limited to placement in the lower lumbar region below the termination of the spinal cord. Epidural catheter placement can occur in the lumbar or thoracic region. Spinal anesthesia is rapidly achieved and produces an intense sensory and motor block. Rapid onset can lead to profound hypotension. Epidural anesthesia onset is gradual, blockade is less profound, and decreases in blood pressure are less intense.[7,9]

Contraindications

Absolute contraindications include patient refusal; cardiovascular diseases such as severe aortic–mitral stenosis and asymmetrical septal hypertrophy; severe uncorrected hypovolemia; documented allergy to local anesthetic; increased intracranial pressure; infection at the site of injection; sepsis or bacteremia;

Table 25-1	Differences Between Spinal and Epidural Anesthesia	
	SPINAL	**EPIDURAL**
Site or mechanism of action	Nerve roots blocked as they pass through the CSF	Nerve roots blocked outside the cerebrospinal fluid
Site of administration	Lower lumbar below the termination of spinal cord	Lumbar or thoracic area
Dose of local anesthetic	Small	Large
Instrument for administration	Needle	Catheter
Ability to repeat dose	No	Yes
Onset	Rapid, intense blockade, may lead to hypotension	Gradual; may have less intense blockade, decrease in blood pressure is more gradual

and coagulopathy.[1,5,7,9] Coagulation-altering medications should be reviewed and current recommendations should be followed to avoid the potentially catastrophic complication of a neuraxial hematoma.[10] Current guidelines related to anticoagulation therapy and regional anesthesia can be accessed and reviewed at http://asra.com/publications-anticoagulation-3rd-edition-2010.php.[11] Relative contraindications include preexisting neurologic disease, musculoskeletal abnormalities, prior back surgery, and untreated hypertension.[1,5,7,9] Placing a neuraxial block through a tattoo is controversial.[12] The perianesthesia nurse should alert the anesthesia provider to potential contraindications.

Spinal Anesthesia

Universal protocol, as outlined by The Joint Commission, should be followed and medications should be labeled before the procedure.[13] An initial set of vital signs should be documented. Patients may be positioned in a lateral decubitus or sitting position with the back flexed to maximize the intervertebral opening (Figs. 25-3 and 25-4). Tuffier's line is generally used to identify the 3rd and 4th lumbar spaces, but may not always be reliable.[14] After the anesthesia provider has identified the desired interspace, he or she will follow sterile technique (mask, sterile gloves, hat) and proceed with preparing and placing sterile drapes. The perianesthesia nurse should maintain verbal contact with the patient to reassure and inform them of what to expect. Local anesthetic is used to anesthetize the skin and underlying tissue. A 25-gauge or smaller spinal needle is used in patients at risk for a postdural puncture headache

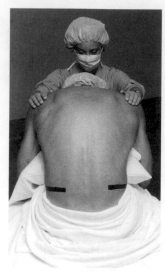

FIG. 25-4 Sitting position for a neuraxial block. The assistant provides the patient with a foot rest (stool) and a pillow and prevents the patient from slumping to either side. (From Miller RD, et al: *Miller's anesthesia*, ed 7, Philadelphia, 2009, Churchill Livingstone.)

(PDPH): patients younger than 50 years, females, pregnancy, and a prior history of PDPH. Needle design is an important consideration in at risk groups, with pencil point needles being less likely to cause a PDPH.[1,15] A 22-gauge cutting tip needle can be used in patients older than 50 years. The spinal needle will transverse the supraspinous and interspinous ligaments, ligamentum flavum, and dura; this is noted by a change in the resistance. The stylet is removed and CSF is noted at the hub of the needle. Procaine, bupivacaine, or tetracaine are commonly used for spinal anesthesia. Epinephrine (0.1 to 0.2 mg) or phenylephrine (2 to 5 mg) can be added to increase duration of action. Local anesthetic is administered and patient positioned. Vital signs should be monitored at 1-minute intervals for the first 10 minutes and then, if stable, every 5 minutes. Blood pressure decreases of 20% or more should be treated with fluids and vasopressors (ephedrine or phenylephrine).[1,5,7,9]

Progression of onset is noted by loss of autonomic or sympathetic function, sense of temperature, pain, touch, movement and proprioception. During recovery, function will return in the opposite order (Box 25-1). Spinal anesthetics are dosed for specific surgical procedures (Table 25-2). Level of anesthesia is monitored by dermatome level (Fig. 25-5). Monitoring regression of spinal anesthetic is aided with the knowledge of the dermatome level and can be assessed by the use of an alcohol wipe, a blunt needle that does not break the skin, or a light pinch.[5,6]

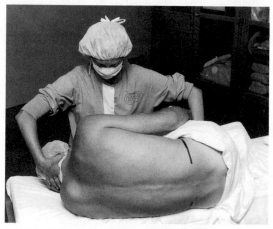

FIG. 25-3 Lateral decubitus positioning for a neuraxial block. The assistant can help the patient assume the ideal position of "forehead to knees." (From Miller RD, et al: *Miller's anesthesia*, ed 7, Philadelphia, 2009, Churchill Livingstone.)

BOX 25-1	Onset and Return of Neuraxial Blockade

Order of Loss of Function	Order of Return of Function
1. Autonomic, sympathetic function	1. Proprioception (sense of body location)
2. Sense of temperature	2. Movement
3. Pain	3. Touch
4. Touch	4. Pain
5. Movement	5. Sense of temperature
6. Proprioception (sense of body location)	6. Autonomic, sympathetic function

From Schick L, Windle PE, editors: *Perianesthesia nursing core curriculum: preprocedure, Phase I and Phase II PACU nursing,* ed 2, St. Louis, 2010, Saunders.

Epidural Anesthesia

Epidural anesthesia or analgesia is similar to spinal anesthesia in regard to positioning, sterile technique, monitoring, progression, and assessment. Epidural anesthesia can be a single shot technique (i.e., caudal anesthesia) or more commonly as an intermittent or continuous technique for anesthesia or analgesia. Anesthesia may be administered for the same type of surgical procedures as spinal anesthetics (see Table 25-2), but may be less effective for procedures of the perineum because of sacral sparing. Epidurals are versatile for analgesic purposes and may be used for labor and delivery or postoperative analgesia for surgical procedures ranging from the thorax to lower extremities. Epidural needles are larger than spinal needles to allow for the insertion of a catheter. The average needle is 9 cm and is marked to indicate the depth of insertion. An epidural needle transverses the supraspinous and intraspinous ligament and seated in the ligamentum flavum. A special loss-of-resistance syringe with preservative-free saline is attached to the hub, and the needle is advanced until a loss of resistance is noted upon entering the epidural space. An epidural catheter is then inserted to a desired depth. Epidural catheters are marked to indicate the depth of insertion.[1,5,7,9,16] A 3-mL test dose of 1.5% lidocaine with 1:200,000 epinephrine is administered to help detect intravascular, subarachnoid, or subdural placement.[17] If positive, the heart rate and systolic blood pressure will increase by at least 20 beats/min and 15 mm Hg, but may not be reliable in the presence of beta blockers, advanced age, and general anesthesia.[18] A subarachnoid injection will result in a spinal anesthetic, whereas a subdural injection can result in an extensive block relative to a small dose of local anesthetic.[19] Common local anesthetics used for epidural anesthesia include 2-chloroprocaine, lidocaine, bupivacaine, and ropivacaine. Epidurals are dosed based on the number of dermatomes that are to be blocked (1 to 2 mL per dermatome). Dosing occurs slowly with no more than 5 mL of local anesthetic administered at a time because there is a risk of local anesthetic toxicity. Epinephrine (1:200,000) can be used to decrease absorption and prolong duration. Epidural catheters should be monitored for signs of drainage or dislodgement. The site is covered with a sterile dressing and connections should be tight. The American Society of PeriAnesthesia Nurses position statement on safe medication administration[20] and local institutional policy should be followed for the administration of medications. When initiating a continuous infusion check dose and concentration of local anesthetic solution and confirm the infusion rate.

Combined spinal-epidural is a versatile technique that allows for the administration of a spinal anesthetic for immediate anesthesia and an epidural to extend the duration of the anesthetic or provide for postoperative analgesia. It is similar to spinal–epidural anesthesia in regard to positioning, sterile technique, monitoring, progression, and assessment.

Table 25-2	Dermatome Level and Surgical Procedure		
SENSORY LEVEL	**SURGICAL PROCEDURE**		**CUTANEOUS LEVEL**
Above T4			Pinky, inner arm, apex of axilla
T4	Cesarean section, upper abdomen, uterine		Nipple
T6-7	Lower abdomen		Xiphoid
T7-8	Tourniquet pain		
T10	Hip and genitourinary		Umbilicus
L1-3	Lower extremities		
S2-5	Perineal region (genitalia/buttocks)		

Modified from Schick L, Windle PE, editors: *Perianesthesia nursing core curriculum: preprocedure, phase I and phase II PACU nursing,* ed 2, St. Louis, 2010, Saunders.

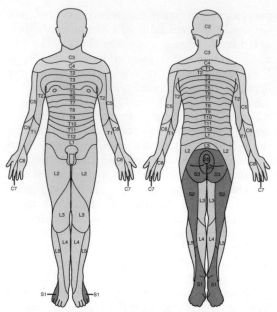

FIG. 25-5 Dermatomes. (From Nagelhout J, Plaus K, editors: *Nurse anesthesia,* ed 4, St. Louis, 2010, Saunders.)

Neuraxial Complications

Complications related to neuraxial blockade can range from minor to life threatening. Anticipation, recognition, and prompt intervention are essential roles of the perianesthesia nurse.

High Spinal Block

Excessive spread of local anesthetic that occurs with spinal or epidural anesthesia is a high spinal block. Signs and symptoms include high sensory block resulting in upper extremity sensory and motor changes, nausea and vomiting, loss of consciousness, anxiety, hypotension, bradycardia or asystole, respiratory distress or apnea. Treatment is dependent on extent of spread. Airway, breathing, and circulation are primary considerations. Supplemental oxygen, assistance with a bag-mask-valve device, or intubation may be required. The patient may be aware of the surrounding environment and verbal reassurance is important to reduce anxiety. Hypotension is caused by an extensive sympathectomy and treated with fluid bolus, elevation of the legs, and vasopressors (see Chapter 11), which may include phenylephrine, norepinephrine, ephedrine, or epinephrine. Bradycardia is treated with ephedrine or atropine. Phenylephrine and norepinephrine administration can cause reflex bradycardia and should be used with caution in the setting of significant bradycardia. Asystole is treated with established ACLS protocol. High

spinal blocks are generally self limiting, and the patient will improve as the concentration of local anesthetic declines.[1,5,7,9]

Local Anesthetic Toxicity

See Chapter 24.

Hypotension

Postoperative hypotension can be caused by sympathectomy and can occur with spinal or epidural anesthesia. Treatment consists of raising the legs, fluid bolus, and vasopressors (i.e., ephedrine or phenylephrine). Refractory hypotension can be treated with a continuous infusion of phenylephrine, norepinephrine, or low-dose epinephrine. It is important to rule out other causes of hypotension during stabilization, including hemorrhage or cardiovascular complications (see Chapter 29).[1,5,7,9]

Nausea and Vomiting

When associated with neuraxial blockade, the precipitating factor of nausea and vomiting is often hypotension. Supplemental oxygen should be applied and blood pressure should be measured. Treat hypotension, and if nausea does not resolve seek other causes.[1,5,7,9]

Urinary Retention

Urinary retention is often caused by autonomic blockade of the sacral nerves, resulting in a hypotonic bladder. Other causes such as surgical genitourinary trauma, pain, opioids, and renal failure should be ruled out. Patients may exhibit restlessness and incoherence. A neurologic insult, electrolyte disorders, hypoxia, pain, and abnormal glucose levels should also be ruled out. A bladder scan can help to confirm retention, and insertion of a urinary catheter is the treatment.[9,21]

Hypothermia

Regional anesthesia results in centrally mediated vasodilatation and inhibits peripheral vasoconstriction, transferring body heat from the core to periphery through radiation, convection, conduction, and evaporation. Recognition of hypothermia and initiation of measures to return the patient to a normal temperature are important considerations.[22] (see Chapter 53).

Postdural Puncture Headache

This condition is caused by leaking CSF through the dura, which can occur with spinal anesthesia or inadvertent dural puncture with an epidural. Symptoms usually occur 24 to 48 hours after dural puncture. Symptoms include a headache in the occipital-frontal region that intensifies when upright and declines when supine, nuchal rigidity, visual and auditory disturbances, and nausea and vomiting. Significant neurologic complications such as meningitis, intracranial tumors, and hemorrhage should be ruled out. Treatment is initially symptomatic and includes bed rest, fluids, caffeine, and analgesics. If persistent, an epidural blood patch is the definitive treatment and is highly successful (95% success rate). The anesthesia provider accesses the epidural space at one space below the dural puncture; 15 to 20 mL of the patient's blood is drawn aseptically and administered through the epidural needle. The patient remains on bed rest for 30 to 60 minutes before ambulation. Complications include back pain, fever, meningitis, and arachnoiditis.[5,9,23,24]

Neurologic Complications

The overall incidence after neuraxial blockade is 0.04%, and permanent injury is rare.[25] Palsies, paralysis, or pain should be reported immediately to the anesthesia provider and surgeon. This complication may be related to traumatic needle placement, bleeding or hematoma formation, surgical trauma, or injury related to a portion of the body being insensate. A neurologic consultation may be required to help diagnose and manage the patient's condition.[5,9]

Transient Neurologic Symptoms

These symptoms are most often associated with spinal lidocaine, although it can occur with any local anesthetic. Signs and symptoms usually appear within 24 hours of block resolution and consist of low back pain with radiation to the lower extremities. It is important to rule out other more serious causes. It is generally self limiting with full recovery occurring in 2 days.[26] Cauda equina syndrome is associated with lidocaine and continuous spinal microcatheters. It manifests with low back pain with radiation to the lower extremities as well as sensory and motor changes. Prospects of recovery are poor.[9] Infectious complications such as meningitis, epidural abscess, and arachnoiditis can occur but are extremely rare.[5,9]

Spinal or Epidural Hematoma

Spinal or epidural hematoma is rare but devastating. It is more likely to occur in patients with altered homeostasis. Symptoms include low back pain, motor changes, and bowel or bladder dysfunction. Treatment is emergent decompression, but recovery is poor if surgery is delayed more than 8 hours. Awareness of coagulation-altering medications and notification of anesthesia personnel may prevent this complication from occurring.[5,10]

Care of Patients After Neuraxial Blockade

In addition to routine PACU Phase I care for patients receiving sedation, the perianesthesia nurse should perform a continual assessment for complications as outlined. Rapid intervention is required for hypotension or bradycardia. Care should be taken not to rapidly change the patient's position, as this may cause hypotension related to residual sympathectomy. Ensure the patient's insensate limbs are positioned in correct anatomic alignment and padded to prevent injury.[27] Any concerns should be reported to the anesthesia provider. Before discharge, the patient should meet the standards for discharge criteria that are applicable to all patients recovering from anesthesia. Additional concerns include a less than 10% decrease in blood pressure with position change and a sensory level equal or less than T10 with evidence that the block is receding by at least two sensory segments. There is no required minimum stay time, but length of stay should be tailored to the individual patient's needs.[28]

PERIPHERAL NERVE BLOCKS

Peripheral nerve blocks may be used as a sole anesthetic, in combination with general or neuraxial anesthesia, or for postoperative analgesia. Advantages include a reduction in postoperative pain, decreased nausea and vomiting, reduces complications associated with general anesthesia, and may reduce time to discharge for outpatient procedures.[29] Generalized absolute contraindications include patient refusal, documented allergy to local anesthetics, coagulopathy, and infection at the site of injection.[30,31] Specific peripheral nerve block contraindications are noted in their descriptions. Relative contraindications include uncooperative patients and neurologic disorders.[30,31] If the perianesthesia nurse identifies contraindications, the anesthesia provider should be notified.

Ultrasound

Ultrasound technology furnishes anesthesia providers with anatomic images. Ultrasound guidance for regional anesthesia was first described in 1978.[32] Technological advancement, affordability of equipment, and research has increased its use and acceptance. Benefits include anatomic identification of structures in real time; confirmation of local anesthetic spread; increased success rate, quality, and faster onset time for sensory blockade;

decrease in number of attempts; and identification of vascular structures. At this time there is no conclusive evidence that it decreases the risk for local anesthetic toxicity. Successful and safe use of ultrasound is user dependent.[33-37]

Ultrasound waveforms are created by piezoelectric crystals. Electrical impulses cause each crystal to produce sound waves, called an *ultrasound beam*, which travel through tissue. Echoes are transmitted back to the transducer, converted to an electrical impulse, and then to an image. Biologic tissue varies in its resistance to sound waves, and echoes are reflected back at varying speeds. In general the best position for a transducer, in relation to an anatomic structure, is 90 degrees because the transducer will capture most of the reflected echoes.[38,39] See Box 25-2 for common terms associated with the use of ultrasound.

Basic Ultrasound Anatomy and Characteristics

Fat is hypoechoic with hyperechoic lines. Fascial layers appear hyperechoic. Muscle appears hypoechoic with several hyperechoic striations more numerous than those seen in fat. Ultrasound waves do not penetrate bone and appear hyperechoic with a dark shadow below. Arteries are round and pulsating, whereas veins are rounded and compressible. Because arteries and veins contain blood, they appear as anechoic (do not reflect echoes; Fig. 25-6). Color Doppler can help to identify vasculature. A red image indicates flow toward the transducer, and blue indicates the opposite. Orientation of the transducer is important because a 90-degree angle might not detect any flow. If the transducer is oriented to the vessel so that the blood flow is going away from the transducer, it will appear blue despite being an artery.[38]

Transducer Orientation

To obtain an optimal image, the anesthesia provider manipulates the transducer by aligning, tilting, rotating, and sliding. Transducer position relative to nerve position is termed *axis*. *In axis* means that the beam is oriented to view the nerve in its length, and *out of axis* indicates that the beam is oriented to view the nerve as a cross section. Transducer-to-needle orientation is termed *plane*. An in-plane orientation uses the ultrasound beam to view the needle in its length, and out-of-plane orientation indicates that the needle is viewed as a cross section. Combining terms of axis and plane define the overall approach to a peripheral nerve block. Approaches include in axis/in plane, in axis/off plane, off axis/in plane, and off axis/off plane. Two of the most common approaches are off axis/off plane (Fig. 25-7) and off axis/in plane.[38,39]

BOX 25-2   Terms Associated with the Use of Ultrasound

Anechoic: Tissue with no reflective index appears gray (fluid filled structures are anechoic).
Curved Array Probe: Ultrasound waves are transmitted in a fanlike fashion.
Echo: The reflection of acoustic impedance is collected by the probe from the tissue.
Hyperechoic: Tissue with a high reflective index appears brightly (bones and tendons).
Hypoechoic: Tissue with a low reflective index appears dark.
In Axis: Ultrasound beam is orientated to view the nerve in its entirety.
In Plane: Ultrasound beam is orientated to view the needle in its entirety.
Linear Array Probe: Ultrasound waves are transmitted in a straight, frontal direction.
Out of Axis or Off Axis: Ultrasound beam is orientated to view the nerve as a cross section.
Out of Plane or Off Plane: Ultrasound beam is orientated to view the needle as a cross section.

(From Chan VWS, et al: *Ultrasound imaging for regional anesthesia: a practical guide,* ed 2, Toronto, 2007, Toronto Printing Company; Falyar CR: Ultrasound in anesthesia: applying scientific principles to clinical practice, *AANA J* 78:332-341, 2010.)

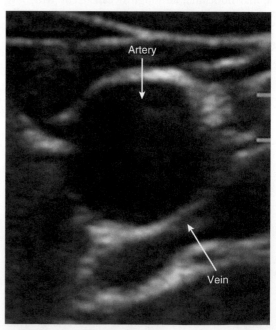

FIG. 25-6 Ultrasound image of artery with vein compressed. (Courtesy Daniel D. Moos.)

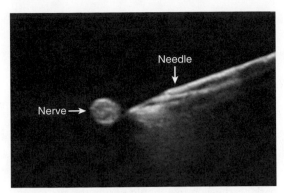

FIG. 25-7 Off-axis, in-plane approach. (Courtesy Daniel D. Moos.)

Assisting with Ultrasound Guided Peripheral Nerve Blocks

Perianesthesia nurses may be involved with placement of peripheral nerve blocks with ultrasound. Sterile preparation and basic ultrasound controls should be understood. Anesthesia providers choose the transducer based on the peripheral nerve block. Low-frequency probes are used to identify anatomic structures that are more than 4 cm below the skin surface (i.e., the sciatic nerve). A frequency of less than 7 MHz allows for deeper penetration at the expense of image quality. High-frequency probes are used for superficial structures (less than 4 cm, brachial plexus or femoral nerve) and have a frequency greater than 7 MHz, limiting tissue penetration but producing a superior image. Transducers are linear or curved. A linear probe will provide better images because waves are transmitted in a linear fashion, allowing transmission of sound waves back to the transducer at the cost of a narrow field of view. Curved probes provide a wide field of vision, but lower resolution because of scattering of returning sound waves.[38-40]

For a single injection, clear sterile occlusive dressings can be applied to the transducer after gel has been applied. Sterile gel should be available for the skin. Alternatively, a sterile sleeve may be applied for single injection techniques or insertion of a peripheral nerve catheter. Meticulous attention to sterile technique is an important role of the perianesthesia nurse to avoid the introduction of contaminants to the injection site. Notify the anesthesia provider of inadvertent breaks in sterility.[40] Knowledge of basic ultrasound controls is important because adjustments to frequency, gain, and depth may be required. Frequency is determined by the transducer; however fine adjustments may improve the image. Gain increases or decreases amplification of ultrasound echoes.

Increases brighten the image but produce artifact, whereas decreasing gain darkens the image. Key anatomic structures may be either more superficial or deep than initially anticipated necessitating adjustments in depth. Application of the color Doppler function may be required to determine whether a structure is a nerve, vein, or artery.[38,40,41]

Peripheral Nerve Stimulators

Peripheral nerve stimulators can be used as a standalone technique or as an adjunct to ultrasound for the placement of peripheral nerve blocks. Electrical stimulation of large alpha motor fibers occur at low intensities (measured in milliamps). Pain is a function of small delta fibers and can be elicited with high-intensity stimulation. Use of low-intensity currents elicits a motor response without patient discomfort. The patient should be forewarned that they will experience involuntary movement of muscles. Insulated needles are used to concentrate electrical current at the tip of the needle. The intensity is decreased as the nerve is located. Positive and negative leads are required to complete the circuit. A negative lead is attached to the needle and a positive lead is attached to the patient with an electrocardiogram pad. Good contact with the skin is important for accurate use.[30,40,42,43]

The perianesthesia nurse may be asked to assist in adjusting the stimulator, subject to state board of nursing regulations and institutional policy. There are three common controls on a nerve stimulator that the perianesthesia nurse should know: current (intensity of stimulation in milliamperes), pulse width (duration of stimulation in milliseconds), and frequency (frequency of stimulation in hertz; Fig. 25-8). A short pulse width of 100 to 200 μs allows the identification of alpha fibers for most peripheral nerves, while the optimal frequency is 2 to 2.5 Hz. The milliampere control is manipulated during block placement; initially it is set at a higher level of intensity. The greater the distance the needle is from the nerve, the greater the intensity required to elicit a response. As the needle is advanced toward the target nerve, the intensity is decreased while still obtaining a motor response. The perianesthesia nurse may be asked to assist in administering the injection under the guidance of the anesthesia provider, subject to state board of nursing regulations and institutional policy. When the nerve is located, aspiration should occur to verify that the needle is not within a vessel. If the needle is not within a vessel, a small test dose of local anesthetic is administered to confirm placement. Injection of 2 to 3 mL of local anesthetic will cause contractions to stop; this is a positive Raj test

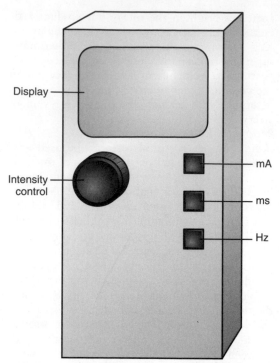

Display

Intensity
control

mA

ms

Hz

FIG. 25-8 Schematic illustration of a peripheral nerve stimulator.

result. Significant resistance to injection may indicate an intraneural injection and should be immediately stopped. Injection should be slow and in increments of 5 mL, with aspiration occurring before each injection. The patient should be closely monitored for signs and symptoms of complications.[30,40,42,43]

Peripheral Nerve Block Catheters

Peripheral nerve catheters are used for postoperative analgesia. Markings on the catheter measure the depth of insertion. The thick black line that indicates the needle length is followed by smaller markings measured in centimeters. Catheters may be stimulating or nonstimulating. Stimulating catheters are used for placement with a peripheral nerve stimulator. The target nerve is located with a needle. After the desired stimulation is achieved, the catheter is placed inside the needle. The negative lead is attached and the catheter is advanced while maintaining muscle contractions at the desired level of stimulation. Catheters can be tunneled under the skin and are inserted to the desired depth. A test dose of local anesthetic helps to determine correct placement. When in place, the catheter is secured and a bolus can be given, followed by a continuous infusion. Nonstimulating catheters can be placed under the guidance of ultrasound. Because the catheter is

placed under direct visualization, nerve stimulation is not required. Some providers use ultrasound and a stimulating catheter to confirm placement. Peripheral nerve catheters may be placed during the preoperative or postoperative periods. Perianesthesia nurses may assist placement. Reassuring the patient, monitoring vital signs, monitoring for inadvertent vascular injection, and attention to sterile technique are important roles.[40]

Peripheral nerve catheters should be monitored for signs of drainage or dislodgement. The perianesthesia nurse should ensure the site is covered with a sterile dressing, and that connections are tight. When initiating a continuous infusion, check the dose and concentration of the local anesthetic solution and confirm the infusion rate. Any concerns should be addressed with the anesthesia provider.[40]

Nursing Considerations for Peripheral Nerve Blocks

Perianesthesia nursing actions are outlined in Box 25-3.

Upper Extremity Peripheral Nerve Blocks
Brachial Plexus

The brachial plexus is created primarily by the ventral rami of C5 to T1 (Fig. 25-9). C5 and C6 form the superior trunk, C7 from the middle trunk, and C8 and T1 from the inferior trunk as they exit their intervertebral foramina. As the brachial plexus continues its course, trunks split into anterior and posterior divisions. The anterior division of the upper and middle trunk forms the lateral cord; posterior division of the upper, middle, and lower trunk will form the posterior cord; and the anterior division of the lower trunk forms the medial cord. The lateral cord divides into musculocutaneous nerve and contributes to the median nerve. The posterior cord divides into the axillary and radial nerves. The medial cord divides into the ulnar and medial antebrachial cutaneous nerves, and contributes to the median nerve. Individual cutaneous nerve supply to the upper extremity and major motor function are noted in Fig. 25-10 and Table 25-3. The anatomy of the brachial plexus allows the placement of local anesthetic at the level of trunks, cords, or terminal branches. The most common blocks include the interscalene, supraclavicular, infraclavicular, and axillary approach. Determining the approach is dependent on the surgical procedure. Basic knowledge of each approach will help the perianesthesia nurse monitor for potential complications. Techniques include anatomic landmarks, patients'

BOX 25-3   General Perianesthesia Nursing Actions for Peripheral Nerve Blocks*

BEFORE PERIPHERAL NERVE BLOCKADE

- Notify the anesthesia provider of potential contraindications.
- Document baseline vital signs.
- Medications in syringes should be clearly labeled.
- Resuscitative equipment (i.e., crash cart, bag-mask apparatus, lipid emulsions) should be immediately available.
- Time out. The anesthesia provider and perianesthesia nurse should confirm that consent has been obtained and identify correct patient, peripheral nerve block, limb, and side.

DURING PERIPHERAL NERVE BLOCKADE

- Use Universal Precautions.
- Patient monitoring should include intermittent blood pressure recordings, continuous electrocardiography, pulse oximetry, mental status, and end tidal carbon dioxide if indicated.
- Fear, anxiety, and pain can cause vasovagal reactions.
- Assist in positioning of the patient.
- Continually reassure and communicate with the patient during and after peripheral nerve blockade.
- Institute meticulous attention to sterile technique and potential breaks.
- Administer sedatives and opioids as directed by the anesthesia provider to decrease anxiety, but not so excessive that the patient can communicate subjective sign and symptoms that may indicate a complication.
- Ensure familiarity with basic controls that may require adjustment during blockade for ultrasound and peripheral nerve stimulator.
- Check for adequate electrogram pad contact with patient skin for the positive lead and a tight connection to the negative lead with peripheral nerve catheters.
- Patients may require verbal reassurance with involuntary muscle movements associated with peripheral nerve stimulator use.
- Administer local anesthetics as directed by the anesthesia provider. The syringe should be clearly labeled with local anesthetic and concentration. Always aspirate before injection. If resistance is encountered, stop immediately and notify the anesthesia provider. Inject slowly in 5-mL increments with aspiration occurring in between.
- Monitor the patient for block-specific complications.

POSTPERIPHERAL BLOCKADE: BEFORE OPERATION

- Monitor vital signs and mental status as directed by the anesthesia provider, with a minimum of every 15 minutes for the first hour after the block and document the information.
- Monitor for complications and report immediately to anesthesia provider.

POSTPERIPHERAL BLOCKADE: RECOVERY

- Institute routine postoperative care. There are no specific time limitations or criteria concerning sensation and motor function with peripheral nerve blocks.
- Monitor for block-specific complications.
- Protect the insensate limb and caution the patient on movement that could lead to injury because of partial motor blockade.
- Avoid direct pressure on injection sites. Assist the patient in repositioning.
- Assess the injection site if possible for hematoma formation.
- For patients with peripheral nerve catheters, ensure that connections are tight and secure.
- Check the insertion site if it can be visualized and ensure that sterile dressings remain intact.
- Report bleeding, dislodgement, or drainage to the anesthesia provider.
- Ensure that the correct local anesthetic solution is infusing at the ordered infusion rate.
- Avoid dislodgement during repositioning or patient transfers.

PATIENT TEACHING

- Patient teaching should be tailored to specific blocks.
- Patients should use slings or braces as ordered to prevent injury because of partial motor blockade and insensate limb.
- Duration of the blockade can be variable and largely dependent on whether single injection or continuous infusion is used.
- As sensation returns, the patient may experience numbness, tingling, and possible burning sensation as well as a return of discomfort.
- Be proactive with pain medications to avoid uncontrollable discomfort as the block resolves.

Compiled from references 13, 28, 30, 38, 40, 41, 43.
*It is essential to ensure that the perianesthesia nurse's participation in various aspects of peripheral nerve blocks is appropriate according the individual's state board of nursing regulations and institutional policy.

CONCEPTS IN ANESTHETIC AGENTS

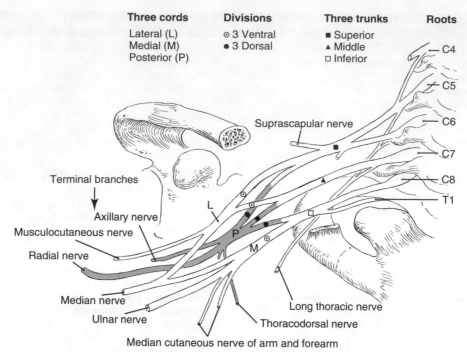

Three cords
Lateral (L)
Medial (M)
Posterior (P)

Divisions
⊙ 3 Ventral
● 3 Dorsal

Three trunks
■ Superior
▲ Middle
□ Inferior

Roots

— C4
— C5
— C6
— C7
— C8
— T1

Suprascapular nerve

Terminal branches

Axillary nerve

Musculocutaneous nerve

Radial nerve

Median nerve

Ulnar nerve

Long thoracic nerve

Thoracodorsal nerve

Median cutaneous nerve of arm and forearm

FIG. 25-9 Deviation of the brachial plexus from the cervical spine. (From Nagelhout J, Plaus K, editors: *Nurse anesthesia,* ed 4, St. Louis, 2010, Saunders.)

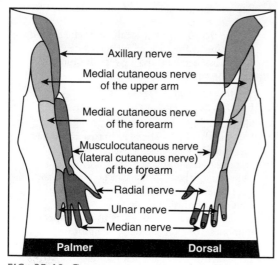

Axillary nerve

Medial cutaneous nerve of the upper arm

Medial cutaneous nerve of the forearm

Musculocutaneous nerve (lateral cutaneous nerve) of the forearm

Radial nerve

Ulnar nerve

Median nerve

Palmer   **Dorsal**

FIG. 25-10 Cutaneous nerve supply to the upper extremities.

Table 25-3	Motor Function of Individual Nerves of the Brachial Plexus
NERVE	**MAJOR MOTOR FUNCTION**
Axillary nerve	Abduction of the shoulder
Musculocutaneous nerve	Flexion of the elbow
Radial nerve	Extension of the elbow, wrist, and finger
Median nerve	Flexion of the wrist and finger
Ulnar nerve	Flexion of the wrist and finger

report of paresthesia, use of a nerve stimulator, and ultrasound guided techniques.[30,31,40,44-46]

Interscalene

Upper, middle, and lower trunks are located in between the anterior and middle scalene muscles. The trunks are named based on their vertical arrangement within this groove. This approach is used for surgical procedures of the shoulder and

spares the ulnar distribution. Surgical procedures of the arm and hand use other approaches to the brachial plexus. Positioning of the patient is dependent on the approach. Patients may be in the supine or sitting position with their head turned 30 degrees toward their nonoperative side. Additional positions include lateral decubitus. Key anatomic landmarks include the sternocleidomastoid muscle, interscalene groove, and cricoid cartilage. Paresthesia techniques rely on subjective description of paresthesias in the upper arm or shoulder. Nerve stimulator techniques rely on identification of muscle contractions of the deltoid, biceps, triceps, pectoralis major, forearm, or hand. Ultrasound techniques help to identify specific nerve roots or trunks to guide placement. Complications include blockade of the phrenic nerve resulting in dyspnea, making it an unsuitable block for patients with chronic respiratory conditions. Vascular structures located in close proximity mandate monitoring for signs and symptoms of local anesthetic toxicity (see Chapter 24). As little as 1 to 3 mL of local anesthetic placed within a vertebral artery can result in seizure activity. Pneumothorax is also a potential complication. Signs and symptoms include dyspnea, decreased or absent breath sounds on the affected side, chest pain with deep inspiration, hyper resonance with percussion, and hypoxemia as indicated by arterial blood gases and pulse oximetry. Immediate notification of the provider, anticipation of a chest radiograph, and possible chest tube insertion should be considered. Blockade of the stellate ganglion results in Horner syndrome. The patient may experience hoarseness of the voice, constriction of the pupil (myosis), drooping of the upper eyelid (ptosis), decreased sweating (anhidrosis), and nasal congestion on the affected side. This experience is disconcerting but self limiting, and reassurance is an important consideration. Local anesthetic may be inadvertently placed with the epidural, spinal, or subdural space, leading to a high spinal block (see High Spinal Block). Additional complications include nerve trauma, hematoma, and infection.[30,31,40,43-46]

Supraclavicular

As the brachial plexus passes between the first rib and clavicle, individual trunks are closely compacted and found slightly posterior to the subclavian artery. This approach is used for surgical procedures of the arm and hand. It is not suitable for shoulder surgery. The patient is placed in a supine position with the head turned at a 30-degree angle toward the nonoperative arm. Anatomic landmarks include the clavicle, sternocleidomastoid, and subclavian artery. A paresthesia of the arm or hand may be sought. With a peripheral nerve stimulator technique, muscle contraction of the fingers is desired. Ultrasound techniques rely on identification of the subclavian artery and trunks of the brachial plexus, which are located posterior to the artery. An in-plane technique is used to identify the needle tip as it is advanced to avoid vasculature and pleura. Complications are similar to interscalene approaches with the addition of hemothorax. Respiratory complications may not be immediate and nursing staff should be sensitive to changes in the patient's respiratory status.[30,31,40,43-46]

Infraclavicular

After the first rib and clavicle, the brachial plexus divides into anterior and posterior divisions and then forms the lateral, medial, and posterior cords (named by their relationship to the subclavian artery). This approach is used for surgical procedures of the arm and hand; it is not suitable for shoulder surgery. Patients may be positioned supine with the head turned slightly toward the nonoperative side and the operative limb abducted at 90 degrees or at their side. Anatomic landmarks include the clavicle, coracoid process, and subclavian artery. Infraclavicular techniques are limited to peripheral nerve stimulator and ultrasound techniques. Peripheral nerve stimulators rely on muscle contraction of the median nerve (wrist–finger flexion), radial nerve (elbow–wrist extension) and ulnar nerve (wrist–finger flexion). Complications are similar to interscalene approaches with the addition of hemothorax and chylothorax (accumulation of lymphatic fluid within the chest and associated with left sided blocks). Signs and symptoms of chylothorax are similar to a pleural effusion.[30,31,40,43-46]

Axillary

Trunks become terminal braches at the pectoralis minor. Blockade here results in anesthesia–analgesia of the median, radial, and ulnar nerves. As the terminal nerves enter the axilla, the musculocutaneous nerve has already left the brachial plexus and is located within the coracobrachialis muscle and must be blocked separately. If a tourniquet is used, a skin wheal of local anesthetic will block the intercostobrachial and medial brachial cutaneous nerves. This approach is acceptable for surgical procedures of the hand, forearm, and elbow. The patient is in the supine or sitting position. The arm is abducted and the elbow is flexed at a 90-degree angle. The primary landmark is the axillary artery. Approaches include transarterial, paresthesia, nerve stimulation, and ultrasound. During a transarterial technique, a needle is inserted through the axillary artery. When blood can no longer be aspirated, local anesthetic is slowly injected with frequent aspirations to ensure that the needle tip is not within the artery. Continuous monitoring of the patient is essential to detect complications such as intravascular injection. Paresthesia techniques rely on subjective reporting by the patient. The anesthesia provider may elect to inject a paresthesia in the surgical distribution or elicit several paresthesias. Nerve stimulator techniques rely on muscle contractions of the hand. Ultrasound techniques identify the axillary artery and vein and the individual nerves that surround them. This approach has a low complication rate but may include intravascular injection, local anesthetic toxicity, nerve

CONCEPTS IN ANESTHETIC AGENTS

trauma leading to neuropathy, hematoma formation, and infection.[30,31,40,43-46]

Bier Block

Bier blocks produce anesthesia by injecting a large volume of 0.5% lidocaine into an exsanguinated limb with an inflated tourniquet. A Bier block is primarily used for the upper extremities, but is also suitable for surgical procedures of the distal forearm and hand. A history of Raynaud or sickle cell disease are contraindications to a Bier block. Before surgery, an intravenous line started in the dorsum of the operative hand is required. A second running intravenous line is started in the nonoperative arm. In the operating room the arm will be exsanguinated, a double tourniquet will be inflated, and 0.5% lidocaine will be injected. Local anesthetic is distributed systemically once the tourniquet is deflated, and anesthesia and analgesia will dissipate. The nurse should anticipate the administration of analgesics for postoperative pain and monitor the patient for signs and symptoms of local anesthetic toxicity.[30,31,40,43-46]

There is a low incidence of complications; however, cardiac arrest, seizures, compartment syndrome, nerve injury, thrombophlebitis, and bruising have been reported in the literature.[47]

Lower Extremity Peripheral Nerve Blocks

Anesthesia of the lower extremities requires blockade of the lumbar or sacral plexus, or both. The lumbar plexus is formed after the anterior rami of T12-L4 and emerges from their intervertebral foramina. It forms several nerves including the iliohypogastric, ilioinguinal, genital femoral, lateral femoral cutaneous, femoral, and obturator nerves (Fig. 25-11). The sacral plexus is formed by the ventral rami of L4-S4 and forms the gluteal and sciatic nerves.[30,31,40,45,46,48]

Femoral

The femoral nerve divides from the plexus and enters lateral to the femoral artery under the inguinal ligament. It is located below the fascia iliaca and lateral to the femoral artery and vein, which are located between the fascia lata and

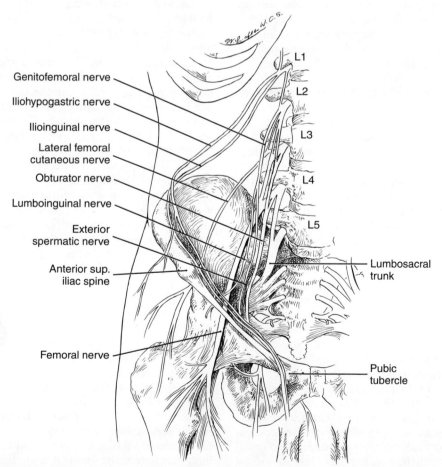

FIG. 25-11 Origin and position of nerves of the lower extremity. (From Nagelhout J, Plaus K, editors: *Nurse anesthesia,* ed 4, St. Louis, 2010, Saunders.)

iliaca. The femoral nerve innervates the quadriceps, pectineus, and sartorius muscles, providing sensation to the anterior and medial thigh as well as medial ankle and foot. Localized groin infections or a history of a femoral vascular graft are contraindications. This block can provide effective anesthesia and analgesia to the anterior portion of the leg including the thigh, knee, and medial ankle and foot along the saphenous nerve distribution. The block can be used in conjunction with a sciatic nerve block to effectively block the remaining portion of the leg innervated by the sacral plexus. Placement of peripheral nerve catheters allow for postoperative analgesia. Common approaches include peripheral nerve stimulator and ultrasound. Peripheral nerve stimulation relies on muscle contraction of the quadriceps and patellar movement. The patient is positioned supine and landmarks are identified, to include the anterior superior iliac spine and superior corner of the pubic tubercle identifying the inguinal ligament and femoral artery. The femoral nerve is located lateral to the artery. Complications include hematoma, local anesthetic toxicity, nerve trauma, and infection. Patients with a femoral nerve block should have a knee immobilizer placed and assisted with ambulation. Local anesthetics block the quadriceps and the patient is at risk for falls.[30,31,40,45,46,48]

Sciatic

The sciatic nerve is the largest nerve in the human body and originates from the sacral plexus (L4-S4). The sciatic nerve leaves the pelvis through the sacrosciatic foramen down the posterior portion of the buttocks and is located between the greater trochanter and ischial tuberosity. It provides innervation to the hamstrings and all the muscles below the knee. Sensory innervation includes the posterior portion of the knee as well as the lower leg with the exception of the medial portion of the lower leg, which is supplied by the saphenous nerve (a branch of the femoral nerve). The sciatic nerve has poor blood supply and is prone to trauma through pressure exerted through large volumes of local anesthetic, tourniquet, and positioning. Solutions containing epinephrine are avoided secondary to vasoconstriction. Diabetes and neuropathies are relative contraindications. Sciatic nerve blocks are placed with ultrasound or peripheral nerve stimulators. Single injection and peripheral nerve catheters may be placed. Nerve stimulator techniques rely on contraction of the hamstring or gastrocnemius muscle or dorsal–plantar flexion of foot, or both. Positioning of the patient varies and can include lateral decubitus position, lithotomy, or supine position. Major landmarks for a posterior approach include the greater trochanter, posterior superior iliac spine, and sacral hiatus. Landmarks for

a lithotomy approach include the ischial tuberosity and greater trochanter, whereas the anterior approach uses the inguinal ligament and greater trochanter. Complications include intraneural injection (resulting in foot drop), local anesthetic toxicity, and hematoma formation. It is important to position the patient so that pressure on the sciatic nerve injection site is reduced.[30,31,40,45,46,48]

Popliteal

The sciatic nerve divides into the common peroneal and tibial nerve 7 to 10 cm above the popliteal crease within the popliteal fossa. The lateral border of the fossa includes the biceps femoris while the semitendinosus and semimembranous form the medial border. Popliteal blocks provide surgical anesthesia and analgesia for the ankle and foot. The saphenous nerve provides sensory innervation to the medial ankle and foot and may be supplemented. Peripheral nerve stimulators and ultrasound are common techniques. Peripheral nerve stimulator use seeks motor movement of the ankle, foot, or toes. Patient positioning is either prone or supine. Local anesthetic solutions containing epinephrine are avoided. Contraindications and complications are similar to sciatic nerve block.[30,31,40,45,46,48]

Ankle

An ankle block is purely sensory and requires blockade of five nerves. Superficial, deep peroneal nerves and posterior tibial and sural nerves originate from the sciatic nerve. The saphenous nerve is a branch of the femoral nerve. Major landmarks include medial and lateral malleolus, posterior tibial artery, Achilles tendon, and flexor hallucis longus tendons. The patient is positioned supine. Ultrasound may be used, but this is a basic block and can be placed easily with landmarks. Solutions containing epinephrine are avoided because they may result in ischemia. Contraindications include infection, severe diabetes, and decreased blood flow to a compromised foot. Serious complications are unlikely. Patients should be cautioned that they can easily injure their foot, and care should be taken to avoid injury.[30,31,43,45,46]

SUMMARY

Regional anesthesia continues to be a mainstay of anesthetic care and postoperative analgesia. Continued progress in the knowledge of neural blockade, advances in pharmacology, and technology should serve to propel the use of regional anesthesia in the future. Perianesthesia nurses with a foundational knowledge of basic anatomy, common techniques, technology, and complications will be well equipped to manage patients under their watchful eyes.

REFERENCES

1. Kleinman W, Mikhail M: Spinal, epidural, & caudal blocks. In Morgan GE, et al, editors: *Clinical anesthesiology*, ed 4, New York, 2006, McGraw-Hill Medical.
2. Greensmith JE, Murray WB: Complications of regional anesthesia, *Curr Opin Anaesthesiol* 19: 531–537, 2006.
3. Venes D, editor: *Tabor's cyclopedic medical dictionary*, ed 20, Philadelphia, 2005, F.A. Davis.
4. Nagelhout J: Autonomic and cardiac pharmacology. In Nagelhout J, Plaus K, editors: *Nurse anesthesia*, ed 4, St. Louis, 2010, Saunders.
5. Olson RL, et al: Regional anesthesia: spinal and epidural anesthesia. In Nagelhout J, Plaus K, editors: *Nurse anesthesia*, ed 4, St. Louis, 2010, Saunders.
6. Brown C: Anesthetic agents and adjuncts. In Schick L, Windle PE, editors: *Perianesthesia nursing core curriculum: preprocedure, phase I and phase II PACU nursing*, ed 2, St. Louis, 2010, Saunders.
7. Drasner K, Larson MD: Spinal and epidural anesthesia. In Stoelting RK, Miller RD, editors: *Basics of anesthesia*, ed 5, Philadelphia, 2007, Churchill Livingstone.
8. Patton KT, Thibodeau GA, editors: *Anatomy & physiology*, ed 7, St. Louis, 2010, Mosby.
9. Reese CA: *Clinical techniques of regional anesthesia*, ed 3, Park Ridge, Ill, 2007, AANA Publishing.
10. Horlocker TT, et al: Regional anesthesia in the patient receiving antithrombotic or thrombolytic therapy, *Reg Anesth Pain Med* 35:64–101, 2010.
11. American Society of Regional Anesthesia (ASRA): *Consensus Statements*, available at http://asra.com/publications-anticoagulation-3rd-edition-2010.php. Accessed December 15, 2010.
12. Welliver D, et al: Lumbar epidural catheter placement in the presence of low back tattoos: a review of the safety concerns, *AANA J* 78:197–200, 2010.
13. The Joint Commission: *Accreditation program: hospital national safety goals*, available at http://www.jointcommission.org/patientsafety/nationalpatientsafetygoals/. Accessed November 29, 2010.
14. Margarido CB, et al: The intercristal line determined by palpation is not a reliable anatomical landmark for neuraxial anesthesia, *Can J Anesth* 58(3):262–266, 2011.
15. O'Connor G, et al: The effect of spinal needle design, size, and penetration angle on dural puncture cerebral spinal fluid loss, *AANA J* 75:111–116, 2007.
16. Fischer B: Techniques of epidural block, *Anaesth Intensive Care* 10: 552–556, 2009.
17. Guay J: The epidural test dose: a review, *Anesth Analg* 102:921–929, 2006.
18. Mulroy MF: Systemic toxicity and cardiotoxicity from local anesthetics: incidence and preventative measures, *Reg Anesth Pain Med* 27:556–561, 2002.
19. Kalil A: Unintended subdural injection: a complication of epidural anesthesia-a case report, *AANA J* 74:207–211, 2006.
20. American Society of PeriAnesthesia Nurses: Position statement 9: a position statement on safe medication administration. In American Society of PeriAnesthesia Nurses: *Perianesthesia nursing standards and practice recommendations 2010-2012*, Cherry Hill, NJ, 2010, ASPAN.
21. Baldini G, et al: Postoperative urinary retention: anesthetic and perioperative considerations, *Anesthesiology* 110:1139–1157, 2009.
22. Burns SM, et al: Unintentional hypothermia: implications for perianesthesia nurses, *J Perianesth Nurs* 24:167–176, 2009.
23. Boyle JAH, Stocks GM: Post-dural puncture headache in the parturient—an update, *Anaesth Intensive Care* 11: 302–304, 2010.
24. Apfel CC, et al: Prevention of postdural puncture headache after accidental dural puncture: a quantitative systematic review, *Br J Anaesth* 105:255–263, 2010.
25. Brull R, et al: Neurological complications after regional anesthesia: contemporary estimates of risk, *Anesth Analg*, 104:965–974, 2007.
26. Zaridc D, Pace NL: Transient neurologic symptoms (TNS) following spinal anesthesia with lidocaine versus other local anesthetics, *Cochrane Database Sys Rev*, 2, Art. No.: CD003006, 2009.
27. Redmond MC: Immediate postoperative assessment and postanesthesia assessment phase II. In Schick L, Windle PE, editors: *Perianesthesia nursing core curriculum: preprocedure, phase I and phase II PACU nursing*, ed 2, St. Louis, 2010, Saunders.
28. Fetzer SJ: Phase I discharge criteria. In Schick L, Windle PE, editors: *Perianesthesia nursing core curriculum: preprocedure, phase I and phase II PACU nursing*, ed 2, St. Louis, 2010, Saunders.
29. Yauger YJ, et al: Patient outcomes comparing CRNA-administered peripheral nerve blocks and general anesthetics: a retrospective chart review in a U.S. Army same-day surgery center, *AANA J* 78:215–220, 2010.
30. Burkard JF, Vacchiano CA: Regional anesthesia: upper and lower extremity blocks. In Nagelhout J, Plaus K, editors: *Nurse anesthesia*, ed 4, St. Louis, 2010, Saunders.
31. Gray AT, et al: Peripheral nerve blocks. In Stoelting RK, Miller RD, editors: *Basics of anesthesia*, ed 5, Philadelphia, 2007, Churchill Livingstone.
32. LaGrange P, et al: Application of the doppler ultrasound bloodflow detector in supraclavicular brachial plexus block, *BJ Anaesth* 50:965–967, 1978.
33. Neal JM, et al: The ASRA evidence based medicine assessment of ultrasound-guided regional anesthesia and pain medicine: executive summary, *Reg Anesth Pain Med* 35: S1–S9, 2010.
34. Liu SS, et al: Evidence basis for ultrasound-guided block characteristics: onset, quality, and duration, *Reg Anesth Pain Med* 35: S26–S35, 2010.
35. Neal JM: Ultrasound-guided regional anesthesia and patient safety: an evidence based analysis, *Reg Anesth Pain Med* 35: S59–S67, 2010.
36. McCartney CJL, et al: Evidence basis for the use of ultrasound for upper extremity blocks, *Reg Anesth Pain Med* 35: S10–S15, 2010.
37. Salinas FV: Ultrasound and review of evidence for lower extremity peripheral nerve blocks, *Reg Anesth Pain Med* 35: S16–S25, 2010.
38. Chan VWS, et al: Basic principles & physics of ultrasound. In Chan VWS, et al: *Ultrasound imaging for regional anesthesia*, ed 2, Toronto, 2008, Toronto Printing Company.

39. Falyar CR: Ultrasound in anesthesia: applying scientific principles to clinical practice, *AANA J* 78:332–341, 2010.

40. Moos DD: Understanding peripheral nerve blocks, *OR Nurse 2011* 5(5):24-32.

41. Brull R, et al: Practical knobology for ultrasound-guided regional anesthesia, *Regional Anesthesia and Pain Medicine* 35(2): S68–S73, 2010.

42. Hadzic A, Vloka JD: Peripheral nerve stimulators and nerve stimulation. In Hadzic A, Vloka JD: *Peripheral nerve blocks: principles and practice,* New York, 2004, McGraw-Hill.

43. McCamant KL: Peripheral nerve blocks: understanding the nurse's role, *J Perianesth Nurs* 21:16–23, 2006.

44. Neal JM, et al: Upper extremity regional anesthesia, essentials of our current understanding, *Reg Anesth Pain Med,* 34:134–170, 2009.

45. Morgan GE, et al: Peripheral nerve blocks. In Morgan GE, et al, editors: *Clinical anesthesiology,* ed 4, New York, 2005, McGraw-Hill.

46. Wedel DJ, Horlocker TT: Peripheral nerve blocks. In Longnecker DE, et al, editors: *Anesthesiology,* New York, 2008, McGraw-Hill Medical.

47. Guay J: Adverse events associated with intravenous regional anesthesia (Bier bock): a systematic review of complications, *J Clin Anesth* 21:585–594, 2009.

48. Enneking FK, et al: Lower-extremity peripheral nerve blockade: essentials of our current understanding, *Reg Anesth Pain Med* 30:4–35, 2005.

CONCEPTS IN ANESTHETIC AGENTS

26 Transition from the Operating Room to the PACU

Kay Ball, BSN, MSA, PhD, RN, CNOR, FAAN

The practice of nursing is directed toward the assessment, planning, implementation, and evaluation of the patient's care through a continuum of patient care services. Often the nurse is involved with the patient's transition from one level of care to another as the patient is transferred from one specialty area to another or from one unit to another. This transition of care is common in the surgical environment as perioperative nurses transfer care from the preoperative holding area to the intraoperative surgical suite, and perioperative nurses and anesthesia providers transfer the patient's care to a perianesthesia nurse at the completion of an operative procedure or treatment. Clear communication among these professionals is critical and directly affects the patient's postoperative response and outcome.

Modern care of the surgical patient is complex because advanced technology, minimally invasive techniques, new anesthetic agents, and increased patient comorbidities challenge perioperative nurses to communicate a comprehensive report when shifting the patient's care to the perianesthesia nurse. This chapter describes the importance of communication and what should be communicated when a patient is transitioned from the operating room to the postanesthesia care unit (PACU).

DEFINITIONS

Documentation of Handoff: Includes information about the patient's status, assessment notes, plan of care, nursing interventions, and a continuous evaluation of nursing care and patient responses.

Patient Handoff: Transfer of information about the patient so that the next health care provider can take responsibility for the patient's safety and care while ensuring that continuity of care is preserved.

Perianesthesia Care: Includes care of a patient undergoing a surgical procedure, intervention, or treatment that requires anesthesia or sedation during

the perianesthesia continuum: before (preanesthesia), after (postanesthesia phase 1, postanesthesia phase 2, extended care).

Perioperative Care: Includes care of a patient before (preoperative), during (intraoperative), and after (postoperative) surgery.

Verbal Report: Used for a "snapshot" or abbreviated synopsis of the patient status and care delivered.

Written Report: Provides a basis for verbal reports and is usually in the form of standardized operative or anesthesia records.

PERIOPERATIVE NURSING

According to the Association of periOperative Registered Nurses (AORN), the goal of perioperative nursing practice is "to assist patients and their designated support person(s) with achieving a level of wellness equal to or greater than that which they had before their operative or other invasive procedures."[1] At the core of the Perioperative Patient Focused Model is the patient surrounded by the four domains of "patient safety, physiological responses, behavioral responses of the patient and support person(s), and the health system in which the perioperative care is delivered."[1] Perioperative care is delivered by a nurse during the preoperative, intraoperative, and postoperative phases of the patient's surgical experience in a variety of environments, including hospital surgical suites, outpatient centers, catheterization suites, endoscopy units, radiation departments, clinics, physician offices, and other sites. The model for competency for perioperative nurses is evidenced through perioperative assessment, diagnosis, outcome identification, planning, implementation, and evaluation. "Standards, knowledge, judgment, and skills based on scientific principles"[1] serve as the solid foundation for perioperative practice. The perioperative nurse, therefore, has the requisite skills and knowledge to use the nursing process to design, coordinate, and deliver care to patients to meet their specific needs when their protective reflexes or self-care abilities are potentially compromised because of an operative or invasive procedure.[1] The care of the surgical patient continues through the transportation to the PACU, where this care is transferred to the perianesthesia nurse.

PERIANESTHESIA NURSING

According to the American Society of Peri-Anesthesia Nurses position statement on perianesthesia safety, characteristics of the culture of safety are identified by activities representing communication, advocacy, competency, efficiency, timeliness, and teamwork.[2] When a patient's care is safely transferred to another provider, these six characteristics are also present. Appropriate communication requires "ensuring a complete and systematic approach to hand-off processes and transfer of care and developing and using effective listening skills."[2] Advocacy mandates protecting the patient from injury and implementing best practices. This requires a complete understanding of the patient's condition and status by actively participating in the hand-off process. Competency involves clinical judgment and critical thinking as the care of the surgical patient is transferred to the perianesthesia nurse postoperatively. Patient hand-offs must be timely so that efficiency of care is encouraged. Finally, teamwork is vital so that the promise of safety can be guaranteed to the recovering patient.

According to the American Society of Peri-Anesthesia Nurses, the scope of perianesthesia nursing practice involves "age-specific assessment, diagnosis, intervention, and evaluation of individuals within the perianesthesia continuum. Those individuals have had or will have sedation/analgesia and/or anesthesia for surgical, diagnostic, or therapeutic procedures." The practice "is systematic, integrative, and holistic and involves critical thinking, clinical decision making, and inquiry. The specialty of perianesthesia nursing encompasses the care of the patient and family/significant other along the perianesthesia continuum of care – Preanesthesia, Postanesthesia Phase I, Phase II, and Extended Care."[3]

"Professional behaviors inherent in perianesthesia practice are the acquisition and application of a specialized body of knowledge and skills, accountability, and responsibility, communication, autonomy, and collaborative relationships with others."[3]

The perianesthesia nurse has a responsibility to the patient to provide quality care and safety. The American Society of PeriAnesthesia Nurses (ASPAN) *Perianesthesia Standards for Ethical Practice* state that the perianesthesia nurse "communicates pertinent information as the patient progresses through the continuum of perianesthesia care."[3] The nurse also has the professional responsibility to collaborate "with appropriate healthcare providers as needed to ensure optimum care."[3]

Evidence-Based Practice

A qualitative detailed observational study of 17 anesthesia providers and 15 nurses was conducted to determine how anesthesia providers hand over information to PACU nurses within a British health care system. The study also described the handover of professional responsibility for the patient. There were 45 handovers that were observed in an event-driven setting that is prone to distractions. The nurses and anesthesia providers had differing views as to the content and timing of the transfer of patient information. The actual transfer of responsibility depended on the patient's condition and the professional relationship between the physician and nurse. The handover information included the patient's intraoperative course and plans for management of the patient's care. Conclusions noted that most handovers in the PACU are largely informal, often with professional and organizational tensions. The nurse usually determines when he or she will take the responsibility from the physician for the care of the recovering patient. Formal standardized handovers usually will work best when the informal elements (trust, balance of power) and cultural factors are identified.

IMPLICATIONS FOR PRACTICE

Although handovers from an anesthesia provider to a postanesthesia care nurse are often standardized and formal, the informal elements and cultural factors must not be overlooked. For example, a PACU nurse usually sets the boundaries of when the responsibility of the patient's care can actually be safely shifted from the physician to the nurse. If the nurse is unsure of the patient's condition or believes that the anesthesia provider cannot safely leave the patient's side, then the PACU nurse intervenes and freely voices these concerns.

Source: Smith AF, et al: Interpersonal handover and patient safety in anaesthesia: observational study of handovers in the recovery room, *Br J Anaesth* 101:332–337, 2008.

NURSING CARE IN THE PACU

According to the *ASPAN Practice Recommendation 2*, "components of initial, ongoing, and discharge assessment and management" provides recommendations for the different phases of perianesthesia patient care. For example, when the patient's care is transferred from the perioperative nurse to the perianesthesia nurse in phase 1, the integration of the information about the patient should include[3]:

- Relevant preoperative status
- Anesthesia or sedation technique and agents
- Length of time anesthesia or sedation was administered; time reversal agents given
- Pain and comfort management interventions and plan
- Medications administered
- Type of procedure
- Estimated fluid and blood loss and replacement
- Complications that occurred during anesthesia course; treatment initiated; response
- Emotional status on arrival to the operating or procedure room

The perioperative nurse or the anesthesia provider should remain in the PACU until the PACU nurse accepts the responsibility of the nursing care of the patient. Patient safety is compromised when a patient is transferred to the PACU and abandoned by the transporting surgical team members before the perianesthesia nurse is able to assume the responsibility for that patient's care.

COMMUNICATION BETWEEN PERIOPERATIVE AND PERIANESTHESIA NURSES

Whether nurses describe their practices or roles as perioperative or perianesthesia, the basic foundation of nursing practice remains the same: high-quality care for the surgical patient. Therefore nurses who provide care during surgical procedures that involve sedation, analgesia, or anesthetics must work closely with nurses who provide care after the procedure to foster continuity, quality services, and desired patient outcomes.

Safe transportation of the surgical patient must be incorporated into the overall patient plan of care. The perioperative nurse must establish a safe environment for the transportation of the surgical patient with use of transportation safety devices, plans for special patient needs during transfer (e.g., oxygen needs), and active participation in the safe transportation of the patient. The patient's individual needs are determined so that the patient can be transferred without injury and without alteration in the patient's condition, such as changes in temperature, respirations, tissue perfusion, discomfort, or pain.

The transportation and transference of care of the surgical patient involves planning, collaboration, and communication between the perioperative and perianesthesia registered nurses. Communication between perioperative and perianesthesia nurses is essential for patient safety and appropriate and consistent nursing care. Both AORN and ASPAN have written recommendations on proper and accepted hand-off procedures.

AORN Recommended Practices for Transfer of Patient Care Information

AORN has published a recommended practice that specifically addresses the transfer of patient care information. This recommended practice provides guidance for perioperative nurses who are responsible for accurately transferring patient information to succeeding healthcare professionals, including perianesthesia nurses. AORN has also created a hand-off tool kit available to all AORN members that provides a companion resource to the recommended practices that are described as follows.[1]

- *Recommended practice I:* "A transfer of patient information process should be developed, standardized, and based upon the best available and most current evidence."[1] Reliability and accuracy of information is improved when standardization is enforced to prevent communication breakdowns. Everyone on the multidisciplinary team (perioperative nurses, perianesthesia nurses, anesthesia providers, surgeons, and others) should be involved with creating a format and process upon which a standardized transfer policy can be created. Written and verbal formats are both included in a successful patient transfer. When nurses use both verbal (like face-to-face interaction) and a standardized written form, data loss is minimal.[4] Actual transfers should be made in an environment that has minimal interruptions and extraneous sounds.
- *Recommended practice II:* "Patients, families, and significant others should have an active role in transfer of patient information processes whenever possible."[1] When families or support persons are kept informed about an impending patient transfer from surgery to PACU, anxiety is reduced and realistic expectations are promoted.
- *Recommended practice III:* "Personnel should receive education, training, and competency validation on effective communication skills and processes for the transfer of patient information."[1] Because communication problems

are often the cause of sentinel events, effective communication techniques and skills are mandatory.

- *Recommended practice IV:* "The perioperative registered nurse should document the process for the transfer of patient information using a standardized documentation format, and the document should be recorded and retained in a manner consistent with the health care organization's policies and procedures."[1] A standardized documentation tool promotes timely and accurate patient information and continuity of care.

- *Recommended practice V:* "Policies and procedures for standardized transfer of patient information processes should be developed, reviewed periodically, readily available in the practice setting,, and reflect the rules and recommendations from regulatory and accreditation bodies."[1] Policies and procedures guide practices within a health care facility, should emanate from evidence-based practices, and may often be used as the basis to validate competencies of practice.

- *Recommended practice VI:* "A quality management program should be implemented to evaluate and monitor the processes for the transfer of patient information. Components should include patient, process, and structural (e.g., format) outcome indicators. A fundamental precept of AORN is that it is the responsibility of professional perioperative registered nurses to provide safe, high-quality nursing care to patients undergoing operative and invasive procedures."[1] Quality review activities help to identify communication problems, practice issues, and practices that may need improvement. Evaluation efforts of transfer activities should be ongoing to ensure patient safety and compliance with evidence-based practices.

These recommended practices can be used when attempting to standardize patient transfer practices. Proper communication and documentation must be explored so that appropriate hand-off practices are accepted and enforced.

Hand-Off Communication

Patient hand-offs today are extremely variable and often lack purpose and structure.[5] In the past, *The Joint Commission's National Patient Safety Goals* included implementation of a standardized approach to hand-off communication. The 2011 National Patient Safety Goals note that communication errors can occur when patient care is transferred from one provider to another.[6] A standardized approach to patient hand-off must include a reconciled list of medications and this communication must also be documented.[6] Accurately communicating the patient's reconciled list of medications to the next provider "reduces the risk of transition-related adverse drug events."[6] The interface between the preoperative nurse to the operating room (OR) nurse and the OR nurse to the PACU nurse are crucial to continuity of care and safety for the patient. Standardizing a process in which all information about patient care is communicated in a consistent manner assures that the information about the patient will be accurate and pertinent.

During a comprehensive literature search, approximately 400 articles were reviewed that identified seven primary functions for patient hand-offs. These include[7]:

1. Information processing (transfer of patient data)
2. Highlighting deviations from stereotypical narratives (e.g., the patient is allergic to the preferred antibiotic that would be used to treat his or her condition)
3. Identification of erroneous assumptions and actions (e.g., a nurse questioning a surgeon or anesthesia provider about a specific patient order)
4. Accountability (e.g., transfer of responsibility and authority over the patient's care)
5. Social interactions (in support of interdisciplinary team communication and actions)
6. Distributed cognition (promoting the ease of transfer of up-to-date information to all professionals involved in the patient's care)
7. Cultural norms (negotiating and educating about hand-off procedures)

Hand-off information needs to be standardized and communicated in a logical and meaningful manner. Current literature notes that hand-off quality measures lack consensus regarding the primary purpose of the hand-off.[7] Basic principles of hand-off practices include written and verbal communication along with the essentials of documentation.

Different standardized documentation formats have been developed that have gained popularity in the United States. These formats are easy to remember as the letters represent the name of the step within the process of handing off a patient from one provider to another. The goal of these standardized formats is to reduce communication breakdowns. Some of these formats include[1]:

- SBAR: situation, background, assessment, recommendation
- I PASS the BATON: introduction, patient, assessment, situation, safety concerns, (the) background, actions, timing, ownership

- SURPASS: surgical patient safety system
- SHARED: situation, history, assessment, request, evaluate, document

The SBAR is one of the most popular and accepted standardized documentation formats today. This format can be used for patient hand-offs during the perioperative experience as shown in Box 26-1.

Written and Verbal Communication

Researchers have documented that approximately 20% to 30% of the information relayed during a patient hand-off is not documented in the medical record.[7] Written documentation provides a basis for verbal reports and is usually in the form of standardized operative or anesthesia records. AORN's recommended practice for *Documentation of Perioperative Nursing Care* notes that the "patient's record should reflect the perioperative patient's plan of care, including assessment, diagnosis, outcome identification, planning, implementation, and evaluation."[1] Documentation should include information about the patient's status, assessment notes, plan of care, nursing interventions, and a continuous evaluation of nursing care and patient responses. The written patient operative

---

BOX 26-1   **Sample of SBAR Format Used for Perioperative Patient Transfers**

PATIENT TRANSFER FROM PREOPERATIVE TO INTRAOPERATIVE PHASE
SITUATION
Patient transferred from holding area to OR #_____
Current surgical plan for patient: _____
BACKGROUND
Preoperative medications administered: _____
History and physical findings (including allergies): _____
ASSESSMENT
Pertinent laboratory findings: _____
NPO since: _____
IV site: _____
Fluids being administered: _____
Other pertinent information: _____
RECOMMENDATION
Chart in order (H & P and operative consent on chart): _____
    Name and phone of RN in Holding Area: _____
    Name of Receiving RN: _____

PATIENT TRANSFER FROM POSTOPERATIVE UNIT TO PATIENT ROOM
SITUATION
Surgeon: _____
Anesthesia: _____
Patient being transferred to patient room #_____
BACKGROUND
Medications administered in PACU: _____
Dressings/drains: _____
Operative notes: _____
ASSESSMENT
Vital signs: _____
O_2 saturation: _____
Pain level: _____
Nausea presence: _____
Comments on recovery course: _____
RECOMMENDATION
Equipment needed: _____
Rehabilitation: _____
Recovery notes: _____
    Name and phone of RN in PACU: _____
    Name of Receiving RN:_____

Modified from Sandlin D: Improving patient safety by implementing a standardized and consistent approach to hand-off communication, *J Perianesth Nurs* 22:289–292, 2007.

record facilitates communication and provides continuity of care and also serves as a legal record of the care provided.

A verbal report is used for a snapshot or abbreviated synopsis of the patient status and care delivered. The perioperative nurse should give direct and concise information about the surgical patient in a consistent and organized manner. The perianesthesia nurse must listen to the report and ask questions when appropriate. Effective listening involves more effort than speaking, because concentration is vital for processing of this critical information. Feedback by the perianesthesia nurse is often needed for clarification so that information is not misinterpreted.

For an examination of the issues of communication and documentation between the perioperative nurse and the perianesthesia nurse, the basic questions of why, when, where, who, how, and what must be explored.

- *Why?* Verbal reports highlight written documentation on the patient record. A written report records the details of the patient care, whereas a verbal report is a quick description or overview used when the patient's care is transferred to another nurse. This communication and documentation is vital so that continuity and safe patient care can be maintained.
- *When?* A formal written report begins with the admission of the patient for the surgical procedure and extends through discharge from the surgical arena. Written reports that document patient information before admission or after discharge may be added to the patient's chart. A verbal report from the perioperative nurse to the perianesthesia nurse begins with the call to the PACU to announce the completion of the surgical procedure and the request to transfer the patient to the PACU. At this time, any special needs must be communicated (i.e., ventilator needed). The verbal report continues when the patient is actually admitted to the PACU.
- *Where?* Ideally the written patient record is kept with the patient during transfer from the operating room into the PACU. The verbal report is given when the patient's care is transferred from the perioperative nurse to the perianesthesia nurse in the PACU. Sometimes with a recovering patient from the obstetric unit, the postanesthesia care can be delivered in an area outside the normal postanesthesia care unit. Wherever the postanesthesia care is given, the standards of care (including communication) are no different than

those used for nonobstetric surgical patients.[8]
- *Who?* Written patient reports are completed by the perioperative nurse, anesthesia provider, and surgeon (or a designee). Usually the verbal report is given by the anesthesia provider and the perioperative registered nurse. In a few surgical environments, the perioperative nurse may phone the perianesthesia nurse to give a report while the anesthesia provider and an orderly (patient care assistant) transfer the patient to the PACU. Ideally the perioperative nurse and anesthesia provider should both accompany the patient to the PACU. Sometimes the surgeon or the surgical assistant may also participate in the patient transportation and verbal report.
- *How?* The written patient record is documented on a health care facility–approved standardized form. The verbal report is usually given in person from one professional to another, but verbal reports have also been given via telephone or computer, depending on the patient acuity and facility protocols.
- *What?* The reporting of specific and appropriate information about the patient's surgical experience is critical. The perianesthesia nurse must receive the full details of the patient's condition, interventions, and plan of care so that continuity and safety can be maintained.

Care of certain patients, such as the patient recovering from cesarean section, can pose unique challenges. Documentation and verbal reports should alert the perianesthesia nurse to watch for signs and symptoms of adverse anesthetic effects, pulmonary problems, hemorrhage, infection, and other specific potential complications.[8] The care of a pregnant patient who is transferred from the operating room presents distinctive challenges because the status of the fetus must also be assessed, documented, and reported verbally.

Patient reporting when care is transferred from one provider to another should include but not be limited to:

- Type of surgery, length of surgery, complications encountered
- Vital signs and airway patency (e.g., oxygen saturation)
- Level of consciousness
- Muscular strength (e.g., mobility limitations)
- Allergies
- Condition of operative site and dressing
- Location and patency of tubes or drains
- Medications given and response to those medications (e.g., anesthetic agents and technique, reversal agents)

NURSING CARE IN THE PACU

- Intake and output (e.g., intravenous, estimated blood loss)
- Tests ordered, with pertinent results, if available
- Pain level
- Nausea and vomiting
- Psychosocial status (e.g., substance abuse, physical or mental impairments, prostheses)
- Discharge orders

Surgical team members, including the anesthesia provider, perioperative nurse, and surgeon (or designee including fellow, resident, or intern) participate in giving the report during transfer of the patient's care to the PACU nurse. Box 26-2 includes suggestions on what each professional should report.[9]

In the hustle and bustle of today's surgical environment, seemingly minor details that may have major effects on the patient's recovery can be disregarded or overlooked in the documentation and reporting during patient care transfer. For example, the perioperative nurse might not realize the importance of reporting the positioning used during a surgical procedure when transferring care to the PACU nurse. The following section explains why the documentation and reporting of patient positioning are so critical.

Documentation and Reporting of Patient Positioning

Documentation and reporting of positioning used during a surgical procedure may seem trivial and insignificant and often may be overlooked by the surgical team members. However, patient injuries from prolonged or improper positioning during the surgical procedure have been assessed and documented by astute PACU nurses. Practices recommended by AORN note that perioperative documentation should include "patient positioning and/or repositioning devices and supports, including immobilization devices used during the surgical procedure."[1]

The effects of improper positioning might not be immediately recognized in the operating room; therefore positioning must be documented and reported to allow the perianesthesia nurse to look for symptoms of potential problems. The results of improper positioning can be discovered during the assessment of various body systems, including the cardiovascular, skin, musculoskeletal, nervous, and respiratory systems. Positioning during a surgical procedure can influence breathing patterns, gas exchange, cardiac output, tactile sensory perception, mobility, and skin integrity. The perianesthesia nurse should assess the patient carefully with an understanding of the different systems that may be compromised from faulty positioning during surgery.

Cardiovascular

Cardiac output can indicate intraoperative positioning injuries and can easily be assessed with measurement of the patient's blood pressure. The

---

BOX 26-2   Suggestions on Topics for Report from Each Professional

ANESTHESIA PROVIDER MAY REPORT
- Patient name, allergies, surgical procedures performed
- Patient medical and surgical histories
- Current medications
- Anesthetic delivered
- Medications administered
- Regional anesthetic
- Intraoperative course (anesthesia-related)
- Lines, fluids, fluid losses
- Blood transfusions
- Pain management
- PACU orders
- Pertinent lab results
- Questions and answers

PERIOPERATIVE NURSE MAY REPORT
- Identify patient
- Preoperative diagnosis
- Procedure performed

- Drains, stomas
- Skin condition
- Surgical complications
- Allergies and reactions
- Patient warming devices used
- Medications, fluids, irrigations delivered by surgeon or RN
- Positioning surgery
- Isolation precautions, if present
- Communication of other pertinent issues (family or support persons waiting for information about the patient, special devices used by patient, patient deficits)
- Questions and answers

SURGEON MAY REPORT
- Immediate orders
- Diagnostic tests for PACU
- Interventions needed in PACU

Modified from Sullivan EE: Handoff communication, *J Perianesth Nurs* 22:275–279, 2007.
PACU, Postanesthesia care unit; *RN,* registered nurse.

following list provides some examples of how positioning in surgery can affect the patient's cardiovascular status after surgery:

- Hypotension or hypertension can be caused by the type of anesthesia administered, but can be intensified by specific positioning during a surgical procedure.
- Regional or general anesthesia may cause peripheral blood vessels to dilate (from the relaxation of the muscle lining of the blood vessels) and may lead to venous pooling, a decrease in circulating blood volume, and a fall in blood pressure if the extremities are in a dependent position.
- Reverse Trendelenburg, lithotomy, or jack-knife positions can contribute to venous pooling because of the dependent position of the lower extremities.
- Pooling of the blood in the trunk may be caused from unusual pressure on the abdomen from the thighs during the lithotomy position, which compresses the external iliac artery that distributes blood to the abdominal wall, external genitalia, and lower limbs.
- Lowered blood pressure may be the result of unusual pressure or tension on the major blood vessels, such as the inferior vena cava, from improper positioning or through the inappropriate positioning of deep retractors.
- Hyperabduction of the arm (greater than 90 degrees) can cause axillary and subclavian vessels to be stretched and compressed between the first rib and the clavicle, which can cause the radial pulse to be undetectable and could result in arterial thrombosis.

Skin

The skin is the largest organ of the body and the first line of defense against infection; therefore the skin must be inspected thoroughly by the perianesthesia nurse for determination of whether any positioning injury has resulted. The four potential positioning injuries that can cause skin problems are described in the following discussion.

Pressure

Pressure injuries are the most common skin injuries caused by inappropriate positioning. A lower pressure on the skin surface sustained for a prolonged time cannot be tolerated as easily as a greater pressure for a shorter time period. The PACU nurse should note the time surgery began to determine the possibility of the formation of pressure ulcers from lengthy surgical procedures.

If the patient's skin is thin, tissue can be easily compromised. With prolonged pressure, blood vessels may constrict and occlude and thus lead to possible ischemia, which is the first step in pressure ulcer formation. In a classic study, researchers showed that pressures of more than 32 mm Hg cause arterioles to constrict and occlude, thus leading to decreased nourishment and oxygenation of the capillary beds. Ischemia and microscopic necrosis can then result and cause pressure ulcerations.[10] Injuries from prolonged pressure may not be evident for hours or even days and may even be missed by the perianesthesia nurse. Because a pressure ulcer starts at a bony prominence and extends to the skin, manifestation at the skin level takes time; therefore a pressure ulcer may not be readily identified. Researchers have noted that one in every 12 patients who undergoes surgery for more than 3 hours can have at least one pressure ulcer develop within 4 days of surgery.[11]

Head injuries from pressure also may not be immediately evident in the PACU. With prolonged pressure on the scalp, localized postoperative alopecia may result. This condition can appear with a reddened area or may not be evident until days or weeks after the surgery. Pain and swelling can occur where the pressure has been applied during surgery. Repositioning of the head every 30 minutes during a procedure and in the PACU can minimize this problem.

Shearing

Shearing injuries occur when the skin stays stationary while the underlying tissue moves during patient positioning. The moving of tissue layers on each other causes the tissue and vessels to be stretched and damaged. The perianesthesia nurse may note that the skin integrity has been broken, or a redness or discoloration may occur when shearing injuries are sustained.

Friction

Friction injuries occur when the skin is moved across a rough surface during positioning or when the skin is rubbed with operating room devices such as a safety strap or face mask. The perianesthesia nurse may note that the skin has become abraded during a potential friction injury that could lead to inflammation, infection, and pain. Friction injuries may involve deeper levels of skin and tissues, which might not be immediately evident during the PACU experience.

Maceration

Maceration injuries are caused by prolonged contact of the patient's skin with fluids (e.g., pooling of preparation solutions, incontinence, sweat, or irrigants) during a surgical procedure. This contact with fluids causes the skin to weaken and become more vulnerable to pressure, shearing, or friction injuries. The perianesthesia nurse should consider maceration injuries if the skin integrity has been compromised.

Musculoskeletal System

The structural framework of the body skeleton consists of more than 200 bones that provide support and allow movement to occur. Unusual pressure or overextension of a joint or extreme positioning coupled with anesthesia agents that lead to relaxation can cause musculoskeletal injuries. Stretching of a joint or ligament can lead to increased pressure on an area, thus compromising the bone by decreasing the blood supply. The perianesthesia nurse may notice discoloration or redness over a bony prominence or joint that could indicate an injury. Moreover, the patient's subjective symptoms of pain in a specific joint might suggest a musculoskeletal problem.

Nervous System

The two components of the nervous system are the central nervous system and the peripheral nervous system. The peripheral nervous system is more vulnerable to positioning injuries with pressure and stretching of structures that leads to pain. These injuries can be temporary or permanent and may result in a disability. Neural injuries from positioning usually are delayed in discovery in the PACU, which makes tracing the original injury back to the surgical experience more difficult.

The most frequently injured nerves from positioning problems are the following:

- The ulnar nerve extends from the upper arm to the lower arm. When the compression of the ulnar nerve is near the elbow, a clawing effect of the fingers may be present.
- Lower extremity nerves in the legs can be injured by improper stirrup use or by improper use of positioning devices.
- The brachial plexus consists of a network of nerves from the clavicle down the upper arm. When the arm is overextended, a numbness or palsy of the hand, arm, or wrist can result.
- Lumbosacral nerves are located in the lower back region. When a patient is placed in the lithotomy position for a long procedure, the lumbosacral nerves can be stretched, thus leading to weakness of the quadriceps muscle or a sensory deficit in the anterior thigh area.

Respiratory System

If the lungs are not allowed to expand well because of positioning problems during a surgical procedure, the alveoli can begin to close, thus decreasing the exchange of respiratory gases. A pulse oximeter applied to the recovering patient in the PACU can be used to note any changes or respiratory problems that might have resulted from prolonged or improper positioning.

SUMMARY

Thorough communication from the perioperative professionals to the perianesthesia nurse is imperative and directly affects the outcomes in the care of the surgical patient. When written and verbal formats are used, continuity of patient care and attention to the details of the surgical event and the patient's responses to the interventions are vital to ensure a smooth transition from the intraoperative surgical suite into the PACU. The perioperative nurse must be diligent in observing what details to document and verbalize, and the perianesthesia nurse must be unfailing in listening and observing patient details that could indicate untoward responses to the surgical event. The importance of this critical part of communication within nursing should never be overlooked.

Florence Nightingale wrote in *Notes on Nursing* in 1860, "In dwelling upon the vital importance of sound observation, it must never be lost sight of what observation is for. It is not for the sake of piling up miscellaneous information or curious facts, but for the sake of saving life and increasing health and comfort."[12]

REFERENCES

1. Association of periOperative Registered Nurses: *Perioperative standards and recommended practices*, Denver, 2011, AORN.
2. American Society of PeriAnesthesia Nurses: *Position statement on perianesthesia safety*, available at https://www.aspan.org/ClinicalPractice/PositionStatements/PerianesthesiaSafety/tabid/3282/Default.aspx. Accessed March 27, 2011.
3. American Society of PeriAnesthesia Nurses: *Perianesthesia nursing standards and practice recommendations, 2010-2012*, Cherry Hill, NJ, 2010, ASPAN.
4. Pothier D, et al: Pilot study to show the loss of important data in nursing handover, *Br J Nurs* 14(20):1090–1093, 2005.
5. Van Eaton E: Handoff improvement: We need to understand what we are trying to fix, *The Joint Commission Journal on Quality and Patient Safety* 36(2):51, 2010.
6. The Joint Commission: *Accreditation program: hospital national patient safety goals, 2011*, available at http://www.jointcommission.org/assets/1/6/2011_NPSGs_HAP.pdf. Accessed March 27, 2011.
7. Patterson E, Wears M: Patient handoffs: Standardized and reliable measurement tools remain elusive, *The Joint Commission Journal on Quality and Patient Safety* 36(2): 52–61, 2010.

8. Torgersen K: Communication to facilitate care of the obstetric surgical patient in a postanesthesia care setting, *J Perianesth Nurs* 20(3):177–184, 2005.

9. Sullivan EE: Handoff communication, *J Perianesth Nurs* 22:275–279, 2007.

10. Kosiak M: Etiology and pathology of ischemic ulcers, *Physiol Med Rehabil* 40:60–69, 1959.

11. American Health Consultants: Are you overlooking your OR in the battle against pressure ulcers? *Wound Care* 3(6):61–63, 1998.

12. Nightingale F: *Notes on nursing* (an unabridged republication of the first American edition published by D. Appleton and Company in 1860), Toronto, 1969, Dover Publications.

27 Assessment and Monitoring of the Perianesthesia Patient

Lois Schick, MBA, MN, RN, CPAN, CAPA

The primary purpose of the postanesthesia care unit (PACU) is the critical evaluation and stabilization of patients after procedures, with an emphasis on the anticipation and prevention of complications that result from anesthesia or the operative or interventional procedure. A knowledgeable, skillful perianesthesia nurse must fully assess the condition of each patient not only at admission and at discharge but also at frequent intervals throughout the postanesthesia period. Assessment must be a continuous and complete process that leads to sound nursing judgment and the implementation of therapeutic care. Assessment includes the gathering of information from direct observation of the patient (the primary source), from the physician, other health care personnel, and from the medical record and the care plan. Traditionally perianesthesia nurses have, with only limited information, performed the role of caring for the surgical and interventional patients in the vulnerable postanesthesia state. However, for assessment of the perianesthesia patient and plan and implementation of appropriate care, preoperative information must be available as a basis for comparison with postoperative data. The perianesthesia nurse has a professional obligation to consider the patient's history, clinical status, and psychosocial state. The necessary data may be gathered with chart review, personal preoperative visit, and consultation with other health care members who provide care to the patient. The collection of such information should be a coordinated effort with all involved members of the health care team. This chapter discusses the assessment of postprocedure patients and their common needs. Specific assessments related to patient age, the type of procedure, and problems that result from complicated diagnoses are addressed in following chapters. The assessment and management of postoperative pain is presented in Chapter 31.

DEFINITIONS

Alveolar Artery Carbon Dioxide Differences: The difference between the $PaCO_2$ and the $ETCO_2$ level is referred to as the *alveolar-arterial CO_2 difference* (a-$ADCO_2$).

Alveolar Dead Space: Alveoli that do not participate in gas exchange because of lack of blood flow.

Anatomic Dead Space: Areas of the tracheobronchial tree not involved in gas exchange.

Capnography: Measurement of end-tidal carbon dioxide at the patient's airway that allows continuous assessment of the adequacy of alveolar ventilation.

Dead Space Ventilation: Includes anatomic, alveolar, and physiologic (total) dead space.

End-Tidal Carbon Dioxide ($ETCO_2$): At the end of exhalation, the peak carbon dioxide occurs, which in the normal lung is the best approximation of alveolar carbon dioxide levels.

Flow-Directed Pulmonary Artery Catheter (FDPAC): Pulmonary artery thermodilution catheter used in hemodynamic monitoring.

Hemodynamic Monitoring (Invasive Monitoring): The monitoring of blood flow through the use of invasive catheters to provide pressure measurements in the systemic and pulmonary circulations, central veins, pulmonary capillary bed, and the right or left atrium, as well as cardiac output.

Hyperthermia: A core temperature greater than 38° C (100.4° F).

Hypothermia: A core temperature less than 36° C (96.8° F).

Left Atrial Pressure: Measured with a catheter placed directly in the left atrium. Usually monitored only in open heart cases when direct access to the left atrium can be reached. In the absence of mitral valve disease or left atrial tumor, left atrial pressure reflects left ventricular end-diastolic pressure and left ventricle preload.

Obstructive Sleep Apnea: Repeated episodes of obstructive apnea during sleep together with daytime sleepiness, mood changes, and altered function.[1]

Physiologic Dead Space: The sum of anatomic and alveolar dead space.

Pulmonary Artery Pressure: Pressure in the pulmonary artery.

Pulmonary Capillary Wedge Pressure (PCWP): Also known as the *pulmonary capillary occlusive pressure;* reflects the pressure in the left atrium.

Pulmonary Vascular Resistance: The resistance, impedance, or pressure that the right ventricle must overcome to eject the blood into the pulmonary artery.

Pulse Oximetry: Pulse oximetry (SpO_2) is used for noninvasive measurement of arterial oxygen saturation (SaO_2) in the blood.

Right Atrial Pressure: Reflects venous return to the right side of the heart and right ventricular end diastolic pressure (preload).

Systemic Vascular Resistance: The resistance, impedance, or pressure the left ventricle must overcome to eject the blood from the left ventricle.

Temporal Artery Temperatures: Scanning of the forehead over the temporal artery with a noninvasive thermometer.

PREOPERATIVE ASSESSMENTS

The preoperative evaluation of both the physical and the emotional status of the surgical patient is extremely important, and nursing brings a unique perspective to this assessment. The scope of perianesthesia nursing practice involves the age-specific assessment, diagnosis, intervention, and evaluation of patients within the perianesthesia continuum. The scope identifies risks for problems that can result from the administration of sedation/analgesia or anesthetic agents for surgical, diagnostic, or therapeutic procedures.[2] Nurses in a number of subspecialties, including perianesthesia nurses, perioperative nurses, and general unit nurses, have advocated this assessment. A preoperative visit from each nurse who will care for the patient seems redundant and can be overwhelming for the patient. More appropriately, nurses should treat each other as colleagues who communicate needs for specific information, coordinate the collection of such information, and document data to be used for planning care. Multidisciplinary communications are instrumental in the education of all those who care for the patient and in the development of communication patterns.

Because many PACUs include preoperative holding areas, the perianesthesia nurse must participate in the patient's preoperative interview and assessment. A complete preoperative nursing assessment should include relevant preoperative physical and psychosocial condition, spiritual and cultural status, medical history (including anesthesia history), length of fasting, understanding of the procedure and postprocedure course, and the need for follow-up services. The preoperative physical assessment should include documentation of temperature, pulse, blood pressure, respirations, oxygen saturation, height, and weight and a review of systems. Nursing diagnoses are established on the analysis of data collected during the assessment phase and generation of an appropriate plan of care.

ADMISSION OBSERVATIONS

Physical assessment of the perianesthesia patient must begin immediately on admission to the PACU. The patient is accompanied from the procedure room to the PACU by the anesthesia provider or monitoring nurse, who reports to the receiving nurse on the patient's general condition, the procedure performed, and the type of anesthesia or sedation used. In addition, the nurse should be informed of any problems or complications encountered during the procedure and anesthesia or sedation (see Chapter 26). Because all anesthetics are depressants, postoperative assessment and care generally are the same, regardless of the specific agent used. For special precautions required for certain agents, review the chapters on anesthesia (see Chapters 19 through 25).

Rapid assessment of the life-sustaining cardiorespiratory system is of initial concern. The nurse ensures that the airway is patent and that respirations are free and easy; check and record the patient's blood pressure, pulse, rate of respiration, temperature, and oxygen saturation level; and quickly inspect all dressings and drains for gross bleeding. These baseline observations, which are made immediately on admission, should be reported to the anesthesia or sedation provider in attendance and recorded in the admission note.

After these initial observations are made, systematic assessment of the patient's total condition is essential. This assessment can be made from head to toe or by a systems review, whichever the individual nurse prefers. These observations are essentially identical, and each system of the body has an integral function, making all observations interrelated.

RESPIRATORY FUNCTION

Because the postanesthesia patient has had some interference with the respiratory system, maintenance of adequate gas exchange is a crucial aspect of care in the PACU. Any change in respiratory function must be detected early so that appropriate measures can be taken to ensure adequate oxygenation and ventilation. The most significant respiratory problems encountered in the immediate postoperative period include hypoventilation, airway obstruction, aspiration, and atelectasis.

Respiratory assessment is coupled with the related responses of the cardiovascular and neurologic systems for total evaluation of the adequacy of gas exchange and ventilatory efficiency. Respiratory function is evaluated with clinical assessment. Pulse oximetry is used for assessment of arterial oxygenation, and capnography is used in evaluation of the adequacy of alveolar ventilation. Arterial blood gas measurements may be a part of the respiratory assessment (see Chapters 12, 29, and 30).

NURSING CARE IN THE PACU

Clinical Assessment

Inspection

The resting respiratory rate of a normal adult is approximately 12 to 20 beats/min. Infants and children have a higher respiratory rate and a lower tidal volume than adults (see Chapter 49). Respirations should be quiet and easy and have a regular rate and rhythm. The chest should move freely as a unit, and expansion should be equal bilaterally. Alterations in symmetry can be caused by many factors, including pain, that may cause splinting at the incision site, consolidation, and pneumothorax. The nurse should note the character of the respirations; intercostal retractions, bulging, nasal flaring, or use of the accessory respiratory muscles, which are signs of respiratory distress. The depth of respiration is as important as the rate. Shallow respirations are the cardinal sign of continuing depression from anesthesia or preoperative medications, but can be caused by many other factors, including incisional pain, obesity, tight binders, and dressings that restrict movements of the thoracic cage or abdomen. Shallow respirations and use of the neck and diaphragmatic muscles may also indicate reparalyzation from the use of skeletal muscle relaxants such as succinylcholine, atracurium, pancuronium, and vecuronium. The presence of chest movements alone does not provide evidence that adequate gas exchange is occurring.

Airway obstruction may be present when the normal duration of inspiration versus exhalation is altered. Restlessness, confusion or anxiety, and apprehension are the earliest signs of hypoxemia and CO_2 retention and should receive immediate attention for determination of cause. The patient's color is regularly evaluated. Although this assessment is difficult to make, the results provide important information about the respiratory function. Cyanosis is a late sign of severe tissue hypoxia, and if it appears, immediate and vigorous efforts must be instituted to determine and correct the cause of hypoxia. The noninvasive monitors that are increasingly used in the PACU provide an effective means of continuous and objective assessment of gas exchange; pulse oximeters are used for monitoring hemoglobin oxygen saturation, and capnographs are used in evaluation of the adequacy of alveolar ventilation. A discussion of these monitors is forthcoming.

The presence of an artificial airway is noted; airways are used primarily to maintain a patent air passage so that respiratory exchange is not hampered. Five types of airways commonly used are: (1) the balloon-cuffed endotracheal tube (extends from the mouth through the glottis to a point above the bifurcation of the trachea); (2) the balloon-cuffed nasotracheal tube (extends from the nose to the trachea); (3) the laryngeal mask airway (inflatable silicone mask and rubber connecting tubing blindly inserted into the pharynx forming a low pressure seal around the laryngeal inlet); (4) the oropharyngeal airway (extends from the mouth to the pharynx and prevents the tongue from falling back and obstructing the trachea); and (5) the nasopharyngeal airway (extends from the nose to the pharynx). The airway must be kept clear of secretions for adequate gas exchange to occur, and suctioning may be needed if gurgling develops. The airway should not be removed until the laryngeal and pharyngeal reflexes return; these reflexes enable the patient to control the tongue, to cough, and to swallow. If the patient "reacts on the airway" (attempts to eject it), and gags, this can progress to retching and vomiting. The airway should be removed as soon as clinically possible in this instance to avoid aspiration.

An endotracheal tube can be removed as soon as the patient's condition is adequately reversed, the patient can maintain an airway without the tube, and the danger of aspiration is over. Determination of this point may be difficult; the decision of when a patient needs an airway is usually much easier than the decision of when such an adjunct is not needed. If PACU policy permits removal of an airway, insertion of an airway should definitely be included and both procedures should be accompanied by appropriate education and skill training for the nurses who perform them.

Listening and Auscultation

First, the perianesthesia nurse should listen unaided to the patient's respirations. Normal respiration should be quiet; noisy breathing indicates a problem. Extraneous sounds always indicate some kind of obstruction; however, quiet breathing does not always indicate the absence of problems. An accumulation of mucus or other secretions, evidenced by gurgling in any of the respiratory passages, can cause airway obstruction and should be removed immediately. Purposeful coughing with good expiratory airflow is the most effective method of clearing secretions. If the patient is not yet reactive enough to do this alone, the secretions must be suctioned orally and nasally. Nasotracheal suctioning may be useful to clear secretions and to stimulate cough, but the catheter is ineffective for reaching secretions distal to the carina. Obstruction can also occur from poor oropharyngeal muscle tone caused by the muscle-relaxant effect of general anesthesia plus the rolling back of the tongue. Patients with obstructive sleep apnea are prone to airway obstruction and should not undergo extubation until they are fully awake.

Tracheal extubation should be performed only when the patient is breathing spontaneously with adequate tidal volumes, oxygenation, and ventilation.[1,3] To relieve airway obstruction, use the jaw thrust maneuver by providing anterior pressure support on the angle of the jaw to open the air passages.

Crowing, a sudden violent contraction of the vocal cords, may indicate laryngospasm and can result in complete or partial closure of the trachea. Other signs and symptoms of laryngospasm include wheezing, stridor, reduced compliance, cyanosis, and respiratory obstruction. If spasms continue and are not broken with jaw thrust and positive pressure, succinylcholine may be administered with subsequent endotracheal tube insertion for maintenance of a patent airway. Total blockage of the airway caused by laryngospasm produces no sound because of the absence of moving air. Equipment and medications for management of a difficult airway should be readily available in the PACU.

Wheezing may indicate bronchospasm caused by a reflex reaction to an irritating mechanism. Bronchospasm occurs most often in patients with preexisting pulmonary disease, such as severe emphysema, reactive airway disease, pulmonary fibrosis, and radiation pneumonitis. Laryngeal edema after endotracheal intubation is not uncommon and can contribute significantly to airway obstruction. Acute changes in the patient's skin condition, cardiovascular status, and bronchospasm after regional anesthesia must alert the nurse to a possible rare allergic reaction.

The perianesthesia nurse should auscultate the patient's chest with a stethoscope for quality and intensity of breath sounds. Any abnormality should be located and identified and then described in the patient's medical record. Total absence of breath sounds on one side may signal the presence of pneumothorax (collapsed lung), obstruction, or fluid or blood within the pleural space. Auscultation of breath sounds in the PACU is often difficult because the patient usually cannot sit up or respond to commands to breathe deeply with the mouth open. Positioning the patient on alternating sides during the stir-up regimen provides an opportunity for examination of the posterior lung field.

Palpation

Palpation and inspection of the chest can be performed simultaneously for validation of observations such as symmetry of expansion. Crepitus and fremitus may be heard and felt. The temperature, the level of moisture and general turgor of the skin, and the presence of any edema should be noted.

Percussion

The normal sound over the lungs is resonance. Dullness heard where normally resonance should be heard indicates consolidation or filling of the alveolar or pleural spaces by fluid.

Monitoring of Oxygenation with Pulse Oximetry

A pulse oximeter is used for noninvasive measurement of arterial oxygen saturation (SaO_2) in the blood (SpO_2 when measured with pulse oximetry) and is a valuable adjunct to the clinical assessment of oxygenation. Many clinical indicators, such as the patient's color and the characteristics of the respirations, are subjective, and the physical signs of cyanosis are not evident until hypoxia is severe. Pulse oximetry monitoring is objective and continuous and provides an early warning of developing hypoxemia, thus allowing intervention before signs of hypoxia appear. Consequently, pulse oximetry has been widely adopted in the PACU as a tool for both safety monitoring and patient management. As a confirmation of the importance of pulse oximetry, the American Society of PeriAnesthesia Nurses (ASPAN) *PeriAnesthesia Nursing Standards and Practice Recommendations 2010–2012* recommends evaluation of all PACU patients with pulse oximetry at admission and discharge, and ASPAN recommends a pulse oximeter for every patient in all phases of perianesthesia nursing levels of care.[2]

A pulse oximeter consists of a microprocessor-based monitor and a sensor (Fig. 27-1). In addition

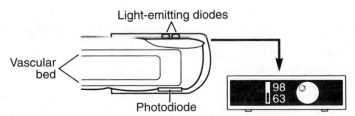

FIG. 27-1 Pulse oximeter uses two light-emitting diodes and photodiode to determine arterial hemoglobin saturation.

NURSING CARE IN THE PACU

to a SpO_2 display, most oximeters display the pulse rate and have an adjustable alarm system that sounds when values register outside a designated range. A variety of sensors is available, each intended for application to specific sites and for use on patients of various sizes (the manufacturer's instructions describe these requirements). The sensor is applied to a site with a good arterial supply. The most common application site is a finger or toe (hand or foot in neonates); other sites include the nose, the forehead, the earlobe, or the temple. Both reusable sensors and disposable adhesive sensors are available, and disposable sensors allow for patient-dedicated monitoring when infection control concerns are present.

Technology Overview

A pulse oximeter uses plethysmography for detection of the arterial pulse and spectrophotometry in determination of SpO_2. The pulse oximetry sensor incorporates a red and an infrared light-emitting diode as light sources and a photodiode as a light detector. In the most common type of sensor, a transmission sensor, the light sources and detector are positioned on opposite sides of an arterial bed, such as around the finger. In a reflectance oximetry sensor, they are positioned on the same surface, such as on the forehead.

With both transmission and reflectance sensors, red and infrared light passes into the tissue, and the detector measures the amount of light absorbed. Because oxyhemoglobin and deoxygenated hemoglobin differ in the absorption of red and infrared light, the detector can determine the percentage of oxyhemoglobin in the arterial pulse.

Applications

Pulse oximetry is used in many clinical settings for safety monitoring and as a patient management tool. As a safety monitor, a pulse oximeter detects hypoxemia caused by unanticipated events such as severe atelectasis, bronchospasm, airway displacement, disconnections or kinks in the breathing circuit, and cardiac arrest. As a patient management tool, pulse oximetry is valuable in titrating oxygen therapy, weaning a patient from mechanical ventilation, and evaluating response to medications or other interventions that are intended for improvement of oxygenation.

In addition to these broad applications, certain uses of pulse oximetry are of particular value in the PACU. For example, patients after surgery can become significantly hypoxemic during transport to or from the PACU. Pulse oximetry during transport can be used to diagnose undetected hypoxemia and to identify a need for supplemental oxygen. As indicated by the ASPAN standards, pulse oximetry is a valuable adjunct to clinical assessments in determination of readiness for PACU discharge. Some patients in the PACU judged to be stable and ready for transfer on the basis of clinical evaluation alone have been found to be hypoxemic after evaluation with pulse oximetry.

Interpretation of Pulse Oximetry Measurements

Consideration of the mechanisms of oxygen transport is essential for adequate interpretation of SpO_2. Approximately 98% of the oxygen in blood is bound to hemoglobin; SaO_2 and SpO_2 reflect this blood oxygen. The remaining blood oxygen is dissolved in plasma; blood gas analysis measures the partial pressure exerted by this oxygen dissolved in plasma ($PaO_2 = 80 - 100$ mm Hg at sea level). The dissolved oxygen is used to meet immediate metabolic needs. The oxygen bound to hemoglobin serves as the reservoir that replenishes the pool of dissolved oxygen (see Chapter 12).

The rate at which oxygen binds to hemoglobin is primarily controlled by two factors: the PaO_2 and the affinity of hemoglobin for oxygen. This relationship between SaO_2 and PaO_2 is represented by the oxyhemoglobin dissociation curve. The curve is sigmoid in shape, and its position is affected by a number of physiologic variables that change the affinity of hemoglobin for oxygen (Fig. 27-2).

Many factors that shift the oxyhemoglobin dissociation curve are commonly seen in patients in the PACU. For example, a patient with hypothermia may have a left-shifted curve. In such a patient, a given SpO_2 as measured with pulse oximetry may correspond to a lower than normal PaO_2. Although oxygen saturation may be adequate, hemoglobin has a greater affinity for oxygen and is less willing to release oxygen to meet tissue needs. Warming the patient to a normothermic range facilitates oxygen unloading from the hemoglobin molecule and helps to maintain adequate tissue oxygenation.

Clinical Issues

As with any technology, important clinical issues must be considered for appropriate use of pulse oximetry. Shifts in the oxyhemoglobin dissociation curve that are caused by abnormal values of pH, temperature, partial pressure of carbon dioxide (PCO_2), and 2,3-diphosphoglycerate must be considered. Consideration of the patient's hemoglobin level is also important because a pulse oximeter cannot detect depletion in the total amount of hemoglobin. When pulse oximetry is used on a postoperative patient with a low hemoglobin level, a high SpO_2 value might not reflect adequate oxygenation. The amount of hemoglobin,

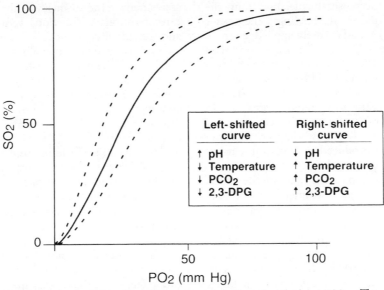

FIG. 27-2 Normal oxyhemoglobin dissociation curve is indicated with the *solid line*. This curve may shift (indicated with *broken lines*) whenever pH, temperature, PCO_2, or 2, 3-DPG values are increased or decreased. SO_2, Oxygen saturation; PO_2, partial pressure of oxygen; PCO_2, partial pressure of carbon dioxide; *2, 3-DPG*, 2, 3-diphosphoglycerate.

although it is well saturated with oxygen, may be inadequate to meet tissue needs because fewer carriers are available to transport oxygen.

Adequate oxygenation is a factor of not only adequate oxygen saturation and hemoglobin values but also of adequate oxygen delivery, which necessitates appropriate cardiac output, and the ability of the tissues to effectively use oxygen. Tissue hypoxia results when oxygen demand exceeds oxygen supply. Pulse oximetry readings therefore should be assessed in conjunction with all other indices of oxygenation.

Dysfunctional hemoglobin, variants of the hemoglobin molecule that is unable to transport oxygen, present a similar problem. Despite the high SpO_2 level, hemoglobin may be insufficient to carry oxygen. Carboxyhemoglobin is hemoglobin that is bound with carbon monoxide and therefore is unavailable for carrying oxygen. Its effect must be considered in patients with burns or in tobacco smokers with carbon monoxide poisoning. In methemoglobinemia, the iron molecule on the hemoglobin is oxidized from the ferrous to the ferric state. This form of iron is unable to transport oxygen. Methemoglobinemia, although rare, can occur in patients who receive nitrate-based and other drugs and in those who are exposed to a variety of toxins. When dysfunctional hemoglobins are suspected, assessment of oxygenation with pulse oximetry must be supplemented with arterial blood gas saturations measured with a laboratory cooximeter to determine whether dyshemoglobins are present and oxygenation is adequate.

Perfusion at the sensor application site must be sufficient for the pulse oximeter to detect pulsatile flow, which is an important consideration for some patients in the PACU, such as those treated with vasoconstrictors, those with marked hypothermia, and those with significantly reduced cardiac output. A well-perfused site should be selected for application of the sensor. If in doubt, the pulse and adjacent capillary refill can be checked.

If the monitor cannot track the pulse, the patient first is evaluated for adverse physiologic changes. Next, the perianesthesia nurse should ensure that blood flow is not restricted, such as by a flexed extremity, a blood pressure cuff, an arterial line, any restraints, or a sensor that is applied too tightly. Local perfusion to the sensor site can be improved by covering the site with a warm towel or with the use of a forced air warming device. Certain sensors, such as nasal sensors, are designed for application to areas where perfusion is preserved even when peripheral perfusion is relatively poor. Finally, some pulse oximeters use an electrocardiographic signal as an aid in identification of the pulse, thus enhancing the instrument's ability to detect a weak pulse.

Patient movement can produce false signals that interfere with the ability of the pulse oximeters to identify the true pulse, thus leading to unreliable SpO_2 and pulse rate readings. The sensor should be properly and securely applied; a sensor that is loosely attached or incorrectly positioned can magnify the effect of motion. If the problem persists, consideration should be given to moving the sensor to a less active site. Pulse oximeters that use the electrocardiographic signal as an aid in identification of the pulse can have an enhanced ability to distinguish between the true pulse and artifacts produced by motion. The result is more reliable SpO_2 readings.

Normally, venous blood is nonpulsatile and is not detected with a pulse oximeter. In the presence of venous pulsations, the SpO_2 value provided by the pulse oximeter may be a composite of both arterial and venous saturations. Venous pulsations can occur in patients with severe right-sided heart failure or other pathophysiologic states that create venous congestion and in patients receiving high levels of positive end-expiratory pressure. They can also occur when the sensor is placed distal to a blood pressure cuff or occlusive dressing and when additional tape is wrapped tightly around the sensor. When venous pulsations are present, the perianesthesia nurse should take care in interpreting the SpO_2 readings and, if possible, attempt to eliminate the cause.

Because pulse oximeters are optical measuring devices, the perianesthesia nurse must be aware of additional factors that can influence the reliability of SpO_2 readings. To ensure good light reception, the sensor's light sources and detector must always be positioned according to the manufacturer's specifications. In the presence of bright lights, such as infrared warming devices, fluorescent lights, direct sunlight, and surgical lights, the sensor must be covered with an opaque material to prevent incorrect SpO_2 readings. In addition, agents that significantly change the optical-absorbing properties of blood, such as recently administered intravascular dyes, can interfere with reliable SpO_2 measurements. The use of pulse oximetry with certain nail polishes, especially those that are blue, green, and reddish-brown in color, can result in inaccurate readings. If nail polish in these shades cannot be removed, the sensor should be applied to an alternate unpolished site.

Monitoring of Ventilation with Capnography

Monitoring of end-tidal carbon dioxide ($ETCO_2$) in respiratory gases provides an early warning of physiologic and mechanical events that interfere with normal ventilation. Capnography, which measures $ETCO_2$ at the patient's airway, is increasingly used in the PACU. It allows continuous assessment of the adequacy of alveolar ventilation, cardiopulmonary function, ventilator function, and the integrity of the airway and the breathing circuit. Consequently, it enables early detection of many potentially catastrophic events, including the onset of malignant hyperthermia, esophageal intubation, hypoventilation, partial or complete airway obstruction, breathing circuit leaks or disconnections, a large pulmonary embolus, and cardiac arrest.

Two variants of the instrument are available. A capnometer provides numeric measurement of exhaled CO_2 levels. A capnograph provides the same numeric information, and it also displays a CO_2 waveform. Both types of instruments usually incorporate an adjustable alarm system and often have trending and printing capabilities. The following discussion focuses on the use of capnographs because they allow more complete and effective patient assessment than do capnometers. As discussed subsequently, changes in the shape of the CO_2 waveform can provide crucial diagnostic information about ventilation, similar to the way in which the waveform provided with an electrocardiogram (ECG) can provide crucial diagnostic information about the heart.

Technology Overview

For measurement of exhaled CO_2, the most common type of capnograph passes infrared light at a wavelength that is absorbed by CO_2 through a sample of the patient's respiratory gas. The amount of light that is absorbed by the patient's gas reflects the amount of CO_2 in the sample.

Capnographs differ in the manner in which they obtain respiratory gas samples for analysis. Sidestream (or diverting) capnographs transport the sample through narrow-gauge tubing to a measuring chamber. Mainstream (or nondiverting) capnographs position a flow-through measurement chamber directly on the patient's airway. Special adapters are available to allow sidestream capnographs to be used on patients who are not intubated. The sample adapter should be placed as close to the patient's airway as possible.

Sidestream capnographs incorporate moisture-control features that are designed to minimize clogging of the sample tube, protect the measurement chamber from moisture-induced damage, and minimize the risk of cross contamination. The design of these moisture-control systems significantly affects a monitor's ease of use. Most systems rely on water traps, which must be emptied routinely. A new technology uses a special system of filters and tubing to dehumidify the sample and thus eliminate the need for water traps.

Capnographs also differ in calibration requirements. Many require removal of the patient from the respiratory circuit and adjustment of the instrument with special mixtures of calibration gases. Advanced capnographic technology includes automatic calibration and does not require any user calibration skills or time.

The Normal Capnogram

For effective use of capnography, it is important to understand the components of the normal CO_2 waveform (capnogram)—a square wave pattern with a plateau (Fig. 27-3). Early in exhalation, air from the anatomic dead space, which is virtually CO_2 free, is measured with the instrument. As exhalation continues, alveolar gas reaches the sampling site, and the CO_2 level increases rapidly. The CO_2 concentration continues to increase throughout exhalation and reaches the alveolar plateau because alveolar gas dominates the sample. At the end of exhalation, the $ETCO_2$ occurs, which in the normal lung is the best approximation of alveolar CO_2 levels. The CO_2 concentration then drops rapidly as the next inhalation of CO_2-free gas begins.

End-Tidal Versus Arterial Carbon Dioxide

In normal conditions, when ventilation and perfusion are well matched, $ETCO_2$ closely approximates arterial CO_2 ($PaCO_2$). The difference between the $PaCO_2$ and the $ETCO_2$ level is the alveolar-arterial CO_2 difference (a-$ADCO_2$). $ETCO_2$ is usually as much as 5 mm Hg lower than $PaCO_2$. When the two measurements differ significantly, an anomaly in the patient's physiology, the breathing circuit, or the capnograph is usually present. Significant divergence between $ETCO_2$ and $PaCO_2$ is often attributable to increased alveolar dead space. CO_2-free gas from nonperfused alveoli mixes with gas from perfused regions, thus decreasing the $ETCO_2$ measurement. Clinical conditions that cause increased

dead space, such as pulmonary hypoperfusion, cardiac arrest, and embolic conditions (e.g., air, fat thrombus, amniotic fluid), can increase the a-$ADCO_2$. Changes in the a-$ADCO_2$ can be used in assessing the efficacy of the treatment; as the patient's dead space improves, the partial pressure of the alveolar carbon dioxide less the partial pressure of arterial carbon dioxide ($PACO_2$ – $PaCO_2$) narrows. Increases in dead space ventilation lower $ETCO_2$ and therefore increase the $PaCO_2$ – $ETCO_2$ gradient. Widened $PaCO_2$ – $ETCO_2$ examples include embolic phenomena, hypoperfusion, and chronic obstructive pulmonary disease. Alternatively, a significant $PACO_2$ – $PaCO_2$ value can indicate incomplete alveolar emptying (e.g., with reactive airway disease), a leak in the gas-sampling system that allows loss of respiratory gas, and contamination of respiratory gas with fresh gas.[4]

Interpretation of Changes in the Capnogram

An abnormal capnogram provides an initial warning of many events that warrant immediate intervention. Abnormalities may be seen on a breath-by-breath basis or when the CO_2 trend is examined. For this reason, visualization is preferable of both the real-time waveform and the CO_2 trend on the monitor display. Examples follow for a look at changes produced by significant events that commonly occur in the PACU.

A sudden decrease in $ETCO_2$ to a near-zero level indicates that the monitor is no longer detecting CO_2 in exhaled gases (Fig. 27-4). Immediate action is crucial for detection and correction of the cause of this loss of ventilation. Possible causes include a completely blocked endotracheal tube, esophageal intubation, a disconnection in the breathing circuit, and inadvertent extubation. The latter three possibilities are particularly likely if the decrease in $ETCO_2$ coincides with movement

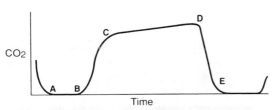

FIG. 27-3 Normal capnogram. **AB,** Beginning exhalation, dead space; **BC,** initial alveolar emptying; **CD,** end-alveolar emptying; **D,** end tidal CO_2; **E,** inspiration (CO_2-free gas).

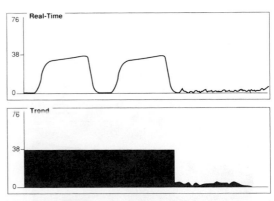

FIG. 27-4 Sudden decrease in $ETCO_2$ to near-zero level.

of the patient's head. First, after elimination of possible clinical causes for this decrease in $ETCO_2$, a clogged sampling tube or instrument malfunction is investigated as the cause of the problem.

An exponential decrease in $ETCO_2$ over a small number of breaths usually signals a life-threatening cardiopulmonary event that has dramatically increased dead space ventilation (Fig. 27-5). Sudden hypotension, pulmonary embolism, and circulatory arrest with continued ventilation must be considered.

A gradual increase in the $ETCO_2$ level while the capnogram retains its normal shape usually indicates that ventilation is inadequate to eliminate the CO_2 that is produced (Fig. 27-6). This situation can be the result of a small ventilator leak or a partial airway obstruction that reduces minute ventilation. It can also reflect increased CO_2 production associated with increased body temperature, the onset of sepsis, or shivering. Of particular importance, a large increase in $ETCO_2$ can be one of the earliest signs of malignant hyperthermia, which may not begin until after emergence from anesthesia.

A gradual decrease in the $ETCO_2$ level commonly occurs in the patient who is anesthetized, narcotized, hyperventilated, or hypothermic (Fig. 27-7).

Assessment of the capnogram can reveal information about the quality of alveolar emptying. For example, the patient with bronchospasm is unable to completely empty the alveoli, and the resulting capnogram does not have an alveolar plateau (Fig. 27-8). The $ETCO_2$ reported by the capnograph in this instance is not a good estimate of alveolar CO_2. Effective administration of bronchodilator therapy commonly improves alveolar emptying and results in a more normal capnogram.

Clinical Issues

In addition to the diagnostic usefulness of changes in the capnogram, some specific applications of capnography are particularly valuable in the PACU. Of primary importance is its ability to provide early warning of hypoventilation that, in the PACU, may be the result of anesthesia, sedation, analgesia, or pain. A falling $ETCO_2$ value may indicate pulmonary hypoperfusion from blood loss

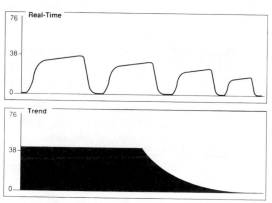

FIG. 27-5 Exponential decrease in $ETCO_2$.

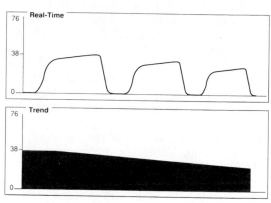

FIG. 27-7 Gradual decrease in $ETCO_2$.

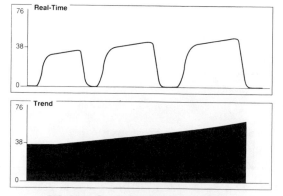

FIG. 27-6 Gradual increase in $ETCO_2$.

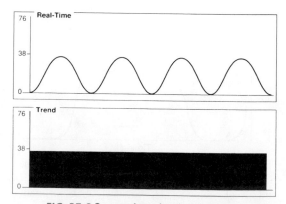

FIG. 27-8 Incomplete alveolar emptying.

or hypotension. During rewarming, $ETCO_2$ values are likely to increase as metabolic activity increases.

Capnography can signal when shivering produces an unacceptable increase in oxygen consumption and metabolic rate. During ventilator weaning, capnography is valuable in assessing adequacy of ventilation. Recent studies have shown the value of capnography in monitoring the course and efficacy of cardiopulmonary resuscitation (CPR). $ETCO_2$ measurements, which decrease during cardiac arrest, typically reach approximately 50% of normal levels during effective CPR. When spontaneous circulation is restored, $ETCO_2$ values increase dramatically. The presence and persistence of normal $ETCO_2$ values are also useful determinants in confirming tracheal intubation, because CO_2 is not normally found in the esophagus. However, capnography cannot be substituted for chest auscultation and radiography in elimination of the possibility of bronchial intubation.

Importantly in the PACU, capnography can provide critical information about the patient's ventilatory status, including an early warning of apnea that results in overall patient safety.[5] Deterioration of a patient is discernable 2 to 3 minutes earlier in a patient with an $ETCO_2$ reading than with oxygen saturation. Therefore capnography is a helpful assessment for patients who are extremely sedated, who require high doses of opioids, or who have obstructive sleep apnea.[6]

The ASPAN does not currently have a practice recommendation requiring continuous monitoring of $ETCO_2$ in the phase I PACU. Practice Recommendation 2, *Components of Initial, Ongoing, and Discharge Assessment and Management,* recommends that vital signs are monitored, to include "end-tidal CO2 (capnography) monitoring if available and indicated."[2,6]

CARDIOVASCULAR FUNCTION AND PERFUSION

The three basic components of the circulatory system that must be evaluated are: (1) the heart as a pump; (2) blood; and (3) the arteriovenous system. The maintenance of good tissue perfusion depends on a satisfactory cardiac output; therefore most assessment is aimed at evaluating cardiac output.

Clinical Assessment

Observe the overall condition of the patient, especially skin color and turgor. Peripheral cyanosis, edema, dilatation of the neck veins, shortness of breath, and many other findings may be indicative of cardiovascular problems. In addition to checking all operative sites for blood loss,

note the amount of blood lost during surgery and the patient's most recent hemoglobin level.

Blood Pressure Monitoring

Arterial blood pressure must be assessed in the preoperative physical assessment, on admission to and discharge from the PACU, and at frequent regular intervals during the PACU stay. Arterial blood pressure is the pressure of blood in the arteries and arterioles. It is a pulsatile pressure because of the cardiac cycle, and systolic (peak) and diastolic (trough) numbers are reported in millimeters of mercury. Arterial blood pressure is regulated by the vasomotor tone of the arteries and arterioles, the amount of blood entering the arteries per systole, and blood volume. The pressure is currently measured either noninvasively (indirectly) or invasively (directly). Noninvasive methods include manual cuff measurement with either an aneroid sphygmomanometer or automatic measurement with an electronic blood pressure monitor. Invasive measurement can be accomplished via an arterial line connected to a transducer. A clear understanding of proper technique is essential to ensure accurate and reliable readings with all the blood pressure measurement methods.

Noninvasive Measurement
Manual Method
An aneroid sphygmomanometer with inflatable cuff and stethoscope is needed for the standard auscultatory blood pressure measurement technique. The cuff is placed on the extremity around the arm or thigh. The pressure may be auscultated over the brachial artery of an arm cuff or popliteal artery at the ankle over the posterior tibial artery (just posterior to the medial malleolus). Systolic pressure in the legs is usually 20 to 30 mm Hg higher than in the brachial artery. Use of the correct cuff size is essential. The width of the inflatable bladder that is encased inside the cuff should be 40% to 50% of the upper arm or thigh circumference. A bladder that is too wide underestimates blood pressure, whereas a bladder that is too narrow overestimates blood pressure. The length of the cuff bladder should be at least 80% of the arm circumference.

The cuff is inflated, and when cuff pressure exceeds the arterial pressure, arterial blood flow ceases and the pulse is no longer palpated. As pressure is released with turning the valve of the inflation bulb, blood flow resumes and audible (Korotkoff) sounds are noted with the stethoscope. These sounds change in quality and intensity throughout further cuff deflation and generally disappear. Systolic pressure is noted as the first audible sound in the cuff-deflating process.[7] The diastolic pressure is marked by the disappearance of sounds in the adult patient and the muffling of sounds in the pediatric patient.

A common cause of error in blood pressure measurement is an auscultatory gap that may be present, especially in patients with hypertension. This gap is a silent interval between the systolic and diastolic pressures. During this gap, the pulse is palpable. Therefore, to avoid mistakenly low systolic readings, the cuff should be inflated until the pulse is obliterated. Blood pressure readings should be recorded completely, including the systolic pressure, the points at which the sounds become muffled and cease, and the range of the auscultatory gap, if present.

Auscultatory blood pressure measurements can be completed quickly and easily in many circumstances. The accuracy and reliability of the readings can be affected by low flow states (including decreased cardiac output and vasoconstriction) or decreased sound transmission caused by factors related to the patient (edema and obesity) or the environment (noise). Cuff size and placement, user error, and improperly calibrated manometers can also contribute to unreliable readings. Because measurements are intermittent and must be initiated by the user, blood pressure changes may go unnoticed in the postoperative patient with labile hemodynamics or sudden blood loss. The use of automatic blood pressure monitors that can be set to measure blood pressure at regular frequent intervals can minimize some of this risk. Single measurements do not adequately reflect a patient's blood pressure. Trending blood pressure readings is essential.

Automatic Method

Automatic blood pressure monitoring with electronic devices has become increasingly prevalent in the PACU. The devices are commonly used for frequent blood pressure measurements over relatively brief periods, when the need for arterial sampling is minimal to absent, and when the risks of arterial lines cannot be justified.

One of the most commonly used automatic noninvasive blood pressure methods is based on oscillometric technology. The cuff is chosen and applied according to conventional technique. Oscillations of the arterial wall are occluded as the cuff is inflated and are detected during cuff deflation. Systolic pressure is indicated at the onset of oscillations. As cuff pressure decreases, oscillations increase in amplitude and peak at the mean arterial pressure. The point at which oscillations disappear is the diastolic pressure (Fig. 27-9). All three pressures are normally reported on oscillometric monitoring devices.

Automatic noninvasive blood pressure monitors can be set to cycle at various measurement periods. The instruments alarm when systolic and diastolic pressures register outside of a preset range.

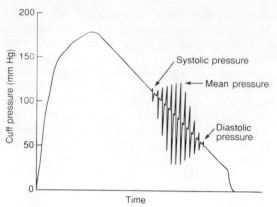

FIG. 27-9 Oscillometric blood pressure measurement. Systolic pressure is indicated at onset of oscillations. Mean arterial pressure occurs when oscillations peak in amplitude. Point at which oscillations disappear is diastolic pressure.

Equipment should be calibrated on a regular basis, and preventive maintenance should include assessment for leaks. The use of automatic devices may be limited in patients with low-flow states or high peripheral vascular resistance and in those who are severely obese or edematous. These devices provide only intermittent measurements and are less desirable for assessment of the patient who is labile.

Newer advances in noninvasive blood pressure technology, currently available for intraoperative monitoring of the patient who is anesthetized, include continuous monitoring capabilities that ensure detection in sudden blood pressure variations. The only other reliable method of continuous blood pressure monitoring currently available is invasive arterial blood pressure technology.

Invasive Measurement

Invasive arterial pressure measurements are most commonly obtained via cannulation of the radial artery, but can also be obtained at brachial or femoral sites. A continuous flush solution is connected to the intraarterial catheter and is slowly infused into the arterial vessel under pressure. The pressure within the artery is transmitted through the column of fluid via noncompliant pressure tubing to the transducer. The transducer then converts this pressure to an electric signal that can be converted to millimeters of mercury and displayed on the monitor. A corresponding arterial waveform, or pressure pulse, is also displayed on the monitor.

Arterial blood pressure measurements are continuous and are indicated for patients at high risk hemodynamically. Changes in patient pressures can be observed on an ongoing basis. This technology may also be chosen for patients in whom indirect measurements fail because of diminished or absent Korotkoff sounds (i.e., patients who are obese or edematous) and for those with high peripheral vascular resistance. The direct arterial access is also beneficial if the patient needs frequent blood samples for laboratory analysis.

To ensure more reliable arterial blood pressure readings, the clinician should level and zero the system according to the manufacturer's specifications. Level the transducer by positioning the open air reference stopcock at the fourth intercostal level at the midaxillary line, known as the *phlebostatic axis*. The air reference stopcock is when the stopcock is turned off to the patient and opened to air. Depressing the *0* button on the monitor balances the transducer to atmospheric pressure so that it reads 0 mm Hg. Once the monitor is zeroed, turn the stopcock so that it is open to the patient and pressure readings will appear. Aseptic technique must always be used during placement and maintenance of the arterial line and transducer.

Damping of the arterial waveform with subsequent unreliable readings may occur for a variety of reasons, including clotting and kinking of the arterial catheter, positioning of the catheter against the arterial wall, and the presence of air bubbles within the arterial line system. Loose connections, calibration error, and equipment failure can also contribute to unreliable readings. A square-wave test evaluates the dynamic response of the pressure monitoring system. To perform a square-wave test, activate the fast flush device for 1 to 2 seconds and note the monitor configuration. The patient wave form will be replaced with a square wave (Fig. 27-10).

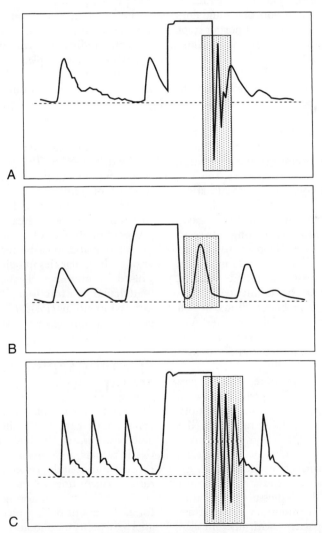

FIG. 27-10 Square wave test using the fast flush valve. **A,** Normal test and accurate waveform. **B,** Overdamped. **C,** Underdamped. (From Dennison RD: *Pass CCRN!* ed 3, St. Louis, 2007, Mosby.)

An Allen test should be performed before radial artery cannulation for minimization of the risk of hand ischemia (see Chapter 11). If arterial lines are discontinued in the PACU, constant pressure should be applied to the site for 5 to 10 minutes or until bleeding has ceased. A pressure dressing should be applied, and the site should be checked frequently for any bleeding and radial pulse palpation.

Complications and risks of invasive arterial blood pressure monitoring include infection, thrombosis, emboli, tissue ischemia, hemorrhage, and vessel perforation. Arterial blood pressure monitoring is generally contraindicated in patients with septicemia, coagulopathies, irradiated arterial sites, anatomic anomalies, inadequate collateral blood flow, or thrombosis. No intravenous solution or medications should be administered through the arterial pressure monitoring system at any time. If the catheter patency is in question, blood and fluid are aspirated from the blood drawing port or stopcock and the system is flushed with the fast flush device, not a syringe.[8]

Clinical Issues

For assessment of significance, blood pressure readings in the postoperative period must be compared with preoperative baseline measurements. A low postoperative blood pressure may be the result of a number of factors, including the effects of muscle relaxants, spinal anesthesia, preoperative medication, changes in the patient's position, blood loss, poor lung ventilation, and peripheral pooling of blood. The administration of oxygen to help eliminate anesthetic gases and to assist the patient in awakening causes an increase in blood pressure. Deep breathing, leg exercises, verbal stimulation, and conversation can be instituted to raise the blood pressure. A low fluid volume may be augmented by increasing the rate of intravenous fluids, which helps to maintain the arterial pressure. Any method designed to raise the pressure must be instituted with consideration for the patient's overall condition.

An increase in blood pressure after surgery is common because of the effects of anesthesia, respiratory insufficiency, or decreased respiratory rate and depth that cause CO_2 retention. The surgical procedure, with the accompanying discomfort, also causes increased blood pressure. Emergence delirium, with its excitement, struggling, and pain, may also be a causative factor in a transient increase in blood pressure. Obviously, determining the cause is important before treatment is instituted. In patients with uncontrolled hypertension, continuous intravenous antihypertensive medications may be necessary. However, diagnosis of the cause of the hypertension is extremely important so that effective therapy can be administered rapidly.

Pulse Pressure Monitoring

Pulse pressure is an important determinant in the evaluation of perfusion. Because of the pulsatile nature of the heart, blood enters the arteries intermittently, causing pressure increases and decreases. The difference between the systolic and diastolic pressures equals the pulse pressure. The pulse pressure is affected by two major factors: the stroke volume output of the heart and the compliance (total distensibility) of the arterial tree. The pulse pressure is determined approximately by the ratio of stroke output to compliance; therefore any condition that affects either of these factors also affects the pulse pressure.

For accurate evaluation of the patient's cardiovascular status, all signs and symptoms must be evaluated individually and within the body system as a whole. For example, cool extremities, decreased urine output, and narrowed pulse pressure may be indicative of decreased cardiac output, even in the presence of normal blood pressure.

Pulses

The rate and character of all pulses should be assessed bilaterally. The pulses should be examined simultaneously for determination of equality at time of arrival. Peripheral arterial occlusion is not uncommon; if it is suspected, a Doppler instrument can be of great value in detecting the presence or absence of blood flow. Occlusion is an emergency and must be reported to the surgeon at once. Irregularities in pulse are most commonly caused by premature beats, generally premature ventricular contractions (PVCs) or premature atrial contractions (PACs). These irregular rhythms should be thoroughly investigated before therapy is initiated.

ELECTROCARDIOGRAPHIC MONITORING

The perianesthesia nurse must have a basic understanding of cardiac monitoring and should be able to interpret the basic cardiac rhythms and dysrhythmias and correlate them with expected cardiac output and its effects on the patient's condition. According to the most recent ASPAN standards, ECG monitoring should be performed for each patient during phase I level of care, and an ECG monitor should be readily available for patients in preanesthesia and phase II level of care areas.[2] Dysrhythmias of any type can occur at any time and in any patient during the postoperative period; therefore accurate ECG monitoring and interpretation are mandatory skills for the perianesthesia nurse. This section is designed to provide an introduction to specific problems of cardiac monitoring in the PACU.

Any type of cardiac dysrhythmia may be seen in the PACU. The causes of specific dysrhythmias must be carefully differentiated before any treatment is instituted. Some commonly encountered problems are reviewed here, but the list is by no means complete.

All abnormal rhythms should be documented with a rhythm strip and recorded in the patient's progress record. Any questionable rhythms should be documented with a complete 12-lead ECG. Electric monitoring of the patient's heart is only one assessment parameter and must be interpreted in conjunction with other salient parameters before therapy is initiated. Cardiac monitors generally depict only a single lead. They do not detect all rhythm disturbances and alterations, and a 12-lead ECG is essential for accurate definition of a conduction problem.

Lead Placement

The skin where the electrode will be placed should be clean, dry, and smooth. Excessive hair is removed; moisture or skin oils are removed with soap and water or alcohol, and the skin is mildly abraded to obtain good adherence of the electrode.

Site selection on the chest is based on a triangular arrangement of positive, negative, and ground electrodes. Placement of electrodes directly over the diaphragm, areas of auscultation, heavy bones, or large muscles is avoided. Adequate space for application of defibrillator paddles is allowed in the event that defibrillation should become necessary. Fig. 27-11 depicts the most commonly used electrode leads. Lead II is the most commonly used in the PACU because it is the most versatile; it is useful in assessing P waves, P-R intervals, and atrial dysrhythmias. The modified chest lead I is useful

for assessing of bundle branch block and differentiation between ventricular dysrhythmias and aberrations. This lead is useful when the patient is known to have preexisting cardiac disease. The Lewis lead is useful when P waves are difficult to distinguish with other leads and is used to detect atrial flutter when it is suspected clinically but not demonstrated on the ECG.

Sinus Dysrhythmias
Sinus Bradycardia

Fig. 27-12 shows a slow heart rate, less than 60 beats/min. Sinus bradycardia is a rhythm with impulses that originate at the sinus node at a rate of less than 60 beats/min. Its rhythm may be irregular because of accompanying sinus dysrhythmias. All other complex features are normal.

Sinus bradycardia is commonly encountered in the PACU because of the depressant effects of anesthesia. It can occur normally during sleep, and young healthy adults, especially those who are normally physically active, often have bradycardia. Usually no treatment is necessary except continuation of the stir-up regimen. Excessive parasympathetic stimulation from pain may cause bradycardia, in which case appropriate analgesics and other pain-relieving measures should be initiated. If the patient shows symptoms of low cardiac output, notify the physician; treatment may be initiated with atropine to block vagal effects or epinephrine and dopamine to stimulate the cardiac pacemaker. If temporary pacing wires are available, either atrial or ventricular pacing can be attempted. Bradycardia in conjunction with hypotension is considered an ominous sign for a pediatric trauma patient in shock, because the major component of cardiac output in small children is the heart rate.[9]

Sinus Tachycardia

Fig. 27-13 shows a fast heart rate (greater than 100 beats/min). The rhythm may be slightly irregular; all other complex features are normal.

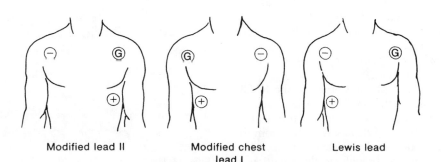

Modified lead II   Modified chest   Lewis lead
                          lead I

FIG. 27-11 Basic electrode placement.

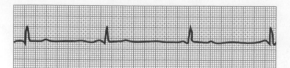

FIG. 27-12 Sinus bradycardia (lead III).

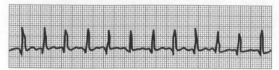

FIG. 27-13 Sinus tachycardia (lead I).

Sinus tachycardia results from any stress and may be encountered in the PACU because of numerous causes, particularly factors relating to an increase in sympathetic tone, including the stress of surgery, anoxia, fever, overhydration, hypovolemia, pain, anxiety, apprehension, or any combination of these factors. Tachycardia is an important postoperative sign and should be fully evaluated before treatment is instituted. Increasing tachycardia is an early sign of shock and must be thoroughly investigated. Treatment must be specific and based on removal of the underlying cause. The patient should be assessed carefully for the ability to tolerate the rapid rate. The deleterious effects of tachycardia are generally related to diminished stroke volume and cardiac output. In general, the patient with previously normal cardiac function can tolerate tachycardia as high as 160 beats/min without manifestation of symptoms. Poor tolerance with a resultant decrease in cardiac output occurs when the diastolic interval, and thus the ventricular filling time, is significantly compromised. Interventions for the compromised condition include beta-adrenergic blockers such as metoprolol and atenolol or calcium channel blockers such as verapamil.

Sinus Arrest (Atrial Standstill)

Sinus arrest is failure of the sinoatrial (SA) node to discharge, with the resulting loss of atrial contraction. The rate remains within normal ranges. The rhythm is regular except when the SA node fails to discharge. P waves and QRS complexes are normal when the SA node is firing and absent when it fails to discharge.

Common causes of sinus arrest in the PACU are the depressant effects of anesthesia or analgesics and electrolyte disturbances. Treatment is aimed at elimination of depressant drugs from the body and correction of electrolyte imbalances. This dysrhythmia must be brought to the attention of the physician immediately, because persistent sinus

arrest constitutes an emergency and CPR must be initiated.

Supraventricular Dysrhythmias

Supraventricular dysrhythmias are abnormalities in the rhythm of the heart caused by ectopic impulses originating from the SA node, atria, and atrioventricular junction. Supraventricular dysrhythmias occur in 10% to 40% of patients after coronary artery bypass graft surgery. These rhythms should be documented with a 12-lead ECG. Their cause has been related to a number of possible factors, such as an inflammatory reaction to surgical trauma, insufficient protection of the atria during surgery, atrioventricular node ischemia, and sudden withdrawal of beta blockers. A correlation exists between persistent atrial activity during cardioplegia and postoperative supraventricular dysrhythmias.

Premature Atrial Contraction

Premature atrial contraction, or atrial premature beat, occurs earlier than expected as a result of an irritable focus in the atrium (Fig. 27-14). Cardiac rate and rhythm are normal except for the prematurity. The P wave configuration of the premature beat usually differs from that of the normal beat. The PAC is followed by a pause that is not fully compensatory. This dysrhythmia results from anxiety and is commonly encountered in the PACU. No treatment is necessary unless the PACs become frequent or the patient becomes symptomatic. Pharmacologic therapy may become necessary with agents such as digitalis, beta blockers, or verapamil if hemodynamic function is impaired.

Atrial Tachycardia

Atrial tachycardia is a rhythm disturbance that is a rapid regular supraventricular heart rate that results from an irritable focus of five or more PACs in succession (Fig. 27-15). The rate is 150 to 200 beats/min with a regular rhythm.

Premature beat

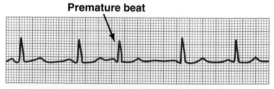

FIG. 27-14 Atrial premature beat (lead I).

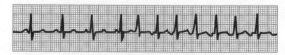

FIG. 27-15 Atrial paroxysmal tachycardia: onset in middle of record (lead I).

This rhythm should be documented with a full 12-lead ECG. The physician should be notified for institution of therapy. Maneuvers that enhance vagal tone such as the Valsalva maneuver and carotid sinus massage may be successful in termination of this dysrhythmia. Antiarrhythmic agents such as digitalis, quinidine, and verapamil may cause atrial tachycardia to revert to normal sinus rhythm. Adenosine can be used to stop atrial tachycardia, and quinidine or procainamide can be used to establish normal sinus rhythm. If these measures are unsuccessful, synchronized cardioversion is necessary.

Atrial Flutter

Atrial flutter consists of rapid supraventricular contractions that result from an ectopic focus with varying degrees of ventricular blocking (Fig. 27-16). Its cause is the same as that of PAC and atrial tachycardia. The rhythm is usually regular; the atrial rate is 250 to 350 beats/min. Treatment is the same as for atrial tachycardia.

Atrial Fibrillation

In atrial fibrillation, one or more irritable atrial foci discharge at an extremely rapid rate that lacks coordinated activity (Fig. 27-17). Atrial fibrillation occurs commonly in patients with atrial enlargement from mitral valve disease or from long-standing coronary artery disease and is often preceded by PACs, tachycardia, or flutter. Clinically, the patient has an irregular heartbeat, pulse rate, and usually, a noticeable pulse deficit. Cardiac output decreases in varying degrees. Normally, atrial filling and contraction account for 30% of ventricular filling. Without this atrial filling, or "atrial kick," of volume into the ventricle, stroke volumes and thus cardiac outputs are diminished. Treatment involves digitalis, quinidine, verapamil, atrial pacing, ablation, or cardioversion.

Ventricular Dysrhythmias

Myocardial ischemia and perioperative myocardial infarction remain the two major causes of ventricular dysrhythmias; however, bradycardia, hypokalemia, hypoxemia, acidosis, and hypothermia are also potential causes.

Premature Ventricular Contraction

Premature ventricular contraction is a rhythm disturbance that involves an earlier-than-expected ventricular contraction from an irritable focus in the ventricle (Fig. 27-18). The rhythm is regular except for the premature beat, and the rate is normal.

The P wave is absent from the premature beat. A wide, bizarre, notched QRS complex that may be of greater-than-normal amplitude is present. A widened T wave of greater-than-normal amplitude is present after the premature beat and is of opposite deflection to that of the QRS complex.

The PVC is followed by a pause that is fully compensatory (i.e., the time of the PVC plus the pause time equals the time of two normal beats). PVCs are commonly encountered in the PACU and can occur in any patient. Occasional PVCs occur normally and need no treatment. Multiple PVCs may indicate inadequate oxygenation; when they occur, the patient's respiratory status should be assessed thoroughly. Other causative factors of PVCs include electrolyte disturbances, acid-base

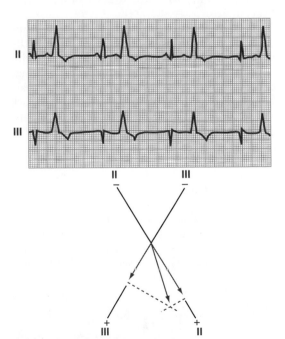

FIG. 27-18 Premature ventricular contractions (leads II and III). (From Hall J: *Guyton and Hall textbook of medical physiology*, ed 12, Philadelphia, 2011, Saunders.)

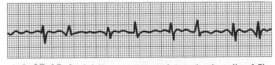

FIG. 27-16 Atrial flutter: 2:1 and 3:1 rhythm (lead I).

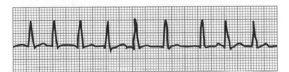

FIG. 27-17 Atrial fibrillation (lead I).

NURSING CARE IN THE PACU

imbalance, drug toxicity, and hypoxemia of the myocardium.

Treatment of PVCs is based on the underlying cause and obliteration of the irritable focus. Occasional isolated PVCs need not be treated. If PVCs occur more frequently than five per minute, if a successive run of two or more occurs, if they are multifocal, or if they occur during the vulnerable period on the ECG complex, they must be treated because they are the precursors of the more lethal ventricular dysrhythmias.

Ventricular dysrhythmias present in the setting of bradycardia should be treated with atropine or with overdrive pacing for elimination of ventricular escape rhythms.

Ventricular Tachycardia

Three or more consecutive PVCs constitute ventricular tachycardia (Fig. 27-19). The rhythm is fairly regular, and P waves are not seen. Occasionally, patients may have ventricular tachycardia and be asymptomatic, but usually they have anxiety, palpitations, fluttering, pounding in the chest, dizziness, faintness, and precordial pain. If ventricular tachycardia is prolonged, cyanosis, mental confusion, convulsions, and unconsciousness develop as a result of decreased blood and oxygen supply to the brain.

The causative factors of ventricular tachycardia are essentially the same as those for PVCs. Most commonly, ventricular tachycardia in the PACU is the result of hypoxia, drug toxicity, or underlying heart disease.

Ventricular tachycardia must be treated immediately. If the patient initially tolerates the dysrhythmia, treatment should be instituted with amiodarone or lidocaine. If the patient has cardiac decompensation and circulatory insufficiency, cardioversion with direct current electric countershock should be immediately instituted. Immediate notification of the physician is essential.

Ventricular Fibrillation

Ventricular fibrillation is characterized by a rapid irregular quivering of the ventricles that is uncoordinated and incapable of pumping blood (Fig. 27-20). This rhythm disturbance is the major death-producing cardiac dysrhythmia. The immediate initial treatment is external direct current countershock (Fig. 27-21). Ventricular fibrillation may

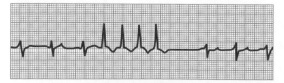

FIG. 27-19 Ventricular paroxysmal tachycardia (lead III).

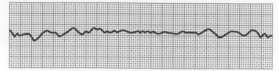

FIG. 27-20 Ventricular fibrillation (lead II).

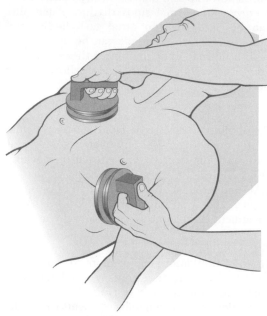

FIG. 27-21 Emergency administration of external direct-current countershock. (From Miller RD, Pardo Jr MC: *Basics of anesthesia*, ed 6, Philadelphia, 2011, Saunders.)

occur spontaneously without any forewarning, or it may be preceded by evidence of ventricular irritability. Patients in whom ventricular fibrillation is likely to develop include those with underlying heart disease, those with ventricular irritability in the operating room during surgery, and those with symptoms of shock. All these patients should be monitored continuously throughout the recovery period. If ventricular fibrillation is not immediately terminated with countershock, CPR and a cardiac code must be initiated without delay (see Chapter 57).

HEMODYNAMIC MONITORING

Although more prominent in cardiac surgery, hemodynamic monitoring using pulmonary artery catheters are commonly used with patients of higher acuity who receive care in many PACUs. Minimally invasive monitoring techniques include use of the esophageal Doppler, arterial pressure-based cardiac output, impedance cardiography, or ultrasound cardiac output monitoring. These minimally invasive techniques reflect cardiac output and assessment of fluid requirements by volumetric means.

Hemodynamic monitoring can be accomplished via the following invasive lines: a flow-directed pulmonary artery catheter, a central venous pressure catheter, a left-atrial or right-atrial catheter, a pulmonary artery thermistor catheter, or a peripheral arterial catheter (A-line). The parameters obtained from these various lines, the catheter insertion sites, and the placement and monitoring methods are presented in Table 27-1 and depicted in Fig. 27-22.

Problems associated with maintenance of these lines are summarized in Table 27-2.

Right-Atrial Pressure

The normal right-atrial pressure ranges from 2 to 6 mm Hg. Pressures that exceed that level can be the result of fluid overload, right-ventricular failure, tricuspid valve abnormalities, pulmonary hypertension, constrictive pericarditis, or cardiac tamponade. Values in the lower range are usually indicative of hypovolemia.

Table 27-1 Methods for Invasive Monitoring of Hemodynamic Parameters

PARAMETERS	CATHETER PLACEMENT	INSERTION SITES	MONITORING METHOD	SPECIAL CONSIDERATIONS
RAP	Proximal port of FDPAC lies in right atrium	Brachial, jugular, subclavian	Water manometer	Intermittent readings at lowest fluctuation*
	Distal end of RAC or CVP lies in right atrium	Direct insertion through right atrial wall[†]	Transducer[‡]	Intermittent or continuous readings on mean[§]
PAP	Distal end of FDPAC lies in right or left branch of pulmonary artery	Brachial, jugular, subclavian	Transducer	Readings on systole and diastole
	Distal end of PATC lies in main pulmonary artery	Direct insertion through pulmonary artery wall[†]		
PCWP	Inflation of balloon on tip of FDPAC allows it to float into wedged position in smaller branch of pulmonary artery	Brachial, jugular, subclavian	Transducer	Intermittent readings on mean[§]
LAP	Distal end of LAC lies in left atrium	Direct insertion through left atrial wall[†]	Water manometer	Intermittent reading recorded at lowest fluctuation*
MAP	Distal end of catheter lies in peripheral artery	Radial, brachial, femoral	Aneroid manometer	Midpoint of needle fluctuation
			Transducer	Continuous readings on mean[§]

Adapted from Dennison R: *Pass CCRN!* ed 3, St. Louis, 2007, Mosby; Schick L, Windle PE, editors: *Perianesthesia nursing core curriculum: preoperative phase I and phase II PACU nursing*, ed 2, St. Louis, 2010, Mosby.

RAP, Right-atrial pressure; *FDPAC*, flow-directed pulmonary artery catheter; *RAC*, right-atrial catheter; *CVP*, central venous pressure; *PAP*, pulmonary artery pressure; *PATC*, pulmonary artery thermistor catheter; *LAC*, left-atrial catheter; *PCWP*, pulmonary capillary wedge pressure.

*Fluctuation indicates patent catheter and good position in thorax.

[†]Direct insertion is achieved during open chest procedure via median sternotomy incision. Exit site is via a stab wound at distal portion of median sternotomy. Catheter is attached to skin with suture. Removal is achieved with removal of the suture and application of gentle traction to the catheter to free it from the chamber wall. The catheter is sutured to the chamber wall with an absorbable suture so that it releases easily. Chest tubes remain in place until such lines are removed because of the possibility of bleeding.

[‡]To convert mm Hg to cm H_2O, multiply mm Hg reading times 1.36.

[§]Biphasic waves are measured on mean.

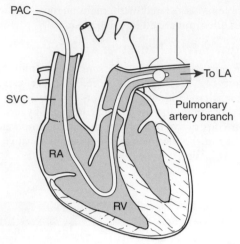

FIG. 27-22 Schematic view of anatomy of pulmonary catheterization. (From Papadakos P, Szalados J: *Critical care: the requisites in anesthesiology*, St. Louis, 2005, Mosby.)

Pulmonary Artery Pressure

Pulmonary artery systolic pressures normally range from 15 to 30 mm Hg, whereas a normal pulmonary artery diastolic pressure is 5 to 15 mm Hg. Mean pulmonary artery pressures range from 10 to 20 mm Hg. Hypovolemia contributes to low pressure readings. Increased volume loads that can develop with an atrial or ventricular septal defect or left-ventricular failure can create elevations in pressure. In addition, obstructions to forward flow that can be caused by mitral stenosis or pulmonary hypertension can lead to an elevation in pulmonary artery pressures.

Pulmonary Capillary Wedge Pressure

Normal pulmonary capillary wedge pressure (PCWP) recordings are between 8 and 12 mm Hg. Values in this range can be caused by an increased volume load, as is seen in left-ventricular failure, or they can be created by an obstruction to forward flow. Such obstructions may be caused by

Table 27-2	Potential Problems Associated with Invasive Hemodynamic Monitoring	
POTENTIAL PROBLEMS	**ETIOLOGY**	**PRECAUTIONS AND TREATMENT**
Alterations in Pressure Wave Configurations		
Dampened tracings	*Technical*	
	Air in system	Check system for bubbles; flush bubbles out of system.
	Disconnection in system	Inspect and tighten all connections. Check that stopcocks are positioned correctly and covered with dead-end stopcock port covers (no holes).
	Kinked catheter	Remove dressing to ascertain whether catheter is kinked externally.
	Catheter tip against wall	Turn patient's head or reposition extremity in which that catheter is inserted; watch for improvement in tracing. Gently aspirate catheter from various angles to determine at which angle best flow is achieved; tape and redress catheter at angle at which best flow is achieved. Gently flush catheter in an attempt to push tip away from vessel wall. Never flush catheter in which clotting is suspected.
	Physiologic	
	Clot on catheter tip	Attempt to aspirate blood from catheter. If possible, keep aspirating until clot is retrieved or blood no longer seems thickened, then flush system until line is cleared and readable tracing reappears. If blood cannot be aspirated, do not flush system and notify physician.
	With FDPAC, this may also indicate that catheter has advanced forward and is in wedged position*	Ensure balloon is deflated. Recheck system and line. If no improvement, obtain chest radiograph and notify physician.

Table 27-2   Potential Problems Associated with Invasive Hemodynamic Monitoring—cont'd

POTENTIAL PROBLEMS	ETIOLOGY	PRECAUTIONS AND TREATMENT
Abrupt exaggeration of pressure tracings	*Technical* Loss of calibration of level of transducer	Re-zero and re-level transducer. Check that balloon has not accidentally inflated. Check for dysrhythmia.
	Physiologic Slippage of catheter out of chamber or vessel	Avoid traction on intravascular lines; tape catheter to skin or secure with suture.
	FDPAC slipping from pulmonary artery to right ventricle; characterized by systolic pressure that remains same while diastolic pressure falls into range of right-ventricular end-diastolic pressure	Inflate balloon in an attempt to let catheter float back into pulmonary artery. If catheter does not migrate back into pulmonary artery, obtain chest radiograph and notify physician.
	RAC, PAC, or PATC has slipped out of vessel wall into thoracic cavity	Attempt to aspirate to see whether catheter is still in vessel. If blood returns, flush system and attempt to obtain readable pressure tracings. If no blood return is achieved, notify physician and remove catheter, per protocol.

Alterations in Vascular Integrity

POTENTIAL PROBLEMS	ETIOLOGY	PRECAUTIONS AND TREATMENT
Venous and arterial spasms	Trauma to vessels during prolonged insertion attempts; artery irritated by catheter	Apply local anesthetic to catheter surface or administer anesthetic via intravenous route. Use guidewire to facilitate insertion. Cool catheter to make it less flexible and easier to insert.
Thrombophlebitis	Irritation to vessels from prolonged insertion attempts or from constant motion of catheter against vessel	See Venous and Arterial Spasms, discussed previously. Secure catheter in place with either tape or suture. Avoid prolonged infusions of chemically irritating medications. Maintain adequate dilutions and observe for signs and symptoms of phlebitis and change flush solution bag before it empties. Notify physician for possible withdrawal of catheter. Distal placement of stopcocks, connecting catheters, and tubing permits atraumatic blood sampling and flushing.
Embolization	Clot embolization from thrombophlebitis or from clot on catheter tip	Always aspirate catheter first if clot is suspected. *Never flush.*
	Pulmonary embolism with infarct from FDPAC	Observe for changes in chest radiograph that indicate pulmonary embolization.
	Cerebral embolization from LAC	Observe for neurologic changes that may indicate embolization from LAC.
	Peripheral embolization with extremity ischemia from peripheral arterial lines	Observe for ischemic changes of extremity in which catheter is located.
Air embolization	Loose connections	Secure and tighten all connections. Vigilantly observe LAC, because even minute amounts of air in this system can lead to serious neurologic complications.
	Rupture of balloon on FDPAC caused by overinflation	Inflate balloon slowly, and do not overinflate. Limit inflations. Allow balloon to empty air passively back into syringe. Avoid aspirating air back because this weakens integrity of balloon. Aspirate only if air fails to return passively. If air does not return and rupture is questioned, sterile saline solution can be injected into balloon and attempts made to aspirate it back. Failure to aspirate fluid back indicates leak; physician should be notified.

NURSING CARE IN THE PACU

Continued

Table 27-2   Potential Problems Associated with Invasive Hemodynamic Monitoring—cont'd

POTENTIAL PROBLEMS	ETIOLOGY	PRECAUTIONS AND TREATMENT
Vessel erosion or hemorrhage	Inadequate hemostasis after insertion	Apply firm pressure for 15 to 20 minutes.
Bleeding from insertion site: Rupture of branch of pulmonary artery	Overinflation of balloon in normal-sized vessel	Do not attempt to inflate balloon if tracing already appears wedged. Inject only prescribed amount of air into balloon.
	Normal inflation of balloon in too-small vessel	Inject air slowly, and stop injecting if resistance is felt. Inject only amount of air necessary to obtain wedge tracing.
	Repeated normal inflations in brittle or susceptible vessel	Limit wedge intervals in patients at high risk, such as patients with pulmonary hypertension or long-standing mitral valve disease.
Atrial dysrhythmias	Irritation of right atrium from RAC or during insertion of FDPAC	Withdraw CVP catheter to level of superior vena cava, and obtain readings from that area. Continue with insertion of FDPAC because dysrhythmias are usually self limiting and stop once catheter tip exits right atrium.
Ventricular dysrhythmias	Irritation of right ventricle from tip of FDPAC during insertion procedure or from catheter tip slipping out of pulmonary artery and back into right ventricle	Continue with insertion of FDPAC because dysrhythmias are usually self limiting and stop once catheter passes into pulmonary artery. If catheter tip falls back into right ventricle from pulmonary artery, inflate balloon because this cushions tip of catheter and may alleviate dysrhythmias. Administer antidysrhythmic if ventricular dysrhythmias continue. Notify physician, obtain chest radiograph, and manipulate catheter, per hospital policy.

Infections

Local infection	Faulty aseptic techniques during insertion or during subsequent dressing changes	Maintain sterility during insertion. Change dressings with sterile technique and tubings, per hospital policy.
Systemic infection	Faulty aseptic technique during insertion	Avoid spasms during insertion. Avoid development of thrombophlebitis along vessel. Change indwelling catheters and insertion sites every 48 to 72 hours, which may be impossible in patients with difficult vascular access sites. In these situations, rethreading new catheter over guidewire at previous insertion site can be done every 48 to 72 hours. However, once site is questionable or patient has symptoms of sepsis develop, such as elevated temperatures and white blood cell count, new line at new site is necessary.
Endocarditis	Extension of local insertion site; infection along catheter and into circulation	Culture per hospital policy. Observe for development of new murmurs.

Adapted from Cole D, Schlunt M: *Adult perioperative anesthesia: the requisites in anesthesiology*, Philadelphia, 2004, Mosby; and Dennison R: *Pass CCRN!* ed 3, St. Louis, 2007, Mosby.
RAC, Right-atrial catheter; *PATC*, pulmonary artery thermistor catheter; *LAC*, left-atrial catheter. *FDPAC*, flow-directed pulmonary artery catheter; *CVP*, central venous pressure.
*Wedging of catheter in postoperative patient may be common occurrence for two reasons: (1) catheter may have advanced forward during operative procedure when chest was open and lungs were not fully inflated, because less resistance to forward advancement was found; and (2) as hypothermia is reversed and patient and catheter rewarm, its increased flexibility may allow it to float forward.

mitral stenosis, mitral regurgitation, or pulmonary embolism. Lower values may result from hypovolemia or indicate an obstruction to left-ventricular filling, which could occur with a pulmonary embolism, pulmonary stenosis, or right-ventricular failure.

Left-Atrial Pressure

Normal left-atrial pressures range from 8 to 12 mm Hg. As is seen with the PCWP, elevations in left-atrial pressure are associated with volume overloads or obstructions to forward flow, the latter of which may consist of left-ventricular failure states, mitral or aortic valve dysfunctions, or constrictive pericarditis. Lower recordings are generally a consequence of hypovolemia from inadequate volume or are related to an obstruction to forward flow. Such an obstruction may be a pulmonary embolism or pulmonic valve stenosis, or it may result from right-ventricular failure.

Mean Arterial Pressure

Normal mean arterial pressures generally range between 80 and 120 mm Hg. In a postoperative cardiac surgical case, pressures less than 60 mm Hg are generally avoided because coronary artery filling may be limited or impeded when parameters reach this level and may contribute to an ischemic or infarction state. Conversely, pressures greater than 120 mm Hg are avoided because they place too much stress on newly created suture lines that could readily rupture with sustained pressures.

Cardiac Output and Cardiac Index

Cardiac output is the amount of blood ejected by the ventricle in 1 minute. Normal cardiac output is 4 to 8 L/min; it is calculated with the following formula:

$$SV \times HR \times CO$$

in which SV is stroke volume, HR is heart rate, and CO is cardiac output.

Cardiac index is calculated with the following formula:

$$CO / BSA = CI$$

in which BSA is body surface area in square meters and CI is cardiac index. Normal CI ranges from 2.5 to 4 Lmin/m^2. Because CI takes body size into consideration, it is a better indicator of the patient's perfusion status.[1,6,8,9]

Systemic Vascular Resistance

Systemic vascular resistance (SVR) is the resistance the left ventricle must work against to eject its volume of blood. Normal SVR is 900 to 1400 dynes/s/cm^{-5}. An elevated SVR can create enough resistance to left-ventricular ejection that cardiac output and cardiac index decrease, which leads to a state of hypoperfusion or shock. Infusion of vasodilators and afterload-reducing agents can counteract this elevation. SVR is calculated with the following formula:

$$SVR = (MAP - CVP) \times 80/CO$$

in which MAP is mean arterial pressure and CVP is central venous pressure.[1,8,10,11]

Pulmonary Vascular Resistance

Pulmonary vascular resistance (PVR) is the resistance the right ventricle must work against to eject blood into the pulmonary bed. Normal PVR is 80 to 240 dynes/s/cm^{-5}. An elevated PVR can create enough resistance to right-ventricular ejection that right-sided failure or infarction can develop. Infusion of vasodilators or pulmonary artery dilators such as aminophylline can counteract these elevations. PVR is calculated with the following formula:

$$PVR = [PAM - (PCWP \text{ or } LAP)] \times 80/CO$$

in which PAM is pulmonary artery mean pressure and LAP is left-atrial pressure.[1,8,10,11]

CENTRAL NERVOUS SYSTEM FUNCTION

All anesthetics affect the central nervous system (CNS), and one can assume for the present, although it is not known exactly how narcosis occurs, that anesthetics are general nonselective depressants. The complexity of the CNS, coupled with our incomplete knowledge of how it functions, makes it a most difficult system to evaluate.

Assessment of the CNS in the PACU generally involves only gross evaluation of behavior, level of consciousness, intellectual performance, and emotional status. A more detailed assessment of CNS function is necessary for patients who have undergone CNS surgery; that discussion occurs in Chapters 10 and 38.

Emergence from Anesthesia

Patients arrive in the PACU at all levels of consciousness, from fully awake to completely anesthetized. With modern anesthesia techniques, however, most patients respond appropriately by the time they are established in the PACU and become oriented quickly when the stir-up regimen is begun (see Chapter 28). With the use of fluorinated and opioid anesthetics, emergence is generally quiet and uneventful. Occasionally, a patient becomes agitated and thrashes about; this situation seems to occur more often in adolescents and young adults than in patients of other age groups. Emergence delirium also tends to occur more frequently in patients who have undergone intraabdominal and intrathoracic procedures (see Emergence Excitement in Chapter 29).

The perianesthesia nurse can facilitate patient orientation by telling the patient where he or she is, that the surgery is over, and what time it is as a part of the stir-up regimen. Reorientation occurs in reverse order from anesthesia; the patient first becomes oriented to person, then place, then time. This order, of course, may not hold true for the patient who was somewhat confused or disoriented before surgery, which emphasizes the importance of recording accurate information about the mental status of the patient before anesthesia.

Alterations in cerebral function are often the first signs of impaired oxygen delivery to the tissues; therefore an orderly and periodic assessment of mental function is necessary for detection of early evidence of abnormal cerebral function. Restlessness, agitation, and disorientation in the PACU can be ascribed to a number of other causes and are often difficult to evaluate. The use of continuous pulse oximetry can assist the perianesthesia nurse in determination of whether symptoms may be related to hypoxemia.

THERMAL BALANCE

The measurement of the patient's body temperature in the PACU is particularly important. The most recent ASPAN standards state that, at minimum, the preoperative assessment, initial postoperative physical assessment, and discharge evaluation of the patient in phases I and II Level of care should include documentation of temperature.[2] Normal body temperature may vary from 36° to 38° C (96.8° to 100.4° F). In the healthy adult, body temperature remains fairly constant because of the balance between heat production and heat loss. Alterations in body temperature occur often in the postoperative patient. Factors that affect the body temperature in the PACU patient are listed in Box 27-1.

Premedications, anesthesia, and the stress of surgery all interact in a complex fashion to disrupt normal thermoregulation. Both hypothermia (temperature less than 36° C) and hyperthermia (temperature greater than 38° C) are associated with physiologic alterations that may interfere with recovery (Box 27-2). Patients at the age extremes and those with extreme debilitation are

---

BOX 27-1	Factors that Influence Body Temperature of the PACU Patient

- Anesthesia
- Preoperative medications
- Age of patient
- Site and temperature of intravenous fluids
- Vasoconstriction (from blood loss or anesthetic agent)
- Vasodilation (from regional anesthesia or use of inhalational agent)
- Body surface exposure
- Temperature of irrigation fluid
- Temperature of ambient air

BOX 27-2	Physiologic Alterations Associated with Hypothermia and Hyperthermia

Hypothermia	Hyperthermia
Bluish tint to skin (cyanosis)	Pale skin (mottled)
Increased metabolic rate with shivering, then decreased metabolic rate	Increased metabolic rate
Decreased oxygen consumption	Increased oxygen consumption
Decreased muscle tone	Decreased muscle tone
Decreased heart rate	Increased heart rate (rapid and bounding)
Dysrhythmias	Dysrhythmias
Decreased level of consciousness	Alterations in central nervous system (patient may be agitated)

---

at even greater risk for postoperative development of temperature abnormalities.

Core temperature (approximate value of temperature of blood perfusing the major metabolically active organs) is measured via the pulmonary artery, distal esophagus, nasopharynx, or tympanic membrane (using infrared thermistor). Monitoring the true core temperature is unrealistic and not clinically feasible for use on all patients in the PACU. Therefore, other measurement techniques (axillary, rectal, tympanic, temporal artery, oral) are required in the PACU even while their correlation to core temperature is debated. Consistency in use of the same method of measurement is required so that trends can be spotted and management of hypothermia begun.

Evidence-Based Practice

ASPAN's evidenced-based clinical practice guideline for the promotion of perioperative normothermia recommends, as supported by strong evidence, that near core measures of oral temperatures best approximate core readings, the same route of temperature measurement should be used throughout the perianesthesia period; and caution should be taken in interpreting extreme values from any site with near core instruments. Temperature measurement recommendations supported by weak evidence suggests that temporal artery measurements approximate core temperature at normothermic temperature but not extremes outside of normothermia; and that infrared tympanic thermometry does not provide accurate temperature measurements during the perianesthesia period. Temperature measurement recommendations supported by conflicting evidence suggests that oral chemical dot thermometers are acceptable near-core alternatives.

IMPLICATIONS FOR PRACTICE

Overall, the research on perianesthesia temperature measurement is weak because of a lack of controls, insufficient statistical analysis, and lack of replication. Perianesthesia nurses should keep up to date with research in the area of accurate temperature measurements during the perianesthesia period. Consideration for the use of oral temperatures is important because that route has the strongest evidence. Consistency of temperature measurement is of utmost importance throughout the perianesthesia period to reflect an accurate picture of the patient's body temperature.

Source: Hooper VD et al: ASPAN's evidence-based clinical practice guideline for the promotion of perioperative normothermia, ed 2, *J Perianesth Nurs* 25:346-365, 2010.

Management of the patient with hypothermia is directed toward the restoration of normothermia and the avoidance of shivering. Warm blankets can be placed over the patient as specific hospital protocol allows. Forced air warming systems provide a safe and effective means of gradually rewarming the patient. Hypothermia and hyperthermia are discussed in greater detail in Chapter 53.

FLUID AND ELECTROLYTE BALANCE

Evaluation of a patient's fluid and electrolyte status involves total body assessment. Imbalances readily occur in the postoperative patient for a number of reasons, including the restriction of food and fluids before surgery, fluid loss during surgery, patient's physical status, and stress. The normal body response to stress of surgery is renal retention of water and sodium. In addition, patients often have abnormal avenues of postoperative fluid loss (see Chapter 14).

Fluid Intake

Each patient must be evaluated for determination of baseline requirements and the fluid needed to replace abnormal losses. The healthy adult who is deprived of oral intake needs 2000 to 2200 mL of water per day to compensate for urinary output and insensible loss.

Intravenous Fluids

Most patients admitted to the PACU from the operating room are receiving intravenous fluids. The anesthesia care provider must have an open intravenous line for the administration of necessary medications and replacement fluids during surgery, and an open line is needed after surgery for supply of necessary fluids, electrolytes, and medications. Because all efforts to substitute for normal oral intake of electrolytes and adequate volumes of fluid are at best temporary and inadequate, the first objective is to return the patient to adequate oral intake as soon as possible. Until this objective can be attained, an intravenous line must be maintained. The nurse should be aware of the type and amount of any fluid administered and any medications that may have been added to it.

The intravenous site should be checked to ensure that the needle or cannula is still in the vein and that no extravasation has occurred. Watch for kinks or disconnected tubing, and ensure that the rate of infusion is accurate. The intravenous site should be positioned comfortably; a board may be helpful in maintaining the intravenous site if the patient should become restless.

Pediatric patients may need a protective device over the site or soft protective devices to prevent dislodging of the needle or cannula. A simple paper cup device can be helpful in preventing dislodgement of the intravenous line from the scalp veins of small infants. Snip the bottom out of the cup; thread the cup over the tubing; place the large opening over the intravenous site; and secure the cup to the baby's head with tape crisscrossed over the entire cup. In addition to providing protection for the intravenous site, this method allows the nurse to check the insertion site frequently.

After ensuring that the intravenous fluids are infusing correctly, check to see what fluids, if any, are to follow or if the infusion is to be

NURSING CARE IN THE PACU

discontinued. If the patient is receiving total parenteral nutrition and intralipids, only feeding solutions should go through this line; another intravenous pathway must be secured for other uses. Multilumen catheters allow for the administration of multiple fluids and medications, and central line catheters can be connected to a transducer to provide continuous hemodynamic monitoring, if indicated.

The flow of intravenous fluids in the patient receiving hyperalimentation, the patient who is fluid-restricted, the infant or small child, and the patient who is receiving intravenous analgesia or vasopressors should always be regulated with electronic fluid administration devices.

Oral Fluids

Oral intake must be prohibited after anesthesia until the laryngeal and pharyngeal reflexes are fully regained, as evidenced by the patient's ability to gag and swallow effectively. If the patient is permitted oral intake, starting with small amounts of ice chips is best because they are less likely to cause nausea and vomiting. Some PACUs use isotonic ice chips that are made from a balanced electrolyte solution, such as Lytren, Pedialyte, and Ricelyte. If ice chips are well tolerated, the patient can progressively increase oral intake to include water and other clear liquids. Kool-Aid and fruit-flavored popsicles are well tolerated and accepted by children and adults. In addition, carbonated beverages may be soothing to a patient who feels slightly nauseated. The management of postoperative nausea and vomiting is discussed in Chapters 16 and 29.

Fluid Output

Normal output in the average adult results from obligatory urinary output and insensible avenues of loss, including evaporation of water from the skin and exhalation during respiration. The amount of urine necessary for the normal renal system to excrete waste products of a day's metabolism is approximately 600 mL. Optimally, 30 mL/h or more of urine should be obtained from an adult who is catheterized to ensure proper hydration and kidney function. Urinary output should be closely monitored in the recovery phase; measurement of urinary output and urine specific gravity yields important clues to the overall status of the patient and may alert the nurse to overhydration or dehydration or the development of shock.

A lower than normal urinary output can be expected in the postoperative patient as a result of the body's normal reaction to stress; however, an unduly small volume of urine (less than 500 mL in 24 hours) may indicate the presence of renal insufficiency, and the physician should be notified.

If a urinary catheter is in place, a more accurate observation of hourly output is available. If urine volume is low and specific gravity remains fixed at a low level, renal insufficiency is indicated. A small urine volume plus a high specific gravity indicates dehydration. In addition to the volume and specific gravity of urinary output noted, the urine should be examined for the presence of pus, blood, or casts.

The perianesthesia nurse must evaluate abnormal and normal avenues of output. Abnormal ways include external losses from vomiting, nasogastric tubes, T-tubes, and fistula or wound drainage and temporary functional losses from fluid shifting within the body, such as hemorrhage into soft tissues and the edema of surgical wounds.

The surgical site should be noted on admission to the PACU, and the dressing should be checked for drainage. The perianesthesia nurse must be aware of the presence of any drains and the expected amount of drainage. Drainage tubes should be checked to ensure patency, and the amount, color, and odor of any drainage should be observed and documented. All tubes should be secure and either clamped shut or connected to drainage apparatus as ordered by the physician. A summary of imbalances that may occur with abnormal avenues of output is presented in Table 27-3. Any deviations from the normally expected drainage in a specific route should be reported promptly to the surgeon.

Obviously, the accurate measurement and recording of all intake and output is vital to the assessment of each patient's fluid and electrolyte status. A running total kept on the postanesthesia flow sheet or online documentation system is essential for quick assessment of fluid status. In addition to observation and assessment of avenues of intake and output, the perianesthesia nurse should be alert to symptoms of fluid and electrolyte imbalance, which are summarized in Table 27-4.

MUSCULOSKELETAL ASSESSMENT

An increase of orthopedic surgical procedures for both ambulatory and hospitalized patients provides a challenge to the perianesthesia nurse. Primary risk factors for complications in those with musculoskeletal injuries include the patient's multiple comorbid conditions, age, and the multiple types of drugs used, including

Table 27-3	Imbalances that May Occur with Abnormal Avenues of Output*		
FLUID	pH	CONTENT (mEq/L)	LIKELY IMBALANCES WITH SIGNIFICANT LOSSES
Gastric juice (fasting) (nasogastric suction)	1-3	Na^+ (60) K^{++} (10) Cl^- (85) HCO^{-3} (0-15)	Metabolic alkalosis Potassium deficit Sodium deficit Fluid volume deficit
Small intestine (suction) jejunum	7-8	Na^+ (111) K^+ (4.6) Cl^- (104) HCO^{-3} (31)	Metabolic acidosis Potassium deficit Sodium deficit
Ileum	7-8	Na^+ (117) K^+ (5.0) Cl^- (105)	Fluid volume deficit
New ileostomy		$Na+$ (129) K^+ (11) Cl^- (116)	Potassium deficit Sodium deficit Fluid volume deficit Metabolic acidosis
Biliary	7.8	$Na+$ (148) K^+ (7.0) Cl^- (80) HCO^{-3} (30)	Metabolic acidosis Sodium deficit Fluid volume deficit
Pancreatic juice	7.8-8.3	Na^+ (130) K^+ (4.6 -7) Cl^- (76) HCO^{-3} (121)	Metabolic acidosis Sodium deficit Fluid volume deficit

Adapted from Bland J: *Clinical metabolism of body water and electrolytes*, Philadelphia, 1963, Saunders; Heitz U, Horne M: *Fluid, electrolyte, and acid-base balance*, ed 5, St. Louis, 2005, Mosby; Hall J: *Guyton and Hall's textbook of medical physiology*, ed 12, Philadelphia, 2011, Saunders.
*Values are approximate.

anticoagulants, steroids, estrogens, and opioids. Assessment and care of these patients include consideration for circulation, reflexes, positioning, transfer, and ambulation. See Chapter 37 for more specifics.

INTEGUMENTARY SYSTEM

Chapters 5 and 17 address aspects of the integumentary system. The integumentary system can be injured by the physical forces used in positioning and maintaining the patient position during and after surgery. Pressure, shear, friction, and maceration can cause damage to tissue integrity. The perianesthesia nurse must assess the patient's skin and positioning to prevent integumentary complications from occurring.

PSYCHOSOCIAL ASSESSMENT

Assessment of the patient's psychological and emotional well being is an important component of perianesthesia nursing. As with any other assessment, this assessment must be made in the context of the whole patient. Illness, hospitalization, surgery, and pain all take on a variety of values, depending on the person. The meaning of the surgery to the person must be explored before surgery and will probably have been obtained by other health care providers; this information should be communicated to the perianesthesia nurse who will care for the patient. Likewise, the perianesthesia nurse must ensure that additional assessment information and psychosocial care in the PACU are shared with those who care for the patient after discharge from the unit.

Almost all surgical patients have a degree of anxiety about anesthesia and the surgical procedure and a fear of postoperative pain. The physical signs and symptoms of anxiety are the same as those produced by any stressor. Reactions are mediated by the sympathetic nervous system and are listed in Box 27-3.

Symptoms of anxiety must be carefully differentiated from those of other causes. Differentiation is particularly difficult while the effects of anesthesia

NURSING CARE IN THE PACU

Table 27-4   Signs and Symptoms of Acute Fluid and Electrolyte Imbalance

IMBALANCE	SYMPTOMS AND FINDINGS
Hyperosmolarity	
Water excess, sodium deficit	Polyuria (if kidneys are healthy), twitching, hyperirritability, disorientation, nausea, vomiting, weakness, serum Na < 120 mEq/L
Isotonic Disturbances	
Dehydration	Weakness, nausea, vomiting, oliguria, postural drop in systolic BP, elevated hematocrit, normal serum Na^+
Circulatory collapse	Shock
Volume excess	Dyspnea, cough, sweating, edema
Hydrogen Ion Imbalances	
Metabolic acidosis	Bicarbonate loss: nausea, vomiting, abdominal discomfort, Weakness, tremors, malaise, headache, Kussmaul respiration, hypotension, tachycardia and other dysrhythmias, confusion, drowsiness, lethargy leading to coma
	Symptoms of K^+ excess, ABG pH < 7.35, $HCO^{-3} < 25$, acid urine with pH < 6.0; increased rate and depth of breathing
Metabolic alkalosis	Increased bicarbonate, slow breathing, nausea, vomiting, diarrhea, paresthesia of mouth and extremities, confusion, dizziness, muscle irritability, tetany, seizures, coma; decreased rate and depth of breathing to retain CO_2 (hypoventilation)
Respiratory acidosis (CO_2 retention)	Hypoventilation: tachycardia, tachypnea initially; bradypnea, hypotension, dysrhythmias, confusion, headache, blurred vision ABG pH < 7.4, $PCO_2 > 40$, HCO^{-3} 25-35
Respiratory alkalosis	Hyperventilation: tachycardia, palpitations, dry mouth, anxiety, profuse perspiration, paresthesia of mouth and extremities, dizziness, vertigo, increased muscle twitching, tetany, inability to concentrate, seizures, coma
	Increased irritability, disorientation, shallow slow respirations, periods of apnea, irregular pulse, muscle twitch, ABG pH > 7.45, $HCO^{-3} > 29$, alkaline urine with pH > 7.0
Potassium Imbalances	
Deficit (hypokalemia)	Weakness, mental confusion, shallow respirations, hypotension, dysrhythmias, serum $K^+ < 3.5$ (measurement of extracellular K^+ and only gives vague reflection of intracellular balance)
	Four common causes of hypokalemia: reduced intake, GI losses, excessive renal loss of K^+, K^+ shifts from extracellular to intracellular, metabolic alkalosis
Excess (hyperkalemia)	Intestinal colic, oliguria, bradycardia, cardiac arrest, serum $K^+ > 5$ mEq/L Metabolic acidosis
Calcium Imbalances	
Deficit (hypocalcemia)	Tingling of fingers, laryngospasm, facial spasms, painful muscle spasms, positive Trousseau sign, positive Chvostek sign, convulsions, palpitations, cardiac dysrhythmias, serum $Ca^{++} < 4.5$ mEq/L
Excess (hypercalcemia)	Drowsiness, lethargy and headaches. Weakness and muscle flaccidity, heart block, anorexia, nausea, vomiting, constipation and dehydration

BP, Blood pressure; *ABG,* arterial blood gas; *GI,* gastrointestinal; *PCO2,* partial pressure of carbon dioxide.

are still present. A quiet and calm environment is important to the postanesthesia recovery of the surgical patient. A calm and confident nurse can do much to allay anxiety for the postoperative patient through both verbal reassurance and touch. Hearing is the first sense to return after anesthesia. Speaking loudly to patients is not necessary; they may not respond even if they can hear. In fact, yelling at patients may increase anxiety early in the PACU period, because the patients may believe they are not recovering as quickly as they should.

BOX 27-3   Signs and Symptoms of Anxiety

- Tachycardia
- Increased blood pressure
- Pale cool skin
- Increased respiratory rate
- Hyperventilation
- Increased muscle tone
- Restlessness or agitation
- Dilated pupils

Attention to comfort, including minimal environmental noise and stimuli, and the reassuring presence of the nurse are calming. When the patient has fully regained consciousness, simply talking may help to allay anxiety. Simple factual statements repeated often are best. At this point, the nurse may be able to explore the cause of the distress with the patient.

For the patient in acute distress from anxiety, a mild tranquilizer, such as diazepam (Valium), midazolam (Versed), or lorazepam (Ativan), may be indicated; however, these benzodiazepines should be used judiciously. One advantage of their use is that they potentiate opioids and often allow a reduction of the analgesic dosage necessary to control pain. Because apnea is a common side effect when benzodiazepines are given to patients receiving opioids, continuous respiratory monitoring with pulse oximetry and capnography is indicated.

Attention to the psychosocial ramifications of specific surgical interventions is provided in each of the following chapters on postanesthesia care. These comments are incorporated into the overall text whenever deemed appropriate. For further discussion of the relationship between pain and anxiety, see Chapter 31.

SUMMARY

Obviously, the perianesthesia nurse must be an expert in assessment. The perianesthesia nurse must not only understand the normal physiologic functioning of the human body but also be able to differentiate and evaluate the variety of pathologic symptoms that may arise in the postprocedure patient. The perianesthesia nurse must be aware of the interrelationships between mind and body and must be sensitive to the psychosocial factors that influence the patient's reactions. Knowledgeable assessment of the postprocedure patient is essential for the provision of safe and effective treatment and nursing care.

REFERENCES

1. Cole D, Schlunt M: *Adult perioperative anesthesia: the requisites in anesthesiology*, Philadelphia, 2004, Mosby.
2. American Society of PeriAnesthesia Nurses: *Perianesthesia nursing: standards and practice recommendations 2010-2012*, Cherry Hill, NJ, 2010, ASPAN.
3. Atlee J: *Complications in anesthesia*, ed 2, Philadelphia, 2007, Saunders.
4. Miller R, et al: *Miller's anesthesia*, ed 7, Philadelphia, 2009, Churchill Livingstone.
5. Odom-Forren J: Capnography and sedation: A global initiative, *J Perianesth Nurs* 26:221–224, 2011.
6. Godden B: Where does capnography fit into the PACU? *J Perianesth Nurs* 26(6):408–410, 2011.
7. Stoelting R, Miller R: *Basics of anesthesia*, ed 6, Philadelphia, 2011, Churchill Livingstone.
8. Urden L, et al: *Priorities in critical care nursing*, ed 5, St. Louis, 2009, Mosby.
9. Litman RS: *Pediatric anesthesia: the requisites in anesthesiology*, Philadelphia, 2004, Mosby.
10. Morton P, et al: *Critical care nursing: a holistic approach*, ed 9, Philadelphia, 2009, Lippincott Williams & Wilkins.
11. Diehl T, editor: *Hemodynamic monitoring made incredibly visual*, ed 2, Philadelphia, 2011, Lippincott Williams & Wilkins.

RESOURCES

Alspach J: *Core curriculum for critical care nursing*, ed 6, Philadelphia, 2006, Saunders.

Arbour R: Impact of bispectral index monitoring on sedation and outcomes in critically ill adults: a case series, *Crit Care Nurs Clin North Am* 18:227–241, 2006.

Barash P, et al: *Clinical anesthesia*, ed 6, Philadelphia, 2009, Lippincott Williams & Wilkins.

Bickley L, Hoekelman R: *Bates' guide to physical examination and history taking*, ed 10, Philadelphia, 2009, Lippincott Williams & Wilkins.

Black J, Hokanson-Hawks J: *Medical-surgical nursing: clinical management for positive outcomes*, ed 8, St. Louis, 2009, Saunders.

Brunton L, et al: *Goodman and Gilman's the pharmacological basis of therapeutics*, ed 12, New York, 2010, McGraw-Hill Professional.

Dennison R: *Pass CCRN!* ed 3, St. Louis, 2007, Mosby.

Fleisher L: *Evidence-based practice of anesthesiology*, ed 2, Philadelphia, 2009, Saunders.

Hall J: *Guyton and Hall textbook of medical physiology*, ed 12, Philadelphia, 2011, Saunders.

Headley JB, et al: *Implementing nurse driven protocols: using arterial based cardiac output technologies* AACN, available at http://www.aacn.org/DM/CETests/Overview.aspx?TestID=33&mid=2864&ItemID=26. Accessed April, 25, 2011.

Heitz U, Horne M: *Fluid, electrolyte, and acid-base balance*, ed 5, St. Louis, 2005, Mosby.

Hickey J: *The clinical practice of neurological and neurosurgical nursing*, ed 6, Philadelphia, 2008, Lippincott Williams & Wilkins.

Katzung BG: *Basic and clinical pharmacology*, ed 11, Los Altos, Calif, 2009, Appleton & Lange.

Mason RJ, et al: *Murry and Nadel's textbook of respiratory medicine*, ed 5, Philadelphia, 2010, Saunders.

NURSING CARE IN THE PACU

McCance K, Huether S: *Pathophysiology: the biologic basis for disease in adults and children*, ed 6, St. Louis, 2010, Mosby.

Nagelhout J, Plaus K: *Nurse anesthesia*, ed 4, Philadelphia, 2009, Saunders.

Rathmell J, et al: *Regional anesthesia: the requisites in anesthesiology*, Philadelphia, 2004, Saunders.

Schick L, Windle PE, editors: *Perianesthesia nursing core curriculum: preoperative phase I and phase II PACU nursing*, ed 2, St. Louis, 2010, Mosby.

Schumacker L, Chernecky C: *Critical care & emergency nursing*, ed 2, St. Louis, 2009, Saunders.

Springhouse: *Critical care nursing made incredibly easy*, ed 2, Ambler, Penn, 2007, Lippincott Williams & Wilkins.

Springhouse: *IV therapy made incredibly easy*, ed 4, Springhouse, Penn, 2009, Lippincott Williams & Wilkins.

Swearingen P: *Manual of medical-surgical nursing care*, ed 7, St. Louis, 2010, Mosby.

28 Patient Education and Care of the Perianesthesia Patient

Denise O'Brien, DNP, RN, ACNS-BC, CPAN, CAPA, FAAN

Patients primarily arrive for operative and interventional procedures on the day of the procedure, unlike many years ago when most patients spent days in the hospital before procedures. This transition necessitated a change in preparation of patients and families for procedures and in focused interest on patient education processes and products. This chapter discusses effective patient education, which supports improved patient outcomes. Nursing care of postanesthesia patients who are emerging from anesthesia is also reviewed in this chapter. Postanesthesia care includes the stir-up regimen, intravenous therapy, maintenance of respiratory function, patient transfers, and general comfort measures.

DEFINITIONS

Affective Learning: Relates to attitude and includes the ability to receive, respond, value, and organize a personal value system and internalize the value system.

Cognitive Learning: The human processing of information; application of knowledge.

Continuous Positive-Pressure Airway (CPAP): Delivers air into the patient's airway and creates enough pressure to keep the airway open during inhalation.

Intermittent Mandatory Ventilation (IMV): Allows patients to breathe on their own as often and as deeply as they like and ensures that a set tidal volume is delivered at a predetermined back-up rate.

Patient Education: Useful information that helps patients and their families or companions become more informed about the medical and nursing care they receive before, during, and after surgical and diagnostic procedures.

Positive End-Expiratory Pressure (PEEP): A technique that can be used to help prevent collapse of the alveoli during the expiratory phase of ventilation, to increase the lung's functional residual capacity, and to reduce the amount of physiologic shunting.

Stir-Up Regimen: Consists of five major activities as the patient is recovering from anesthesia: deep-breathing exercises, coughing, positioning, mobilization, and pain management.

Sustained Maximal Inspiratory (SMI) Maneuver: The patient inhales as close to total lung capacity as possible and, at the peak of inspiration, holds that volume of air in the lungs for 3 to 5 seconds before exhaling.

Synchronous Intermittent Mandatory Ventilation (SIMV): Allows the patient to control the inspiratory time and the size of the spontaneous tidal volumes.

PATIENT EDUCATION CONCEPTS AND PERIANESTHESIA CARE

Patient preparation for surgical and interventional procedures includes not only preanesthesia assessment and appropriate testing, but also education individualized for the patient and the family or companion. The goals of patient education are to increase the patient's sense of self worth, decrease anxiety, and reduce facility and provider liability by ensuring that the patient and family or companion receive information in a form that they can comprehend and use to enhance the operative experience. Ideally, the patient and family or companion has an opportunity to review the educational content and ask questions of the health care provider before the day of surgery.

The purpose of preoperative education is to empower patients, give them greater decision-making authority related to their care, and enable them to better manage their health. The patient benefits from learning before the surgery with decreased preoperative fear and anxiety, postoperative complications, recovery time, and postoperative pain.[1,2] Education also increases patient compliance with instructions and improves coping mechanisms for the patient and preparation. Preoperative education is for the patient and the family or companion and is a responsibility of the professional registered nurse.

Before providing education for patients, perianesthesia nurses complete a self-assessment that reflects on strengths and weaknesses such as knowledge base, understanding of the information to teach, and whether they like or dislike teaching. Consideration should be given to personal biases: does the nurse react negatively to patients with a history of alcohol use or who are obese? Does the nurse dislike children or the elderly? Do the religious or ethnic preferences of the nurse conflict with the patient population served? Sensitivity to diversity and cultural awareness of patients improve the professional registered nurse's ability to provide appropriate education for the patients and families or companions. The nurse may need to work on improving knowledge and teaching skills while preventing biases from affecting the duty to provide patient education.

Learning Environment and Learning Needs

If possible, education should take place in an environment that is conducive to learning. Unfortunately, the nurse is often challenged by noise, lack of privacy, and limited space. A quiet private space should help to reduce the patient's anxiety and facilitate learning. An area that is family oriented and lacks physical barriers is best, especially when the population consists of children or elderly patients.

Methods for identifying learning needs of the patient and the family or companions include asking open-ended questions, directly observing the patient and family, and hearing the verbal cues that indicate learning and knowledge. Nonverbal cues are also observed and noted. The patient's and family's or companion's current knowledge level can be identified through questionnaires, telephone conversations, observation, or interview. Patient education is more effective when the content and methods are individualized for the patient and family; the nurse should determine what the patient and family or companion want and need to know and teach them accordingly.[1]

Learner Characteristics

Patient demographic information includes age; primary language; reading level; sensory limitations; physical condition; developmental level; mental, emotional, or educational limitations; and motivation and attitude. Identification of how the patient prefers to learn is also essential in individualization of learning materials for the patient. For the pediatric patient, developmental stage is evaluated. Age-related challenges need to be considered with older patients.

Types of Learners

The adult learner is internally motivated, self directed, and self governed; uses experience as a resource; may have difficulty accepting new concepts; and has a problem-centered orientation to learning. The child learner does not assume responsibility for learning, is totally dependent on adults, relies on a transmittal method of learning, is open to new concepts, and is subject centered.

When a child is the patient, the parents often begin education at home, depending on the age of the child and the preparation needed. Therefore parent preparation is essential and requires knowledge of adult learning characteristics by the nurse. Typically the younger the child, the closer to the day of the procedure the education occurs. Parents' and caregivers' understanding of the child's behavior and developmental stage should guide the nurse in choosing appropriate teaching tools and techniques. Even with preparation, separation anxiety for both child and parent occurs and may be especially difficult for the 1- to 5-year-old child. See also Chapter 49 for specific information about caring for the pediatric patient.

The older adult may have had less formal education, and comprehension may be limited. However, the learning challenges of older patients may be related to sensory deficiencies that can interfere with the ability to learn, and not educational level or intellect. Chapter 50 reviews the care of the geriatric patient and the specific challenges of this population.

Influences on Learning

Physiologic, emotional, cultural, and environmental barriers can hinder the learning process for all ages and developmental levels.[1] Language barriers can decrease the patient's ability to understand instructions and limit compliance with instructions because of a lack of comprehension. Inadequate or poor teaching can also be a barrier to the learning process, and the professional registered nurse works on improving knowledge and skills of teaching and learning for the patient populations encountered. Another consideration is evaluation of the learner's present knowledge, previous experience, prior education, perceptions, expectations, and potential misinformation. The patient's health beliefs, attitudes, level of stress, coping skills, anxiety, and social support also influence learning.

Retention of information is dependent on how the information is presented. The reading of an educational pamphlet is less effective than hearing the same information while reading the material and talking about it. Content that is visually appealing, perhaps with photographs or diagrams, may also help the learner retain the information. Demonstration and return demonstration with the learner talking through the process is probably the most effective way to help the learner retain new information.

Teaching Characteristics and Planning

The professional registered nurse needs to have knowledge of teaching-learning principles, to recognize that anxiety and pain impede learning, and to value reinforcement of learning. Common language, not medical terminology, should be used. Knowledge of the teaching tools available and the content to teach is essential for successful patient education.

Content knowledge guides the development of an individualized teaching plan for the patient and family or companion. The plan is based on assessment of learning needs. As part of the plan, one should consider developing a verbal or written contract with the patient or family or companion that helps to meet the purpose of empowering the individual patient in the health care environment.

Learning goals focus on the domains of learning. Cognitive learning involves knowledge. Intellectual abilities such as the recall of facts and understanding of concepts, the application and analysis of learned ideas, and synthesis and evaluation fall in the cognitive domain. The affective learning domain relates to attitude and includes the ability to receive, respond, value, and organize a personal value system and internalize the value system. Skills are in the psychomotor domain. This domain includes imitation, manipulation, development of precision, skill integration, and expertise.

Content of Teaching Plan

The teaching plan includes generic content, with general information about preoperative preparation, day of surgery activities, and postoperative issues. The environment is described, as is the usual sequence of events. Individualized content is also integrated into the teaching plan to meet needs identified by the nurse's assessment of learning, review of the patient's history, and information requested by the patient or family.[1]

Preoperative teaching content describes the procedure on the day of surgery, including expected behaviors to prepare the patient, possible alterations in comfort after the procedure, and strategies for pain reduction. Recommendations for fasting from solids and liquids are reviewed, as are medications to be held or taken on the day of surgery. Patients should be instructed to leave valuables and jewelry at home. Bathing or showering with an antibacterial cleanser can help to reduce the risk of surgical infection; patients should be reminded to do this the evening before and the morning of the procedure if possible. For patients undergoing outpatient or ambulatory procedures, the requirement for a responsible adult companion and, if needed, a ride home at discharge should be reinforced.

Facility policies vary regarding transportation requirements (e.g., whether the companion must stay in the facility during the procedure or if the companion may be called to pick up the patient). The professional registered nurse is responsible for knowing the facility policies; awareness of resources such as risk management or legal counsel is beneficial should questions arise regarding patient transportation or responsible adult companion issues.

Discussion related to possible alterations in comfort helps to prepare the patient for what to expect after surgery. Common concerns include pain, sore throat, nausea, and vomiting. The patient's past experience may influence expectations. Descriptions of strategies for pain reduction, including request of pain medication and use of positioning, ice, or other techniques, may ease the patient's concerns about pain and discomfort. Postoperative nausea and vomiting may be minimized or controlled with medications, aromatherapy, hydration, and slow movements. Additional information on pain management can be found in Chapter 31; nausea and vomiting are discussed in Chapter 29.

A demonstration of equipment that the patient will see or hear during or after the procedure may ease fears of the unknown or unusual sounds and sights, especially for children.

The surgeon may discuss procedure-specific educational information for the patient. Brochures, booklets, videos, or group classes can be used. The anesthesia care provider may offer educational material for the planned anesthesia on the basis of the type of procedure and the patient's needs for the nurse to review or may provide the education personally.

Finally, postoperative behaviors are reviewed to complete the patient's preparation for surgery. The content includes passive exercises to reduce the risk of venous thromboembolism; safe ambulation; effective deep breathing and coughing to reduce the risk of respiratory complications; dressing, drain, or cast care; diet and fluid needs or restrictions; signs and symptoms that indicate complications; follow-up care; and emergency contact information for use after leaving the facility.

Teaching Strategies

The nurse's primary objectives when teaching are establishing a rapport to reduce anxiety and fear, assessing patient and family knowledge and expectations for learning, and assessing patient and family learning style to enhance the learning process. These objectives can apply to teaching before the day of surgery in a structured setting, patient education that occurs at the bedside while the patient is in the postanesthesia care unit (PACU), or teaching during preparation for discharge. The level of detail provided should be based on these assessments, with the education tailored specifically to the patient and family or companion. Teaching should be directed to the patient, but the family decision-maker or primary caregiver should also be considered as important to educational success. Ample opportunity for the patient and family to voice concerns and ask questions should be provided. If language is a barrier, interpreter services can assist in the teaching process. Short simple explanations are best, with the importance of the instructions and expected benefits of compliance with the instructions stressed. Jargon should be avoided and all terms should be clarified. Teachable moments should be used to take advantage of times when the patient and family are most likely to accept new information (e.g., symptoms are present).

The incorporation of more than one teaching method can enhance learning and reinforce teaching. A variety of teaching methods should be used, including written material and demonstration of skills. Formal education can occur in a classroom setting and involve lecture, group discussion, or audiovisual materials. Written material should be readable at a grade 5 or 6 level. Other options include play therapy, tours of the facility, films or videos, web-based learning activities, or games.

For children, factors that affect the choice of teaching method include the child's age and developmental level, the family's available resources, and the cognitive ability of the child and parent. The facility tour can be effective for 4 to 12 year olds and can be combined with puppets or models. Play therapy provides an opportunity for the 3- to 7-year-old child to draw, act out, or describe events. Puppets or dolls can be used. Films or videos can be viewed in multiple places and are most effective if the patient is the same age, race, and gender as the children shown in the video. This method is most effective in the 7- to 12-year-old age group, but requires quiet time for viewing. Models allow visualization and manipulation of equipment such as breathing masks, circuits, splints, intravenous tubing, and anatomic parts. Although models are most effective with 3 to 6 year olds, they can be used with all ages.

Written material may include a description of events to be expected on the day of surgery and should be easy to understand. This material can be taken home for referral throughout the preparation period and after the procedure. Instead of text, picture or coloring books may be helpful to 4 to 8 year olds or to patients with low literacy or language barriers. An advantage of preprinted instructions is the standardized information. Any written material needs to be legible with larger print size for the visually impaired and elderly. The use of internationally recognized symbols is also helpful.

Patient Education on the Day of Surgery

The patient's greatest need on the day of surgery is psychosocial. Less emphasis should be placed on information and skills, and more on reassurance and support. Any information given is limited to the essential information for safe transitioning of the patient to the operative suite. The family or companion may have additional informational needs and need support during this time.

Discharge Instructions

Ideally, the patient and family or companion have had an opportunity to review any discharge instructions before the day of surgery to help prepare the home with any needed supplies or alterations (e.g., removal of rugs that increase fall risk, sleeping area moved closer to the bathroom) for minimization of safety concerns or enhancement of care. Discharge instructions are reviewed with the patient and family or companion before the patient is discharged. Included in the instructions are recommended diet; medications (new prescriptions, resumption of regular medications); pain management (when to take medications, when to call if pain not relieved); bowel habit (increase in dietary fiber and fluids, use of stool softener); wound, dressing, or drain care (when to change, supplies needed, when to call physician); follow-up plan and visit; resumption of activities of daily living and return to work; and emergency instructions (who to call, where to go).

Documentation

Patient education completed by the nurse is documented as a record of education provided to the patient. Forms vary by institution and may be paper or electronic. Standardized care plans include documentation of individualized education. Checklists or flow sheets may be used. Whatever the form, teaching should be documented to support the work of the nurse and record what the patient was told and the response to the educational information. This documentation protects the patient, the nurse, and the facility should concerns arise over educational content and patient preparation. Additional information on documentation can be found in Chapter 7.

CARE OF THE PERIANESTHESIA PATIENT

Stir-Up Regimen

The stir-up regimen is an important aspect of postanesthesia nursing care, especially for the patient who has received general anesthesia. Patients transition to an awake state more quickly than in the past or arrive in the PACU awake and alert; however, prevention of complications remains important and elements of the stir-up regimen can help to minimize complications. Like most other PACU activities, the basics of the stir-up regimen are aimed at preventing complications, primarily atelectasis and venous stasis. Five major activities constitute the stir-up regimen: deep breathing exercises, coughing, positioning, mobilization, and pain management.

Deep-Breathing Exercises

The primary factor that contributes to postoperative pulmonary complications is decreased lung volumes. The major factor that contributes to low lung volumes in the PACU patient is a shallow, monotonous, sighless breathing pattern caused by general anesthesia, pain, and opioids. Full inflation of the lungs prevents small areas of patchy atelectasis from developing and assists in the elimination of inhalation anesthetics, thus hastening the awakening process. Intravenous anesthesia differs from inhalation anesthesia in that, once injection has occurred, little can be done to expedite removal of the drug; however, the prevention of atelectasis with deep breathing remains just as important. The patient should be stimulated to take three or four deep breaths every 5 to 10 minutes. Full expansion is important but can be impeded by a number of factors. Every effort must be made to enhance the patient's ability to expand the lungs. Patients who are emerging from anesthesia may have difficulty participating in the activity because of reduced levels of consciousness and awareness.

The sustained maximal inspiratory (SMI) maneuver is a method for enhancement of lung volumes after surgery. The SMI maneuver consists of the patient inhaling as close to total lung capacity as possible and, at the peak of inspiration, holding that volume of air in the lungs for 3 to 5 seconds before exhaling. Ideally the patient has received instruction and coaching in the postoperative use of this maneuver. The patient may use an incentive spirometer that provides visual or auditory feedback and observation of inspiratory volume.

Incentive spirometry is used to prevent or assist reversal of atelectasis, promote normal lung expansion, and improve oxygenation. Instruction and practice before surgery provide patients the opportunity to master the device and establish a baseline for before anesthetic and surgical interventions. Devices currently available include disposable flow-oriented and volume-oriented incentive spirometers that are inexpensive and can be used by the patient at home. Incentive spirometry may have greater use after the immediate postanesthesia period, because patients are more awake and capable of manipulating the devices than they are in the PACU.

Coughing

The patient must be instructed to cough in addition to the SMI maneuvers. The best way to clear the air passages of obstructive secretions is a purposeful cough. Cough effectiveness depends on the inspired tidal volume and the velocity of expired airflow. For the patient who is recovering from anesthesia, the cascade cough is the most effective cough maneuver. The patient should be taught to take a rapid deep inspiration to increase the volume of air in the lungs, which in turn dilates the airways, thus allowing air to pass beyond the retained secretions. On exhalation, the patient should perform multiple coughs at subsequently lower lung volumes. With each cough during exhalation, the length of the airways that undergo dynamic compression increases and cough effectiveness is enhanced.

Coughing is most effective when the patient is sitting. Splinting of incisions and adequate analgesia facilitate a good cough. If the patient is unable to sit upright, the side-lying position with hips and knees flexed or a semi-Fowler position with head and arms supported with pillows and with knees flexed decreases abdominal tension and allows maximal movement of the diaphragm, thereby improving the effectiveness of the cough.

Preoperative teaching of postoperative breathing exercises and coughs and their importance is effective and should be included in the preoperative regimen whenever possible. Patients scheduled for surgery may attend formal teaching sessions before surgery or may receive instructions for coughing, deep breathing, and incentive spirometry through educational booklets, video programs, and visits to preoperative testing departments.

Positioning

When possible, patients in the PACU should maintain a semiprone or side-lying position. The semiprone position promotes maintenance of a patent airway, prevents aspiration of vomitus into the trachea, and permits optimal ventilation of the lower lung lobes. Frequent repositioning of patients (at least every hour) is essential to prevent atelectasis and peripheral stasis. The patient's position should be changed from side to side. Care must be taken to ensure that all drainage tubes and intravenous catheters remain in place and patent and that no tension on any of these lines is created. As soon as they are able, patients should be encouraged to turn and change positions alone.

Mobilization

For prevention of venous stasis, patients are encouraged to move the legs and arms rhythmically. Patients should flex and extend the extremities. Mobilization and flexion of the muscles aid venous return, automatically cause deep breathing, and improve cardiac function.

Pain Management

Achievement of the stir-up regimen's first four activities is difficult if adequate pain relief is not provided. Opioids depress the cough reflex and ciliary action and may lower alveolar ventilation with direct depression of the respiratory center. If breathing is painful and splinting occurs or if the patient refuses to cough or move because of pain, respiratory or embolic complications can occur. Pain management is discussed in detail in Chapter 31.

Modifications of the Stir-Up Regimen

Modifications of the stir-up regimen may be needed depending on the type of anesthesia used and the operative procedure performed. Ketamine may cause emergence excitement during the initial recovery period. When ketamine is used, a rigorous stir-up regimen is eliminated from routine PACU care, and verbal and tactile stimulation of the patient is minimized as much as possible. Cough must be eliminated after eye surgery and other delicate plastic surgery procedures. Stimulation of the patient with increased or potentially increased intracranial pressure must be undertaken carefully to avoid dangerous and potentially life-threatening pressure changes. If any doubt exists regarding purposeful coughing after a procedure, check with the surgeon for specific instructions.

Positioning is probably the activity most often modified in the stir-up regimen. Positioning of the patient and modifications of the stir-up regimen after specific surgical procedures and anesthetics are discussed in related chapters.

Intravenous Therapy

Postoperative parenteral fluid requirements vary with the patient's preoperative status and with the surgical procedure. For a discussion of fluid and electrolyte imbalance, see Chapter 14.

Maintenance of Respiratory Function
Oxygen Therapy

The optimization of the oxygen-carrying capacity of arterial blood is the goal of oxygen therapy. All anesthetized patients have had some interference with respiratory processes, and most experts suggest routine oxygen administration to all patients after anesthesia. However, oxygen is a drug and should be treated as such, with full prescription information provided by the anesthesia care provider. This information may be contained in standard orders that are individualized for each patient. Low-flow oxygen administration assists the patient in maintenance of adequate oxygenation of all tissues. Optimal arterial oxygen tension should be between 70 and 100 mm Hg. Patients with chronic lung disease may have maintenance with low-flow oxygen administration, which keeps the oxygen tension in the range of 50 to 70 mm Hg. Pulmonary processes should be monitored carefully in the PACU. Pulse oximetry monitoring of all patients who have received an anesthetic is recommended in the initial postanesthesia period.

Pulse oximetry, a noninvasive technique, is used to measure arterial oxygen saturation of functional hemoglobin. In the postanesthesia setting, continuous monitoring of a patient's oxygen saturation assists in manipulation of the fraction of delivered oxygen (F_DO_2) levels and in identification of episodes of desaturation and hypoxemia.[3] Normal pulse oximetry values are 97% to 100%. Oxygen saturation as measured with pulse oximetry (SpO_2) values of 95% or greater are acceptable. Preanesthetic baseline SpO_2 values should be noted; patient levels may normally fall below the normal range in room air. Attempts to maintain higher oxygen saturation levels than the baseline level can result in prolonged oxygen therapy and PACU stays.

Evidence-Based Practice

The Cochrane Collaboration conducted a review to assess the use of pulse oximetry in the perioperative period and to identify adverse outcomes that could be prevented or improved by its use. Results from five studies showed that the use of pulse oximetry reduced hypoxemia by 1.5 to 3 times in those who were monitored with pulse oximetry. However, there was no evidence that the use of pulse oximetry affects the anesthetic outcomes of patients. The use of pulse oximetry did not reduce patient mortality or transfers to the intensive care unit.

IMPLICATIONS FOR PRACTICE

Pulse oximetry monitoring can reduce the degree of perioperative hypoxemia, enabling the detection and treatment of hypoxemia and related respiratory events. The implementation of perioperative pulse oximetry monitoring does not, however, reduce the number of postoperative complications. The question remains whether pulse oximetry improves outcome in other situations. Pulse oximetry can be a tool that guides the perianesthesia management in teaching situations, emergencies, and especially in caring for children. Although inconclusive, the data suggest that there may be a benefit for patients at high risk of postoperative pulmonary complications.

Source: Pedersen T, et al: Pulse oximetry for perioperative monitoring, *Cochrane Database Syst Rev* 4 (CD002013):2009.

Sensor site selection and application, ambient light, motion, electric interference, and impaired blood flow (low perfusion states, excessive edema) can influence SpO_2 levels. Temperature, pH, partial pressure of carbon dioxide ($PaCO_2$), hemodynamic status, and anemia affect accurate measurement. These factors alter the oxyhemoglobin dissociation curve and oxygen delivery. In addition, dysfunctional hemoglobins (carboxyhemoglobin, a byproduct of smoking and smoke; methemoglobin, formed from drugs such as lidocaine and nitroglycerin) can result in false elevation of oximetry values. Newer oximeters that measure eight wavelengths, rather than the two-wavelength pulse oximetry that has been in use, are now available and measure these dyshemoglobins.

Nurses may need to draw arterial blood gases to aid in the assessment of a patient's status. For discussion of arterial blood gases and the method for measurement, see Chapter 12.

Perianesthesia nurses should be aware of complications that can occur with oxygen therapy. Oxygen-induced hypoventilation, atelectasis, substernal chest pain, and toxicity can occur when high concentrations are administered over prolonged periods (fraction of inspired oxygen concentration [FiO_2] > 0.5 for more than 24 hours). Clinical detection of decreased oxygen saturation levels is difficult without pulse oximetry or arterial blood gas sampling.

Methods of Administration

Routine oxygen administration in the PACU can be accomplished with nasal cannula (prongs) or face masks. Table 28-1 lists commonly used oxygen delivery methods. Nasal cannulas are advantageous for routine short-term oxygen administration in the PACU. The cannula is made of plastic tubing with two soft plastic tips that insert into the nostrils about 1.5 cm. The prongs deliver 100% oxygen and thus yield a final inspired oxygen concentration of approximately 30% to 40% when a flow of 4 to 6 L/min is used. The prongs are easily inserted, comfortable, inexpensive, and disposable. Simple clear plastic disposable face masks can be used for oxygen administration in the PACU. They are also easy to apply and comfortable. The oxygen concentration inspired depends on the mask fit and the patient's inspiratory flow rate; however, an oxygen flow rate of 10 L/min yields an FiO_2 of up to 60%. A higher flow rate keeps the patient from rebreathing exhaled carbon dioxide (CO_2). Face masks in the PACU must be clear to provide adequate observation of the patient's nose and mouth. The mask should be removed intermittently to dry the face.

Humidity

Surgery and anesthesia often interrupt the normal functioning of the nose in heating and humidifying inspired air. When oxygen is administered via nasal cannula at flow rates of less than 4 L/min or with a Venturi mask, humidification is generally unnecessary because adequate amounts of humidified room air are inspired. At higher flow rates, humidification or nebulization may be needed in the PACU.

Humidifiers convert water from the liquid to the gaseous state, whereas nebulizers produce tiny water particles. Humidifiers are used to add water vapor to the airway; a nebulizer can provide both water vapor and particulate water or medication or saline aerosols to the airway. Aerosol therapy can be used to administer antibiotics, bronchodilators, and corticosteroids. Care when filling humidifiers, avoidance of contamination of the water in the humidifier, and proper disposal of humidifiers after use helps to avoid the spread of infectious agents.

Capnography

Capnography is used to measure ventilatory status at the end of expiration thereby measuring the adequacy of ventilation at the alveolar level. End-tidal carbon dioxide can be measured via an endotracheal

METHOD	FIO$_2$	FLOW (L/MIN)	COMMENTS
Low-Flow Method			
Nasal cannula (prongs)	0.24-0.4	5-6	Comfortable to wear; patient can breathe orally or nasally and still raise FiO$_2$; humidification unnecessary
Simple face mask	0.4-0.6	10	Adjustable to fit face; may be hot for patients; poorly tolerated; potential for skin irritation from tight fit and oxygen contact
Face tent	0.3-0.55	4-10	Less confining; useful when extra humidity is needed
Partial rebreathing mask	0.35-0.6	6-10	Mask with attached reservoir bag; no valves on mask (exhalation ports open)
High-Flow Method			
Nonrebreathing mask	0.4-1	6-15	Mask with reservoir bag; one-way valves on mask; side ports of mask; one-way valve between mask and bag for inhalation
Venturi mask	0.24-0.55	2-14	Believed accurate delivery of desired FiO$_2$; may be less if patient is hyperpneic or unable to keep mask in position on face
T-piece or Brigg's	0.21-1	2-10	Used with endotracheal or tracheostomy tube; provides accurate delivery of desired FiO$_2$ and humidification; most often used in weaning patients from ventilator assistance before endotracheal tube removal
Mechanical ventilator	0.21-1	Direct from supply	Pressure, volume, flow, and oxygen percentage all adjustable

FiO$_2$, Fraction of inspired oxygen concentration.

tube or via a sensor as part of a nasal cannula that also delivers oxygen. A patient in the PACU may require assessment of ventilatory status with the use of capnography. See Chapter 27 for a detailed discussion of capnography.

Mechanical Ventilation

Rarely, some patients who are recovering from anesthesia may need some form of mechanical ventilation in the PACU. Various techniques such as positive end-expiratory pressure (PEEP), continuous positive airway pressure (CPAP), and intermittent mandatory ventilation (IMV) are used to improve the respiratory status of the patient. Table 28-2 gives the terminology of the common ventilatory modes.

Positive End-Expiratory Pressure

PEEP is a technique that can be used to help prevent collapse of the alveoli during the expiratory phase of ventilation, to increase the lung's functional residual capacity, and to reduce the amount of physiologic shunting. PEEP also increases the PaO$_2$, which usually enables the FiO$_2$ to be reduced, thus lessening the chances of oxygen toxicity. In patients with preexisting obstructive lung disease, PEEP should be used cautiously because it can overexpand relatively normal alveoli. When PEEP is used in such circumstances, the dead space increases and occasionally causes a decrease in the PaO$_2$ and an increase in the PaCO$_2$.

Table 28-2 Terminology: Common Ventilatory Modes

ABBREVIATION	TERM
Mechanical Ventilation with Positive Airway Pressure	
A/C	Assist–control ventilation
CMV	Continuous mandatory ventilation
IMV	Intermittent mandatory ventilation
SIMV	Synchronized intermittent mandatory ventilation
PSV	Pressure support ventilation
PEEP	Positive end-expiratory pressure
APRV	Airway pressure-release ventilation
Spontaneous Breathing with Positive Airway Pressure	
CPAP	Continuous positive airway pressure
BiPAP	Bilevel positive airway pressure

When a patient receives PEEP therapy, hemodynamic status should be monitored because this ventilatory technique decreases venous return and may cause a decrease in cardiac output, especially in the patient with hypovolemia. In some instances, the reduced cardiac output can cause a decrease in systolic blood pressure. Other parameters to be monitored are vital signs, skin perfusion, and urine output.

Continuous Positive Airway Pressure

Continuous positive airway pressure helps to keep the lungs expanded. The patient breathes out against increased pressure as high as 10 to 20 cm H_2O, but the mechanics of ventilation do not change. The lung performs at a larger, more inflated volume, thereby increasing the functional residual capacity and decreasing the tendency to atelectasis. CPAP is a technique that can be used for weaning a patient from a ventilator. When CPAP is used, the patient should be monitored for tachypnea, tachycardia, increases in blood pressure, dysrhythmias, or generalized distress, which should be reported to the physician, if detected.

Bilevel Positive Airway Pressure

Bilevel positive airway pressure (BiPAP) is another form of noninvasive positive-pressure ventilation that provides continuous high-flow positive airway pressure that cycles between a high positive pressure and a lower positive pressure. Gas exchange improves with BiPAP because of an increase in alveolar ventilation. Monitoring is similar to that for CPAP.

Synchronous Intermittent Mandatory Ventilation

Synchronous intermittent mandatory ventilation allows the patient to control the inspiratory time and the size of the spontaneous tidal volumes depending on patient effort and muscle strength, lung compliance, airway resistance, and whether pressure support is present to increase spontaneous tidal volume delivery. The patient receives three different types of breath: controlled (mandatory), assisted (synchronized), and spontaneous. Synchronized intermittent mandatory ventilation (SIMV) can be combined with pressure support ventilation to provide both a back-up support ventilation strategy and can also be implemented as SIMV (pressure mode).

Intermittent Mandatory Ventilation

Intermittent mandatory ventilation was originally devised for facilitation of the weaning process from mechanical ventilation. It is currently used when a patient is first given mechanical ventilation. This technique allows patients to breathe on their own as often and as deeply as they like; it also ensures that every minute a set tidal volume is delivered at a predetermined back-up rate. IMV allows gradual progression from complete ventilatory support with the ventilator to spontaneous provision of ventilation by the patient.

Nursing Responsibilities

All PACU nurses must be familiar with the specific types and modes of operation of ventilators used in the area (Fig. 28-1; see Table 28-2);

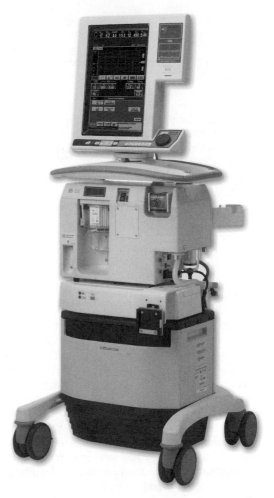

FIG. 28-1 840 Ventilator system. Volume ventilator used either to assist or to control a patient's respirations. (Image used by permission from Nellcor Puritan Bennett LLC, Boulder, Colorado, doing business as Covidien.)

however, some nursing responsibilities remain the same regardless of mechanical ventilator. The following list discusses these responsibilities.

1. Ascertain that the patient's lungs are ventilated with frequent observation of the chest for bilateral synchronous and equal expansion and by listening for bilaterally present and equal breath sounds.

2. Check the airway frequently for complete patency. See that the patient's ventilator system is free of significant leaks by listening for air gurgling in the upper airway during ventilation and by comparing the exhaled volume with the tidal volume set on the ventilator.

3. Ensure that the cuff is never overinflated. Inflate the cuff until no leak is identified on tidal ventilation and a small barely audible leak occurs on sigh volume.

4. Empty the ventilatory hoses frequently of excess water from condensation.

5. Ensure that proper humidification is delivered to the patient by noting the presence of water droplets in the ventilator hoses.

6. Check the humidifier and fill frequently to ensure proper humidification.

7. Ensure that the temperature gauge is between 32.2° and 36.6° C, and that the ventilator hoses and humidifier are warm to the touch and never cold or hot.

8. Position the patient's endotracheal or tracheostomy tube so that there is never any pull.

9. Perform the tracheostomy wound care as needed during the postanesthesia phase.

10. Ascertain frequently that all alarms on the ventilator are on, set appropriately, and functioning properly.

The observations and checks of mechanical devices often seem simple and routine but are an important part of nursing the patient who requires mechanical ventilation. Ideally all these checks, along with measured parameters of the patient's respiratory status, should be recorded either on a flow sheet attached to the patient's bed or to the ventilator or electronically as defined by the facility. Frequently, respiratory therapists maintain and manage the ventilator in the PACU. The respiratory therapist is available to assist the nurse caring for the patient who requires a ventilator and to complete the appropriate documentation of ventilator and patient status.

Suctioning

When large amounts of secretions accumulate that cannot be handled effectively with coughing, suctioning must be instituted to assist the patient in clearing air passages.

Oral and Nasal Suctioning

Suctioning the nose and mouth is simple and safe. This procedure is commonly used to assist patients in eliminating secretions when they have not yet regained full consciousness and cannot spit out secretions. The catheter should be soft and pliable. The technique should be clean but need not be strictly sterile. A Yankauer or tonsil suction tip can be used to remove oral secretions from the mouth and over the tongue; however, care must be used to avoid breaking or chipping the teeth.

Tracheal Suctioning

Tracheal suctioning can be performed through the mouth or nose, via endotracheal tube, or through a tracheostomy tube (Fig. 28-2). Tracheal suctioning must be accomplished atraumatically with aseptic technique. A selection of sterile suctioning catheters in a variety of sizes should be

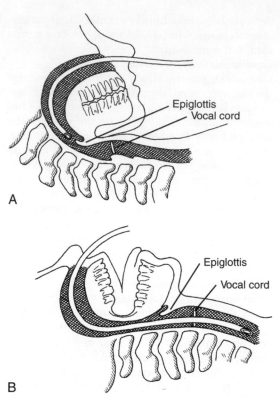

FIG. 28-2 Cross section through the airway showing nasotracheal suctioning. **A,** The patient's head may be kept in a neutral position as the catheter is advanced through a nostril to the back of the throat. **B,** The patient's head is carefully moved to the sniff position. During inspiration, the catheter is advanced into the trachea. The patient will cough, and secretions can be suctioned out. (From Sills JR: *The comprehensive respiratory therapist exam review*, ed 5, St. Louis, 2010, Mosby.)

kept at the bedside of every patient in the PACU along with sterile gloves and sterile water or normal saline solution. The catheter chosen for suctioning should not have an external diameter that exceeds by one third the internal diameter of the tube to be suctioned. Most commonly, a 14 or 16 F size is used for adult patients. The catheter must not completely occlude the trachea or endotracheal tube.

The procedure should be explained to the patient even if the patient appears unconscious. Explaining the procedure alleviates fear and also helps to gain cooperation from the patient.

Before suctioning, ensure proper ventilation. In most patients, suctioning lowers the arterial pressure of oxygen 30 to 35 mm Hg. Because suctioning removes oxygen, which can in turn initiate cardiac dysrhythmias, the nurse should assess the total physiologic condition of the patient before beginning the procedure. Is the patient restless, agitated, or disoriented? Although these conditions can be caused by other factors, they often indicate inadequate oxygenation. Conscious patients should be asked to take four or five deep breaths. The patient who cannot cooperate must undergo preoxygenation with a bag-mask unit or anesthesia bag. A bag-mask device delivers variable oxygen concentrations (FiO_2 between 30% and 95%) and volumes. Flow rates should be at least 10 to 15 L/min for higher FiO_2. Higher volumes can be obtained with the use of two hands to compress the bag. If the patient has an endotracheal airway in place and is using a ventilator, several sigh volumes can be delivered at 1 FiO_2 before suctioning.

For suctioning in a patient with no airway adjunct, the nurse should instruct the patient to stick out the tongue and then should grasp the tongue with a gauze pad and apply gentle traction to make the glottis open and move in line with the trachea. The nurse then lubricates the catheter tip with a small amount of water-soluble jelly and gently inserts the catheter into the nostril. A slight curvature in the tubing may facilitate intubation of the larynx. The catheter is advanced until intubation of the trachea is accomplished. The nurse listens through the catheter or feels for air movement against the cheek through the proximal end of the catheter. An increasing intensity of breath sounds or more air against the cheek indicates nearness to the larynx. If the breath sounds decrease or the patient begins to gag, the catheter is in the hypopharynx and the nurse needs to draw back and advance again. A sudden cough indicates the presence of the catheter in the larynx; the nurse should advance quickly with the next breath.

When the catheter is positioned in the trachea, intermittent suction is applied with alternate occluding and opening of the vent of the Y-connector with the thumb and withdrawal of the catheter in a spiral motion. If an airway adjunct is present, suctioning can be accomplished through it.

Suction should never be applied until the catheter is in the trachea and never for longer than 15 seconds. One useful trick is for the nurse to hold his or her breath while suctioning the patient as a reminder of the time limits. The patient is monitored carefully during all suctioning procedures. Any form of suctioning can lead to dysrhythmias, and prolonged suctioning can produce hypoxia, asphyxia, and cardiac arrest. Suctioning removes oxygen and secretions; therefore the patient should undergo oxygenation before and after the procedure.

Suctioning is not without risk of complication, nor should it be done routinely. Risks include bradycardia and vagal responses. Appropriate indications for suctioning are the presence of bronchial secretions, identified visually or with auscultation or, in the patient with mechanical ventilation, with rising airway pressures from retained secretions. Hypoxemia is the most common complication that can lead to atelectasis and dysrhythmias. Other complications include mucosal trauma, infection, paroxysmal coughing, and increased systemic and intracranial pressures.

Tracheostomy care is discussed in Chapter 32.

General Comfort and Safety Measures

General comfort and safety measures are important parts of postanesthesia care. For safety, at least two nurses (one of whom is a registered nurse competent in phase I perianesthesia nursing care) should always be present in the same room or unit whenever patients in PACU Phase I level of care are recovering.[4] An unconscious patient should never be left alone, and side rails should be raised on the bed or stretcher whenever direct patient care is not being provided. The wheels of the bed or stretcher should be locked to prevent sliding when care is rendered.

General physical measures such as cleanliness should not be overlooked in the PACU. Comfort measures, important to the total well being of the patient, are often forgotten in the hustle of caring for postanesthesia patients. As soon as the patient is settled into the unit and assessment has been accomplished, all excess skin preparations and electrodes should be removed; in addition to providing comfort, washing off excess skin preparations gives the nurse an excellent opportunity to further assess the patient's general condition. The stretcher or bed linen should be dry and wrinkle free to minimize risk of skin irritation or breakdown. This time is also good for changing the patient's position, assisting with range-of-motion exercises, and encouraging deep breathing. Frequent position changes help to prevent atelectasis, promote circulation, and prevent pressure from developing on the skin surfaces.

Mouth care with moistened Toothettes or swabs may be comforting to the patient who has been without oral fluids or breathing dry gases. When patients are fully conscious and laryngeal reflexes have returned, they can rinse the mouth with water. Ice chips and small sips of water or juice can be offered to the patient who can tolerate fluids. Ointment should be applied to the lips after mouth care to prevent drying and consequent cracking.

NURSING CARE IN THE PACU

Patients often are cold when they return from the operating suite. This condition is caused in part by the effects of anesthesia and the cool atmosphere of the operating suite and the PACU. These reasons must be explained to the patient. Active warming measures, such as a convective warming device, should be instituted on arrival to the PACU if the patient is hypothermic.[5] Devices should be used according to the manufacturers' recommendations to avoid patient injury.

The patient who is normothermic may shiver or feel cold; warm blankets may provide psychologic comfort, and active warming interventions may be needed to reduce or eliminate shaking. Blankets of any type should not, however, obscure the intravenous lines, arterial lines, or other monitoring apparatuses from the direct view of the attending nurse. The patient's body temperature must be monitored closely to avoid overheating. Shivering may be treated with low doses of meperidine, 12.5 to 25 mg intravenously, which attenuates the shivering response. Hypothermia is discussed in Chapter 53.

In addition to physical comfort measures, remember to provide psychologic comfort. Reorientation, especially to time and place, is important to the postanesthesia patient, as is constant reassurance that the surgery is completed and that all went well. The nurse's presence at the bedside or gentle touch may also be comforting to the patient.

Transfer of the Patient from the Postanesthesia Care Unit

When the patient has recovered from the effects of anesthesia, vital signs are stabilized; if no surgical complications have arisen, the patient is ready for transfer to the nursing unit or discharge area. The patient's postanesthesia recovery score, if a scoring system is used, should meet preestablished minimums, unless criteria for exceptions are noted. The patient should have regained a satisfactory level of consciousness to the point of being oriented and able to call for assistance, if necessary, and should be clean, dry, and dressed in appropriate hospital garb. All dressings should be dry and intact, and all drainage receptacles should be emptied. A licensed practitioner should see the patient before discharge, or the name of the responsible physician should be documented in the patient's record. The PACU nurse should discharge the patient when the patient meets medically approved discharge criteria.

No patient should be discharged immediately after receiving an initial dose of an opioid medication. Discharge should be delayed to assess pain relief and adverse side effects of the medication. Pain assessment and management should be documented in the patient's record for ongoing evaluation of pain intensity and treatment effectiveness.

A summarizing PACU discharge note should be written on the patient's progress record or entered into the electronic health record to indicate condition and time of transfer. The nurse should alert the receiving unit that the patient is being transferred and request the preparation of any specialized equipment for care and the assignment of a receiving nurse.

Patients can be transferred on a stretcher or bed as required by condition and operative procedure. The patient should be adequately covered with bed linens, including a warmed blanket if hallways are kept cool. The side rails of the stretcher should be locked in place. Ideally, two persons should wheel the stretcher to the receiving unit. Transport personnel vary by institution, and decisions regarding who transports can vary based on the patient's condition, staffing, and unit needs. Practice Recommendation 6, in the American Society of PeriAnesthesia Nurses' *2010-2012 Perianesthesia Nursing Standards and Practice Recommendations*, address required elements for the safe transfer of care.[4] The handoff between providers should allow communication of patient status and care needs; the opportunity to ask questions of the transferring caregiver is required. The form of that transfer varies by facility policy and practice, but must minimize patient risk.

A receiving nurse should meet the patient on arrival to the unit and direct the transfer to the patient's room. The patient is transferred to the bed along with all apparatuses. Safety precautions must be strictly followed. At least two people should always transfer the patient. A third person may be necessary to assist with the patient transfer if extra equipment or multiple drainage tubes are present. Use of transfer devices such as slider boards, roller tubes, or mechanical lifts facilitates the transfer and minimizes the risk of injury for both the patient and the nursing staff. Both the bed and the stretcher should be stabilized by locking the wheels when transferring the patient from one to the other. The nurse should ensure that all drainage tubes and catheters are safely transferred, that no kinking occurs, and that they do not become tangled underneath the patient. All drainage receptacles should remain below the level of the patient. Intravenous tubing and solution must be carefully transferred from the portable stand attached to the stretcher to the bedside stand or holder. Drainage tubes should be connected to suction or gravity drainage as indicated, and their proper functioning checked. The patient's call light should be positioned within the patient's reach, along with any other items that may be needed. The intravenous infusion rate should be assessed and adjusted as necessary. Side rails on the bed should be raised.

The report can be written, telephoned, faxed, printed from the electronic health record, or reviewed online before or at the time of transfer. It can be given in person to the receiving nurse. The PACU nurse should give a complete report to the receiving nurse, including pertinent facts about the following: patient demographic information; pertinent health history; the operative procedure performed; the type of anesthesia or sedation used and any reversal agents given; the patient's general condition and postanesthesia course; incision; any drains placed and the dressing; any drainage tubes or catheters; intake and output, including intravenous fluids given, estimated blood loss, and time of void or catheterization; any medications given in the PACU, especially analgesics; and the patient's response and level of comfort. As appropriate, orders are reviewed with the receiving nurse, the location of sensory aids and valuables is discussed, and social support availability is reviewed.

SUMMARY

This chapter discussed patient education concepts including learner characteristics and teaching strategies. Nursing care of postanesthesia patients who are emerging from anesthesia is also reviewed in this chapter. Postanesthesia care discussed included the stir-up regimen, intravenous therapy, maintenance of cardiopulmonary function, and general comfort measures.

REFERENCES

1. Suhonen R, Leino-Kilpi H: Adult surgical patients and the information provided to them by nurses: a literature review, *Patient Educ Couns* 61(1):5–15, 2006.
2. Fredericks S, et al: Postoperative patient education: a systematic review, *Clin Nurs Res* 19(2):144–164, 2010.
3. Pedersen T, et al: Pulse oximetry for perioperative monitoring, *Cochrane Database Syst Rev* 4(CD 002013):2009, doi: 10.1002/14651858.CD002013.pub2. Accessed December 6, 2011.
4. American Society of PeriAnesthesia Nurses (ASPAN): *Perianesthesia nursing standards and practice recommendations 2010–2012*, Cherry Hill, NJ, 2010, ASPAN.
5. Hooper VD, et al: ASPAN's evidence-based clinical practice guideline for the promotion of perioperative normothermia, *J Perianesth Nurs* 24(5):271–287, 2009.

RESOURCES

American Association of Critical-Care Nurses: *AACN procedure manual for critical care*, ed 6, St. Louis, 2011, Saunders.

Black JM, Hawks JH: *Medical-surgical nursing: clinical management for positive outcomes*, ed 8, St. Louis, 2008, Saunders.

Finucane BT, et al: *Principles of airway management*, ed 4, New York, 2011, Springer.

Godden B: Where does capnography fit into the PACU? *J Perianesth Nurs* 26(6):408–410, 2011.

Johansson K, et al: Surgical patient education: assessing the interventions and exploring the outcomes from experimental and quasiexperimental studies from 1990 to 2003, *Clin Effectiveness Nurs* 8(2):81–92, 2004.

Pasquina P, et al: Respiratory physiotherapy to prevent pulmonary complications after abdominal surgery: a systematic review, *Chest* 130(6):1887–1899, 2006.

Sjoling M, et al: The impact of preoperative information on state anxiety, postoperative pain and satisfaction with pain management, *Patient Educ Couns* 51:169–176, 2003.

Stern C, Lockwood C: Knowledge retention from preoperative patient information, *International Journal of Evidence-Based Healthcare* 3:45–63, 2005, doi: 10.1111/j.1479-6988.2005.00021.x. Accessed December 6, 2011.

Zhang CY, et al: Impact of nurse-initiated preoperative education on postoperative anxiety symptoms and complications after coronary artery bypass grafting, *J Cardiovasc Nurs* 27(1):84–88, 2012.

NURSING CARE IN THE PACU

29 Postanesthesia Care Complications

Denise O'Brien DNP, RN, ACNS-BC, CPAN, CAPA, FAAN

Complications can occur during any phase of the patient's perianesthesia experience. From allergic reactions to preoperative medications in the holding area to postanesthesia airway obstruction, situations occur that require the perianesthesia nurse's vigilance, prompt action, and appropriate treatment. The postanesthesia period is a precarious time for the patient; prevention of complications is an essential role for the perianesthesia nurse. The perianesthesia nurse, whether in an inpatient or outpatient setting, must be prepared to respond to rapidly evolving potentially life-threatening situations. Complications that more commonly occur in the postanesthesia setting are addressed in this chapter, including respiratory and cardiovascular complications; thermoregulation; and complications associated with anesthesia medications, techniques, and procedures.

DEFINITIONS

Acute Myocardial Infarction: Occurs when an area of heart muscle dies or is permanently damaged because of an inadequate supply of oxygen to that area.

Anaphylactic Reactions: Anaphylaxis is a severe whole-body allergic reaction that occurs rapidly and causes a life-threatening response that involves the whole body.

Aspiration: The inhalation of either oropharyngeal or gastric contents into the lungs.

Awareness During Anesthesia: Occurs when a person is aware of some portion of the procedure (sometimes even pain) during general anesthesia; can cause long-term psychologic effects and symptoms of posttraumatic stress.

Bradycardia: A heart rate of less than 60 beats/min (adult) with a regular rhythm and P waves present.

Bronchospasm: Narrowing of the bronchi and bronchioles from smooth muscle contraction that results in wheezing, coughing, and decreased oxygen exchange.

Delayed Emergence (Awakening): Patient emergence from anesthesia is delayed; failure to emerge can be classified as the result of drug effects, metabolic disorders, or neurologic disorders.

Dilutional Hyponatremia: Absorption of irrigating solutions through open blood vessels (during prostate resection) or perforation of the uterine or bladder wall that leads to circulatory overload from water intoxication. May also be caused by excessive free water intake, excess sodium losses, or inappropriate antidiuretic hormone secretion.

Emergence Excitement: A condition characterized by restlessness, disorientation, crying, moaning, irrational talking, and inappropriate behavior.

Hemolytic Transfusion Reactions: An ABO-incompatible blood reaction that precipitates a hemolytic reaction that results in agglutination, or clumping, of red blood cells, which blocks the patient's capillaries and thus obstructs the flow of blood and oxygen to vital organs.

Hemorrhage: Rapid, copious blood loss.

Hypertension: A blood pressure increased 20% to 30% above the baseline blood pressure.

Hyperthermia: A core temperature of more than 38° C.

Hypotension: A blood pressure that is less than 20% to 30% of the baseline blood pressure.

Hypothermia: A core temperature of less than 36° C.

Hypoventilation: A decrease in respiratory rate and tidal volume that leads to an increase in partial pressure of carbon dioxide ($PaCO_2$).

Hypoxemia: A PaO_2 of less than 60 mm Hg.

Laryngospasm: An involuntary partial or complete closure of the vocal cords, caused by secretions, or stimulation or irritation of the laryngeal reflexes during emergence.

Malignant Hyperthermia (MH): A pharmacogenetic (autosomal dominant inheritance) disorder of muscle metabolism involving hypermetabolism that can be triggered by succinylcholine or the volatile anesthetics.

Noncardiogenic Pulmonary Edema: Respiratory disorder that most commonly occurs after an obstructive event that results in pulmonary capillary leakage and pulmonary edema.

Nonhemolytic Febrile Reactions: Most often caused by sensitivity to leukocytes and platelets and seen most often in patients who have received multiple transfusions.

Perforated Viscus: Internal organs perforated during the operative procedure.

Plasma Cholinesterase Deficiency: An uncommon genetic disorder that renders the patient with an inability to metabolize succinylcholine, resulting in prolonged skeletal muscle paralysis and apnea of 2 hours or more.

Pneumothorax: An accumulation of air or gas in the pleural space.

Postdischarge Nausea and Vomiting (PDNV): Nausea or vomiting that occurs after discharge from the health care facility after ambulatory surgery.

Postdural Puncture Headache: A headache that typically develops 24 to 48 hours after lumbar puncture from a spinal needle placement or unintentional dural puncture during an epidural placement.

Postoperative Nausea and Vomiting (PONV): Nausea or vomiting that occurs within the first 24 hours after inpatient surgery.

Pulmonary Edema: Increase in lung fluid as a result of leakage from pulmonary capillaries into the interstitium and alveoli of the lung; leads to impaired gas exchange and may cause respiratory failure.

Pulmonary Embolism: A sudden blockage of an artery in the lungs by fat, air, clumped tumor cells, or a blood clot; usually a blood clot that traveled to the lung from the leg.

Spinal Epidural Hematoma: A hematoma after spinal procedures or surgery; blood accumulates between the spinal dura and bone compressing nerves; without prompt treatment, it can cause permanent neurologic deficits.

Tachycardia: A heart rate greater than 100 beats/min (adult) with a regular rhythm and P waves present.

Transfusion-Related Acute Lung Injury (TRALI): Rare but devastating complication of blood component therapy; findings are similar to adult respiratory distress syndrome and consist of hypotension, fever, dyspnea, and tachycardia.

RESPIRATORY COMPLICATIONS

Airway management and respiratory care are first in the mind of the perianesthesia nurse when patients arrive in the postanesthesia care unit (PACU). Avoidance of postoperative pulmonary complications, including atelectasis, pneumonia, respiratory failure, and exacerbation, helps to reduce patient morbidity and mortality rates. The perianesthesia nurse works to prevent these serious longer-term complications by maintaining and improving the patient's respiratory function in the immediate postanesthesia period of care. Some patients are at greater risk for developing these complications. Primarily these risk factors are related to the patient or the procedure. Box 29-1 lists the most common risk factors supported by evidence.[1]

Airway Obstruction

One of the most commonly occurring complications in the postanesthesia care setting is airway obstruction. Airway obstruction can be upper or lower in origin, from the simple problem of the tongue falling back and obstructing the upper airway to complete laryngospasm with no air movement.

Upper airway obstruction can be caused by tongue relaxation, which is most common, and is seen in the patient who has not fully recovered from anesthesia, who has received opioid or sedative drugs, or who has residual neuromuscular blocking

---

BOX 29-1   Risk Factors for Postoperative Pulmonary Complications

PATIENT-RELATED RISK FACTORS
- Advanced age
- American Society of Anesthesiologists class greater than or equal to II
- Congestive heart failure
- Functional dependence
- Chronic obstructive pulmonary disease
- Weight loss
- Impaired sensorium
- Cigarette use
- Alcohol use
- Abnormal findings on chest examination

PROCEDURE-RELATED RISK FACTORS
- Aortic aneurysm repair
- Thoracic surgery
- Abdominal surgery
- Upper abdominal surgery
- Neurosurgery
- Prolonged surgery
- Head and neck surgery
- Emergency surgery
- Vascular surgery
- General anesthesia

Data from Smetana GW, et al: Preoperative pulmonary risk stratification for noncardiothoracic surgery: systematic review for the American College of Physicians, *Ann Intern Med* 144:581–595, 2006.

---

agents on board. Other causes include swelling or edema of the airway, airway injury, bleeding (hemorrhage), or obstructive sleep apnea. Treatment includes verbal or tactile stimulation of the patient, airway repositioning with chin lift or jaw thrust, placement of an oral or nasopharyngeal airway adjunct, and application of positive pressure with a bag-valve-mask device. If the patient's airway cannot be maintained with these methods, oral or nasal placement of an endotracheal tube may be necessary, or emergency cricothyroidotomy or tracheostomy may be performed. Positioning the patient in the recovery position (side-lying with head down to facilitate drainage) can also help to maintain a patent airway in the patient at risk for soft tissue obstruction or significant oral drainage that interferes with the airway.

Laryngospasm

Laryngospasm is an involuntary partial or complete closure of the vocal cords, caused by secretions or stimulation or irritation of the laryngeal reflexes during emergence. Wheezing, reduced compliance, stridor (partial), paradoxical chest or abdominal movements, and absence of ventilation (complete) are signs and symptoms of laryngospasm. Ventilation is decreased or absent, and oxygenation of the patient is difficult as carbon dioxide builds ($PaCO_2$ increases). Treatment includes airway maneuvers (chin lift/jaw thrust), elevation of the head of bed to maximize respiratory excursion, and application of a bag-valve-mask for continuous positive pressure with oxygen. Secretions need to be carefully removed with suction. The patient may need reintubation to secure the airway if mask ventilation is difficult. Medications include succinylcholine and can include other neuromuscular blocking agents and lidocaine. When the patient has received a neuromuscular blocking agent, the patient may need sedation to reduce anxiety related to apnea, muscle relaxation, and awareness.

Subglottic Edema

For the pediatric patient, obstruction may be caused by subglottic edema, usually observed in children 1 to 4 years of age. Traumatic intubation, tight fit of the endotracheal tube, coughing with the tube in place, position change with the tube inserted, surgery of the head or neck, and procedures that last more than 1 hour can result in subglottic edema. Crowing respirations, stridor, and rocking chest wall respiratory attempts may signal subglottic edema. Postoperative supplemental humidified oxygen can diminish airway swelling. Initial treatment includes humidified oxygen and nebulized mist treatment with racemic epinephrine. Further treatment can include inhalation of a helium–oxygen mixture, administration of dexamethasone, and calming with analgesics and parental or caregiver presence. Ambulatory surgery patients with subglottic edema who are treated with racemic epinephrine may be considered for overnight admission because of the risk of rebound edema. Extended observation for up to 8 hours may be sufficient if the parents are comfortable and emergency resources are readily available.

Bronchospasm

Narrowing of the bronchi and bronchioles from smooth muscle contraction results in bronchospasm. Bronchospasm may be the result of preexisting asthma; allergy or anaphylaxis; histamine release; mucous plugging; aspiration; pulmonary edema; wheezing with acute heart failure, but without any other acute pulmonary pathology (cardiogenic asthma); or foreign body aspiration. Signs and symptoms include cough, expiratory wheezing, dyspnea, use of accessory muscles, and tachypnea. Treatment of the patient includes removal of the identified cause, oxygen administration, inhaled bronchodilators, and epinephrine. Depending on cause, an antihistamine or dexamethasone may be appropriate. Secretions should be suctioned. If the condition results from foreign body aspiration, such as a tooth, emergent bronchoscopy is needed. Ventilatory support may be necessary, and the patient may need reintubation for maintenance of oxygenation and ventilation.

Aspiration

Identified as a high-risk low-frequency occurrence, aspiration may be observed in the postanesthesia setting. The patient with a nasal or oropharyngeal airway in place and returning gag reflexes may become nauseated and vomit. In a nonresponsive state and supine position, the patient is at greater risk for aspiration. Types of aspirates include large particle, clear acidic or nonacidic fluid, foodstuff or small particle, and contaminated material. In addition, foreign bodies such as teeth or blood may be aspirated. Symptoms include unexplained tachypnea and tachycardia, cough, bronchospasm, hypoxemia, atelectasis, interstitial edema, hemorrhage, and acute respiratory distress syndrome. The aspiration can trigger laryngospasm, infection, and pulmonary edema. Prevention of aspiration is preferred. Patients at risk should be identified before surgery and premedicated. Patients at risk are patients with emergent procedures, known full stomachs, or history of gastroesophageal reflux disease; those older than age 65 years; and women in labor. Medications include histamine blockers, nonparticulate antacids, and anticholinergic agents. During surgery, rapid sequence induction and nasogastric tube placement may help to minimize the risk of aspiration. After surgery, maintenance of the endotracheal tube until airway reflexes have returned and positioning of the patient with the head to the side or in a left lateral decubitus position can aid in decreasing the risk of aspiration. If aspiration occurs, hypoxemia should be corrected and hemodynamic stability maintained. The patient may need reintubation and suctioning and mechanical ventilation. Arterial blood gases assist in planning respiratory management of the patient. A chest radiograph is obtained, but findings may be inconclusive initially; radiographic findings may lag behind clinical signs by 24 hours after the suspected aspiration event. Prophylactic antibiotics or steroids are not recommended. Tracheal secretions should be cultured; if results are positive, antibiotics can be prescribed.

Hypoventilation

Hypoventilation may be the result of residual anesthetic agents; opioids; neuromuscular blocking agents; inadequate reversal of opioids, sedatives, or neuromuscular blocking agents; thoracic or abdominal incisions and procedures; or neuromuscular diseases.

Signs and symptoms include decreased respiratory rate, shallow respirations, increased end-tidal carbon dioxide ($ETCO_2$), and increased $PaCO_2$ (>45 mm Hg [hypercarbia]). Treatment includes identification and management of the cause of the hypoventilation, supplemental oxygen administration, verbal and tactile stimulation, deep breathing exercises, repositioning, and cautious use of analgesics or sedatives. Oxygen saturation monitoring is necessary, and capnographic monitoring may be appropriate for patients at risk.

Hypoxemia

Unidentified hypoxemia in the postanesthesia patient is not as common since the advent of noninvasive oxygen saturation monitoring with pulse oximetry. Hypoxemia may be the result of a low inspired concentration of oxygen, hypoventilation, ventilation–perfusion inequality, increased intrapulmonary right to left shunt, or pneumothorax. It can also be caused by diffuse airway collapse, pulmonary edema, and pulmonary embolism. Treatment includes identification and correction of the cause, stimulation of the patient, supplemental oxygen administration, and continuous positive airway pressure (CPAP), which can be used in the spontaneously breathing patient. Patients who cannot maintain oxygen levels may need tracheal intubation and mechanical ventilation and positive end-expiratory pressure (PEEP) support.

Pneumothorax

Pneumothorax, an accumulation of air or gas in the pleural space, can occur during the perianesthesia period. It may be the result of percutaneous internal jugular and subclavian vein cannulation, hemodynamic monitoring line placement, certain upper extremity blocks (supraclavicular and infraclavicular approaches to the brachial plexus), or operative procedures of the chest. The patient may have sharp ipsilateral chest pain and dyspnea. Assessment findings include decreased breath sounds and hyperresonance on the affected side of the chest. Treatment includes supplemental oxygen administration and ordering of a chest radiograph. If a less than 20% pneumothorax is diagnosed based on the chest radiograph, the treating physician may want to observe the patient for a period of time until the pneumothorax either resolves or increases. If the pneumothorax is greater than 20% or the patient has cardiovascular compromise, a chest tube may be needed.

Pulmonary Edema

Fluid overload, congestive heart failure, or acute pulmonary injury can result in pulmonary edema. Signs and symptoms include hypoxemia, crackles (rales), and decreased pulmonary compliance. Pulmonary infiltrates are seen on chest radiograph results.

Identification and treatment of the cause of the pulmonary edema is the first step in treatment. In addition, diuretics and fluid restriction to decrease afterload and supplemental oxygen administration may be ordered. Patients with an inability to maintain oxygenation or adequate ventilation may undergo intubation and mechanical ventilation and PEEP.

Noncardiogenic Pulmonary Edema

Noncardiogenic pulmonary edema may be the result of upper airway obstruction, laryngospasm, bolus dosing with naloxone, incomplete reversal of neuromuscular blockade, or a significant period of hypoxia. When the cause is obstructive in origin, two types of postobstructive pulmonary edema (POPE) have been identified: type I and type II.[2] Both are present with acute respiratory distress. Type I usually occurs within 60 minutes of a precipitating event, but onset can be delayed up to 6 hours. Type I POPE may follow postextubation laryngospasm, epiglottitis, croup, choking or foreign body, strangulation, hanging, endotracheal tube obstruction, laryngeal tumor, goiter, mononucleosis, postoperative vocal cord paralysis, migration of the urinary catheter balloon used for tamponade epistaxis, near drowning, and intraoperative direct suctioning of an endotracheal tube adapter.[3] Type II POPE develops soon after relief of chronic upper airway obstruction, such as after tonsillectomy or adenoidectomy, removal of upper airway tumor, choanal stenosis, and hypertrophic redundant uvula.[3]

Signs and symptoms include hypoxemia, cough, failure to maintain oxygen saturation levels, tachypnea, and frothy sputum. Treatment includes supplemental oxygen administration and maintenance of a patent upper airway. CPAP may be used. Patients with an inability to maintain a patent airway may need intubation and mechanical ventilation with PEEP. For patients with significant compromise, hemodynamic support and continued observation in an intensive care unit may be needed. Patients with noncardiogenic pulmonary edema typically recover rapidly after the intense initial phase and leave the critical care unit within approximately 24 to 36 hours and without permanent sequelae from the event.

Pulmonary Embolism

Patients predisposed to development of pulmonary emboli include patients who are obese or immobile, who are undergoing pelvic or long bone procedures, and who have a history of congestive heart failure or malignant disease.[4] Signs and symptoms can include tachypnea, pleuritic chest pain, hemoptysis, breathlessness, and a sense of impending doom. Treatment is supportive for correction of hypoxemia and hemodynamic instability. Intravenous heparin and morphine sulfate can be given to help stabilize the pulmonary capillary membrane. Prevention of venous thromboembolism and subsequent pulmonary emboli development includes subcutaneous unfractionated heparin, low–molecular-weight heparins, or intermittent or sequential compression devices.

CARDIOVASCULAR COMPLICATIONS

Cardiovascular complications that occur in the PACU range from relatively benign ectopic beats to hemodynamic collapse from an acute myocardial infarction. The perianesthesia nurse monitors the patient continuously in phase I, observing rate and rhythm and blood pressure and noting any signs or symptoms of hemodynamic compromise. The following section briefly discusses the more common cardiovascular complications seen in the perianesthesia setting.

Major cardiovascular perioperative risks are identified as myocardial infarction, heart failure, and death. Clinical predictors of increased perioperative cardiovascular complications are listed in Box 29-2.[5]

Dysrhythmias

Dysrhythmias can occur as the result of hypoxia, hypercarbia, electrolyte abnormalities, acid-base alterations, myocardial ischemia, drug effects, pain, hypovolemia, bladder distention, and hypothermia. Occasional ectopic beats may be seen in healthy patients. Significant dysrhythmias necessitate immediate identification and treatment; these include premature ventricular contractions (more than five per minute, coupled [more than two together], or multifocal), ventricular tachycardia, ventricular fibrillation, asystole, heart block, pulseless electric activity, and new onset atrial fibrillation. Treatment includes identification and treatment of the cause, supplemental oxygen administration, ventilatory and hemodynamic support, and pharmacologic therapy. Advanced

---

BOX 29-2	Clinical Predictors of Increased Perioperative Cardiovascular Complications

ACTIVE CARDIAC CONDITIONS—MAJOR (DELAY OR CANCEL SURGERY UNLESS EMERGENT)
- Unstable coronary syndromes: recent myocardial infarction with evidence of important ischemic risk, unstable or severe angina
- Decompensated heart failure
- Significant dysrhythmias: atrioventricular block, symptomatic ventricular dysrhythmias, supraventricular dysrhythmias with uncontrolled ventricular rate
- Severe valvular disease

CLINICAL RISK FACTORS
- History of ischemic heart disease
- Compensated or prior heart failure
- History of cerebrovascular disease
- Diabetes mellitus
- Renal insufficiency

MINOR (RECOGNIZED MARKERS FOR CARDIOVASCULAR DISEASE BUT NOT PROVEN TO INCREASE RISK INDEPENDENTLY)
- Advanced age (older than 70 years)
- Abnormal electrocardiogram
- Rhythm other than sinus
- Uncontrolled systemic hypertension

Data from Fleisher LA, et al: 2009 ACCF/AHA focused update on perioperative beta blockade incorporated into the ACC/AHA 2007 guidelines on perioperative cardiovascular evaluation and care for noncardiac surgery, *J Am Coll Cardiol* 54(22):e13–e118, 2009.

---

cardiac life support (ACLS) or pediatric advanced life support (PALS) protocols are initiated when appropriate.

Bradycardia

Sinus bradycardia can occur as the result of vagal responses, hypoxia, drug effects, increased intracranial pressure (ICP), or distended bladder. Treatment is dependent on the cause and can include anticholinergic agents (e.g., atropine), supplemental oxygen administration, and stimulation. If the condition is the result of elevated ICP, hyperventilation and pharmacologic therapy may be indicated.

Tachycardia

Sinus tachycardia occurs commonly in the postanesthesia setting. Causes include hypoxia, hypercarbia, hypovolemia, sepsis, hyperthermia, heart failure, pain, drugs, and psychologic stress.

Treatment includes administration of supplemental oxygen, ventilation support, and evaluation of fluid and cardiac status. If the condition results from pain, medication with analgesics is the treatment. Sedatives may be needed if the condition is from anxiety or stress. If the patient is hyperthermic, the patient's core temperature is lowered with recommended cooling devices. Tachycardia in patients with coronary artery disease can increase the risk of myocardial ischemia.

Hypotension

Hypotension is defined as blood pressure that is less than 20% to 30% of the baseline blood pressure.[6] Causes range from use of an inappropriately sized cuff, to hypovolemia, myocardial dysfunction, and a decrease in systemic vascular resistance (Fig. 29-1). Management and treatment of hypotension in the PACU includes use of a cuff of the appropriate size, administration of supplemental oxygen, initiation of fluid resuscitation, stoppage of drug infusions if causative, and elevation of the legs. Inotropic agents or vasopressor or vasoconstrictive agents may be ordered.

Hypertension

Hypertension is defined "as persistent elevation of systolic blood pressure greater than 140 mm Hg or a diastolic blood pressure greater than 90 mm Hg or requires an antihypertensive treatment."[7] Too small or narrow of a cuff can result in abnormally elevated blood pressures. Pain, stress, hypoxemia, hypercarbia, fluid overload, delirium, drugs, bladder, bowel or stomach distention, or hypothermia can cause hypertension. Many of the patients in PACU in whom hypertension develops have preexisting hypertension. The elevation in blood pressure is usually benign and short lived; however, the hypertension can precipitate myocardial ischemia in the patient with coronary artery disease as a result of stimulation of the sympathetic nervous system. Treatment for hypertension includes use of an appropriately sized cuff and identification and management of the underlying cause first. This condition may necessitate ventilatory support and oxygen administration, analgesics or sedatives, bladder decompression, and antihypertensive agents.

Patients who have had a cervical or thoracic spinal cord injury (above T6) are at risk for developing autonomic dysreflexia, which is a massive uninhibited sympathetic cardiovascular response to noxious stimuli (e.g., bowel or bladder overdistention) characterized by paroxysmal hypertension, pounding headache, facial flushing, sweating, temporal or neck vessel engorgement, nasal congestion, blurred vision, chill bumps, chills, nausea, and occasional bradycardia. Treatment includes elimination of the precipitating stimuli if known and elevation of the head of bed. Pharmacologic treatment may be needed to reduce the blood pressure if the blood pressure remains elevated after these measures. Medications for the treatment of hypertension include nifedipine, nitrates, captopril, prazosin, phenoxybenzamine hydrochloride, prostaglandin E2, and sildenafil.[8]

Acute Myocardial Infarction

The patient with a history of preexisting coronary artery disease, diabetes, and significant dysrhythmias is at risk for perioperative cardiac events (see Box 29-2). The pathology of perioperative myocardial infarction is shown in Fig. 29-2.[9]

When a patient has chest pain in the PACU, the cause needs to be evaluated, with the first consideration for the source as cardiac in origin (Box 29-3). The signs and symptoms of myocardial infarction include chest pain, tachypnea, tachycardia or other dysrhythmias, hypotension or hypertension, pallor,

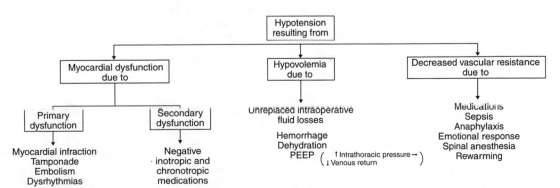

FIG. 29-1 Causes of hypotension. (From Litwack K: *Postanesthesia care nursing*, ed 2, St. Louis, 1995, Mosby.)

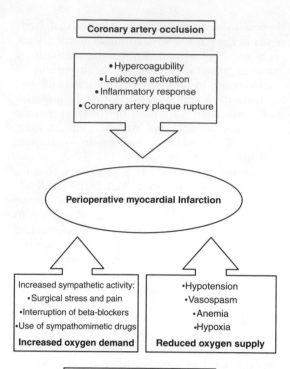

FIG. 29-2 Pathology of perioperative myocardial infarction. (From Kertai MD, et al: Predicting perioperative cardiac risk, *Progress Cardiovasc Dis* 47(4):240–257, 2005.)

BOX 29-3	Differential Diagnosis of Chest Pain

- Anxiety
- Aortic dissection
- Cardiac arrhythmia
- Esophageal spasm or rupture
- Gastroesophageal reflux disease
- Musculoskeletal pain
- Myocardial ischemia or infarction
- Pericardial tamponade
- Pericarditis
- Pneumonia
- Pneumoperitoneum
- Pneumothorax
- Pulmonary embolism
- Thoracic aneurysm

Data from Anderson JL, et al: 2011 ACCF/AHA focused update incorporated into the ACC/AHA 2007 guidelines for the management of patients with unstable angina/non-st-elevation myocardial infarction, *Circulation* 123:e426–e579, 2011; Klingensmith ME, Washington University Department of Surgery in St. Louis: *The Washington manual of surgery*, ed 6, Philadelphia, 2011, Lippincott Williams & Wilkins; Ruskin K, Rosenbaum SH: *Anesthesia emergencies*, New York, 2011, Oxford University Press.

diaphoresis, cool extremities, nausea, vomiting, and generalized weakness. New Q waves or increasing prominence of existing ones, ST segment elevations, and T wave inversions may be seen on electrocardiogram (ECG) results. Initial treatment is aimed at relieving chest pain, reducing cardiac workload, stabilizing cardiac rhythm, limiting infarct size, preventing further damage, and detecting and treating complications. The first response is to order a 12-lead ECG; initiate supplemental oxygen to maintain arterial oxygen saturation (SaO_2) above 90%[10]; administer morphine, nitrates, and antiplatelet or anticoagulant agents; and continuously monitor the ECG. Laboratory blood studies are obtained, including troponin-I, troponin-T, MB fraction of creatine kinase (CK-MB), and CK-MB isoforms. The patient is evaluated and transferred to a critical care unit as indicated by diagnosis for continued monitoring and possible interventional procedures and management.

THERMOREGULATION

For a more detailed discussion of thermoregulation, see Chapter 53.

Hypothermia

Hypothermia is defined as a core temperature of less than 36° C.[11] Signs and symptoms of hypothermia include shivering, restlessness, discomfort, and cold pale cyanotic extremities and distal appendages from peripheral vasoconstriction. This state can lead to delayed drug clearance, myocardial ischemia, unexplained hypertension, and residual paralysis from neuromuscular blocking agents. The American Society of Peri-Anesthesia Nurses *Evidence-Based Clinical Practice Guideline for the Promotion of Perioperative Normothermia* offers the perianesthesia nurse guidance for assessment and management of the patient who is hypothermic during the perianesthesia period.[11] Recommendations for treatment of the patient include active rewarming, supplemental oxygen administration, and ventilatory support if necessary.

Hyperthermia

Hyperthermia is defined as a core temperature of more than 38° C.[11] Temperature elevations may be the result of blood transfusion reactions, warm environment, drug-induced fever, use of anticholinergic drugs, overcorrected hypothermia, endocrine disorder, hypothalamic injury, or malignant hyperthermia (MH). Signs and symptoms include fever, tachycardia, and warm flushed skin and other sign and symptoms depending on the cause of the hyperthermia (shaking, chills or rigors, agitation). The cause should be identified and corrected when possible. Cooling blankets or pads may be used, and an antipyretic agent may be given.

Malignant Hyperthermia

MH is a drug-induced hypermetabolic state of genetic origin (autosomal dominant inheritance) that can be triggered by succinylcholine or the volatile anesthetics. It can occur on induction, during emergence, or up to 24 hours after anesthesia. The exact incidence rate is unknown but is thought to be approximately 1:15,000 in children and less common in adults older than 30 years. Patients with central core disease and other muscle diseases may be at added risk for developing MH.

The signs and symptoms of MH include the earliest sign of an unanticipated doubling or tripling of end-tidal CO_2 in the anesthetized patient. This sign may be followed by unexpected tachycardia, tachypnea, and jaw muscle rigidity. Respiratory acidosis and, after severe temperature increase, metabolic acidosis are present. Body rigidity is a specific sign of MH syndrome. Fever, when it develops, is a late sign of MH; the temperature may rise at a rate of 1° C every 3 to 5 minutes. The urine may become dark and cola colored from the breakdown of myoglobin.

Early recognition of MH is essential; additional help needs to be summoned. If it occurs in the operating suite, discontinue all volatile anesthetics, hyperventilate the patient's lungs with 100% oxygen with a new circuit, and end the operative procedure as soon as safely possible. Dantrolene sodium (Dantrium should be available in sufficient quantities [36 vials recommended in all locations where volatile anesthetics or succinylcholine are administered]) as should diluent. Dosing begins at 2.5 mg/kg of dantrolene sodium, up to 10 mg/kg. Laboratory blood studies including coagulation profile, creatine, electrolytes, arterial blood gas, and creatinine kinase should be obtained. Acidosis not reversed with dantrolene sodium can be treated with sodium bicarbonate. The patient's body temperature should be monitored, and cooling measures should be initiated if the temperature is more than 38.5° C. Dysrhythmias can be treated with standard antiarrhythmics, but calcium channel blockers should be avoided. Elevated potassium levels are treated with intravenous (IV) insulin, glucose, and calcium. Hydration and diuretics ensure urine output of at least 2 mL/kg/h.

After the MH crisis is treated and the patient's condition is stabilized, the patient should be transferred to a critical care unit for continued monitoring, including temperature, for at least 24 hours because recrudescence can occur and does in approximately 25% of MH cases.

Patients who have had an MH episode during a previous surgery or have a family history of MH are treated as MH susceptible; triggering agents are avoided. Dantrolene sodium prophylaxis is not recommended for these patients. The patient who undergoes an uneventful anesthetic and is scheduled as an outpatient may be discharged home on the day of surgery; this patient should be monitored in the phase I PACU for a minimum of 1 hour and in the phase II PACU for an additional 1.5 hours.

Diagnosis of MH susceptibility involves a skeletal muscle biopsy specimen from the thigh. Only eight medical centers in the United States and Canada perform the test on fresh muscle. Genetic testing is available, but not all the genes responsible for MH have been identified; therefore risk may still exist for the patient whose test results are negative and who has unidentified genes.

When an MH crisis occurs, consultation is available from the MH Hotline at 1-800-MH-HYPER (1-800-644-9737) in the United States or 1-315-464-7079 outside the United States. Additional information and resources can be found at www.mhaus.org.

ANESTHESIA-RELATED COMPLICATIONS

Awareness Under Anesthesia

One to two per thousand patients at low risk has an ability to recall some aspect of the surgical experience. The effects of awareness with anesthesia vary from pleasant recall to terror that leads to posttraumatic stress disorder. Difficulty in diagnosis of awareness adds to the challenge of this event. Patient recall can include events such as conversations, pain, or anxiety related to perception of an inability to breathe. Risk factors include a history of drug or alcohol abuse, extreme anxiety, or a previous episode of awareness. Patients undergoing cardiac, major trauma, and obstetric procedures are at greatest risk of awareness. Patients who are defined as sicker by the American Society of Anesthesiologists status appear to be at higher risk for awareness under anesthesia.

When patients arrive in the postanesthesia care unit, nurses tell the patients that surgery is over, they are in the PACU or wake-up room, they are doing well, and the nurses are going to take care of them while they are awakening. This reassurance can minimize fears of waking up while still in the operating suite. Frequent reminders to the patients

NURSING CARE IN THE PACU

of status and safety help reduce anxiety related to awareness or awakening. If a patient indicates recall of events from the operating suite, the perianesthesia nurse should contact the anesthesia care provider to come to the bedside and interview the patient. Telling the patient an event did not occur or was a dream is inappropriate. If an awareness event is suspected, the nurse should sympathize and apologize to the patient, explain and answer questions as appropriate, and notify the anesthesia care provider, surgeon, and risk management department.

Anesthesia care providers, when interviewing patients after procedures, may use a structured interview tool, such as the Brice questionnaire (Box 29-4).[12] This interview may dispel concerns and identify awareness events with greater frequency.

Emergence Excitement

Most patients emerge from general anesthesia in a calm tranquil manner. Some patients, however, emerge in a state of excitement, a condition characterized by restlessness, disorientation, crying, moaning, irrational talking, and inappropriate behavior. In the extreme form of excitement, which is also called *emergence delirium* (Fig. 29-3) or agitation, the patient screams, shouts, and wildly thrashes. Postoperative delirium or emergence excitement is defined as responsive or unresponsive agitation.

The incidence rate of emergence excitement is higher among children, the elderly, and those with a history of drug dependency or psychiatric disorders. Medications administered before or during surgery, including ketamine, droperidol, opioids, benzodiazepines, large doses of metoclopramide, and atropine or scopolamine, may precipitate delirium. Patients who are emotional or anxious before induction of anesthesia or who awaken restrained are at increased risk of emergence excitement or delirium.

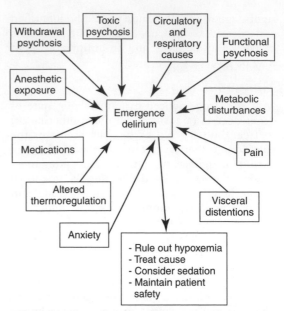

FIG. 29-3 Emergence delirium in the postanesthesia care unit: contributing factors and treatment. (From Nagelhout JJ, Plaus KL: *Nurse anesthesia*, ed 4, St. Louis, 2010, Saunders.)

The PACU nurse should assess the patient's status if emergence excitement is encountered. The patient's cardiopulmonary function, airway patency, and oxygen saturation should be checked first because restlessness and agitation are well-known manifestations of hypoxemia. Other causes include bladder distention, cramped or sore muscles and joints from prolonged abnormal positioning on the operating table, the presence of pain, incomplete reversal of neuromuscular blockade, withdrawal from alcohol and other drugs, central anticholinergic syndrome, acid-base disturbances, and electrolyte abnormalities.

The restless patient needs constant careful observation. Gentle physical restraint may be necessary for prevention of injury. Several nurses or attendants may be needed to provide safety for the patient, and for the caregivers too. Treatment is symptomatic. If hypoxia, pain, and full bladder are ruled out, a change in position may have a quieting effect. Physostigmine can be used to reverse central anticholinergic drug effects. Anxiolytics, such as midazolam, usually calm the patient. If sedative treatment is instituted, the patient should be monitored for respiratory depression. Nurses should be alert to increased agitation after benzodiazepine administration. These agents may contribute to restlessness rather than decreasing

---

BOX 29-4   Original Brice Questionnaire

1. What was the last thing you remember before you went to sleep for your operation?
2. What was the first thing you remember after your operation?
3. Can you remember anything in between those two periods?
4. Did you dream during your operation?
5. What was the worst thing about your operation?

From Brice DD, et al: A simple study of awareness and dreaming during anesthesia, *Br J Anaesth* 42:535–542, 1970.

it; a paradoxical reaction to benzodiazepines can occur.

Anticholinergic syndrome (ACS), or central anticholinergic syndrome, is rare but occurs most frequently with atropine and scopolamine. Other agents that cause ACS are glycopyrrolate, antihistamines, and antipsychotics. This syndrome or response to anticholinergic agents may present as emergence excitement in the PACU. It is produced by the inhibition of cholinergic neurotransmission at muscarinic receptor sites. It can manifest before surgery or in the PACU when patients are given atropine or have applied transdermal scopolamine patches. Signs and symptoms include sinus tachycardia, agitation, flushing, dry skin and mucous membranes, mydriasis with loss of accommodation, altered mental status, fever, decreased bowel sounds, functional ileus, urinary retention, hypertension, tremulousness, and myoclonic jerking. Patients with central ACS may have ataxia, disorientation, short-term memory loss, confusion, hallucinations (visual, auditory), psychosis, agitated delirium, seizures (rare), coma, respiratory failure, and cardiovascular collapse. Supportive care, removal of scopolamine patches, and administration of IV physostigmine constitute initial treatment of ACS.

Physostigmine is a reversible acetylcholinesterase inhibitor that directly antagonizes the central nervous system manifestations of anticholinergic toxicity. Increased acetylcholine allows for stimulation at muscarinic and nicotinic receptors. The drug crosses the blood-brain barrier and reverses the central effects of coma, seizures, severe dyskinesias, hallucinations, agitation, and respiratory depression.

Adverse effects include vomiting, diarrhea, abdominal cramps, diaphoresis, and rare bradyasystole in the presence of prolonged PR or QRS intervals on the ECG.

Delayed Emergence (Awakening)

Occasionally patients awaken from anesthesia more slowly than expected. Causes include prolonged action of anesthetic and other drugs; metabolic problems such as hypoglycemia, hypocalcemia, hyponatremia, and hypermagnesemia; hypovolemia; hypothermia; and neurologic injury. Respiratory inadequacy with resultant hypercarbia and hypoxemia can result from opioids, sedatives, other anesthetic agents and adjuncts, or neurologic causes. The most common cause of delayed awakening is prolonged drug effects (Fig. 29-4).

Treatment consists of thorough assessment and identification of the cause or causes of the delayed arousal. Oxygenation and ventilation along with adequate cardiac output must be maintained. Residual anesthetic agents may be treated with maintenance of ventilation. Residual opioids, sedatives, neuromuscular blocking agents, and anticholinergic drugs can be reversed with the appropriate antagonists. Metabolic disturbances should be corrected. If hypothermia is the suggested cause, warming measures are instituted with appropriate temperature monitoring. Neurologic evaluation may be needed if other causes of delayed arousal have been excluded.

Evaluation of the patient for possible cerebrovascular accident (stroke) should be included in the immediate assessment of the postanesthesia patient. Observe facial symmetry assessing for droop, evaluate speech assessing for slurring of

NURSING CARE IN THE PACU

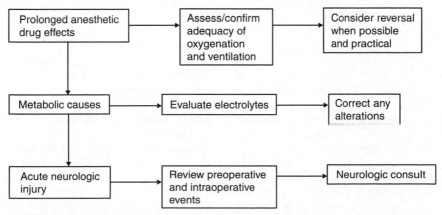

FIG. 29-4 Delayed emergence (awakening). (From Litwack K: *Postanesthesia care nursing,* ed 2, St. Louis, 1995, Mosby.)

words and abnormal speech, and assess arm drift. In addition, neurologic assessment including level of orientation, pupillary response, movement, and muscle strength can assist in determining variations and need for intervention to avoid further neurologic deterioration.

Nausea and Vomiting

A common problem for the postanesthesia patient is postoperative nausea and vomiting (PONV). The incidence rate of nausea and vomiting has remained between 20% and 30% of all patients undergoing anesthesia and rises up to 80% in patients at high risk. PONV contributes to postoperative complications, increases the costs of care, and delays patient recovery and return to work. PONV is a major source of patient discomfort and fear.

Mechanism of Action

The vomiting (emetic) center is located in the medulla near the dorsal nucleus of the vagus nerve. It can be excited by reflex impulses that arise in the pharynx, stomach, or other portions of the gastrointestinal tract. Foreign materials, such as blood and mucus or irritant gases in the stomach or other portions of the gastrointestinal tract, can produce nausea and subsequent vomiting. The vomiting center can be excited by impulses received from cerebral centers, because the vomiting center is located close to the fourth cerebral ventricle (see Chapter 10) and receives impulses from the chemoreceptor trigger zone (CTZ), cerebral cortex, and vestibular center. Of these physiologic centers, the CTZ has the greatest effect on the vomiting center. In fact, when stimulated by the appropriate stimuli, the CTZ can initiate vomiting independent of the vomiting center. The CTZ is rich in serotonin, dopamine, histamine, and opioids and is not protected by the blood-brain barrier. This lack of protection allows the CTZ to be directly stimulated by chemical stimuli from the systemic circulation or the cerebral spinal fluid.

Drugs such as anesthetic agents and opioids sensitize the vestibular apparatus, the organ of balance. This sensitization explains why two of the principal causative factors of nausea and vomiting are rough handling of the patient during transportation and regular changes of position in the immediate recovery period.

The vomiting center and the CTZ can be excited by chemical materials carried in the blood. Drugs such as morphine and meperidine directly excite the vomiting center, which is designated as central vomiting. The vomiting center can be

excited by interference with its blood supply. Severe cerebral anoxia and increased intracranial pressure are such examples. Finally, the vomiting center can be excited by dehydration and electrolyte imbalance.

Incidence of Postoperative Nausea and Vomiting

Primary risk factors for postoperative nausea and vomiting fall into three categories: patient-specific, anesthetic-related, and surgery-related.[13] Patient-specific risk factors include female gender, nonsmoking status, history of PONV, and history of motion sickness. Use of volatile anesthetics, nitrous oxide, and postoperative opioids are the anesthetic-related factors. Duration of surgery and anesthesia and the type of surgery are the surgery-related factors.

Simplified risk factor assessment tools are used to identify patients at greatest risk for development of PONV. Risk can be predicted depending on the number of factors that are present. The factors in these tools include female gender, nonsmoking status, history of PONV or motion sickness, postoperative opioid use, or duration of surgery greater than 60 minutes.

The presence of each additional factor predicts increased risk of development of PONV and guides antiemetic prophylaxis for the prevention of PONV. Patients with zero to one factor have a low level risk of PONV; those with two are at moderate risk, with an approximately 40% chance of PONV. With three or more factors, patients have a 60% chance of development of PONV. Very severe risk, a more than 80% risk of PONV, can be found in patients with four to five risk factors. See Fig. 29-5 for recommendations for preoperative antiemetic prophylaxis from the American Society of PeriAnesthesia Nurses *Evidence-Based Clinical Practice Guideline for the Prevention and/or Management of PONV/PDNV.*[14]

Care of the Patient with Nausea and Vomiting

In most cases, vomiting is preceded by nausea. Nausea is a feeling of impending vomiting. Several signs accompany the feelings of nausea. The patient usually has excessive salivation, dilated pupils, tachypnea, swallowing, pallor, sweating, and tachycardia. If the patient's nausea worsens, retching usually occurs and the tachycardia may change to bradycardia. If patients have nausea, they should be encouraged to breathe deeply. A cool washcloth placed on the patient's forehead and words of encouragement sometimes help to ease the nausea. The nurse remains with the

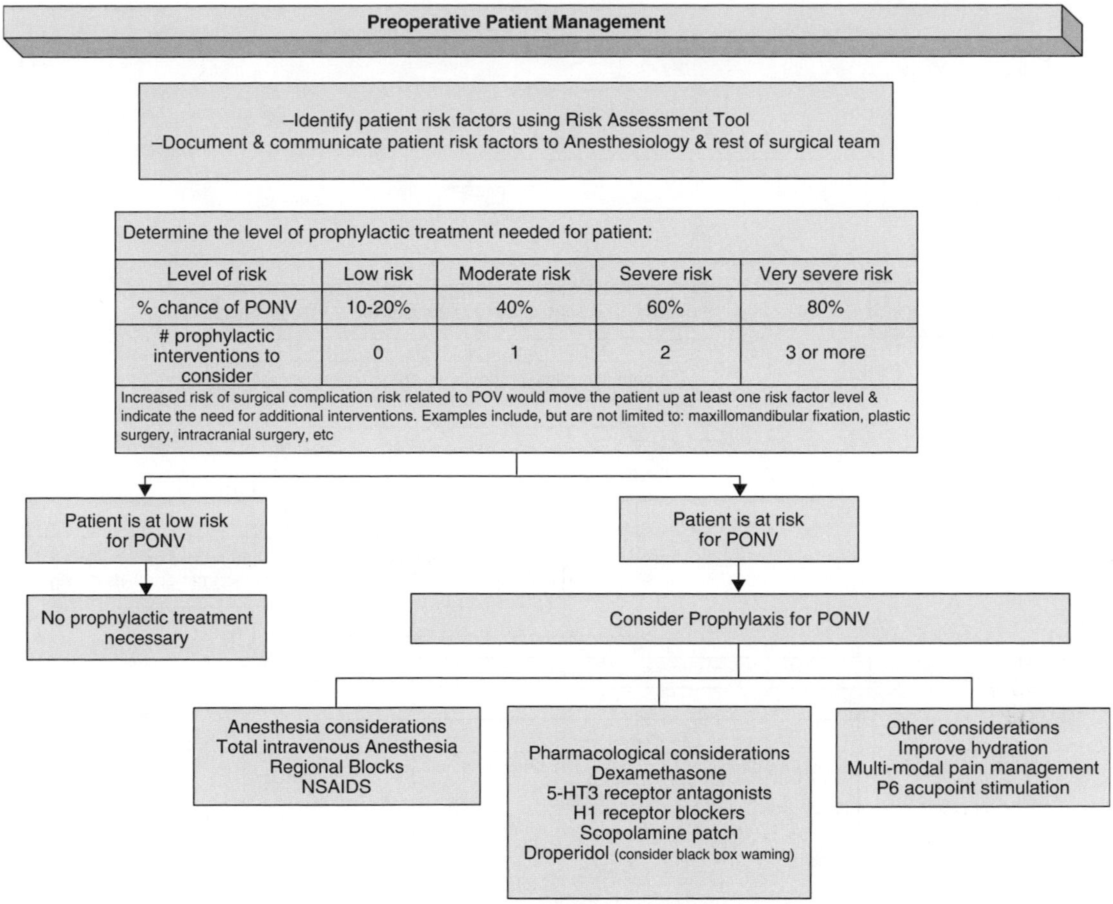

Preoperative Patient Management

–Identify patient risk factors using Risk Assessment Tool
–Document & communicate patient risk factors to Anesthesiology & rest of surgical team

Determine the level of prophylactic treatment needed for patient:

Level of risk	Low risk	Moderate risk	Severe risk	Very severe risk
% chance of PONV	10-20%	40%	60%	80%
# prophylactic interventions to consider	0	1	2	3 or more

Increased risk of surgical complication risk related to POV would move the patient up at least one risk factor level & indicate the need for additional interventions. Examples include, but are not limited to: maxillomandibular fixation, plastic surgery, intracranial surgery, etc

Patient is at low risk for PONV

Patient is at risk for PONV

No prophylactic treatment necessary

Consider Prophylaxis for PONV

Anesthesia considerations
Total intravenous Anesthesia
Regional Blocks
NSAIDS

Pharmacological considerations
Dexamethasone
5-HT3 receptor antagonists
H1 receptor blockers
Scopolamine patch
Droperidol (consider black box warning)

Other considerations
Improve hydration
Multi-modal pain management
P6 acupoint stimulation

FIG. 29-5 Preoperative patient management. (From American Society of PeriAnesthesia Nurses: Evidence-based clinical practice guideline for the prevention and/or management of PONV/PDNV, *J Perianesth Nurs* 21:230–250, 2006.)

patient because the patient may begin vomiting without notice, and the danger of aspiration of vomitus and an obstructed airway is always present.

Pharmacologic Interventions

If the previous intervention does not relieve the nausea and vomiting, a pharmacologic intervention is needed (Fig. 29-6; Table 29-1). As previously discussed, the following receptors are in the CTZ: serotonin (5-HT_3), dopamine (D_2), histamine, and muscarinic. Drugs that block serotonin (5-HT_3) receptors are ondansetron (Zofran), dolasetron (Anzemet), granisetron (Kytril), or palonosetron (Aloxi) and the drugs that block the dopamine (D_2) receptors are droperidol (Inapsine), prochlorperazine (Compazine), or metoclopramide (Reglan). For the

histamine receptors, promethazine (Phenergan) or diphenhydramine (Benadryl) can be given. For the muscarinic receptors, atropine, glycopyrrolate (Robinul), or scopolamine patches can be used. Dexamethasone (Decadron) is often administered in combination with a serotonin (5-HT_3)–blocking drug and dopamine (D_2)–blocking agent. Another neurotransmitter of interest is substance P, which belongs to the tachykinin family of neurotransmitters, known as *neurokinins*. Substance P has the greatest affinity for neurokinin 1 (NK-1) receptors, which are found centrally in the brainstem vomiting center and peripherally in the gastrointestinal tract. Currently, the only available medication that targets these neurokinin 1 receptors is aprepitant (Emend), available orally for prophylaxis of PONV.

NURSING CARE IN THE PACU

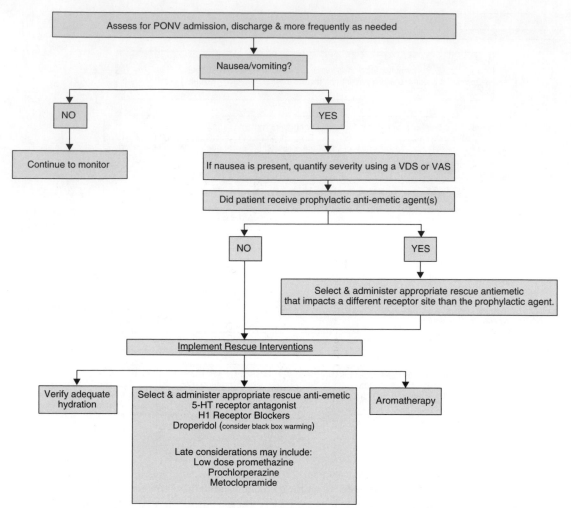

FIG. 29-6 Postoperative management of postanesthesia nausea and vomiting (PONV): PACU Phase I and Phase II. (From American Society of PeriAnesthesia Nurses: Evidence-based clinical practice guideline for the prevention and/or management of PONV/PDNV, *J Perianesth Nurs* 21:230–250, 2006.)

Evidence-Based Practice

The use of steroids in the perianesthesia period has been linked to reduced pain and nausea after ambulatory surgery. It was unknown whether the use of steroids would influence the quality of recovery after surgery. The researchers in this study hypothesized that perioperative dexamethasone would enhance the quality of recovery in patients who had undergone laparoscopic cholecystectomy. The 120 patients were randomized to receive either a placebo or 8 mg of dexamethasone. Nausea, vomiting, fatigue, and pain scores were collected. Global quality of recovery scores were higher in the treatment group compared with the placebo group. Nausea, fatigue, pain scores, and analgesic requirements were reduced in the dexamethasone group during hospitalization. Total length of stay in the hospital was also reduced.

IMPLICATIONS FOR PRACTICE

The use of preoperative steroids in patients who have had laparoscopic cholecystectomy surgery improved quality-of-recovery scores in all areas, including pain, fatigue, and nausea. More research needs to be conducted in this area to determine whether the use of steroids affects quality of recovery in other patient populations.

Source: Glenn S, et al: Preoperative dexamethasone enhances quality of recovery after laparoscopic cholecystectomy, *Anesthesiology* 114:882–890, 2011.

Table 29-1   Pharmacologic Interventions

DRUG (TRADE NAME; *RECEPTOR SITE AFFINITY*)	DOSE*	DURATION OF ACTION	ADVERSE EFFECTS	COMMENTS AND RECOMMENDATIONS FOR USE
Droperidol (Inapsine; *dopamine*)	*Adult:* 0.625-1.25 mg IV *Pediatric:* 20-50 mcg/kg IV	12-24 hours	Sedation, hypotension (especially in patients with hypovolemia), EPS	Higher doses and doses that are repeated too soon can cause sedation, EPS, and QT prolongation (U.S. FDA black box warning; ECG monitoring) Effective first-line agent
Prochlorperazine (Compazine; *dopamine*)	*Adult:* 5-10 mg IM or IV; 25 mg PR *Pediatric‡:* 0.13 mg/kg IM; 0.1 mg/kg PO; 2.5 mg PR	2-6 hours (12 hours when given PR)	Sedation, hypotension (especially in patients with hypovolemia), EPS	Good for patients with motion sickness or undergoing surgery affecting vestibular apparatus (U.S. FDA black box warning; Respiratory depression; severe tissue injury, gangrene with IV/IM administration)
Promethazine (Phenergan; *dopamine, histamine, acetylcholine*)	*Adult:* 6.25-25 mg IM, IV, or PR *Pediatric (>2 years of age):* 0.25-0.5 mg/kg IV, IM, or PR‡	4 hours	Sedation, hypotension (especially in patients with hypovolemia), EPS	Good for patients with motion sickness or undergoing surgery affecting vestibular apparatus
Diphenhydramine (Benadryl; *histamine, acetylcholine*)	*Adult:* 12.5-50 mg IM or IV *Pediatric:* 1 mg/kg IV or PO (maximum, 25 mg for <6 years old)	4-6 hours	Sedation, dry mouth, blurred vision, urinary retention	
Metoclopramide (Reglan; *dopamine*)	*Adult:* 10-20 mg IV *Pediatric:* 0.15-0.25 mg/kg	6-8 hours	Sedation, hypotension, EPS	Increases gastric motility; good if nausea or vomiting is from gastric stasis; reduce dose to 5 mg in renal impairment; consider diphenhydramine to prevent EPS in children
Ondansetron (Zofran; *serotonin*)	*Adult:* 4 mg IV; 4, 8 mg ODT *Pediatric:* 0.05-0.1 mg/kg	Up to 24 hours	Headache, lightheadedness	Much more effective for vomiting than nausea; 2 mg may be sufficient to treat PONV in PACU
Dolasetron (Anzemet; *serotonin*)	*Adult:* 12.5 mg IV *Pediatric:* 0.35 mg/kg	Up to 24 hours	Headache, lightheadedness	Much more effective for vomiting than nausea
Granisetron (Kytril; *serotonin*)	*Adult:* 1 mg IV over 30 sec *Pediatric:* N/A	Up to 24 hours	Headache, lightheadedness	Much more effective for vomiting than nausea
Palonosetron (Aloxi; *serotonin*)	*Adult:* 0.075 mg IV	24 hours	Headache, constipation	Prolonged during of action; given immediately before induction of anesthesia

Continued

Table 29-1   Pharmacologic Interventions—cont'd

DRUG (TRADE NAME; *RECEPTOR SITE AFFINITY*)	DOSE*	DURATION OF ACTION	ADVERSE EFFECTS	COMMENTS AND RECOMMENDATIONS FOR USE
Scopolamine (Transderm Scop; *acetylcholine*)	*Adult:* 1.5 mg transdermal patch *Pediatric:* N/A	72 hours§	Sedation, dry mouth, visual disturbances, dysphoria, confusion, disorientation, hallucinations	Good for patients with motion sickness or undergoing surgery affecting vestibular apparatus; apply 4 hours before exposure
Dexamethasone (Decadron; *none—works by another mechanism*)	*Adult:* 4-8 mg IV *Pediatric:* 0.5-1 mg/kg	Up to 24 hours	Watch blood sugar in patients with diabetes; watch for fluid retention, especially in cardiac patients	Generally well tolerated in healthy patients; may take time (hours) to work
Aprepitant (Emend)	*Adult:* 40 mg PO 1-3 hours before anesthesia	Up to 24 hours	Generally well tolerated	Oral prophylaxis only; caution with patients taking warfarin; can reduce effectiveness of oral contraceptives

Adapted from *AHFS Drug Information*,® Bethesda, MD, 2012, American Society of Health-System Pharmacists, Inc.; *Drug Facts and Comparisons 2012*, ed 66, St. Louis, 2011, Wolters Kluwer Health. *IV*, Intravenous; *EPS*, extrapyramidal symptoms, such as motor restlessness or acute dystonia; *FDA*, Food and Drug Administration; *ECG*, electrocardiogram; *IM*, intramuscular; *ODT*, orally disintegrating tablets; *PR*, per rectum; *PO*, orally; *PONV*, postoperative nausea and vomiting; *PACU*, postanesthesia care unit.

*Unless otherwise indicated, pediatric doses should not exceed the adult dose for each antiemetic agent.

†Children weighing more than 10 kg or older than 2 years of age only. Change from IM to PO as soon as possible. With administration PR, dosing interval varies from 8 to 24 hours depending on child's weight.

‡Maximum of 12.5 mg in children younger than 12 years.

§Remove after 24 hours when used to prevent or treat PONV. Instruct patient to wash the patch site and hands thoroughly.

Nonpharmacologic Interventions

In addition to pharmacologic interventions to manage nausea and vomiting, nonpharmacologic interventions are useful adjuncts. Adequate hydration with IV fluids and modified fasting protocols can help to minimize PONV.[15] Aromatherapy (e.g., isopropyl alcohol, peppermint oil) is equal in benefit and risk, and it is easy for the nurse to perform or administer. P6 acupoint stimulation with acupuncture or acupressure techniques has been shown to be effective and is recommended for use.[16]

Airway Management

Perianesthesia care of the patient who is vomiting focuses on airway management. The patient should be placed in a head-down position so that the vomitus drains away from the lungs. Oral suctioning should be instituted if the patient is not completely able to control the airway. Oxygen should be administered when any question of compromise of the respiratory status arises. Rapid assessment of the patient's respiratory status should be made during and after the vomiting episode. This assessment is done with bilateral auscultation of the chest for adventitious sounds. Any possible aspiration of vomitus should be reported immediately to the physician. If the airway becomes obstructed, place the patient in a head-down position, turn the head to one side, and try to remove foreign material with suctioning or with the finger. While performing this maneuver, the nurse should send another person for an anesthesia care provider.

Postdischarge Nausea and Vomiting

After discharge, up to 30% to 50% of patients undergoing outpatient surgery have postdischarge nausea and vomiting (PDNV).[17] PDNV affects the quality of recovery, increases the potential for patient morbidity and hospitalization of patients at high risk, and decreases patient satisfaction. PDNV is defined as nausea and vomiting that occurs up to 24 hours after the patient is discharged from the facility. See Fig. 29-7 for rescue and treatment recommendations. More research is needed to establish the scope of the PDNV problem and the effectiveness of these recommendations.

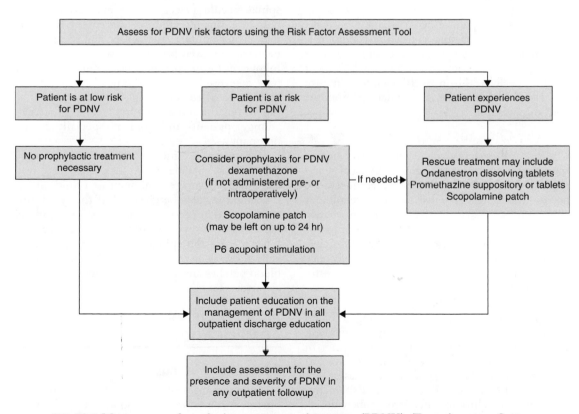

FIG. 29-7 Management of postdischarge nausea and vomiting (PDNV). (From American Society of PeriAnesthesia Nurses: Evidence-based clinical practice guideline for the prevention and/or management of PONV/PDNV, *J Perianesth Nurs* 21:230–250, 2006.)

NURSING CARE IN THE PACU

OTHER COMPLICATIONS

Spinal Epidural Hematoma

Particular attention should be paid to patients who have undergone spinal or epidural anesthesia who are seen in the PACU with severe back pain and symptoms of cord compression. The severe pain is a cardinal symptom of an emergent situation: spinal epidural hematoma. Typically, a rapid onset of sensory and motor deficits progresses to paralysis if not identified and promptly treated. Rapid action is needed to prevent permanent neurologic sequelae.

Patients at greatest risk for developing this serious complication are female and older, may have had a traumatic needle or catheter placement, and have indwelling epidural catheters. Also at risk are patients who received low-molecular-weight heparin therapy near the time of the epidural placement. In addition, concomitant dosing with anticoagulants or antiplatelet agents contributes to risk.

If the patient has severe back pain during recovery and has received epidural or spinal anesthesia, the nurse should immediately notify the anesthesia care provider to evaluate the patient. Definitive diagnosis of an epidural hematoma is with magnetic resonance imaging. When the condition is determined to be a hematoma, emergency laminectomy and hematoma evacuation needs to occur quickly, ideally within 6 to 8 hours, to minimize the risk of permanent neurologic damage from the cord compression.

Plasma Cholinesterase Deficiency

Plasma cholinesterase deficiency is an uncommon genetic disorder that creates unusual sensitivity to succinylcholine and ester local anesthetic agents. The typical response to succinylcholine is skeletal muscle paralysis that lasts approximately 5 to 10 minutes. The patient with abnormal or deficient plasma cholinesterase may remain apneic and paralyzed for 2 hours or more. The deficiency renders the patient unable to hydrolyze the ester bonds in succinylcholine, which leads to the prolonged skeletal muscle paralysis.

Questioning the patient regarding a blood relative's history of any anesthetic events may help to identify the patient at risk. The deficiency in plasma cholinesterase may also be acquired as the result of liver disease, malignant disease, pregnancy, collagen vascular disease, malnutrition, hypothyroidism, chronic infections (tuberculosis), extensive burn injuries, organophosphate pesticide poisoning, or uremia. Neonates and older patients are at risk. Other causes of lower plasma cholinesterase activity include plasmapheresis and medications such as anticholinesterase inhibitors, contraceptives, echothiophate eye drops, esmolol, glucocorticoids, metoclopramide, monoamine oxidase inhibitors, and pancuronium.

Care is supportive, with mechanical ventilation until the patient regains spontaneous respiratory effort, because succinylcholine is not reversible. After recovery, the patient should be counseled to carry identification that indicates plasma cholinesterase deficiency and to alert blood relatives that they may also have this genetic variant.

Testing for plasma cholinesterase deficiency can be accomplished with dibucaine, an amide local anesthetic agent, combined with the patient's blood, which reflects the ability of plasma cholinesterase to metabolize succinylcholine. This test does not measure levels of the enzyme in the plasma. Also available is a simplified screening test of plasma cholinesterase enzyme activity that can be performed with specialized test paper (i.e., Acholest Test Paper).

Postdural Puncture Headache

Postdural puncture headache typically develops 24 to 48 hours after lumbar puncture from spinal needle placement or inadvertent dural puncture during epidural placement. Patients may either contact the facility reporting severe headache relieved by lying down or respond on follow-up by the perianesthesia nurse that they have a severe headache. The headache is caused by leakage of cerebrospinal fluid. The incidence rate of postdural puncture headache is greater in younger patients and women, especially during pregnancy.

Treatment is initially conservative; recommendations include mild analgesics, bed rest, caffeinated beverages, and increased fluid intake. Caffeine may also be given IV. If the symptoms continue, definitive treatment is an epidural blood patch, in which fresh autologous blood is injected into the epidural space until the headache resolves or fullness or pain is felt. Epidural blood patches are effective in greater than 95% of symptomatic patients.

PROCEDURE-RELATED COMPLICATIONS

Perforated Viscus

Internal organs may be perforated during the operative procedure. Commonly caused by various types of endoscopic procedures (e.g., laparoscopy, gastroscopy), perforations can appear as pain out of proportion to the procedure; a distended, firm abdomen; hypotension, or bleeding. The esophagus, stomach, bladder, uterus, or bowel may be damaged and not noticed until after the patient arrives in the PACU and becomes symptomatic. The nurse should call the surgeon immediately, provide hemodynamic support as ordered (fluid resuscitation, blood component therapy, vasoactive medications, positioning, additional line placement), and analgesia or sedation if appropriate. The nurse may need to prepare for emergent transfer to the operative suite for repair of the perforation.

Hemorrhage

Bleeding after operative procedures should be minimal. Dressings remain dry with minimal bloody drainage. However, hemorrhage can and does occur in the PACU and requires the attentive nurse to respond promptly to avert potential serious events. Any operative site may bleed if hemostasis is inadequate. Some sites may be more prone to bleeding, such as the tonsillar beds, nasopharynx resulting in epistaxis, the cervix after conization, and the uterus after dilatation and curettage vaginal/cervical. Signs and symptoms of overt or hidden hemorrhage include bright red bleeding; saturation of more than one pad per hour after uterine, cervical, or vaginal procedures, hypotension, tachycardia, restlessness, hematoma formation, and pain. Initial treatment for minor bleeding may be the application of ice or reinforcement of dressings or binders. More severe bleeding requires immediate action by the nurse. Pressure is applied depending on the location of the bleeding, the surgeon is called, fluid resuscitation is initiated, and preparations are made to return the patient to the operative suite for ligation of bleeding veins or arteries, hematoma evacuation, or other necessary surgical interventions to stop the bleeding.

Dilutional Hyponatremia

Referred to as *TURP syndrome* when primarily seen in men undergoing prostate resections, dilutional hyponatremia can also occur in women undergoing hysteroscopic procedures. The usual cause is absorption of irrigating solutions through open blood vessels or perforation of the uterine or bladder wall that leads to circulatory overload from water intoxication. Signs and symptoms include hyponatremia, hypertension, bradycardia, agitation, nausea, central nervous system aberrations, muscle twitching, visual disturbances, excessive sedation, obtundation, increased ICP, seizures, coma, cardiovascular compromise including hemodynamic instability, pulmonary edema, and cardiovascular

collapse. Patients may behave in a confused manner, have difficulty seeing, or be difficult to arouse. Treatment includes diuresis with loop diuretics and IV normal saline solution administration. If the serum Na^+ level is less than 120 mEq/L, 3% to 5% saline solution should be given and hemodynamic support should be provided. Visual disturbances generally resolve with prompt treatment. Permanent blindness can occur if the severe hyponatremia is left untreated.

OTHER EMERGENCIES

Allergic Reactions or Anaphylaxis

Although allergic reactions to anesthetics are rare, they can occur. Patients also react to antibiotics, latex products, analgesics, and other agents while in the perianesthesia setting. The target organs in an allergic response are the cutaneous, gastrointestinal, respiratory, and cardiovascular.

Cutaneous responses include erythema, flushing, and pruritus, especially of the palms, soles, and groin. Nausea, cramping, abdominal pain, vomiting, and diarrhea are the gastrointestinal responses. The respiratory responses involve laryngeal edema with hoarseness, dysphonia or a "lump in throat," chest tightness, shortness of breath, coughing, and wheezing. Cardiovascular responses may be most significant with hypotension, tachycardia, lightheadedness, faintness, syncope, myocardial infarction, dysrhythmias, and cardiovascular collapse experiences. Other symptoms may include nasal, ocular, and palatal pruritus, sneezing, diaphoresis, disorientation, and incontinence.

The nurse should respond immediately when a patient exhibits signs and symptoms of an allergic or potential anaphylactic reaction. The nurse should stop the administration of drugs, attempt to reduce the absorption of the offending agent, maintain the airway, and administer 100% oxygen. Intubation may need to be considered, particularly if significant respiratory distress or laryngeal swelling is present. Fluid bolus for volume expansion is initiated. Epinephrine should be administered. Start with 0.1 mL/kg of 1:1000 subcutaneously (subcut) or intramuscularly (IM) or 0.1 mL/kg of 1:10,000 IV (maximal dose, 5 mL) and titrate to effect on the basis of physician orders. Secondary treatment includes antihistamines, glucocorticoids, continuous catecholamine infusion, and sodium bicarbonate if acid-base status indicates the need. With supportive care, and especially if the patient is not intubated and symptoms continue, continually reevaluate the airway to ensure adequate oxygenation and ventilation.

Transfusion Reactions

The exact incidence rate of transfusion reactions is unknown. Reports of the incidence rate vary from 0.2% to 10%, and some reactions are undoubtedly unrecognized and unreported.

Nurses in the PACU must be especially adept at assessing the patient receiving blood, because many of the signs and symptoms of an adverse reaction to blood may be difficult to separate from those caused by other variables, such as the patient's illness, surgery, or medications (including anesthesia). In addition, the patient who is not fully conscious may not report symptoms. Blood transfusion reactions or complications may be either immediate or delayed.[18] Immediate reactions include hemolytic, nonhemolytic febrile, and anaphylactic reactions. Other reactions include transmission of infectious disease (acquired disease), graft-versus-host disease, and transfusion-related acute lung injury.

Hemolytic Reactions

Fifty to 75 mL of ABO-incompatible blood can precipitate a hemolytic reaction that results in agglutination, or clumping, of red blood cells (RBCs), which blocks the patient's capillaries, thus obstructing the flow of blood and oxygen to vital organs. In time, hemolysis of the RBCs occurs, thus releasing free hemoglobin into the plasma. Free hemoglobin may plug the renal tubules and disrupt the work of the nephrons and result in renal failure. Improper storage, overheating, or freezing of blood can also cause hemolysis of the cells and the release of free hemoglobin.

The clinical signs of the hemolytic reaction occur quickly and include sudden hypotension; tachycardia; chest tightness; abdominal, leg, and back pain; dyspnea; and sensorium changes, most often restlessness and apprehension. Headache may be one of the awakened patient's first symptoms. Pain may occur along the vein path. Fever and chills develop later, along with hemoglobinuria, which leads to oliguria. The patient may also have nausea and flushing of the skin. Many of these symptoms may be significantly masked by the influence of anesthesia. Bleeding from the wound strongly suggests that the patient has received incompatible blood; it is also a poor prognostic sign.

Nonhemolytic Febrile Reactions

Febrile reactions are most often caused by sensitivity to leukocytes and platelets and are seen most often in patients who have received multiple transfusions. The thought now is that these reactions stem from the formation of cytokines during blood storage. A febrile reaction may also be attributed to bacterial contamination. The symptoms do not occur as rapidly as in hemolytic reactions. In febrile or bacterial contamination reactions, the patient may have headache and chills, followed by a rapid rise in temperature. Backache, nausea, vomiting, diarrhea, and abdominal pain follow. Hypotension and tachycardia develop quickly. Pyrogenic reactions caused by the polysaccharide products of bacterial metabolism are manifested by the same symptoms, except that blood pressure does not drop and the temperature usually returns to normal within 12 hours. Patients at risk for febrile responses can be premedicated with acetaminophen and diphenhydramine to minimize the discomfort associated with this reaction.

Anaphylactic Reactions

Anaphylactic reactions occur in approximately 1 in 20,000 of all transfusions and are most often seen in patients who have a history of allergy. The reactions are more frequently seen in transfusions of large plasma amounts, as found in whole blood, pooled platelets, and fresh frozen plasma. Symptoms, which can occur after transfusion of as little as 10 mL of blood, include chills, abdominal cramps, dyspnea, vomiting, and diarrhea. Minor allergic reactions are associated with urticaria. Wheezing, laryngeal edema, and hypotension are associated with more severe reactions.

Transfusion-Related Acute Lung Injury

Patients who receive blood products, particularly plasma-containing products, may be at risk for transfusion-related acute lung injury (TRALI), a serious pulmonary syndrome that can lead to death if not recognized and treated appropriately. The syndrome may be confused with noncardiogenic pulmonary edema, which can be a symptom of TRALI. Symptoms typically begin 1 to 2 hours after transfusion and are fully manifested within 1 to 6 hours. Any transfusions should be stopped immediately. The condition is poorly understood and underdiagnosed. Patients may have dyspnea, hypoxemia, fever, and hypotension. Care is supportive; the condition can be mild to fatal, with a mortality rate of approximately 10%. Most cases resolve within 72 hours.

Treatment of Immediate Reactions

At the first sign of a reaction, the transfusion must be stopped and the physician should be notified. The donor blood is replaced with a new infusion set and normal saline solution. Recheck the patient's identity and blood label information match. The donor blood unit and administration set, along with a sample of the recipient's blood (drawn atraumatically from a site other than the IV catheter where the blood was administered), should be sent to the blood bank for transfusion reaction investigation. Urine output must be monitored carefully. Ideally, a urinary catheter should be inserted and hourly output is recorded. Vital signs must be monitored, and the patient is treated according to symptoms. Blood transfusion with properly matched blood may be needed to correct blood volume deficits and control shock. Vasopressors may be necessary to control blood pressure, but must be used with caution because they can contribute to renal damage, especially if blood volume has not been restored. Oxygen and epinephrine may be used to treat dyspnea and wheezing. Steroids and broad-spectrum antibiotics may be necessary to treat reactions caused by bacterial contamination. Antihistamines and antipyretics are given to the patient with an allergic reaction. Diuretic therapy (e.g., furosemide) and the infusion of 0.9% sodium chloride or 5% dextrose in 0.45% sodium chloride may be prescribed to maintain hydration and urine flow of more than 100 mL/h.

Delayed Reactions

Delayed reactions include the transmission of disease (hepatitis, cytomegalovirus, HIV, human T cell lymphotropic virus I and II), graft-versus-host disease, circulatory overload, citrate intoxication, cardiac dysrhythmias, and bleeding caused by depleted coagulation factors. Delayed hemolytic reactions commonly occur 4 to 8 days after blood transfusion, but can develop up to 1 month later. Symptoms are generally mild and can include a mild elevation in serum bilirubin or fever.

Circulatory overload results when fluid is infused into the circulatory system either too rapidly or in too great a quantity. Elderly patients and those with minimal cardiac reserve are particularly susceptible. The use of packed RBCs in these patients should be considered carefully. Symptoms of circulatory overload include cough, dyspnea, edema, tachycardia, hemoptysis, and frothy pink-tinged sputum. If the patient is conscious, the patient may have a pounding headache, a feeling of constriction around the chest, back pain, and chills. If these symptoms develop, the transfusion should be stopped and the physician should be notified.

When large amounts of banked blood are transfused, citrate intoxication may occur. If the blood is infused rapidly, the liver cannot metabolize the citrate ions, which combine with the calcium in the blood and cause calcium deficit symptoms such as tingling of the fingers, muscular cramps, and nervousness. If the calcium deficit is not corrected, cardiac dysrhythmias, including ventricular fibrillation, can occur. Treatment consists of slow IV administration of calcium gluconate, 1 g for every 1000 mL of blood the patient received. If calcium gluconate is unavailable, calcium chloride can be used, but this is more irritating to the veins.

The rapid infusion of cold blood can result in cardiac dysrhythmias or cardiac arrest. Blood should be warmed to room temperature or passed through a warming infuser, with care taken not to overheat it, which would cause hemolysis of the RBCs.

In cases of massive blood replacement, bleeding from dilution of coagulation factors and platelets can occur. If massive transfusions are necessary, several fresh blood infusions (<4 hours old) are suggested to be used along with banked blood.

Blood must be properly stored and refrigerated at 5° C, except for platelets. In most instances, blood should be stored in the blood bank until needed. If blood is to be kept in the PACU, proper storage requirements must be met. When units of blood prepared for a given recipient are not used, they should be promptly returned to the blood bank.

Following blood bank protocols for acquiring blood specimens, proper handling and storage of the blood products, checking patient identification with blood products before transfusion, and managing transfusion reactions are necessary for safe blood product administration.

SUMMARY

The perianesthesia nurse in the postanesthesia care unit monitors the patient, vigilant and mindful of the potential for complications and adverse events. Proactive and responsive, the nurse reacts with sound clinical judgment to intervene quickly and assertively for the patient. Some complications are minor, transitory, and easily resolved; others are life threatening and require skillful intervention by the nurse and the anesthesia care team to save the patient's life or avoid permanent injury. All perianesthesia nurses, regardless of the facility size or location, need competence in managing potential postanesthesia complications.

NURSING CARE IN THE PACU

REFERENCES

1. Smetana GW, et al: Preoperative pulmonary risk stratification for noncardiothoracic surgery: systematic review for the american college of physicians, *Ann Intern Med* 144(8):581–595, 2006.
2. Udeshi A, et al: Postobstructive pulmonary edema, *J Crit Care* 25(3):538.e531–538.e535, 2010.
3. Van Kooy MA, Gargiulo RF: Postobstructive pulmonary edema, *Am Fam Physician* 62(2):401–404, 2000.
4. Desciak MC, Martin DE: Perioperative pulmonary embolism: diagnosis and anesthetic management, *J Clin Anesth* 23(2):153–165, 2011.
5. Fleisher LA, et al: 2009 ACCF/AHA focused update on perioperative beta blockade incorporated into the ACC/AHA 2007 guidelines on perioperative cardiovascular evaluation and care for noncardiac surgery, *J Am Coll Cardiol* 54(22):e13–e118, 2009.
6. Bijker JB, et al: Incidence of intraoperative hypotension as a function of the chosen definition: literature definitions applied to a retrospective cohort using automated data collection, *Anesthesiology* 107(2):213–220, 2007.
7. Kheterpal S, et al: Preoperative and intraoperative predictors of cardiac adverse events after general, vascular, and urological surgery, *Anesthesiology* 110(1):58–66, 2009.
8. Krassioukov A, et al: A Systematic review of the management of autonomic dysreflexia after spinal cord injury, *Arch Phys Med Rehabil* 90(4):682–695, 2009.
9. Kertai MD, et al: Predicting perioperative cardiac risk, *Prog Cardiovasc Dis* 47(4):240–257, 2005.
10. Anderson JL, et al: 2011 ACCF/AHA focused update incorporated into the ACC/AHA 2007 guidelines for the management of patients with unstable angina/non-stelevation myocardial infarction, *Circulation* 123(18):e426–e579, 2011.
11. Hooper VD, et al: ASPAN's evidence-based clinical practice guideline for the promotion of perioperative normothermia: second edition, *J Perianesth Nurs* 25(6):346–365, 2010.
12. Brice DD, et al: A simple study of awareness and dreaming during anaesthesia, *British Journal of Anaesthesiology* 42:535–542, 1970.
13. Murphy MJ, et al: Identification of risk factors for postoperative nausea and vomiting in the perianesthesia adult patient, *J Perianesth Nurs* 21(6):377–384, 2006.
14. American Society of PeriAnesthesia Nurses (ASPAN): Evidence-based clinical practice guideline for the prevention and/or management of PONV/PDNV, *J Perianesth Nurs* 21(4):230–250, 2006.
15. Couture DJ, et al: Therapeutic modalities for the prophylactic management of postoperative nausea and vomiting, *J Perianesth Nurs* 21(6):398–403, 2006.
16. Mamaril ME, et al: Prevention and management of postoperative nausea and vomiting: a look at complementary techniques, *J Perianesth Nurs* 21(6):404–410, 2006.
17. Odom-Forren J, et al: Evidence-based intervention for post discharge nausea and vomiting: a review of the literature, *J Perianesth Nurs* 21(6):411–430, 2006.
18. Eder AF, Chambers LA: Noninfectious complications of blood transfusion, *Arch Pathol Lab Med* 131(5):708–718, 2007.

RESOURCES

Ali SZ, et al: Malignant hyperthermia, *Best Pract Res Clin Anaesthesiol* 17(4):519–533, 2003.

American Association of Critical-Care Nurses: *AACN procedure manual for critical care*, ed 6, St. Louis, 2011, Saunders.

American Society of Anesthesiologists Task Force on Intraoperative Awareness: Practice advisory for intraoperative awareness and brain function monitoring, *Anesthesiology* 104:847–864, 2006.

American Society of PeriAnesthesia Nurses: *Perianesthesia nursing standards and practice recommendations 2010–2012*, Cherry Hill, NJ, 2010, ASPAN.

Atlee JL: *Complications in anesthesia*, ed 2, Philadelphia, 2007, Saunders.

Bruns JJ, Jr: *Anticholinergic toxicity*, available at www.emedicine.com/EMERG/topic36.htm. Accessed December 21, 2011.

Bycroft J, et al: Autonomic dysreflexia: a medical emergency, *Postgrad Med J* 81:232–235, 2005.

Cullen DJ, et al: Spinal epidural hematoma occurrence in the absence of known risk factors: a case series, *J Clin Anesth* 16(5):376–381, 2004.

Finucane BT, et al: *Principles of airway management*, ed 4, New York, 2011, Springer.

Joint Commission: Preventing, and managing the impact of, anesthesia awareness, *Sentinel Event Alert* 32:2004, available at www.jointcommission.org/sentinel_event_alert_issue_32_preventing_and_managing_the_impact_of_anesthesia_awareness/. Accessed December 21, 2011.

Kardon E: *Transfusion reactions*, available at www.emedicine.com/emerg/topic603.htm. Accessed December 21, 2011.

Klingensmith ME, Washington University Department of Surgery in St. Louis: *The Washington manual of surgery*, ed 6, Philadelphia, 2011, Lippincott Williams & Wilkins.

Lepouse C, et al: Emergence delirium in adults in the postanaesthesia care unit, *Br J Anaesth* 96(6):747–753, 2006.

Osborne GA, et al: Crisis management during anaesthesia: awareness and anaesthesia, *Qual Saf Health Care* 14(3):e16, 2005.

Ruskin K, Rosenbaum SH: *Anesthesia emergencies*, New York, 2011, Oxford University Press.

Vlajkovic GP, Sindjelic RP: Emergence delirium in children: many questions, few answers, *Anesth Analg* 104(1):84–91, 2007.

Valchanov K, et al: *Anaesthetic and perioperative complications*, Cambridge, 2011, Cambridge University.

30 Assessment and Management of the A

Suzanne M. Wright, PhD, CRNA

Airway management is a fundamental skill essential to all personnel in perianesthesia nursing. Airway assessment and airway management are crucial for providing safe and effective care to patients after surgery. As these vulnerable patients enter the postanesthesia care unit (PACU), they are extremely susceptible to many events that can compromise ventilation and adequate oxygenation of vital body tissues. Of particular concern are the residual effects of many potent and potentially life-threatening medications given by anesthesia personnel during the intraoperative period. These medications include, but are not limited to, opioids, sedatives, hypnotics, inhalational gases, neuromuscular blockers, insulin, intravenous fluids, and blood products. In addition, predisposing factors have the potential to affect the patency of the postsurgical airway. These factors include histories of obstructive sleep apnea, obesity, snoring, smoking, asthma, and ear, nose, and throat surgery and neck surgery.[1] Anticipation and early recognition of respiratory distress coupled with adequate airway assessment and management skills are paramount in assuring the best possible patient outcome.

DEFINITIONS

Airway Obstruction: A mechanical impediment to the delivery of air to the lungs or to the absorption of oxygen in the lungs.

Auscultate: To listen, most commonly with a stethoscope, for sounds within the body to aid in assessment of the frequency, intensity, duration, and quality of sounds.

Blind Nasotracheal Intubation: Nasotracheal intubation performed without the use of a laryngoscope.

Cricothyrotomy: A puncture through the cricothyroid membrane with a large-bore cricothyrotomy catheter or large-bore intravenous catheter for immediate access to the airway.

Extubate: The removal of an endotracheal or nasotracheal tube from the trachea.

Laryngoscopy: Use of a laryngoscope to view the anatomy of the larynx.

Laryngospasm: An involuntary, spasmodic closure of the vocal cords of the larynx.

Nasopharyngeal Airway: A device, usually a flexible tube, placed through the nares to create an air passage between the nose and the nasopharynx.

Nasotracheal Intubation: Insertion of a breathing tube through the nose into the trachea for facilitation of a patent airway.

Oropharyngeal Airway: A device placed in the oropharynx to conduct air or gases into the trachea; commonly referred to as an *oral airway*.

Oropharynx: One of three anatomic components of the pharynx; it extends behind the mouth from the soft palate to directly above the hyoid bone. The oropharynx contains the palatine and lingual tonsils and lies between the nasopharynx and the laryngopharynx.

Orotracheal Intubation: The insertion of a breathing tube through the mouth into the trachea for facilitation of a patent airway.

Sellick Maneuver: Also referred to as *cricoid pressure*, it is the application of external pressure to the cricoid bone before and during laryngoscopy in an effort to compress the esophagus, preventing regurgitation through the esophagus during intubation of the trachea.

Tracheostomy: An opening through the neck into the trachea that provides a conduit for the placement of an indwelling tube to establish a patent airway.

AIRWAY MANAGEMENT

Patients arrive in the PACU still experiencing the depressant effects of anesthesia. They may be obtunded, which renders them unable to maintain their own airway. Loss of important airway reflexes soon leads to airway obstruction. In some instances, the obtunded patient's tongue and epiglottis fall back on the posterior pharyngeal wall, further occluding the airway. Indications of airway obstruction include increased respiratory effort, retraction of the muscles of respiration, a rocking chest motion, abnormal or absent breath sounds, cyanosis, and signs associated with hypoxemia and hypercarbia.[2] Upon recognizing an airway obstruction, the nurse should place the patient supine, position a pillow beneath the head, tilt the head backward, and extend the neck, unless contraindicated. The nurse should then lift the lower jaw upward using moderate pressure (Fig. 30-1). Often this maneuver is all that is necessary for spontaneous respiratory effort to be effective. If the airway obstruction does not clear, the oral cavity should be inspected for foreign material and the oral pharynx should be suctioned

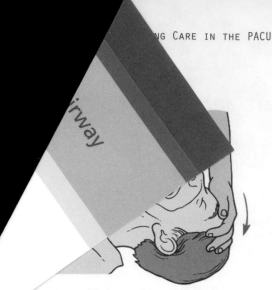

Opening of airway with head-chin-lift maneuver. (From Lewis S, et al: *Medical-surgical nursing: assessment and management of clinical problems*, ed 8, St. Louis, 2011, Mosby.)

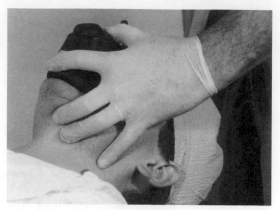

FIG. 30-2 Holding of mask with one hand. (From Miller R, et al: *Miller's anesthesia*, ed 7, Philadelphia, 2010, Churchill Livingstone.)

if necessary. If large particles are present, the nurse should turn the patient's head to the side and remove the particles manually.[3]

If spontaneous respiratory effort is absent, positive pressure breathing must be initiated. A bag-mask unit that is connected to an oxygen source should be used. The requirements for a bag-mask unit are addressed in Box 30-1.[3] For optimal airway management, the perianesthesia nurse should be positioned behind the patient's head. The mask should be securely placed over the patient's mouth and nose with the neck extended. The lower jaw should be lifted at its angle with the other fingers of the hand holding the mask. The thumb of that hand should be placed at the top of the mask. Moderate downward pressure provides compression over the bridge of the nose and reduces air leaks (Fig. 30-2).

After the mask is properly placed, ventilation of the patient's lungs should be attempted. While the perianesthesia nurse is ventilating the lungs, an assistant should auscultate the chest and assess the quality of breath sounds. If an assistant is unavailable, the perianesthesia nurse should check to determine whether the chest rises with inspiration and falls with expiration. This observation is merely a crude estimate of ventilation.[4] If breath sounds are not audible during auscultation, or if the crude estimate of ventilation is inconclusive, an appropriately sized oropharyngeal airway should be inserted and bag-valve-mask ventilation should be resumed (Fig. 30-3). The oral airway is noxious to

---

BOX 30-1	Requirements for Bag-Mask Unit

- Self-refilling but without sponge rubber inside
- Nonjam valve system at 15 L/min oxygen inlet flow
- Transparent plastic face mask with an air-filled or contoured resilient cuff
- Standard 15-mm inside/22-mm outside diameter fittings
- No pop-off valve, except in pediatric models
- System for delivery of high concentrations of oxygen through an ancillary oxygen outlet at the back of the bag or via an oxygen reservoir
- True nonrebreathing valve
- Oropharyngeal airway
- Availability of adult and pediatric sizes
- Satisfactory practice on mannequins

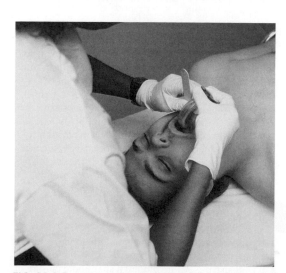

FIG. 30-3 Insertion of oral airway. Airway is inserted with use of tongue blade to displace tongue forward. (From Sanders MJ: *Mosby's paramedic textbook*, ed 3, St. Louis, 2007, Mosby.)

conscious or lightly sedated patients and should be used with extreme caution in this population.[5] The untoward consequences associated with inappropriate use of the oral airway include bradycardia, retching, vomiting, and laryngospasm.[6]

The oropharyngeal airway relieves an airway obstruction by providing a mechanical conduit for air to pass between the base of the tongue and the posterior oropharynx.[3] For placement of an oropharyngeal airway, the perianesthesia nurse should first open the patient's mouth with the right hand and place a tongue blade toward the posterior aspect of the tongue with the left hand. Slight pressure should then be applied to draw the tongue forward. With the oropharyngeal airway held in the right hand, the nurse should slip the airway in over the tongue blade into the oropharynx. The airway should not be twisted or forced into place, and placement should be accomplished quickly with careful avoidance of trauma to the soft tissue and teeth.

In comparison with the oropharyngeal airway, the nasopharyngeal airway is less stimulating to the irritant receptors in the upper airway, especially in awake or lightly sedated patients.[7] The nasopharyngeal airway should be lubricated with a local anesthetic water-soluble lubricant, such as 1% lidocaine gel or ointment, and gently passed with the right hand through the nostril along the curvature of the nasopharynx into the oropharynx. The nasopharyngeal airway should never be forced. If resistance is encountered on placement, the other nostril should be considered unless otherwise indicated. When positioned properly, the nasopharyngeal airway should rest between the base of the tongue and the posterior pharyngeal wall.[7] This airway should not be used in a patient with a nasal-septal deformity, a leakage of cerebrospinal fluid from the nose, or a coagulation disorder.[6]

After the oropharyngeal or the nasopharyngeal airways has been placed properly, ventilation should be attempted. Assessment of ventilatory effort should be continuous. With insertion of the oropharyngeal airway, the airway obstruction often clears. In this instance, the patient should be given a breath via the bag-valve-mask unit to assist with the spontaneous ventilatory effort and to help with removal of accumulated carbon dioxide. If apnea persists, positive-pressure breathing should be initiated via bag-mask with adequate tidal volumes. For a normal healthy adult, the perianesthesia nurse should consider tidal volumes of 8 to 12 mL/kg at a rate of 12 to 14 breaths/min as initial settings. For prevention of oxygen delivery into the stomach, pressure on the bag-mask device should not exceed 25 cm H_2O.[6]

INTUBATION OF THE TRACH

Intubation of the trachea is a proficien for only those nursing personnel with airway management training and who a erly credentialed to intubate. Nurses sho familiar with their states' Nurse Practice A well as their hospitals' policies regarding int tion privileges. The perianesthesia nurse shou be familiar with the technique of intubation an capable of performing it quickly and efficiently should it be necessary and if it is in his or her scope of practice to do so. Airway management skills, such as endotracheal intubation, can be developed in the operating room setting under the mentorship of a certified registered nurse anesthetist or a physician anesthesiologist. With the same mentor, the perianesthesia nurse should continue to practice intubation skills on a monthly basis in the operating room. In an airway emergency, the properly trained perianesthesia nurse should intubate the trachea if ventilation of the patient's lungs is unsuccessful. Endotracheal intubation indicates the placement of an endotracheal tube directly into the trachea. When the endotracheal tube is placed through the mouth, the method is called *orotracheal intubation*. When the endotracheal tube is placed through the nose, the method is called *nasotracheal intubation*. Other indications for endotracheal intubation in the PACU include the inability of the patient to protect the airway, prolonged mechanical ventilation, and cardiac and respiratory arrest.[8]

The perianesthesia nurse should be familiar with the technique of endotracheal intubation with the recognition that the conditions in which intubation is performed in the PACU may be less than ideal. The patient's position in the bed, excess upper airway secretions, and intact airway reflexes contribute to the degree of difficulty in performance of this maneuver in the PACU.

Equipment for Endotracheal Intubation

Adult and pediatric intubation equipment should be kept in the PACU at all times. This equipment should be inspected daily and after each use for proper functioning. For a list of the suggested airway management items to be kept in the PACU, see Box 30-2. Table 30-1 shows the recommended sizes for endotracheal tubes given the patient demographic. The formula *age / 4 + 4* may be used as a guide when preparing endotracheal tubes for pediatric patients.[9] For example, a size 5.0 mm endotracheal tube may be prepared for a 4-year-old child. Because of their importance, the laryngoscope and endotracheal tubes are discussed in detail.

blades
ys
sizes
tubes
nge for inflation of an
tube cuff
ngle endotracheal tubes
racheal and oral suction catheters
pe for securing endotracheal tube
- Appropriate sized stylets
- Plastic thin-walled tube
- Pediatric Magill forceps
- Water-based lubricant

PEDIATRIC LMA EQUIPMENT
- LMA-Classic: sizes 1, 1½, 2, 2½, and 3
- LMA-Unique: sizes 1, 1½, 2, 2½, and 3
- 20-mL syringes for inflation of LMA
- Pediatric oral airways
- Tongue blades

ADULT ENDOTRACHEAL EQUIPMENT
- Laryngoscope handles
- C Batteries
- Laryngoscope blades
  - Nos. 2, 3, and 4 Miller
  - No. 3 Macintosh
- Stylets
- Sterile gauze with topical water-soluble lubricant
- Sizes 6-mm through 9-mm cuffed tracheal tubes
- Endotracheal and oral suction catheters
- Tape for securing endotracheal tube
- 10-mL syringe for inflation of the endotracheal tube cuff
- Small hemostatic clamp
- Tongue blades for airway insertion
- Assorted-sized oropharyngeal airways
- Assorted-sized nasopharyngeal airways

ADULT LMA EQUIPMENT
- LMA-Classic: sizes 3, 4, and 5
- LMA-Unique: sizes 3, 4, and 5
- 60-mL Syringes for inflation of LMA

PACU, Postanesthesia care unit; *LMA,* laryngeal mask airway.

Laryngoscope

The laryngoscope is used for visualization of the larynx and the anatomic structures in close proximity to the larynx (Fig. 30-4). The laryngoscope has two main parts: the handle and the blade. The handle holds the blade and houses batteries that

Table 30-1	Recommended Sizes for Endotracheal Tubes
GROUP	**INTERNAL DIAMETER (mm)**
Pediatric	
Premature	2.0
Newborn	2.5
6 months	3.5
1 year	4.0
2 years	4.5
4 years	5.0
6 years	5.5
8 years	6.0
10 years	6.0-6.5
12 years	6.5-7.0
14 years	7.0-7.5
Adult	
Female	7.0-7.5
Male	7.5-8.0

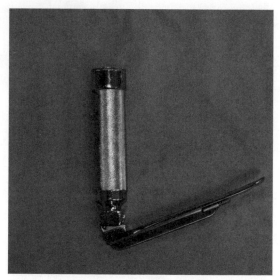

FIG. 30-4 Laryngoscope. (Courtesy Suzanne M. Wright.)

provide electricity for the light on the side of the blade. The blade consists of three sections: the spatula, the flange, and the tip. The spatula can be straight or curved; it is the long main shaft of the blade. It compresses and moves the soft tissue of the lower jaw for facilitation of direct vision of the larynx.[10] The flange, which is on the side of the spatula, deflects tissue that may obstruct the direct vision of the larynx. The tip, at the distal end of the spatula, is either curved or straight and serves to elevate the epiglottis, either directly or indirectly. The blade is attached to the handle at a connection called the *hook-on fitting.* The perianesthesia nurse is strongly encouraged to practice connecting the blade to the handle before using the laryngoscope in an emergency.

The Macintosh and Miller blades are the most popular types of laryngoscope blades in clinical use. The Macintosh is a curved blade with the flange on the left side for aid in moving the tongue, which enhances visual exposure of the larynx. The Macintosh blade (Fig. 30-5) comes in four sizes: No. 1 for the infant, No. 2 for the child, No. 3 for the medium adult, and No. 4 for the large adult. For most adults, the No. 3 medium adult is the blade of choice. The Miller blade (see Fig. 30-5) has a straight spatula with a slightly curved tip. This blade has five sizes: No. 0 for the premature infant, No. 1 for the infant, No. 2 for the child or small adult, No. 3 for the medium adult, and No. 4 for the large adult. The Miller Nos. 0 and 1 are the blades of choice for premature and full-term infants, whose anatomic structures are more receptive to the use of a straight blade.[9] Many anesthesia practitioners use the No. 2 Miller for intubation of adults. The perianesthesia nurse is encouraged to use both the straight and the curved blades if learning the technique. In most instances, the curved blade is easier to use than the straight blade; however, the exposure of the vocal cords might not be as good as with the straight blade.

Endotracheal Tube

The endotracheal tube is also called the *tracheal tube*, *intratracheal tube*, or *ET tube*; it is usually made from natural or synthetic rubber or plastic. The proximal end, or machine end, protrudes from the patient's mouth and receives the adaptor of the ventilating device. The distal end, or patient end, has a slanted portion called the *bevel*. Endotracheal tubes are numbered according to the internal diameter in millimeters. Endotracheal tubes are available in many variations; some with inflatable cuffs and some without. Uncuffed endotracheal tubes are usually seen in the pediatric population. Near the distal end of the endotracheal tube is the inflatable cuff. Leading away from the cuff is a long, thin inflating tube with a pilot balloon at its proximal end. The pressure within the pilot balloon indicates whether the cuff is inflated. Above the pilot balloon is a one-way valve to which the inflation syringe is attached.

The cuff is an inflatable sleeve that provides a leak-resistant fit between the tube and the trachea when inflated. It also prevents aspiration and allows positive-pressure ventilation of the lungs. The cuff is permanently attached to the endotracheal tube at the distal end. High-volume or low-volume cuffs are available. The high-volume cuff is also referred to as a *low-pressure cuff*. The low-volume cuff is also referred to a *high-pressure cuff*. The arterial pressure in the tracheal wall is approximately 30 torr, and the venous pressure in that area is approximately 20 torr.[11] Most clinicians agree that a low-pressure (high-volume) thin-walled cuff should be inflated to a pressure of 17 to 23 torr.[4] Local tracheal damage is associated with high cuff pressures, especially after long periods of intubation. Excessive cuff pressure is a primary factor that leads to ulceration, necrosis, and tracheal stenosis. These complications occur because high cuff pressure reduces the blood supply to the tracheal mucosa. For long-term ventilation, the cuff should be long, with a large residual volume (low-pressure).

In an emergency, the perianesthesia nurse should prepare a cuffed endotracheal tube that is one size smaller than the size normally recommended for the patient. In making this choice, many clinicians look at the little finger of the patient; a smaller than normal little finger indicates that the patient has an opening at the vocal cords that is smaller than normal. In addition, a stylet made of malleable metal or plastic should be inserted inside the endotracheal tube to improve its curvature and maintain its shape on insertion. A stylet should never be used with nasotracheal intubation.[3] Before the stylet is placed inside the tracheal tube, it must be covered with a water-soluble lubricant to ease its withdrawal from the tube after placement. The end of the stylet should be approximately 3 cm from the distal end of the tracheal tube and should not protrude beyond the bevel because damage to the vocal cords can occur. If a cuffed endotracheal tube will be used, an empty 10-mL syringe should be available for inflation of the cuff.

Oral Endotracheal Intubation

Before oral endotracheal intubation is attempted, additional equipment should be immediately

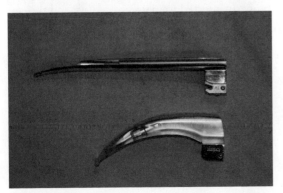

FIG. 30-5 Most frequently used laryngoscope blades: Miller *(top)* and Macintosh *(bottom)*. (Courtesy Suzanne M. Wright.)

available and ready for use. Such equipment includes a tonsil suction connected to a working suction device, McGill forceps, 1-inch tape, a 10-mL empty syringe, an anesthesia bag system or bag-mask unit, and an oxygen source. Throughout the procedure, the patient's oxygen saturation should be monitored continuously with a pulse oximeter.[12]

The essential steps in the technique of oral endotracheal intubation include proper positioning of the patient, proper positioning of the patient's head, insertion of the laryngoscope blade, lifting of the epiglottis, visualization of the vocal cords, placement of the endotracheal tube, and assessment of the patient for correct endotracheal tube placement. The methods for accomplishing these steps are discussed in the following sections.

Positioning the Patient

Position the patient so that the head is at the top of the bed. Raise the entire bed so that the patient's face is approximately at the level of the standing laryngoscopist's xiphoid process.

Positioning the Head

Place a firm 4-inch pillow or blanket under the patient's occiput. Flex the patient's head at the neck. This position is called the *sniffing position* (Fig. 30-6). Extend the patient's head unless contraindicated.

Insertion of the Laryngoscope Blade

With the fingers of the right hand, open the jaw, ensuring that the lips are not entangled in the teeth. With the laryngoscope in the left hand, insert the blade between the upper and lower teeth at the right side of the patient's mouth. Advance the blade slowly inward, past the tonsillar pillars and toward the midline of the oral cavity. Sweep the tongue toward the left side of the mouth. The key to successful intubation is moving

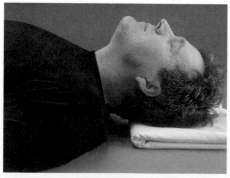

FIG. 30-6 Sniffing position. (From Sanders MJ: *Mosby's paramedic textbook,* ed 3, St. Louis, 2007, Mosby.)

the tongue to the left, out of the visual path to the vocal cords. At this point, the right hand can be placed under the patient's occiput to lift the head further. The epiglottis should now be visualized and appears as a red, leaf-shaped structure seen behind the tip of the blade as the laryngoscope is advanced down the oral cavity.

Raising the Epiglottis and Visualizing the Vocal Cords

With the epiglottis in direct vision, slip the straight blade just beneath the tip of the epiglottis, gently lift the blade forward and upward at a 45-degree angle, and hold the wrist rigid (Fig. 30-7). If a curved blade is used, slip the tip of the blade between the epiglottis and the base of the tongue (see Fig. 30-7). With the left hand, lift forward and upward on the handle at a 45-degree angle. The epiglottis folds onto the blade, and the vocal cords should then be visible.

Regardless of whether a curved or straight blade is used, the handle should not be used as a lever, nor should the upper teeth be used as a fulcrum because the tip of the blade will push the larynx up and out of sight and the teeth can become chipped or broken.

At this point, if the vocal cords cannot be visualized, an assistant should apply gentle external downward pressure on the larynx (the Sellick maneuver). The vocal cords should come into view. If the blade is inserted too deeply, it enters the esophagus. At this point, withdraw the blade, ventilate the patient's lungs with 100% oxygen, and attempt the procedure again. While ventilating the lungs, review the initial attempt and design an alternative strategy to facilitate successful intubation of the trachea.

Placing the Endotracheal Tube

When the vocal cords are visualized, an assistant should place the endotracheal tube, with a stylet properly inserted to maintain a curve and the cuff deflated, in the laryngoscopist's right hand. The laryngoscopist should never lose sight of the cords once they are visualized. Pass the endotracheal tube with the right hand along the right side of the tongue and blade and through the vocal cords until the cuff disappears beyond the vocal cords or until the tip of the endotracheal tube protrudes 2 or 3 cm into the trachea.

Assessing the Patient for Proper Endotracheal Tube Placement

After the endotracheal tube is placed, correct placement must be verified. Remove the blade with the left hand while holding onto the endotracheal tube with the right hand. Slowly remove

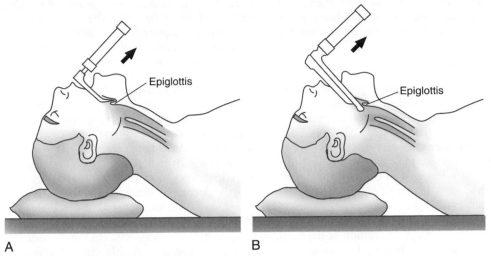

A   B

FIG. 30-7 Proper positioning of laryngoscope blade for facilitation of endotracheal intubation. **A,** With curved blade (e.g., Macintosh), tip is placed into space between base of tongue and pharyngeal surface of epiglottis, which is called *vallecula*. **B,** With straight blade (e.g., Miller), tip is placed on laryngeal surface of epiglottis. Regardless of type of blade used, after the blade is in position, forward and upward movements on handle *(arrows)* exert pressure on long axis of blade, which serves to elevate epiglottis and expose vocal cords. (Redrawn from Miller R, et al: *Miller's anesthesia,* ed 7, Philadelphia, 2010, Churchill Livingstone.)

the stylet without dislodging the tracheal tube and place the laryngoscope blade in an emesis basin or other container for cleaning. With a 10-mL syringe, inject a volume of air (4 to 6 mL) into the pilot balloon of the endotracheal tube cuff until leakage around the cuff is minimal or stops. A cuff leak is assessed with placement of the bell of the stethoscope over the larynx.[5] The end of the endotracheal tube should be connected to a bag-mask unit or an anesthesia bag system and ventilated while an assistant auscultates the chest for breath sounds. Breath sounds should be assessed in all four quadrants, and the stomach should also be auscultated. If no breath sounds are audible or if a gurgling sound is heard over the stomach, deflate the cuff, remove the endotracheal tube, and ventilate the patient's lungs by mask with 100% oxygen. These signs indicate an esophageal intubation. While ventilating the lungs, consider why the attempt was unsuccessful, review the procedure, and reintubate the patient. If breath sounds are audible on only the right side of the chest, a right endobronchial intubation should be suspected.[6] If this condition occurs, withdraw the tube at 1-cm intervals and auscultate until breath sounds are bilateral. Confirmation of endotracheal intubation is also verified with bilateral and symmetric chest rise and the presence of expiratory carbon dioxide. The gold standard for assessing proper placement of an endotracheal tube is the measurement of expired carbon dioxide.[6] Expired carbon dioxide can be measured with spectroscopy, often found only in the operating room, or disposable carbon dioxide detectors used specifically for this purpose. Disposable carbon dioxide detectors are placed between the ventilating device and the endotracheal tube. If carbon dioxide is present, indicating proper placement of the endotracheal tube, the pH-sensitive indicator on the device changes color.[3] When correct endotracheal tube placement and cuff pressure are confirmed, insert an oral airway and secure the tube with adhesive tape or another appropriate device.

Documentation of the procedure should include the number of attempts, the degree of visualization of the vocal cords, whether the intubation was traumatic or atraumatic, the quality and distribution of breath sounds, the presence of carbon dioxide as indicated by a carbon dioxide detector, the amount of air injected into the cuff, the cuff pressure, the endotracheal tube size, and the laryngoscope blade type and size.

Ventilating the Lungs

The adult patient's lungs should be ventilated approximately 12 to 14 times per minute at a tidal volume of 8 to 12 mL/kg.[6] Infants should be ventilated at approximately 26 to 30 times per minute at a volume large enough to raise the chest on inspiration. However, when time permits, a tidal volume of 7 mL/kg should be used.

Children's lungs should be ventilated at a rate of 18 to 24 breaths/min. The tidal volume to be delivered can be determined in the same manner for infants.[9]

Nasotracheal Intubation

When the endotracheal tube is inserted through the nose, the method is called *nasotracheal intubation*. When nasotracheal intubation is attempted without the use of a laryngoscope, the method is called a *blind nasotracheal intubation*. Direct-vision intubation is the insertion of an endotracheal tube with the aid of a laryngoscope. Using the direct-vision method of a nasotracheal intubation, the laryngoscopist can use Magill forceps designed to direct the tip of the endotracheal tube to the glottic opening (Fig. 30-8). A description of the nasal intubation technique can be found in many anesthesia textbooks.

Tracheal intubation has many advantages. It provides a route for mechanical ventilation, reduces the amount of anatomic dead space, and protects the patient from aspiration of blood, mucus, or foreign material into the tracheobronchial tree. It also relieves upper airway obstruction and provides an access route for removal of excess secretions in the airways.

The disadvantage of intubation is that it can produce trauma to the teeth, lips, soft palate, epiglottis, vocal cords, and other tissues in that region. Tracheal intubation is best left to those who are properly trained in the procedure.

Emergency Airway Management

At times, the perianesthesia nurse must care for a patient with a documented or undocumented difficult airway. A difficult airway implies an inability to ventilate or intubate under optimal conditions by an airway expert. The perianesthesia nurse must be familiar with methods to manage this life-threatening event. The American Society of Anesthesiologists (ASA) Difficult Airway Algorithm is a helpful tool that can be easily referenced for decision support while managing this complex patient.[13] Patients at increased risk of a difficult airway in the PACU include, but are not limited to, those who are obese; patients recovering from ear, nose, and throat surgery or neck surgery; and those who have a history of a difficult airway. Patients at increased risk for difficult ventilation can include those who have a beard, are edentulous, have a history of snoring, and are elderly. A copy of the ASA Difficult Airway Algorithm, or one like it, should be available in the PACU at all times.

Cricothyrotomy is a last attempt at securing an airway; it is instituted only after all other viable options of securing the airway have been exhausted. Cricothyrotomy is a puncture through the cricothyroid membrane with a large-bore cricothyrotomy catheter or large-bore intravenous catheter.[14] The perianesthesia nurse should become familiar with locating the cricothyroid membrane, which falls midline between the thyroid

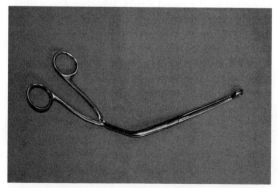

FIG. 30-8 Magill forceps. This equipment is often used to direct the endotracheal tube to the glottis opening during nasal intubation. (Courtesy Suzanne M. Wright.)

Evidence-Based Practice

The American Society of Anesthesiologists (ASA) Difficult Airway Algorithm was originally developed in 1993, with its most recent update published in 2003. This practice guideline was developed based on a thorough review of scientific evidence and input from airway management experts. The algorithm was designed for use by health care professionals with advanced training in management of the airway as a decision support tool when encountering a patient with a difficult airway. The information provided in this guideline is embraced by anesthesia providers as a best evidence approach to managing this complex clinical situation.

IMPLICATIONS FOR PRACTICE

Perianesthesia nurses are in an ideal position to make a significant contribution to patient safety. Through knowledge and application of the ASA Difficult Airway Algorithm, nurses can perform more effectively should a patient require immediate assistance with ventilation and oxygenation in the perioperative period.

Source: Caplan RA, et al: Practice guidelines for management of the difficult airway: an updated report by the American Society of Anesthesiologists Task Force on Management of the Difficult Airway, *Anesthesiology* 98(5):1269–1277, 2003.

cartilage and the cricoid cartilage on the anterior portion of the neck around the level of the sixth cervical vertebra. Before ventilating through this *temporary* airway, the nurse should confirm correct placement into the trachea, which is evidenced by the aspiration of air through the catheter into an attached syringe. A jet ventilator, which delivers oxygen at high pressure, is ideal for ventilating through this type of airway because the resistance is difficult to overcome. Witnessing the egress of air after each inspiration with the jet ventilator is crucial to avoid excessive accumulation of pressure in the lungs. For this procedure to be successful, the nurse must know where the requisite supplies are located and how the equipment functions. Cricothyrotomy is merely a bridge until a more definitive airway can be established, such as a surgical cricothyrotomy or tracheostomy.

Perianesthesia Care of the Intubated Patient

Nursing care of the intubated patient involves: (1) frequent auscultation of the chest for bilateral breath sounds to ensure correct placement of the endotracheal tube; (2) frequent suctioning of the oral cavity and, if clinically necessary, suctioning inside the endotracheal tube to remove secretions (delivery of at least five maximal ventilations of 100% oxygen before endotracheal suctioning is performed should be considered); and (3) maintenance of communication between patient and nurse to reduce anxiety.[12] The perianesthesia nurse must reassure the patient of continuous observation and monitoring and provide the patient with a means to effectively communicate his or her needs and concerns.

Extubation of the Patient

After determining that the patient can be safely extubated, the perianesthesia nurse should first ensure that all intubation, suction, and ventilation equipment is functioning properly and is at the patient's bedside. The entire procedure should be explained to the patient. Depending on the amount and location of secretions, the trachea and the nasopharynx should be suctioned. All secretions must be aspirated from the upper airway to reduce the incidence of coughing and laryngospasm. The patient should be ventilated with 100% oxygen for several breaths before extubation. A syringe is then placed into the side valve of the pilot balloon, and the endotracheal tube cuff is deflated completely. The patient should be asked to take a deep breath, and at the end of inspiration, the tube should be removed gently. If the patient is completely awake and responding,

the oral airway should also be removed. Oxygen (100%) should be administered via mask, and the patient assessed for dyspnea, stridor, and airway obstruction. Oxygenation should be assessed continuously by the pulse oximeter and the clinical picture.

Adverse Sequelae after Tracheal Intubation

Hoarseness and Sore Throat

On emergence from anesthesia, some patients who have been intubated during surgery may complain of a sore throat. Although the duration of sore throat after intubation is short, it can be a significant discomfort, especially after long surgeries.[15] The incidence of sore throat may increase dramatically when the patient's head is turned frequently or is placed in an abnormal position during surgery.

Assessment of the patient with a sore throat should include observation of the oropharynx and auscultation of the chest. Abnormal findings should be reported to the anesthesia provider. Counseling the patient is probably the most important nursing intervention. The nurse should review the anesthesia record to determine whether the patient was intubated and whether the procedure was traumatic (e.g., multiple attempts and difficult intubation). A sore throat can result from a traumatic intubation.

Interventions consist of communicating to the patient that an endotracheal tube was placed in the throat during surgery to help with breathing and that throat discomfort may persist for 1 to 3 days. When the patient understands the reason for the discomfort and learns that it is not life threatening, the perception of the discomfort often becomes less severe. If treatment is necessary, medications such as dexamethasone can be given to reduce the inflammation. An ice bag or ice chips can also be given to the patient to relieve symptoms.

Laryngospasm

Partial or complete closure of the vocal cords can occur because of increased secretions or as a reflex caused by stimulation of the irritant receptors.[6] Assessment reveals reduced or no breath sounds. If partial laryngospasm is present, the patient may make crowing sounds, especially on inspiration. Interventions include the administration of 100% oxygen under positive pressure with a bag-mask unit. If the patient's lungs cannot be ventilated, the perianesthesia nurse should call for help; intravenous administration of succinylcholine and reintubation of the trachea may be mandated (see Chapter 23).

Aspiration of Gastrointestinal Contents

Aspiration of gastrointestinal contents is a complication that may be seen in the PACU in weak and debilitated patients, those with neurologic disease, or those with an intestinal obstruction. See Chapters 16 and 29 for a complete discussion of this syndrome.

Airway Adjuncts

Laryngeal Mask Airway

The laryngeal mask airway (LMA) was developed in the 1980s by a British anesthesiologist named Archie Brain. The product became available in the United States in 1992. During the last 15 years, modifications have been made to the design of the original LMA, known as the *LMA-Classic,* that have resulted in numerous LMA products that are useful for a variety of patient airway needs. The LMA can be useful in obtaining an adequate airway when attempts at mask ventilating or intubating have failed.

Laryngeal Mask Airway–Classic

The LMA-Classic was designed to provide an alternative method of airway management that is intermediate in invasiveness between the face mask and the endotracheal tube (ETT; Fig. 30-9). The reusable latex-free device consists of three basic components. The first component is the soft inflatable cuff that, when inserted correctly, conforms to the hypopharynx with its opening facing the patient's laryngeal opening. At the proximal end, on the inside of the cuff, is a set of aperture bars located at the junction of the cuff and airway tube. The aperture bars allow passage of air into the cuff yet prevent airway anatomy, such as the epiglottis, from entering the tube and blocking the airway passage. The cuff is connected to the second component, an airway tube, which is a large-bore tube with a 15-mm standard connector

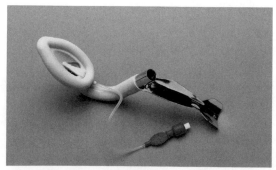

FIG. 30-9 LMA-Classic. (Used with permission of The Laryngeal Mask Company Limited, United Kingdom.)

on the end. The tube acts as a gas conduit for ventilation and, if needed, an endotracheal tube can be passed through the LMA through the vocal cords for intubation. The size of the ETT able to pass through the LMA depends on the size of the LMA inserted. Last, a long thin inflation tube is attached to a pilot balloon that permits inflation and deflation of the LMA cuff.

The LMA-Classic is used for a variety of patient circumstances during general anesthesia and is commonly reserved for patients who will be spontaneously breathing throughout the surgical procedure. The LMA is often well tolerated in the patient who is lightly anesthetized and semiconscious. The LMA is available in eight sizes and can be used in patients ranging in size from neonates to more than 100 kg. More importantly, the LMA has been used routinely in management of difficult and emergent airway situations. The device has proved successful in providing a bridge or temporary airway in patients in whom a permanent airway has not been obtained. Recently, the LMA has been included in two nationally recognized association protocols: the ASA Difficult Airway Algorithm and the American Heart Association Guidelines for Cardiopulmonary Resuscitation and Emergency Cardiovascular Care for Advanced Cardiac Life Support.[3,13]

Insertion of the LMA is simple, and most providers find the learning curve to be gentle. After the cuff is deflated so that it is flat and free of wrinkles, the anterior portion of the cuff is lubricated with a water-soluble product. The patient then is placed in the preferred position, the sniffing position, although a neutral position can be used in patients with actual or suspected cervical spine injury. The provider places the dominant index finger at the junction between the cuff and the airway tube while ensuring that the solid black line on the tube faces the patient's upper lip. The cuff is placed against the patient's hard palate and is moved back and forth against the palate to effectively lubricate the airway and prevent the cuff from folding over on insertion. Without forcing, the LMA is advanced as far down into the pharynx as possible. The nondominant hand holds the tube, and the dominant finger is withdrawn from the LMA device. Without the nurse holding onto the device, the LMA is inflated following the recommended maximum cuff inflation volumes. Correct placement of the LMA may be observed during inflation; a slight and upward movement of the LMA in the airway and notable swelling in the neck may occur after cuff inflation. Insertion of an oral airway next to the LMA tube may be necessary to prevent occlusion of the airway tube as the patient regains consciousness.

Auscultation of bilateral breath sounds and the presence of end-tidal carbon dioxide confirm placement of the LMA device.

Other Laryngeal Mask Airway Products

Additional LMA products are available for management of the patient's airway. The LMA-Unique is the disposable version of the LMA-Classic. This product is often found in prehospital settings and in code carts and other airway management carts. The LMA-Flexible has a mask similar to the LMA-Classic but with a flexible, wire-reinforced tube. The LMA-Flexible is used primarily for procedures that involve the head or neck area. The flexible airway tube permits the airway product to be positioned away from the surgical field while an adequate seal is maintained. The LMA-Fastrach is designed to facilitate endotracheal intubation (Fig. 30-10). The reusable device differs from the classic LMA design primarily in its rigid anatomically curved airway tube that is connected to a metal handle. The handle is used to facilitate one-handed insertion and removal and to adjust the LMA cuff position and the glottic alignment of the ETT. The aperture bars of the classic LMA have been replaced in the LMA-Fastrach with an epiglottic elevating bar. The elevating bar is designed to lift the epiglottis as the ETT passes through the LMA device, which may decrease the risk of arytenoid trauma or esophageal placement.

The LMA-ProSeal is designed specifically for separation of the alimentary and respiratory tracts with improvement of the laryngeal seal. The enhanced seal offers a higher airway seal pressure during positive-pressure ventilation and may be used in the patient who is either spontaneously breathing or paralyzed. A built-in bite block provides protection from occlusion by the patient, and a removable introducer allows insertion of the product without the need to place fingers directly in the patient's mouth. Another unique feature of this product is the ability to blindly pass a gastric tube through the device, which allows for stomach decompression and drainage. The LMA Supreme is a disposable device that offers the rigidity of the LMA-Fastrach for easy placement, a drain tube for emptying stomach contents, and a built-in bite block that helps to avoid obstruction caused by biting on the tube.

The following guidelines are for the perianesthesia nurse caring for patients in the PACU who have or have had an LMA inserted for surgery. If an LMA is present in the patient arriving in the PACU, a few important points should be remembered. The LMA is designed to be removed in either a conscious awake patient or a deeply anesthetized one. Removal of the LMA while the patient is awake is the most common and preferred technique, especially in adult patients. Most patients are able to open their mouths on command for removal of the LMA. Because cuff deflation before the return of effective swallowing and coughing reflexes may allow secretions in the upper airway to enter the larynx and cause laryngospasm, the LMA cuff should not be deflated until the LMA is being removed. Also, any existing bite block or oral airway should be removed along with the LMA device and not before, in order to prevent occlusion of the airway from the patient biting on the LMA tube. For patients in the PACU who still have an LMA present, manual support of the airway is usually not necessary. In fact, lifting of the jaw may actually displace the LMA cuff and cause laryngospasm, malposition, or possibly, obstruction of the airway.

Although LMA products may differ regarding indications for use in patient airway management, there are important similarities in their use. The LMA products are contraindicated in patients at risk for aspiration and regurgitation, because the devices do not protect the airway from gastric secretions. LMA products are not used in patients undergoing surgery requiring muscle relaxation. The LMA is intended to be used in patients who will remain spontaneously breathing throughout the surgical procedure.

The LMA products are also contraindicated in patients with upper airway pathology or obstruction.

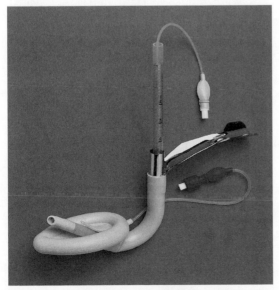

FIG. 30-10 LMA-Fastrach. (Used with permission of The Laryngeal Mask Company Limited, United Kingdom.)

LMA devices are advantageous for use in patients who are professional speakers or singers who need a general anesthetic. Because LMA devices do not come in contact with the vocal cords, voice changes caused by vocal cord trauma are less likely. The devices are especially useful in patients who have a difficult mask airway because of distorted facial anatomy or the presence of a beard. LMA products have gained acceptance in many areas of health care. The ease of insertion combined with a variety of different products has allowed health care professionals to offer a greater degree of airway management and safety for surgical patients.

Video Laryngoscope

One of the newest airway management tools to make its way into surgical suites around the country is the video laryngoscope. Video laryngoscopes, of which there are many types, provide a direct and often superior view of the glottis under suboptimal intubating conditions. A video laryngoscope system involves the use of a rigid laryngoscope along with a video screen for visualization of airway structures. The perianesthesia nurse should be familiar with the availability and operation of this type of airway management tool.

SUMMARY

Throughout the postoperative period, surgical patients remain vulnerable to the respiratory effects of anesthetic medications and the surgical procedure. The perianesthesia nurse should be vigilant at all times in monitoring the postoperative patient's respiratory status. It is essential for the nurse to be prepared to respond immediately to airway problems that may arise in the PACU. Knowledge of airway management techniques coupled with early recognition of difficulties are key in optimizing patient outcomes in the perioperative setting.

REFERENCES

1. Atlee J: *Complications in anesthesia*, ed 2, Philadelphia, 2007, Saunders.
2. Dolenska S: *Basic science for anaesthetists*, London, 2006, Cambridge University Press.
3. Sinz E, et al: *American Heart Association advanced cardiac life support provider manual*, Dallas, 2011, American Heart Association.
4. Miller RD, Pardo MC, Jr: *Basics of anesthesia*, ed 6, New York, 2011, Churchill Livingstone.
5. Nagelhout J, Plaus K: *Nurse anesthesia*, ed 4, St. Louis, 2009, Saunders.
6. Barash P, et al: *Clinical anesthesia*, ed 6, Philadelphia, 2009, Lippincott Williams & Wilkins.
7. Miller R, et al: *Miller's anesthesia*, ed 7, Philadelphia, 2009, Churchill Livingstone.
8. Alspach J: *Core curriculum for critical care nursing*, ed 6, Philadelphia, 2006, Saunders.
9. Davis PJ, et al: *Smith's anesthesia for infants and children*, ed 8, St. Louis, 2011, Mosby.
10. Hagberg C: *Benumof's airway management*, ed 2, St. Louis, 2007, Mosby.
11. Hall J: *Guyton & Hall's textbook of medical physiology*, ed 12, Philadelphia, 2010, Saunders.
12. Schick L, Windle PE: *Perianesthesia nursing core curriculum: preprocedure, phase I and phase II PACU nursing*, ed 2, Philadelphia, 2010, Saunders.
13. Caplan RA, et al: Practice guidelines for management of the difficult airway: an updated report by the American Society of Anesthesiologists Task Force on Management of the Difficult Airway, *Anesthesiology* 98(5):1269–1277, 2003.
14. Orebaugh SL: *Atlas of airway management: techniques and tools*, Philadelphia, 2007, Lippincott Williams & Wilkins.
15. Biro P, et al: Complaints of sore throat after tracheal intubation: a prospective evaluation, *Eur J Anaesthesiol* 22(4): 307–311, 2005.

31 Pain Management

Chris Pasero, MS, RN-BC, FAAN

Pain is one of the most common reasons people seek health care. Despite an abundance of research and improvements in analgesics and drug delivery technology, pain continues to be undertreated and costly for patients and the health care system in general.[1,2] Nurses are experts in assessment, drug administration, and patient education and are the only members of the health care team who are at the patient's bedside around the clock. These characteristics have led to their distinction as the patient's primary pain manager.[3] Nurses are critical to ensuring that their patients receive the best possible pain relief available.

DEFINITIONS

Addiction: A chronic, neurobiologic disease characterized by impaired control over drug use, compulsive use, continued use despite harm, and craving.

Multimodal Analgesia: Combinations of drugs with different underlying mechanisms administered to allow lower doses of each of the drugs, reduce the potential for analgesic adverse effects, and provide comparable or greater pain relief than can be achieved with any single analgesic.

Neuropathic Pain: Pain that results from abnormal processing of sensory input by the nervous system because of damage to the peripheral or central nervous systems or both.

Nociceptive Pain: Pain that results from the normal functioning of physiologic systems that leads to the perception of noxious stimuli (tissue injury) as being painful.

Opioid Naive: An individual who has not recently taken enough opioid on a regular enough basis to become tolerant to the effects of an opioid.

Opioid Tolerance: An individual who has taken opioids long enough at doses high enough to develop tolerance to many of the effects of the opioid, including analgesia and sedation; a timeframe for development of tolerance has not been established.

Physical Dependence: Potential for withdrawal symptoms if the opioid is abruptly stopped or an antagonist is administered; not the same as addiction.

Pseudoaddiction: A mistaken diagnosis of addiction in which the patient exhibits behaviors often seen in addictive disease, such as asking for analgesics on time or early, but actually reflect undertreated pain.

Titration: The process of adjusting the amount of the dose of an analgesic.

Tolerance: A process characterized by decreasing effects of a drug at its previous dose, or the need for a higher dose of drug to maintain an effect; not the same as addiction.

DEFINITION OF PAIN

The American Pain Society defines pain as "an unpleasant sensory and emotional experience associated with actual or potential tissue damage, or described in terms of such damage."[4] This definition describes pain as a complex, multifactoral phenomenon that affects a person's psychosocial, emotional, and physical functioning. The definition of pain that is applied in the clinical setting reinforces that pain is a highly personal and subjective experience: "Pain is whatever the experiencing person says it is, existing whenever he says it does."[5] All accepted guidelines consider the patient's report to be the most reliable indicator of pain and the gold standard of pain assessment.[2,4]

TYPES AND CATEGORIES OF PAIN

Pain is usually described as being *acute* or *chronic* (*persistent*).[6] Acute pain and chronic pain differ from one another primarily in their duration. For example, tissue damage as a result of surgery, trauma, or burns produces acute pain that is expected to have a relatively short duration and to resolve with normal healing. Chronic pain can occur from an underlying medical condition, such as peripheral neuropathy from diabetes, cancer pain from tumor growth, or osteoarthritis pain from joint degeneration, and it can persist throughout the course of a person's life. Some medical conditions can produce both acute and chronic pain. For example, some patients with cancer have continuous chronic pain and also experience acute exacerbations of pain periodically (called *breakthrough pain*) or endure repetitive painful procedures during cancer treatment.

Pain is increasingly classified by its inferred pathology as being either *nociceptive pain* or *neuropathic pain* (Table 31-1).[6] *Nociceptive pain* refers

Table 31-1	Classification of Pain by Inferred Pathology		
	NOCICEPTIVE PAIN	**NEUROPATHIC PAIN**	**MIXED PAIN**
Physiologic processes	Normal processing of stimuli that damages tissues or has the potential to do so if prolonged; is somatic or visceral	Abnormal processing of sensory input by the peripheral or central nervous system or both	Components of both nociceptive and neuropathic pain; poorly defined
Categories and examples	A. Somatic pain: Arises from bone joint, muscle, skin, or connective tissue. It is usually described as aching or throbbing in quality and is well localized. *Examples*: Surgical, trauma; wound, and burn pain; cancer pain (tumor growth) and pain associated with bony metastases; labor pain (cervical changes and uterine contractions); osteoarthritis and rheumatoid arthritis pain; osteoporosis pain; pain of Ehlers–Danlos Syndrome; ankylosing spondylitis B. Visceral pain: Arises from visceral organs, such as the GI tract and pancreas. This may be subdivided: 1. Tumor involvement of the organ capsule that causes aching and fairly well-localized pain 2. Obstruction of hollow viscus, which causes intermittent cramping and poorly localized pain *Examples*: Organ-involved cancer pain, ulcerative colitis, irritable bowel syndrome, Crohn's disease, pancreatitis	A. Centrally generated pain 1. Deafferentation pain: Injury to either the peripheral or central nervous system; burning pain below the level of a spinal cord lesion reflects injury to the central nervous system *Examples*: Phantom pain as a result of peripheral nerve damage; post-stroke pain; pain following spinal cord injury 2. Sympathetically maintained pain: Associated with dysregulation of the autonomic nervous system *Example*: Complex regional pain syndrome B. Peripherally generated pain 1. Painful polyneuropathies: Pain felt along the distribution of many peripheral nerves *Examples*: Diabetic neuropathy; postherpetic neuralgia; alcohol-nutritional neuropathy; some types of neck, shoulder, and back pain; pain of Guillain–Barre syndrome 2. Painful mononeuropathies: Usually associated with a known peripheral nerve injury; pain felt at least partly along the distribution of the damaged nerve *Examples*: Nerve root compression, nerve entrapment; trigeminal neuralgia; some types of neck, shoulder, and back pain	No identified categories *Examples*: Fibromyalgia; some types of neck, shoulder, and back pain; some headaches; pain associated with HIV; some myofascial pain; pain associated with Lyme disease
Pharmacologic treatment	Most responsive to nonopioids, opioids, and local anesthetics.	Adjuvant analgesics, such as antidepressants, anticonvulsants, and local anesthetics, but there is wide variability in terms of efficacy and adverse-effect profiles	Adjuvant analgesics, such as antidepressants, anticonvulsants, and local anesthetics, but there is wide variability in terms of efficacy and adverse-effect profiles

From Pasero C, McCaffery M: *Pain assessment and pharmacologic management*, St. Louis, 2011, Mosby. Copyright 1999, Chris Pasero, Margo McCaffery. Used with permission.
GI, Gastrointestinal.

to the normal functioning of physiologic systems that leads to the perception of noxious stimuli (tissue injury) as being painful. This explains why nociception is described as "normal" pain transmission. Pain from surgery, trauma, burns, and tumor growth are examples of nociceptive pain. Patients often describe this type of pain as "aching," "cramping," or "throbbing."

Neuropathic pain is pathologic and results from abnormal processing of sensory input by the nervous system as a result of damage to the peripheral nervous system (PNS) or central nervous system (CNS), or both.[6] Examples include postherpetic neuralgia, diabetic neuropathy, phantom pain, and post-stroke pain syndrome. Patients with neuropathic pain describe their pain with distinctive words, such as "burning," "sharp," and "shooting."

Some patients have a combination of nociceptive and neuropathic pain. For example, a patient may have nociceptive pain as a result of tumor growth and also report radiating sharp and shooting neuropathic pain if the tumor is pressing against a nerve plexus. Sickle cell pain is usually a combination of nociceptive pain from the clumping of sickled cells and resulting perfusion deficits, and neuropathic pain from nerve ischemia.

Some painful conditions and syndromes are not easily categorized as either nociceptive or neuropathic. These are sometimes referred to as *mixed pain syndromes* and include fibromyalgia and some low back and myofascial pain.

NOCICEPTION AND ANALGESIC ACTION SITES

Nociception includes four specific processes: transduction, transmission, perception, and modulation.

Figure 31-1 illustrates these processes, and an overview of each follows.

Transduction

Transduction refers to the processes by which noxious stimuli activate primary afferent neurons called *nociceptors,* which are located throughout the body in the skin, subcutaneous tissue, and visceral and somatic structures (see Fig. 31-1).[6] These neurons have the ability to respond selectively to noxious stimuli generated as a result of tissue damage from mechanical (e.g., incision, tumor growth), thermal (e.g., burn, frostbite), chemical (toxins, chemotherapy), and infectious sources.[7,8] The noxious stimuli cause the release of a number of excitatory compounds (e.g., serotonin, bradykinin, histamine, substance P, prostaglandins), which facilitate the movement of pain along the pain pathway.[6] These substances are collectively referred to as *inflammatory soup.*[8]

Prostaglandins are a particularly important group of compounds that accompanies tissue injury and initiates inflammatory responses that increase tissue swelling and pain at the site of injury.[9] They are formed when the enzyme phospholipase breaks down phospholipids into arachidonic acid, and arachidonic acid, in turn, is acted upon by the enzyme cyclooxygenase (COX) to produce prostaglandins (Fig. 31-2). The two best characterized isoenzymes of COX are COX-1 and COX-2; they have an important role in producing the effects of the nonopioid analgesics, which act peripherally and centrally to inhibit the COX isoenzymes. Nonsteroidal antiinflammatory drugs (NSAIDs) work primarily by blocking the formation of prostaglandins in the periphery. The nonselective NSAIDs,

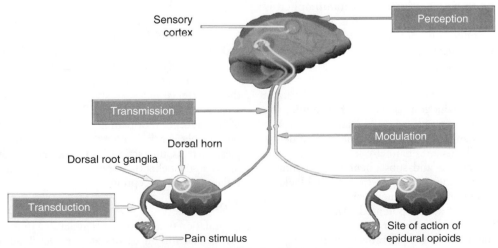

FIG. 31-1 Modern model of pain: sensory pathway.

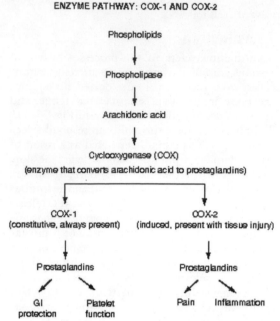

ENZYME PATHWAY: COX-1 AND COX-2

Phospholipids
↓
Phospholipase
↓
Arachidonic acid
↓
Cyclooxygenase (COX)
(enzyme that converts arachidonic acid to prostaglandins)

COX-1
(constitutive, always present)
↓
Prostaglandins

GI protection   Platelet function

COX-2
(induced, present with tissue injury)
↓
Prostaglandins

Pain   Inflammation

FIG. 31-2 Enzyme pathway: COX-1 and COX-2. *GI,* Gastrointestinal. (From Pasero C, McCaffery M: *Pain assessment and pharmacologic management*, St. Louis, 2011, Mosby. Copyright Pasero C, McCaffery M. Used with permission.)

such as ibuprofen, naproxen, diclofenac, and ketorolac, inhibit both COX-1 and COX-2, and the COX-2 selective NSAIDs, such as celecoxib, inhibit just COX-2. As Fig. 31-2 illustrates, both types of NSAIDs produce antiinflammatory and pain relief through the inhibition of COX-2. Although the exact underlying mechanisms of action of acetaminophen continue to be investigated,[10] acetaminophen is a known COX inhibitor that has minimal peripheral effect, is not antiinflammatory, and can both relieve pain and reduce fever by preventing the formation of prostaglandins in the CNS.[6]

Other types of analgesics work by partially blocking transduction as well. For example, sodium channels are closed and inactive at rest, but undergo changes in response to membrane depolarization. Transient channel opening leads to an influx of sodium and subsequent nerve conduction.[11] Local anesthetics are capable of blocking sodium channels and reducing the nerve's ability to generate an action potential. Anticonvulsants also affect the flux of other ions, such as calcium and potassium, to reduce transduction and produce pain relief.

Transmission

Transmission is the second process involved in nociception. Effective transduction generates an action potential that is transmitted along the A-delta (δ) and C fibers.[6] A-δ fibers are lightly myelinated and faster conducting than the unmyelinated C fibers. The endings of A-δ fibers detect thermal and mechanical injury and allow relatively quick localization of pain and a rapid reflex withdrawal from the painful stimulus. Unmyelinated C fibers are slow conductors and respond to mechanical, thermal, and chemical stimuli. They yield poorly localized, often aching or burning pain. A-beta (β) fibers are the largest of the fibers and do not normally transmit pain, but do respond to touch, movement, and vibration.[6]

Afferent information passes through the cell body of the dorsal root ganglia (see Fig. 31-1), which lie outside of the spinal cord, to synapse in the dorsal horn of the spinal cord. An action potential is generated and the impulse ascends up to the spinal cord and transmits information to the brain, where pain is perceived. Extensive modulation occurs in the dorsal horn via complex neurochemical mechanisms. The primary A-δ fibers and C fibers release a variety of transmitters including glutamate, neurokinin, and substance P. Glutamate binds to the *N*-methyl-D-aspartate (NMDA) receptor and promotes pain transmission. Ketamine is an NMDA receptor antagonist that provides pain relief by preventing glutamate from binding to the NMDA receptor sites. Endogenous and therapeutically administered opioids bind to opioid receptor sites in the dorsal horn to block substance P and thereby produce analgesia.[6]

Perception

The third broad process involved in nociception is perception. Perception, the result of the neural activity associated with transmission of noxious stimuli,[6] involves the conscious awareness of pain and requires activation of higher brain structures for the occurrence of awareness, emotions, and drives associated with pain (see Fig. 31-1). The physiology of the perception of pain is poorly understood, but presumably can be targeted by mind-body therapies, such as distraction and imagery, which are based on the belief that brain processes can strongly influence pain perception.[6]

Modulation

Modulation of afferent input generated in response to noxious stimuli occurs at every level from the periphery to the cortex and involves dozens of neurochemicals.[9] For example, serotonin and nor-epinephrine are central inhibitory neurotransmitters that are released in the spinal cord and brainstem by the descending fibers of the modulatory system (see Fig. 31-1). Some antidepressants provide pain relief by blocking the body's reuptake of serotonin and norepinephrine, extending their availability to fight pain. Endogenous opioids are located throughout the peripheral and central nervous systems, and like therapeutically administered opioids they inhibit neuronal activity by binding to opioid receptors. As an example, Fig. 31-1 shows that the dorsal horn of the spinal cord, which is densely populated with opioid receptors, is the primary action site of epidural opioids.

PATHOPHYSIOLOGY OF NEUROPATHIC PAIN

Neuropathic pain is sustained by mechanisms that are driven by damage to, or dysfunction of, the PNS or CNS. In contrast to nociceptive pain, neuropathic pain is abnormal processing of stimuli.[7,12] Whereas nociceptive pain involves tissue damage or inflammation, neuropathic pain can occur in the absence of either. Neuropathic pain, even when acute, reflects a pathophysiology that serves no useful purpose.[6] A discussion of some of the peripheral and central mechanisms that initiate and maintain neuropathic pain follows. Extensive research is ongoing to better define these mechanisms.

Peripheral Mechanisms

At any point from the periphery to the CNS, the potential exists for the development of neuropathic pain. For example, when nociceptors are injured, changes in the number and location of ion channels, particularly sodium channels, can abnormally accumulate.[6] The threshold for nerve depolarization is then lowered, which leads to an increased response to stimuli and ectopic discharges. Hyperexcitable nerve endings in the periphery can become damaged, leading to abnormal reorganization of the nervous system, an underlying mechanism of some neuropathic pain states.[7] Chemically mediated connections can form between nerve fibers and cause abnormal activation of neurons and ultimately pain. These processes lead to a phenomenon called *peripheral sensitization*, which is thought to contribute to the maintenance of neuropathic pain. Topical local anesthetics, such as lidocaine patch 5%, are an example of analgesics that produce effects in the tissues under the site of application by "dampening" neuropathic pain mechanisms in the peripheral nervous system.[13]

Central Mechanisms

Central mechanisms also have a role in establishing neuropathic pain. *Central sensitization* is defined as abnormal hyperexcitability of central neurons as a result of complex changes induced by incoming barrages of nociceptors.[6] Extensive release and binding of excitatory neurotransmitters, such as glutamate, activate the NMDA receptor and cause an increase in intracellular calcium levels into the neuron, resulting in pain. As noted, the NMDA antagonist ketamine directly antagonizes this activity. An increase in the influx of sodium is thought to lower the threshold for nerve activation, increase response to stimuli, and enlarge the receptive field served by the affected neuron. The accumulation of intracellular ions causes spinal neurons to become highly sensitized and fire rapidly in a process called *wind-up*.[9] As mentioned, local anesthetics and anticonvulsants can block ion channels and inhibit abnormal pain sensation.

As with injured peripheral neurons, synaptic reorganization and anatomic changes can also occur in the CNS. These are thought to be sustained by an increased responsiveness of central neurons to relatively mild peripheral stimuli.[12] For example, injury to a nerve route can lead to reorganization in the dorsal horn of the spinal cord. Nerve fibers can invade other areas and create abnormal sensations in the area of the body served by the injured nerve. Allodynia, or pain from a normally nonnoxious stimulus (e.g., touch), is one such type of abnormal sensation and a common feature of neuropathic pain. In patients with allodynia, the mere weight of clothing or bed sheets can be excruciatingly painful. The ability of the nervous system to change structure and function as a result of noxious stimuli is called *neuroplasticity*.[6]

Another underlying mechanism called *central disinhibition* occurs when control mechanisms along inhibitory (modulatory) pathways are lost or suppressed, leading to abnormal excitability of central neurons.[6] Possible causes of disinhibition include dysfunction of the gamma-aminobutyric acid (GABA) pathways. GABA is the most abundant neurotransmitter in the CNS and composes a major inhibitory neurotransmitter system. Increased GABA function may help to relieve neuropathic pain. Benzodiazepines, such as midazolam, enhance GABA function, resulting in analgesia for pathologic conditions like muscle spasm.[6,13]

HARMFUL EFFECTS OF UNRELIEVED PAIN

Literally every system in the body is affected by unrelieved pain; the harmful effects are numerous

(Table 31-2). Unrelieved pain triggers and prolongs the stress response causing the release of excessive amounts of hormones, such as cortisol, catecholamines, and glucagon; insulin and testosterone levels decrease.[14,15] This increased endocrine activity initiates a number of metabolic processes that can result in weight loss, tachycardia, increased respiratory rate, shock, and even death.[14] Persistent unrelieved pain has been linked to increased tumor growth[16] and a higher incidence of health care–associated infections.[17]

Effects on the cardiovascular (CV) system include increased postoperative blood loss[18] and hypercoagulation,[14] which can lead to myocardial infarction and stroke. The respiratory system is affected by small tidal volumes and decreases in functional lung capacity, which can lead to pneumonia, atelectasis, and an increased need for mechanical ventilation.[19,20]

Every surgical procedure has the potential to produce persistent (chronic) postsurgical pain; however, inguinal hernia repair, amputation, and thoracic, cardiac, and breast surgery are among those identified as high risk for this complication.[6,21,22] Multiple factors are thought to contribute to the development of persistent postsurgical pain, including nerve injury from the surgical procedure, preexisting pain, and genetic

susceptibility.[23] Persistent postsurgical pain may have nociceptive, inflammatory, and neuropathic components indicating a need for a multimodal treatment approach.[22] Similar to other complex pain syndromes, it can be difficult to treat and last a lifetime.

PAIN ASSESSMENT: THE GOLD STANDARD

The gold standard for assessing the existence and intensity of pain is the patient's self report.[2] A comprehensive pain assessment includes obtaining the following information from the patient:
- *Location of pain:* Ask the patient to state or point to the areas of pain on the body.
- *Intensity:* Ask the patient to rate the intensity of the pain using a reliable and valid pain assessment tool. A number of scales in several language translations have been evaluated and made available for use in clinical practice and for educational practice.[2] See Box 31-1 for practical tips on using self-report pain rating tools. The most common are:
  - *Numeric Rating Scale (NRS):* The NRS is most often presented as a horizontal 0-to-10 point scale, with word anchors of "no pain" at one end of the scale, "moderate pain"

Table 31-2	Harmful Effects of Unrelieved Pain
DOMAINS AFFECTED	**SPECIFIC RESPONSES TO PAIN**
Endocrine	$\uparrow$ ACTH, $\uparrow$ cortisol, $\uparrow$ ADH, $\uparrow$ epinephrine, $\uparrow$ norepinephrine, $\uparrow$ GH, $\uparrow$ catecholamines, $\uparrow$ renin, $\uparrow$ angiotensin II, $\uparrow$ aldosterone, $\uparrow$ glucagon, $\uparrow$ interleukin-1, $\downarrow$ insulin, $\downarrow$ testosterone
Metabolic	Gluconeogenesis, hepatic glycogenolysis, hyperglycemia, glucose intolerance, insulin resistance, muscle protein catabolism, $\uparrow$ lipolysis
Cardiovascular	$\uparrow$ Heart rate, $\uparrow$ cardiac workload, $\uparrow$ peripheral vascular resistance, $\uparrow$ systemic vascular resistance, hypertension, $\uparrow$ coronary vascular resistance, $\uparrow$ myocardial oxygen consumption, hypercoagulation, deep vein thrombosis
Respiratory	$\downarrow$ Flows and volumes, atelectasis, shunting, hypoxemia, $\downarrow$ cough, sputum retention, infection
Genitourinary	$\downarrow$ Urinary output, urinary retention, fluid overload, hypokalemia
Gastrointestinal	$\downarrow$ Gastric and bowel motility
Musculoskeletal	Muscle spasm, impaired muscle function, fatigue, immobility
Cognitive	Reduction in cognitive function, mental confusion
Immune	Depression of immune response
Developmental	$\uparrow$ Behavioral and physiologic responses to pain, altered temperaments, higher somatization, infant distress behavior, possible altered development of the pain system, $\uparrow$ vulnerability to stress disorders, addictive behavior, and anxiety states
Future pain	Debilitating chronic pain syndromes: postmastectomy pain, postthoracotomy pain, phantom pain, postherpetic neuralgia
Quality of life	Sleeplessness, anxiety, fear, hopelessness, $\uparrow$ thoughts of suicide

From Pasero C, McCaffery M: *Pain assessment and pharmacologic management*, St. Louis, 2011, Mosby. Copyright Pasero C, McCaffery M. Used with permission.
ACTH, Adrenocorticotrophic hormone; *ADH,* antidiuretic hormone; down arrow ($\downarrow$), decreased; *GH,* growth hormone; up arrow ($\uparrow$), increased.

BOX 31-1   Practical Tips on the Use of Self-Report Pain Rating Scales

- Try using a standard pain assessment tools such as the 0-to-10 numerical rating scale; verbal descriptor scale with simple adjectives such as *mild, moderate, severe,* and *worst possible* pain; or the FACES Pain Scale-Revised.
- Increase the size of the font and other features of the scale.
- Ensure that eyeglasses and hearing aids are functioning.
- Try using alternative words, such as *ache, hurt,* and *sore* when discussing pain.
- Provide a written example of the scale and clear instructions on how to use it.
- Present the tool vertical format (rather than the frequently used horizontal).
- Ask about pain in the present.
- Repeat instructions and questions more than once.
- Allow ample time to respond.
- Ask awake and oriented ventilated patients to point to a number on the numerical scale if they are able.
- Repeat instructions and show the scale each time pain is assessed.

From Pasero C, McCaffery M: *Pain assessment and pharmacologic management,* St. Louis, 2011, Mosby. Copyright 2008, Pasero C, McCaffery M. Used with permission.

in the middle of the scale, and "worst possible pain" at the end of the scale.

- *Wong-Baker FACES Pain Rating Scale:* The FACES scale consists of six cartoon faces with word descriptors, ranging from a smiling face on the left for "no pain (or hurt)" to a frowning, tearful face on the right for "worst pain (or hurt)". The faces are most commonly numbered using a 0, 2, 4, 6, 8, 10 metric; however 0 to 5 can also be used. Patients are asked to choose the face that best describes their pain. The FACES scale is used in adults and children as young as 3 years old.[2] Figure 31-3 provides the Wong-Baker FACES scale combined with the NRS.
- *Faces Pain Scale-Revised (FPS-R):* The FPS-R has seven faces to make it consistent with other scales using the 0-to-10 metric. The faces range from a neutral facial expression to one of intense pain and are numbered 0, 2, 4, 6, 8, and 10. Patients are asked to choose the face that best describes their pain. It is important for clinicians to understand that the scale is reliable and valid in children as young as 3 years old, but the ability to optimally quantify pain (identify a number) is acquired at approximately 8 years of age.[24] The FPS-R has

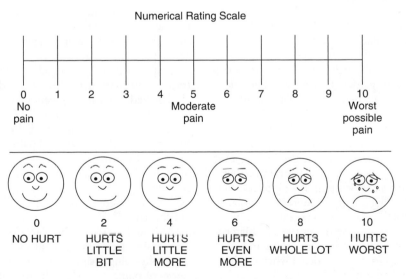

FIG. 31-3 Pain rating scales. A numeric rating scale or visual analog scale is useful for evaluation of adult pain status. The Wong-Baker FACES pain rating scale is useful in rating of pain in the pediatric population. (From Hockenberry MJ, Wilson D: *Wong's essentials of pediatric nursing,* ed 8, St. Louis, 2009, Mosby. Used with permission.)

been shown to be preferred by both cognitively intact and impaired elders[25,26] and minority populations.[25,27]

- *Verbal Descriptor Scales (VDS):* A VDS uses different words or phrases to describe the intensity of pain, such as *no pain, mild pain, moderate pain, severe pain, very severe pain,* and *worst possible pain.* The patient is asked to select the phrase that best describes the pain intensity. The scale can be presented horizontally or vertically and can be helpful for patients who have difficulty using a numeric scale.[2]
- *Quality:* Ask the patient to describe how the pain feels. Descriptors such as *sharp, shooting,* or *burning* may help to identify the presence of neuropathic pain.
- *Onset and duration:* Ask when the pain started and whether it is constant or intermittent.
- *Aggravating and relieving factors:* Ask the patient what makes the pain worse and what makes it better.
- *Effect of pain on function and quality of life:* It is particularly important to ask patients with persistent pain about how pain has affected their lives; what could they do before the pain began that they can no longer do, or what do they want to do but cannot do because of the pain?
- *Comfort-function (pain) goal:* For patients with acute pain, identify short-term functional goals and reinforce the link between good pain control and successful achievement of the goals. For example, surgical patients are told that they will be expected to cough, deep breathe, turn, and ambulate or participate in physical therapy postoperatively. Patients with chronic pain can be asked to identify their unique functional or quality-of-life goals, such as being able to work, walk the dog, or garden. Patients are then asked to identify (using a 0-to-10 scale) a level of pain that will allow accomplishment of the identified functional or quality-of-life goals with reasonable ease. A realistic goal for most patients is 2 or 3, and pain intensity ratings that are consistently above the goal warrant further evaluation and consideration of an intervention and possible adjustment of the treatment plan.[2]
- *Other information:* The patient's culture, past pain experiences, and pertinent medical history, such as comorbidities, laboratory tests, and diagnostic studies, are considered when establishing a treatment plan.[28]

Challenges in Assessment

Many patients are unable to provide a report of their pain using the customary self-report pain rating tools, placing them at higher risk for undertreated pain than those who can report.[2] These patients are collectively called *nonverbal patients*[29] and include infants, toddlers, and patients who are cognitively impaired, critically ill (intubated, unresponsive), comatose, or imminently dying. Patients who are receiving neuromuscular blocking agents or are sedated from anesthesia and other drugs given during surgery are also among this at-risk population.

When patients are unable to report pain using traditional methods, an alternative approach based on the Hierarchy of Pain Measures is recommended.[2,29,30] The key components of the hierarchy are to: (1) attempt to obtain self-report; (2) consider underlying pathology or conditions and procedures that might be painful (e.g., surgery); (3) observe behaviors; (4) evaluate physiologic indicators; and (5) conduct an analgesic trial. See Box 31-2 for detailed information on each component of the Hierarchy of Pain Measures.

Self report is at the top of the hierarchy and should be attempted, even in patients who present challenges in assessment.[2] Many patients with mild to moderate cognitive impairment can provide self-report when clinicians implement fairly simple measures (see Box 31-1).

Several behavioral pain assessment tools exist to facilitate assessment in nonverbal patients; however, patients must be carefully evaluated for their ability to respond with the requisite behaviors in the selected tool.[2] For example, tools that require assessment of body movement as a pain indicator should not be used in patients who are unable to move, such as those receiving a neuromuscular blocking agent. According to the hierarchy, pain can be assumed to be present in these patients, justified by research showing that endotracheal intubation, ventilation, and suctioning—all required in patients receiving a neuromuscular blocking agent—are painful.[31,32] It is equally important to understand that the score obtained from the use of a behavioral pain assessment tool helps to identify the presence of pain, but the score is a behavioral score and not a pain intensity rating. Simply put, if the patient cannot report the intensity of the pain, the intensity is not known.[2,33]

Although nurses who care for patients with acute pain often rely on vital signs to assess pain, these physiologic signs are considered poor indicators of pain.[2,34,35] Many factors other than pain can influence changes in vital signs, and patients quickly adapt physiologically despite the presence of pain. The primary message is that the absence of an elevated blood pressure or heart rate does not mean the absence of pain.[2]

BOX 31-2   Hierarchy of Pain Measures

1. Attempt to obtain the patient's self-report, which is the single most reliable indicator of pain. Do not assume that a patient cannot provide a report of pain; many cognitively impaired patients are able to use a self-report tool, such as the FACES Pain Scale-Revised or Verbal Descriptor Scale.
2. Consider the patient's condition or exposure to a procedure that is thought to be painful. If appropriate, assume that pain is present and document it when approved by institution policy and procedure.
3. Observe behavioral signs such as facial expressions, crying, restlessness, and changes in activity. There are many behavioral pain assessment tools available that will yield a pain behavior score and may help to determine whether pain is present. However, it is important to remember that a behavioral score is not the same as a pain intensity score. Pain intensity is unknown if the patient is unable to provide it.
   - A surrogate who knows the patient well (e.g., parent, spouse, caregiver) may be able to provide information about underlying painful pathology or behaviors that may indicate pain.
4. Evaluate physiologic indicators with the understanding that they are the least sensitive indicators of pain and may signal the existence of conditions other than pain or a lack of it (e.g., hypovolemia, blood loss). Patients may have normal or below normal vital signs in the presence of severe pain. The absence of an elevated blood pressure or heart rate does not mean the absence of pain.
5. Conduct an analgesic trial to confirm the presence of pain and to establish a basis for developing a treatment plan if pain is thought to be present. An analgesic trial involves the administration of a low dose of nonopioid or opioid and observing patient response. The initial low dose may not be enough to illicit a change in behavior and should be increased if the previous dose was tolerated, or another analgesic may be added. If behaviors continue despite optimal analgesic doses, other possible causes should be investigated. In patients who are completely unresponsive, no change in behavior will be evident and the optimized analgesic dose should be continued.

From Pasero C, McCaffery M: *Pain assessment and pharmacologic management,* St. Louis, 2011, Mosby. Copyright 1999, McCaffery M, Pasero C. Used with permission.

Reassessment of Pain

Following initiation of the pain management plan, pain is reassessed and documented on a regular basis as a way to evaluate the effectiveness of treatment. At a minimum, pain should be reassessed with each new report of pain and before and after the administration of analgesics.[2] The frequency of reassessment depends on the stability of the patient's pain and is guided by institutional policy. For example, in the postanesthesia care unit (PACU) reassessment may be necessary as often as every 10 minutes when pain is unstable during opioid titration, but can be done every 4 to 8 hours in patients with stable pain 24 hours after surgery.

Pain Control on a Continuum

The quality of patients' pain control should be addressed when patients are discharged from one clinical area to another. Many PACUs establish the criterion that patients must achieve a pain rating of 4 on a scale of 0 to 10 or better before discharge; however, the expectation that all patients must be discharged from a given clinical unit with pain ratings less than an arbitrary number is unrealistic and can lead to the unsafe administration of additional opioid doses to patients who are excessively sedated and is widely discouraged.[28,36-38]

Instead, achieving optimal pain relief is best viewed on a continuum with the primary objective being to provide both effective and safe analgesia.[28] Optimal pain relief is the responsibility of every member of the health care team and begins with analgesic titration in the PACU followed by continued prompt assessment and analgesic administration after discharge from the PACU to achieve pain ratings that allow patients to meet their functional goals with relative ease.

Although it may not always be possible to achieve a patient's pain rating goal within the short time the patient is in an area like the PACU, this goal provides direction for ongoing analgesic care. Important information to give to the nurse assuming care of the patient on the clinical unit is the patient's pain rating goal, how close the patient is to achieving it, what has been done thus far to achieve it (analgesics and doses), and how well the patient has tolerated analgesic administration (adverse effects).[28]

PHARMACOLOGIC MANAGEMENT OF PAIN: MULTIMODAL ANALGESIA

Pain is a complex phenomenon involving multiple underlying mechanisms as described earlier in this chapter. This characteristic underscores the importance of using more than one analgesic to manage pain.[28] This approach is called *multimodal analgesia* and is recommended for the treatment of all types of pain.[4,28,39,40] A multimodal regimen combines drugs with different underlying mechanisms; this allows lower doses of each of the drugs in the treatment plan, which reduces the potential for each to produce adverse effects.[28] Furthermore, multimodal analgesia can result in comparable or greater pain relief than can be achieved with any single analgesic. The use of multimodal analgesia should be the rule, rather than the exception in pain treatment.

The most common analgesics used for postoperative pain management are nonopioid analgesics (e.g., acetaminophen, NSAIDs), opioid analgesics (e.g., morphine, hydromorphone, fentanyl, nd oxycodone), local anesthetics, and anticonvulsants. A multimodal approach in the perioperative setting may combine agents from each of these analgesic groups to provide effective pain relief and help minimize adverse effects. Unless contraindicated, all surgical patients should routinely be given acetaminophen and an NSAID in scheduled doses throughout the postoperative course (preferably initiated preoperatively). Opioid analgesics are added to manage moderate-to-severe postoperative pain in most patients. For some major surgical procedures, a local anesthetic is administered with an opioid epidurally or alone by continuous peripheral nerve block. An anticonvulsant may be added to the treatment plan as well to control severe pain or prevent a chronic postsurgical pain syndrome, such as persistent pain after thoracotomy or mastectomy.[6]

Routes of Administration

One principle of pain management is to use the oral route of administration whenever feasible.[28] When the oral route is not possible, such as in patients who cannot swallow, can receive nothing my mouth, or are nauseated, other routes of administration are used. In the perioperative setting, the intravenous (IV) route is the first-line route of administration for analgesic delivery; patients are transitioned postoperatively to the oral route as tolerated. Some of the methods used to manage pain are accomplished via catheter techniques, such as intraspinal analgesia and continuous peripheral nerve block infusions. Nurses have an extensive role in the successful management of these therapies, and the American Society for Pain Management Nursing (http://www.aspmn.org) provides guidelines for care.[3]

Although drugs are rarely administered rectally in adults in the perioperative setting in the United States, this route of analgesic administration has a long history of safety in children undergoing surgery and is an alternative when oral or IV analgesics are not an option.[28,41] The rectum allows passive diffusion of medications and absorption into the systemic circulation. This route of administration can be less expensive and does not involve the expertise required of the parenteral route of administration. Drawbacks are that drug absorption can be unreliable and depends on many factors, including rectal tissue health and administrator technique. The rectal route is contraindicated in patients who are neutropenic or thrombocytopenic because of potential rectal bleeding.[28] Diarrhea, perianal abscess or fistula,

---

Evidence-Based Practice

In a prospective, randomized-controlled study, 80 patients undergoing total knee replacement were assigned to receive morphine via intravenous (IV) patient-controlled analgesia (PCA) alone or as a single 400-mg dose of celecoxib 1 hour before surgery followed by 200 mg of celecoxib every 12 hours for 5 days postoperatively along with IV PCA morphine. Resting pain scores were better, and active range of motion increased significantly in those who received celecoxib compared with those who did not. Celecoxib demonstrated a 40% morphine dose-sparing effect, which resulted in a lower incidence of nausea and vomiting in those who received celecoxib (28%) than in those who did not (43%). Other important findings were that intraoperative and postoperative blood loss was comparable among patients in

both groups and celecoxib resulted in no significant increase in the need for blood transfusions.

IMPLICATIONS FOR PRACTICE

Multimodal analgesia is the recommended approach for the management of postoperative pain. As the patient's primary pain managers, perianesthesia nurses can ensure the prescription of analgesics, such as nonopioids, that are appropriate for the multimodal pain treatment plan. Perioperative administration of the nonopioid celecoxib can improve postoperative pain control, reduce opioid requirements and opioid-induced nausea and vomiting, and facilitate patient participation in important recovery activities, without increasing the risk of bleeding in the surgical patient.

Source: Huang YM, et al: Perioperative celebrex administration for pain management after total knee arthroplasty—a randomized, controlled study, *BMC Musculoskelet Disord* 9:77, 2008.

and abdominoperineal resection are also relative contraindications.[28]

Topical local anesthetics are used for acute procedural pain, but the other second-line routes of administration, such as transdermal and subcutaneous, are generally reserved for the management of chronic pain. The primary disadvantages of transdermal drug delivery are that the skin serves as both a barrier and a reservoir. There is significant lag time before the effects of the drug are felt after transdermal patch application, and the drug continues to enter the systemic circulation for a variable period after the patch is removed.[42]

Nonopioid Analgesics

The nonopioid analgesic group includes acetaminophen and NSAIDs. There are two categories of NSAIDs: the nonselective NSAIDs (e.g., ibuprofen, naproxen, diclofenac, ketorolac), which inhibit both COX-1 and COX-2, and the COX-2 selective NSAIDs (e.g., celecoxib), which inhibit just COX-2 (see Fig. 31-2).

Nonopioids are flexible analgesics used for a wide spectrum of painful conditions. They are appropriate alone for mild to some moderate nociceptive-type pain (e.g., from surgery or trauma) and are added to opioids, local anesthetics, or anticonvulsants as part of a multimodal analgesic regimen for more severe nociceptive pain.[28,43] Acetaminophen and an NSAID can be given concomitantly, and there is no need for staggered doses.[43]

Acetaminophen is versatile in that it can be given by multiple routes of administration, including oral, rectal, and IV. IV acetaminophen is approved for treatment of pain and fever in adults and children 2 years of age and older and is given by a 15-minute infusion in single or repeated doses. It can be given alone for mild to moderate pain or moderate to severe pain with adjunctive opioid analgesics and has been shown to be well tolerated and to produce a significant opioid dose-sparing effect and superior pain relief compared with placebo.[44] The maximum daily dose for IV acetaminophen is the same as for oral acetaminophen (e.g., 1000 mg every 6 hours, for maximum of 4000 mg in adults and adolescents weighing more than 50 kg; 15 mg/kg every 6 hours in adults, adolescents, and children weighing less than 50 kg).

There is evidence that oral NSAIDs are more effective than oral acetaminophen. A randomized controlled trial ($n = 151$) showed that oral ibuprofen 800 mg taken three times a day provided better pain relief than 1000 mg of oral acetaminophen taken two times a day following anterior cruciate ligament repair.[45] For many painful conditions, such as osteoarthritis, oral NSAIDs are tried for mild to moderate pain if oral acetaminophen has been unsuccessful in controlling the pain.[43] For surgical pain, an NSAID is added to both acetaminophen and an opioid as part of a multimodal plan.

Ketorolac and ibuprofen are available in IV formulation. An abundance of research has shown ketorolac to be effective for postoperative pain following a wide variety of surgical procedures.[43] Although further clinical experience and research are needed with IV ibuprofen, the drug is less COX-1 selective than ketorolac,[43] which may result in fewer adverse effects than ketorolac (see Fig. 31-2). A randomized, placebo-controlled study ($n = 185$) found that orthopedic surgery patients who were given preoperative followed by postoperative IV ibuprofen reported better pain relief, used 31% less morphine, and experienced similar adverse effects and complications, including blood loss, compared with placebo.[46]

Adverse Effects of Nonopioids

Acetaminophen is widely considered one of the safest and best tolerated analgesics.[47,48] Its most serious complication is hepatotoxicity (liver damage) as a result of overdose. In the healthy adult, a maximum daily dose below 4000 mg is rarely associated with liver toxicity.[49] Its lack of effect on platelet aggregation and low incidence of gastrointestinal (GI) adverse effects make acetaminophen the analgesic of choice in individuals with renal insufficiency, advanced chronic kidney disease, and end-stage renal disease.[50,51] Acetaminophen has been shown to increase the International Normalized Ratio when administered with warfarin, but the likelihood of surgical bleeding as a result of perioperative acetaminophen intake is thought to be low.[52,53]

The NSAIDs have significantly more adverse effects than acetaminophen, with gastric toxicity and ulceration being the most common.[43] The primary underlying mechanism of NSAID-induced gastric ulceration is the inhibition of COX-1, which leads to a reduction in GI-protective prostaglandins (see Fig. 31-2).[47] This effect is systemic, rather than local, and can occur regardless of the route of administration of the NSAID.[43] Risk factors include advanced age (older than 60 years), presence of prior ulcer disease, and CV disease and other comorbidities. The use of a COX-2 selective NSAID (e.g., celecoxib) is recommended if not contraindicated by CV risk or the least ulcerogenic nonselective NSAID (e.g., ibuprofen).[43] GI adverse effects are also related to the dose and duration of NSAID therapy; the higher the NSAID dose and the longer the duration of NSAID use, the higher the risk of cumulative GI toxicity.[43] This fact underscores the importance of administering the lowest dose for the shortest time necessary.

All NSAIDs carry a risk of CV adverse effects through prostaglandin inhibition, and the risk is increased with COX-2 inhibition, whether it is produced by those labeled COX-2 selective NSAIDs (e.g., celecoxib) or those that are nonselective inhibitors of both COX-1 and COX-2 (e.g., ibuprofen, naproxen, ketorolac).[43] One proposed underlying mechanism for this adverse effect is that any drug that inhibits COX-2 will have prothrombotic effects, and those that inhibit COX-2 to a much greater extent than COX-1 will promote thrombosis more than others because of a disturbance in the physiologic balance between thromboxane A_2, which promotes platelet aggregation, and prostacyclin, which antagonizes platelet aggregation.[54,55] Postoperative studies showing elevated CV risk with NSAIDs[56,57] led to a recommendation from the U.S. Food and Drug Administration against the use of any NSAIDs after high-risk open heart surgery.[58]

Most nonselective NSAIDs increase bleeding time though inhibition of COX-1. This is both drug and dose-related; therefore the lowest dose of nonopioids with minimal or no effect on bleeding time should be used in patients or procedures with high risk for surgical bleeding. Options include acetaminophen, celecoxib, choline magnesium trisalicylate, salsalate, and nabumetone.[43] There is abundant research showing the safety of both preoperative and postoperative administration of nonopioids with minimal effect on bleeding time.[43,59,60]

NSAID-induced renal toxicity is relatively rare in otherwise healthy adults who are given NSAIDs during the short-term perioperative period.[43] A Cochrane Collaboration Review could find no cases of renal failure or serious kidney problems in individuals with normal preoperative kidney function who were given NSAIDs after surgery in any of the 23 trials (1459 patients) reviewed.[61]

In contrast, individuals with acute or chronic volume depletion or hypotension rely on prostaglandin synthesis to maintain adequate renal blood flow, and NSAID inhibition of prostaglandin synthesis in such patients can cause acute renal failure (ARF).[62] Patients at increased risk for ARF include those with cardiac failure, liver cirrhosis, ascites, diabetes, preexisting hypertension, preexisting renal impairment, advanced age, or left ventricular dysfunction, and those being treated with ACE inhibitors.[62] It is generally recommended that NSAIDs are avoided in patients with chronic renal failure and in any patient with a creatinine clearance less than 30 mL/min.[50] ARF can develop with the first NSAID dose in patients with elevated risk, and higher doses carry greater risk.[49,50] Older adults and anyone with risk factors for ARF should be assessed frequently for adverse renal effects during perioperative NSAID therapy.[43] Acetaminophen and opioids (e.g., fentanyl) would be better choices in patients with significant risk.[43]

The inflammatory process is initiated when bone is fractured, just as it is with any other tissue trauma. Prostaglandins have a central role in bone healing, providing a balance between bone formation and resorption.[62] Despite the safe use of NSAIDs for decades to control pain associated with fracture, concerns have been raised about their use under these circumstances.[62] Unfortunately, there are few well-designed studies that examine the effects of NSAIDs on bone healing in humans.[43] The studies that have been done are retrospective in design and present conflicting findings. There have also been no adequate studies evaluating NSAIDs and spinal fusion. In an effort to offer a balanced appraisal of the existing, limited data, several researchers have agreed that short-term use of an NSAID after skeletal surgery, for a period less than 2 weeks, probably is safe and might be considered an option unless a patient has a comorbid condition that could negatively affect fracture healing, such as smoking, glucocorticoid use, or metabolic bone disease.[62-64]

Opioid Analgesics

The first-line opioids for the treatment of immediate postoperative pain are morphine, hydromorphone, and fentanyl. At steady state (when equal amounts of a drug are entering and exiting the body), all opioids have similar characteristics; however, differences are noted when administration is by bolus technique (Table 31-3).[28] For example, fentanyl is a lipophilic drug (soluble in fatty tissue), which allows it to move rapidly through membranes, a characteristic that produces a relatively fast onset and peak and short duration of action. By bolus technique, blood levels decline rapidly with fentanyl, but with repeated, regular dosing the drug can accumulate and redistribute from fatty tissue back into the blood. Under these circumstances, the terminal half-life of fentanyl (3 to 4 hours) can be extended by as much as fivefold.[65] Morphine is a hydrophilic drug (soluble in water) and has a slower onset and peak and longer duration compared with other first-line opioids. Hydromorphone is

Table 31-3	Characteristics of the First-Line IV Opioid Analgesics			
DRUG	**ONSET (MINUTES)**	**PEAK (MINUTES)**	**DURATION (HOURS)**	**IV EQUIANALGESIC DOSE***
Morphine	5-10	15-30	3-4	10 mg
Fentanyl	3-5	10-15	2	100 mcg
Hydromorphone	5	10-20	3-4	1.5 mg

From Pasero C, McCaffery M: *Pain assessment and pharmacologic management,* St. Louis, 2011, Mosby.

IV, Intravenous.

*Doses are approximately equal to one another in terms of pain relief.

less hydrophilic than morphine but less lipophilic than fentanyl, which produces pharmacokinetics intermediate between morphine and fentanyl.

Patient characteristics must be considered when selecting the appropriate opioid for pain treatment. For example, fentanyl is the recommended opioid for patients with end-stage organ failure because it has no clinically relevant metabolites.[66] It also produces minimal hemodynamic adverse effects[66] and is often preferred in patients who are hemodynamically unstable, such as the critically ill.[28]

The goals of care are also considered when selecting an opioid. A general principle of initial titration in patients with acute pain is to keep in mind the patient's ongoing pain treatment plan. As an example, consider the patient who will have hydromorphone by intermittent IV boluses for ongoing postoperative pain management after discharge from the PACU. Unless the patient has severe, rapidly escalating pain on admission to the PACU, it makes sense to begin titration with hydromorphone so that the effects (both pain relief and adverse effects) of the drug that will be used for the next day or so can be evaluated more easily.[28] The fast action of fentanyl makes the IV route the best choice when it is necessary to control quickly escalating, severe pain on admission to the PACU. In ambulatory surgery where the goal is to initiate oral analgesia as soon as possible to facilitate a rapid discharge to home, an oral opioid is often administered preoperatively followed by IV fentanyl for immediate pain relief in the PACU. The oral opioid that will be taken in the home setting can be administered before discharge to help ensure adequate pain relief during the ride home.

The nonopioid-opioid analgesics, such as acetaminophen or ibuprofen in combination oxycodone or hydrocodone, are highly popular for the treatment of mild to moderate acute pain and are the most common choice after invasive pain management therapies are discontinued and for pain treatment after discharge. However, it is important to remember that these combination drugs are not appropriate for severe pain because the maximum daily dose of the nonopioid limits the escalation of the opioid dose.[28]

Safe Opioid Titration

Research has shown that the relationship between pain intensity scores and dose requirements during and after titration in postoperative patients is not linear, suggesting that there is no specific dose that will relieve pain of a specific intensity.[67] Many factors, such as sedation level, respiratory status, and previous analgesic and sedative intake, in addition to pain intensity must be considered when selecting an opioid dose. Some institutions have guidelines that require dosing based on a specific pain intensity (e.g., set orders that mandate the administration of 2 mg of IV morphine for pain ratings of 1 to 3 on a scale of 0 to 10; 4 mg for pain ratings of 4 to 6; and 6 mg for pain ratings of 7 to 10). This practice can be extremely dangerous and is strongly discouraged.[28,38]

The goal of titration is to use the smallest dose that provides satisfactory analgesia with the fewest adverse effects.[28] At all times, nurses must strive to achieve a balance between pain relief and adverse effects. In opioid-naive patients (those who do not take regular daily doses of opioids) with moderate to severe pain, recommended starting IV doses are given, for example, 2 to 3 mg of morphine, 0.3 to 0.5 mg of hydromorphone, or 25 to 50 mcg of fentanyl.[4,28] When an increase in the opioid dose is necessary and safe, this can be done by percentages. When a slight improvement in analgesia is needed, a 25% increase in the opioid dose may be sufficient; a 50% increase for moderate improvement; and a 100% increase may be indicated for strong improvement, such as when treating severe pain.[28] The time when the dose can be increased is determined by the onset or peak effect of the opioid. The frequency of IV opioid doses during initial titration may be as often as every 5 to 15 minutes. Doses should not be increased in patients who are excessively sedated (e.g., unable to keep eyes open and falling asleep midsentence). In such cases, nonopioid analgesics should be added or increased (e.g., full doses of an NSAID and acetaminophen). Safe pain management is a primary objective.

Selected Opioid Therapies

The oral route for analgesic administration is generally reserved for later in the postoperative course when patients can tolerate oral intake; however, there has been a trend over the past few years to use modified-release (long-acting) oxycodone, initiated preoperatively, as a component in multimodal postoperative pain treatment plans.[28] One study randomized 40 patients to receive either 20 mg of modified-release oxycodone or placebo preoperatively and every 12 hours postoperatively, in addition to IV morphine via PCA plus IV acetaminophen (1000 mg) for two days following lumbar discectomy.[68] Those who received oxycodone consumed significantly less morphine; had significantly lower pain scores during rest, when coughing, and with movement; experienced less nausea and vomiting and earlier recovery of bowel function; and reported higher satisfaction with their pain treatment than those who received placebo.

One of the most common methods for administering opioid analgesia in the postoperative setting is via IV patient-controlled analgesia (PCA), whereby patients manage their own pain by pressing a button attached to an infusion pump to deliver a preset bolus dose of pain medication. The concept of PCA recognizes that only the patient can feel the pain and only the patient knows how much analgesic will relieve it.[28] This concept underscores the importance of telling family members and friends that PCA is for patient use only. Patients who use PCA must be able to understand the relationships between pain, pushing the PCA button, and pain relief. They must also be able to cognitively and physically use the PCA equipment.[28] Table 31-4 provides starting IV PCA prescription ranges in opioid-naive adults.

The use of a basal rate (continuous infusion) during IV PCA is controversial in opioid-naive patients.[4,28] The primary safeguard in PCA therapy is that a patient must be awake to self-administer a PCA dose. Patients who are excessively sedated are likely to drop the PCA button, thereby preventing further sedation and clinically significant respiratory depression. However, with a basal rate, the patient has no control over the delivery of a continuous infusion, and the built-in safeguard is gone. As a result, the American Pain Society recommends extreme caution in using basal rates for acute pain management in opioid-naive individuals.[4] Absolutely essential to the safe use of a basal rate with PCA is close monitoring by nurses of sedation and respiratory status and prompt decreases in opioid dose (e.g., discontinue basal rate) if increased sedation is detected.[28,69,70]

Intraspinal analgesia has a long history of safety and effectiveness for major surgical procedures, and extensive guidelines for the nursing care of patients receiving this therapy are available.[3,28] Delivery of analgesics via the intraspinal route is accomplished by inserting a needle into the subarachnoid space (for intrathecal analgesia) or the epidural space and injecting the analgesic (usually opioid and local anesthetic), or by threading a catheter through the needle and taping it in place temporarily for bolus dosing or continuous administration. Intrathecal catheters for acute pain management are used more often for providing anesthesia or a single analgesic bolus dose. Temporary epidural catheters for acute pain management are removed after 2 to 4 days.[28] Epidural analgesia is administered by clinician-administered bolus, continuous infusion (basal rate), and patient-controlled epidural analgesia. The most common opioids administered intraspinally are morphine, fentanyl, and hydromorphone. These opioids are usually combined with a local anesthetic, most often ropivacaine or bupivacaine, to improve analgesia and produce an opioid dose-sparing effect.

Table 31-4	Starting IV PCA Prescription Ranges for Acute Pain in Opioid Naive Adults				
DRUG	COMMON CONCENTRATION	LOADING DOSE	PCA DOSE	LOCKOUT (MINUTES)	BASAL RATE
Morphine	1 mg/mL	2.5 mg, may repeat PRN	0.5-2 mg	8	0-0.5 mg/h
Hydromorphone	0.2 mg/mL	0.4 mg, may repeat PRN	0.1-0.4 mg	6-8	0-0.1 mg/h
Fentanyl	10-20 mcg/mL	25 mcg, may repeat PRN	5-25 mcg	5-6	0-5 mcg/h

From Pasero C, McCaffery M: *Pain assessment and pharmacologic management,* St. Louis, 2011, Mosby.
IV, Intravenous; *PCA,* patient-controlled analgesia; *PRN,* as needed.

Transition to Oral Analgesics

Providing adequate oral analgesia and avoiding gaps in pain control after invasive therapies are discontinued are keys to optimizing patient outcomes. Equianalgesic dose charts are widely available[4,28] and helpful when switching from one drug or route of administration to another to ensure that patients receive approximately the same pain relief that they were receiving before the switch. Table 31-5 provides equianalgesic dosing guidelines when transitioning a patient from IV to oral analgesia.

Nurses can be instrumental in helping patients maintain adequate pain control after discharge from the inpatient setting by teaching patients about the importance of maintaining pain control. Discharge pain management instructions should focus on reminding patients to take their prescribed pain medication before pain becomes severe and out of control. The goal is to stay on top of the pain so that functional goals of recovery (e.g., self care, physical therapy) can be achieved with relative ease.

Adverse Effects of Opioid Analgesics

The most common adverse effects of opioid analgesics are nausea, vomiting, constipation, pruritus, and sedation.[28] Respiratory depression is less common but the most feared of the opioid adverse effects. In surgical patients, postoperative ileus can become a major complication as well. A common perception is that opioids cause hypotension, but research shows that the opioid doses commonly used for pain management rarely cause

Table 31-5	Making the Transition from IV to Oral Analgesia	
DAILY DOSE IV ANALGESIA		
MORPHINE (MG)	**HYDROMORPHONE (DILAUDID; MG)**	**SUGGESTED DAILY ORAL DOSE (MG)***
15	2.2	Hydrocodone 5/APAP 500 (Vicodin) 1 tab every 4 hours (8 tabs maximum)†
20	3	Hydrocodone 7.5/APAP 500 (Lortab) 1 tab every 4 hours (8 tabs maximum) or Oxycodone 5/APAP 325 (Percocet 5/325) 1 tab every 4 hours (12 tabs maximum)
25	3.75	Hydrocodone 10/APAP 325 (Norco) 1 tab every 4 hours (12 tabs maximum) or Percocet 5/325 1 or 2 tabs every 4 hours (12 tabs maximum)
30	4.5	Percocet 5/325 2 tabs every 4 hours (12 tabs maximum) or Percocet 7.5/325 1 tab every 4 hours (12 tabs maximum) or Oxycodone controlled release (OxyContin) 20 every 12 hours plus Percocet 5/325 1 tab every 4 hours PRN (12 tabs maximum)
35	5.25	Percocet 5/325 2 tabs every 4 hours (12 tabs maximum) or OxyContin 20 every 12 hours plus Percocet 5/325 1 tab every 4 hours PRN (12 tabs maximum)
45	6.75	OxyContin 20 every 12 hours plus Percocet 7.5/325 1 or 2 tabs every 4 hours PRN (12 tabs maximum)
50	7.5	OxyContin 20 every 12 hours plus Percocct 10/325 1 tab every 4 hours PRN (12 tabs maximum) or OxyContin 30 every 12 hours plus Percocet 7.5/325 1 tab every 4 hours PRN (12 tabs maximum)

From Pasero C, McCaffery M: *Pain assessment and pharmacologic management*, St. Louis, 2011, Mosby. Copyright 2003, McCaffery M. May be duplicated for use in clinical practice. *APAP*, Acetaminophen; *PRN*, as needed.

*In calculating the oral dose, acetaminophen is given the following opioid values: acetaminophen 325 mg = hydrocodone 2.5 mg or oxycodone 1.5 mg; acetaminophen 650 mg = hydrocodone 5 mg or oxycodone 3 mg. For example, Vicodin (hydrocodone 5 mg/acetaminophen 500 mg) = hydrocodone 7.5 to 8 mg.

†Maximum acetaminophen dosage is 4000 mg/day. For some patients, such as older adults or heavy consumers of alcohol, the dose should be 2000 mg or less per day.

NOTE: Recommend a laxative to patients receiving daily opioids.

This table provides a guideline to help ensure approximately the same pain relief when switching from IV to oral opioid analgesia. It can be posted in clinical units where opioid orders are written for the clinician's quick reference.

NURSING CARE IN THE PACU

this adverse effect.[71] Many other factors, including pain, can cause hypotension, underscoring the importance of promptly addressing unrelieved pain. When hypotension is a concern, it can be minimized by administering the opioid slowly, keeping the patient supine, and optimizing intravascular volume.[71]

There is great individual variation in the development of opioid adverse effects, which is why most must be managed with an individualized approach. Prevention rather than treatment of opioid adverse effects is a key principle of pain management.[28] Most opioid adverse effects are dose related. Therefore a practical approach includes the use of nonsedating analgesics that have an opioid dose-sparing effect, such as nonopioids and local anesthetics, so that the lowest effective opioid dose can be given. For many patients, simply decreasing the opioid dose is sufficient to eliminate or make an adverse effect tolerable.[28]

Postoperative nausea and vomiting (PONV) are among the most unpleasant of the adverse effects associated with surgery, and it can have a negative effect on patient outcomes and increase the burden on nursing staff.[72] Consensus guidelines have identified opioids as a primary risk factor for the PONV.[73-75] Other risks are female sex, nonsmoking status, and history of PONV or motion sickness. Guidelines recommend that all patients are evaluated for risk, baseline risk factors are reduced if possible, multimodal analgesia is provided so that no opioid or the lowest effective opioid dose can be given, and prophylactic treatment (e.g., dexamethasone and a serotonin receptor antagonist such as ondansetron at the end of surgery) is given to patients with moderate risk.[73-75] More aggressive interventions should be used in patients with high risk.[28]

Postoperative ileus is the temporary impairment of GI motility following surgery. It has been described as part of the normal pathophysiologic response to surgical injury, characterized by delayed gastric emptying and inability to pass gas or stool and exacerbated by opioid consumption.[76] Unresolved ileus is a postoperative complication that can cause significant discomfort and patient morbidity.[76] The incidence is particularly high with colorectal surgery. A major advance in the management of postoperative ileus is the approval of alvimopan for the acceleration of time to upper and lower GI recovery after partial large or small bowel resection.[28]

Constipation is an almost universal opioid adverse effect (i.e., tolerance rarely develops) and requires a preventive approach and aggressive management if symptoms are detected. Risk is elevated with opioid use, advanced age, and immobility.[28] The usual initial daily therapy is a combination of stool softener and mild peristaltic stimulant, such as senna. Patients should be instructed to continue this regimen as long as they are taking opioids.

Pruritus is an adverse effect, not an allergic reaction to opioids.[71] It is one of the most common adverse effects when opioids are delivered by intraspinal routes.[77] Numerous pharmacologic strategies have been tried for relief of pruritus. IV serotonin receptor antagonists (e.g., ondansetron, dolasetron) are effective for the prevention of pruritus from intraspinal opioids.[78] Although antihistamines such as diphenhydramine are commonly used, there is no strong evidence that they relieve opioid-induced pruritus.[79] Patients may report being less bothered by itching after taking an antihistamine, but this is likely the result of sedating effects.[71] Sedation can be problematic in those already at risk for excessive sedation, such as postoperative patients, as this can lead to life-threatening respiratory depression.[80] A common clinical observation is that patients with postoperative opioid-induced pruritus usually have well-controlled pain.[28] This may be because painful stimuli can inhibit itching and inhibition of pain processing may enhance itching.[71] This helps to explain why the single most effective, safest, and least expensive treatment for pruritus is opioid dose reduction. Opioid orders should include the expectation that the opioid dose will be decreased by 25% before or in conjunction with pharmacologic management.[28]

Sedation and Respiratory Depression

Most patients experience sedation at the beginning of opioid therapy and whenever the opioid dose is increased significantly.[28] In addition to adversely affecting the patient's ability to participate in the postoperative recovery process, if left untreated, excessive sedation can progress to clinically significant respiratory depression.[28,69] The observation that excessive sedation precedes opioid-induced sedation indicates that systematic sedation assessment is an essential aspect of the care of opioid-naive patients receiving opioid therapy.[69,70] Nursing assessment of sedation is convenient and inexpensive and takes minimal time to perform. A simple, easy-to-understand and communicate sedation scale, developed for assessment of unwanted sedation and that includes what should be done at each level of sedation is widely recommended to enhance accuracy and consistency of assessment, monitor trends, and communicate effectively between members of the health care team (Box 31-3).[28,69,70] The use of scales that include agitation assessment and other

BOX 31-3   Pasero Opioid-Induced Sedation Scale (POSS) with Interventions

S = Sleep, easy to arouse
   Acceptable; no action necessary; may increase
      opioid dose if needed
1 = Awake and alert
   Acceptable; no action necessary; may increase
      opioid dose if needed
2 = Slightly drowsy, easily aroused
   Acceptable; no action necessary; may increase
      opioid dose if needed
3 = Frequently drowsy, arousable, drifts off to sleep
   during conversation
   Unacceptable; monitor respiratory status and
      sedation level closely until sedation level is
      stable at less than 3 and respiratory status is
      satisfactory; decrease opioid dose 25% to
      50%* or notify primary[†] or anesthesia

provider for orders; consider administering a
nonsedating, opioid-sparing nonopioid, such
as acetaminophen or an NSAID, if not contraindicated; ask patient to take deep breaths
every 15-30 minutes.
4 = Somnolent, minimal or no response to verbal
   and physical stimulation
   Unacceptable; stop opioid; consider adminis-
      tering naloxone[‡,§]; call Rapid Response
      Team (Code Blue); stay with patient,
      stimulate, and support respiration as indi-
      cated by patient status; notify primary[†] or
      anesthesia provider; monitor respiratory
      status and sedation level closely until
      sedation level is stable at less than 3 and
      respiratory status is satisfactory.

NSAID, Nonsteroidal antiinflammatory drug.

*Opioid analgesic orders or a hospital protocol should include the expectation that a nurse will decrease the opioid dose if a patient is excessively sedated.

[†]For example, the physician, nurse practitioner, advanced practice nurse, or physician assistant responsible for the pain management prescription.

[‡]For adults experiencing respiratory depression, mix 0.4 mg of naloxone and 10 mL of normal saline in syringe and administer this dilute solution slowly (0.5 mL over 2 minutes) while observing the patient's response (titrate to effect).

[§]Hospital protocols should include the expectation that a nurse will administer naloxone to any patient suspected of having life-threatening opioid-induced sedation and respiratory depression.

From Pasero C, McCaffery M: *Pain assessment and pharmacologic management,* St. Louis, 2011, Mosby. Copyright 1994, Pasero C. Used with permission.

parameters are appropriate when sedation is desirable but are not appropriate for assessment when sedation is undesirable, such as during opioid administration for pain management.[28,69] Many hospitals adopt two scales and distinguish their use according to these goals of care. All opioid orders and titration protocols should include the expectation that nurses will stop titration or decrease the opioid dose immediately if excessive sedation is detected.

Respiratory depression is assessed on the basis of what is normal for a particular individual and is usually described as clinically significant when there is a decrease in the rate, depth, and regularity of respirations from baseline, rather than just by a specific number of respirations per minute.[24,69] There are many risk factors for opioid-induced respiratory depression including opioid naivety, older age (65 years or older), obesity, obstructive sleep apnea, and preexisting pulmonary disease or dysfunction or other comorbidities.[28] Risk is elevated during the first 24 hours following surgery and in patients who require a high dose of opioid in a short period of time (e.g., greater than 10 mg of IV morphine or equivalent in the PACU).

Clinically significant opioid-induced respiratory depression can be prevented by careful titration and close nurse monitoring of sedation and respiratory status.[28] Administration of the lowest effective opioid dose is critical, and this is best accomplished with the use of a multimodal analgesic approach that includes nonopioid analgesics. A comprehensive respiratory assessment constitutes more than counting a patient's respiratory rate.[69] A proper assessment requires the nurse or nurse technician to watch the rise and fall of the patient's chest to determine rate, depth, and regularity of respirations. Listening to the sound of the patient's respiration is critical as well.[69] Snoring indicates airway obstruction and must be addressed promptly with repositioning, and depending on severity, a request for respiratory therapy consultation and further evaluation.[81]

Hospital protocols and opioid orders should include the expectation that nurses will administer the opioid antagonist naloxone intravenously for the treatment of clinically significant respiratory depression.[28] The goal is to reverse just the sedation and respiratory depressant effects of the opioid. To this end, it should be diluted and titrated slowly to prevent severe pain and other adverse effects, which can include hypertension, tachycardia, ventricular dysrhythmias, pulmonary edema, and cardiac arrest (see the third footnote in Box 31-3 for correct technique).[4,28] Sometimes more than one dose of naloxone is necessary, because naloxone has a shorter duration of action (1 hour in most patients) than most opioids.[28]

Addiction, Physical Dependence, and Tolerance

The terms *physical dependence* and *tolerance* often are confused with *addiction;* therefore clarification of definitions is important.[28] The definitions proposed in a 2001 consensus statement by the American Academy of Pain Medicine, the American Pain Society, and the American Society of Addiction Medicine are[82]:

- *Physical dependence* is a normal response that occurs with repeated administration of the opioid for more than two weeks and cannot be equated with addictive disease. It is manifested by the occurrence of withdrawal symptoms when the opioid is suddenly stopped or rapidly reduced or when an antagonist such as naloxone is given. Withdrawal symptoms may be suppressed by the natural, gradual reduction of the opioid as pain decreases or by gradual, systematic reduction, referred to as *tapering.*[82]

- *Tolerance* is also a normal response that occurs with regular administration of an opioid and consists of a decrease in one or more effects of the opioid (e.g., decreased analgesia, sedation, respiratory depression). Tolerance cannot be equated with addictive disease. Tolerance to analgesia usually occurs in the first days to 2 weeks of opioid therapy, but is uncommon after that. It may be treated with increases in dose. However, disease progression, not tolerance to analgesia, appears to be the reason for most dose escalations. Stable pain usually results in stable opioid doses; therefore tolerance poses few clinical problems.[82]

- *Opioid addiction,* or addictive disease, is a chronic neurologic and biologic disease. The development and characteristics of addiction are influenced by genetic, psychosocial, and environmental factors. No single cause of addiction, such as taking an opioid for pain relief, has been found. Addiction is characterized by behaviors that include one or more of the following: impaired control over drug use, compulsive use, continued use despite harm, and craving.[82] This statement reinforces that taking opioids for pain relief is not addiction, no matter how long a person takes opioids or at what doses.

- *Pseudoaddiction* is a mistaken diagnosis of addictive disease.[83] When a patient's pain is not well controlled, the patient may begin to manifest symptoms suggestive of addictive disease. In an effort to obtain adequate pain relief, the patient may respond with demanding behavior, escalating demands for more or different medications, and repeated requests for opioids on time or before the prescribed interval between doses has elapsed. Pain relief typically eliminates these behaviors and is often accomplished by increasing opioid doses or decreasing intervals between doses.

The incidence of addiction as a result of taking an opioid for therapeutic reasons, such as postoperative pain management, is thought to be rare.[84,85] An evidence-based review of all available studies on the development of addiction and aberrant drug-related behaviors in patients with persistent non–cancer-related pain being treated with opioids calculated the percentage of abuse and addiction to be 0.19%.[86] These data suggest that patients with no past or present history of abuse or addiction usually remain responsible medication users over time. Similarly, a registry study of 227 patients who were treated with modified-release oxycodone and followed for up to 3 years after participating in a clinical trial also showed a low occurrence of problematic drug-related behavior—there were just six cases of misuse and no cases of new addiction.[87] Again, this number is reassuring in terms of the rate of iatrogenic addiction among those with no history of abuse.

Opioid Administration to Patients with Addictive Disease

Opioids, if they are appropriate, should not be withheld from patients with pain who also have addictive disease.[28,88] The perioperative period is not the optimal time to attempt detoxification or rehabilitation of a patient who is abusing opioids or other substances.[88] Furthermore, there is no research showing that providing opioid analgesics to a person with addictive disease will worsen the disease, or that withholding opioid analgesics when needed will increase the likelihood of recovery.[28] In fact, withholding opioids in this situation may cause significant pain, which can increase the patient's stress level and lead to increased craving for drugs of abuse. Clearly, providing pain relief to the patient with addictive disease, even when it includes opioids, is preferable to withholding opioids.[28]

Management of the Opioid-Dependent Surgical Patient with Chronic Pain

The management of postoperative pain in patients with underlying chronic pain can be extremely challenging. The key to success in the postoperative period is optimizing the management of the chronic pain before the surgical procedure.[28] If preexisting pain is poorly controlled preoperatively, the primary care provider or anesthesia provider should be contacted for evaluation and appropriate orders.

A multimodal postoperative pain treatment plan, initiated preoperatively whenever possible, is essential in patients with underlying chronic pain. NSAIDs that do not affect bleeding time (see earlier in chapter) do not need to be discontinued preoperatively.[52] Anticonvulsants and antidepressants, which are often administered for treatment of persistent neuropathic pain, should also be initiated or continued if taken preoperatively.[52] Guidelines recommend the continuation of opioid analgesics to prevent opioid withdrawal syndrome in patients who are taking them preoperatively for preexisting pain.[28,52,89]

Patients who have been taking opioids on a long-term basis preoperatively are likely to be opioid tolerant and may require higher postoperative opioid doses in the postoperative period compared with opioid-naive patients. Unfortunately there are no evidence-based guidelines for predicting postoperative opioid requirements on the basis of the opioid dose consumed before surgery. One suggestion is to expect opioid requirements postoperatively in the opioid-tolerant patient to be twofold to fourfold the dose required in an opioid-naive person[90]; however, individualization of care is essential.[28] Occasionally patients are underdosed by clinicians who are fearful of the high doses often required by patients who are opioid tolerant. Tolerance to the adverse effects of opioids develops more rapidly than to analgesia, which means that opioids can be safely titrated to relatively high doses to provide adequate analgesia.[89] It is reassuring to know that, although respiratory depression can occur in opioid tolerant patients, the occurrence is rare when doses are carefully titrated and the patient is monitored appropriately for effect.

Local Anesthetics

Local anesthetics have a long history of safe and effective use for acute pain management. They are given by a variety of routes of administration for both procedural and postoperative pain treatment and are generally well tolerated by most individuals.[13]

For many years regional anesthesia has been administered via single injection peripheral nerve blocks to target a specific nerve or nerve plexus. Although extremely effective, this method has limited usefulness for postoperative pain treatment because of a short duration of action (4 to

12 hours for bupivacaine and ropivacaine).[13] Continuous peripheral nerve block is a relatively new pain management technique that offers an alternative. It involves establishment of an initial block followed by placement of a catheter through which an infusion of local anesthetic is administered continuously, with or without PCA capability. Advances in technology have allowed the expansion of this technique to the outpatient setting where catheters can be removed by patients or families and small disposable pumps can be discarded easily at the end of therapy.[13] Another therapy, continuous local anesthetic wound infusion, involves the surgeon's placement of a catheter subcutaneously into the surgical wound at the end of the surgical procedure to be used for infusion of a local anesthetic to control postoperative pain.[13] There is extensive research supporting both continuous peripheral nerve blocks and wound infusions as primary postoperative analgesic strategies following a wide variety of surgical procedures.[13,91,92] Guidelines for the nursing care of patients receiving these therapies are available.[3,13]

IV lidocaine is occasionally used for acute pain that has been refractory to first-line treatment approaches. One of its major benefits is its ability to reduce postoperative GI complications[93] A metaanalysis of eight studies involving patients who underwent abdominal surgery revealed that IV lidocaine compared with placebo was associated with better pain control as well as decreases in the duration of ileus, nausea, and vomiting and length of hospital stay.[94] Guidelines for the use of IV lidocaine for postoperative pain are provided elsewhere.[13]

Anticonvulsants

The anticonvulsants gabapentin and pregabalin are first-line analgesics for neuropathic pain and are increasingly being added to postoperative pain treatment plans to address the neuropathic component of surgical pain. Although further research is needed,[95] anticonvulsants have been shown to improve analgesia, allow lower doses of other analgesics, and help to prevent persistent neuropathic postsurgical pain syndromes.[96] There is no consensus on an optimal dosing regimen; both single and multiple dosing have been described.[97-99] Generally, preoperative doses range between 400 and 1200 mg, and postoperative doses are typically 400 to 600 mg every 6 to 8 hours.[13] Treatment varies from 24 hours to several days. The most concerning adverse effect of anticonvulsants is sedation; therefore sedation levels should be watched closely during therapy (see Box 31-3).

NONPHARMACOLOGIC METHODS

Research shows that most individuals want to be offered alternative self-management strategies for their health care.[100,101] Nonpharmacologic methods that are used to provide comfort and pain relief include the body-based (physical) modalities, such as massage, acupuncture, and application of heat and cold, and the mind-body (cognitive-behavioral) methods, such as relaxation breathing, imagery, and meditation. There are also biologically-based therapies that involve the use of herbs and vitamins, as well as energy therapies such as reiki and tai chi.[100] Biologically based and energy therapies are used most often in the outpatient setting.

Nonpharmacologic methods may be effective alone for mild to some moderate-intensity pain and are used to complement, but not replace, pharmacologic therapies for more severe pain.[102] The effectiveness of nonpharmacologic methods can be unpredictable, and although not all have been shown to relieve pain, they offer many benefits to patients with pain. For example, researchers have demonstrated that nonpharmacologic methods can facilitate relaxation and reduce anxiety and stress.[102-104] Many patients find that the use of nonpharmacologic methods helps them cope better with their pain and feel greater control over the pain experience.

Although time is limited in the acute care setting for implementation of nonpharmacologic interventions,[102] nurses have an important role in providing them and teaching patients about their use.[105] The following list includes some examples of nonpharmacologic interventions for acute pain that are relatively easy to incorporate into daily clinical practice; they can be used individually or in combination with other non-drug therapies.

- *Proper body alignment* achieved through optimal positioning and regular repositioning can help to prevent or relieve pain. Pillows can be used to maintain the position and support the patient's back and extremities.
- *Thermal measures* such as the application of localized, superficial heat and cooling may relieve pain and provide comfort by decreasing sensitivity to pain and muscle spasms and alleviating joint and muscle aches. The two can be used interchangeably.
- *Mind-body therapies* are designed to enhance the mind's capacity to affect bodily function and symptoms and include music therapy, distraction techniques, meditation, prayer, hypnosis, guided imagery, relaxation techniques, and pet therapy.

SUMMARY

With advances in pain research and technology over the past several years, the role of the perianesthesia nurse has rapidly expanded in regard to pain. Although assessment and management of pain are the responsibilities of all members of the health care team, perianesthesia nurses are recognized as the patient's primary pain managers by virtue of their unique assessment and monitoring abilities, knowledge of drug delivery, and constant presence. They educate patients about pain before it is experienced and are the first to treat it after surgery. They strive to tailor the application of their pain interventions to meet the needs of the individual patient, which is the hallmark of high-quality pain care. In summary, perianesthesia nurses are the link between safe and effective pain control and optimal patient outcomes and are essential to ensuring that every surgical patient receives the best possible pain relief.

REFERENCES

1. Abouleish AE, Ranganathan G: Economics and costs: a primer for acute pain management specialists. In Sinatra RS, et al, editors: *Acute pain management*, New York, 2009, Cambridge University Press.
2. McCaffery M, et al: Assessment. In Pasero C, McCaffery M: *Pain assessment and pharmacologic management*, St. Louis, 2011, Mosby.
3. Pasero C, et al: The nurse's perspective on acute pain management. In Sinatra RS, et al, editors: *Acute pain management*, New York, 2009, Cambridge University Press.
4. American Pain Society (APS): *Principles of analgesic use in the treatment of acute and cancer pain*, ed 6, Glenview, IL, 2008, APS.
5. McCaffery M: *Nursing practice theories related to cognition, bodily pain, and man-environment interactions*, Los Angeles, 1968, University of California, Los Angeles.
6. Pasero C, Portenoy RK: Neurophysiology of pain and analgesia and the pathophysiology of neuropathic pain. In Pasero C, McCaffery M: *Pain assessment and pharmacologic management*, St. Louis, 2011, Mosby.
7. Argoff CE, et al: Multimodal analgesia for chronic pain: rationale and future directions, *Pain Med* 10(Suppl 2):S53–S66, 2009.
8. Marchand S: The physiology of pain mechanisms: from the periphery to the brain, *Rheum Dis Clin N Am* 34(2):285–309, 2008.
9. Vadivelu N, et al: Pain pathways and acute pain processing. In Sinatra RS, et al, editors: *Acute pain management*, New York, 2009, Cambridge University Press.
10. Pasero C, et al: Nonopioid analgesics. In Pasero C, McCaffery M: *Pain assessment and pharmacologic management*, St. Louis, 2011, Mosby.
11. Dib-Jajj SD, et al: Voltage-gated sodium channels: targets for pain, *Pain Med* 10(7):1260–1269, 2009.
12. Adler JE, et al: Modulation of neuropathic pain by a glial-driven factor, *Pain Med* 10(7):1229–1236, 2009.

13. Pasero C, et al: Adjuvant analgesics. In Pasero C, McCaffery M: *Pain assessment and pharmacologic management*, St. Louis, 2011, Mosby.

14. Ghouri MK, et al: Pathophysiology of acute pain. In Sinatra RS, et al, editors: *Acute pain management*, New York, 2009, Cambridge University Press.

15. Beilin B, et al: The effects of postoperative pain management on immune response to surgery, *Anesth Analg* 97:822–827, 2003.

16. Page GG: Acute pain and immune impairment, *Pain Clinical Updates* 12(1):1–4, 2005.

17. Weatherstone KB, et al: Are there opportunities to decrease nosocomial infection by choice of analgesic regimen? *Arch Pediatr Adolesc Med* 157:1108–1114, 2003.

18. Guay J: Postoperative pain significantly influences postoperative blood loss in patients undergoing total knee replacement, *Pain Med* 7(6):476–482, 2006.

19. Erb J, et al: Interactions between pulmonary performance and movement-evoked pain in the immediate postsurgical period: implications for perioperative research and treatment, *Reg Anesth Pain Med* 33(4):312–319, 2008.

20. Shea RA, et al: Pain intensity and postoperative pulmonary complications among the elderly after abdominal surgery, *Heart Lung* 31:440–449, 2002.

21. Hanley MA, et al: Chronic pain associated with upper-limb loss, *Am J Phys Med Rehabil* 88(9):742–751, 2009.

22. Kehlet H, et al: Persistent postsurgical pain: risk factors and prevention, *Lancet* 367(9522):1618–1625, 2006.

23. Hanley MA, et al: Preamputation pain and acute pain predict chronic pain after lower extremity amputation, *J Pain* 8(2):102–109, 2007.

24. Spagrud LJ, et al: Children's self-report of pain intensity. The faces pain scale—revised. *Am J Nurs* 103(12):62–64, 2003. Scale is available for free for clinical and research use: www.painsourcebook.ca.

25. Ware L, et al: Evaluation of the revised faces pain scale, verbal descriptor scale, numeric rating scale and Iowa pain thermometer in older minority adults, *Pain Manage Nurs* 71:117–125, 2006.

26. Herr KA, et al: Pain intensity assessment in older adults: use of experimental pain to compare psychometric properties and usability of selected pain scales with younger adults, *Clin J Pain* 20:207–219, 2004.

27. Li L, et al: Postoperative pain intensity assessment: a comparison of four scales in Chinese adult, *Pain Med* 8(3):223–234, 2007.

28. Pasero C, et al: Opioid analgesics. In Pasero C, McCaffery M: *Pain assessment and pharmacologic management*, St. Louis, 2011, Mosby.

29. Herr K, et al: Pain assessment in the nonverbal patient: position statement with clinical practice recommendations, *Pain Manag Nurs* 7(2):44–52, 2006.

30. Pasero C: Challenges in pain assessment, *J Perianesth Nurs* 24(1):50–54, 2009.

31. Puntillo KA, et al: Patient's perceptions and responses to procedural pain: results from Thunder Project II, *Am J Crit Care* 10(4):238–251, 2001.

32. Stanik-Hutt JA, et al: Pain experiences of traumatically injured patients in a critical care setting, *Am J Crit Care* 10(4):252–259, 2001.

33. Pasero C, McCaffery M: No self report means no pain intensity, *Am J Nurs* 105(10):50–53, 2005.

34. Gelinas C, Arbour C: Behavioral and physiologic indicators during a nociceptive procedure in conscious and unconscious mechanically ventilated patients: similar or different? *J Crit Care* 24(4):628e.7–17, 2009.

35. Arbour C, Gelinas C: Are vital signs valid indicators for the assessment of pain in postoperative cardiac surgery ICU adults? *Intensive Crit Care Nurs* 26(2):83–90, 2010.

36. Blumstein HA, Moore D: Visual analog pain scores do not define desire for analgesia in paitents with acute pain, *Acad Emerg Med* 10(3):211–214, 2003.

37. Lucas CE, et al: Kindness kills: the negative impact of pain as the fifth vital sign, *J Am Coll Surg* 205(1):101–107, 2007.

38. Vila H, et al: The efficacy and safety of pain management before and after implementation of hospital-wide pain management standards: is patient safety compromised by treatment based solely on numerical pain ratings, *Anesth Analg* 101(2):474–480, 2005.

39. Ashburn MA, et al: Practice guidelines for acute pain management in the perioperative setting. An updated report by the American Society of Anesthesiologists task force on acute pain management, *Anesthesiology* 100(6): 1573–1581, 2004.

40. Dworkin RH, et al: Pharmacologic management of neuropathic pain: evidence-based recommendations, *Pain* 132(3): 237–251, 2007.

41. Pasero C: Perioperative rectal administration of nonopioid analgesics, *J Perianesth Nurs* 25(1):5–6, 2010.

42. Kaestli LZ, et al: Use of transdermal drug formulations in the elderly, *Drugs Aging* 25(4):269–280, 2008.

43. Pasero C, et al: Nonopioid analgesics. In Pasero C, McCaffery M: *Pain assessment and pharmacologic management*, St. Louis, 2011, Mosby.

44. Sinatra RS, et al: Efficacy and safety of single and repeated administration of 1 gram intravenous acetaminophen injection (paracetamol) for pain management after major orthopedic surgery, *Anesthesiology* 102(4):822–831, 2005.

45. Dahl V, et al: Ibuprofen vs. acetaminophen after arthroscopically assisted anterior cruciate ligament reconstruction, *Eur J Anaesthesiol* 21(6):471–475, 2004.

46. Singla N, et al: A multi-center, randomized, double-blind placebo-controlled trial of intravenous-ibuprofen (IV-ibuprofen) for treatment of pain in post-operative orthopedic adult patients, *Pain Med* 11(8):1284–1292, 2010.

47. Burke A, et al: Analgesic-antipyretic agents: pharmacotherapy of gout. In Brunton LL, et al, editors: *Goodman & Gilman's the pharmacological basis of therapeutics*, ed 11, New York, 2006, McGraw-Hill.

48. Schug SA, Manopas A: Update on the role of non-opioids for postoperative pain treatment, *Best Prac Res Clin Anesth* 21(1):15–30, 2007.

49. Laine L, et al: COX-2 selective inhibitors in the treatment of osteoarthritis, *Semin Arthritis Rheum* 38(3):165–187, 2008.

50. Launay-Vacher V, et al: Treatment of pain in patients with renal insufficiency: the World Health Organization three-step ladder adapted, *J Pain* 6(3):137–148, 2005.

51. Leo RJ: Safe analgesic use in patients with renal dysfunction, *Pract Pain Manage* 12:22, 27, 2008.

52. Ashraf W, et al: Guidelines for preoperative administration of patients' home medications, *J Perianesth Nurs* 19(4):228–233, 2004.

NURSING CARE IN THE PACU

53. Munsterhjelm E, et al: Dose-dependent inhibition of platelet function by acetaminophen in healthy volunteer, *Anesthesiology* 103(4):712–717, 2005.

54. FitzGerald GA: Coxibs and cardiovascular disease, *N Engl J Med* 351(17):1709–1711, 2004.

55. Scheiman JM: *Cardiovascular risks associated with cyclooxygenase-2 selective inhibitors and traditional nonsteroidal antiinflammatory drugs, 2006,* available at www.medscape.com/viewarticle/543804_1. Accessed February 20, 2011.

56. Nussmeier NA, et al: Complications of the COX-2 inhibitors parecoxib and valdecoxib after cardiac surgery, *N Engl J Med* 352(11):1081–1091, 2005.

57. Ott E, et al: Efficacy and safety of the cyclooxygenase 2 inhibitors parecoxib and valdecoxib in patients undergoing coronary artery bypass surgery, *J Thorac Cardiovasc Surg* 125(6):1481–1492, 2003.

58. United States Food and Drug Administration (FDA): *Medication guide for non-steroidal anti-inflammatory drugs (NSAIDs), 2007,* available at www.fda.gov/cder/drug/infopage/COX2/NSAIDmedguide.htm. Accessed February 10, 2011.

59. Dorr LD, et al: Multimodal analgesia without parenteral narcotics for total knee arthroplasty, *J Arthrop* 23(4):502–508, 2008.

60. Sun T, et al: Perioperative versus postoperative celecoxib on patient outcomes after major plastic surgery procedures, *Anesth Analg* 106(3):950–958, 2008.

61. Lee A, et al: Effects of nonsteroidal anti-inflammatory drugs on postoperative renal function in adults with normal renal function, *Cochrane Database Syst Rev* 18(2)(CD002765):2007.

62. Helstrom J, Rosow CE: Nonsteroidal anti-inflammatory drugs in postoperative pain. In Shorten G, et al, editors: *Postoperative pain management: an evidence-based guide to practice,* Philadelphia, 2006, Saunders.

63. Einhorn TA: Cox-2 inhibitors and fracture healing: arguments for such an effect and a suggestion about caution in use, *J Bone Miner Res* 18(3):584, 2003.

64. Langford RM, Mehta V: Selective cyclooxygenase inhibition: its role in pain and anaesthesia, *Biomed Pharmacother* 60(7):323–328, 2006.

65. Liu LL, Gropper MA: Postoperative analgesia and sedation in the adult intensive care unit: a guide to drug selection, *Drugs* 63(8):755–767, 2003.

66. Fukuda K: Intravenous opioid anesthetics. In Miller RD, editor: *Miller's anesthesia,* ed 6, St. Louis, 2005, Churchill Livingstone.

67. Aubrun F, Riou B: In reply to correspondence, *Anesthesiology* 100(3),745, 2004.

68. Blumenthal S, et al: Postoperative intravenous morphine consumption, pain scores, and side effects with perioperative oral controlled-release oxycodone after lumbar discectomy, *Anesth Analg* 105(1):233–237, 2007.

69. Pasero C: Assessment of sedation during opioid administration for pain management, *J Perianesth Nurs* 24(3):186–190, 2009.

70. Nisbet AT, Mooney-Cotter F: Selected scales for reporting opioid-induced sedation, *Pain Manage Nurs* 10(3):154–164, 2009.

71. Ho KT, Gan TJ: Opioid-related adverse effects and treatment options. In Sinatra RS, et al, editors: *Acute pain management,* New York, 2009, Cambridge University Press.

72. Miaskowski C: A review of the incidence, causes, consequences, and management of gastrointestinal effects associated with postoperative opioid administration, *J Perianesth Nurs* 24(4):222–228, 2009.

73. American Society of PeriAnesthesia Nurses (ASPAN): ASPAN's evidence-based clinical practice guideline for the prevention and/or management of PONV/PDNV, *J Perianesth Nurs* 21(4):230–250, 2006.

74. Gan TJ, et al: Consensus guidelines for managing postoperative nausea and vomiting, *Anesth Analg* 97(1):62–71, 2003.

75. Gan TJ, et al: Society for Ambulatory Anesthesia guidelines for the management of postoperative nausea and vomiting, *Anesth Analg* 105(6):1615–1628, 2007.

76. Kehlet H: Preventive measures to minimize or avoid postoperative ileus, *Sem Colon Rec Surg* 16(4):203–206, 2005.

77. Ganesh A, Maxwell LG: Pathophysiology and management of opioid-induced pruritus, *Drugs* 67(6):2323–2333, 2007.

78. Iatrou CA, et al: Prophylactic intravenous ondansetron and dolasetron in intrathecal morphine-induced pruritus: a randomized, double-blinded, placebo-controlled study, *Anesth Analg* 101(5):1516–1520, 2005.

79. Grape S, Schug SA: Epidural and spinal analgesia. In Macintyre PE, et al, editors: *Clinical pain management: acute pain,* ed 2, London, 2008, Hodder Arnold.

80. Anwari JS, Iqbal S: Antihistamines and potentiation of opioid induced sedation and respiratory depression, *Anaesthesia* 58(5):494–495, 2003.

81. American Society of Anesthesiologists: Practice guidelines for the perioperative management of patients with obstructive sleep apnea, *Anesthesiology* 104(5):1081–1093, 2006.

82. American Society of Addiction Medicine: *Definitions related to the use of opioids for the treatment of pain, 2001,* available at www.painmed.org/pdf/definition.pdf. Accessed March 10, 2009.

83. Weissman DE, Haddox JD: Opioid pseudoaddiction—an iatrogenic syndrom. *Pain* 36(3):363–366, 1989.

84. Jackson KC: Opioid pharmacology. In Smith HS, editor: *Current therapy in pain,* Philadelphia, 2009, Saunders.

85. Rowbotham DJ, et al: Clinical pharmacology: opioids. In Macintyre PE, et al, editors: *Clinical pain management: acute pain,* ed 2, London, 2009, Hodder Arnold.

86. Fishbain DA, et al: What percentage of chronic nonmalignant pain patients exposed to chronic opioid analgesic therapy develop abuse/addiction and/or aberrant drug-related behaviors? A structured evidence-based review, *Pain Med* 9(4):444–459, 2008.

87. Portenoy RK, et al: Long-term use of controlled-release oxycodone for noncancer pain: results of a 3-year registry study, *Clin J Pain* 23(4):287–299, 2007.

88. Mitra S, Sinatra RS: Patients with opioid dependence and substance abuse. In Sinatra RS, et al, editors: *Acute pain management,* New York, 2009, Cambridge University Press.

89. Mehta V, Langford RM: Acute pain management for opioid dependent patients, *Anaesthesia* 61(3):269-272, 2006.

90. Carroll IR, et al: Management of perioperative pain in patients chronically consuming opioids, *Reg Anesth Pain Med* 29(6):576–591, 2004.

91. Richman JM, et al: Does continuous peripheral nerve block provide superior pain control to opioids? A meta-analysis, *Anesth Analg* 102(1):248–257, 2006.

92. Liu SS, et al: Efficacy of continuous wound catheters delivering local anesthetic for postoperative analgesia: a quantitative and qualitative systematic review of randomized controlled trials, *J Am Coll Surg* 203(6):915–932, 2006.

93. Wright JL, et al: A brief review of innovative uses for local anesthetics, *Curr Opin Anaesthesiol* 21(5):651–656, 2008.

94. Marret E, et al: Meta-analysis of intravenous lidocaine and postoperative recovery after abdominal surgery, *Br J Surg* 95(11):1331–1338, 2008.

95. Wiffen PJ, et al: Anticonvulsant drugs for acute and chronic pain, *Cochrane Database Syst Rev* 3(CD001133): 2005.

96. Dauri M, et al: Gabapentin and pregabalin for the acute post-operative pain management. A systematic-narrative review of the recent clinical evidences, *Curr Drug Targets* 10(8):716–733, 2009.

97. Ho KY, et al: Gabapentin and postoperative pain—a systematic review of randomized controlled trials, *Pain* 126(1–3): 91–101, 2006.

98. Peng PWH, et al: Use of gabapentin for perioperative pain control—a meta-analysis, *Pain Res Manage* 12(2): 85–91, 2007.

99. Tiippana EM, et al: Do surgical patients benefit from perioperative gabapentin/pregabalin? A systematic review of efficacy and safety, *Anesth Analg* 104(6): 1545–1556, 2007.

100. Bruckenthal P: Integrating nonpharmacologic and alternative strategies into a comprehensive management approach for older adults with pain, *Pain Manage Nurs* 11(2):S23–S31, 2010.

101. National Center for Complementary and Alternative Medicine (NCCAM): *What is CAM?* available at nccam.nih.gov/health/whatiscam/overview.htm. Accessed February 23, 2010.

102. McCaffery M: What is the role of nondrug methods in the nursing care of patients with acute pain? *Pain Manage Nurs* 3(3):77–80, 2002.

103. Kwekkeboom KL, et al: Mind-body treatments for the pain-fatigue-sleep disturbance symptom cluster in persons with cancer, *J Pain Symptom Manage* 39:126, 2010.

104. Allred KD, et al: The effect of music on postoperative pain and anxiety, *Pain Manage Nurs* 11:15, 2010.

105. Gatlin CG, Schulmeister L: When medication is not enough: nonpharmacologic management of pain, *Clin J Onc Nurs* 11:699, 2007.

NURSING CARE IN THE PACU

Candace N. Taylor, BSN, RN, CPAN

The patient with ear, nose, and throat (ENT) dysfunction presents many challenges to the perianesthesia nurse. These patients often have a difficult airway for management (see Chapter 30), which in itself can be challenging. These patients also often have abnormal or dysfunctional anatomy that presents major concerns and requires enhanced awareness of the "normal" anatomy of the structures associated with ENT surgical procedures. In addition, the patient emerging from maxillofacial surgery, which usually consists of dental or plastic surgery, needs close monitoring of airway patency and clearance along with management of the pain associated with those surgical procedures in a way that does not depress respiratory status. The perianesthesia nurse who manages these types of surgical procedures needs a strong knowledge of airway anatomy and physiology and excellent skills in the management of a difficult airway. Finally, the perianesthesia nurse must also manage the behavioral component of patients who undergo ENT or maxillofacial surgery. These patients have all kinds of emotions: from fright because of wiring of the jaw to fear because of the tight bandaging and pain. Because patients who undergo ENT and maxillofacial surgery present a great challenge to the perianesthesia nurse, a complete review of this category of surgical patients is presented. The reader is encouraged to read Chapters 12 and 30 as follow-up; they present more information on the respiratory system and airway management.

DEFINITIONS

Ankyloglossia (Tongue Tied): A short lingual frenulum that may cause difficulty with suckling in the infant and subsequent speech impairment. It is treated surgically with clipping of the frenulum.

Cochlear Implant: A prosthesis with an internal electrode is surgically implanted into the cochlea so that an external microphone later can be applied for stimulation of the eighth cranial nerve and provision of sound for a deaf person.

Electrocautery Unit: A snare heated with electricity for the purpose of cauterization of small vessels to bleeding or for cutting tissue, without blood loss.

Endoscopy: Nasal surgery performed with direct vision with endoscopic equipment.

Ethmoidectomy: Removal of ethmoid bone.

Fenestration: Reconstruction of the outer and middle parts of the ear by means of a new drum or skin flap; creation of a new window into the internal ear mechanism with a newly established drum or skin flap.

Glossectomy: Removal of the tongue.

Intranasal Antrostomy (Antral Window): Creation of an opening in the lateral wall of the nose under the middle turbinate and the removal of the anterior end of the inferior turbinate.

Labyrinthectomy: Opening of the labyrinth to destroy the inner ear in an attempt to relieve medically uncontrollable symptoms of unilateral Meniere disease.

Laryngectomy: Removal of the larynx; total laryngectomy is the complete removal of the cartilaginous larynx, the hyoid bone, and the strap muscles connected to the larynx and the possible removal of the preepiglottic space along with the lesion.

Laryngofissure: Opening of the larynx for exploratory, excisional, or reconstructive procedures.

Laryngoscopy: Direct examination of the interior of the larynx with a laryngoscope.

Mastoidectomy: Removal of mastoid air cells and of the tympanic membrane. Radical mastoidectomy also involves removal of the malleus, incus, chorda tympani, and mucoperiosteal lining.

Myringotomy: Incision of the tympanic membrane with direct vision and insertion of tubes for facilitation of drainage.

Ossiculoplasty: Reconstruction of the ossicular chain.

Palatouvuloplasty: The reconstruction of the posterior section of the palate and the uvula.

Radical Antrostomy (Caldwell-Luc Operation): Use of an incision into the canine fossa of the upper jaw and exposure of the antrum for removal of bony diseased portions of the antral wall and contents of the sinus; establishment of drainage by means of a counteropening into the nose through the inferior meatus to create a large opening in the nasoantral wall of the inferior meatus, which ensures adequate gravity drainage and aeration and permits removal of all diseased tissue in the sinus with direct vision.

Semi-Fowler Position: The patient is in an inclined position, with the upper half of the body raised with elevation of the head of the bed by approximately 30 degrees.

Sensorineural Hearing Loss: The sound is conducted normally through the external and middle ear, but a defect in the inner ear or auditory nerve results in a loss or deficit in hearing.

Serosanguineous: A discharge from the body that is composed of serum and blood.

Stapedectomy: Removal of the stapes, followed by the placement of a prosthesis.

Stents: A rod for supporting tubular structures.

Submucosal Resection: Removal of either cartilaginous or osseous portions of the septum that lie between the flaps of the mucous membrane and the perichondrium for establishing an adequate partition between the left and right nasal cavities, thereby providing a clear airway for both the internal and the external cavities and the parts of the nose.

Tonsillectomy and Adenoidectomy (T&A): Surgical removal of the tonsils and adenoids.

Tracheostomy: Opening of the trachea and insertion of a cannula through a midline incision in the neck below the cricoid cartilage.

Tympanoplasty (Myringoplasty): Reconstruction of the tympanic membrane.

SURGERY ON THE EAR

Otologic surgery has been revolutionized by antibiotics, the operating microscope, new and more delicate instruments, and an increased understanding of the anatomic structures involved (Fig. 32-1). New methods have been devised for the surgical treatment of hearing loss with correction of conduction apparatus abnormalities, and selected patients can now be surgically relieved of the disabling symptoms of sensorineural hearing loss.

Most otologic procedures are performed in the day surgery arena. The immediate postanesthesia care for patients who have undergone surgery on the ear is generally the same, regardless of the procedure. Immediate postoperative complications are rare. Occasionally excessive bleeding may occur, especially if a large blood vessel has been entered during the operation. If bleeding has occurred, the incident should be reported to the postanesthesia care unit (PACU) nurse who provides care for the patient on admission. Immediate postanesthesia assessment should follow the same format as for any patient who undergoes general anesthesia.[1] In addition, postanesthesia assessment should include testing for function of the facial nerve. The patient should be instructed to frown, smile, wrinkle the forehead, close the eyes, bare the teeth, and pucker the lips.[2] An inability to perform these actions indicates injury to the facial nerve and should be appropriately indicated in the patient's medical record and reported to the surgeon.

If surgery has been performed near the brain (e.g., the inner ear), check for clear fluid in the ear or on the dressings that may indicate cerebrospinal fluid leakage. Aseptic technique for all dressings and protection from infection are especially important elements in the care of the patient who has undergone surgery on the ears, because infection can be transmitted easily to the meninges and the brain. The outer ear is highly vascular and susceptible to circulatory damage and excoriation.

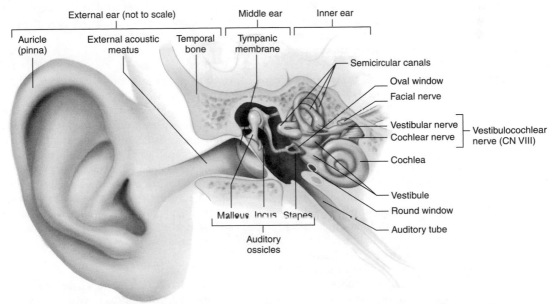

FIG. 32-1 Frontal section through outer, middle, and internal ear. *CN,* Cranial nerve. (From Thibodeau GA, Patton KT: *Anatomy and physiology,* ed 7, St. Louis, 2010, Mosby.)

The outer ear may even become necrotic if circulation is impaired by poor positioning or excessive pressure of a dressing. Assessment of the dressing should therefore include proper positioning.[2,3]

Positioning of the postanesthesia patient who has undergone ear surgery should be indicated by the surgeon. If position is unimportant, the patient should be allowed to assume a position of comfort, usually with the head of the bed elevated to facilitate drainage. This position also decreases the need to move the head to see. Generally, lying on the unoperated side is most comfortable for the patient.

Nausea, vertigo, and nystagmus commonly occur in patients after ear surgery. The patient may minimize discomfort by remaining in the position ordered, moving slowly, and avoiding quick jerky movements.[2,3] The patient should be advised to take slow, deep breaths through the mouth to minimize nausea. Antiemetic drugs and sedatives, such as a 5-HT$_3$ antagonist (e.g., ondansetron [Zofran]) may be ordered for prevention or treatment of nausea and vertigo. The nurse should avoid jarring the bed. When approaching the patient, the nurse should place a hand on top of the patient's head as a reminder not to turn suddenly when the nurse speaks. Sudden turns should be avoided, and movement should be slow in patient transport. Particular attention must be paid to maintaining the integrity of the airway should nausea and vomiting occur.

Patient education should include not allowing water in the ears, such as with swimming. Special ear plugs can be purchased. Some surgeon's offices have someone who can make ear plugs so that they are a custom fit. Instructions should also include not blowing the nose forcefully, especially in the case of myringotomy with tube placement. Surgeons have varying preferences regarding these instructions; therefore care should be made to give instructions pertinent to that specific practitioner.

Special Considerations
Myringotomy
Myringotomy is the most common procedure performed on infants and small children; it is performed for eustachian tube dysfunction. Often these children will exhibit frequent ear infections or symptoms of pain, poor coordination, hearing loss, or speech delays.[4] After a hole in the tympanic membrane is created with a myringotomy blade, the surgeon will place a tube to maintain patency. There are several types of tubes and are placed according to the surgeon's preference.[5]

Special pediatric considerations must be given in the immediate postanesthesia phase to airway management, safety, parental involvement, and outpatient teaching.[3] This procedure is commonly bilateral in children; however in adults it is commonly unilateral.[4] A small piece of sterile cotton can be placed loosely in the external ear to absorb the drainage that commonly occurs. The cotton should be changed when saturated to avoid contamination.

Mastoidectomy
A firm bulky dressing is placed over the ear and held in place with a circular head bandage after mastoidectomy.[5] This dressing may be reinforced, if necessary, but should be changed only by the physician. Minimal serosanguineous drainage may be expected, but bright bloody drainage should be reported to the surgeon.

The patient should be placed in a position of comfort, usually on the nonoperative side. Grafts are often taken from the arm or leg for radical mastoidectomy, and the donor sites should be assessed for drainage and treated according to facility or department policy and surgeon preference. Dizziness and vertigo are common after mastoidectomy and can be treated with the previously mentioned measures.[2,3]

Tympanoplasty
Patients are usually positioned on the unoperated side after tympanoplasty. Care must be taken to keep bandages and grafts in place. Patients should be instructed not to blow the nose or cough and to avoid sneezing to prevent disruption of the grafts. Instruct the patient to open his or her mouth if sneezing occurs so that the force of the sneeze has a larger exit opening, keeping the pressure out of the eustachian tubes.

Fenestration
Fenestration is not commonly performed; however, it may occasionally be the procedure of choice for patients who have lost effective hearing in both ears. Fenestration is a major surgical procedure and is usually performed with general anesthesia. Nausea, vertigo, and pain on moving the jaws can be expected after fenestration. The patient is usually placed on the operated side to keep drainage from the operative site from entering the ear. The patient may be allowed to change position from the operated side to the back for nursing care and comfort.

Stapedectomy
Patients who have undergone stapedectomy are usually admitted to the PACU with ear packing in place; this packing should not be disturbed[5] (Fig. 32-2). Occasionally patients have vertigo

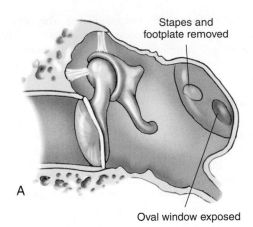

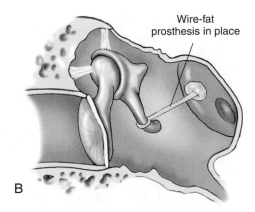

FIG. 32-2 Stapedectomy. **A,** Stapes is removed. **B,** Prosthesis is in place. (From Brooks ML: *Exploring medical language: a student-directed approach,* ed 7, St. Louis, 2009, Mosby.)

after surgery. Patients should be advised to avoid blowing the nose, coughing, and sneezing.

Cochlear Implant

Patients who have undergone a cochlear implant need the same postanesthesia care as any other patient for ear surgery. Verification of the integrity of the facial nerve is important. These patients do not have hearing immediately after surgery and need emotional support and a means of communication such as pen and paper, white board and markers, or a sign language interpreter.[3]

SURGERY ON THE NOSE AND SINUSES

Nasal and sinus surgery can be accomplished with local or general anesthesia. The disposition of the patient is determined by the nature and type of surgery and anesthesia and by the perianesthesia course related to complications and sedation required in the PACU.[6] Although no longer common with the use of endoscopic procedures, overnight observation of the patient in an inpatient setting may be necessary before discharge from the hospital. An inpatient stay may be considered for patients with comorbidities such as obstructive sleep apnea because they will have some difficulty with use of the CPAP machine owing to the nasal splints or packing.[7] The anatomy of the nasal cavity is shown in Fig. 32-3.

Nasal Surgery

Conscious patients admitted to the PACU after nasal surgery, such as septoplasty or functional endoscopic sinus surgery, should be placed in a semi-Fowler position to promote drainage, reduce local edema, minimize discomfort, and facilitate

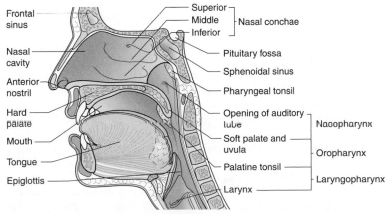

FIG. 32-3 Sagittal section of the nose, mouth, pharynx, and larynx. (From Watson R: *Anatomy and physiology for nurses,* ed 13, London, 2011, Baillière Tindall.)

NURSING CARE IN THE PACU

respiration. Some postoperative serosanguineous drainage is expected; however, the nurse should observe closely for gross bleeding.[2] Loss of vision is a complication that may indicate orbital hematoma required immediate attention by the surgeon. The patient is usually admitted with one or both nostrils packed and a mustache dressing in place to catch any drainage from the packing.[5] The position of the nasal packs and the amount of drainage should be checked frequently. The mustache dressing may be changed as necessary; two or three changes within a 4-hour period are not unusual. Another method commonly used to facilitate postoperative drainage is the insertion of nasal stents. This approach affords more comfort and permits nasal breathing.

The back of the patient's throat should be checked frequently for blood. Frequent belching (from the accumulation of blood in the stomach), frequent swallowing, and the classic signs of hemorrhage, such as tachycardia, are additional signs of unusual bleeding.[3] The patient should be instructed not to blow the nose or swallow secretions, but to spit them into a basin. An ample supply of disposable tissues along with an emesis basin should be placed within easy reach of the patient.

Airway obstruction or laryngeal spasm can occur if a postnasal pack accidentally slips out of place.[1] A flashlight, scissors, and a hemostat for emergency removal of nasal packing and emergency airway equipment must be kept readily available at the patient's bedside.

Fluids are withheld until bleeding is controlled, vomiting and nausea have subsided, and independent airway management has been established. Occasionally an antiemetic may be ordered to alleviate nausea and vomiting.

Mouth breathing, bleeding, and postnasal drainage create dryness and an offensive taste and odor in the patient's mouth; therefore, once the gag reflex has returned, oral hygiene is a priority. Lemon-glycerin swabs or mouthwash may be used for mouth care and to make the patient more comfortable. An ointment may be applied to the lips to prevent drying and cracking.

Ice packs across the nose or to the cheeks may be ordered to minimize pain, edema, discoloration, and bleeding. These ice packs should be small and lightweight.

Oxygen should be delivered via cool mist mask through a face tent, because dry mucous membranes often produce coughing, dyspnea, and decreased respiratory exchange. Ice chips may be a comfort measure if intake is warranted.

When assessing the patient for pain and discomfort, the nurse should inquire about pain to the roof of the mouth and front teeth; this occurs from the edema underneath the septum. Most patients will complain of burning in the nose and a headache that is similar to the pain they experienced with sinus pressure before surgery.

Sinus Surgery

After surgery on the sinuses, the patient is usually admitted to the PACU with packing or splints in place. Reports of feelings of numbness in the upper lip and teeth are not unusual. After general anesthesia, the patient should be positioned well on one side to prevent aspiration of drainage. The conscious patient should be placed in a semi-Fowler position, with the head elevated 45 degrees to promote drainage and minimize edema. The same general care, including oral hygiene and instructions to the patient not to blow the nose, should be followed as for the patient with nasal surgery.[1-3]

SURGERY ON THE TONGUE

The tongue occupies a large portion of the floor of the mouth. Surgery on the tongue generally involves excision of benign or malignant lesions, correction of congenital anomalies, or repair of traumatic lacerations. Lesions may be excised without associated neck dissection; however, when the lesion is malignant, surgical treatment usually involves a combined operation that may include radical neck dissection and resection of both the mandible and the tongue.[2,5]

Local anesthesia is used for minor surgical procedures, such as incision and longitudinal closure of the frenulum in ankyloglossia. Local infiltration is also used to repair lacerations caused by trauma. More extensive surgical procedures on the tongue require general anesthesia with endotracheal intubation.

After surgery, the patient must be placed in a side-lying position with the head slightly dependent to allow for the drainage of secretions out of the mouth. When protective reflexes have returned, the patient should be placed in a sitting position to promote venous and lymphatic drainage.

Maintenance of the airway is the most crucial nursing concern. Suctioning equipment with soft-tipped catheters must be immediately available at the bedside.[1,3] The patient should be instructed to allow saliva to run out of the mouth. A wick of gauze is placed in the patient's mouth to assist in the elimination of secretions. Swelling of the tongue can occur and obstruct the airway; therefore an intubation tray should be readily available.

Because of the vascular nature of the tongue and oral cavity, postoperative bleeding may be a problem. If excessive bleeding occurs, local pressure should be applied until the surgeon can be notified and repair can be performed in the operating room.

THROAT SURGERY

Surgery on the throat and neck is generally accomplished with general anesthesia.[6] Aside from routine care and assessment, specific postanesthesia care for the patient who has undergone surgery on the throat involves: (1) close observation for bleeding from the surgical site; (2) maintenance of a patent airway; (3) prevention of aspiration of secretions; and (4) awareness of possible cerebral neurologic complications that may develop.

The most common procedures are tonsillectomy, either alone or in combination with adenoidectomy, and tracheostomy.[8] Other procedures that are performed on the throat include laryngoscopy with or without biopsies and laryngectomy.

Tonsillectomy and Adenoidectomy

Most patients who undergo tonsillectomy (Fig. 32-4) and adenoidectomy (T&A) are children and young adults. However, the number of the young children

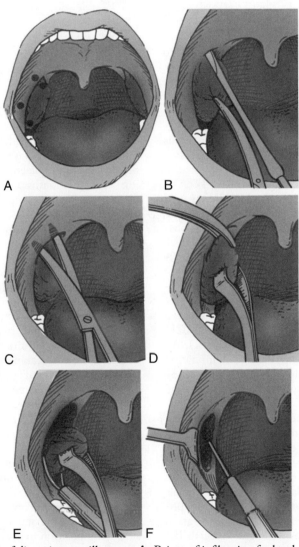

FIG. 32-4 Method of dissection tonsillectomy. **A,** Points of infiltration for local anesthesia. **B,** Start of incision with tonsil knife at attachment of anterior pillar to tonsil superiorly. **C,** Separation with scissor dissection of superior pole of tonsil. **D,** Continuation of dissection of tonsil from its attachment to pillars and bed of tonsillar fossa. **E,** Separation of tonsil with snare at lower pole, including plica triangularis. **F,** Hemostasis. (From Luckman J, Sorenson KC: *Medical-surgical nursing,* ed 3, Philadelphia, 1987, Saunders.)

for T&A continues to be reduced each year as a result of excellent antibiotic treatment. Patients who have undergone T&A and are admitted to the PACU fully conscious can be positioned on their backs with the head elevated 45 degrees. Patients who return after general anesthesia and who are unconscious or semiconscious must be placed in the tonsillar position—well over on the side with the face partially down. The Trendelenburg position can be used to facilitate drainage. The patient's airway and chest expansion must be in full view of the nurse to ensure maximal respiratory integrity at all times. In this position, secretions are easily drained from the mouth.[2] An oral airway should be left in place until the swallowing reflex has returned and the patient can handle secretions. The patient should be advised to spit out secretions as much as possible and to try not to cough, clear the throat, blow the nose, or talk excessively. An ice collar can be applied to minimize pain and postoperative bleeding. The administration of cool humidified air to the patient after T&A provides comfort, helps to minimize swelling, and supplies oxygen. As soon as oral intake is permitted, ice chips should be offered to moisten the throat and reduce swelling.

The most common complication of T&A is postoperative bleeding, for both children and adults. Frequent swallowing, clearing of the throat, and vomiting of dark blood are indications of possible bleeding. The nurse should frequently check the back of the throat with a flashlight for trickling blood. If any of the cardinal symptoms of hemorrhage occur, such as decreased blood pressure, tachycardia, pallor, and restlessness, the surgeon should be notified.[3] Because the surgeon may want to treat a bleeding episode in the PACU, a tonsil tray should be available (Box 32-1). An electrocautery unit and appropriate illumination with a headlight should also be available, along with suction equipment. Postoperative bleeding after T&A can often be controlled with the application of vasoconstrictors via nasal packing with pressure. If significant bleeding occurs, however, the patient may have to return to the operating room for suturing or cauterizing of blood vessels.

With the advent of laser dissection of tonsils and adenoids, swelling of the tissue in the hypopharyngeal area is increased. Close observation and measures to alleviate swelling are crucial. The advantage of laser dissection is that the potential for bleeding is significantly decreased.[9]

Once the patient is conscious and the reflexes have returned, ice chips and fluids may be offered. Oral liquids should be started with caution as

---

BOX 32-1   Contents of Tonsil Tray

- Tongue depressors
- Hurd retractor (1)
- Mouth gags (2)
- Allis clamp (1)
- Tonsil hemostats (2)
- Short sponge forceps (1)
- Pair of scissors (1)
- Sterile towels
- Epinephrine hydrochloride (adrenalin) 1:1000
- Set of tonsil suture needles (1)
- Needle holder (1)
- Glass medicine cup (1)
- Sterile basin (1)
- Cotton balls
- Tonsil tampons
- Soft rubber catheter (1)
- Petrolatum

---

the tonsillar beds were infiltrated with a local anesthetic. Have suction readily available in the case of choking or difficulty swallowing. Some practitioners prefer patients not to use straws so not to precipitate bleeding. Oral hygiene, including alkaline mouthwash, may provide comfort. Ointment should be applied to the lips to prevent drying and cracking.

Patients who have undergone T&A are especially prone to laryngospasms and must be observed closely for patency of the airway.[1] Airway obstruction may be created by swelling of the palate or nasopharynx, swelling in the retropharyngeal space, or swelling of the tongue and nose. If laryngospasm does occur, positive pressure via a bag-mask device and 100% fraction of inspired oxygen (FiO_2) is administered. If this method is not effective in breaking the spasm, reintubation and administration of succinylcholine and opioids as prescribed may be necessary.[1,6]

Laryngoscopy

Laryngoscopy can be accomplished with local or general anesthesia. If the patient's gag and cough reflexes have been obliterated, the patient should not be given anything orally until these reflexes have fully returned.[2,3] The conscious patient may be placed in a semi-Fowler position on either side. If unconscious, the patient should be placed in the side-lying position to avoid aspiration. Cool mist, sips of water, and intravenous opioids may help to relieve the coughing that often occurs.

These patients are especially susceptible to the development of laryngospasm, and the most important observations in the patient after laryngoscopy

Evidence-Based Practice

Hadden and colleagues evaluated complications of pain, postoperative nausea and vomiting (PONV), and respiratory depression. The sample included 102 children with an American Society of Anesthesiologists classification I to III, who were neurologically intact, younger than 17 years, and undergoing tonsillectomy and adenoidectomy (TA). All children received at least one opioid and antiemetic perioperatively; 67% of the children had moderate to severe pain in the PACU and received rescue opioids. Respiratory events were experienced by 27%, which included 24% experiencing oxygen desaturation, 11% with obstruction, 5% with bronchospasm, and 3% with laryngospasm. Postoperative vomiting occurred in 7% of the children. One quarter of these patients experienced respiratory depression. and, although treated preemptively with opioids, postoperative pain was high.

IMPLICATIONS FOR PRACTICE

The perianesthesia nurse should be diligent in the assessment and management of pain for the TA patient. Use of multimodal approaches should include opioids, nonopioids, and nonpharmacologic therapies. This approach may lessen the risk of respiratory depression, pain and PONV.

Source: Hadden SM, et al: Early postoperative outcomes in children after adenotonsillectomy, *J Perianesth Nurs* 26:89–95, 2011.

BOX 32-2   Contents of Tracheostomy Tray

- Adson or Poole suction (without guard; 1)
- No. 3 knife handle with no. 15 blade (1)
- No. 11 blade (1)
- Metzenbaum scissors (1)
- One-point sharp scissors (1)
- Curved tenotomy scissors (1)
- Collier needle holder (1)
- Six-inch needle holder (1)
- Adson forceps (2)
- Tissue forceps (1)
- Dressing forceps (1)
- Curved mosquito forceps (4)
- Straight mosquito forceps (2)
- Allis clamps (2)
- Small towel clips (4)
- Sponge stick (or forceps; 1)
- Probe (1)
- Grooved director (1)
- Goiter right-angle retractor (1)
- Tracheostomy hook (1)
- Vein retractors (2)
- Army-Navy retractors (2)
- Tonsil suction with tip screwed on (1)
- Ten-mL, three-ring syringe (1)
- Needle, 25 gauge, ⅝ inch (1)
- Prep cup (1)
- Medicine glass (1)
- Tracheostomy tubes, sizes 00 to 8 (1 each)
- Hand towels (4)
- Trousseau tracheal dilator (1)

---

are aimed at ascertaining the patency of the airway. Laryngeal stridor, dyspnea, decreased oxygen saturation, or shortness of breath should alert the nurse to respiratory impairment, and the anesthesiologist should be notified.[1-3] Equipment for endotracheal intubation and emergency tracheostomy should be immediately available at the bedside should laryngeal edema or laryngospasm develop (Box 32-2).

A certain amount of throat discomfort can be expected and may be relieved with the use of an ice collar. The administration of high-humidity oxygen via face tent or mask decreases throat irritation. After the cough and gag reflexes have returned, the patient may be allowed sips of warm normal saline solution, which is soothing to irritated tissues. If severe pain occurs in either the throat or the chest, the physician should be notified. The nurse should watch for signs of hemorrhage, including coughing or regurgitation of blood, apprehension, and the classic signs of tachycardia and lowered blood pressure.

In patients who have undergone laryngoscopy (with biopsy) or removal of polyps, vocal rest is important. Coughing should be avoided if possible, and paper and pencil or a white board with markers should be made available so that the patient can communicate without talking. If intractable coughing occurs, the anesthesiologist may need to be consulted for further measures of control, including pharmacotherapeutics such as codeine and lidocaine, to suppress the cough reflex.[3]

Because laser surgery is common in ENT surgery and the technology has improved to a significant degree, Chapter 47 is devoted to the care of the patient after laser and laparoscopic surgery. Patients for ENT surgery, especially involving the upper airway, may undergo laser surgery because lasers enable a precise excision of tissue without significant edema and bleeding. Lasers emit one wavelength, whereas light emits multiple wavelengths. Lasers with shorter wavelengths allow for less absorption by water and therefore less tissue penetration.[9] Patients who are received in the

PACU after laser surgery may still have the endotracheal tube in place. Table 32-1 describes the advantages and disadvantages of the laser-resistant tracheal tubes. A debate between cuffed and uncuffed tracheal tubes continues. However, from a perianesthesia point of view, when a patient who has had laser surgery arrives in the PACU, the nurse must inquire whether the tube is cuffed or uncuffed. If the tracheal tube is cuffed, the cuff was possibly inflated with a methylene blue-tinged normal saline solution. This solution is used because it absorbs and disperses heat and does not act as a reservoir of combustion-supporting gas.[5,9] Extubation should be handled as described in this chapter and in Chapter 30. Chapter 47 also provides an excellent description of the use of lasers during surgery.

Tracheostomy

A tracheostomy, an incision into the trachea and the insertion of a cannula, may be done as either an emergency or an elective procedure (Fig. 32-5). Ideally, a tracheostomy is performed in the operating suite with controlled conditions. Tracheostomies are performed to improve the airway and to provide access for suctioning of secretions from the trachea and bronchi. The PACU nurse should know what condition necessitated the tracheostomy.

The PACU personnel should anticipate the arrival of a patient with a tracheostomy and have the necessary items at the bedside (Box 32-3). A variety of tracheostomy tubes are available, and the nurse should be familiar with those used in the particular institution. Several common types are shown in Fig. 32-6.

Immediate postanesthesia care of the patient with a new tracheostomy includes a complete assessment of the patient's general condition and detailed attention to respiratory status and tracheostomy wound care.[3] Because of the many nursing needs and the necessity of intensive ongoing respiratory assessment, the patient with a new tracheostomy needs constant attendance.

Assessment of respiratory function should include all parameters mentioned in previous chapters. The nurse should auscultate the patient's chest frequently for normal bilateral breath sounds and report any adventitious sounds or indications of pulmonary congestion. Pulse oximetry should be used to assist in assessment.

Suctioning and Tracheostomy Care

Patency of the newly created airway is vital, and frequent suctioning is necessary because of increased secretions from the tracheobronchial tree caused by trauma. Suctioning of the tracheostomy must be sterile and atraumatic; a sterile disposable catheter and glove should be used for each procedure. A suction catheter in a plastic sleeve provides a means of suctioning without the use of gloves and is most convenient for use in the PACU. Catheters should be smooth and small enough to pass easily into the lumen of the tracheostomy tube without obstructing it.

Table 32-1	Advantages and Disadvantages of Commonly Available Laser-Resistant Tracheal Tubes	
TUBE TYPE	**ADVANTAGES**	**DISADVANTAGES**
Metal	Atraumatic external surface Double cuff maintains seal even if punctured with laser Kink resistant	Thick-walled nonflammable cuff reflects laser and transfers heat Cuff difficult to deflate if punctured Metal may reflect beam onto nontargeted tissue
Polyvinyl chloride (PVC)	Inexpensive Nonreflective Maintains shape well Double cuff maintains seal after proximal cuff puncture	Burns vigorously and yields pulmonary toxin (hydrogen chloride) Cuffed version contains flammable material
Red rubber	Wrapping protects flammable material but dries tube Maintains structure Nonreflective	Highly flammable Thick-walled tubes
Silicone rubber	Wrapping protects flammable material Methylene blue aids in detection of cuff perforation Nonreflective	Contains flammable material Turns to toxic ash Single cuff is vulnerable to laser damage

From Nagelhout J, Plaus K: *Nurse anesthesia*, ed 4, St. Louis, 2009, Saunders.

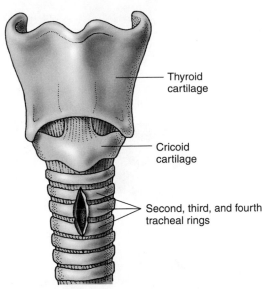

Thyroid cartilage

Cricoid cartilage

Second, third, and fourth tracheal rings

FIG. 32-5 Incision for tracheostomy. (From Ignatavicius DD, Workman ML: *Medical-surgical nursing: patient-centered collaborative care,* ed 6, St. Louis, 2010, Saunders.)

BOX 32-3	Bedside Equipment Needed for a Patient with Tracheostomy

- Suction equipment
- Respirator
- Ambu or anesthesia bag
- Extra sterile tracheostomy tray, including tracheostomy tubes of proper size, sterile forceps, tracheal hook, and Trousseau tracheal dilator (see Box 32-2)
- Sterile gauze squares
- Sterile scissors
- Tracheostomy ties
- Cleaning solutions for the tracheostomy tube and the incision
- Syringe
- Hemostat (for inflation of the tracheostomy tube cuff)

As with any suctioning technique, the patient should undergo hyperventilation with increased FiO_2 both before and after the procedure. For suctioning, insert the catheter 6 to 8 inches into the tracheostomy tube. Do not apply suction during insertion. Apply suction intermittently by occluding the air valve with the thumb and at the same time slowly withdrawing the catheter in a twisting motion. Suctioning should not continue for longer than 5 seconds. Time should

be allotted between each suctioning for adequate oxygenation of the patient. Suctioning often stimulates forceful coughing, which is effective in producing secretions; therefore the nurse should be prepared to wipe expelled secretions away from the tracheostomy tube orifice with plain gauze squares. To determine the effectiveness of the suctioning, the chest should be auscultated immediately afterward.

If deep suctioning is indicated, a coudé tip catheter should be used. Insert the catheter with the tip pointing in the direction of the main stem bronchus to be suctioned. Recent evidence indicates that positioning the patient's head to the left or the right has little effect, if any, on which bronchus is entered.

If the patient's secretions are exceptionally thick, the physician may order instillation of 3 to 5 mL of sterile normal saline solution into the tracheostomy tube to help loosen secretions and promote coughing. Although this procedure is common, whether it is actually effective is questionable; if the normal saline solution is not immediately removed with suctioning, it may produce the effects of any inhaled fluid and act as a contaminant. More effective measures to ensure liquefaction of secretions include providing inspired air that is well humidified and ensuring that the patient is well hydrated.[2,3]

Immediate postanesthesia care of the patient with a new tracheostomy also includes care and cleaning of the tracheostomy tube, which may be necessary as often as every hour. A variety of methods can be used to clean the inner cannula of the tracheostomy tube, including normal saline solution and hydrogen peroxide or 2% sodium bicarbonate solution. A small test tube brush or pipe cleaners can be used to scrub sticky crusts of mucus. Regardless of the method, the procedure must be sterile, and no supplies should be used that may leave on the cannula any lint or other debris that may be inhaled by the patient.

Wound drainage from the tracheostomy is generally minimal; however, soiling of the tracheostomy dressing occurs from secretions and sweating.[2] The dressings should be changed as often as necessary, and the skin should be kept clean and dry to prevent maceration and infection. The skin around the stoma should be cleansed with hydrogen peroxide and normal saline solution and dried with sterile gauze pads, and an antibiotic ointment such as bacitracin should be applied. The tracheostomy dressing should be plain gauze with the edges bound and should have no cotton filling or loose strings. Special tracheostomy "pants" that fit over the tracheostomy tube and have all edges sewn make the best dressing. Sterile gauze may be

A

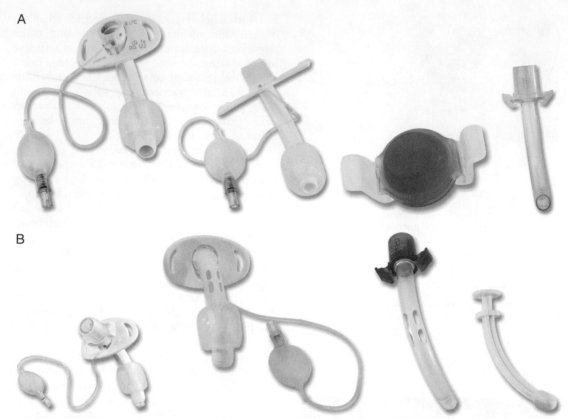

B

FIG. 32-6 Tracheostomy tubes. **A,** Dual-lumen cuffed tracheostomy tubes, disposable decannulation plug, and disposable inner cannula. **B,** Dual-lumen cuffed fenestrated tracheostomy tubes, disposable fenestrated inner cannula, and obturator. (Images used by permission from Nellcor Puritan Bennett LLC, Boulder, Colorado, doing business as Covidien.)

cut halfway to the center and fitted over the tube (Fig. 32-7); however, this approach has the disadvantage of cut edges that may fray and allow bits of gauze to enter the wound or the trachea.

Fabric tapes or ties or Velcro devices are used to secure the tracheostomy tube in place; these should be checked frequently to ensure the proper tension. If they are too tight, they are uncomfortable for the patient and may compress the external jugular veins. If they are too loose, the cannula slides up and down in the trachea or is even expelled. When the tapes are tied so that one finger can easily slip underneath, the tension is right.

Complications

When complications of a tracheostomy occur, PACU nurses should be especially astute in observing for signs of danger. The most common complication is respiratory obstruction caused by

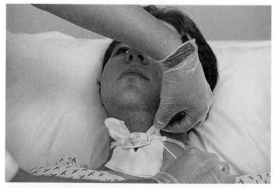

FIG. 32-7 Applying tracheostomy dressing. (From Potter PA, et al: *Fundamentals of nursing,* ed 8, St. Louis, 2013, Mosby.)

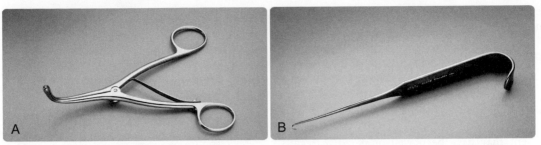

FIG. 32-8 **A,** Tracheal dilator. **B,** Tracheal hook. (From Wells MP: *Surgical instruments: a pocket guide,* ed 4, St. Louis, 2011, Saunders.)

external pressure, foreign bodies, tracheal edema, or excessive secretions. If suctioning does not relieve airway obstruction, the tracheostomy tube may be removed immediately, the tracheal stoma held open with a tracheal dilator and hook or forceps (Fig. 32-8), and the surgeon or anesthesia provider should be summoned.

Occasionally a tube is coughed out either because the ties are not sufficiently tight or because the tube is too short. If a tube is accidentally expelled, it must be reinserted by persons qualified to do so. In some institutions, nurses practice changing tracheostomy tubes under the supervision of physicians so that if accidental expulsion should occur in the PACU, the nurse is skilled in replacement. If the tube cannot be inserted easily, the stoma should be held open and the surgeon should be called.[2] Misplacement or displacement of the tube is a common complication and must be corrected immediately (Fig. 32-9).

Obstruction below the tracheostomy tube can create respiratory insufficiency. Respiratory adventitious sounds, unequal lung expansion, and marked respiratory efforts, including supraclavicular, intercostal, and substernal retractions, should alert the nurse to this problem and the physician should be notified.

Some bloody secretions from the tracheal stoma may be expected in the immediate postoperative period, but frank bleeding is abnormal and the surgeon should be notified.[2] Sometimes bleeding from a thyroid vein or other neck vessel next to the tube occurs and blood, which runs down into the trachea, is sprayed about with every cough. This situation is usually not serious and can often be controlled with local packing with petrolatum gauze. Occasionally, however, serious bleeding occurs and the patient must be taken back to the operating room, where the wound is reopened and the bleeding vessel ligated.

Subcutaneous emphysema can occur as a complication of tracheostomy if the wound is sutured

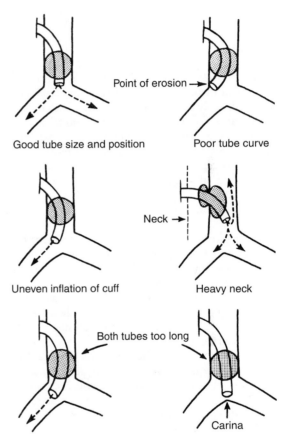

FIG. 32-9 Tracheostomy tube positions and factors that affect them. (From Murphy ER: Intensive nursing care in a respiratory unit, *Nurs Clin North Am* 3:433, 1968.)

too tightly about the tracheostomy tube, thus allowing air to enter the subcutaneous tissues, or it can result from an overly large incision or a partially obstructed tube. Although subcutaneous emphysema is annoying, it is usually not serious and generally clears after several days. If the nurse notices a crackling sensation under the skin of the neck, chest, or face of the patient, it should be

NURSING CARE IN THE PACU

reported to the surgeon because removal of a suture or two may readily correct this problem.

The complications of tracheostomy in infants and children are almost always more serious because the relative size of the airway is smaller and tolerance for any obstruction is lessened. Emotional support of the patient with a new tracheostomy is important and begins immediately on the patient regaining consciousness.[3] Although the patient may have been well prepared in regard to the loss of ability to speak, awakening in that state is still a traumatic event. A pad and pencil should be readily available to allow the patient to communicate.

Laryngectomy

Partial laryngectomy (Table 32-2) is the surgical treatment of choice for patients with a limited malignant process of the vocal cords. It is commonly performed through a laryngofissure, and tracheostomy is usually performed concomitantly to ensure a good airway during the immediate postoperative period. Postanesthesia nursing care is essentially the same as that for a patient after tracheostomy.[5]

Postoperative subcutaneous emphysema is not uncommon and should be reported to the surgeon. After laryngectomy, patients have trouble swallowing and need frequent suctioning and reassurance.

Supraglottic laryngectomy is performed for carcinoma of the epiglottis and adjacent structures above the level of the true vocal cords. A tracheostomy is mandatory for these patients; they also have a great deal of difficulty swallowing and need close observation and assistance with elimination of saliva and other secretions.[2,3]

Total laryngectomy is reserved for patients with advanced carcinoma of the true cords (Fig. 32-10). Tracheostomy is always performed.[5] Some means of communication should be established before surgery for postoperative use. Speech and language consultations should be performed preoperatively to determine the patients ability to care for a voice prosthetic.[2]

The primary nursing concern after laryngectomy is maintenance of an adequate airway.[3] Tracheostomy care, as previously discussed, should be deftly performed and the air well should be humidified. In the immediate postanesthesia period, patients need frequent suctioning, not only of the tracheostomy but also of the nose and mouth, because they cannot blow the nose and may have difficulty spitting.[2] Frequent mouth care provides additional comfort, and an ointment should be applied to the lips to prevent drying and cracking.

After surgery, the patient should be positioned on the side until full consciousness is regained.

While positioning, care should be taken not to cover the stoma. These patients are unable to breathe through the mouth or nose; they can breathe though only the newly created stoma.[2] When conscious, the patient may be positioned in a low semi-Fowler position with the head elevated approximately 30 degrees. This position promotes drainage, minimizes edema, prevents uncomfortable pressure on suture lines, and facilitates respirations.

Dressings should be checked frequently for excessive drainage and reinforced or changed as necessary. Sometimes drainage catheters are placed under the wound flaps for removal of fluid from the potential dead space left after removal of the larynx and related structures.[2] Drainage catheters must be connected to a constant vacuum source at 40 to 60 mm Hg, and free drainage must be maintained within the system, which can be accomplished with a Hemovac drainage device (Fig. 32-11). Excessive bloody drainage should be reported to the surgeon. The most common site of hemorrhage is the base of the tongue.

After laryngectomy, patients are frequently apprehensive on awakening and should have someone in close attendance at all times. Although patients may be prepared for the postoperative loss of the voice, the first experiences of being voiceless and unable to call for help are always extremely frightening. A bell to ring or other noisemaker is more reassuring in this instance than the routine pencil-and-paper communication system.

RADICAL NECK SURGERY

The radical neck procedure itself is relatively simple; it involves removal of all the subcutaneous fat, lymphatic channels, and some of the superficial muscles within a prescribed area of the neck (Fig. 32-12). Generally, the procedure involves the removal of the sternocleidomastoid muscle, omohyoid muscle, internal and external jugular veins, and all lymphatic tissue on one side of the neck.[2,5] The purposeful resection of the cranial nerve XI (spinal accessory) causes atrophy of the large trapezius muscle. In the modified neck dissection, the accessory nerve and the internal jugular vein are spared.

Postanesthesia nursing care of the patient after radical neck surgery is somewhat less demanding than that after laryngectomy, because these patients do not have a tracheostomy and can talk and eat normally. The patient should be placed in a low semi-Fowler position with the head elevated 30 to 45 degrees to improve venous return. Pillows must be used cautiously when patients are positioned to

Table 32-2   Laryngectomy

STRUCTURES REMOVED	STRUCTURES REMAINING	POSTOPERATIVE CONDITIONS
Total Laryngectomy		
Hyoid bone	Tongue	Loss of voice; breathing through tracheostomy; no problem swallowing
Entire larynx (epiglottis, false cords, true cords)	Pharyngeal walls	
Cricoid cartilage	Lower trachea	
Two or three rings of trachea		
Supraglottic or Horizontal Laryngectomy		
Hyoid bone	True vocal cords	Normal voice; occasional aspiration may occur, especially with liquids; normal airway
Epiglottis	Cricoid cartilage	
False vocal cords	Trachea	
Vertical (or hemi-) Laryngectomy		
One true vocal cord	Epiglottis	Hoarse but serviceable voice; normal airway; no problem swallowing
False cord	One false cord	
Arytenoid	One true vocal cord	
One half thyroid cartilage	Cricoid	
Laryngofissure and Partial Laryngectomy		
One vocal cord	All other structures	Hoarse but serviceable voice; occasionally almost normal voice; no airway problem; no swallowing problem
Endoscopic Removal of Early Carcinoma		
Part of one vocal cord	All other structures	Possibility of normal voice; no other problems

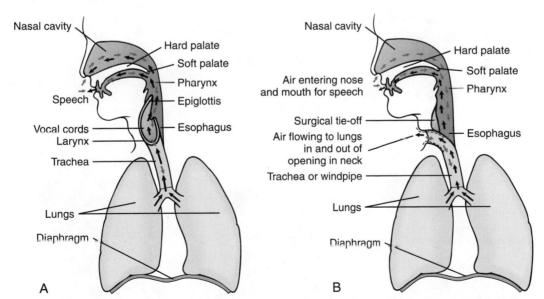

FIG. 32-10 Total laryngectomy. **A,** Normal airflow in and out of lungs. **B,** Airflow in and out of the lungs after a total laryngectomy. (From Lewis SL, et al: *Medical-surgical nursing: assessment and management of clinical problems*, ed 8, St. Louis, 2011, Mosby.)

NURSING CARE IN THE PACU

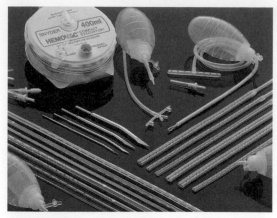

FIG. 32-11 Silicone evacuator (Snyder Hemovac drainage) device is closed suction apparatus and blood receptacle for facial and neck surgery. (Courtesy Zimmer, Inc., Warsaw, Ind.)

avoid restriction of venous return or compression of the bases of pedicle flaps. Venous congestion, when present, gives the patient's face a purplish hue. This hue can be differentiated from cyanosis caused by inadequate ventilation with observation of the color of the extremities to confirm good circulation and close monitoring of oxygen saturation. Postoperative pain is usually minimal after radical neck dissection and can be managed with the usual analgesics.

Dressings are minimal. Skin flaps are secured over drainage tubes, which should be connected to constant suction at 40 to 60 mm Hg.[5] The suction catheters constantly working under the skin flaps suck them firmly against the neck. Approximately 70 to 120 mL of serosanguineous drainage can be expected the day of operation. This amount drastically decreases the second day and becomes minimal (less than 30 mL) the third day. If the dressing soaks through with blood, the surgeon should be notified immediately.

Edema of the recurrent laryngeal nerve and of the nerves to the pharynx may cause difficulty in swallowing and in expectorating secretions; therefore frequent, gentle suctioning of oral secretions

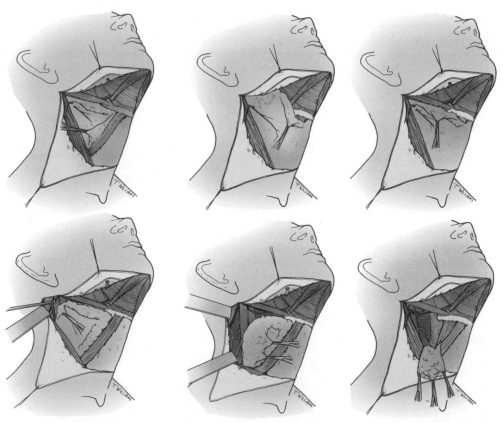

FIG. 32-12 Steps of modified radical neck dissection with preservation of spinal accessory nerve, internal jugular vein, and sternocleidomastoid muscle. (From Rothrock J: *Alexander's care of the patient in surgery,* ed 14, St. Louis, 2011, Mosby.)

may be needed. Extreme care must be taken to avoid any trauma to the internal suture lines. A gauze wick placed in the corner of the patient's mouth can alleviate the annoyance of constant dribbling of mucus and saliva. Mouth care is important for the comfort of this patient and can be accomplished with any of the conventional methods.

Complications

Edema of the lower part of the face on the same side as the surgery is to be expected. Lower facial paralysis may occur because of injury of the facial nerve during dissection. The most common complication after radical neck dissection is hemorrhage, which is most often the result of inadequate hemostasis in the immediate postoperative period.[3] The most serious complication is rupture of the carotid artery ("carotid blowout"). This event is uncommon and occurs almost exclusively when radical neck dissection is combined with total laryngectomy. It is more likely to occur in a patient who before surgery has had a course of radiation therapy or who has a fistula that bathes the carotid artery in secretions. If the danger of a rupture of the carotid artery is present, all personnel should be aware of it and know what to do if it occurs.

If a carotid rupture occurs, digital pressure with gauze pads, bath towels, or anything available should be applied immediately and help should be summoned. Intravenous fluids must be started immediately if they are not already infusing. Fluids should be administered at an increased rate to replace loss and combat shock. The nurse should inflate the cuff on the tracheostomy tube and perform tracheal suctioning to prevent aspiration of blood. Most importantly, a patent airway needs to be maintained and oxygen needs to be administered. Patients requiring carotid precautions—that is, those who may have this complication—should be typed and cross-matched for whole blood, and appropriate emergency equipment, including gauze pads, vascular clips, and suture ties, should be immediately available at the bedside.

Reconstruction Surgery in Head and Neck Cancer

A large variety of reconstructive procedures can be used to reestablish both contour and function after the removal of large areas of the head and neck for malignant disease. Skin grafts have largely been replaced with skin flaps or muscle-skin combined flaps that can cover extensive areas both inside and outside the neck. These flaps provide a lining of the throat or mouth and can also replace excised skin on the external surfaces.[2] The commonly used flaps are the pectoralis major muscle-skin unit and the deltopectoral flap, both from the anterior chest area. In rare instances, a free flap may be used. This flap is usually a muscle-skin flap that is moved a long distance from one area of the body to another. For this procedure to be successful, this type of flap requires the microsurgical repair of its tiny artery and vein with an artery and vein in its new location. In general, these reconstructive flaps must be free of any pressure or dressings. A light coat of antibacterial ointment is usually applied along the suture lines, and the area is frequently observed for color, warmth, and bleeding. Because these flaps depend on a single small artery and vein, any kinking or external pressure may result in the death of the flap.

MAXILLOFACIAL SURGERY

The care of patients with extensive maxillofacial surgery follows the principles outlined earlier for tracheostomy care and care after laryngectomy or radical neck dissection. The care of these patients is extremely demanding, and attention to detail is the basis for the prevention of complications.

Maxillofacial surgery may be needed to correct trauma and fractures or congenital skeletal deformities. After this type of surgery, the patient is in intermaxillary fixation (IMF) with the jaws wired shut.[2] Care revolves around protection of the airway and includes wire cutters at the bedside.[3] Maxillofacial surgery is lengthy, and the anesthesia time can exceed 3 hours. As a result, the patient usually arrives in the PACU in a rather sleepy condition and has a slow emergence from the anesthesia; yet in most cases, the patient is able to respond to stimuli and verbal commands.

Some additional emergency equipment is needed at the bedside of patients who are admitted with IMF, including wire cutters, a suture set, additional nasal airways, small suction catheters, and gauze pads.[2] On admission of the patient, the surgeon should review placement of the IMF wires with the nurse.[3] A line drawing of these wires that indicates which to cut in case of extreme emergency (e.g., cardiac or respiratory arrest) should be posted at the head of the bed.

Preoperative preparation of the patient who is undergoing IMF is particularly important and should include instructions on how to clear secretions or remove vomitus while remaining in IMF. The patient should also be taught how to use the suction catheter. These instructions have to be repeated frequently in the PACU as the patient recovers. Having the jaws wired closed is a frightening experience for any patient, no matter how

NURSING CARE IN THE PACU

well prepared that patient is. Blood, emesis, lingual and pharyngeal edema, hematoma formation, or laryngospasm may further compromise the oral airway, which is already obstructed as much as 90% by fixation of the jaws. Reassurance is provided with proximity to the patient, ensuring a means to attract attention, and explaining fully all treatments and procedures.

The patient arrives in the PACU with a nasotracheal tube in place. Extubation should not be considered until the patient is fully awake and reflexes have returned sufficiently to allow handling of secretions. A soft nasal airway may be inserted after extubation to assist in maintenance of a patent airway.

The patients should be observed closely for bleeding. Some oozing of blood is normal, but excessive amounts should be reported to the surgeon. Frequent gentle suctioning with a small catheter assists in keeping the airway clear by removing blood and saliva. The patient may be more comfortable doing this independently when able. A suction catheter in hand for use as necessary is reassuring to these patients.

Vomiting and subsequent aspiration is a significant risk for this patient. A nasogastric tube is frequently used to reduce the likelihood of nausea and vomiting.[3] The nurse should ensure that the tube is correctly positioned and patent. Antiemetics should be administered as necessary, and pain should be treated promptly to prevent nausea and vomiting.

Despite all efforts at prevention, vomiting may occur. If still drowsy, the patient should be turned immediately to the lateral or semiprone position, and the emesis should be suctioned via the nose or mouth. If the patient is awake, the nurse should help the patient sit up, lean over, and allow emesis to flow from the mouth and nose. The cheeks are retracted by holding them out with the fingers. Most importantly, instructions and reassurances need to be repeated quietly but confidently to keep the patient calm. Rarely is cutting the wires necessary, but if any question exists, an anesthesia practitioner should be notified immediately; with a team approach, airway management and resolution of the postoperative nausea and vomiting (PONV) should be initiated.

The patient should be positioned with the head of the bed elevated 30 degrees to assist in maintaining the airway with control of edema. Ice packs are usually ordered after surgery to assist in control of edema and to promote comfort. A surgical glove partially filled with cracked ice can be used, or ice collars can be molded to the jaws, chin, or nose. Iced saline solution gauze pads may be applied to the eyes.

Ointment or other emollient cream should be applied to the lips and corners of the mouth to relieve tenderness and prevent drying and cracking. Dental wax can be molded and applied to protruding wires, which are highly irritating to the oral mucosa.

When the patient is fully awake and protective reflexes have sufficiently returned, rinsing the mouth with warm saline solution provides additional comfort. The patient may then also have small sips of liquids.

SUMMARY

Perianesthesia care of the patient after ENT and maxillofacial surgery requires basic knowledge of the pathophysiology of the face and neck. Advanced airway management skills are important in rendering nursing care to these patients. The perianesthesia nurse must also use enhanced behavioral techniques to aid the patient through the initial fear and anxiety generated by the many appliances and devices that can be placed about the oral airway. Patients who undergo maxillofacial surgery may have serious complications from the possibility of the jaw being wired or rubber bands placed to stabilize the jaw. As a result, complications such as delayed emergence from lengthy surgery and anesthesia time, possible airway obstruction from bleeding, edema, and the possibility PONV all become serious.

REFERENCES

1. Hamlin L, et al: *Perioperative nursing: an introductory text*, Sydney, Australia, 2009, Mosby.
2. Stannard D, Krenzischek D: *Perianesthesia nursing care: a bedside guide for safe recovery*, Sudenbury, Mass, 2012, Jones and Bartlett Learning.
3. Schick L, Windle PE: *Perianesthesia nursing core curriculum: preprocedure, phase I and phase II PACU nursing*, ed 2, St. Louis, 2010, Saunders.
4. Burton M, et al: Extracts from the Cochrane library: grommets (ventilation tubes) for hearing loss associated with otitis media with effusion in children, *Otolaryngol Head and Neck Surg* 14:657–651, 2011.
5. Rothrock J: *Alexander's care of the patient in surgery*, ed 14, St. Louis, 2011, Mosby.
6. Stoelting R, Miller R: *Basics of anesthesia*, ed 6, Philadelphia, 2011, Churchill Livingstone.
7. Lakdawala L: Creating a safer perioperative environment with an obstruction sleep apnea screening tool, *J Perianesth Nurs* 26(1):15–24, 2011.
8. Nelson M, et al: Pathologic evaluation of routine pediatric tonsillectomy specimens: analysis cost-effectiveness, *Otolaryng Head and Neck Surg* 144(5):778–783, 2011.
9. Ball K: *Lasers: the perioperative challenge*, ed 3, Denver, 2004, AORN.

RESOURCES

Aitkenhead A, et al: *Textbook of anaesthesia*, ed 5, London, 2007, Churchill Livingstone.

Alspach J: *Core curriculum for critical care nursing*, ed 6, Philadelphia, 2006, Saunders.

Atlee J: *Complications in anesthesia*, ed 2, Philadelphia, 2007, Saunders.

Balkany TJ: The Cochlear implant, *Otolaryngol Clin North Am* 19:217–449, 1986.

Barash P, et al: *Clinical anesthesia*, ed 5, Philadelphia, 2005, Lippincott Williams & Wilkins.

Bickley L, Szilagy P: *Bates' guide to physical examination and history taking*, ed 9, Philadelphia, 2005, Lippincott Williams & Wilkins.

Cote C, et al: *A practice of anesthesia for infants and children*, ed 3, Philadelphia, 2001, Saunders.

Drake R, et al: *Gray's anatomy for students*, ed 2, Philadelphia, 2009, Churchill Livingstone.

Fisher L: *Benumof's anesthesia and uncommon diseases*, ed 5, Philadelphia, 2007, Saunders.

Frost CM, Frost DE: Nursing care of patients in intermaxillary fixation, *Heart Lung* 12(5):524–528, 1983.

Gallager C, Issenberg B: *Simulation in anesthesia*, Philadelphia, 2007, Saunders.

Ganong W: *Review of medical physiology*, ed 22, New York, 2005, McGraw-Hill Medical.

Miller R, et al: *Miller's anesthesia*, ed 7, Philadelphia, 2009, Churchill Livingstone.

Murray J, Nadel J: *Textbook of respiratory medicine*, ed 4, Philadelphia, 2005, Saunders.

Nagelhout J, Plaus K: *Nurse anesthesia*, ed 4, St. Louis, 2009, Saunders.

Pop RS, et al: Perianesthesia nurses' pain management after tonsillectomy and adenoidectomy: pediatric patient outcomes, *J Perianethes Nurs* 22:91–101, 2007.

Rook JL, Rook M: Head and neck cancer, *J Post Anesth Nurs* 4(6):263–277, 1989.

Shorten G, et al: *Postoperative pain management: an evidence-based guide to practice*, Philadelphia, 2006, Saunders.

Smalley PJ: Lasers in otolaryngology, *Nurs Clin North Am* 25(3):645–655, 1990.

Townsend CM, et al: *Sabiston textbook of surgery: the biological basis of modern surgical practice*, ed 19, Philadelphia, 2012, Saunders.

Carolyn G. Baddeley, BSN, MSN, APN, CRNA

Caring for the ophthalmic surgical patient offers unique challenges to the perianesthesia nurse. It requires a thorough understanding of not only the surgical aspect of the patient's care, but also the pharmacologic, physiologic, and emotional concerns. As the need for maintaining quality patient care and controlling overall medical costs continues to grow, many surgical advances have taken the most complex of ophthalmic procedures from hospital-based operating rooms to free-standing ambulatory surgery centers, thus enabling more patients to return home within 24 hours of surgery.[1] This trend alone necessitates that the perianesthesia nurse have a fundamental knowledge base to anticipate an array of patients' preoperative and postoperative needs. Recognizing and treating a variety of complex symptoms and complications, providing sufficient patient education, and planning discharge are just a few of the many needs with which the perianesthesia nurse will have to contend on a daily basis. Ophthalmic surgical patients vary widely in age. Any age-appropriate special needs or medical concerns should be identified by the perianesthesia nurse during the preadmission evaluation time. Knowledge of comorbidities in elderly patients becomes even more important when the amount of time with each patient is limited. Hypertension, diabetes mellitus, coronary artery, cerebral vascular, and renal disease are just a few examples. Despite the fact that ophthalmic surgery is most common in the elderly, advances in anesthesia, surgical techniques, and surgical instrumentation have allowed the most sophisticated procedures to be performed on the most fragile of the pediatric population (i.e., premature infants and neonates).[2] Normal growth and development in the pediatric patient should be assessed and any variances should be noted. These comorbidities and other factors may predispose patients to sudden and potentially life-threatening postoperative complications.[3] Close attention to the preoperative assessment is of utmost importance. Working with this wide range in patient population, certifications in advanced cardiac life support (ACLS) and pediatric advanced life support (PALS) are essential in the educational foundation for the perianesthesia nurse.

DEFINITIONS

Amblyopia: Condition in which there is a lack of development of central vision in one eye because of a failure in using both eyes simultaneously ("lazy eye"). It primarily develops before 6 years of age and can have complete recovery with early diagnosis and treatment. Treatment is a combination therapy approach with prescriptive lenses, eye patching, prisms, and vision therapy.

Anterior Segment: The anterior one-third segment of the globe, extending from the anterior hyaloid face filled with aqueous fluid.

Blepharophimosis: Abnormal narrowing of the palpebral fissures or eye lids.

Blepharoplasty: Removal of excess tissue, fatty deposits, or tightening of the skeletal muscle from the upper or lower eyelids to increase range of vision by reduced sagging of excess skin.

Cataract: An opacity clouding that is found most commonly in the lens and the cortex of the eye.

Chalazion: A small eyelid cyst that is a result of chronic inflammation of a meibomian gland.

Choroid: The spongelike vascular membrane in the globe between the sclera and the retina, supplying nutrients to the retina.

Choroidal Melanoma: A rare form of cancer found in the spongelike vascular membrane of the eye. It is the most common form of cancer of the eye in the adult population.

Ciliary Body: A ring of tissue that encircles the lens of the eye, containing smooth muscle fibers and capillaries.

Ciliary Muscle: Smooth muscle fibers located in the ciliary body that control the shape of the lens.

Ciliary Process: Pigmented ridges located in the smooth muscle fibers surrounding the lens that contain capillaries that secrete aqueous humor into the anterior segment of the eye.

Dacryocystitis: Infection of the lacrimal sac.

Dacryocystorhinostomy: A procedure in which a new pathway is created from the lacrimal sac to the nasal passageway.

Deep Lamellar Endothelial Keratoplasty: Transplantation of the cornea in which the epithelium of the cornea is replaced without an incision in the anterior corneal surface.

Dermatochalasis: Excess tissue, fatty deposits, or excess relaxation of the skeletal muscle of the upper or lower eyelids.

Descemet's Stripping Endothelial Keratoplasty: Transplantation of the corneal inner endothelium and its underlying membrane via two small incisions.

Ectropian: Eversion of the eyelid (typically the lower lid). Surgical correction is performed by horizontally shortening the lid.

Entropian: Inversion of the eyelid (typically the lower lid), which causes the eyelashes to continually rub against the surface of the eye. Surgical treatment is performed by one of two ways, both of which anastomose the lid after removing a small section of the skin, muscle, and tendon.

Enucleation: Complete removal of the eye globe.

Epiphora: Excessive tear production. Can be caused by secondary lacrimal duct obstruction.

Evisceration of the Eye: Removal of the entire contents of the eye globe, leaving the sclera and extraocular muscles intact.

Glaucoma: A family of eye diseases characterized by increased intraocular pressure resulting in permanent optic nerve damage and visual loss. Surgical treatment is aimed at reestablishing the outflow of aqueous fluid. Nearly all procedures are so-called filtration operations (e.g., trabeculectomy or tube shunt procedures).

Goniotomy: A surgical procedure for congenital glaucoma in which a 90- to 120-degree arc incision is made within the anterior trabecular meshwork of the eye.

Hydroxyapatite Implant: An implant that is a complex calcium phosphate salt made from coral. Placed after an enucleation, the implant is less likely to be rejected because of its resemblance of human bone in its chemical and porous properties. The orbital tissues are attached directly and a prosthesis placed over it. The implant becomes integrated over time with blood vessels and tissue, thus allowing for a more realistic appearance and movement.

Intraocular Lens Implant (IOL): An artificial lens implanted to replace the crystalline lens after removal in cataract surgery. IOLs are made in a variety of styles and from a variety of materials. One of the newest and smallest multifocal IOLs is a pliable, foldable lens that can be inserted through an incision of 1.4 mm or smaller.

Keratoplasty: Replacement of the diseased, central portion of the cornea with donor tissue. A cookie-cutter–like trephine is used on both the donor and recipient cornea.

Lacrimal Punctum: The opening of the lacrimal duct at either the upper or lower eyelid at the inner canthus of the eye.

Laser-Assisted In Situ Keratomileusis (LASIK): A surgical procedure used to correct nearsightedness (myopia), farsightedness (hyperopia), and astigmatism in which an excimer laser is used to remove inner layers of cornea tissue, thereby reshaping it.

Miosis: Contraction of the pupil induced by light or eye drops.

Mydriasis: Dilation of the pupils usually induced by eye drops, but also induced by lack of light.

Oculocardiac Reflex (OCR): A sudden onset bradycardia elicited by traction on the extraocular muscles, especially the medial rectus, or by direct pressure on the eye globe. This reflex is a trigeminovagal reflex arc. It can also cause cardiac dysrhythmias such as ventricular ectopy, sinus arrest, and ventricular fibrillation. The pediatric population is especially sensitive to OCR.

Phacoemulsification: Fragmentation and removal of the lens with ultrasonic vibrations while aspirating during cataract surgery.

Plaque Therapy: A highly concentrated radiation implant most commonly used in the treatment of choroidal melanoma.

Presbyopia: A condition associated with aging whereby the lens loses its flexibility and the ability to focus on objects up close.

Proliferative Diabetic Retinopathy: The latter stages of diabetic retinopathy in which a proliferative growth of abnormal new blood vessels develop from the retina. These vessels can lead to vitreous hemorrhages and detachment of the retina.

Proptosis or Exophthalmos: Protrusion of the eyeball.

Pterygium: A benign growth of the conjunctiva that extends to the cornea at approximately a 3 o'clock or a 9 o'clock position. It is caused by excessive exposure to ultraviolet light (sunlight) or wind. Excision becomes necessary when visual disturbances become present.

Ptosis: Drooping of the upper eyelid. Surgery involves various procedures on the upper eyelid and/or the levator muscle.

Retinoblastoma: A malignant tumor of the retina that occurs predominantly in early childhood.

Retinopexy: Surgical procedure to correct a retinal tear. This is done by causing scar formation to occur with the use of laser photocoagulation, electric current, or cryotherapy.

Scleral Buckle: A piece of silicone plastic or sponge material that is surgically sewn onto the sclera in order to correct a retinal detachment via compression of the sclera against the retina. This procedure is often used in conjunction with a retinopexy, often with a pars plana vitrectomy.

Strabismus: A condition in which the eyes are not properly aligned and the extraocular muscles lack coordinated muscle movements. Inward deviation is called *esotropia*, and outward deviation is called *exotropia*. Surgical correction is performed by either shortening and removal of part of the tendon or lengthening a muscle via transfer of the muscle insertion site posterior to the original attachment point on the eye. It is occasionally treated with glasses or drops; however, it can lead to amblyopia if not treated in a timely manner.

Tonometer: An instrument used for the measurement of intraocular pressure. Can be hand-held or mounted to a slit lamp microscope. Requires topical anesthesia via eye drops, unless a noncontact "air pull" instrument is used.

Trabecular Meshwork: A ring of spongelike tissue through which aqueous humor drains to control the intraocular pressure.

Trabeculectomy: A surgical procedure to create a drainage channel from the anterior chamber to the subconjunctival space to lower intraocular pressure, for treatment of uncontrolled glaucoma.

NURSING CARE IN THE PACU

Vitrectomy: Surgical removal of the vitreous gel within the eye. Performed to clear blood that is occluding vision, to sever vitreous traction bands that are pulling on the retina, or to help with the repair of a retinal detachment. The removed vitreous is replaced with fluid, specialized gas, or silicone oil.

Vitreous Fluid: A clear, jellylike substance that fills the posterior chamber of the eye.

Vitreous Hemorrhage: Bleeding within the vitreous fluid that is usually the result of proliferative diabetic retinopathy, a retinal tear, detachment, or trauma.

Zonule of Zinn: A ring of fibrous strands that connects the ciliary processes with the crystalline lens of the eye. The eye focuses (accommodates) by the ciliary muscle exerting traction on the zonules, thereby changing the shape of the lens.

PREOPERATIVE EVALUATION

Preadmission evaluations are a critical tool for the perianesthesia nurse. Many hospitals and free-standing ambulatory surgery facilities have established preadmission testing clinics with guidelines designed for this purpose. The goals of the preoperative evaluation in the surgical patient is to obtain informed consent, perform physical assessments, arrange for laboratory tests and any necessary consultations, prescreen for any diseases, and provide patient education to reduce patient and caregiver anxiety. Upon evaluation, if the need for further medical testing arises, the patient can then be referred to their primary care physician or to a subspecialty to obtain medical clearance.[4] A preadmission evaluation can decrease cancellations, provide ample time to establish rapport, and assess for any psychological or psychosocial needs that can be addressed before the actual day of surgery. In a 10-year observational study, Jiménez and colleagues[5] concluded that 57.1% of surgical cases that were cancelled had a preventable or possibly preventable cause. With preadmission evaluations, this percentage can be greatly reduced, thereby decreasing the anxiety and frustration level of patients, caregivers, and health care team members on the day of surgery.

OPHTHALMIC MEDICATIONS

Most ophthalmic medications are administered topically in highly concentrated solutions (Table 33-1). Because of the highly vascular nature of the conjunctival sac and the nasolacrimal duct leading to the vascular mucosa of the nasopharynx, undesirable systemic effects can be caused by the rapid systemic absorption of topical solutions that are administered.[6] These medications

can also significantly alter a patient's reaction to anesthetic drugs, thus causing changes in the intraocular dynamics.[1] It is essential that the perianesthesia nurse learn to identify these medications and their potential systemic effects. The elderly patient is at higher risk for these severe systemic effects. This age group takes a higher number of prescription medications and undergoes a higher percentage of eye surgeries than any other age group.[7]

In order to easily identify the specific classifications of topical ocular medications, the American Academy of Ophthalmology (AAO), with input from pharmaceutical companies and the U.S. Food and Drug Administration (FDA), developed a universal color-coding system to distinguish between all topical ophthalmic medications. The color-coded system identifies every pharmaceutical class with its own unique cap-and-label color scheme (Table 33-2). With the introduction and implementation of the voluntary color-coding system, the AAO expects to "decrease the amount of serious adverse events resulting from patients (and medical personnel) difficulty in distinguishing between various ocular medications."[8] The threefold partnership of voluntary cooperation between the FDA, the pharmaceutical industry, and the AAO has proved effective and advantageous in the primary interest of patient safety since its inception.

PREOPERATIVE PHASE

Patients undergoing eye surgery have more apprehension and will need more constant verbal communication and reassurance.[9] Using this opportunity, the perianesthesia nurse should review any preoperative education and postoperative instructions with the patient and any caregivers present. Expectations regarding the operative procedure's outcome should also be explored. It is important that the patient and caregiver have realistic expectations. The more information and education that can be given to a patient and caregiver about the anticipated perioperative and postoperative course, the less amount of anxiety the patient will have and the fewer antianxiety medications that will be required.[10] All preoperative lab work, medical tests, and clearance letters should be reviewed to ensure that all paperwork is in order and placed on the chart. The nurse should also verify each patient's name, the operative eye, and procedure to be performed. Planned preoperative medications should be discussed. Depending on the type of ophthalmic procedure to be performed, ophthalmic medications may be administered in the preoperative holding area. A

Table 33-1	Ophthalmic Medications		
PHARMACOLOGIC CATEGORY	**NAME OF MEDICATION**	**CLINICAL INDICATION**	**SYSTEMIC EFFECTS**

Adrenergic agonists	Alphagan P
	Combigan
		Decreases IOP via
		  decrease in aqueous
		  humor production
			Oral dryness
			Visual disturbance, dizziness
			Bradycardia, hypotension,
			  nausea

α-Adrenergic agonist β-Adrenergic agonist	Epinephrine Apraclonidine Phenylephrine	Mydriasis Decreases IOP Potent vasoconstrictor	Hypertension, bradycardia, tachycardia Headache, sedation Dysrythmias

Anticholinergic
Muscarinic agonist
	Cyclopentolate
	Tropicamide
	Atropine
	Scopolamine
		Cycloplegia
		Prolonged Mydriasis
			Central anticholinergic
			  syndrome
			Tachycardia, flushing, dry skin,
			  thirst
			Elderly may display agitation
			  or CNS excitation

Anticholinesterases	Echothiophate
	Phospholine Iodide
		Induce miosis
		Increased aqueous
		  drainage
			Bradycardia, bronchospasm
			Reduction in plasma
			  cholinesterase for up
			  to 3-7 wk after being
			  discontinued
			Prolonged duration of action
			  for procaine, chloroprocaine,
			  and succinylcholine

Nonsteroidal
  antiinflammatory
	Diclofenac
	Nevanac
	Ketorolac
		Decrease postoperative
		  inflammation and
		  pain
			Burning sensation
			Headache
			Rhinitis, facial edema
			Abdominal pain, nausea
			Delayed wound healing

Steroidal antiinflammatory	Alrex Maxidex Pred Forte Zylet	Decrease inflammation	Increased IOP Delayed wound healing Rare hypercorticoidism

β-Adrenergic antagonist	Betimol
	Combigan
	Cosopt
	Timolol
		Mydriasis	Lightheadedness, fatigue,
			  disorientation
			General CNS depression
			Bradycardia, palpitations,
			  syncope, increase in heart
			  block, and CHF
			Bronchospasm

Carbonic anhydrase
  inhibitor
	Azopt
	Acetazolamide
	Diamox
		Decreases IOP via
		  decreased production
		  of aqueous humor
			Confusion, tinnitus
			Flushing, headache, polyuria
			Electrolyte imbalance
			Dyspepsia after long-term
			  use
			IV administration can cause
			  acute hypotension

Cholinergic agonist	Acetylcholine
	Pilocarpine
	Miochol-E
		Induce miosis	Headache, bradycardia,
			  hypotension, flushing,
			  and bronchospasm
			May inhibit focusing

Prostaglandin	Lumigan
	Tavatan Z
	Xalatan
		Decreases IOP via
		  increasing outflow
		  of aqueous humor
			Ocular dryness, visual
			  disturbances
			Headache, increased risk of
			  infections

Miscellaneous	Fluorescein	Intravascular dye for
		  evaluation of retinal
		  vasculature
			Urticaria, rhinorrhea, dizziness,
			  pharyngoedema
			Nausea and vomiting

From Physician's Desk Reference: *PDR for ophthalmic medicines*, ed 36, Montvale, NJ, 2008, Thomson Healthcare.
IOP, Intraocular pressure; *CNS*, central nervous system; *CHF*, congestive heart failure; *IV*, intravenous;

NURSING CARE IN THE PACU

Table 33-2	Ophthalmic Medication Color-Coding System
CLASS	**COLOR**
Adrenergic agonists	Purple
Antiinfectives, antimicrobials, antivirals, antifungals	Tan
Antiinflammatories, steroids	Pink
β-Blockers	Yellow
β-Blocker combinations	Dark Blue
Carbonic anhydrase inhibitors	Orange
Miotics	Dark Green
Mydriatics and cycloplegics	Red
Nonsteroidal antiinflammatories	Gray
Prostaglandin analogues	Turquoise

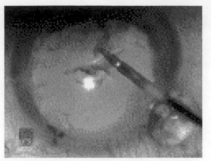

FIG. 33-1 Microincision phacoemulsification is a technologic advance that allows surgeon to operate through wounds nearly half the size of usual phacoemulsification. (From Alio J, et al: Outcomes of microincision cataract surgery versus coaxial phacoemulsification, *Ophthalmology* 112(11):1999, 2005.)

significant reduction of systemic absorption can be achieved by occluding the nasolacrimal duct by pressing on the inner canthus of the eye or closing the eyelids for at least 3 minutes immediately following the administration of ophthalmic medications. Doing so will reduce the chances of undesirable systemic side effects.[1]

ANESTHETIC OPTIONS

The determination of the type of anesthesia to be used belongs to the surgeon, the anesthesia provider and, most importantly, the patient. Factors that influence this decision are the type and length of the procedure to be performed, the physical status of the patient, and the ability of the patient to remain still. Local anesthesia can appear less stressful and more beneficial to some patients, but to others the thought of being awake while having eye surgery is terrifying. For those patients, general anesthesia is safer and more acceptable. Children and other uncooperative adults also benefit from general anesthesia. Lack of patient cooperation and head or body movements could result in poor outcomes.

Local anesthesia can range from the topical instillation of 0.5% tetracaine anesthetic drops to an injection of a local anesthetic. A patient with a relatively quick surgeon performing a simple anterior chamber cataract removal (Fig. 33-1), intraocular lens implantation (Fig. 33-2), or glaucoma procedure (Fig. 33-3) could have a topical anesthetic, provided the patient is cooperative. Intracorneal anesthesia is also used for cataract surgery. The surgeon injects a local anesthetic directly into the anterior chamber of the cornea where anesthesia is needed. The most common regional anesthetic techniques used in eye surgical cases are the peribulbar and retrobulbar blocks. These blocks

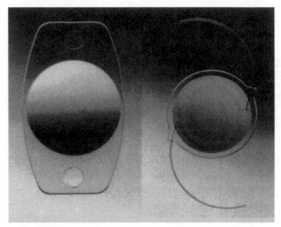

FIG. 33-2 Examples of intraocular lens implants used today. (Courtesy Wills Eye Hospital, Philadelphia, Penn.)

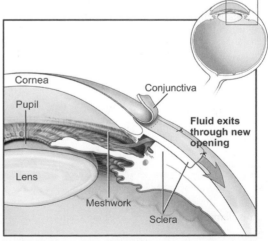

FIG. 33-3 Presurgical illustration of an anterior chamber in a glaucoma patient. (Courtesy National Eye Institute, National Institutes of Health, Bethesda, Md.)

are performed by the surgeon or the anesthesia provider after sufficient sedation has been given. A 23- to 25-gauge retrobulbar (blunt-tipped) needle is used to inject 2 to 5 mL of local anesthetic either into the peribulbar or retrobulbar space. Lidocaine 2% and bupivacaine 0.75% are the most common local anesthetics used. Epinephrine (1:200,000 or 1:400,000) may be premixed into the local anesthetic to cause vasoconstriction of the blood vessels, thus reducing bleeding and decreasing the absorption rate of the local anesthetic. It is important that the perianesthesia nurse be aware of these techniques and potential side effects, because assistance may be needed with the application of a local anesthetic. An eye that has had a successful retrobulbar block will not move during head turning. Complications are rare but can include: hemorrhage, globe perforation, optic nerve injury, oculocardiac reflex, instantaneous convulsions, and respiratory arrest. Other local blocks used alone or in conjunction with the peribulbar or retrobulbar blocks are the subtenon block and the facial nerve block. It is imperative that the patient be closely monitored for any signs or symptoms of any complications while they are in the preoperative area.[6]

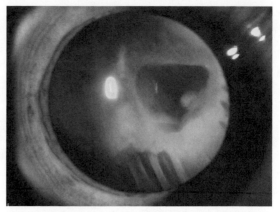

FIG. 33-4 Retinal detachment in Von Hippel-Lindau disease. (Courtesy National Eye Institute, National Institutes of Health, Bethesda, Md.)

PERIOPERATIVE PHASE

Numerous ophthalmic procedures are performed routinely. Most procedures are performed on an outpatient basis. A few exceptions include true ophthalmic emergencies such as chemical burns of the cornea, central retinal artery occlusion, open-globe injuries, endophthalmitis, acute narrow-angle glaucoma, acute retinal detachment (Fig. 33-4), corneal foreign body, and lid lacerations. These emergencies require surgical treatment within one to several hours. However, these procedures do not always necessitate an overnight admission to the hospital. If the patient is stable and able to meet discharge criteria, most physicians will discharge the patient, and schedule an appointment the following morning in the office. Semiurgent situations would include ocular tumors, blowout fractures of the orbit, congenital cataract (Fig. 33-5), and chronic retinal detachment. Treatment for these types of situations is usually started within days of the initial injury, but can be rescheduled for several weeks after an incident. Another reason for an overnight hospital admission would be for a prolonged procedure on a pediatric patient or a patient with an extensive medical history.[2]

Whatever the procedure to be performed, the risk of stimulating the oculocardiac reflex (OCR) is present. This reflex is a trigeminovagal reflex arc. It is elicited by traction on the extraocular

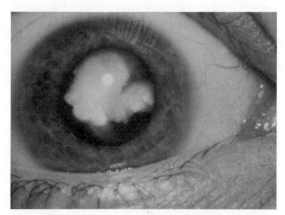

FIG. 33-5 A white congenital cataract. (Courtesy National Eye Institute, National Institutes of Health, Bethesda, Md.)

muscles, especially the medial rectus muscle, or by placing pressure directly on the globe. This reflex causes a sudden bradycardia and cardiac dysrhythmias, such as ventricular ectopy, sinus arrest, or ventricular fibrillation. Hypotension will usually accompany this sudden decrease in heart rate. Atropine or glycopyrrolate given before surgery intravenously (IV) can often aid in preventing the reflex. OCR is most commonly seen during strabismus surgery in the pediatric population. The reflex can occur during certain retinal or glaucoma procedures during which traction is applied to the rectus muscles. Nevertheless, the reflex is still present at any age and can be triggered by any ophthalmic procedure. When the reflex occurs, cessation of the surgical stimulation should provide relief within 10 to 20 seconds. Atropine (10 to 20 mcg/kg) or glycopyrrolate (10 mcg/kg) can also be administered if bradycardia persists. The use of retrobulbar blocks can aid in reducing the incidence of OCR; however, the reflex can also be triggered at the time of placement of the regional blockade. OCR is self-limiting, in that when the stimulation has ceased, the bradycardia will end. When normal sinus rhythm has return within 10% of the baseline heart rate, it is safe to proceed.[10]

POSTOPERATIVE PHASE

Upon arrival to the postanesthesia care unit (PACU), the anesthesia provider will give report to the PACU nurse. Report should include the procedure that was performed, any pertinent medical history of the patient, and any significant perioperative medications or events that have occurred. The PACU nurse will administer oxygen to the patient via a face mask and monitor the patient's heart rate and rhythm, blood pressure, oxygen saturation, temperature, and level of consciousness. The patient's condition will continually be monitored during this initial phase of recovery. The patient will typically respond to verbal stimuli and begin to follow commands within a short period of time. The level of postoperative care that a patient is required to have is determined by the "degree of underlying illness, the duration and complexity of anesthesia and surgery, and the risk of postoperative complications."[11]

As the patient emerges from general or regional anesthesia with sedation, the incidence of postoperative nausea and vomiting (PONV) is higher in the ophthalmic surgical patient than in other surgical procedures.[6,11] Other factors that can cause PONV are dehydration, hypotension, and pain. PONV avoidance should be a high priority. Antiemetics given perioperatively assist in decreasing the amount of PONV; however, ondansetron (2 to 4 mg IV) can be given as prophylaxis in the PACU, if not previously given.

If PONV persists, patients will not respond to a second dose of ondansetron because targeting an already blocked receptor is ineffective.[2] Promethazine (12.5 to 25 mg IV) is the next optimal choice. Another virtually unknown alternative treatment was studied by Pellegrini and colleagues.[12] In this comparison study, the inhalation of 70% isopropyl alcohol (IPA) from a standardized alcohol pad was used to successfully treat breakthrough PONV, after prophylactic treatment with ondansetron. The IPA group reported a faster time in reduction of PONV and an overall decrease in the antiemetic requirements. The implications of this study are fascinating, and the option of using IPA inhalational therapy for PONV is a viable one.

Evidence-Based Practice

In a randomized controlled study, Pellegrini and colleagues[12] evaluated the efficacy of using 70% isopropyl alcohol (IPA) in the treatment of postoperative nausea and vomiting (PONV) in two separate groups of patients that were high-risk for PONV. Patients were selected and randomly assigned into two different groups. Both groups received general anesthesia using similar medications and intravenous (IV) ondansetron intraoperatively before extubation. When the patients arrived in the postanesthesia care unit (PACU), the control group was given promethazine (12.5 to 25 mg IV) upon complaints of nausea. This dose could be repeated in 30 minutes up to a total dose of 50 mg IV. The experimental group of patients was treated with a commercially available 70% IPA pad upon complaints of nausea. The IPA pad was folded in half and placed 0.5 inches from the nares of the patient. The patient was then instructed to deeply inhale three times through their nose. The IPA treatments were to be given every 15 minutes for three applications. Demographics, a verbal numeric rating scale (VNRS) for nausea, the time it took to achieve a 50% reduction in the VNRS scores, and the overall antiemetic incidence of PONV per group were measured. The results showed no differences in the demographic variables or the baseline measurements between groups. There was a similar incidence in PONV between groups. However, the IPA group reported a faster overall time to 50% reduction in VNRS scores when compared to the control group. In addition, a decrease in the overall antiemetic requirements of the IPA group was noted.

IMPLICATIONS FOR PRACTICE

The overall effectiveness of IPA therapy in the treatment of PONV in high-risk postoperative patients is clearly shown in this study. The perianesthesia nurse should endeavor to seek the latest research information in regard to practical treatment modalities that would be beneficial to the patient. It is evident that IPA inhalation therapy can assist in alleviating PONV.

Source: Pellegrini J, et al: Comparison of inhalation of isopropyl alcohol vs promethazine in the treatment of postoperative nausea and vomiting (PONV) in patients identified as at high risk for developing PONV, *AANA J* 77:293–299, 2009.

Not all ophthalmic surgical patients will have postoperative pain. Patients who receive examinations under anesthesia, cataract removal, nasolacrimal duct probing, and some glaucoma surgery, pain is usually minimal. Topical and regional anesthetics are beneficial in that they will typically last throughout the procedure and into the immediate postoperative period. This will allow the patient to progress rapidly into phase II of recovery, from which discharge will be possible within a short amount of time. These patients typically arrive in the PACU awake and alert.[13] It is expected for those having longer ophthalmic procedures under general anesthesia to experience a moderate amount of pain. Opioid analgesics can cause nausea and vomiting, but the importance of controlling pain in the postoperative period takes priority. Opioid analgesics can also help to reduce coughing and decrease the incidence of emergence delirium in pediatric patients. Giving intravenous nonsteroidal antiinflammatory medications can also be a feasible option for controlling postoperative pain. Ketorolac (0.5 mg/kg) IV can be as effective as fentanyl (1 mcg/kg) or morphine (0.1 mg/kg) for postoperative pain in strabismus surgery patients without increasing PONV. Ketorolac has several advantages over opioids, in that it does not cause respiratory depression, sedation, or nausea and vomiting. A single dose will last approximately 6 to 8 hours. Conversely, ketorolac is eliminated through the kidneys and should not be given to patients with renal disease.[11]

Depending on the procedure, the patient will usually have some type of sterile dressing or patch covered by an eye shield over the operative eye (Fig. 33-6). It is imperative that this dressing is not disturbed by the patient. Damage can be done to delicate sutures, resulting in excessive bleeding and possibly an unexpected return to the operating room. Continual reorientation and vigilant observation of the patient is necessary to prevent rubbing the eyes or removing the dressing. A small amount of serosanguineous drainage can be expected. Reinforcement of the initial sterile dressing is appropriate. If the dressing becomes saturated or is removed in any way, the surgeon will need to be notified immediately to assess the operative eye and to replace the dressing.

Observation of patients until discharge criteria have been met is more beneficial than having a standard minimum time that each patient must remain in the PACU. Post anesthesia discharge scoring systems have been developed and used in many facilities to judge a patient's readiness for discharge. A standardized patient scoring system cannot substitute for a physical assessment by the perianesthesia nurse that accounts for the individual patient's needs. Before discharge, all of the patient's vital signs should be within normal limits. Pain, nausea, and vomiting should also be under control. Discharge criteria

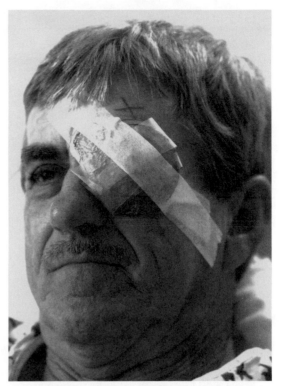

FIG. 33-6 Patient with lead shield after surgical application of iodine plaque. (Courtesy Wills Eye Hospital, Philadelphia, Penn.)

should be based on the patient's physical assessment, the severity of underlying disease, the anesthetic and recovery course, the last dose of opioids, and the level of continued care after discharge. Discharge criteria should be developed in consultation with the anesthesia department and approved by the medical staff.[14] Whenever a doubt exists regarding the patient's condition or safety, discharge should be delayed and the surgeon notified. Patients that meet predefined discharge criteria can bypass PACU and be fast-tracked to the Phase II recovery area directly from the operating room.[15]

SUMMARY

The perianesthesia nurse has a role that encompasses various modalities. Being a patient advocate, educator, and collaborative health care team member will prove invaluable. Perianesthesia nurses can participate in and use evidence-based approaches that will provide a higher level of care and an advanced knowledge base to rely upon. By optimizing and streamlining patient care, the benefits in postoperative ophthalmic outcomes will have a direct physical, psychologic, and financial effect on the patient and their families.

NURSING CARE IN THE PACU

REFERENCES

1. McGoldrick KE, et al: Anesthesia and the eye. In Barash PG, et al: *Clinical anesthesia*, ed 5, Philadelphia, 2006, Lippincott Williams & Wilkins.
2. Feldman MA, Patel A: Anesthesia for eye, ear, nose, and throat surgery. In Miller RD, editor: *Miller's anesthesia*, ed 7, St. Louis, 2009, Churchill Livingstone.
3. George EE, Bigatello LM: The postanesthesia care unit. In Hurford WE, et al, editors: *Clinical anesthesia procedures of the Massachusetts General Hospital*, ed 6, Philadelphia, 2002, Lippincott Williams & Wilkins.
4. Gomillion MC: Ambulatory surgery. In Yao FF, editor: *Anesthesiology: problem-oriented patient management*, ed 5, Philadelphia, 2003, Lippincott Williams & Wilkins.
5. Jiménez A, et al: Cancellations in ambulatory day surgery: ten years observational study, *J Ambulatory Surgery* 12(3): 119–123, 2006.
6. Morgan GE, Jr, et al: *Clinical anesthesiology*, ed 4, New York, 2006, McGraw-Hill.
7. Cook-Sather SD: Pediatric ophthalmologic complications. In Atlee JL, editor: *Complications in anesthesia*, Philadelphia, 1999, Saunders.
8. American Academy of Ophthalmology: *Policy statements: color codes for topical ocular medications, 2010*, available at www.aao.org/about/policy/upload/color-codes-for-topical-ocular-medications-2010.pdf. Accessed June 23, 2011.
9. Lydon A, Acquadro MA: Anesthesia for head and neck surgery. In Hurford WE, et al, editors: *Clinical anesthesia procedures of the Massachusetts General Hospital*, ed 6, Philadelphia, 2002, Lippincott Williams & Wilkins.
10. Hauser MW, et al: Anesthesia for pediatric ophthalmic surgery. In Motoyama EK, Davis PJ, editors: *Smith's anesthesia for infants and children*, ed 7, Philadelphia, 2006, Mosby.
11. Mecca RS: Postoperative recovery. In Barash PG, et al, editors: *Clinical anesthesia*, ed 5, Philadelphia, 2006, Lippincott Williams & Wilkins.
12. Pellegrini J, et al: Comparison of inhalation of isopropyl alcohol vs promethazine in the treatment of postoperative nausea and vomiting (PONV) in patients identified as at high risk for developing PONV, *AANA J* 77(4):293–299, 2009.
13. Morgan GE, Jr, et al: *Clinical anesthesiology*, ed 4, Philadelphia, 2006, McGraw-Hill.
14. American Society of PeriAnesthesia Nurses (ASPAN): *2010-2012 Standards of perianesthesia nursing practice*, Cherry Hill, NJ, 2010, ASPAN.
15. Apfel CC: Postoperative nausea and vomiting. In Miller RD, editor: *Miller's anesthesia*, ed 7, Philadelphia, 2005, Churchill Livingstone.

RESOURCES

Feldman MA, Patel A: Anesthesia for eye, ear, nose, and throat surgery. In Miller RD, et al, editors: *Miller's anesthesia*, ed 7, St. Louis, 2009, Churchill Livingstone.

National Institutes of Health, National Eye Institute: *Eye health information*, available at www.nei.nih.gov/health/. Accessed September 23, 2011.

34 Care of the Thoracic Surgical Patient

Jan Odom-Forren, PhD, RN, CPAN, FAAN

Thoracic surgery involves procedures in the structures within the chest cavity, including the lungs, heart, great vessels, and esophagus. In this chapter, discussion focuses on procedures of the lungs and respiratory system. Postanesthesia care after cardiac surgery is discussed in Chapter 35, care after surgery of the great vessels is discussed in Chapter 36, and care after surgery of the esophagus is discussed in Chapter 40.

Lung surgery may be recommended for the diagnosis and treatment of:
- Persistent cough
- Hemoptysis
- Wheezing
- Obstruction
- Abnormal chest radiograph results
- Cancer
- Tumors (solitary pulmonary nodules)
- Small areas of long-term infection (highly localized tuberculosis or mycobacterium)
- Pockets of infection (abscess)
- Permanently enlarged (dilated) bronchus (bronchiectasis)
- Permanently enlarged (dilated) section of lung (lobar emphysema)
- Permanently collapsed lung tissue (atelectasis)
- Injuries with collapsed lung tissue (atelectasis, pneumothorax, hemothorax)
- Correction of congenital or acquired chest wall deformities

DEFINITIONS

Atelectasis: Collapse of the alveoli, caused primarily by obstruction of lower airways. Most commonly, this obstruction is caused by accumulation of respiratory secretions, but it may also be caused by diminished lung volumes, tumors, prolonged bronchospasm, and foreign bodies.

Bronchoscopy: Direct visualization of the tracheobronchial tree with use of a lighted scope. It is used for diagnostic and therapeutic interventions for visualization of structures of the tracheobronchial tree; removal of secretions, washings, mucous plugs, or foreign bodies; and performance of a tissue biopsy or application of medication. Bronchoscopy can be combined with yttrium aluminium garnet (YAG) laser therapy for

ablation of tracheal and bronchial obstructions. It can be performed in the operating room, special procedures unit, or at the patient's bedside, depending on the degree of urgency and the patient's status.

Chest Tube: A drainage tube into the intrapleural space to remove air, fluid, or blood with the goal of restoring normal negative pressure and to allow reexpansion of the lung. The tube is placed on the operative side after open chest procedures.

Chest Wall Reconstruction: Repair of chest wall defects caused by trauma, tumor, or chest wall deformities, with the use of muscle or omentum (underlying abdominal tissue). It provides for protection of underlying structures and organs and provides support for respiration.

Decortication of the Lung: Removal of fibrous deposits or restrictive membranes on the visceral or parietal pleura that interfere with ventilatory action. The goal is restoration of normal lung function.

Endobrachial Ultrasound: A procedure that may be performed during a bronchoscopy, to provide further information to diagnose or determine the stage of a lung cancer. This allows visualization of the lungs and surrounding chest area, which have traditionally required more invasive surgical procedures to evaluate.

Hemothorax: Accumulation of blood or serosanguineous fluid or both within the pleural cavity, compromising lung expansion.

Lobectomy: Removal of one or more lobes of the lung. Lobectomy is the preferred procedure when a cancerous lesion involves a single lobe of the lung. It is used primarily in the treatment of bronchial cancer and is also used in the treatment of bronchiectasis, emphysematous blebs, large benign tumors, fungal infections, and congenital anomalies.

Mediastinoscopy: Direct visualization of lymph nodes or tumors at the tracheobronchial junction, subcarina, or upper lobe bronchi via a lighted scope. This procedure is done by passing the mediastinoscope through a small incision at the suprasternal area and then down along the anterior course of the trachea. It is a diagnostic procedure for patients with identified changes on chest radiograph results.

Needle Biopsy: Insertion of a needle with subsequent aspiration of lung tissue or fluid for diagnostic purposes. It is generally performed with local anesthesia via a percutaneous approach.

Pneumonectomy: Removal of an entire lung, most commonly for lung cancer when lobectomy cannot be performed for total removal of bronchial cancer. It is occasionally indicated for removal of a lung destroyed by chronic infections.

Pneumothorax: Accumulation of air or gas within the pleural cavity, thus compromising lung expansion. Pneumothorax can occur as a direct result of a thoracotomy incision or after chest wall trauma, such as a stab wound.

Segmentectomy (Segmental Resection): Excision of individual bronchovascular segments of the lobe of the lung with ligation of segmental branches of the pulmonary artery and vein and division of the segmental bronchus. Segmentectomy conserves healthy tissue while allowing for removal of localized lesion.

Sleeve Resection: Surgical removal of part of the bronchi, with healthy tissue left for reanastomosis, thus preserving some tissue and lung function. Sleeve resection is used primarily for metastatic disease in either the right or left upper bronchus.

Sternotomy: Incision through the sternum.

Thoracentesis: Insertion of a needle through the chest wall into the pleural space to remove either air or fluid to relieve lung compression or for diagnostic purposes. Removed fluid is evaluated for chemical, bacteriologic, and cellular composition. This procedure can be performed at the bedside, generally with local anesthesia.

Thoracoplasty: Removal of ribs or portions of the ribs to reduce the size of the thoracic space and to collapse a diseased lung.

Thoracoscopy: The insertion of an endoscope, a narrow-diameter tube with a viewing mirror or camera attachment, through a small incision in the chest wall for examination of the lungs or other structures in the chest cavity, without a large incision. The procedure may be diagnostic or therapeutic.

Thoracostomy: An incision of the chest wall for the purpose of drainage. Closed thoracostomy is used to place chest tubes or catheters for drainage of air or fluid to restore normal negative pressure within pleural space. It also can be used to create a surgical access port for video-assisted lobectomy and other endoscopic procedures. Open thoracostomy (partial rib resection) allows healing and reinflation of an infected lung.

Thoracotomy: Incision into the chest cavity that can be used as a diagnostic tool to diagnose or stage cancer. It allows the surgeon access to the thoracic organs including the heart, esophagus, great vessels, or the lungs. Surgery can result from benign or malignant conditions.

Transplantation: Removal of a diseased recipient lung with an immediate replacement of a cadaveric donor lung.

Volume Reduction Surgery: Incision and removal of the parts of the lung that are the most destroyed, most commonly from emphysema, to allow for full function of remaining lung structures.

Wedge Resection: Excision of a small wedge-shaped section from the peripheral portion of the lobe of a lung. It is commonly used to remove cancerous growths in the outer section of the lung to spare lung tissue and function.

ANESTHESIA

Invasive surgery that involves the chest cavity is generally performed with general anesthesia, although diagnostic procedures such as bronchoscopy, needle biopsy, and thoracentesis are commonly performed with local (topical) anesthesia, often with small titrated amounts of intravenous sedation.[1] Epidural catheters can also be placed before surgery for use during surgery and for extended postoperative pain control after pneumonectomy or lobectomy. Because these procedures all involve the airway in addition to anesthesia, patients are given nothing by mouth before any procedure.

Topical anesthesia involves the instillation or spray of a local anesthetic, commonly 4% lidocaine hydrochloride (Xylocaine), onto the laryngeal and pharyngeal surfaces. Although uncommon, toxic reactions or bronchospasm can occur; therefore emergency equipment should be readily available. Recovery of the patient after topical anesthesia requires airway assessment, ready availability of emergency resuscitation equipment, and the administration of humidified oxygen after the procedure. The patient must be given nothing by mouth until the pharyngeal and laryngeal reflexes have returned (2 to 4 hours). Patients should be advised to rest their voices after the procedure; in fact, the surgeon may prescribe a time interval for voice rest. When the gag reflex has returned, throat lozenges and warm drinks may help to relieve the sore throat that inevitably follows bronchoscopy.

Epidural anesthesia involves placement of a catheter into the epidural space of the thoracic vertebrae with subsequent instillation of an infusion combination of an opioid and local anesthetic to achieve sensory blockade of pain without compromising motor function needed for coughing, deep breathing, and ambulating. Thoracic epidural anesthesia can be used in combination with either sedation or general anesthesia.[1] The catheter can be left in place for up to 3 days after surgery for pain control and may be regulated solely by medical personnel or controlled by the patient. Epidural anesthesia is commonly used as an adjunct to general anesthesia.

Paravertebral or intercostal blockade is a regional technique used for the thoracic surgery patient. The advantage of these blocks is neural blockade; the disadvantage is that they last only until the local anesthetic is metabolized.[1] The most commonly used anesthetics for these blocks are lidocaine, bupivacaine, and ropivacaine. Intrapleural local anesthetic instillation can be used for postoperative analgesia, but has the potential for systemic absorption and toxicity.[1] See Chapters 24 and 25 for information on local anesthetics and regional anesthesia.

General anesthesia involves the administration of some combination of inhalation anesthetics, intravenous anesthetics, benzodiazepines, opioids, muscle relaxants, and reversal agents and aims to render the patient amnestic and pain free. Somatic, autonomic, and endocrine reflexes are eliminated, and skeletal muscle relaxation is achieved. Because of the effects of general anesthesia on respiratory function and effort, in conjunction with a preexisting compromise in the respiratory system that necessitates surgery, nursing care must emphasize respiratory assessment, monitoring, and application of prompt intervention if evidence of compromise is noted after surgery.

The patient and family should receive detailed information preoperatively. When possible, taking time to improve the patient's pulmonary, physical, and nutritional status is desirable.[2] Smoking cessation is an important preoperative aspect of surgery; however, the effects of smoking linger after cessation with benefits noted after a year. Smokers who have recently quit have no difference in pulmonary complications than current smokers.[3] Preoperative medications should be continued with the exception of anticoagulant medications.[2] The perianesthesia nurse should review the diagnostic and laboratory tests preoperatively. Preoperative evaluation of the patient who will undergo thoracic surgery may include laboratory tests and pulmonary function tests listed in Table 34-1.

Table 34-1   Laboratory Studies for Assessment of Patients Undergoing Thoracic Procedures

LABORATORY STUDY	NORMAL RESULTS	SIGNIFICANCE OF ABNORMAL FINDINGS
Perfusion Studies—Arterial Blood Gases		
pH	7.35-7.45	Changes indicate metabolic or respiratory acidosis.
$PaCO_2$	35-45 mm Hg	Elevations indicate possible COPD, asthma, pneumonia, anesthetic effects, or use of opioids (respiratory acidosis). Decreased levels indicate hyperventilation/respiratory alkalosis.
HCO_3^-	21-28 mEq/L	Elevations indicate possible respiratory acidosis as compensation for primary metabolic alkalosis. Decreased levels indicate possible respiratory alkalosis as compensation for primary metabolic acidosis.
PaO_2	80-100 mm Hg	Elevations may indicate possible excessive oxygen administration. Decreased levels indicate possible COPD, asthma, chronic bronchitis, cancer of bronchi and lungs, respiratory distress syndrome, or any other cause of hypoxia.
O_2 saturation	95%-100%	Decreased levels indicate possible impaired ability of hemoglobin to release oxygen to tissues.
Complete Blood Count		
RBCs	*Male:* 4.7-6.1 million/mm³ *Female:* 4.2-5.4 million/mm³	Elevated levels may be due to excessive production of erythropoietin, which occurs in response to a hypoxic stimulus, such as COPD. Decreased levels may indicate anemia, hemorrhage, or hemolysis.
Hemoglobin	*Male:* 14.8 g/dL *Female:* 12-16 g/dL	Same as for RBCs.
Hematocrit	*Male:* 42%-52% *Female:* 37%-47%	Same as for RBCs.
WBCs	5000-10,000/mm³	Elevations indicate possible acute bacterial infections or inflammatory conditions (smoking). Decreased levels may indicate overwhelming infection or immunosuppression.

Continued

NURSING CARE IN THE PACU

Table 34-1	Laboratory Studies for Assessment of Patients Undergoing Thoracic Procedures—cont'd	
TEST	**PURPOSE**
FVC (forced vital capacity): Records maximum amount of air that can be exhaled as quickly as possible after maximum inspiration.	Provides an indication of respiratory muscle strength and ventilatory reserve. Often reduced in obstructive disease (because of air trapping) and in restrictive disease.
FEV_1 (forced expiratory volume in 1 sec): Records maximum amount of air that can be exhaled in first second of respiration.	Effort dependent and declines with age. Reduced in certain obstructive and restrictive disorders.
FEV_1/FVC: Ratio of expiratory volume in 1 sec to FVC	Provides a more sensitive indicator of obstruction to airflow. Ratio is normal or increased in restrictive disease.
$FEF_{25\%-75\%}$: Records forced expiratory flow over 25%-75% volume (middle half) of FVC.	This measure provides a more sensitive index of obstruction in smaller airways.
FRC (functional residual capacity): Amount of air remaining in lungs after normal expiration.	Increased FRC indicates hyperinflation or air trapping, which can result from obstructive disease.
TLC (total lung capacity): Amount of air remaining in lungs at end of maximum inhalation	Increased TLC indicates air trapping associated with obstructive pulmonary disease. Decreased TLC indicates restrictive disease.
RV (residual volume): Amount of air remaining in lungs at end of a full, forced exhalation	RV is increased in obstructive pulmonary disease, such as emphysema.
DL_{co} (diffusion capacity of carbon monoxide): Reflects surface area of alveolocapillary membrane	DL_{co} is reduced when alveolocapillary membrane is diminished, such as in emphysema, pulmonary hypertension, and pulmonary fibrosis.

From Pagana KD, Pagana TJ: *Mosby's diagnostic and laboratory test references*, ed 9, St. Louis, 2009, Mosby; Rees HC: Assessment of the respiratory system. In Ignatavicius DD, Workman ML, editors: *Medical-surgical nursing: patient-centered collaborative care*, ed 6, Philadelphia, 2010, Saunders.
COPD, Chronic obstructive pulmonary disease; *HCO_3*, bicarbonate ion; *$PaCO_2$*, partial pressure of arterial carbon dioxide; *PaO_2*, partial pressure of arterial oxygen; *RBC*, red blood cell; *WBC*, white blood cell.

SURGICAL PROCEDURES

Surgical procedures can be diagnostic or therapeutic in nature. Diagnostic procedures can include bronchoscopy, mediastinoscopy, laryngoscopy, and thoracoscopy. Bronchoscopies are performed to visualize the airway or remove abnormal tissue, mucous plugs, or foreign bodies. They also aid in evaluating lung lesions and staging of lung cancer. Complications can include airway obstruction, hypoxemia, pneumothorax, hemorrhage, or cardiovascular problems such as dysrhythmias or hypotension (Fig. 34-1).

Mediastinoscopy is performed for direct visualization of lymph nodes or tumors at the tracheobronchial junction, subcarina, or upper lobe bronchi via a lighted scope. The potential for hemorrhage is present because of the close proximity of the innominate vessels and aortic arch to the mediastinoscope. Other complications can include venous air embolism; vagally mediated reflex bradycardia from compression of the trachea or great vessels; airway or esophageal injury, including subcutaneous emphysema; chest pain; or pneumothorax. Recurrent laryngeal nerve

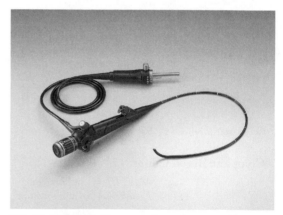

FIG. 34-1 Flexible fiber-optic bronchoscope. (Courtesy Olympus America, Melville, NY.)

injury can occur and manifest symptoms such as hoarseness or vocal cord paralysis.[4] A laryngoscopy is performed to visualize or biopsy the oropharynx, laryngopharynx, larynx, or proximal trachea. Complications include trauma to the lips, mucous membranes, teeth, or eyes; rupture of the esophagus; hypoxemia; or laryngospasm. Endobronchial ultrasound (EBUS) is a new minimally invasive technique that allows the proceduralist to see beyond the lumen of the airway. There are two EBUS systems currently available—the radial probe EBUS allows for evaluation of central airways, accurate definition of airway invasion, and facilitates the diagnosis of peripheral lung lesions; and the linear EBUS guides transbronchial needle aspiration of hilar and mediastinal lymph nodes.[5]

Thoracoscopy is the insertion of an endoscope, a narrow-diameter tube with a camera attachment, through a small incision in the chest wall for examination of the lungs or other structures in the chest cavity, without a large incision. It is performed for basic diagnostic (undiagnosed pleural fluid or pleural thickening) and therapeutic procedures (pleurodesis). Complications can include bleeding, infection of the pleural space, and injury to intrathoracic organs, atelectasis, and respiratory failure.[6] This procedure is different from video-assisted thoracoscopic surgery (VATS), an invasive procedure that uses a high-level access platform and multiple ports for separate viewing and working instruments to access pleural space.[6] VATS can be diagnostic or therapeutic and is used often for biopsy of mediastinal masses, to perform wedge resections, to obtain hemostasis, or to evacuate blood clots. A variety of procedures can be performed via thoracoscopy, from lung volume reduction to a biopsy and excision of mediastinal lesions. Robotic-assisted thoracic procedures can enhance the speed and safety of VATS. Smaller incisions are used for robotic surgery which may contribute to less postoperative pain and morbidity.[7]

A significant advantage of thoracoscopy is that it is minimally invasive and results in less incisional pain. It can also decrease recovery time and length of hospital stay. In some facilities, patients come to the PACU with a small chest tube that is pulled if chest radiograph results are clear; the patient then is allowed to go home in a few hours. VATS may be converted to an open surgery if there is an inability to achieve one-lung ventilation, extensive pleural adhesions, uncontrolled or significant intraoperative bleeding, an inability to identify target lesion for biopsy, or technical difficulties with or rarely, primary failure of video equipment and/or endoscopic instruments.[8]

Therapeutic thoracic surgeries may include pectus excavatum, chest wall reconstruction, wedge resection of a lung lesion, segmentectomy, lobectomy, or pneumonectomy. Excision of the right lung is less tolerated than removal of the left lung because of the larger vascular bed and breathing capacity. Other thoracic surgeries include lung volume reduction, for removal of emphysematous lung tissue, or lung transplant.

PERIANESTHESIA NURSING CARE AFTER THORACIC PROCEDURES

Admission assessment in the PACU is the same as for any other surgical patient (see Chapters 27 and 28). Common problems that lead to delayed discharge from the hospital for the patient who has undergone a thoracic procedure include inadequate pain control, prolonged air leak, severe nausea, fever, debility, and arrhythmias.[2] Postoperative care should target prevention or speedy treatment of these complications. Some specific issues for the patient after thoracic surgery are discussed.

Positioning

Positioning after thoracic procedures varies; therefore, medical orders must be checked. The patient may be kept in a side-lying position until awake, and then the head of the bed is elevated 30 to 45 degrees to facilitate ventilation. This position allows the diaphragm to drop into normal position, thus enhancing lung expansion and, if present, facilitating chest tube drainage. After lobectomy, segmentectomy, and wedge resection, the patient can be turned freely from side to side to allow full expansion of lung tissue on both the operative and nonoperative side. After pneumonectomy, the patient may be placed on the back or on the operative side.[9] The patient is *not* positioned side lying on the nonoperative side because the mediastinum is no longer confined by lung tissue and may move freely, thereby compressing the remaining lung or creating traction or torsion of the vena cava. In addition, if the bronchial stump ruptures and bleeds profusely, the unaffected lung is compressed by secretions from the pneumonectomy site.

Position changes are important after thoracic surgery. If the patient undergoes an outpatient procedure, such as bronchoscopy, position changes are made independently. If the patient has a chest tube in place, the perianesthesia nurse needs to assist with position changes to ensure system patency and patient comfort. Position changes also include early return to ambulation, with the goal of promoting patient comfort, drainage of secretions, and prevention of venous stasis and atelectasis.

Respiratory Assessment and Care

On arrival, the patient is placed on oxygen via the delivery system required per the extent of the patient's surgery, preexisting medical conditions, and need for continued assistance. Continued assistance may include a nasal cannula after bronchoscopy, face mask or face tent, or mechanical ventilation. Delivered oxygen should be given with humidification to help thin tracheobronchial secretions and thus permit the ciliary mechanism and coughing to clear the airway.

The perianesthesia nurse should assess respiratory function on arrival, beginning with inspection of the patient's respiratory effort and ease of effort. Respiratory rate is noted; a rate of 10 to 20 breaths per minute is considered normal. A rate of greater than 20 is considered to be tachypnea and may be caused by pain, hypoxemia, hypoventilation, or secretions. The use of pulse oximetry helps in the quick assessment for hypoxemia. A respiratory rate of less than 10 is considered bradypnea, which may occur as a result of anesthetic and opioid administration. The patient should also be assessed for the quality of respirations. The patient may have a respiratory rate within normal limits but not deep enough to blow off the carbon dioxide of normal respirations. Some PACUs have the capability to monitor end-tidal CO_2 with a capnograph. The nurse should auscultate the patient's lungs to assure that respirations are of good quality. Appropriate pain management can promote effective ventilation. The patient may also arrive in the PACU intubated with either a T piece, if respiratory effort is sufficiently present but loss of airway patency is a concern, or mechanical ventilation, if airway and ventilation are concerns.

Breath sounds should be assessed for depth, clarity, and the presence of adventitious sounds, including crackles, rhonchi, or a pleural friction rub. The use of accessory muscles should be noted. Accessory muscle actions include nasal flaring, suprasternal retractions, diaphragmatic breathing, and intercostal retractions.

The regularity of breathing is assessed as regular, irregular, or ventilated. Ventilator settings are confirmed. If arterial blood gases are drawn, adjustments are made, if necessary, after assessment of results. Ongoing pulse oximetry monitoring is necessary for any patient who has undergone a thoracic surgical procedure with capnography available if needed.

Intubation might have been used to protect the airway, to assist ventilation, or to provide a means for management of secretions through suctioning. Tracheal suctioning of the patient after thoracic surgery may be necessary to assist in removal of accumulated secretions.

Respiratory Management

The modified stir-up regimen, including positioning, mobilization, sustained maximal inspiration (SMI), cascade coughing, and pain relief, is especially important for a patient recovering from a thoracic surgical procedure. Positioning and mobilization have already been discussed. The SMI and cascade coughing exercises are the easiest ways to maintain a patent airway after the patient is reactive to verbal commands. Preoperative teaching is extremely important; the patient who has been well educated and knows what is expected after surgery can cooperate by taking a deep breath, holding it for 3 seconds, exhaling (the SMI), taking a deep breath, and coughing throughout exhalation (the cascade cough). Effective preoperative teaching enhances the effectiveness of the modified stir-up regimen even if the patient is not fully reactive.

When the patient is fully conscious, rigorous SMIs and cascade coughing are continued every hour. This regimen is most effective with the patient sitting to allow full lung expansion. If the patient cannot sit, raise the head of the bed and have the patient bend the knees to relax the abdominal muscles. The patient is instructed to inspire deeply and hold the breath for 3 seconds to expand the lungs and relax the abdominal muscles so that the belly pouches out. Four to five SMIs are taken, and the patient is instructed to perform the cascade cough to clear the tracheobronchial tree of accumulated secretions. After the patient performs about three cascade coughs, a forceful cough is then usually produced spontaneously, thus clearing the airways of secretions. Endotracheal secretions are usually excessive after thoracic surgery because of manipulation and irritation of the tracheobronchial tree during the operation and intubation, decreased lung ventilation, and a decreased cough reflex. Pain or fear, or both, may interfere with the patient's ability to perform the SMI and cascade cough.

Pain Management

Although pain after bronchoscopy is usually limited to a sore throat, the patient undergoing thoracic surgery should be told before surgery to expect a fair amount of postoperative incisional pain. The patient should also be told that pain relief measures are available and may include epidural analgesia, patient-controlled analgesia, and nurse-administered opioids. The thoracotomy incision is an extremely painful incision because of irritation from respiratory effort and any upper body movement (Fig. 34-2).[1] Because acute pain after thoracic surgery has been linked to chronic

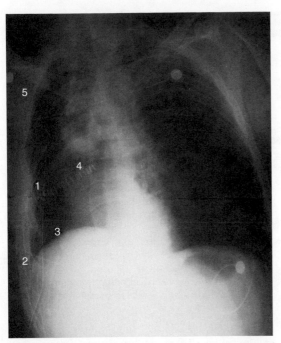

FIG. 34-2 Multiple sources of afferent transmission of pain sensations after thoracotomy. *1,* Intercostal nerves at the site of the incision (usually T4-6); *2,* intercostal nerves at the site of chest drains (usually T7-8); *3,* phrenic nerve afferents from the dome of the diaphragm; *4,* vagal nerve innervation of the mediastinal pleura; *5,* brachial plexus. (From Miller RD, et al: *Miller's anesthesia,* ed 7, Philadelphia, 2010, Churchill Livingstone.)

thoracic pain months later, appropriate pain relief must occur. Severe pain during the first couple of days after surgery is predictive of chronic post-thoracotomy pain with as many as 67% of patients who underwent a thoracotomy developed persistent postsurgical pain.[10]

An effective modality for postsurgical thoracotomy pain is nerve conduction blockade with local anesthetics.[1] Pain management via epidural catheter has been shown to provide more effective pain relief after thoracotomy. Of best benefit is epidural analgesia with an opioid and local anesthetic that has begun at least 30 minutes before induction of anesthesia. Pain medications should be given in adequate doses and in a timely manner because pain interferes with needed activities after surgery, including deep breathing, coughing, and progressive mobilization. Because opioids can diminish respiratory function, care must be taken in their administration, especially after general anesthesia. However, a patient whose pain is not adequately controlled is unable to deep breath effectively to maintain oxygenation and prevent atelectasis (Box 34-1).

In addition to analgesics, pain relief measures can include use of a pillow to splint the incision while the patient coughs. Because coughing is the most effective way to clear secretions, pain medication should be offered and given regularly. See Chapter 31 more detailed information about pain management in the PACU.

Fluid Management

Optimal hydration after thoracic surgery is important to prevent the increased viscosity of mucus to facilitate the removal of secretions. Oral fluids may be started as soon as the patient recovers from anesthesia and the danger of nausea and vomiting has passed. Intravenous fluids are also used after more extensive surgery to ensure hydration and to continue fluid replacement for losses in the operating room. Removal of large segments of lung or of a total lung (pneumonectomy) significantly reduces the size

NURSING CARE IN THE PACU

Evidence-Based Practice

Mathews and colleagues conducted an evidence-based study to determine whether patient-controlled analgesia with ketamine and morphine (PCA-MK) or PCA with morphine alone (PCA-MO) was best for postoperative analgesia in patients who have had thoracic surgery. All identified studies found that morphine requirements were reduced with use of PCA-MK. The authors conclude that adding low-dose ketamine to morphine PCA is safe and may provide better pain control than PCA-MO. Pain scores were lower with PCA-MK as well as improved oxygen saturations and $PaCO_2$ levels.

IMPLICATIONS FOR PRACTICE

The use of ketamine postoperatively in conjunction with an opioid provides safe and effective pain management for patients after thoracic surgery. The incidence of hallucination requiring intervention was 2.9%. Other randomized controlled trials found no hallucination or psychological side effects. The perianesthesia nurse should know the indications and side effects for the use of ketamine for acute postoperative pain in thoracic surgery patients.

Source: Mathews TJ, et al: Does adding ketamine to morphine patient-controlled analgesia safely improve post-thoracotomy pain? *Interact Cardiovasc Thorac Surg,* 2011 [Epub ahead of print].

BOX 34-1   Postoperative Analgesia Modalities

SYSTEMIC ANALGESIA

- Opioids
  - Can control background pain, but pain control usually poor with interrupted sleep patterns when opioid levels fall below therapeutic range
  - Amount needed to control pain during movement causes sedation and hypoventilation in most patients
- NSAIDs
  - Can reduce opioid consumption after thoracotomy
  - Has an antiinflammatory and analgesic effect, but can be associated with decreased platelet function, gastric erosions, increased bronchial reactivity, and decreased renal function
- Acetaminophen
  - Is an antipyretic and analgesic that can be administered orally or rectally in doses up to 4 g/day
  - Has a low toxicity compared with cyclooxygenase-inhibiting NSAIDs
- Ketamine
  - Low-dose intramuscular ketamine (1 mg/kg) is equivalent to the same dose of meperidine and causes less respiratory depression
  - Can also be administered as a low-dose intravenous infusion
  - Psychomimetic effect with ketamine is a concern, but is rarely seen with analgesic, subanesthetic doses
- Dexmedetomidine
  - A selective adrenergic α2-receptor agonist can significantly decrease the requirement for opioids when used in combination with epidural local anesthetics
  - Associated with some hypotension, but seems to preserve renal function

LOCAL ANESTHETICS AND NERVE BLOCKS

- Intercostal nerve blocks
  - An effective adjunct to methods of postthoracotomy analgesia
  - Duration of analgesia limited to the duration of action of the local anesthetic used
  - Indwelling intercostal catheters are an option, but can be difficult to position reliably percutaneously
  - Useful supplements for the pain associated with the multiple small port incisions and chest drains following video-assisted thoracoscopic surgery
- Intrapleural analgesia
  - Produces a multilevel intercostal block that is dependent on patient position, infusion volume, chest drains, and the type of surgery
  - Reliability of intrapleural techniques inadequate to justify their use on a routine basis

OTHER TECHNIQUES

- Application of a −60°C probe to the exposed intercostal nerves intraoperatively
  - Produces an intercostal block that can persist for up to 6 months
  - Moderately efficient to decrease postoperative pain, but is associated with an incidence of chronic neuralgia
- Transcutaneous electrical nerve stimulation
  - May be useful in mild to moderate pain, but ineffective for severe pain

EPIDURAL ANALGESIA

- Spinal injection of opioids can have a duration of analgesia that approaches 24 hours after thoracotomy.
- Epidural techniques reduce the incidence of respiratory complications.
- The majority of thoracotomies received a thoracic epidural between T3 and T8, with infusions of bupivacaine plus either fentanyl or hydromorphone.
- Risks of respiratory depression and hemodynamic instability are due to the use of bolus injection techniques.
- Use of epidural infusions has an excellent record for patient safety when used on routine postoperative surgical wards.
- The majority of thoracotomies receive a thoracic epidural between T3 and T8, with infusions of bupivacaine plus either fentanyl or hydromorphone.

PARAVERTEBRAL BLOCK

- Paravertebral local anesthetics provide a reliable multilevel intercostal blockade. Clinically, the analgesia is comparable to that from epidural local anesthetics.
- Advantages over epidural include comparable analgesia, fewer failed blocks, decreased risk of neuraxial hematoma, and less hypotension, nausea, or urinary retention.

From Slinger PD, Campos JH: Anesthesia for thoracic surgery. In Miller RD, et al: *Miller's anesthesia*, ed 7, Philadelphia, 2010, Churchill Livingstone.
NSAID, Nonsteroidal antiinflammatory drug.

of the pulmonary circulation, thus predisposing the patient to the development of pulmonary edema if fluids are administered too rapidly or in too large a volume. The surgeon writes postoperative fluid orders. Accurate intake and output records are particularly important.

Chest Tube Management

Surgery that involves entry into the thoracic cavity results in air entry and the development of a pneumothorax (atmospheric pressure admitted into the pleural cavity and collapse of the lung). Placement of a pleural chest tube after open-chest procedures allows for drainage of air and blood, restoration of normal negative pressure, and reexpansion of the collapsed lung. Because blood is heavier than air, blood pools in the lower portion of the pleural space, whereas air accumulates in the upper portion. Therefore one or two chest tubes are placed through the chest wall via a stab wound or incision. Most surgeons still place one tube anteriorly and one posteriorly.[2] The upper or anterior chest tube is placed in the second intercostal space to allow for air removal. The lower or posterior chest tube is placed in the sixth to eighth intercostal space to allow for drainage from the pleural space (Fig. 34-3). The chest tubes are sutured in place with pursestring sutures and covered with a dressing. The chest tube insertion site should be palpated for the presence of crepitus (also known as *subcutaneous emphysema*) caused by air trapping in subcutaneous tissue. Crepitus feels like crunchy cereal under the skin. If noted,

the surgeon should be notified for probable repeated securing of the chest tube.

The goal of chest tube drainage is to use positive pressure, gravity, and suction to facilitate evacuation of air and fluid that surrounds the lung for reexpansion of the collapsed lung. The air trapped in the chest creates the positive pressure. Gravity assists primarily in fluid evacuation, and suction, when applied, facilitates removal of both air and fluid. Suction is generally established at 20 cm negative pressure, unless specifically ordered differently. Wall units have a manometer in place to allow for correct setting of suction pressure. Some surgeons now prefer to use no suction if the lung is fully expanded.[2] When the air and fluid are removed, the visceral and parietal pleura are brought back together again, and the pressure in the interpleural space becomes negative again, thus reexpanding the lung. Disposable prefabricated chest drainage units such as the Pleur-Evac or Atrium systems are used for chest drainage (Fig. 34-4). The chest tubes can be connected to chest drainage with a wet seal or a dry seal. Either dry or wet seal chest drainage has its positive attributes and is capable of evacuating air or fluid. The air flow and negative pressure depends on the type of chest drainage system. The dry seal system is optimal when the transporting the patient.[11]

The pleural drainage system has three basic compartments, each with its own specific function. The first compartment, the collection chamber, receives air and fluid from the chest cavity. This compartment is vented to the second chamber, known as the water-seal chamber. This chamber acts as a one-way valve so that air can enter from, but not back into, the collection chamber. If bubbling is noted in this chamber, the lung has not reexpanded. The third chamber is the suction control chamber, which is used to apply controlled suction to the system to facilitate evacuation of air and fluid and to promote reexpansion of the lung. Some of these units have even been designed to allow for reinfusion of collected drained blood for autotransfusion.

Because the goal of chest tube placement is evaluation of air and fluid, the system must remain patent. The perianesthesia nurse must ensure patency of the chest tubes, drainage tubing, and the system through periodic regular assessments. A chest radiograph is often performed on admission to the PACU to ensure placement and lung function. Proper functioning of the system is evidenced by fluctuation or bubbling of the fluid in the water seal tubing in response to the patient's respiration.[2] If no fluctuation is noted, the system should be evaluated for proper

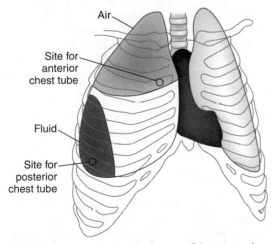

FIG. 34-3 Because air rises to the top of the cavity, chest tube placement for treatment of pneumothorax is at the second intercostal space, close to the sternum. Chest tube placement for fluid removal is generally at level of sixth to eighth lateral intercostal space because this is where fluid collects.

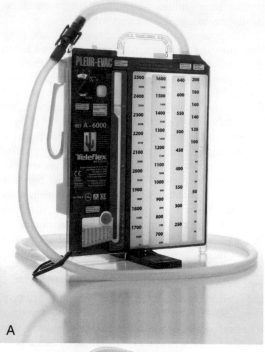

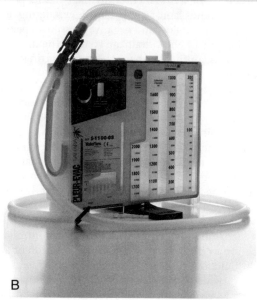

FIG. 34-4 Pleur-Evac chest drainage systems. **A,** Dry and wet seal. **B,** Dry suction and dry seal. (Courtesy Teleflex Medical, Research Triangle Park, NC.)

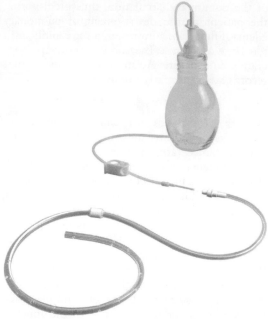

FIG. 34-5 PleurX catheter system. (Courtesy CareFusion Corp., San Diego, Calif. 2010. All rights reserved.)

functioning. The tubing must not kink and should form a straight line from patient to collection unit to allow for unobstructed gravitational flow. *Milking* or *stripping* of the chest tube may dislodge clots of blood that block the tubing.[2] This procedure should be done in the direction away from the patient, toward the drainage system, to prevent forcing clots back into the pleural space.

If the system shows no fluctuation or bubbling with respiration and the tubing has been deemed clear, the physician should be notified, especially in the immediate postoperative period. In the latter days of recovery, the absence of fluctuation or bubbling signals reexpansion of the lung, with further evidence provided by full return of breath sounds and chest radiograph results. However, in the PACU, failure of the system prevents lung reexpansion. Any acute respiratory difficulty or pain should be referred immediately to the surgeon.

New modalities exist for use at home when a patient requires palliation of symptoms associated with recurrent pleural effusions (Fig. 34-5). The PleurX catheter system can be used for patients who require minimal intervention. After placement, usually outpatient surgery, the tunneled catheter eliminates the need for thoracentesis.[12]

Complications
Risks of General Anesthesia

The risks of general anesthesia for any patient, regardless of the underlying medical condition and surgical procedure, include the potential for respiratory and cardiovascular compromise. In the presence of underlying pulmonary disease and surgery that involves the thoracic cavity, the potential for respiratory compromise, including hypoxemia, hypoventilation, and atelectasis, increases greatly. The perianesthesia nurse should be prepared to evaluate for respiratory and ventilatory adequacy and to intervene with appropriate interventions if compromise is noted. This intervention can include the need to simply stimulate the patient to take deep breaths, to increase the concentration of oxygen delivered, or to anticipate and assist with reintubation if necessary.

Wound Infection

As with any surgical procedure, the risk of infection is possible. Prophylactic antibiotics may be given for major thoracic surgical procedures, including lobectomy and pneumonectomy, and are used if prolonged postoperative mechanical ventilation is anticipated.

Bleeding

After bronchoscopy, bleeding should be limited to no more than lightly pink-tinged or slightly blood-streaked sputum. Grossly bloody sputum and coughing of frank blood should be reported to the surgeon and anesthesia provider immediately. After a more invasive procedure such as lobectomy or pneumonectomy, the surgical site must be inspected for bleeding and the chest tube for the presence of bloody drainage. Postoperative hemorrhage occurs in approximately 3% of thoracotomies and may be associated with up to 20% mortality. Signs of hemorrhage include increased chest tube drainage (>200 mL/h), hypotension, tachycardia, and a low hematocrit.[5] If chest tube drainage seems excessive (>100 mL/h) or does not decrease in volume over time or if fresh bleeding is noted, the physician should be notified to evaluate for hemorrhage. Even if drainage is excessive, the chest tube should never be clamped unless specifically ordered. Clamping of the chest tube may result in the development of a tension pneumothorax, which is considerably more dangerous than an open pneumothorax.

Pneumonia

Although pneumonia is unlikely to develop in the immediate postoperative period, diminished ventilatory effort and prolonged bedrest are strong predictors of pneumonia potential. The patient should be encouraged on arrival to the PACU to take deep breaths, to cascade cough, and to use the incentive spirometer to prevent atelectasis and pneumonia, if ordered. The use of sterile technique when suctioning is essential.

Worsening of Existing Heart Problems

Underlying cardiac disease should be carefully evaluated and documented before surgery. In any patient with preexisting cardiac disease, close attention to continuous ECG monitoring in the PACU is of vital importance, because cardiac dysrhythmias commonly develop in these patients. These dysrhythmias can range from benign to life threatening. Sinus tachycardia and atrial fibrillation are the most commonly seen dysrhythmias in the early recovery phases.

SUMMARY

Care of patients undergoing thoracic surgery or procedures of the lungs and respiratory system was discussed in this chapter. These procedures range from minimally invasive procedures to open thoracotomies. The procedures are performed on patients with underlying conditions such as emphysema or malignant disease that must be surgically treated. Care of these patients in the PACU involves respiratory function, observation for complications, and promotion of oxygenation and ventilation.

REFERENCES

1. Barrick BP, Kyle RW: Conduct of anesthesia. In Shields TW, et al: *General thoracic surgery*, ed 7, Philadephia, 2009, Lippincott Williams & Wilkins.
2. Shaw JP, LoCicero III J: General principles of postoperative care. In Shields TW, et al: *General thoracic surgery*, ed 7, Philadephia, 2009, Lippincott Williams & Wilkins.
3. Barrera R, et al: Smoking and timing of cessation: impact on pulmonary complications after thoracotomy, *Chest* 127:1977-1983, 2005.
4. Morgan Jr GE, et al: Anesthesia for thoracic surgery. In Morgan G, et al: *Clinical anesthesiology*, ed 4, New York City, 2006, McGraw-Hill.
5. Gomez M, Silvestri GA: Endobronchial ultrasound for the diagnosis and staging of lung cancer, *Proc Am Thorac Soc* 6(2):180-186, 2009.
6. Ernst A, et al: Interventional pulmonary procedures: Medical thoracoscopy/pleuroscopy, available at www.medscape.com/viewarticle/455720_16. Accessed December 30, 2011.
7. Blanchard B: Thoracic surgery. In Rothrock JC: *Alexander's care of the patient in surgery*, ed 14, St. Louis, 2001, Mosby.
8. Yim APC, et al: Video-assisted thoracic surgery as a diagnostic tool. In Shields TW, et al: *General thoracic surgery*, ed 7, Philadephia, 2009, Lippincott, Williams & Wilkins.
9. Marley RA, Hoyle BL: Respiratory care. In Schick L, Windle PE: *Perianesthesia nursing core curriculum: preprocedure, phase I and phase II PACU nursing*, ed 2, St. Louis, 2010, Saunders.
10. Pasero C: Persistent postsurgical and posttrauma pain, *J Perianesth Nurs* 26:38-42, 2011.
11. Manzanet G, et al: A hydrodynamic study of pleural drainage systems: some practical consequences, *Chest* 127:2211-2221, 2005.
12. Warren K, et al: Identification of clinical factors predicting PleurX catheter removal in patients treated for malignant pleural effusion, *Eur J of Cardio-Thoracic Surg* 33:89-94, 2008.

NURSING CARE IN THE PACU

RESOURCES

Atlee J: *Complications in anesthesia*, ed 2, Philadelphia, 2007, Saunders.

Barash PG, et al: *Clinical anesthesia*, ed 5, Philadelphia, 2005, Lippincott Williams & Wilkins.

Coughlin AM, Parchinsky C: Go with the flow of chest tube therapy, *Nursing* 36(3):L36-42, 2006.

Fibla JJ, et al: Early removal of chest drainage and outpatient program after videothoracoscopic lung biopsy, *Eur J Cardiothor Surg* 28:604–606, 2005.

Fleisher LA: *Anesthesia and uncommon diseases*, ed 5, Philadelphia, 2007, Saunders.

Gotoda Y, et al: The morbidity, time course and predictive factors for persistent post-thoracotomy pain, *Eur J Pain* 5:89–96, 2001.

Mason RJ, et al: *Murray and Nadel's textbook of respiratory medicine*, ed 5, Philadelphia, 2010, Saunders.

Miller R, et al: *Miller's anesthesia*, ed 7, Philadelphia, 2009, Churchill Livingstone.

Pasero C, McCaffery M: *Pain assessment and pharmacologic management*, St. Louis, 2011, Mosby.

Rieker M: Anesthesia for thoracic surgery. In Nagelhout J, Plaus K: *Nurse anesthesia*, ed 4, Philadelphia, 2010, Saunders.

Senturk M, et al: The effects of three different analgesia techniques on long-term postthoracotomy pain, *Anesth Analg* 94:11–15, 2002.

Slinger P: *Principles and practice of anesthesia for thoracic surgery*, New York, 2011, Springer.

Stoelting R, Miller R: *Basics of anesthesia*, ed 6, Philadelphia, 2011, Churchill Livingstone.

35 Care of the Cardiac Surgical Patient

Patricia C. Seifert, MSN, RN, CNOR, CRNFA, FAAN

The first suture repair of a right ventricular stab wound in 1896 demonstrated that the heart could be manipulated and sutured without causing ventricular fibrillation and without entering the pleural cavity, thereby creating a pneumothorax. The introduction of positive-pressure endotracheal anesthesia obviated the dangers of a pneumothorax because clinicians could access the heart and enter the pleural cavities without causing the lungs to collapse. Gibbon's introduction in 1953 of extracorporeal circulation (i.e., cardiopulmonary bypass) enabled surgeons to isolate the heart and lungs from the circulation without producing irreversible tissue anoxia.[1] The development of electric defibrillation and induced chemical cardiac arrest made stopping and restarting the heart possible with consistent predictability; myocardial protection techniques protected and conserved myocardial energy resources during the period of induced cardiac arrest. Newer diagnostic imaging and monitoring devices have allowed clinicians to visualize the heart, identify specific pathoanatomic changes, record the heart's electric activity, measure blood pressure and flow, and assess ventricular function. These imaging and monitoring improvements, along with the refinement of mechanical and bioprosthetic materials, improved anesthetic agents, percutaneous and newer minimally invasive surgical techniques, and additional technologic advances have made development of more effective procedures possible to revascularize the myocardium, repair and replace valves, treat aneurysms, alter conduction disturbances, and assist and replace a failing heart.[1] The reader will find related information in Chapters 11, 34, and 36.

DEFINITIONS

Allograft (Homograft): Tissue from another human, commonly procured from cadaver aortic valves with a portion of the attached aorta. The aortic allograft is obtained in a sterile manner; tested to rule out communicable disease, malignant disease, diabetes, and other pathologic conditions; treated with antibiotics; measured; placed in a sterile bag; and cryopreserved in a special freezer. When needed for surgery to replace the aortic valve or a portion of the ascending aorta and valve, the correct size of allograft is thawed and implanted.

Annuloplasty: The surgical repair of a dilated valve annulus, which causes valvular regurgitation. A cloth-covered prosthetic annuloplasty ring is sewn to the valve annulus (usually mitral or tricuspid) to reduce the overall circumference of the annular tissue, thereby reducing the amount of regurgitant blood flow.

Aortic Aneurysm: A localized or diffuse dilation of the arterial wall. Weakening and degeneration of the medial layer of the aortic wall leads to progressive enlargement of all layers of the aorta. Thoracic aortic aneurysms can occur in the ascending aorta, the aortic arch, or the descending aorta and extend into the abdominal aorta and branch vessels.

Aortic Dissection: A unique condition that affects the aortic media in which repeated stress (often from hypertension) and a congenital predisposition produce a tear in the intimal layer. Blood enters the tear, creating a dissecting hematoma within the tunica media and forming a false lumen. As the false lumen enlarges, with more blood entering the tear, the true lumen compresses and eventually compresses branches of the aorta. The intimal tear usually forms in the ascending aorta, although it can originate in any portion of the thoracic aorta. Surgery (excision of the aorta that contains the tear and replacement with a graft) is indicated for ascending aortic and transverse aortic arch dissections.

Aortic Insufficiency (AI): Also called *aortic regurgitation;* a condition that occurs when the aortic valve leaflets do not close properly (or have tears) and the valve becomes incompetent, thereby allowing regurgitation of blood from the aorta back into the left ventricle during diastole. AI can be the result of a primary valve disorder or aortic root disease. Valve disorders may be the result of congenital or rheumatic heart disease, infective endocarditis, torn leaflets, or trauma; aortic root disease may include aneurysmal dilatation, aortic dissection, Marfan syndrome, or some other condition that predisposes the root to dilatation (e.g., ectasia).

Aortic Stenosis (AS): The development of stiff and fibrotic valve leaflets or a narrowing of the orifice of the aortic valve itself. Valvular AS is often characterized by a fusion of the commissures of the valve leaflets that leaves only a small opening. A calculated aortic valve orifice of less than 1 cm^2 is considered critical AS. Cardinal symptoms are syncope, angina pectoris, and dyspnea; these symptoms are related to insufficient cerebral blood flow, myocardial blood flow, and impaired left ventricle function, respectively.

AS can occur as a congenital process, as in the bicuspid valve (a common congenital anomaly first diagnosed in adulthood), as an acquired disease process related to a history of rheumatic heart disease, or as calcific AS.

Aortocoronary Bypass Grafts: See Myocardial Revascularization.

Atrial Septal Defect (ASD): An opening in the atrial septum, ASDs are among the frequently seen congenital anomalies in adulthood. The most common form in the adult is the ostium secundum defect. Depending on the size of the defect (commonly the size of a quarter coin), there is a shunting of blood from the left atrium to the right atrium and subsequent increased pulmonary flow.

Balloon Valvotomy or Valvuloplasty: A catheter-based interventional (i.e., nonsurgical) procedure to enlarge a (stenotic) valve opening. For aortic valvuloplasty, the balloon tip is positioned across the aortic valve, and the balloon is inflated to dilate the aortic valve orifice. Balloon valvotomy for the mitral valve is performed with a catheter percutaneously inserted into a large vein and threaded to the right atrium, where a septal puncture is made to allow access to the mitral valve.

Bicuspid Aortic Valve: See Aortic Stenosis.

Cardioplegia: Literally, "paralysis of the heart"; pharmacologically induced cardiac arrest during surgery on the heart. Potassium is the most commonly used arresting agent, but the solutions may also contain electrolytes, buffers to maintain appropriate pH, glucose, metabolic substrates, calcium antagonists, tromethamine, heparin, and antiarrhythmic agents; the carrying solution may be crystalloid or blood (preferable for its oxygen carrying capacity). The purposes of cardioplegia are protection of the myocardium against irreversible ischemic injury during the aortic cross-clamp period when the heart is arrested and conservation of energy resources that can be used after removal of the cross clamp.

Cardiopulmonary Bypass (CPB): A temporary substitution for the heart and lungs with a mechanical device that drains systemic venous return (thereby decompressing the heart) into an oxygenator that removes excess carbon dioxide and adds oxygen (simulating the lungs) and pumps arterialized blood into the systemic circulation (simulating the heart). The development of CPB enabled surgeons to isolate the heart by cross clamping the aorta and to pharmacologically induce cardiac arrest to create a dry, quiet operative field in which to perform the surgical repairs. During the period of cardiac arrest, the rest of the body can be adequately perfused via CPB.

Coarctation of the Aorta: A congenital narrowing of the thoracic aorta, usually in the area of the ligamentum arteriosum (formerly the fetal patent ductus arteriosus, which shunts blood from the pulmonary artery to the aorta).

Commissurotomy: The opening or separation of fused valve leaflet commissures (in the adult, generally the mitral or pulmonary valve).

Congenital Heart Disease: Cardiac anomalies apparent at birth or later in life. In this section, some of the congenital anomalies that may be seen in adulthood are discussed.

Dysrhythmia Surgery for Atrial Fibrillation (AF): Surgery designed to block or redirect aberrant atrial fibrillatory impulses toward the atrioventricular node to achieve normal sinus rhythm.

Hybrid Suite: Procedure or operating room that integrates interventional and traditional surgical equipment and supplies, and imaging and monitoring capability.

Hypothermia: Cooling of the patient during cardiac surgery. Hypothermia can be induced (elective) or inadvertent. Induced systemic hypothermia is achieved with a heat exchanger incorporated into the cardiopulmonary bypass circuit; induced cardiac hypothermia is achieved with infusion of cooled cardioplegia solution into the coronary circulation. Topical cardiac cooling is achieved by pouring cold solutions onto the heart.

Implantable Cardioverter-Defibrillator (ICD): A device that provides a shock to the heart for tachycardia above a predetermined rate or ventricular fibrillation and also has the capability to provide bradycardia therapy. The device is usually inserted transvenously in the electrophysiology or cardiac catheterization laboratory. Patients with ICDs who undergo surgery have a magnet placed over the generator (usually in the right or left upper chest) to turn off the device and avoid frequent shocks during induced cardiac arrest. After surgery, the magnet is removed and the ICD is again activated.

Minimally Invasive Cardiac Surgery: Operations that use smaller incisions, percutaneous and or endoscopic access, endovascular techniques, or off-pump (i.e., no cardiopulmonary bypass) procedures. A common procedure in minimally invasive surgery is the endoscopic video-assisted excision of saphenous vein coronary bypass grafts. In other cases, smaller sternal or thoracic chest incisions or ports may be used for target areas of the heart that can be accessed through these minimal incisions (e.g., certain coronary bypass operations for single vessel disease and some valve procedures).

Mitral Regurgitation (MR): A condition that occurs when one or more components of the mitral valve apparatus prevents competent closure of the valve, with subsequent regurgitation of blood into the left atrium.

Mitral Stenosis (MS): A narrowing of the mitral valve orifice that creates an impedance to flow across the valve.

Myocardial Protection Techniques: Techniques or procedures designed to conserve myocardial energy resources and limit the amount of ischemic tissue injury that can occur. The use of cardioplegia and induced hypothermia (see previous definition) to arrest and preserve the heart form the foundation of myocardial protection. Additional myocardial protective measures can include minimization of the risk of an air embolus from ambient room air trapped inside the heart with insufflation of CO_2 gas through a catheter into the pericardial well. The CO_2 gas not only displaces ambient air but also dissolves approximately

25 times faster in the blood than room air and is less harmful to cardiac tissue.

Myocardial Revascularization: Also called *coronary artery bypass grafting.* Surgical procedure performed for coronary artery disease in which conduits of the patient's own tissue (autograft), most commonly the internal mammary artery or other arteries (e.g., radial artery, gastroepiploic artery) and the greater saphenous vein, are attached directly to the affected coronary artery at a site distal to the narrowed atherosclerotic lesion. Generally, coronary narrowing of 70% or greater in arteries that are 1 mm or larger is an indication for bypass grafting; narrowing of less than 70% can create competitive flow between the conduit and the native artery and reduce the amount of blood that perfuses the bypass graft (and the anastomosed coronary artery).

Patent Ductus Arteriosus (PDA): A duct between the pulmonary artery and the aorta, present in fetal life. The duct usually closes within 1 or 2 weeks after birth and becomes the ligamentum arteriosum.

Percutaneous Transluminal Coronary Angioplasty (PTCA) with Stent Insertion: A catheter-based interventional technique performed with fluoroscopy in the cardiac catheterization (see previous definition) laboratory for acute or chronically obstructed coronary arteries. A percutaneously inserted balloon catheter is threaded to the right or left coronary os, where the catheter is positioned across the coronary artery at the site of the narrowing. The balloon is inflated to compress the atherosclerotic lesion and enlarge the coronary lumen. A stent (bare metal or coated) is commonly inserted in conjunction with the PTCA to maintain coronary artery patency.

Pericardiectomy, Pericardial Window: Pericardiectomy is the partial excision of an adhered, thickened fibrotic pericardium to relieve constriction of the heart and great blood vessels. In patients with chronic cardiac effusions, the creation of a pericardial window (excision of a portion of the pericardial or pleural wall) between the pericardial sac and the pleural space drains the fluid. In patients with chronic effusions, the window to the pleural space generally allows future fluid accumulation to be reabsorbed.

Pulmonary Stenosis: Fusion of the pulmonary valve cusps at the commissures, which creates an obstruction to the right-ventricular outflow tract. Another form of pulmonary stenosis occurs in the infundibular portion where fibromuscular obstruction occurs proximal to the valve, creating right ventricular outflow tract obstruction.

Tetralogy of Fallot (TOF): A congenital entity with four distinctive features: (1) a high ventricular septal defect (VSD); (2) pulmonary stenosis that affects the valve or the infundibular region; (3) overriding of the ventricular septal defect by the aorta; and (4) hypertrophy of the right ventricle. In the adult and commonly in the child, correction includes closure of the VSD with a patch and enlargement of the pulmonary valve (or stenosed infundibular region) with dilators, via commissurotomy, valve replacement, infundibular resection, or insertion of an allograft, depending on the underlying pathology.

Transplantation: Replacement of the patient's heart with a human donor heart; replacement of one or both lungs with lungs from a donor, or one lung from a living donor). Heart donors are persons with irreversible catastrophic brain injury who do not have atherosclerotic heart disease; age limitations have become less restrictive, and donors and recipients may be 60 years or older in certain cases. Severe pulmonary disease is a contraindication for lung donation.

Tricuspid Regurgitation: A condition that occurs when the tricuspid valve does not totally close because the leaflets do not completely approximate in diastole.

Tricuspid Stenosis: A narrowing of the orifice of the tricuspid valve.

Valve Replacement: A surgical procedure in which the native valve is replaced with a mechanical or biologic prosthesis; allograft valve replacement also may be performed.

Valvuloplasty: The repair of one or more components of the right (tricuspid) or left (mitral) atrioventricular valve complex that consists of the valve annulus (see Annuloplasty), the valve leaflets, the chordae tendineae, the papillary muscles, and the endoventricular wall.

Ventricular Assist Device (VAD): Mechanical devices to support the left ventricle (LVAD), the right ventricle (RVAD), or both ventricles (BiVAD) can be used long term as a bridge to transplant or destination therapy, depending on the underlying pathology. VADs decrease the workload of the heart by diverting blood from the ventricle to an artificial pump that maintains systemic (LVAD) or pulmonary (RVAD) perfusion. Currently, patients can be ambulatory with implantable VADs powered by batteries, which has substantially improved the quality of life for many VAD patients.

Ventricular Septal Defect (VSD): Consists of a hole through the ventricular septum. VSDs may be congenital or acquired (i.e., postinfarction VSD).

PREOPERATIVE CONSIDERATIONS

Before surgery, documentation of the history and physical examination, surgical consents, the results of diagnostic and laboratory tests, and additional pertinent information are reviewed by the nurse. Among the significant factors are estimates of left ventricle (LV) function (e.g., ejection fraction), a history of medications that may affect perioperative bleeding (e.g., aspirin, anticoagulants), oxygen-carrying capacity (e.g., hematocrit, hemoglobin), renal function (creatinine), pulmonary function (spirometry), cardiac anatomy (e.g., of the valves, coronary arteries), and the presence of concomitant carotid artery disease.[2] Many patients are admitted the morning of surgery, which shortens the period of time for teaching. Often preoperative laboratory testing and requests for packed red blood cells are performed a few days before the scheduled surgery; patient teaching can be accomplished at this time (Table 35-1).

Table 35-1   Patient Teaching for Coronary Artery Bypass Graft Surgery and Valve Surgery

TOPIC	CABG SURGERY	VALVE SURGERY
Perioperative Pointers		
Medical diagnosis	Coronary artery occlusive disease	Valve regurgitation, stenosis, or mixed lesion
Diagnostic tests	ECG, chest radiograph, nuclear imaging, cardiac catheterization, carotid duplex studies	Same, plus echocardiogram
Routine preoperative tests	CMP, ECG, T&C, pulmonary function, PT, PTT, INR, urinanalysis	Same
Incision site	Midsternal or anterior thoracotomy; multiple leg incisions for vein harvest, arm incision for radial artery harvest	Mini-sternotomy, full sternotomy, or mini-thoracotomy
Resumption of eating	After removal of ET and NG tubes (postoperative day 1) clear liquids, then advance to high calorie/high protein diet	Same
Pain control	IM, PO, PCA	Same
Estimated length of procedure	3-6 hours	Same
Estimated length of hospital stay	4-6 days	5-7 days
Long-term effects of surgery	Possible loss of saphenous vein or internal mammary or radial arteries; possible intermittent lower leg ischemia	Possible chronic anticoagulation therapy; differences between biologic and mechanical prostheses, valve repair
Drains or tubes	2 days: mediastinal chest tube, pleural tube; 2-3 days: leg drains, urinary drainage catheter; remove tubes when drainage >100 mL for 8 hours	2 days: mediastinal and pleural tubes, urinary catheter
Postoperative Pointers and Home Instructions		
Food	Cardiac diet	Same
Wound care	Wounds covered if draining; redress after shower or bath; contact clinician if signs of infection	Same
Bathing	Daily	Same
Driving	4-6 weeks (automatic shift only)	Same
Sex	Restricted by limits of ability to bear weight on upper arms and chest	Same
Return to work	8-12 weeks	Same
Medications	Aspirin anticoagulant, cardiac drugs	Warfarin (Coumadin), cardiac drugs
Follow-up	7-14 days	Same, plus laboratory tests for determination of bleeding times
Special restrictions	Upper body movement restricted for 6 weeks for sternal healing	Same
Lifestyle changes	Reduction of coronary risk factors; cardiac rehabilitation	Risk factor reduction; cardiac rehabilitation
Worrisome but normal	Fatigue, swelling in leg; leg discomfort 4-6 weeks; weakness; emotional let down	Fatigue; sound of mechanical valve; weakness; emotional let down

Adapted from Lemmer JH, Vlahakes GJ: *Handbook of patient care in cardiac surgery,* ed 7, Philadelphia, 2010, Lippincott Williams & Wilkins; Bojar RM: *Manual of perioperative care in adult cardiac surgery,* ed 5, Oxford, 2011, Wiley-Blackwell.
ECG, Electrocardiogram; *CMP,* comprehensive metabolic panel (includes glucose, blood urea nitrogen, sodium, potassium, chloride, creatinine, albumin, bilirubin, calcium, alkaline phosphatase, total protein); *T&C,* type and cross match (blood); *PT,* prothrombin time; *PTT,* partial thromboplastin time; *INR,* International Normalized Ratio; *ET,* endotracheal; *NG,* nasogastric; *IM,* intramuscular; *PO,* by mouth; *PCA,* patient-controlled analgesia.

Table 35-2 Hemodynamic Effects of Anesthetic Drugs

DRUG	CI	BP	SVR	LVEDP	HR	CONTRACTILITY
Tubocurarine	↓	↓	↓	↓	↑	↔
Diazepam	↓	↓	↓	↓	↔	↔
Dimethyl tubocurarine	↑	↔↑	↔↓	↔↓	↑	↔
Droperidol	↔↑	↓	↓	↓	↑	↔
Enflurane	↓	↓	↓	↔↓	↔↓	↓
Fentanyl	↔	↓	↓	↔	↔	↔
Halothane	↓	↓	↔↓	↔↑	↔↑↓	↓
Innovar	↔↑	↓	↓	↓	↔	↔
Isoflurane	↔	↓	↓	↔	↑	↓
Ketamine	↑	↑	↑	↑	↑	—
Methoxyflurane	↓	↓	↓	↔	↔	↓
Midazolam	↔	↔	↔↓	↓	↑	↔↓
Morphine	↔↑	↔↓	↓	↔↑	↓	↔
Nitrous oxide	↓	↔↓	↔↑	↑	↔↓	↓
Pancuronium	↑	↑	↔	↑	↑	?
Succinylcholine	↓	↔↓	↓	↑	↑↓	?
Thiopental	↔↓	↔	↑	↔	↑	↓
Vecuronium	↔	↔	↔	↔	↔	↔

Adapted from Rothrock JC: *Alexander's care of the patient in surgery*, ed 14, St. Louis, 2011, Mosby; Lemmer JH, Vlahakes GJ: *Handbook of patient care in cardiac surgery*, ed 7, Philadelphia, 2010, Lippincott Williams & Wilkins; Bojar RM: *Manual of perioperative care in adult cardiac surgery*, ed 5, Oxford, 2011, Wiley-Blackwell.

↓, Decrease; ↑, increase; ↔, no change; ?, insufficient data; *BP*, blood pressure; *CI*, cardiac index; *SVR*, systemic vascular resistance; *LVEDP*, left ventricular end-diastolic pressure; *HR*, heart rate.

ANESTHESIA

Anesthesia for cardiac surgery varies by hospital and can also vary by the type of cardiac repair. Ideally, anesthetic management includes drugs that have rapid onset and termination, minimize ischemia, and are nontoxic to myocardial and other tissue.[3] For example, in patients with significant pulmonary involvement, agents that increase pulmonary vascular resistance should be avoided.[2] Hemodynamic effects of some anesthetic drugs are shown in Table 35-2.

PROCEDURES

Monitoring

Monitoring (Table 35-3) of the patient's electrocardiogram (ECG) and direct blood pressure (commonly via the radial artery in the nondominant wrist) results is initiated when the patient arrives in the preoperative area. Central lines are usually inserted after transport into the operating room (OR), but occasionally are inserted in another designated location, such as the preoperative area. Whether the patient first undergoes intubation before insertion of central lines (i.e., central venous pressure, pulmonary artery catheter) or after line insertion is at the discretion of the anesthesia provider; the sequence varies among institutions. Increasingly, an anesthesia provider inserts a transesophageal echocardiography (TEE) probe to illustrate cardiac function. Use of TEE for valve surgery and for patients with compromised LV function is routine.[2,3]

Incisions

After the patient has been anesthetized, positioned, and washed (prepared), the chest is opened. The most commonly used chest incision in cardiac surgery is the median sternotomy; this is the preferred incision when a thorough assessment of, and complete access to, the heart (as with global coronary artery disease) is needed. However, ministernotomy, anterolateral or posterolateral thoracotomy incisions, or transverse sternotomy also may be used (Fig. 35-1). The surgeon splits the sternum with a saw from the sternal

Table 35-3   Physiologic Monitoring

MONITORING DEVICE	LOCATION	ASSESSES/MEASURES
Cardiovascular System		
Electrocardiogram (ECG)	Electrodes placed on shoulders, hips, and left axillary line	Electrical activity of heart: lead II useful to monitor cardiac rhythm (good visualization of P wave and QRS) and myocardial ischemia (inferior surface); lead V5 useful to detect myocardial ischemia (anterior surface)
Intraarterial catheter	Radial artery (also femoral artery) aorta, bypass circuit; in children, may use superficial temporal or dorsalis pedis arteries; in neonates, may use umbilical artery	Direct arterial BP; blood gases; blood chemistries
Blood pressure cuff	Right or left arm	Indirect BP
CVP line	RA	RA pressure (CVP); RV filling pressure; RV preload
PA catheter (addition of fiberoptics provides additional information about mixed venous oxygen saturation [SvO$_2$])	PA (proximal and distal)	PA pressures: systolic, diastolic, mean, wedge; pulmonary vascular resistance; LV filling pressure; LV preload; CO; assessment of stroke volume, stroke work, systemic vascular resistance; mixed venous saturation (continuous indirect assessment of CO and reflection of tissue oxygenation); RV function
LA catheter (when used)	LA	LA pressure (direct); LV filling pressure; LV preload
TEE	Esophagus	Valve function before and after repair; LV wall motion, failure; intracardiac air bubbles
Urinary drainage catheter	Urinary bladder	Urinary output, renal perfusion; indirect measure of CO
Respiratory System		
Mass spectrometry	Anesthesia circuit	Inspired or expired O$_2$, CO$_2$, and anesthetic gases; used to avoid hypoxia, hypercarbia, anesthetic overdose
Pulse oximeter	Finger or toe cot; earlobe, nose	Oxygen saturation of arterial hemoglobin; tissue oxygenation
Capnography	Anesthesia circuit	End-tidal CO$_2$; used to detect integrity of anesthesia circuit; avoid disconnections of monitor, endotracheal tube; detect spontaneous ventilation, rebreathing, obstructive pulmonary disease
Central Nervous System		
Temperature	Esophagus, nasopharynx, urinary bladder, rectum, ventricular septum, bypass circuit, PA catheter	Core, and peripheral temperature of heart, brain, and other organs
Electroencephalogram	Scalp electrodes	Detect cerebral ischemia, embolus; indication of depth of anesthesia
Renal System		
Urinary discharge catheter	Bladder	Urinary output; indirect measure of cardiac output

Adapted from Lemmer JH, Vlahakes GJ: *Handbook of patient care in cardiac surgery,* ed 7, Philadelphia, 2010, Lippincott Williams & Wilkins; Bojar RM: *Manual of perioperative care in adult cardiac surgery,* ed 5, Oxford, 2011, Wiley-Blackwell.
BP, Blood pressure; *CVP,* central venous pressure; *RA,* right atrial; *RV,* right ventricular; *PA,* pulmonary artery; *LA,* left atrial; *CO,* cardiac output; *TEE,* transesophageal echocardiography.

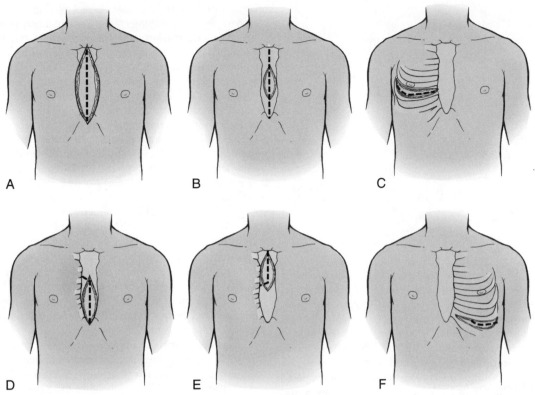

FIG. 35-1 Traditional and less invasive thoracic incisions (*dotted lines* represent chest wall incisions). **A,** Traditional sternotomy. **B,** Full sternotomy with limited skin incision. **C,** Parasternal incision (infrequently used). **D** and **E,** Partial lower and upper sternotomy incisions used mainly for valve procedures. **F,** Right thoracotomy incision can be used for mitral valve procedures. Left anterior thoracotomy (*not shown*) can be used for single coronary bypass graft to left anterior descending coronary artery. (From Braunwald E, et al, editors: *Heart disease,* ed 6, Philadelphia, 2001, Saunders.)

notch to the xiphoid process. After the sternum is opened, the exposed pericardial sac is incised anteriorly, and the pericardial edges are tacked up along the chest wall incision to allow complete access to the entire pericardium without the necessity of entering the pleural cavities. Minimally invasive surgery uses smaller incisions and can speed patient recovery, enable the patient to return faster to normal activities, and reduce costs.

Cardiopulmonary Bypass

Systemic venous return to the heart flows by gravity drainage (the level of the patient needs to be above that of the bypass machine to facilitate drainage) into one or two large-bore (e.g., 32F to 36F) cannulas inserted into the right atrium. With the single two-stage cannula (Fig. 35-2), openings in the distal tip drain blood returning from the inferior vena cava (IVC) and openings in the middle portion of the cannula drain venous blood from the superior vena cava (SVC) and the coronary circulation exiting from the coronary sinus. Some blood enters the right atrium (RA) and the pulmonary circulation. With double cannulation (Fig. 35-3), individual cannulas are inserted into the IVC and the SVC, thereby forcing all venous return into the cannulas. Generally the two-stage cannula is used for coronary artery bypass grafting and aortic valve surgery when total right side decompression is not generally needed and blood entering the right side of the heart does not obscure the surgical field. Individual (double) venous cannulation can be used for procedures in the right side (e.g., tricuspid valve repair) to keep the right heart free of blood. Occasionally, two cannulas can be used when greater decompression of the RA is necessary (e.g., mitral valve surgery).

After the blood is oxygenated, it is pumped into the systemic circulation via an arterial cannula,

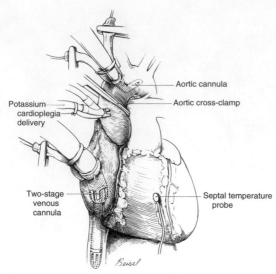

FIG. 35-2 Antegrade cardioplegia infusion catheter is inserted proximal to aortic cross clamp and arterial infusion cannula. Two-stage (single) venous cannula drains sysemic venous return. Openings in distal end of cannula drain blood from lower body; openings in midportion of cannula (within right atrium) drain blood returning from upper body and coronary venous drainage exiting from coronary sinus. Septal temperature probe monitors myocardial septal temperature. (From Waldhausen JA, et al: *Surgery of the chest,* ed 6, St Louis, 1996, Mosby.)

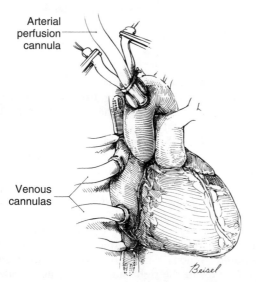

FIG. 35-3 Double venous cannulation. One cannula is inserted into inferior vena cava, and the other into superior vena cava. Also shown is arterial infusion catheter. (From Waldhausen JA, et al: *Surgery of the chest,* ed 6, St. Louis, 1996, Mosby.)

commonly located in the aorta (see Fig. 35-3). When aortic pathology (e.g., aortic aneurysm) prevents cannulation, the femoral artery can be cannulated (retrograde flow) for arterial return. The axillary artery may be needed when the aorta or both of the femoral arteries are unavailable.

In addition to the standard cannulation techniques for cardiopulmonary bypass (CPB), minimally invasive systems use endovascular catheters (Fig. 35-4). A venous catheter is inserted into the femoral vein, and the arterial cannula is placed into the femoral artery. The ipsilateral femoral artery is also used for insertion of a multilumen catheter. One lumen serves as an endovascular cross clamp that occludes the aorta with inflation of an intraaortic balloon at the tip of the catheter, and the other lumen can be used for infusion of antegrade cardioplegia. Pressure lines, venting catheters, and a coronary sinus retrograde cardioplegia catheter can be inserted via the jugular vein. This system does not require median sternotomy and is an important adjunct for minimally invasive surgery.[4]

A number of risks are associated with the use of CPB (e.g., particulate or air embolus), and some form of checklist is often used before CPB is instituted (Box 35-1) and before the patient is weaned from CPB (Box 35-2). Such checklists help to enhance the safety of CPB. In addition, the clinical sequelae of CPB can affect all body systems. Caregivers in the postoperative period should be aware of the possible effects of CPB (Table 35-4).

CPB is not always required. So-called off-pump procedures for myocardial revascularization can be performed while the heart is beating with the use of special devices to isolate the section of the coronary artery to be grafted. For procedures that require entry into the chambers of the heart (e.g., valve replacement), CPB and myocardial protection are necessary for perfusion of the body, avoidance of air emboli that originate from the open cardiac chamber, and myocardial preservation.

Myocardial Protection

The goal of myocardial protection is to conserve cardiac energy resources; the goal is achieved with induced hypothermia and rapid diastolic arrest. Hypothermia reduces the metabolic rate (and therefore the energy demands) of the tissue being cooled; effective intraoperative myocardial protection positively affects the patient's postoperative recovery. For most cardiac procedures of less than 1 hour of induced cardiac arrest (e.g., coronary artery bypass grafting), the

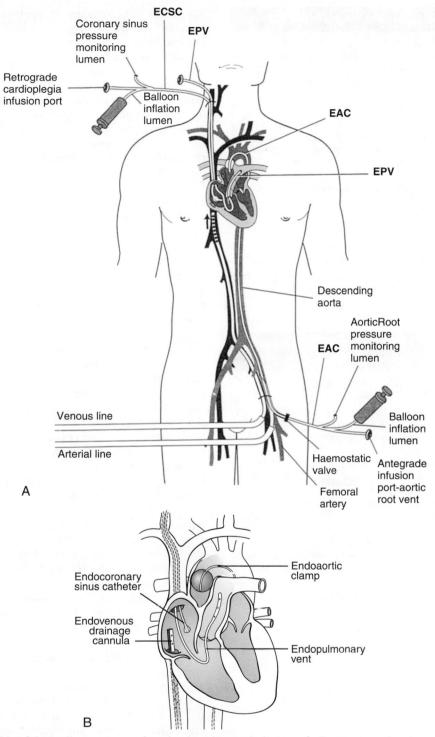

FIG. 35-4 Minimally invasive cardiopulmonary bypass technique. **A,** Positioning of endovascular catheters). **B,** Correct positions of endocoronary sinus catheter, endoaortic clamp, endovenous drainage cannula, and endopulmonary vent for port-access cardiopulmonary bypass. *EAC,* Endoaortic clamp; *ECSC,* endocoronary sinus catheter; *EPV,* cardiopulmonary vent. (**A,** From Toomasian M, et al: Extracorporeal circulation for port-access cardiac surgery, *Perfusion* 12:83, 1997. **B,** From Kaplan J, editor: *Kaplan's cardiac anesthesia,* ed 5, Philadelphia, 2006, Saunders.)

NURSING CARE IN THE PACU

BOX 35-1   Checklist for Initiation of Pump

- Heparin administered
- Activated coagulation time checked and at least 350 to 400 seconds
- Muscle relaxant adequate (or infusion turned on for maintenance)
- Inotropic infusions turned off
- Pupil symmetry assessed for later comparison (unilateral dilation may indicate unilateral carotid perfusion on cardiopulmonary bypass)
- Pulmonary artery catheter (if used) pulled back 5 cm
- Urinary output emptied before bypass (start anew with initiation of bypass)
- Proper functioning of all monitors ensured

From Lemmer JH, Vlahakes GJ: *Handbook of patient care in cardiac surgery,* ed 7, Philadelphia, 2010, Lippincott Williams & Wilkins; Bojar RM: *Manual of perioperative care in adult cardiac surgery,* ed 5, Oxford, 2011, Wiley-Blackwell.

BOX 35-2   Checklist for Weaning from the Pump

- Patient is warm (to at least 36° C)
- Heart rhythm has returned
- All monitors are functioning; electrocardiogram, pulmonary artery tracing, arterial line tracing, central venous pressure reflect heart filling
- Heart rate is 70 to 100 beats/min (<60 beats/min is reduced cardiac output; ≥120 beats/min is detrimental to left ventricular filling)
- Infusions are prepared as necessary
- Lungs are inflated, but kept out of the surgeon's field
- Pressure becomes pulsatile as ventricles fill
- Blood is drawn for measurement of electrolytes, hematocrit, arterial blood gases, and activated clotting time
- The surgeon clamps venous drainage cannula and removes the cannula
- Patient is off pump

From Lemmer JH, Vlahakes GJ: *Handbook of patient care in cardiac surgery,* ed 7, Philadelphia, 2010, Lippincott Williams & Wilkins; Bojar RM: *Manual of perioperative care in adult cardiac surgery,* ed 5, Oxford, 2011, Wiley-Blackwell.

perfusionist cools the systemic circulation from a normal temperature of 37° C (98.6° F) to approximately 32° C (89.6° F). The cardioplegia solution is cooled to a lower temperature (near freezing) for intracardiac cooling as a method of myocardial protection. For procedures with a longer cross-clamp time, the systemic temperature

may be further reduced to protect the brain, kidneys, and other organs while the heart is arrested by reducing energy demands and limiting ischemic injury. Topical cooling of the heart with cold lavage or frozen "slush" placed on the heart and in the pericardial well helps to achieve transmural cooling. Although induced hypothermia plays an important role in minimization of tissue ischemia during selected portions of cardiac procedures, inadvertant hypothermia has become an important consideration for cardiac patients because of associated risks for perioperative complications. Before surgery, shivering increases myocardial oxygen demands and further taxes hearts that have diminished myocardial energy supplies. During surgery, before and after CPB, inadvertent cooling of the patient is associated with increased surgical bleeding and a diminished immune response. After surgery, hypothermia contributes to patient discomfort, impaired wound healing, prolonged bleeding, longer lengths of stay, and cardiac events such as ischemia and tachyarrhythmias.[2,3] Active measures, such as the application of warm blankets before surgery and during the intraoperative period (before and after induced hypothermia), the postoperative use of forced warm air devices and intravenous fluid warmers, and an increased ambient room temperature, can help to maintain normothermia.

Rapid diastolic arrest conserves existing cellular energy resources (e.g., adenosine triphosphate) by avoiding the energy-expensive state of ventricular fibrillation before the heart achieves an arrested state. Quick arrest of a beating heart (e.g., 10 to 20 seconds) enhances myocardial energy conservation. Potassium is the most commonly used arresting agent, but the solutions may also contain electrolytes, buffers to maintain appropriate pH, glucose, metabolic substrates, calcium antagonists, tromethamine, heparin, and antiarrhythmic agents. The carrying solution can be crystalloid or blood (preferable for its oxygen carrying capacity).[4]

Methods of infusing cardioplegia include the antegrade and retrograde routes and the direct coronary ostial route of infusion. With the antegrade method, a needle catheter is inserted into the anterior aorta proximal to the aortic cross clamp (see Fig. 35-2). The cardioplegia solution is infused with sufficient pressure to close the aortic valve. With the cross clamp applied distally and a competent aortic valve proximally, the only paths for the solution to travel are the right and left coronary ostia lying between the cross-clamped aorta and the closed aortic valve. In patients with aortic valve insufficiency, cardioplegia flow into

Table 35-4 Effects of Cardiopulmonary Bypass	
EFFECTS	**CONTRIBUTING FACTORS**
Cardiovascular System	
Perioperative myocardial infarction	Inadequate myocardial protection and emboli
Low cardiac output syndrome after surgery	Preexisting heart disease, inadequate myocardial protection, alteration in colloidal osmotic pressure, left ventricular dysfunction, hypoperfusion injury, hypothermia, long pump run
Increased afterload	Catecholamine release
Hypertension	Elevated rennin, angiotensin, and aldosterone levels
Hypotension	Postoperative diuresis, sudden vasodilation (rewarming), third spacing
Pulmonary System	
Respiratory insufficiency	Alterations in colloidal osmotic pressure, interstitial pulmonary edema, decreased perfusion, alterations in ventilatory patterns, decreased surfactant production, pulmonary microemboli
Atelectasis	Complement activation and inflammatory response, emboli, alveolar-capillary membrane damage
Neurologic System	
Cerebrovascular accident	Cerebral emboli
Transient motor defects	Decreased cerebral blood flow
Cerebral hemorrhage	Systematic heparin administration
Neuropsychological deficits	Microemboli, ischemia, altered perfusion flow of bypass
Gastrointestinal System	
Gastrointestinal bleeding	Hormonal stress and coagulation diatheses
Intestinal ischemia or infarction	Emboli and decreased perfusion
Acute pancreatitis	Pancreatic vasculature emboli
Renal System	
Acute renal failure	Decreased renal blood flow, microemboli, and myohemoglobin release
Hemoglobinuria	Red blood cell hemolysis
Fluid and Electrolyte Balance	
Interstitial edema, weight gain	Increased extravascular fluid and organ dysfunction, fluid shifts, decreased plasma protein concentration, increased capillary permeability
Intravascular hypovolemia	Decreased intravascular volume, bleeding, and interstitial edema
Hypokalemia	Dilution, polyuria, intracellular shifts of potassium ions
Hyperkalemia	Potassium cardioplegia and increased intracellular exchange of glucose and potassium, cellular destruction
Hyponatremia, hypocalcemia, and hypomagnesemia	Dilution, fluid shifts, diureses
Endocrine System	
Water and sodium retention	Increase in antidiuretic hormone
Hypothyroidism	Increased levels of thyroxine (T4) and decreased levels of triiodothyronine (T3) and thyroid-stimulating hormone
Hyperglycemia	Depressed insulin response, stimulation of glycogenesis
Immune System	
Infection	Exposure to multiple pathogens, decreased immunoglobin levels, and hypothermia
Postperfusion syndrome	Release of anaphylactic toxins, complement activation
Hematologic Factors	
Bleeding	Blood cell hemolysis, heparin rebound, reduction in platelet count and coagulation factors, coagulopathy, systemic heparin administration, depressed liver function from hypothermia

Adapted from Lemmer JH, Vlahakes GJ: *Handbook of patient care in cardiac surgery,* ed 7, Philadelphia, 2010, Lippincott Williams & Wilkins; Bojar RM: *Manual of perioperative care in adult cardiac surgery,* ed 5, Oxford, 2011, Wiley-Blackwell.

NURSING CARE IN THE PACU

the coronary ostia is significantly reduced because the incompetent aortic valve provides a lower pressure pathway into the inner ventricular chamber, thereby distending the heart and increasing myocardial wall tension. Retrograde delivery is indicated in the presence of coronary artery lesions that impair the transmural distribution of the cardioplegia when delivered solely by the antegrade route. For the retrograde route, the surgeon inserts a catheter through a stab wound into the right atrial wall and threads the catheter into the coronary sinus. The cardioplegic solution infused into the coronary sinus flows retrograde through the cardiac veins and arteries. The solution exits via the coronary ostia, where it is removed by suction.

In addition to thermal and pharmacologic interventions, other strategies to achieve adequate myocardial energy conservation include implementing actions that consistently maximize myocardial energy supplies and minimizing myocardial energy demands. Surgeons and assistants use caution in touching the heart before bypass to lessen the risk of ventricular fibrillation. Anesthesia providers pharmacologically decrease cellular oxygen demand and increase cellular oxygen supply. Other considerations in protecting the heart include minimization of cross-clamp time with availability of the appropriate supplies and equipment, a plan for surgery (jointly developed by surgeons, anesthesia providers, perfusionists, and nursing personnel), anticipation and ability to respond to potential risks and complications applicable to one's professional responsibilities and skills, implementation of safety procedures, and frequent and collaborative communication.

Surgery for Coronary Artery Disease

Coronary artery disease remains the leading cause of death among men and women.[5] Left heart cardiac catheterization is commonly performed for identification of areas affected by obstructive atherosclerotic coronary artery disease. Selective coronary angiography with an injection of contrast medium into the right and left coronary ostia illustrates coronary anatomy, distal coronary perfusion, the location of atherosclerotic lesions, the status of coronary collateral circulation, and the percentage of narrowing of coronary arteries affected by coronary artery disease (CAD). Dye is injected into the LV (ventriculography) to determine wall motion (e.g., hypokinesia, dyskinesia, paradoxic motion), and valvular function (e.g., mitral regurgitation, prosthetic valve function). Generally, a right-heart catheterization

yields data concerning the inferior and superior vena cava, the right atrium and ventricle, tricuspid and pulmonary valves, and the pulmonary artery.

Percutaneous coronary interventions, specifically percutaneous coronary interventions angioplasty (PTCA) with stent insertion, can be performed for discrete lesions. Equalized pressure measurements above and below the lesion indicate a successful angioplasty. The restenosis rate for angioplasty at 6 months has been approximately 30%, necessitating additional angioplasties or surgery. Complications from the interventional procedure include prolonged chest pain, myocardial infarction, coronary spasm, or coronary artery dissection that can necessitate emergency coronary artery bypass grafting (CABG). Evidence supports surgical revascularization (i.e., CABG) over percutaneous coronary interventions in patients with left main coronary artery disease.[6,7]

When CABG is recommended for patients, the number and type of bypass grafts (e.g., saphenous vein, internal mammary artery) are assessed. Fig. 35-5 illustrates possible arterial and venous

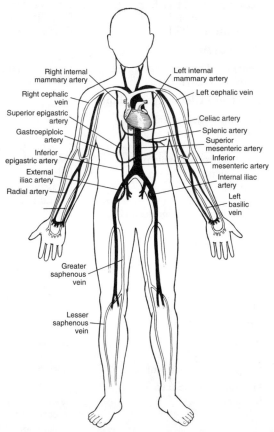

FIG. 35-5 Arterial and venous conduits for coronary bypass surgery. (From Seifert PC: *Cardiac surgery*, St. Louis, 2002, Mosby.)

autologous conduits. Grafts from cadaver human saphenous vein, human and bovine umbilical vein, and synthetic grafts have been used when other conduits were unavailable. CABG does not cure CAD; its purpose is to increase blood flow to the myocardium beyond the obstructive lesions. CAD is a progressive disease, and retardation of the atherosclerotic process requires life style changes and pharmacologic support (e.g., statins). Gender-based differences in CABG outcomes are under scrutiny, and guidelines have been published to provide evidence for the selection of techniques.[5]

Once the sternum is opened, the surgeon dissects the required length of the internal mammary artery (Fig. 35-6). The internal mammary artery (IMA) is dissected from its retrosternal bed to the required length, leaving intact the proximal attachment to the left subclavian artery. The assistant harvests additional bypass conduits, such as the saphenous vein (Fig. 35-7) or the radial artery.[8] Greater saphenous vein is commonly harvested with video-assisted endoscopic techniques.[9] Because leg veins have valves that facilitate flow toward the right heart, reversal of the vein is necessary so that flow as a

Evidence-Based Practice

In an effort to resolve the numerous inconsistencies that surround the issue of gender-based differences between the outcomes of women and men who undergo coronary artery bypass grafting (CABG), the Society of Thoracic Surgeons Workforce on Evidence-Based Surgery reviewed published information on this subject.

IMPLICATIONS FOR PRACTICE

The following guidelines focus specifically on perioperative management and are based on the evidence available to the authors of the Guidelines.

1. Use of the internal mammary artery (IMA)
   - The IMA is underused in women.
   - Use of the IMA is associated with a significant reduction in mortality rate (compared with CABG with venous conduits alone).
   - At least one IMA is used to bypass stenotic coronary artery.
2. Management of hyperglycemia
   - Diabetes is more common in women than in men who undergo CABG.
   - The adverse effects of diabetes are more pronounced in women.
   - Hyperglycemia produced an incremental risk in CABG.
   - Blood glucose levels should be maintained at less than 150 mg/dL (range, 100-150 mg/dL).
3. Intraoperative management of anemia
   - Hematocrits of less than 22% are associated with operative mortality.
   - Strategies to increase red blood cell concentration include hemoconcentration, ultrafiltration,

minimization of pump prime volume, rapid autologous priming.
   - Adequate hematocrit levels should be maintained at or greater than 22%.
4. Use of off-pump CABG (OPCAB)
   - Improved outcomes after OPCAB versus on-pump CABG may be related to increased use of IMA with OPCAB.
   - No major differences in outcomes are associated with valve surgery.
   - With the absence of firm evidence that OPCAB is superior, the guidelines suggest that the indications for OPCAB are the same for women as for men.
5. Optimization of thyroxine treatment for women with hypothyroidism
   - Hypothyroidism is associated with impaired contractility and increased risk of myocardial infarction.
   - A greater incidence rate is seen of women with hypothyroidism (compared with men) undergoing CABG.
   - A euthyroid state should be maintained during surgery.
6. Consideration of preoperative hormone replacement therapy (HRT)
   - HRT is not a significant predictor of mortality rate in multivariate analyses.
   - HRT is associated with complications such as thromboembolism.
   - HRT is not used for postmenopausal women undergoing CABG.

Source: Edwards FH, et al: Gender-specific practice guidelines for coronary artery bypass surgery: perioperative management, *Ann Thorac Surg* 79:2189-2194, 2005; Puskas JD, et al: Off-pump techniques benefit men and women and narrow the disparity in mortality after coronary bypass grafting, *Ann Thorac Surg* 84:1447-1456, 2007; Toumpoulis IK, et al: Assessment of independent predictors for long-term mortality between women and men after coronary artery bypass grafting: are women different from men? *J Thorac Cardiovasc Surg* 131:343-351, 2006; Mosca L, et al: Effectiveness-based guidelines for the prevention of cardiovascular disease in women, *Circulation* 123:1243-1262, 2011; Coulter SA: Heart disease and hormones, *Texas Heart Inst J* 38(2):137-141, 2011.

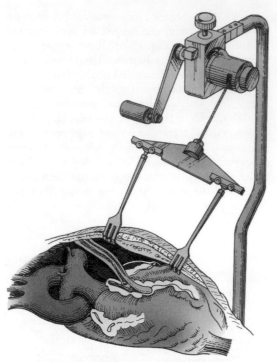

FIG. 35-6 Dissection of left internal mammary artery from retrosternal bed with use of special retractor that elevates sternal border. (Courtesy Rultract, Inc., Cleveland, Ohio.)

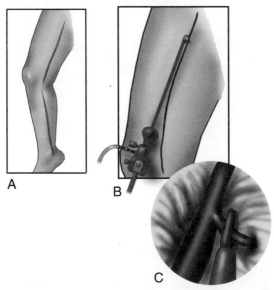

A

B

C

FIG. 35-7 Minimally invasive approach to saphenous vein harvesting. **A,** Traditional open incision. **B,** Insertion of endoscopic camera and dissector. **C,** Venous tributaries cut and clipped, cauterized, or ligated to prevent leaking of blood. (From Zipes DP, et al: *Braunwald's heart disease: a textbook of cardiovascular medicine*, ed 7, Philadelphia, 2005, Saunders.)

bypass graft is not impeded. After conduit harvesting is completed, or if another procedure is planned (e.g., valve repair), the surgeon proceeds to cannulate for CPB. The body is cooled to the desired temperature, and the heart is arrested with cardioplegia. The surgeon then proceeds to attach the grafts to the heart. The left IMA is commonly used in bypass of the left anterior descending coronary artery. The distal anastomosis is created with attaching the end of the graft conduit to the side of the coronary artery; proximally, the IMA graft remains attached to the subclavian artery. For vein grafts, the surgeon attaches the proximal end of the vein to an opening created in the side of the proximal aorta. Veins grafts may be attached to the diagonal, obtuse marginal, posterior descending, or right coronary arteries, as indicated (Fig. 35-8).

In operations that necessitate entry into the heart (valve repair or replacement), CPB is required for perfusion of the body while the heart is arrested and opened. During CABG, the procedure is performed on the epicardial coronary arteries that lie on the surface of the heart, not inside the heart. Coronary bypass surgery can be performed without the use of CPB (off-pump CABG), thereby avoiding the deleterious effects associated with extracorporeal circulation (see Table 35-4). *Off-pump* surgery may be feasible when pulmonary function is poor but LV function is not severely compromised, and access to the target coronary arteries does not require excessive manipulation of the heart.[2,3] During

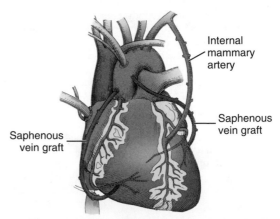

Internal mammary artery

Saphenous vein graft

Saphenous vein graft

FIG. 35-8 Coronary artery bypass grafts with left internal mammary artery to left anterior descending coronary artery, and saphenous vein grafts to obtuse marginal and distal right coronary arteries. (From Braunwald E, et al, editors: *Heart disease*, ed 6, Philadelphia, 2001, Saunders.)

off-pump procedures, the heart beats to perfuse the systemic, pulmonary, and coronary circulations. This *beating heart* surgery has been facilitated with the use of stabilizing devices that isolate and reduce the motion of the portion of the artery to be anastomosed (Fig. 35-9, *1*). An attachment applies suction to the LV apex and allows the heart to be retracted for access to the lateral (i.e., obtuse marginal branches) and posterior (i.e., posterior descending or distal right coronary artery) portions of the heart (see Fig. 35-9, *2*). Patient teaching considerations related to on-pump or off-pump surgery are listed in Table 35-5.

Other technical advances have brought together interventional procedures and traditional surgical treatments. This combination is seen in the hybrid cardiovascular suite, which enables patients to receive both percutaneous coronary stent placement and traditional surgical revascularization.[10]

Left Ventricular Aneurysm Repair

Another form of myocardial revascularization is repair of an LV aneurysm. An LV aneurysm most often results from a large myocardial infarction or numerous smaller adjacent infarctions that cause a portion of the myocardial wall to become scarred, necrotic, thin, and weak. Scar tissue does not contract during systole but instead bulges outward (paradoxic motion or dyskinesia), which decreases the patient's cardiac

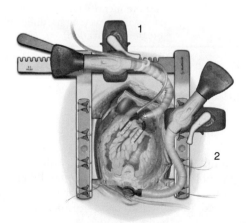

FIG. 35-9 *1*, Octopus® Evo AS off-pump cardiac stabilizer minimizes motion at the coronary anastomotic site. *2*, Starfish® Evo suction positioning device attaches to the apex of the heart and exposes the lateral and posterior coronary arteries for bypass. (Courtesy Medtronic Inc., Minneapolis, Minn.)

output. Thrombus can form within the trabeculations of the LV, and pieces of thrombus can break off and embolize to the systemic circulation. In addition, the perimeter around the scarred fibrotic aneurysmal area can alter conduction pathways and create reentrant ventricular dysrhythmias. Surgical repair consists of excision of the aneurysmal tissue, removal of existing thrombus, and insertion of a patch into the LV in a manner that restores a more normal (i.e., elliptic) ventricular geometry. If the patient continues to have recurrent ventricular tachycardia, electrophysiologic mapping and possible insertion of an implantable cardioverter-defibrillator (ICD) may be performed after surgery in the electrophysiologic laboratory.[3]

Valvular Heart Surgery

Valve surgery is performed more commonly on valves in the left side of the heart (i.e., aortic and mitral valves), because the higher pressures on the left side aggravate traumatic, infectious, or other preexisting injury to the valves and valve components. Repair of the native valve is preferred to replacement when possible. A left heart catheterization yields information concerning the left atrium and ventricle, the proximal aorta, aortic and mitral valves, and the coronary arteries. Echocardiography increasingly is the gold standard for the diagnosis of valvular heart disease. Other imaging processes include aortography that displays the size and function of the aorta and can be used to identify the location of the intimal tear in a dissection. Computed tomographic (CAT) scan and magnetic resonance arteriography have largely replaced aortography for imaging of aortic disease.[11]

When surgery for valve replacement or repair is indicated, the surgeon selects and inserts the appropriate prosthesis. Valve replacement can be accomplished with biologic (Fig. 35-10) or mechanical (Fig. 35-11) prostheses. Newer, percutaneous aortic valve prostheses (Fig. 35-12) are increasingly available, mainly to patients who may be unable to withstand surgical replacemtnt.[12] Allografts (Fig. 35-13) can serve as biologic valve replacements. Allografts are advantageous because they do not require warfarin anticoagulation, are resistant to infection, and have excellent hemodynamics. They are also useful in patients with small aortic roots, because no sewing ring exists to decrease the size of the aortic valve orifice, unlike prosthetic biologic or mechanical valves. Disadvantages include less availability and technical difficulties associated with insertion. Bioprostheses have the advantage of not requiring chronic anticoagulation

Table 35-5	Patient Teaching Considerations for Minimally Invasive Surgery (On/Off Pump)	
	BEATING HEART/OFF-PUMP	**ARRESTED HEART**
Definition	CABG without CPB or induced cardiac arrest; HR and contractile force may be pharmacologically reduced; stabilizer used at anastomotic site; apical retractor used to expose lateral and posterior coronary arteries	CABG with CPB and endovascular technique for CPB and induced cardiac arrest
Indications	Multiple-vessel disease, angioplasty contraindicated, medical problems, poor anatomy, accessible target arteries, previous CABG with blocked grafts	Multiple-vessel disease; angioplasty contraindicated, need to stop heart to enhance technical precision, accessible target arteries, mitral valve disease
Contraindications	Intramyocardial lesions, hemodynamic instability	High complex lesions, posterior targets
Incisions	Sternotomy or ministernotomy (cephalad or caudad); 1-3 small right or left, rib or submammary incisions	1-4 small rib incisions, 1 or 2 groin incisions
CPB	No, available on standby	Yes
Cardioplegia	No	Yes
Procedure time	2 hours or more	2 hours or more
Hospital LOS	3-5 days (versus 4-6 days for sternotomy)	3-5 days (versus 4-6 days for sternotomy)
Advantages	Avoids CPB, ischemic arrest, and hypothermia; may enable more complete revascularization with postoperative insertion of intracoronary stents into posterolateral coronary arteries in cardiac catheterization laboratory (hybrid procedure)	Allows repair of more complex lesions without technical challenge of moving heart; better ability to produce more complete revascularization
Potential complications and disadvantages	Learning curve technically more challenging; may cause VF; may have to revert to standard sternotomy with CPB and induced arrest	Learning curve technically more challenging; may have to revert to standard sternotomy; potential for endovascular injury to cannulated blood vessels
Discharge planning	Anticipated faster recovery of 1-2 weeks (versus 4-12 weeks for sternotomy), earlier ambulation, need to identify reportable signs and symptoms (angina, difficulty breathing, infection)	Anticipated faster recovery of 1-2 weeks (versus 4-12 weeks for sternotomy), earlier ambulation, need to identify reportable signs and symptoms (angina, difficulty breathing, infection)

Adapted from Rothrock JC: *Alexander's care of the patient in surgery,* ed 14, St. Louis, 2011, Mosby; Lemmer JH, Vlahakes GJ: *Handbook of patient care in cardiac surgery,* ed 7, Philadelphia, 2010, Lippincott Williams & Wilkins; Bojar RM: *Manual of perioperative care in adult cardiac surgery,* ed 5, Oxford, 2011, Wiley-Blackwell.
CABG, Coronary artery bypass grafting; *CPB,* cardiopulmonary bypass; *HR,* Heart rate; *LOS,* length of stay; *VF,* ventricular fibrillation.

postoperatively unless there are other indications, such as chronic atrial fibrillation; their disadvantage is that they do not last as long as mechanical prostheses. Bioprostheses are stored in glutaraldehyde before implantation; the solution must be rinsed off the prosthesis, usually in three baths of normal saline solution.

The advantage of mechanical valves is their durability. The disadvantage is that they require continuous anticoagulation therapy after surgery because mechanical prostheses are thrombogenic.

Minimally invasive techniques are increasingly popular. For example, a catheter-based interventional (i.e., nonsurgical) procedure can be performed in a hybrid suite for percutaneous insertion of a balloon-tipped catheter (commonly inserted into the femoral artery or femoral vein) that is threaded through the aorta or IVC to the intended location to enlarge a (stenotic) valve opening. For aortic valvuloplasty, the balloon tip is positioned across the aortic valve, and the balloon is inflated to dilate the aortic

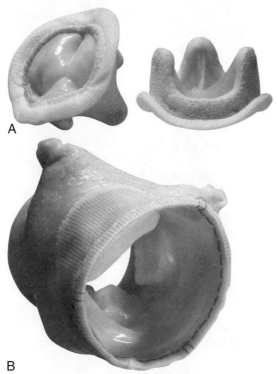

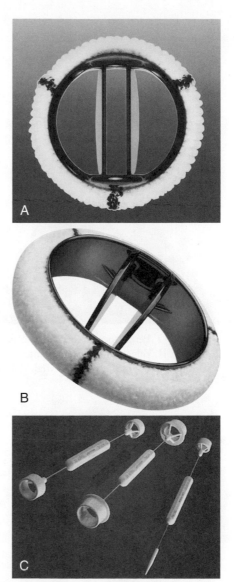

FIG. 35-10 Biologic valves. **A,** Medtronic Hancock II® porcine bioprosthesis (side view and top view). **B,** Freestyle® Aortic Root bioprosthesis. Stentless porcine aortic root bioprosthesis. Use of porcine stentless valves has reduced demand for cadaver allografts. These valves are especially useful in patients with small aortas. (Courtesy Medtronic Inc., Minneapolis, Minn.)

FIG. 35-11 Mechanical valves. **A,** St. Jude Medical bileaflet tilting disk valve prosthesis. **B,** Medtronic Open Pivot™ mechanical valve. **C,** Double-ended obturators (*left* and *center*) for sizing patient's valve; probe (*right*) used to test prosthetic leaflet motion. Sizing obturators are specific to prosthesis. (**A,** Courtesy St. Jude Medical, St. Paul, Minn. **B** and **C,** Courtesy Medtronic Inc., Minneapolis, Minn.)

valve orifice. Complications of valvotomy include development of aortic or mitral regurgitation (depending on the affected valve), cardiac perforation, pulmonary edema, and cerebral embolus. Percutaneous aortic valve implantation also can be performed along with traditional aortic valve replacement.[12]

Aortic Valve Surgery

The closing mechanism of the aortic valve makes repair difficult; aortic stenosis or aortic insufficiency (AI) generally require valve replacement, although some reparative techniques (e.g., suture plicating dilated aortic leaflet commissures) may be performed.

Aortic Insufficiency

The regurgitating blood in AI creates an increased volume load on the LV. Mild chronic AI can be tolerated by the LV for almost 20 years with more

forceful dilation and contraction to eject the additional regurgitant volume. Eventually the LV is stimulated to hypertrophy and decompensates if corrective therapy is not implemented. Symptoms include dyspnea from pulmonary edema and fatigue and other symptoms associated with LV

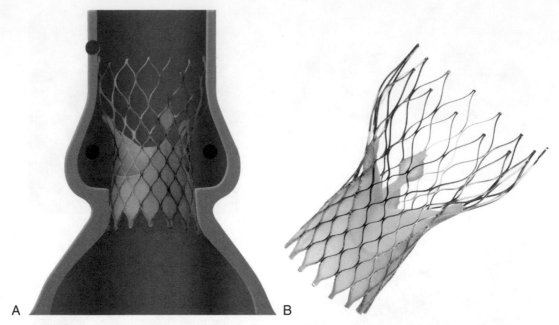

FIG. 35-12 Percutaneous aortic valve. **A,** Diagram of bioprosthesis situated in the aortic valve annulus. **B,** Valve frame with implanted bioprosthesis. (Used with permission from Medtronic Inc., Minneapolis, Minn. Copyright Medtronic 2009.)

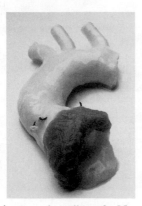

FIG. 35-13 Aortic valve allograft. Note aortic arch branches (*top*), tissue from left ventricle (red-brown tissue in lower portion of graft), and attached anterior leaflet of mitral valve (white smooth tissue in lower right portion of graft). Depending on graft material required, surgeon trims excess or unneeded tissue. (Courtesy CryoLife Inc., Marietta, Ga.)

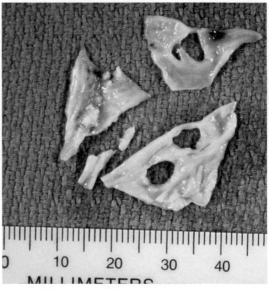

FIG. 35-14 Perforated aortic valve leaflets resulting from bacterial endocarditis. Patient had aortic insufficiency. (From Seifert PC: *Cardiac surgery*, St. Louis, 2002, Mosby. Courtesy Edward A. Lefrak, Md.)

failure. Sudden acute AI (e.g., from bacterial endocarditis that causes tearing of the leaflets [Fig. 35-14] or acute aortic dissection that dilates the aortic annulus) is poorly tolerated, because the normal-sized LV cannot accommodate the sudden increased volume and the lowered diastolic pressure that results from a portion of the cardiac output (CO) being regurgitated into the LV impairs coronary filling. Emergency aortic

valve replacement is indicated for acute AI. Aortic valve replacement (see the definition of valve replacement) is generally indicated for AI; some reparative techniques are available for the aortic valve, but they tend to have less successful outcomes.

Aortic Stenosis

Aortic stenosis (AS) can occur as a congenital process, as in the bicuspid valve (a common congenital anomaly first diagnosed in adulthood),[13] as an acquired disease process related to a history of rheumatic heart disease, or as calcific AS (Fig. 35-15). An inflammatory process has been associated also with the development of aortic stenosis.[2]

AS represents an increased pressure load on the LV (increased afterload). The LV responds by developing LV hypertrophy, which results in decreased LV compliance. The LV cavity becomes reduced because of the hypertrophying muscle invading the ventricular cavity. During cardiac catheterization for study of the aortic valve stenosis,

calculated pressure gradients between the LV and the aorta may exceed 50 mm Hg. As an example, the aortic pressure may be 100 mm Hg, but the LV pressure may be 150 mm Hg, which shows the work required by the LV to eject an adequate cardiac output. LV dilatation and failure can develop when the myocardium is no longer capable of generating sufficient pressure to eject an adequate CO.

Other forms of AS include narrowing of the outflow tract below or above the valve. Subvalvular stenosis occurs when the intraventricular septum becomes hypertrophied and creates an obstruction to LV outflow. This lesion is known as *idiopathic hypertrophic subaortic stenosis* or *hypertrophic*

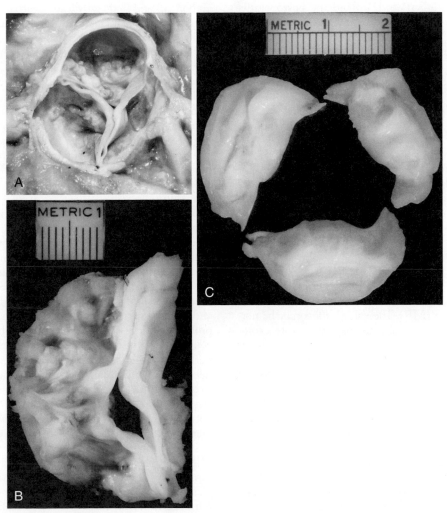

FIG. 35-15 **A,** Bicuspid aortic valve with calcified stiffened leaflets producing stenosis. Note greatly reduced orifice area. **B,** Rheumatic trileaflet (e.g., morphologically normal) aortic valve. Thickened, glistened, and smooth leaflets are typical of rheumatic changes. **C,** Calcific aortic stenosis of trileaflet aortic valve. (From Seifert PC: *Cardiac surgery,* St. Louis, 2002, Mosby. Courtesy William C. Roberts, MD; Michael Spencer, photographer.)

obstructive cardiomyopathy; surgical treatment for subaortic stenosis with a hypertrophied septum involves excision of a portion of the hypertrophied septum; cardiomyopathy may require heart transplantation. Supraaortic valvular stenosis occurs when the aorta above the valve is narrowed from a congenital anomaly. Repair involves opening the affected portion of the aorta and inserting a patch graft to enlarge the narrowed vessel.

Procedure

For aortic valve replacement (Fig. 35-16), the leaflets are excised, the annulus is sized with obturators (i.e., sizers) specific to the prosthesis desired (Fig. 35-17), and the selected prosthesis is implanted. After surgery, anticoagulation therapy is usually initiated 3 to 5 days after surgery, when the patient's intravascular lines and chest tubes are discontinued and immediate postoperative hemorrhage is no longer a concern. Oral warfarin therapy is then started and titrated appropriately to achieve an international normalized ratio of 2.0 to 3.0 times normal (target, 2.5 for mechanical valves); a target international normalized ratio of 2.5 to 3.5 may be sought in the first 3 months following mechanical valve replacement.[3,14]

Mitral Valve Surgery

The structure of the mitral valve often enables the surgeon to repair rather than replace the valve. Most of the components of the mitral valve—the annulus, leaflets, chordate tendineae, papillary muscles, and the endoventricular wall—are amenable to repair. Reparative procedures may be performed for either mitral valve regurgitation or stenosis.

Mitral Regurgitation (MR)

Any of the mitral valve components may be affected. An enlarged annulus is a common cause of mitral regurgitation (MR). The valve leaflets may be normal, but they are unable to coapt and create a competent valve because the dilated annulus pulls the leaflet edges away from one another. The causes of MR may be inflammatory, degenerative, infective, ischemic, structural, or congenital.[15-17] The myxomatous mitral valve (Fig. 35-18) reflects leaflet degeneration from fibroelastic changes. MR also may be related to fibrosis, calcification, or tears in a previously implanted valve prosthesis (Fig. 35-19). Chordae tendineae may be ruptured or excessively elongated or shortened and fused from bacterial endocarditis, one or more papillary muscle heads may have ruptured as a result of ischemic heart disease, or the ventricular endocardium may be dilated.

Chronic MR produces an enlarged atria where stasis of blood can lead to thrombus formation and subsequent thromboembolism; the dilated atrium can also lead to conduction disturbances such as atrial fibrillation. Pulmonary overloading occurs and eventually can produce pulmonary hypertension; the subsequent increased pulmonary pressures may produce functional tricuspid valve regurgitation. Acute MR is poorly tolerated because the left atrium is unable to contain the sudden regurgitant volume overload and pulmonary overload ensues rapidly; emergency valve replacement or repair (if possible) is indicated.

Mitral Stenosis (MS)

Unlike AS, AI, or MR, stenosis of the mitral valve is the only lesion that does not place either a volume or a pressure load on the LV. However, chronic mitral stenosis (MS; like MR) produces an enlarged atria and stasis of blood (with the risk of thromboembolism) and frequently leads to atrial fibrillation. Functional tricuspid regurgitation may develop. MS is the result of changes in one or more of the components of the mitral apparatus. The causes of MS may be inflammation, calcification, tumors (i.e., left atrial myxoma), and infection. Bacterial vegetations and the sequelae of rheumatic fever continue to be significant causes of MS.[15] With MS the leaflets become progressively more fibrotic and stenotic. Fig. 35-20 illustrates the classic "fish mouth" appearance of a rheumatic mitral valve: smooth fibrotic thickened leaflets, commissural fusion, and shortened thickened chordae tendineae.

Procedure

Most of the components of the mitral valve apparatus—valve leaflets, the annulus, chordae tendineae, papillary muscles, and the endoventricular wall—are amenable to repair. The tricuspid valve is similarly configured. Open commissurotomy can be performed by exposing the affected valve (with the use of CPB and induced cardiac arrest) and sharply incising the fused commissures. The procedure is performed often for children or young adults with a history of rheumatic fever. Performed at an earlier age, commissurotomy can delay the inevitable future need for more extensive valve repair or replacement; this is a significant consideration because the patient can avoid the potential complication of prosthetic valve replacement. Balloon valvulotomy also may be performed in some instances.

Annuloplasty and valvuloplasty may be performed on the affected component. An annuloplasty procedure commonly is performed on the mitral or tricuspid valve or both. A cloth-covered prosthetic annuloplasty ring (Fig. 35-21) in a size smaller than the dilated native annulus is sutured to the valve annulus (Fig. 35-22). When the stitches are tied, excess annular tissue is pulled up against the ring, thereby reducing the overall

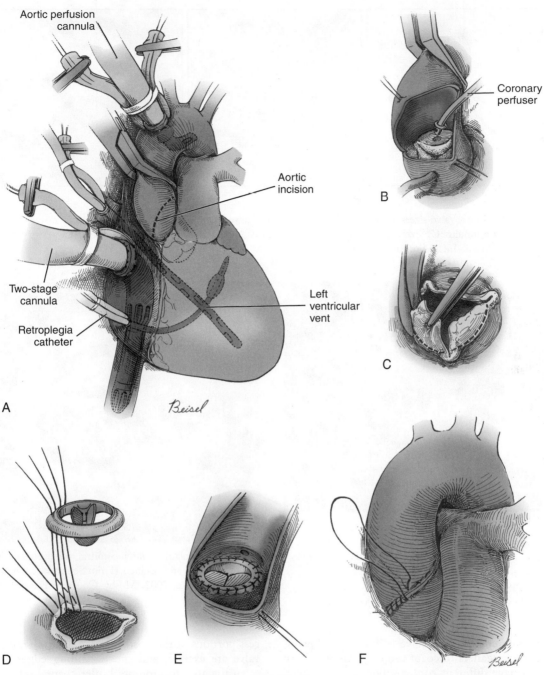

FIG. 35-16 **A,** Aortic valve replacement. Cardiopulmonary bypass cannulation, retrograde cardioplegia, and left ventricular vent (inserted via right superior pulmonary vein) are shown. Note incision site on aorta (*dotted line*). **B,** If retrograde cardioplegia is not used, handheld ostial catheters may be used for cardioplegia infusion. **C,** Valve leaflets are completely excised. **D,** Sutures are placed in aortic annulus and prosthetic sewing ring. **E,** Stitches are tied and cut. **F,** Aorta is closed. (From Waldhausen JA, et al: *Surgery of the chest*, ed 6, St. Louis, 1996, Mosby.)

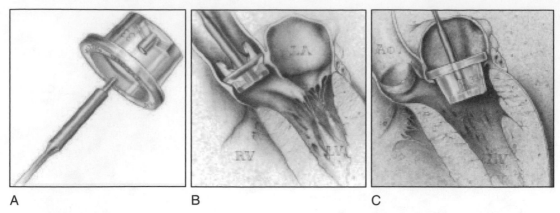

A   B   C

FIG. 35-17 Valve sizers in use. **A,** Obturator/sizer is screwed onto handle. **B,** Obturator used to size aortic annulus. **C,** Sizing mitral valve annulus. *Ao,* Aorta; *LA,* left atrium; *RV,* right ventricle. (Courtesy Medtronic Inc., Minneapolis, Minn.)

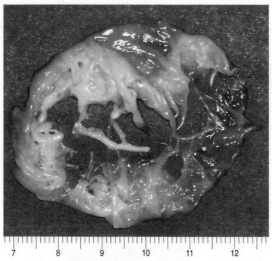

FIG. 35-18 Myxomatous mitral valve producing regurgitation. Thin elongated leaflets are rarely amenable to valve repair and usually require valve replacement. (From Seifert PC: *Cardiac surgery,* St. Louis, 2002, Mosby. Courtesy Edward A. Lefrak, MD.)

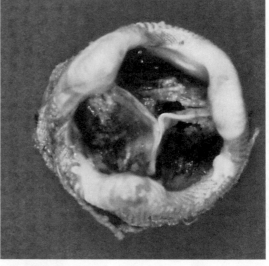

FIG. 35-19 Explanted porcine mitral valve prosthesis. Leaflets are torn and calcified. (From Seifert PC: *Cardiac surgery,* St. Louis, 2002, Mosby. Courtesy Edward A. Lefrak, MD.)

circumference of the valve orifice and allowing the valve leaflets to coapt properly. Annuloplasty rings have different configurations (e.g., circular, almond shaped, C shaped) and are flexible, rigid, or semirigid. The surgeon's selection of the prosthesis is based on factors such as the underlying pathology, anatomy, annular dynamics, remodeling of the annular geometry, and preservation of valve function. Prosthetic valvular annuloplasty itself does not require postoperative long-term anticoagulation therapy.

In addition to insertion of a prosthetic annuloplasty ring for annular dilation (see Figs. 35-21 and 35-22), valvuloplasty can be performed. Ex-cess portions of the posterior leaflet of the mitral valve are excised, and the remaining edges are sewn together to promote leaflet coaptation and to reduce the annular circumference. Torn leaflets can be repaired with a patch of pericardium. Ruptured chordae tendineae can be replaced with suture or reattached to the valve leaflet; shortened thickened chordae can be incised to increase length and improve flexibility; and excessively lengthened chordae can be shortened by implanting a portion of the chord into a papillary muscle head. Debridement of calcific nodules can be done, although valve replacement may be needed with severe calcification.

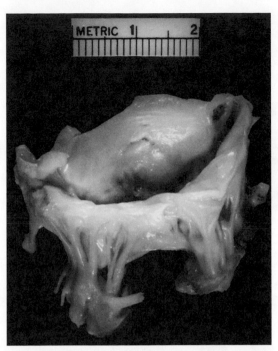

FIG. 35-20 Stenotic rheumatic mitral valve with classic "fish mouth" appearance. Leaflets are smooth and thickened; chordae tendineae arising from papillary muscle tips are shortened and fused. (From Seifert PC: *Cardiac surgery*, St. Louis, 2002, Mosby. Courtesy William C. Roberts, MD; Michael Spencer, photographer.)

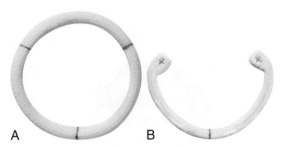

FIG. 35-21 Annuloplasty rings. **A,** Duran AnCore® ring. **B,** CG Future® ring. (Courtesy Medtronic Inc., Minneapolis, Minn.)

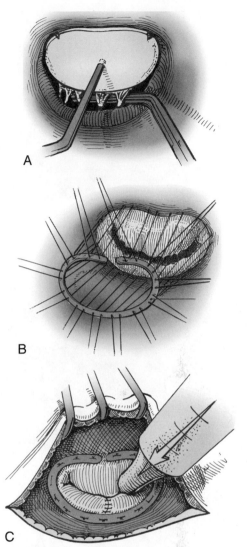

FIG. 35-22 **A,** Annuloplasty ring bean-shaped sizer with handle used to measure annulus (note retraction of chordae tendineae to facilitate sizing). **B,** Stitches are inserted into annulus and into prosthetic ring. **C,** Sutures are tied and cut; bulb syringe squirts saline solution into orifice to determine whether repair has produced competent valve. Portion of excess posterior leaflet tissue has been resected. (From Waldhausen JA, et al: *Surgery of the chest*, ed 6, St. Louis, 1996, Mosby.)

Balloon valvotomy for the mitral valve is performed with a catheter percutaneously inserted into a large vein and threaded to the RA, where a septal puncture is made to allow access into the left atrium and to the mitral valve. This technique is useful for children, young adults, and patients who are too elderly or medically compromised to withstand an operation. Occasionally the catheter is threaded up the aorta and through the aortic valve into the LV and then placed across the mitral valve where the balloon is inflated. Percutaneous mitral valve repair can be performed, but the procedure is less effective than surgery for reducing mitral regurgitation.[18]

When valvular deformation injury is severe, prosthetic replacement may be required. For mitral valve replacement (Fig. 35-23), the anterior

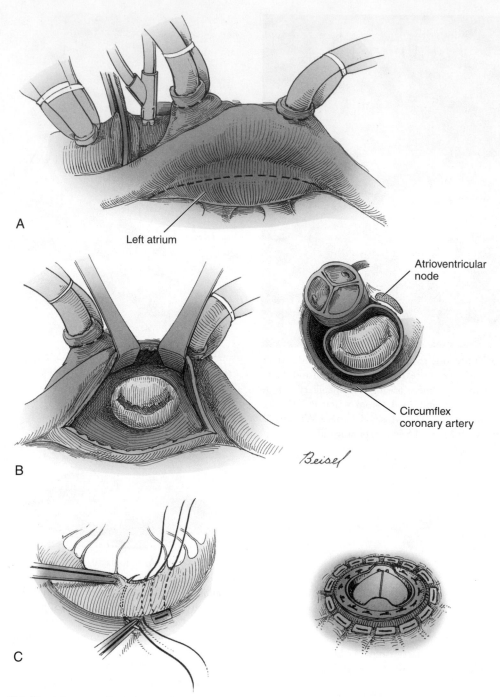

A

Left atrium

Atrioventricular
node

Circumflex
coronary artery

Beisel

B

C

FIG. 35-23 Mitral valve replacement. **A,** Incision (*dotted*) line in left atrium, exposure of mitral valve, and illustration of relationship between mitral and aortic valves and atrioventricular node. Double venous cannulas shown for cardiopulmonary bypass; antegrade cardioplegia catheter inserted into aorta below the cross clamp and aortic cannula are shown. **B,** Sutures are placed in native valve annulus and then prosthetic. **C,** Completed valve replacement. (From Waldhausen JA, et al: *Surgery of the chest,* ed 6, St. Louis, 1996, Mosby.)

Chapter 35 - CARE OF THE CARDIAC SURGICAL PATIENT   513

leaflet is usually excised, but often all or part of the posterior leaflet and its attached chordae are retained to preserve the LV geometry and enhance LV function. Although valve replacement improves cardiac function by removing the stresses associated with volume or pressure overloading, transient symptoms of ventricular failure can exist after mitral valve replacement for chronic MR because the LV no longer has the release valve represented by the incompetent valve. With the insertion of a competent mitral prosthetic valve, the LV must develop sufficient pressure to push all the LV end-diastolic volume forward through the aortic valve. Afterload reduction (e.g., with sodium nitroprusside) assists LV ejection. Potential complications associated with prosthetic valve replacement are thromboembolism, anticoagulation-related hemorrhage, prosthetic valve endocarditis, perivalvular leak, and prosthetic failure.[2,3]

Tricuspid Valve Repair

Tricuspid regurgitation may be the result of severe mitral stenosis that produces significant back pressure that affects the right side of the heart. It can develop also as a result of rheumatic changes, a right ventricle (RV) infarction, infection, or annular dilatation from right atrial remodeling that occurs with RV failure. Although tricuspid stenosis occurs infrequently in adults, it can occur as a result of rheumatic heart disease or bacterial endocarditis.

Annuloplasty repair is generally performed, although tricuspid valve replacement is performed if a repair to the native valve cannot be accomplished. During ring insertion for tricuspid annulus repair (Fig. 35-24), the surgeon is especially cautious when inserting stitches near the atrioventricular node and the bundle of His (in the area of the tricuspid septal leaflet) to avoid creating complete heart block or other injury to the conduction system. A suture annuloplasty (i.e., without the insertion of a prosthetic ring) can be used also for some tricuspid valve repairs (see also the definition of *valvuloplasty*).

Surgery for Thoracic Aortic Aneurysms and Dissections

Localized or diffuse dilation of the aortic wall leads to progressive enlargement of all layers of the aorta. Surrounding tissue may be compressed by the enlarging vessel, and eventual rupture with exsanguination can occur without treatment. Diagnosis is made with CT scan and magnetic resonance arteriography, which display the size and shape of the aorta and can be used to identify the location of the intimal tear in a dissection.[19] Surgical treatment consists of excision of the aneurysmal tissue with insertion of a prosthetic graft (e.g., Dacron; Fig. 35-25). An endovascular stented graft made from expanded polytetrafluoroethylene (PTFE) can be used to repair f descending (and abdominal) aortic aneurysms. The prosthesis is initially compressed, inserted percutaneously into the femoral artery, and guided into the aorta where it is expanded and deployed in the desired position.

Aortic dissection is a unique condition affecting the aortic media. Surgery is indicated for ascending aortic and transverse aortic arch dissections and involves excising the portion of the aorta that contains the tear and replacing excised tissue with a graft. Uncomplicated descending thoracic aortic dissections are more commonly managed medically

NURSING CARE IN THE PACU

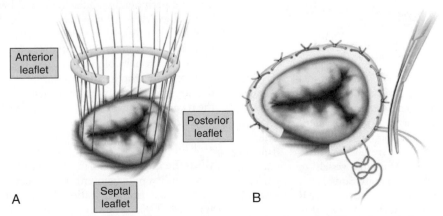

A   B

FIG. 35-24 **A,** Tricuspid valve repair is similar to mitral valve repair. Note that stitches are not inserted in area of atrioventricular conduction tissue (see text). **B,** Completion of tricuspid valve repair. (Courtesy Medtronic Inc., Minneapolis, Minn.)

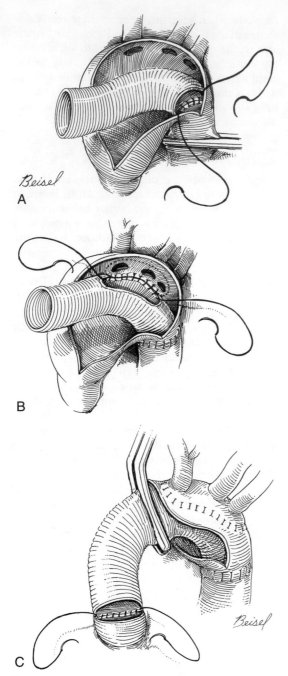

A

B

C

FIG. 35-25 Resection of aneurysmal portion of ascending aorta and transverse arch and insertion of prosthetic patch. Circulatory arrest is instituted until arch vessels are repaired. **A,** Graft anastomosed to distal portion of aorta. **B,** Arch vessels are anastomosed as island to prosthetic graft. **C,** After arch vessels are connected, cross clamp is placed on graft, cardiopulmonary bypass is resumed, and proximal anastomosis is completed. (From Waldhausen JA, et al: *Surgery of the chest,* ed 6, St. Louis, 1996, Mosby.)

with antihypertensive medications and analgesics. Surgery, with a traditional incision or an endovascular prosthesis, is indicated with impending rupture.[20,21]

Blunt trauma to the thoracic aorta can lead to aortic rupture. Newer imaging techniques have enabled clinicians to intervene more promptly in these cases, thereby improving survival.[11] Endovascular graft insertion or traditional repair may be performed.[22]

Ventricular Assistance

Ventricular assist devices (VADs) decrease the workload of the heart by diverting blood from the ventricle to an artificial pump that maintains systemic (left VAD [LVAD]) or pulmonary (right VAD [RVAD]) perfusion. A BiVAD supports both right and left ventricles. Placement of a cardiac transplant candidate on a VAD enhances anabolism, ambulation, and improved organ function; these physiologic improvements enable the patient to become a stronger transplant candidate. In this case, the VAD is used as a bridge to transplantation. Improvements in VAD therapy have significantly reduced the incidence rate of infection and thromboembolism. VADs have been especially valuable in the treatment of heart failure.[23,24] A vented electric LVAD for destination therapy or permanent replacement for the LV enables patients to be relatively independent by reducing the reliance on in-line power sources.[25]

Short-term assist devices include the intraaortic balloon pump (IABP), a sausage-shaped balloon mounted on a catheter percutaneously inserted into the aorta distal to the left subclavian artery via the femoral artery. The balloon inflates during diastole, propelling blood proximally to the aortic root and into the coronary ostia to enhance coronary perfusion. Distally, blood is propelled into the peripheral vascular bed to enhance organ blood flow. When the balloon deflates during LV systole, LV afterload is reduced by the movement of blood during balloon inflation. With the increase in coronary blood flow and the decrease in afterload, the total work of the heart is reduced, thereby providing an environment that supports the recovery of a failing myocardium and improves peripheral vascular perfusion.[24]

Transplantation

With the improvement in pharmacologic therapy, comorbidity management and infection prophylaxis, cardiac transplantation 1-year survival rates approach 90%.[26] Potential candidates are patients who are considered to be in the New York Heart Association Functional Classification System's class

IV, which denotes the most compromised cardiac status, and who have less than a 10% chance of survival for 6 months. Heart donors are persons with irreversible catastrophic brain injury who do not have atherosclerotic heart disease. Age limitations have become less restrictive, and donors and recipients may be 60 years or older in certain cases.

Removal of the donor heart is accomplished with transection of the venae cavae, the pulmonary artery, the left atrium, and the aorta. The donor heart is placed in a sterile bag with cold preservation fluid and transported to the recipient's institution. The surgeon places the recipient on CPB and removes the recipient's heart surgically after the donor heart has been judged acceptable and has arrived in the recipient's operating room. The pulmonary artery, the SVC and the IVC, the pulmonary veins, and the aorta of the donor are anastomosed to the comparable tissue of the recipient. This technique has been modified from the traditional technique, in which a right atrial anastomosis was performed. The newer technique reduces some of the dysrhythmias and tricuspid valve dysfunction associated with the previously created RA connections. After surgery, transplant patients receive the same care provided other cardiac surgery patients with the addition of immunosuppression-related infection and rejection monitoring.

Two new cardiac transplantation subpopulations include patients with previously repaired congenital heart disease and transplantation recipients requiring retransplantation. Ten-year survival after transplantation in the former group is excellent.[26] Retransplantation patient survival improves in the absence of primary allograft failure and refractory rejection within the first 6 months after retransplantation. Guidelines for this subpopulation remain vague and are undergoing refinement.[26,27]

Lung transplantation involves replacement of one or both lungs with lungs from a donor or a single lung from a living donor. Newer allograft organ protective strategies have contributed to improved outcomes in lung transplantation candidates. Contraindications for transplantation include significant pulmonary hypertension, the presence of systemic disease, a recent pulmonary infarction, or active systemic infection.[28,29]

Surgery for Adult Congenital Heart Disease

A number of congenital anomalies might not be treated until adulthood. These congenital lesions tend to be less severe and therefore asymptomatic

(or mildly symptomatic) in childhood. Some of the most common are listed in the following sections.[30]

Atrial Septal Defect

A frequently seen congenital anomaly in adulthood is the atrial septal defect (Fig. 35-26).[31] The most common form of atrial septal defect in the adult is the ostium secundum defect, located in the midportion of the septum in the vicinity of the fossa ovalis (formerly the intrauterine shunt known as the foramen ovale). Less common is the sinus venosus defect located near the entrance of the SVC in the high RA. Sinus venosus defects are associated with partial anomalous pulmonary venous return (commonly of the right superior pulmonary vein), whereby the anomalous pulmonary vein enters the RA (rather than the left atrium) and returns oxygenated blood from the lungs into the SVC or the upper RA. Closure of the secundum and sinus venosus septal defects is accomplished with suturing or patching the defect with a patch of pericardium or prosthetic

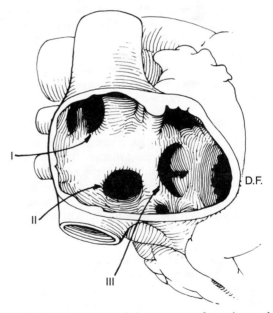

FIG. 35-26 Location of three types of atrial septal defect. Sinus venosus defect (*I*) is shown with anomalous drainage of right upper pulmonary vein. Ostium secundum defect (*II*) is in midportion of septum in area of fossa ovalis. Ostium primum defect (*III*) is located in base of septum, with its inferior edge formed by continuity of tricuspid and mitral valves. Often a cleftlike anomaly is seen in anterior leaflet of mitral valve visible through defect. (From Miller TA, editor: *Physiologic basis of modern surgical care*, St. Louis, 1988, Mosby.)

material. During repair of a sinus venosus defect, the patch is placed in such a way that anomalous pulmonary venous drainage is diverted into the left atrium.

Coarctation of the Aorta

There are two types of coarctation: preductal and postductal. The postductal type is more likely to be seen in adults because the heart in utero has been stimulated to develop extensive collateral circulation in response to the increased afterload represented by the coarctation's position distal to the aortic exit of the patent ductus arteriosus. (In preductal coarctations, the fetal heart is not stimulated to develop collaterals, because blood flow from the heart to the aorta via the patent ductus arteriosus is not restricted.) In adults, a coarctation may be identified when preoperative bilateral arm blood pressure measurements are unequal. A common repair in adults is accomplished by excising the coarctation and interposing a prosthetic graft.

Patent Ductus Arteriosus

If the ductus does not close within 1 or 2 weeks after birth, closure can be achieved surgically with ligation of the ductus or with division of the ductus followed by oversewing of the ductal edges. Failure of the ductus to close can predispose the patient to developing pulmonary hypertension, endocarditis, or cardiac failure.

Pulmonary Stenosis

The fused pulmonary valve commissures are sharply divided to improved leaflet motion. Balloon angioplasty in the cardiac catheterization laboratory also may be performed. Repair of the infundibular portion involves opening the RV outflow tract and inserting a patch to enlarge the outflow tract.

Ventricular Septal Defects

A ventral septal defect (VSD) is a defect (i.e., opening) in the ventricular septum. Congenital VSDs may be small enough to close spontaneously; VSDs that persist necessitate surgical closure before irreversible pulmonary hypertension develops. Adult-acquired VSDs usually develop suddenly after myocardial infarction (MI) of one or more coronary arteries perfusing the ventricular septum. These postinfarction VSDs create pulmonary overloading rapidly and require emergency surgery to close the defect (commonly with a prosthetic patch).

Dysrhythmia Surgery

The atrial contribution to cardiac output becomes especially important to maintain an adequate preload and forward flow of blood and to contribute to a more forceful ventricular contraction. Loss of this atrial contribution, or kick, through the development of supraventricular dysrhythmias (e.g., atrial fibrillation) can result in a marked decrease in cardiac output with resultant pulmonary edema.

Atrial fibrillation (AF) is associated with significant morbidity and mortality rates. In 1991, the Cox Maze procedure[32] showed excellent results in redirecting the impulses of AF with incisions made and the sutured closed. Electric impulses cannot cross sutured (or ablated) tissue. Because electric impulses can travel only through normal tissue, the surgeon locates the various incisions to create a pathway for impulses that direct those impulses toward the atrioventricular node, thereby returning the heart to normal sinus rhythm.[32] More recent research has shown that the source of 90% of the aberrant impulses comes from the area that surrounds the pulmonary veins.[33] Ablation of the targeted tissue (with cold energy, radiofrequency, or other energy sources) has been successful, with a more than 90% success rate in achieving sinus rhythm.[34] Further improvement in outcomes has been seen in patients who are followed with a protocol that coordinates treatments by cardiologists, surgeons, and nurse coordinators.[35]

Completion of Surgery

After the cardiac repair is completed, temporary pacing wires are attached to the right atrial and ventricular surface, brought out through the chest below the sternal incision, and connected to an external pacemaker generator. One or more chest tubes are placed anteriorly, laterally, or posteriorly in the pericardium to facilitate drainage. The tubes exit via stab wounds below the sternal incision. If either of the pleurae were opened during the procedure, the tip of one of the pericardial chest tubes is inserted into the affected pleura. The pericardial sac is rarely closed so that any remaining blood or fluid can drain freely into the chest tubes, avoiding the creation of a cardiac tamponade. Occasionally, when a repeated operation is anticipated (e.g., after a biologic valve replacement in a young person), the upper (cephalad) portion of the pericardium may be closed so that less scar tissue forms over the cannulation sites for CPB (e.g., the aorta). The lower portion of the sac remains open to drain fluid. The sternum is closed with stainless steel wires, and the fascia, subcutaneous tissue, and skin are closed with suture. Before transfer from the OR to the postanesthesia care unit (or intensive care unit [ICU]), portable monitoring lines for heart rate and rhythm, arterial blood pressure, and oxygen saturation are connected for transport to the postoperative unit. Patients can have acute circulatory instability develop, because of either the normal recovering physiologic state or inadvertent movement or displacement of the numerous invasive lines and tubes needed. A portable defibrillator is often placed on the transport bed for use if ventricular tachycardia or ventricular fibrillation develops during transport.

Postanesthesia Care

Cardiac surgery patients commonly go to a specialized cardiovascular surgery ICU or postanesthesia care unit (PACU). Whether a critical care nurse or a postanesthesia nurse, a caregiver should be aware of the level of knowledge, understanding, and anxieties of both the patient and the family before surgery. When possible, and depending on the individual institution's policies and procedures, the postoperative caregiver nurse can provide preoperative instruction for the patient and family or make an introductory visit before surgery. Teaching content for coronary or valve surgery (see Table 35-1) can be initiated in the preoperative period and reinforced after surgery. Discharge from the cardiovascular surgery ICU or open heart PACU to a step-down unit increasingly occurs within hours. A reduction has also been seen in the overall length of stay (LOS) from 1 or longer to a few days. The movement toward rapid postoperative endotracheal extubation and shortened LOS has been spurred not just by costs but also by improved pain control that facilitates earlier extubation and by fundamental shifts in anesthetic management from a high-dose opioid technique to a more balanced approach with moderate-dose opioids, shorter acting muscle relaxants, and volatile anesthetics. The so-called fast-track approach (i.e., extubation immediately after or within a few hours of surgery)[2] is becoming a standard of care in a number of centers.[3] The longer LOS sometimes seen in the rapidly growing number of patients 80 years and older may be the result of comorbid conditions such as peripheral vascular disease, renal pathology, diabetes mellitus, hyperlipidemia, and hypertension, but advances in anesthetic techniques and myocardial protection during surgery have improved morbidity and mortality rates in older and younger patients. This chapter is designed to familiarize the PACU nurse with the perioperative care for the adult cardiac patient. Understanding what the patient has experienced before and during surgery assists the nurse to tailor care after surgery to the patient's needs and to strengthen the continuity of that care.

All patients in the cardiac PACU or cardiovascular surgery ICU need intensive continuous hemodynamic monitoring and rapid intervention to prevent complications from the surgery and CPB. Patients are routinely monitored for dysrhythmias, pleural effusion, bleeding, and cardiovascular, neurologic, renal, pulmonary, respiratory, and temperature alterations. The nurse's role is critical to ensure that anticipated clinical changes (e.g., temperature, fluid shifts) do not progress to more serious complications that can jeopardize optimal patient outcomes. In addition, nurses in the postoperative unit and the step-down unit educate patients about the plan of care and involve patients and family members to implement the plan designed for patients and their families.

On admission to the postoperative unit, the nurse immediately assesses the parameters currently monitored. If any of these parameters indicates circulatory or ventilatory dysfunction, immediate resuscitative measures are instituted. If circulatory and ventilatory statuses appear adequate on entry to the postoperative unit, then admission routines are initiated. The respiratory therapist or anesthesia care provider usually attaches the patient to the ventilator, establishes the initial ventilator settings, and sets the alarms. After the patient is attached to the ventilator, the nurse auscultates both lung fields and repeats the assessment often until discharge from the PACU.

Invasive monitoring lines are attached to transducers or manometers. Patency is ascertained, and values and wave tracings are continuously displayed and recorded. Commonly measured intravascular parameters include mean arterial, right atrial, mean pulmonary artery, pulmonary artery systolic, pulmonary artery diastolic, pulmonary capillary wedge, and left atrial pressures. In addition to these directly measured parameters, these values assist in calculation of indirect or derived hemodynamic parameters, such as cardiac output and cardiac index, systemic vascular resistance, and pulmonary vascular resistance. These parameters assist in the assessment of both LV and RV status and are used in determination of pharmacologic, fluid, and mechanical therapies for the postoperative patient. Once these invasive lines are connected, the nurse reviews and assesses with the anesthesia provider the intravascular lines and solutions in regard to type, drugs infused, flow rates, patency, and expiration times. Intake and output recordings with running totals are made and documented hourly or more often as clinically indicated. Volume administration and replacement treatments are largely determined by the individual patient's hemodynamic parameters, and responses can vary greatly from hour to hour.

Chest tube drainage systems inserted in the OR are connected in the postoperative unit to suction systems to achieve 15 to 20 cm of negative suction. The amount and the type of chest tube drainage are frequently assessed and recorded on an hourly basis. Drainage that exceeds 100 mL/h should be brought to the attention of the physician (e.g., intensivist, surgeon, or anesthesiologist, depending on institutional practice). Chest tubes are usually removed on the first or second postoperative day, as long as intracardiac lines have been removed, no evidence of fluid accumulation is present on chest radiograph results, and drainage has been less than 200 mL in the last 6 hours. Most patients have one or two mediastinal chest tubes that facilitate pericardial drainage after surgery. If the pleural spaces were opened during the procedure or the internal mammary arteries were dissected off the chest wall, or both, then pleural chest tubes are also present to facilitate drainage and to prevent a pneumothorax.

Arterial blood gas values are determined on admission and as needed thereafter. Intubated patients retain their breathing tubes until the effects of anesthesia subside and hemodynamic stability is achieved and maintained. Controlled ventilation is used initially. As patients begin to generate their own respirations, they are switched to intermittent mandatory ventilation modes, in which they gradually increase their spontaneous respirations to maintain adequate minute ventilations. Once patients maintain an adequate respiratory rate, they are switched to continuous positive airway pressure (CPAP) systems. With CPAP, the patient determines the respiratory rate, and the ventilator provides the positive pressure to the airway that the glottis normally provides when the patient is not intubated. The use of CPAP prevents microatelectasis and increases the functional residual capacity of the lung by increasing lung expansion. Once the patient maintains adequate arterial blood gas levels on CPAP, extubation usually follows quickly. After extubation, face masks or nasal cannulas are used to deliver supplemental oxygen.

A continuous ECG recording is established, alarm limits are set, and a strip recording is obtained. A 12-lead ECG may be obtained for complex or unusual dysrhythmias. Cardiac rhythm is assessed frequently and documented at least every 2 hours. Lead selection varies, but modified chest lead one (MCL_1), in which the left-atrial and right-atrial leads are in their respective places and the third lead is placed on the fourth right intercostal space, is commonly used. Electrode placement with this lead does not interfere with defibrillation procedures or with mediastinal or chest tube dressing placement. The apical pulse is auscultated and validated with the ECG recording. Most patients have a temporary external pacer, and the nurse checks and records the type of pacer, the mode, the rate, and the milliamperage and determines whether the pacer is functioning adequately. If the patient is not being paced, the nurse needs to ensure that the unused pacemaker wires are covered with gauze, placed in a plastic covering (e.g., a finger cot), and securely dressed and attached to the chest to protect the patient from electrical hazard. Usually two ventricular and two atrial pacing wires are attached to the epicardium with a fine suture before the chest is closed. These wires then exit the chest via stab wounds on either side of the sternal incision. Wires are most often left in place for a few days after surgery and may be used to assist in cardiac rate and rhythm control. Before the patient is discharged from the hospital, the wires are totally removed with gentle traction or they are clipped off at the skin level (with a portion left attached to the epicardium and residing in the subcutaneous tissues).

The patient's neurologic status is assessed on admission and every 30 to 60 minutes and thereafter until arousal from anesthesia. Neurologic complications can affect the central or the peripheral nervous system and include cerebral or peripheral thromboembolism, encephalopathy, coma, impaired intellectual function. Use of off-pump (versus on-pump) techniques for patients undergoing CABG have not shown improvements in neurocognitive outcomes.[3,36] Once the patient has been aroused, neurologic assessments are decreased to every 2 hours.

An admission temperature is obtained and active rewarming therapies are instituted. Temperatures are recorded hourly during this period, and rewarming devices are discontinued when the patient's condition reaches normothermia. One temperature-related condition is hypothermia-related hypocarbia. The body temperature usually remains lower than normal during the early postoperative hours. The body temperature returns to normal slowly; rebound hyperthermia occurs occasionally. As rewarming takes place, carbon dioxide is produced. Consequently, hypercarbia can develop, and ventilator settings should be adjusted to produce a minute volume necessary to facilitate normocarbia. In addition, if rebound hyperthermia occurs or if rewarming devices are not regulated and monitored appropriately, a hyperthermic overshoot can occur, which increases myocardial oxygen demand and consumption.[3]

An abdominal assessment is performed on admission and every 2 hours thereafter until bowel sounds return. A nasogastric or orogastric tube inserted after induction of anesthesia relieves gastric distention and facilitates removal of gastric contents.[2] It is usually attached to low intermittent suction or gravity drainage and removed at the time of extubation. Analysis of pH and tests for the presence of occult blood can be performed on gastric secretions if they begin to resemble coffee grounds. After the nasogastric tube is removed, the patient is given ice chips and resumes a clear liquid diet within the first 24 hours.

Urinary drainage from the catheter inserted in the OR should be recorded on admission to the PACU and then hourly. The appearance of the urine is also monitored closely. During the first few hours after surgery, massive diuresis of 2 to 3 L of pale dilute urine is usually common from diuretics that are generally administered during the discontinuation of CPB to facilitate the removal of fluid that has sequestered during surgery in the interstitial space. When this initial diuresis resolves, urine color and consistency return to normal. Urinary output should be more than 0.5 mL/kg/h; a lower urine output is commonly the result of decreased renal perfusion.[3]

Peripheral pulses and skin color and temperature are assessed and recorded hourly. All incisions and intravascular and tube insertion sites are observed. The patient is placed in a 30-degree position with the legs supported at the knees and the calves slightly elevated to reduce the incidence of ventilator associated pneumonia. This position facilitates venous return from the legs and limits swelling, particularly in patients with saphenous vein excision. Legs are wrapped from toes to hips with elastic leg wraps or antiembolism stockings.

Cardiopulmonary bypass affects every body system, and a brief review of some of the effects on the patient seen in the postoperative period is useful to the nurse. For example, epinephrine and norepinephrine levels are markedly elevated during CPB. Hyperglycemia and impaired insulin responses are present and result in use of fat stores for energy until carbohydrate metabolism returns to normal levels. Secretion of antidiuretic hormone and aldosterone is also increased, stimulated by different mechanisms associated with the physiologic components of stress. Serum complement that is activated when blood contacts the inner surfaces of the bypass circuit cause an inflammatory response with a marked increase in total body water and interstitial edema. Postoperative fluid requirements are affected by rewarming because rewarming itself causes fluid shifts. This excess fluid usually redistributes itself by the second or third day after surgery and is excreted spontaneously or with diuretic therapy. CPB and hypothermia also alter coagulation factors, platelet formation, and the immune system.[2]

In addition, when exposed to the foreign surfaces of the CPB circuit, platelets clump together. A decrease in the number of functional platelets occurs along with a decrease in the aggregative and adhesive functions of remaining platelets. Release of vasoactive substances occurs as platelets are destroyed. In addition, exposure to the CPB circuit (and suctioning devices) causes a breakdown of plasma proteins, including gamma globulin, which in turn can cause fat microemboli release, microcoagulation, clotting factor consumption, and increased vascular permeability. The shear stresses caused by suction catheters and the tubing and connectors within the circuit also damage the formed elements of the blood (e.g., erythrocytes, leukocytes).

A written assessment is performed after admission routines. The frequency of assessment and documentation of the hemodynamic parameters and routines is dictated by the patient's response to and recovery from surgery. Recovery time varies from among patients but generally occurs within 12 to 24 hours, except with impaired cardiac, pulmonary, renal, or other organ function. During that time numerous expected postoperative physiologic alterations occur, largely because of the techniques of CPB, hypothermia, anesthesia, and surgical manipulation of the myocardium. With correct interventions, these physiologic responses are short lived and reversible; however, two problems exist. First, although these alterations are reversible, they can lead to complications if not identified early and treated quickly. Such is the case with uncontrolled hypertension, which can develop into hemorrhage if fresh suture lines are disrupted. Second, these alterations often resemble complications and thus may be missed in the early stages. For example, the initial absence of a pedal pulse may be attributed to hypothermia and vasoconstriction only to be traced later to a vascular embolism. For these reasons, the PACU nurse must be knowledgeable about the causes, assessment factors, and interventions for both expected physiologic alterations and complications that can occur after cardiac surgery. These alterations and potential complications are reviewed briefly in the following section.

NURSING CARE IN THE PACU

COMPLICATIONS

Cardiovascular System

A number of predisposing factors are known to increase the incidence rates of postoperative complication and early mortality. These factors include preoperative cardiac conditions, such as myocardial dysfunction, recent MI, and previous CABG surgery or systemic conditions such as advanced age, obesity, diabetes mellitus, and chronic obstructive pulmonary disease. The surgical risks of CABG can be assessed before surgery, and complications can be anticipated with these preoperative risk factors taken into consideration.

Complications related to CABG and valvular surgery can generally be classified as either cardiac or noncardiac. Cardiac complications include myocardial infarction, congestive heart failure, tamponade, dysrhythmias, and postoperative hypertension. Each of these complications can contribute to decreased cardiac output.

These complications also contribute to increased costs. One multiyear, statewide study of isolated CABG patients demonstrated the greatest additive costs for prolonged ventilation ($40,704), renal failure ($49,128), and mediastinitis ($62,773).[37] Noncardiac complications include hemorrhage, wound dehiscence and infection, and neurologic, renal, pulmonary, and gastrointestinal problems. Each complication is addressed individually.

Cardiac Complications of Coronary Artery Bypass Grafting and Valvular Surgery

Myocardial Infarction

Despite improved myocardial protection with induced hypothermia, cardioplegic arrest, and topical hypothermia during surgery, MI still remains the most common and serious postoperative complication and the main cause of early death after surgery. Suboptimal myocardial protection can result from uneven distribution of cardioplegic solutions in the coronary arteries. Subendocardial ischemia can occur from a distended or hypertrophic LV and incomplete revascularization. Sudden bypass graft closure (from thrombus) may be a contributing factor. The patient's own underlying heart disease may be too severe for reversal with attempted revascularization. Some patients with CAD are treated medically (e.g., pharmacologically, lifestyle changes) for prolonged periods. Because CAD is a progressive disease, cardiac function can deteriorate significantly without catheter-based (PTCA with stent) or surgical (CABG)

revascularization. In patients with valvular heart disease, the degree of ventricular dysfunction is difficult to gauge accurately, because the heart is capable of performing work by relying on compensatory mechanisms and patients may not be symptomatic until serious myocardial injury has occurred.

Another contributing factor may be reperfusion injury from sudden reperfusion of an ischemic area causing necrosis as a result of a rapid influx of calcium ions, oxygen-free radicals, and other metabolic waste products into the ischemic myocardial cells. The appearance of new Q waves after surgery also has been shown to adversely affect early and late survival. Other predictors of perioperative MI include left main coronary artery stenosis, multivessel disease, minimal collateral circulation, and the duration of CPB.[2,3]

Congestive Heart Failure (Alterations in Myocardial Contractility)

Alteration in myocardial contractility with resultant low cardiac output and shocklike states also can develop after surgery and may be the result of a perioperative ischemia, MI, incomplete revascularization or repair, myocardial edema from surgical manipulation, metabolic disturbances, and depression from hypothermia and anesthesia. The patient has a decrease in CO and cardiac index, hypotension, elevated systemic vascular resistance, elevated filling pressures, acidosis, tachycardia, and decreased urine output. If the condition occurs during surgery after the surgical repair and the discontinuation of CPB, an IABP may be inserted or CPB may be reinstituted for approximately 30 to 60 minutes to rest the heart, relieve myocardial ischemia, and improve ventricular contractility to a level that allows smooth weaning with low doses of inotropic support. (CPB decompresses the heart and removes cardiac volume and pressure work.) If the heart cannot be weaned from CPB, even with IABP support, insertion of a ventricular device may be necessary to support one or more ventricles.

After surgery, treatment can include a combination of pharmacologic and mechanical circulatory support throughout the period of recuperation. Depending on the hemodynamic status of the patient, different combinations of inotropic and vasopressor agents are used as initial therapy, with the addition of mechanical support (i.e., IABP) if cardiac output remains low despite inotropic stimulation and optimal filling pressures, as indicated by a pulmonary capillary wedge pressure greater than 22 to 25 mm Hg.[2,3]

Cardiac Tamponade

Cardiac tamponade develops when the amount of blood or fluid accumulated in the pericardial cavity is sufficient to compress the heart. Cardiac compression produces ineffective filling and ejection of an adequate CO. Signs of tamponade consist of low CO and cardiac index, hypotension, tachycardia, equalization of the RA and LA pressures, development of pulsus paradoxus, narrowed pulse pressure, muffled heart sounds, widening of the mediastinum on chest radiograph, and alteration in neurologic status. Observation of the quality of chest tube drainage is critical, especially in the first 6 hours when tamponade is more likely to occur. Generally, chest tube drainage in cardiac surgical patients is thin, red, or serosanguineous and not clotted, because blood is exposed to the mechanical effects of the contracting heart and the motion of the lungs. Blood in the pericardium that normally begins to clot is defibrinated by this mechanical trauma and becomes thin, nonclotted chest tube drainage.[3] When clots begin to appear in the chest tubes, relatively fresh bleeding may be indicated. In this situation, the incidence rate of tamponade is higher because clot can occlude the chest tube lumen, preventing chest drainage. Sudden cessation of previously and heavily clotted drainage should be promptly investigated for signs of tamponade. The specific cause can be either rapid, active bleeding from a suture line or continuous, slow oozing from a coagulopathy. Mediastinal exploration in the OR, or in the postoperative unit if the patient's condition is unstable, may be necessary to control surgical bleeding. Treatment for coagulopathy is determined with assessment of the underlying cause of the bleeding (e.g., insufficient number of functional platelets) and treatment of the specific problem.

Dysrhythmias

Rhythm disturbances of the atria or ventricles are common after surgery and may be caused by ischemia, hypoxia, hypotension, or pharmacologic or metabolic factors. Inotropic drugs (with their contractile and chronotropic effects), acid-base imbalances, and electrolyte abnormalities can also cause dysrhythmias. The high incidence rate of dysrhythmias necessitates continuous monitoring for the first 48 hours in the critical unit and the stepdown unit. Correction of electrolyte imbalances and hypoxia are basic requirements. Massive diuresis can precipitate hypokalemia, promoting the development of dysrhythmias; potassium replacement should be aggressive to maintain serum potassium concentrations at levels higher than 4 mEq/L. An intravenous infusion of magnesium may reduce premature atrial contractions and promote atrial contraction to enhance preload and CO.[2,3]

Premature ventricular contractions necessitate electrical (cardioversion) or pharmacologic (amiodarone, magnesium) intervention. If the ventricular rhythm deteriorates into ventricular tachycardia or fibrillation, cardiopulmonary resuscitation with defibrillation should be initiated promptly.

AF is common after cardiac surgery.[2,3] Amiodarone may be infused to promote new onset AF conversion to sinus rhythm. For patients with persistent or permanent AF, the goal is rate control of the ventricular response to the atrial ectopic impulses. If cardioversion is considered, a TEE first should be performed to identify the presence of left atrial thrombus, which that could break off and embolize.[3] If thrombus is present, there is an increased risk for thromboembolism after cardioversion.

Patients with transient heart block (e.g., from edema of conduction tissue during valve surgery) can be paced sequentially (in patients with an intact atrioventricular node) with the temporary pacemaker wires until the edema resolves. For patients with bradycardia, temporary pacing at a rate of 90 beats/min can be initiated to maintain an acceptable CO.

Peripheral Vasoconstriction (Postoperative Hypertension)

Factors that contribute to the development of peripheral vasoconstriction include the patient's own sympathetic drive triggered by anxiety, surgical manipulation of the heart and the great vessels with the attached pressor receptors, vasoactive drugs, and systemic hypothermia. Patients may appear pale, with cool extremities and body temperature less than 37° C (98.6° F). Patients may also display increased systemic vascular resistance, weak or impalpable pulses, tachycardia, and varying degrees of hypertension. Hypertension needs to be controlled so that the elevated pressure does not disrupt the surgical anastomoses. Increased systemic vascular resistance increases ventricular afterload and stresses the myocardium. Treatment approaches include active rewarming and administration of vasodilating agents (e.g., intravenous sodium nitroprusside, nitroglycerin, nicardipine, clevidipine).[3,38] These agents have relatively immediate effects and can be easily reversed when use is discontinued. Dosages should be titrated to achieve a mean arterial blood pressure of 70 to 80 mm Hg.

Noncardiac Complications of Coronary Artery Bypass Grafting and Valvular Surgery
Hemorrhage

Coagulation disorders and hemorrhage pose a potential threat to the cardiac surgical patient. Coagulation dysfunction is often the result of CPB,[2,3] from direct trauma to the blood components from solid synthetic surfaces and inline tubing connectors in the CPB circuit, inadequate surgical hemostasis, coagulation disorders, preoperative use of antiplatelets or anticoagulants, inadvertent hypothermia, or insufficient heparin reversal with protamine sulfate. Preoperative evaluation can be used to detect some coagulation disturbances that can be treated before surgery (e.g., discontinuation of anticoagulant medications or switching from warfarin to heparin). Previous health problems such as uremia and hepatic disease also should be considered as possible causes of coagulation disturbances. Adequate heparin reversal with confirmation with a whole-blood activated coagulation time (ACT) or activated partial thromboplastin time (APTT) should be performed. Even if the results of these studies are normal, heparin may still be released from body stores (e.g., adipose tissue) and cause a heparin rebound phenomenon. An initially normal ACT or APTT result does not guarantee that subsequent bleeding is unrelated to the effects of heparin.

Indications for transfusion based on the hematocrit and other clinical factors have undergone reassessment. One study has demonstrated that using a hematocrit value of 24% (versus 30%) as a trigger for transfusion did not result in increased morbidity and mortality.[39] Another study demonstrated that red blood cell transfusion was associated with more adverse outcomes (compared to patients not receiving red blood cell transfusion.[40]

Most postoperative bleeding can be prevented with effective surgical hemostasis at the end of the surgical procedure. Particular attention is paid to the internal mammary artery sites because of the extensive dissection from the chest wall, but all areas incised and sutured during operation are assessed for hemostasis. In patients undergoing reoperation, extensive adhesion and neorevascularization increases the risk of bleeding.

Mediastinal exploration is indicated when signs of cardiac tamponade develop with bleeding of more than 500 mL/h or less or more than 300 mL/h for 6 hours or longer. The decision to operate again should be made before the patient's condition becomes hemodynamically unstable. On reexploration for bleeding, oozing from the mediastinal wound or active bleeding may be found. During exploration, clots and hematoma are removed, the heart and pericardium are explored, and active bleeding is controlled. The pericardium is irrigated, and the chest is closed. Occasionally, no discrete source of bleeding can be found, even after extensive exploration of the surgical site.[2,3]

Bleeding from minimally invasive endoscopic sites (e.g., saphenous vein incision site) may not be noticeable until increased swelling from the leg is seen. The leg may need exploration to find and repair the bleeding site. With endovascular thoracic aneurysm repair, identification and confirmation of bleeding sites may require a CT scan, with severe bleeding necessitating a return to the OR for an open exploration to control bleeding.

Sternal Wound Dehiscence and Infection

Superficial wound infection, sternal osteitis, and mediastinitis can occur after surgery, although superficial wound problems are the most common. Predisposing factors for impaired sternal healing include advanced age, obesity, diabetes mellitus, long-term steroid use, and chronic obstructive pulmonary disease. Postoperative bleeding that necessitates reexploration also contributes to sternal wound infection. Infection can occur at any time, but is usually diagnosed 6 to 12 days after surgery. Treatment consists of intravenous antibiotics, opening of the wound, removal of clot, debridement, and irrigation. After the sternal wound has been debrided, primary closure may be performed. In more severe cases, sternal reconstruction (occasionally with muscle flaps)[2] may be needed and be performed about 1 or 2 weeks after debridement. Intravenous antibiotics are continued for at least 1 week after wound closure.

Inadequate Volume Status

Inadequate volume status can easily develop in postoperative patients. Hypovolemia can be induced by inadequate volume management during rewarming with rapid vasodilatation. Hypovolemia can also be associated with diuretic and vasodilator therapies, hemorrhage, coagulopathies, or inadequate reversal of systemic heparinization required for CPB.

Hypervolemia develops as interstitial fluid moves back into the intravascular space or if over-aggressive volume replacement occurs. Assessment of these states requires extensive hemodynamic monitoring and understanding of the numerous processes involved. Signs and symptoms specific to hypovolemia or hypervolemia should be investigated. Interventions for hypovolemia initially consist of replacement with crystalloid fluids. Colloidal solutions may be more appropriate in patients with significant peripheral edema because colloidal solutions can pull fluid more aggressively into the vascular bed where excess fluid can be excreted through the kidneys. If persistent hemorrhage from coagulopathies exists, transfusion with fresh-frozen plasma, platelet concentrates, or other factors may be indicated. If hemorrhage is related to technical (i.e., surgical) factors, reoperation is necessary. Replacement solutions in the interim can consist of blood, whole blood, or packed cells; however, blood transfusion is generally avoided unless oxygen-carrying capacity is significantly compromised.[39,40]

Respiratory System

The effects of anesthesia, sedation, and the deflation of the lungs during CPB commonly create moderate episodes of impaired gas exchange with concurrent alterations in the arterial blood gas values. These episodes, largely atelectatic in nature, are usually self limiting or easily resolved with sustained maximal inspiration, chest physiotherapy, and administration of supplemental oxygen. If a hemothorax or a pneumothorax develops, more negative pressure may be added to the drainage systems, or additional chest tubes may be inserted. A volume overload from overaggressive replacement or mobilization of fluid from the third spaces may exist and can hamper gas exchange; diuretic therapy is indicated.[2,3]

Nervous System

Temporary and permanent sensory, motor, perceptual, and cognitive deficits can occur during the perioperative period. Permanent deficits can usually be attributed to a low cerebral perfusion state from inadequate cardiac output or to an embolic phenomenon from intracardiac thrombi, calcified valve fragments, aortic plaque dislodgement and subsequent embolization from application of the aortic crossclamp, or air embolization from intracardiac chambers of invasive lines. The magnitude of the deficit is determined by the degree of neurologic involvement. Deficits are usually identified early in the postoperative period when the effects of anesthesia have resolved. Some of these deficits may not be identified until after extubation. Transient deficits, lasting from hours to days, can range in degree from slowness to arousal to confusion and delirium. Deficits can be caused by microemboli from tissue debris, air bubbles, or platelet aggregation and are associated with CPB.[3]

Renal System

Prerenal and acute renal failure states can develop after cardiac surgery. Inadequate CO from myocardial depression or inadequate volume replacement can lead to prerenal oliguria. Blood urea nitrogen and serum sodium levels increase, and serum creatinine levels remain the same. Low sodium content is seen in the urine as the body attempts to save sodium and thus increase its intravascular volume. If these states continue for prolonged periods, acute renal failure can ensue. Treatment focuses on maintenance of adequate volume replacement and increase in CO, with an inotropic agent if necessary. In addition, renal emboli from intracardiac thrombi or hemolysis from blood transfusions or prolonged CPB runs (from trauma to the formed elements of the blood producing hematuria) can also lead to the development of acute renal failure. In acute renal failure, serum creatinine and urea levels elevate and remain in a 10:1 ratio, urine sodium levels increase, and the plasma urine osmolality ratio falls to 1:1. Transient hematuria is usually short lived and may resolve after infusion of an osmotic diuretic (e.g., mannitol).[2,3]

Gastrointestinal System

Gastrointestinal complications are similar to those for general surgery.[41] After extubation, the patient may remain on nothing by mouth (i.e., NPO) status for a few hours. Small amounts of ice or water are then allowed. Gastric distention can occur if air enters the stomach and can cause cardiac problems and pulmonary complications. A nasogastric tube can be inserted to decompress the stomach. Rarely, mesenteric or splenic ischemia or infarction from intracardiac thrombi or air emboli may occur; surgical revascularization can be performed.

Peripheral Vascular System

Vascular complications can include both venous and arterial thrombus formation and embolism development. Venous thrombus can develop as a result of blood stasis from immobilization and inactivity in the immediate postoperative period. Arterial complications are largely associated with various intravascular devices such as intraarterial lines and intraaortic balloon catheters, when present. Assessment of pulses should be ongoing, and a Doppler pencil may be used to confirm the patency of the radial artery after removal of the intraarterial pressure monitoring line. The status of lower extremity pulses, skin color and temperature, and motor activity should be monitored closely, particularly in the presence of an intraaortic balloon catheter and particularly during insertion and removal. Passive and active range-of-motion exercises and early ambulation are advocated and encouraged in these patients to prevent complications. Patients are instructed and assisted in performing active dorsiflexion and extension of the feet and ankles. These maneuvers facilitate venous return and decrease stasis.[2,3]

SUMMARY

This chapter is intended to familiarize the PACU nurse with the perioperative care for the adult cardiac patient. The cardiac surgery patient has complex needs and may have resulting complications. Knowledge of the patient's experiences before and during surgery assists the nurse after surgery to tailor the care to the patient's needs and to strengthen the continuity of that care.

REFERENCES

1. Stoney WS: *Pioneers of cardiac surgery*, Nashville, 2008, Vanderbilt University Press.
2. Lemmer JH, Vlahakes GJ: *Handbook of patient care in cardiac surgery*, ed 7, Philadelphia, 2010, Lippincott Williams & Wilkins.
3. Bojar RM: *Manual of perioperative care in adult cardiac surgery*, ed 5, Oxford, 2011, Wiley-Blackwell.
4. Seifert PC: Cardiac surgery. In Rothrock JC, editor: *Alexander's care of the patient in surgery*, ed 14, St. Louis, 2011, Mosby.
5. Mosca L, et al: Effectiveness-based guidelines for the prevention of cardiovascular disease in women, *Circulation* 123: 2011.
6. Wijns W, et al: Guidelines on myocardial revascularization: the task force on myocardial revascularization of the European Society of Cardiology (ESC) and the European Association for Cardio-Thoracic Surgery (EACTS), *Eur Heart J* 31: 2501-55, 2010.
7. Park SJ, et al: Randomized trial of stent versus bypass surgery for left main coronary artery disease, *New Eng J Med*, 364:1718-1727, 2011.
8. Goldman S, et al: Radial artery grafts vs. saphenous vein grafts in coronary artery bypass surgery, *JAMA* 305(2): 167-174, 2011.
9. Dacey LJ, et al: Long-term outcomes of endoscopic vein harvesting after coronary artery bypass grafting, *Circulation* 123:147-153, 2011.
10. Kpodonu J: Hybrid cardiovascular suite: The operating room of the future, *J Card Surg* 25(6): 704-709, 2010.
11. Zamorano JL, et al: *The ESC textbook of cardiovascular imaging*, New York, 2010, Springer.
12. Coeytaux RR, et al: Percutaneous heart valve replacement for aortic stenosis: State of the evidence, *Ann Intern Med* 153: 314-324, 2010.
13. Aboulhosn J, Child JS: Left ventricular outflow obstruction, *Circulation* 114:2412–2422, 2006.
14. Salem DN, et al: Valvular and structural heart disease: American College of Chest Physicians evidence-based practice guidelines, ed 8, *Chest* 133 (6 Suppl): 593S-629S, 2008.
15. Foster E: Mitral regurgitation due to degenerative mitral-valve disease, *N Eng J Med* 363: 156-65, 2010.
16. Yosefy C, et al: Mitral regurgitation after anteroapical myocardial infarction: New mechanistic insights, *Circulation* 123:1529-1536, 2011.
17. Darke M, et al: Rheumatic mitral and aortic stenosis: To replace or not to replace – That is the question – Part 1, *J Cardiothorac Vasc Anes* 24(1):191-192, 2010.
18. Feldman T, et al: Percutaneous repair or surgery for mitral regurgitation, *N Eng J Med* 364:1395-1406, 2011.
19. Hiratzka L, et al: 2010 ACCF/AHA/AATS/ACR/ASA/SCA/ SCAI/SIR/STS/SVM guidelines for the diagnosis and management of patients with thoracic aortic disease, *Circulation* 121:e266-e369, 2010.
20. Braverman AC: Acute aortic dissection, *Circulation* 122: 184-188, 2010.
21. Cozijnsen L, et al: What is new in dilatation of the ascending aorta? Review of current literature and practical advice for the cardiologist, *Circulation* 123:924-928, 2011.
22. Propper BW, Clouse D: Thoracic aortic endografting for trauma: A current appraisal, *Archives of Surgery* 145(10): 1006-1011, 2010.
23. Birks EJ, et al: Reversal of severe heart failure with a continuous-flow left ventricular assist device and pharmacological therapy: A prospective study, *Circulation* 123: 381-390, 2011.
24. Naidu SS: Novel percutaneous cardiac assist devices: The science of and indications for hemodynamic support, *Circulation* 123:533-543, 2011.
25. Patel-Raman SM, Chen EA: Past, present, and future regulatory aspects of ventricular assist devices, *J of Cardiovasc Trans Res* 3:600-603, 2010.
26. Mancini D, Lietz K: Selection of cardiac transplantation candidates in 2010, *Circulation* 122: 173-183, 2010.
27. Davies RR, et al: Listing and transplanting adults with congenital heart disease, *Circulation* 123:759-767, 2011.
28. Thabut G, et al: Survival differences following lung transplantation among US transplant centers, *JAMA* 304(1): 53-60, 2010.
29. Mascia L, et al: Effect of a lung protective strategy for organ donors on eligibility and availability of lungs for transplantation, *JAMA* 304(23):2620-2627, 2010.
30. Sable C, et al: Best practices in managing transition to adulthood for adolescents with congenital heart disease: the transition process and medical and psychosocial issues: a scientific statement from the American Heart Association, *Circulation* 123:1454–1485, 2011.
31. Webb G, Gatzoulis MA: Atrial septal defects in the adult: recent progress and overview, *Circulation* 114:1645–1653, 2006.
32. Cox JL, et al: The surgical treatment of atrial fibrillation; development of a definitive surgical procedure, *J Thoracic Cardiovasc Surg* 101:569–583, 1991.
33. Haisaguerre M, et al: Spontaneous initiation of atrial fibrillation by ectopic beats originating in the pulmonary veins, *N Engl J Med* 339:659–666, 1998.
34. Seifert PC, et al: Surgery for atrial fibrillation, *AORN J* 86(1):23-40, 2007.
35. Ad N, et al: The implementation of a comprehensive clinical protocol improves ling-term success after surgical treatment of atrial fibrillation, *J Thorac Cardiovasc Surg* 139: 1146-52, 2010.
36. Marasco SF, et al: No improvement in neurocognitive outcomes after off-pump versus on-pump coronary revascularization: a meta-analysis, *Eur J Cardiotorac Surg* 33: 961-970, 2008.
37. Speir AM, et al: Additive costs of postoperative complications for isolated coronary artery bypass grafting patients in Virginia, *Ann Thorac Surg* 88:40-6, 2009.
38. Singla N, et al: Treatment of acute postoperative hypertension in cardiac surgery patients: an efficacy study of

clevidipine assessing its postoperative antihypertensive effect in cardiac surgery-2 (ESCAPE-2), a randomized, double-blind, placebo controlled trial, *Anesth Analg* 107:59-67, 2008.

39. Hajjar LA, et al: Transfusion requirements after cardiac surgery: The TRACS randomized controlled trial, *JAMA* 304(14):1559-1567, 2010.
40. Murphy GJ, et al: Increased mortality, postoperative morbidity, and cost after red blood cell transfusion in patients having cardiac surgery, *Circulation* 116(22): 2544-2552, 2007.
41. Khan JH, et al: Abdominal complications after heart surgery, *Ann Thorac Surg* 82: 1796-1801, 2006.

RESOURCES

Coulter SA: Epidemiology of cardiovascular disease in women: risk, advances, and alarms, *Texas Heart Inst J* 38(2): 145-147, 2011.

Coulter SA: Heart disease and hormones, *Texas Heart Inst J* 38(2):137-141, 2011.

Ferraris VA, et al: Special report: STS workforce on evidence based surgery 2011, update to the society of thoracic surgeons and the society of cardiovascular anesthesiologists blood conservation clinical practice guidelines, *Ann Thorac Surg* 91:944-982, 2011, available at doi:10.1016/j.athoracsur.2010.11.078.

Kolh P: Guidelines on myocardial revascularization, *Eur J Cardio-Thorac Surg* 38:S1-S52, 2010.

Moraca RJ, et al: Strategies and outcomes of cardiac surgery in Jehovah's Witnesses, *J Card Surg* 26:135-143, 2011.

Rahimtoola SH: Choice of prosthetic heart valve in adults: an update, *J Amer Coll Cardiol* 55(22):2413-2426, 2010.

Sable C, et al, on behalf of the American Heart Association Congenital Heart Defects Committee of the Council on Cardiovascular Disease in the Young, Council on Cardiovascular Nursing, Council on Clinical Cardiology, and Council on Peripheral Vascular Disease: Best practices in managing transition to adulthood for adolescents with congenital heart disease: the transition process and medical and psychosocial issues: a scientific statement from the American Heart Association, *Circulation* 123:1454-1485, 2011.

NURSING CARE IN THE PACU

36 Care of the Vascular Surgical Patient

Melody Heffline, MSN, RN, ACNS-BC, ACNP-BC

Peripheral arterial disease (PAD) is a "diverse group of disorders that lead to progressive stenosis or occlusion, or aneurysmal dilatation of the aorta and its noncoronary branch arteries."[1,2] PAD is the preferred clinical term, and the definition includes the carotid arteries, upper extremity, visceral and lower extremity arterial branches.[1,2] It is estimated that PAD affects 8 million people in the United States.[2] Men are more affected than women, and the disease is age-related. As many as 20% of the population older than 70 years may have PAD.[2] The consequences of PAD include a decrease in quality of life with reduction in everyday activities and a greater risk of cardiovascular morbidity and mortality.[2] Treatment is aimed at prevention or reduction of long-term complications.

Venous insufficiency is estimated to affect as many as 25% of women and 15% of men and is a chronic, debilitating disease that consumes much of the health care budget.[3] The treatment of venous disease is aimed at preventing long-term complications such as chronic edema and ulceration.

DEFINITIONS

Aneurysm: A localized abnormal dilation, distention, or sac in an artery. True aneurysm involves all arterial layers. Dissecting aneurysm allows blood to dissect between the vessel layers. False aneurysm (pseudoaneurysm) develops as a result of disruption of the vessel wall that allows blood to escape from the lumen into a contained sac.[4]

Angiography (Arteriography): The injection of radiopaque dye into the arteries followed by rapid sequential radiographs of the vascular tree for determination of abnormalities in a specific region.[5]

Atherectomy: Procedure performed with a special catheter that contains a shaver device at the distal tip. The rotating blade shaves the plaque from the inner lining and removes it from the vessel through a suction device.[5]

Bypass: Performed to reroute blood flow around an area of stenosis in a blood vessel.[5]

Cryoplasty: A technique that uses cooling and balloon angioplasty to open stenotic vessels.[6]

Embolectomy: Extraction of an embolus from an artery to restore blood flow.[4]

Endarterectomy: Surgical removal of atheromatous plaque from a stenotic vessel.[5]

Endograft: Device designed to exclude an area of a blood vessel and provide a new conduit through which blood flows. It is primarily used to exclude aneurysmal vessels.[7]

Fibrinolytic (Thrombolytic) Therapy: Technique that uses clot-dissolving agents to dissolve clot material in a blood vessel.[7]

Ischemia: Lack of adequate blood flow to an area to meet the needs of the tissues.[8]

Ligation: Transection and tying off of a blood vessel.[8]

Stent: Device made of metal or other material used to maintain patency of a blood vessel after angioplasty. The device may be balloon expandable or self expanding.[7]

Sympathectomy: Interruption of the sympathetic nerve chain performed to produce vasodilation of blood vessels distal to the surgical site.[7,9]

Thrombectomy: Surgical removal of a thrombus.[7]

Thrombus: Stationary blood clot or atheromatous plaque that partially or totally occludes a blood vessel.[7]

Transluminal Angioplasty: Use of a special catheter with a balloon at the distal tip that is passed through the vessel to area of stenosis and inflated to compress stenosis and widen the vessel lumen. The balloon is deflated before removal of the catheter from the vessel. The procedure may be done percutaneously, with only a puncture site, or open through an incision in the vessel, and may be done in conjunction with a stent, atherectomy, or cryoplasty.[5]

GENERAL CONSIDERATIONS

Persons with PAD commonly have other underlying disease processes, some of which may contribute to the development of disease and increase the morbidity and mortality rates associated with surgery. Among the underlying conditions are chronic tobacco use with chronic obstructive pulmonary disease, diabetes, peripheral neuropathy, hypertension, dyslipidemia, obesity, and advancing age.[2]

The progression of atherosclerosis, which leads to most vascular surgical procedures, is a systemic disease that affects all arterial beds, including those in the extremities, heart, kidneys, and brain.[2] A vital part of treatment of arterial disease is risk factor modification to include smoking cessation and control of underlying comorbidities such as diabetes, hypertension, and dyslipidemia.[10] Venous surgical procedures have also increased in number as a result of improvements in technology and the use of minimally invasive techniques.[3] This chapter is limited to care of the patient undergoing surgery on blood vessels outside the heart.

DIAGNOSTIC PROCEDURES

Noninvasive diagnostics, such as the ankle-brachial index (ABI), ultrasonography, computed tomography angiogram, magnetic resonance angiography and imaging, have contributed greatly to the early treatment of vascular disease.[5,7] These procedures do not usually require sedation.

The ABI is a ratio of ankle to brachial blood pressure. PAD is present if the ABI is 0.90 or less.[2] Box 36-1 describes the calculation of an ABI. This test may also be used postoperatively to assess patency of vessels following stent placement, percutaneous transluminal angioplasty (PTA), bypass graft placement, or endarterectomy. In patients with diabetes who have developed calcification of the large vessels, an ABI might not be obtainable because of the inability to fully compress the vessels to obtain a pressure. In these patients, toe-brachial index is a useful tool for assessing distal blood flow.[8]

Arteriography continues to be the gold standard for invasive diagnostic testing and usually requires intravenous (IV) sedation. This test requires direct injection of contrast media into the arterial bed and is used to examine the arterial supply of a specific region. Arteriography can also be done in conjunction with various treatment methods, including angioplasty, cryoplasty, atherectomy, and stenting.[5] Computed tomographic angiography (CTA) and magnetic resonance angiography (MAR) may also be used in the diagnosis of vascular disease.[8]

INTERVENTIONAL PROCEDURES

Interventional treatments for peripheral vascular disease include PTA, PTA with stent placement, atherectomy, cryoplasty, and fibrinolytic therapy.[5] These endovascular procedures are performed by a variety of specialists, including interventional radiologists, vascular surgeons, and cardiologists. These procedures may require only local anesthetic and IV sedation depending on the patient's condition and physician's preferences. The procedures can also be performed alone or in conjunction with other vascular surgical procedures in the operating room and may be done with local plus IV sedation, epidural, spinal, or general anesthesia.[7]

BOX 36-1	Obtaining an Ankle Brachial Index

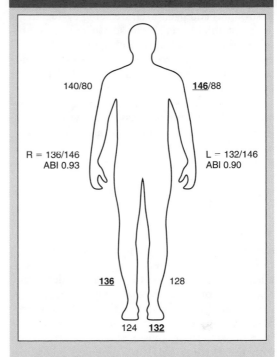

1. Obtain the blood pressure in both arms with the patient lying supine.
2. Obtain the blood pressure with a Doppler scan at the dorsalis pedis and posterior tibial pulses on each ankle.
3. Calculate the ABI with the highest ankle pressure divided by the highest arm pressure. (Example: Right BP 140/80 mm Hg; left BP 146/88 mm Hg; right DP 136 mm Hg; right PT 124 mm Hg; left DP 128 mm Hg; left PT 132 mm Hg; right ABI = 136 mm Hg/146 mm Hg [0.93]; left ABI = 132 mm Hg/146 mm Hg [0.90].)

ABI, Ankle brachial index.

Percutaneous transluminal angioplasty may be performed on carotid, aortic, mesenteric, renal, iliac, femoral, popliteal, and tibial vessel stenosis. This procedure may be used alone or in conjunction with stent placement. Major complications after PTA or stenting include bleeding, hematoma, thrombus formation, and intimal tears (disruption of the inner lining of the vessel).[5] Other complications may occur specific to the vascular bed being treated, such as transient ischemic attack or stroke for carotid stenting[11] and worsening renal failure in treatment of renal artery stenosis.[5] Stents are used to compress and hold the plaque against the vessel wall and are associated with longer patency rates of the vessel.[5] They can also be used to treat an intimal tear in the vessel wall. Stents and balloons with drug coating, such as sirolimus and paclitaxel, are being evaluated for their potential to reduce in-stent stenosis as a result of their effects on smooth muscle cell proliferation. The goal is to increase long-term patency rates. Long-term data will help to determine whether these will be an effective tool for PAD.[12]

Atherectomy is a technique designed for removing plaque from the vessel wall with a special rotating blade and suction apparatus. Angioplasty or stenting may follow atherectomy.[13,14] Cryoplasty uses a freezing technique with nitrous oxide inside a balloon for the opening of occluded vessels and theoretically carries the advantage of less risk of intimal hyperplasia, vessel recoil, and dissection.[6]

After these procedures, patients are monitored for recovery from IV sedation and for bleeding and hematoma formation at the puncture site. Distal pulses are assessed bilaterally to detect any change in blood flow that may be related to formation of an embolism or thrombus for procedures that involve the abdominal vessels or extremities.[7] These pulses should be compared with the baseline pulses documented before the procedure. Intake and output should be monitored closely and adequate hydration should be maintained after any procedure with IV contrast. IV contrast can be toxic to the renal system leading to contrast-induced nephropathy; this is characterized by an increase in creatinine of 25% from baseline within 48 hours of contrast administration. This is of greater concern in patients with preexisting diabetic nephropathy.[15] Treatments such as additional IV fluids, N-acetylcysteine, diuretics, sodium bicarbonate, and fenoldopam can be used to provide additional protection against contrast-induced nephropathy.[15]

Bed rest is maintained for 6 to 8 hours after the procedure with the extremity in a straight position to prevent bleeding at the puncture site. If a closure device is used at the puncture site, the patient may be allowed out of bed sooner.[5,16] Any patient who undergoes an arteriogram, angioplasty, or stenting that involves the carotid or cranial circulation should undergo frequent neurologic assessment after the procedure. Special protection devices are used during angioplasty and stenting to trap any free-floating particles of plaque or thrombus that may be dislodged during the procedure. These devices serve to minimize postprocedural complications such as stroke.[11]

Fibrinolytic therapy is used when an embolus or thrombus has occluded a vessel. Special catheters are placed in the area of the thrombus, and agents such as alteplase, tenecteplase, or reteplase are used to lyse the clot.[5] This process can be done by initial bolus and then completed via infusion and may take hours for complete lysis of the thrombus. These patients need close observation throughout the infusion for signs of bleeding, bruising, anaphylaxis, hematoma at the puncture site, and hematuria. Blood pressure should be monitored closely to decrease the risk of cerebral hemorrhage.[17] Assessing for signs of cerebral bleeding is critical. If treatment is needed, aminocaproic acid (Amicar) can be used to inhibit the fibrinolytic process.[5] Frequent assessment of the limb is also needed as reperfusion occurs. As the limb reperfuses, pain may actually worsen initially as microemboli break away from the thrombus and move distally to smaller vessels. As the infusion continues, pain improves as these emboli are dissolved. Frequent laboratory work includes serial monitoring of complete blood count, fibrinogen, prothrombin time and international normalized ratio (PT/INR), and partial thromboplastin time.[18] Periodic assessment in radiology is done to follow the progress of the lytic agent. The infusion is discontinued when lysis is complete, fibrinogen levels drop to less than 100, bleeding occurs that necessitates transfusion, or no response to the agent is found.[19]

MEDICATIONS USED IN VASCULAR SURGERY

Anticoagulants are among the most commonly used medications in the treatment of the patient for vascular surgery. Unfractionated heparin can be administered before, during, and after surgery. Its actions occur at multiple points in the coagulation cascade to ultimately inactivate thrombin and prevent conversion of fibrinogen to fibrin. Heparin has a short, 60- to 90-minute half-life and may be administered IV or subcutaneously. The response to heparin is measured with the activated partial thromboplastin time and is targeted at 1.5- to 2.5-fold greater than normal to obtain a therapeutic response and prevent thromboembolism.[20] Complications associated with the use of heparin include increased risk of bleeding and heparin-induced thrombocytopenia (HIT). Platelet counts should be monitored for decrease of 40% to 50% from baseline or any decrease to less than 100,000. If HIT develops, heparin must be discontinued and alternative anticoagulants should be used.[20] Protamine is the antidote for heparin; its action occurs within 5 minutes of administration. Care must be taken to avoid overly rapid administration of protamine. When administration is too rapid, side effects can include hypotension, pulmonary hypertension, shortness of breath, and flushing. The usual target dose for reversal is 1 mg of protamine for every 90 units of heparin.[20]

Low-molecular-weight heparins (LMWHs), such as enoxaparin (Lovenox), dalteparin (Fragmin), and tinzaparin (Innohep), may also be used in the care of the patient for vascular surgery. These drugs are administered subcutaneously and have a significantly lower molecular weight than unfractionated heparin, which gives them improved predictability in the dose response and a longer half-life. This advantage greatly reduces the need for laboratory monitoring. If testing is needed, anti-factor Xa level is the test of choice for monitoring. The LMWHs are administered subcutaneously and have a significantly lower incidence rate of HIT associated with their use; they are primarily used to prevent thromboembolism after surgery, but are also approved in the treatment of deep vein thrombosis (DVT) and pulmonary embolism (PE). They may also be used to bridge patients before and after surgery who require long-term anticoagulation with warfarin (Coumadin). The decision to bridge is based on diagnosis and thromboembolic risk. Patients with renal disease may need a dose reduction depending on the severity of their disease. Complications are similar to those of unfractionated heparin. Laboratory testing should be monitored for signs of HIT, although it occurs much less frequently with the use of LMWH.[20]

Warfarin is an oral anticoagulant that inhibits vitamin K–dependent coagulation factors and the anticoagulant proteins C and S; it has a half-life of 36 to 42 hours. Monitoring of warfarin is done with the PT and the international normalized ratio.[20] The PT/INR is laboratory dependent, and specific methods vary among institutions. Caregivers should be familiar with institutional methods. Warfarin is used to treat a variety of thromboembolic disorders, and it can be used to promote long-term patency of infrainguinal bypass grafts, particularly following thrombosis of previously placed grafts. Complications include increased risk of hemorrhage and skin necrosis. Patients receiving warfarin must be counseled to discontinue the drug several days before any invasive procedure to allow time for the PT/INR levels to decrease to normal. Reversal of warfarin is achieved with vitamin K or fresh-frozen plasma.[20]

Two additional oral anticoagulants are currently available. Dabigatran (Pradaxa), a direct thrombin inhibitor, and rivaroxaban (Xarelto), a direct factor Xa inhibitor, are currently approved for the prevention of stroke in nonvalvular atrial fibrillation. Rivaroxaban is also approved for short-term thrombophyphylaxis after elective hip or knee surgery.[20] Dabigatran has a shorter half-life

than warfarin and requires twice daily dosing. Patients receiving dabigatran should be counseled to discontinue its use the day before surgery if renal function is normal. Earlier discontinuation may be needed in patients with creatinine clearance less than 30 mL/min.[21] Rivaroxaban is administered 10 mg daily. There are no reversal agents for dabigatran and rivaroxaban.[20]

IV direct thrombin inhibitors act at the active site of thrombin. These drugs provide an alternative to heparin in the patient with HIT. Current drugs available in this category are lepirudin (Refludan), bivalirudin (Angiomax), and argatroban (Acova).[5,20] Desirudin (Iprivask) is a direct thrombin inhibitor that is administered subcutaneously. It may be used in patients who cannot use fondaparinux (Aristra) or LMWH.[22]

Parenteral factor X inhibitors currently include only fondaparinux (Arixtra). Fondaparinux activates antithrombin III, leading to inactivation of factor X. It is administered subcutaneously and requires no laboratory monitoring. Its primary use is preventing DVT and treating acute coronary syndromes. There is no reversal agent for fondaparinux.[20]

Antiplatelet agents, such as aspirin, clopidogrel (Plavix), prasugrel (Effient), dipyridamole (Persantine), dipyridamole ER/aspirin (Aggrenox), ticlopidine (Ticlid), and cilostazol (Pletal), may also be used in the patient with vascular disease as a preventative measure for myocardial infarction and stroke or as part of medical management for patients following placement of infrainguinal bypass grafts, carotid endarterectomy, and peripheral and carotid stenting.[5,20,23] These drugs exhibit an irreversible permanent effect on the platelet for its lifespan and produce a qualitative effect on the platelet that is measured with the bleeding time. Platelet counts are not affected by these agents. Cilostazol also has some vasodilatory effects and is contraindicated in patients with heart failure. Patients should be counseled regarding the discontinuation of these drugs 7 to 10 days before invasive procedures to decrease the risk of bleeding.[20] Patients at moderate to high risk for cardiovascular events may continue their antiplatelet agents to the time of surgery.[20]

Glycoprotein IIb/IIIa inhibitors are parenteral agents that also interfere with platelet aggregation and include abciximab (Reopro), eptifibatide (Integrilin), and tirofiban (Aggrastat). These agents are administered by IV infusion. Patients who have had drug-eluting coronary stent placement within the previous 12 months of a surgical procedure may need to be bridged with a GP IIb/IIIa inhibitor to discontinue their antiplatelet drugs for surgery or may be instructed to continue their aspirin and clopidogrel (Plavix) up to surgery.[20]

Perioperative use of beta blockers has been associated with decreased morbidity and mortality in the high-risk vascular surgery patient, particularly those undergoing lower extremity bypass or open abdominal procedures.[24,25] There is evidence that, although cardiac events are decreased, there may be an increased risk of stroke.[25,26] There is also some indication that atenolol may be associated with reduced mortality compared with metoprolol.[27] Incidence of preoperative myocardial infarction ranges from 14% to 17.8% for open abdominal procedures and 5% to 15% for lower extremity bypass procedures.[26,28] Preoperative stress testing has assisted in determining a plan of care before surgery, including coronary intervention or beta blockade, and may help to lower the risk of cardiac events postoperatively.[29] Women are at particular risk for complications after vascular surgery and also have lower survival rates. Their responses to beta blockade may also be less beneficial than in men.[29]

ARTERIAL SURGICAL PROCEDURES

Extremity Vessels and Extraanatomic Procedures

Arterial surgical procedures that involve the extremities include bypass, endarterectomy, embolectomy, and thrombectomy.[7] A bypass is performed to reroute blood flow around an area of stenosis and is named for the vessels it arises from and connects into. Examples of these in the lower extremities are femoral-popliteal, femoral-tibial, and femoral-peroneal. The distal anastomosis for femoral-popliteal bypass procedures may be above the knee or below the knee depending on the location of the stenosis (Fig. 36-1). Distal bypasses may also connect into the anterior tibial or posterior tibial artery.[7] Bypass procedures may also be performed in the upper extremities, but are much less common and may include bypass to circumvent lesions of the axillary artery, such as carotid-axillary bypass. Extraanatomic bypass procedures route blood in a more unusual fashion and may be done based on a patient's condition or inability to tolerate a more major procedure. Examples of these types of bypass include axillofemoral, axillary-axillary, and femoral-femoral (Fig. 36-2).[7] Endarterectomy can be done alone or in conjunction with a bypass and involves removal of plaque from a stenotic vessel. The most commonly endarterectomized vessels are the carotid, subclavian, iliac, and femoral arteries. Embolectomy and thrombectomy can also be performed to remove a clot from a vessel.[7]

Materials used for bypass procedures can be autogenous (vein) or synthetic (artificial). The use of the greater saphenous vein can be accomplished

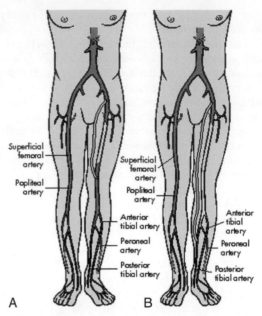

FIG. 36-1 **A,** Femoral-popliteal bypass graft around an occluded superficial femoral artery. **B,** Femoral-posterior tibial bypass graft around occluded superficial femoral, popliteal, and proximal tibial arteries. (From Lewis SL, et al: *Medical-surgical nursing: assessment and management of clinical problems,* ed 8, St. Louis, 2011, Mosby.)

in a reversed fashion or in situ. In the reverse method, the vein is reversed, and the small end is attached to the proximal artery and the large end to the smaller artery distally. Arm veins can be used, but this is much less common. Synthetic grafts that can be used include polytetrafluoroethylene (PTFE), which can be with or without supporting rings and knitted or woven Dacron. PTFE is commonly used in the lower extremities and for other low flow states such as extraanatomic bypass. In some cases, a combination of autogenous and synthetic grafts may be used.[7]

Choice of anesthesia is based on the type of procedure and patient and physician preference. General endotracheal, epidural, and spinal anesthesia have all been used safely in lower extremity vascular surgery procedures.[28] Some upper extremity procedures can be performed using regional block. Many procedures that involve smaller incisions or the use of endovascular techniques can be done with local plus IV sedation. Epidural and spinal anesthesia can be used, but in some situations are not the preferred choice because of the effects on the sympathetic nervous system that result in vasodilation of the vasculature in the lower extremities. This vasodilation can lead to hypotension, which places the patient at risk for thrombosis of the graft after surgery. General anesthesia is associated with more postoperative cardiac events.[28,30]

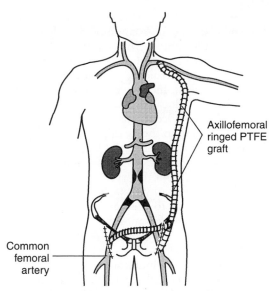

FIG. 36-2 Axillofemoral bypass and femoral-femoral bypass. *PTFE*, polytetrafluoroethylene. (From Fahey V: *Vascular nursing*, ed 4, Philadelphia, 2004, Saunders.)

Positioning

Immediately after surgery, the patient is supine with the head of the bed elevated. Care should be taken to place the limb in a position of comfort. For the patient with lower extremity surgery, care must be taken to prevent compression of the popliteal area and avoid flexion of the extremity. The limb should not be significantly elevated unless edema is present. Turn the patient to the operative side only to avoid external pressure on the graft. Both heels should be protected from pressure, and the toes should be protected from heavy bed linens. Bed rest is usually maintained for the first 24 hours after surgery.[7,19]

Cardiopulmonary Status

Vital signs are monitored at least hourly initially. Because of the atherosclerosis, patients who undergo vascular procedures have much higher mortality rates. Myocardial ischemia is most common in this patient population and occurs more often in the postoperative period than during surgery. Continuous cardiac monitoring and pulse oximetry are standard monitoring parameters for these patients. Arterial lines and pulmonary artery catheters may be used selectively in this patient population. The perianesthesia nurse should observe for signs of shock and monitor wound sites for hemorrhage or hematoma.[19]

Neurovascular Status

The dorsalis pedis pulses and the posterior tibial pulses should be assessed frequently following lower extremity procedures. For extraanatomic bypass procedures such as the axillofemoral bypass, monitor pulses in the donor arm and the revascularized limb.[7] Recommendations are for every 1 to 2 hours in the first 24 hours after surgery. These results should be compared with baseline pulses documented before surgery. Pulses should be assessed based on a scale of 0 to 3 (Box 36-2).[7] In some cases of distal bypass procedures, the position of the palpable pulse may be in a different location than before surgery. This information should be provided by the physician. A Doppler scan should be available for assessment of pulses because pulses are commonly present but not palpable. Routine assessment of Doppler-scanned pulses also provides a method of early detection of a change in blood flow. Normal blood flow is heard as a triphasic (three whooshing sounds) or biphasic (two whooshing sounds) flow. If assessment indicates a change from a triphasic or biphasic sound to a

Evidence-Based Practice

Rich evaluated the effects of positioning on transcutaneous oxygen ($TcPO_2$) measurements as a means of estimating the underlying circulation and tissue oxygenation in a convenience sample of patients who underwent arterial revascularization of the lower extremity. A repeated-measures experimental design was used, and subjects served as their own controls. Patients were randomly assigned to one of two leg positions, sitting upright with legs extended or positioned with the foot of the bed elevated 20 degrees. Assessments were made preoperatively and on postoperative days 1 and 2. Skin temperatures, $TcPO_2$, limb volumes, and other physiologic data were evaluated. The study found that neither position significantly affected the postoperative $TcPO_2$ measurements in patients with PAD.

IMPLICATIONS FOR PRACTICE

Perianesthesia nurses can be involved in ongoing studies to determine the effects of positioning on the postoperative limb. Proper positioning postoperatively has an effect on control of edema, tissue perfusion, and pain control.

Source: Rich K: The effects of leg/body positioning transcutaneous oxygen measurements after lower-extremity arterial revascularization, *J Vasc Nurs* 26:6–14, 2008.

monophasic sound (one whooshing sound), blood flow may have changed in the extremity and the physician should be notified. Establishment of a baseline includes knowledge of whether the patient had monophasic flow before surgery.[19]

Assessment of ABIs is a vital part of assessment for the vascular patient. This measurement is an indicator of blood flow to the lower extremities. The steps for assessing an ABI are listed in Box 36-1. ABIs are not assessed in the patient with a distal bypass graft, because it can cause an occlusion of the graft. Report any ABI that decreases more than 0.15.[19]

Assess for changes in motor and sensory function, the presence of foot drop, and pain out of proportion for surgical procedure. These symptoms may be indicative of compartment syndrome, which occurs as a result of bleeding into the muscle compartment and leads to a decrease in arterial perfusion.[7,19] Color and temperature changes should also be assessed. The extremity should be warm and dry and of normal color. Acute ischemia is recognized quickly with assessment for the six *P*'s: pain, paralysis, paresthesia, pulselessness, poikilothermia, and pallor (Box 36-3).[7,19]

Dressings

Dressings should be dry and intact throughout the postanesthesia care unit stay. After distal bypass procedures, dressings may extend the full length of the extremity. Frequent observation for bleeding or hematoma at the area of the incisions is critical. Signs of bleeding should be reported to the physician as soon as possible.[7,19]

Pain Relief

Pain and discomfort are common after lower extremity arterial surgery. This pain must, however, be assessed and differentiated from ischemic pain and that of compartment syndrome. Sudden severe pain may be indicative of graft occlusion, especially when located across the foot at the metatarsal heads. Occlusions usually result in pain out of proportion to the usual postoperative pain. Patients may have pain in the thigh and medial aspect of the leg away from the incision that could characterized as a burning type of pain; this pain is related to neuropathy that can occur as a result of operative injury to the nerve. Most neuropathies resolve after a few months.[19]

Intake and Output

Renal status must be monitored closely after surgery. Intake and output should be monitored every 1 to 2 hours in the first 24 hours. Hydration is important in the patient with vascular disease because of the potential for renal insufficiency; the use of contrast during the procedure increases the risk of contrast-induced nephropathy. Electrolytes, blood urea nitrogen, glomerular filtration rate, and creatinine should be monitored closely to detect changes in renal status.[7]

Carotid Vessels

The most common procedure performed on the carotid arteries is endarterectomy. Other procedures performed on the carotid arteries include bypass, angioplasty, and stenting. Endarterectomy is performed for the removal of plaque from the carotid artery bifurcation and internal carotid artery. This removal is done to improve cerebral circulation and decrease the risk of embolization to the brain, which can result in a stroke. On completion of the endarterectomy, the carotid artery can be closed in a primary fashion by suturing of the edges of the artery together or with a patch graft. This procedure can be performed using general anesthesia or IV sedation with a field block at the site of operation.[8,31]

For lesions located in the common carotid artery closer to the aortic arch, a bypass to the subclavian artery may be the only means of restoring sufficient blood flow to the brain. A bypass from one carotid to another can also be performed.[7]

Carotid stenting is usually performed using IV sedation and can be done in the operating room or radiologic suite. A major difference in the procedure for carotid angioplasty and stenting is that the procedure uses distal protection devices designed to trap any debris that may be dislodged during the procedure. These devices trap debris in a basket-type apparatus that removes the debris at the conclusion of the procedure as the catheter is withdrawn. This debris, if not trapped, can lead to cerebral embolism and increase the risk of a stroke. Other complications of stenting include acute stent thrombosis, arterial dissection of the common or internal carotid, contrast-induced encephalopathy, and hyperperfusion syndrome.[32] In addition, the patient preparing to undergo carotid stenting begins antiplatelet therapy 4 to 5 days before the procedure or is administered a loading dose of clopridogrel (Plavix; 300 mg) 24 hours before and the day of the procedure.[33]

Positioning

Immediately after the procedure, the patient is positioned supine with the head of the bed elevated for airway protection and prevention of venous pooling at the incision. This positioning is maintained until vasopressors are discontinued.[7,31] Activity is progressed as tolerated. Most patients are ambulatory 6 to 8 hours postoperatively and are discharged the day following surgery.[31]

Cardiopulmonary Status

Vital signs, including oxygen saturation, and neurologic checks are assessed every hour during the first 24-hour period. Intake and output are initially monitored every 4 hours. Uncontrolled hypertension can threaten the anastomosis and is also believed to contribute to the development of hyperperfusion syndrome. Agents that cause

vasodilation should be avoided in the treatment of hypertension, because these may worsen hyperperfusion syndrome. Hypotension may predispose the patient to carotid artery thrombosis. Changes in the baroreceptors as a result of surgery can lead to hypotension. Underlying cardiac disease may also be aggravated by extremes in blood pressure. Vasoactive infusions may be necessary to control blood pressure and maintain the levels at less than 140 mm Hg systolic and 90 mm Hg diastolic after endarterectomy. Patients should also be monitored for respiratory distress and hematoma formation.[7,31]

Neurologic Status

Level of consciousness, movement of extremities, and cranial nerve assessment are included in the assessment of vital signs after endarterectomy. Because of the close proximity of cranial nerves to the operative site, risk of injury during the procedure exists. Cranial nerve assessment is summarized in Table 36-1. Cranial nerve injuries are usually temporary and heal over time as the patient recovers from surgery.[7] Transient focal neurologic deficits may be indicative of embolization, hyperperfusion syndrome, and contrast encephalopathy after stenting. In the case of hyperperfusion syndrome, if intracerebral hemorrhage occurs, the patient may experience vomiting along with changes in level of consciousness. This complication may prove fatal if not treated immediately.[33,34]

Table 36-1   Cranial Nerve Assessment

CRANIAL NERVE	FUNCTION	ABNORMAL RESPONSE
Facial (VII)	Facial expression, saliva secretion	Inability to smile symmetrically Contralateral asymmetry = possible stroke Ipsilateral asymmetry = nerve injury
Glossopharyngeal (IX)	Swallowing, pharyngeal muscle	Difficulty swallowing with ipsilateral, Horner syndrome (ptosis, exophthalmos, reduced sweating)
Vagus (X)	Swallowing Pharyngeal muscle Phonation Sensory, motor and autonomic functions of viscera	Minor swallowing problems and fatigued voice
Superior laryngeal branch or recurrent laryngeal branch	Pharyngeal and laryngeal muscles	Vocal cord paralysis, hoarseness, inadequate gag reflex
Spinal accessory (XI)	Shoulder muscles	Ipsilateral weakness in neck and shoulder with shrugging
Hypoglossal (XII)	Muscles of tongue	Tongue droops to ipsilateral side, difficulties with speech and chewing, hoarseness, difficulty with high-pitched sounds

Dressings

Immediately after surgery, the incision can be covered with a dressing. Some physicians use a drain if oozing is seen in the wound bed at the time of surgical closure. Drainage should be measured and recorded during each shift. Bruising, discoloration, and swelling around the incision are common. However, changes in the patient's respiratory status or increasing hematoma around the incision require immediate attention. Tracheal compression can lead quickly to respiratory compromise. Reoperation may be necessary to locate and correct a suture line bleed and drain the hematoma.[7,31]

Pain Relief

Most patients need little for pain relief after endarterectomy. Opioids are avoided as much as possible because of their effects on level of consciousness and interference with accurate assessment of neurologic function. Acetaminophen is commonly used for postoperative pain. Dosing should not exceed 650 mg per dose or the maximum daily dose of 4000 mg.[31] Over-the-counter guidelines have been revised to a limit of 3000 mg daily for acetaminophen products to reduce the risk of acute liver failure.[32] Close attention should be paid to symptoms of severe headache, because these may indicate hyperperfusion syndrome or cerebral hemorrhage. This is more likely to occur early in the postoperative period for carotid stenting, within 24 hours of the procedure, and 5 to 7 days after endarterectomy as a result of impaired cerebral autoregulation. Severe cases may need treatment with steroids, anticonvulsants, and vasoconstrictors for prevention of seizures and stroke. Patients should be instructed to report headache that is not controlled by routine analgesia after discharge.[34,35]

Large Vessels

Surgical procedures that involve the aorta and iliac vessels may be performed for atherosclerotic disease, aneurysmal disease, dissection, or trauma. Bypass procedures include aortoiliac, aortofemoral, and femoral-femoral procedures and those that involve the renal arteries and the mesenteric vessels. Endarterectomy can also be performed on these vessels.[7,8]

The development of endovascular techniques has led to the use of devices designed to reduce extensive surgical procedures, operative time, blood loss, and anesthesia. Endovascular aneurysm repair (EVAR) procedures (Fig. 36-3) are used to repair thoracic and abdominal aortic aneurysms. Patients must meet certain inclusion criteria to qualify for EVAR. These devices consist of a metal stent with graft material, Dacron, or PTFE attached to the stent. The graft material may be on the outside or the inside of the stent depending on the manufacturer. Some devices are a unibody (one part to the device) design; others are modular in design. Physician preference and individual patient anatomy are used to determine the best design for each patient. These procedures can be performed with local plus IV sedation and are performed most often through a cutdown into the femoral arteries in each groin. In some instances, these procedures can be performed percutaneously.[7,36-38]

Open abdominal procedures that involve the large vessels usually involve a midline incision. Some procedures may be done from a retroperitoneal approach, and laparoscopic techniques have also been used in procedures that involve the aorta.[38,39] These procedures usually require general anesthesia. However, supplemental epidural anesthesia can be used to allow a lighter level of general anesthesia.[7]

Positioning

Immediately after the procedure, the patient is positioned supine with the head of the bed elevated to assist with respiratory function and decrease stress on suture lines.[7] Bed rest is maintained for the initial 24 hours after open procedure. After endovascular surgery, bed rest is maintained for at least 2 hours after the sheath is removed for percutaneous procedures. Activity is advanced as tolerated in patients with surgical approach to endovascular repair. Endovascular surgery patients are usually discharged within 24 to 48 hours.[8,37]

Cardiopulmonary Status

Because of the high risk associated with aortic procedures, cardiopulmonary assessment is of the utmost importance. Many patients receive beta blockers in the perioperative period to decrease left ventricular workload and the risk of myocardial ischemia.[25-27] Cardiac stress is greatly increased as a result of cross-clamping and declamping. The workload of the heart increases with cross-clamping as a result of the increased resistance the heart must pump against.[8] The leading cause of death in postoperative patients after open aneurysm repair is myocardial infarction. At declamping, the patient may experience hypotension and shock.[4] Arterial pressure monitoring, electrocardiography, pulse oximetry, arterial blood gas analysis, pulmonary artery pressure, and central venous pressure measurements are all tools that may be used during the immediate postoperative period. Normotension reduces the stress on suture lines and decreases

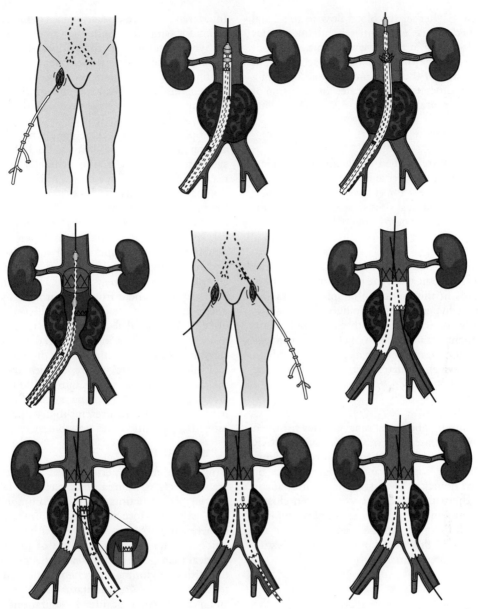

FIG. 36-3 Endovascular repair (ipsilateral and contralateral) of abdominal aortic aneurysm with a modular endograft. (From Phillips N: *Berry & Kohn's operating room technique,* ed 12, St. Louis, 2013, Mosby.)

the risk of thrombosis in a graft limb. Vasoactive medications may be used to normalize blood pressure. Dysrhythmias can occur as a result of hypoxemia, myocardial ischemia, and electrolyte imbalances. Some patients may need mechanical ventilation after surgery. Because of underlying pulmonary disease in many vascular patients, pulmonary status must be monitored closely for atelectasis as a result of incisional pain and decreased lung function.[8]

Neurovascular Status

The level of cross clamp of the aorta, if necessary during the procedure, influences greatly the potential for complications after surgery. Neurologic checks should be monitored with hourly vital signs for assessment of any signs of paralysis as a result of spinal cord injury related to cross clamp. Lower extremity pulses, color, temperature, and motor and sensory function should be assessed every 4 hours initially. ABIs are the best tool for determining whether the blood flow to the distal arterial bed of the extremities is adequate after surgery. Ischemia in the lower extremities can occur as a result of embolization, graft occlusion, or hypoperfusion of the extremity. Any absence of a previously palpable pulse indicates an occlusion of the vessel or graft and necessitates immediate intervention.[7]

Dressings

Dry dressings are applied to the abdominal incision for open procedures and to one or both groins at the site of access for endovascular procedures. Dressings and surgical sites should be assessed for signs of bleeding or hematoma.[8]

Pain Relief

Adequate analgesia is critical to reducing the workload of the heart in the postoperative period. It also aids in the reduction of splinting, tachycardia and hypertension.[7] Epidural analgesia is commonly used to assist with pain relief.[4] Pain management strategies can include pharmacologic and nonpharmacologic measures and should be reassessed at regular intervals to determine effectiveness.[8]

Intake and Output

Cross-clamping above the renal arteries for open repair and increased use of contrast with EVAR may predispose the renal bed to injury and acute renal failure.[8,15] Intake and output should be monitored hourly in the first 24 hours after aortic surgery. The patient should be monitored closely for mobilization of fluids in the initial postoperative period. Diuretics can be used to assist in removing excess fluids and reducing the risk of congestive heart failure.[8]

Temperature

Because of the length of open procedures and the exposure of the peritoneal cavity, hypothermia may be present after surgery. Active rewarming techniques are vital after aortic procedures to return the patient to a normothermic state.[7]

Sympathectomy

Sympathectomy is performed to interrupt the sympathetic nerve chain.[7] It can be performed with radiofrequency ablation, electrocautery, chemical injection, or dissection and excision of a segment of the sympathetic chain.[9,40] Newer techniques used for sympathectomy include the use of laparoscopic and thoracoscopic instruments to allow for minimally invasive surgical options.[41] The procedure is performed to increase blood flow by reducing sympathetic tone in the skin and subcutaneous tissue.

In arterial occlusive disease, pain relief is one indication for sympathectomy.[7]

Sympathectomy in the cervical and thoracic regions can be used to treat upper extremity conditions, such as Raynaud phenomenon (hyperactive response to cold exposure or emotional stress) and hyperhidrosis (excessive sweating of the hands, axilla, or face). It involves excision of the lower portion of the stellate ganglion and T2 and T3 ganglion.[9,40] Complications include Horner syndrome, postsympathetic neuralgia, hemothorax, pneumothorax, bleeding, and impaired functioning of the hand muscles as a result of injury to the first thoracic nerve.[19]

Lumbar sympathectomy is used to treat critical lower limb ischemia when vascular reconstruction is not an option and may also aid in wound healing after amputation. Patients with complex regional pain syndrome and neuropathic pain may also benefit from sympathectomy. Complications can include damage to the vena cava or ureter, paralytic ileus, and postsympathectomy neuralgia. A dry dressing is placed over the surgical site. Assess for urine on the dressing, which may indicate ureteral injury, or bleeding, which may indicate lumbar vessel injury. Mild analgesics are usually sufficient to manage pain. Severe pain may be indicative of ureteral injury and requires immediate attention and possible reexploration.[7]

Amputation

Amputation may be performed as a result of gangrene, infection, trauma, malignancy, or failure of arterial reconstruction. It is more common in men than women. More than half of amputees have diabetes, and 80% have PAD.[7,8] Although amputation is often seen as a failure of medical and surgical management of disease, this procedure is the critical beginning for rehabilitation and is essential to maximizing the status of the patient and enhancing quality of life. Amputations can be done at many levels depending on the patient's level of disease, infectious processes, joint function, and blood supply. Types of amputations are listed in Box 36-4. The more tissue preserved, the

---

BOX 36-4	Types of Amputations

- Toe amputation (ray amputations)
- Transmetatarsal (incision made across the center of the metatarsal bone)
- Transtibial (below knee)
- Transfemoral (above knee)
- Hip disarticulation

higher the functioning of the patient and the lower the morbidity and mortality rate.[8]

Postoperative Care

Immediately after the procedure, the patient is positioned supine with the head of the bed elevated. Elevation of the extremity to assist with edema control and pain management aids wound healing.[19] Epidural analgesia may be used to assist with pain relief. Some pain may also be related to phantom limb sensations that may require long-term pain management. Dressings and surgical sites should be assessed for signs of bleeding or hematoma and kept clean and dry. Patients who undergo amputation may also have multiple comorbidities that require close observation of cardiopulmonary and renal status. Stump dressings will aid in reduction of flexion contracture and improve the ability to be fitted with a prosthesis.[4,8]

VENOUS SURGICAL PROCEDURES

Chronic venous insufficiency affects approximately 15% of men and 25% of women[42] and occurs when valves within the veins of the lower extremities become incompetent, leading to an increase in the venous pressure in the lower extremities. This condition may develop as a result of venous obstruction as from DVT, congenitally absent valves or veins, or failure of the calf muscle pump.[8] Varicose veins often develop as a result of chronic venous insufficiency and significantly affect quality of life.[43] Ulcers may occur in up to 4% of patients older than 65 years and is the most serious consequence of venous insufficiency. Traditional procedures for treating venous disease include high ligation of the greater saphenous vein with stab avulsion, stripping of the vein, and perforator vein ligation.[44] These procedures can be performed alone or in combination with each other, typically in the operating room.[8] Advances in the treatment of venous disease have added procedures that include liquid and foam sclerotherapy, ambulatory phlebectomy, radiofrequency closure, and endovascular laser. These procedures are usually performed in an outpatient setting and may be done in the physician's office. Many patients undergo more than one type of procedure because of the complexity of venous disease.[40,43]

Ligation of the greater saphenous vein is performed to limit pressure on the distal saphenous vein to decrease the risk of further incompetence and distal varices. Ligation is performed at the level of the saphenofemoral junction; the vein can then be removed through stripping of the vein from the groin to the knee or to the ankle if the distal portion of the vein is involved. Individual varicose veins can be treated with stab avulsion, a technique in which individual varicose veins are removed through tiny incisions at the point of valvular reflux. Complications include wound infection, DVT, nerve injury that results in numbness in the lateral foot, and hematoma formation.[8,43,44]

Perforator (communicating) vein ligation is performed to interrupt incompetent perforator veins and can be performed as an open procedure or with a minimally invasive endoscopic technique.[8] Perforator veins serve to channel blood from the superficial to the deep veins and may become incompetent, leading to reflux of blood into the superficial veins. Interruption of these incompetent perforators decreases the pressure in the superficial system and may be performed in conjunction with other procedures.[44] Many patients with incompetent perforator veins also have ulcers in the lower extremities. This procedure may enhance wound healing as a result of the decreased venous pressure over the gaiter area, where most venous ulcers are located.[8]

Sclerotherapy uses a sclerosing agent and is injected directly into the vein, which causes the vessel to swell and seal itself. This action prevents blood from reentering the vessel. Foam sclerotherapy has advantages over traditional sclerotherapy in that it has fewer side effects, requires fewer treatments, and usually yields better results. This technique involves the mixing of oxygen into the sclerosant to produce the foam. The foam forces blood from the vein and as the oxygen bubbles dissolve, the vein deflates. The most commonly used agent is sodium tetradecyl sulfate. Hypertonic saline has also been used, but is associated with a higher risk of cutaneous necrosis. Associated complications include allergic reaction, intraarterial injection, multiple needle punctures, pigment discoloration, hematoma, and ulceration.[45]

Ambulatory phlebectomy is a technique that is performed with tumescent anesthesia, which is produced by diluting lidocaine. It is performed with a phlebectomy hook, and large varicosities are removed through small incisions that do not require suturing. Complications include hemorrhage, superficial hematoma, blisters, hyperpigmentation, nerve injury, scarring, contact dermatitis, and superficial phlebitis.[45]

Radiofrequency (RF) closure of varicose veins can be performed with local or tumescent anesthesia and involves the use of RF energy through an endovenous electrode that causes controlled heating of the vessel, producing collapse of the vessel from heat-induced vasospasm and collagen shrinkage as the electrode is slowly withdrawn from the vessel.[44] Endovenous laser ablation is the most common method for saphenous vein ablation and uses laser energy with an electrode that is painless, bloodless, and shorter duration of procedure than RF. No scarring and a shorter recovery period are seen with this procedure. Rather than shrinking the vessel wall, this procedure leads to thrombotic occlusion from heating of the blood components and thermal damage to the endothelium. Adverse postoperative events include ecchymosis, skin burns, phlebitis, vessel perforation, DVT, PE, hematoma, infection, and paresthesias.[44,45]

Postoperative Care

After venous procedures, most patients are placed in a compression dressing with elastic bandage. Position the extremity to avoid severe joint flexion and assess dressings for signs of bleeding. Circulation should be assessed to ensure adequate blood flow and to be certain that the elastic bandages are not wrapped too tightly. Elevation of the extremities can be used to assist in the management of edema. Ambulation is encouraged as soon as possible after surgery to reduce the risk of thromboembolic events.[7,43,45]

VENA CAVAL FILTERS

Inferior vena caval (IVC) filters are placed to prevent PE, which is a life-threatening complication of DVT. According to the 2012 *ACCP Evidence-Based Clinical Practice Guidelines*,[20] indications for placement of an IVC filter include inability to use anticoagulation therapy in a patient with proximal DVT or acute PE and/or documented progression of the thrombus. This procedure can be performed percutaneously in the operating room or in the radiology suite with fluoroscopy, and local anesthesia and can be inserted via the jugular or femoral vein.[7] Traditionally, these filters were placed permanently. A new generation of devices now allows some devices to be removed after the high-risk period is over. Retrievable filters are used in situations where patients are found to have a short-term risk of PE. Safe indwelling times are still under evaluation, and there is some evidence to suggest that even when retrievable filters are used they may not be removed.[46] Placement of an IVC filter does not eliminate the need for concurrent means of prophylaxis for thromboembolic events.[47] Complications of filter placement include perforation of the vena cava with retroperitoneal bleeding, migration of the filter, and improper deployment of the filter. Occlusion of the vena cava as a result of a large embolus is also a possibility.[48]

SUMMARY

The patient undergoing vascular surgery presents many challenges to the perianesthesia nurse. Most patients have multiple comorbidities that require extensive preparation before surgery and critical thinking to prevent complications after surgery. New medications and technology have enabled these patients to survive longer with a higher quality of life than ever before. The perianesthesia nurse plays a vital role in the care and survival of these patients.

REFERENCES

1. Hirsch AT, et al: ACC/AHA 2005 practice guidelines for the management of patients with peripheral arterial disease (lower extremity, renal, mesenteric, and abdominal aortic): a collaborative report from the AAVS/SVS, SCAI, SVMB, SIR, and the ACC/AHA Task Force on Practice Guidelines (Writing Committee to Develop Guidelines for the Management of Patients with Peripheral Arterial Disease), *Circulation* 113: e463–654, 2006.
2. Olin JW, et al: ACCF/AHA/ACR/SCAI/SIR/SVM/SVN/SVS 2010 performance measures for adults with peripheral arterial disease: a report of the ACCF/AHA Task Force on Performance Measures, the American College of Radiology, the SCAI, the SIR, the SVM, the SVN, and the SVS (Writing Committee to Develop Guidelines for the Management of Patients with Peripheral Arterial Disease), *J Am Coll Cardiol* 56:2147–2181, 2010.
3. Frasier K, Latessa V: Minimally invasive vein therapy and treatment options for endovenous heat-induced thrombus, *J Vasc Nurs* 26:53–57, 2008.
4. Rothrock J: *Alexander's care of the patient in surgery*, ed 14, St. Louis, 2011, Mosby.
5. Levine B, Miller K: *Cardiac vascular nursing review and resource manual*, ed 2, Silver Spring, Md, 2006, ANCC.
6. Gonzalo B, et al: Cryoplasty and endovascular treatment in the femoropopliteal region: hemodynamic results and follow-up at one year, *Ann Vasc Surg* 24:680–685, 2010.
7. Lisberger ME: Peripheral Vascular Care. In Schick L, Windle PE, editors: *Perianesthesia nursing core curriculum: preprocedure, phase I and phase II PACU nursing*, ed 2, St. Louis, 2010, Saunders.
8. Lewis P, et al: *Core curriculum for vascular nursing*, Beverly, Mass, 2007, Society for Vascular Nursing.
9. Durai R, Hoque H: Chemical sympatholysis: indications, technique and complications, *Br J Hosp Med* 69:635–638, 2008.
10. Muir R: Peripheral arterial disease: pathophysiology, risk factors, diagnosis, treatment and prevention, *J Vasc Nurs* 27:26–30, 2009.
11. Custer N: What nurses should know about carotid stents, *MedSurg Nurs* 18:277–282, 2009.
12. Ansel GM, Lumsden AB: Evolving modalities for femoropopliteal interventions, *J Endovasc Ther* 16: 1182–1197, 2009.

13. Korabathina R, et al: Orbital atherectomy for symptomatic lower extremity disease, *Catheter Cardiovasc Interv* 76:326–332, 2010.

14. Shrikhande GV, et al: Lesion types and device characteristics that predict distal embolization during percutaneous lower extremity interventions, *J Vasc Surg* 53:347–352, 2011.

15. Prevention of contrast-induced nephropathy: an update, *Prescriber's Letter* 24:detail document 240577, 2008.

16. Van den berg J: A close look at closure devices, *J Cardiovasc Surg* 47:285–295, 2006.

17. Agle SC, et al: The association of periprocedural hypertension and adverse outcomes in patients undergoing catheter-directed thrombolysis, *Ann Vasc Surg* 24:809–814, 2010.

18. Morris J, Neaton M: Continuous improvement process for a high-risk population: catheter-directed thrombolytic infusions, *J Vasc Nurs* 27:8–12, 2009.

19. Fahey V: *Vascular nursing*, ed 4, Philadelphia, 2004, Saunders.

20. American College of Chest Physicians: Antithrombotic therapy and prevention of thrombosis, ed 9: American College of Chest Physicians evidence-based clinical practice guidelines, *Chest,* 141(2 Suppl), 2012.

21. New Drug: Pradaxa (Dabigatran), *Prescriber's Letter* 27:detail document 270101, 2011.

22. Comparison of injectable anticoagulants, *Prescriber's Letter* 26:detail document 260512, 2010.

23. Antiplatelet agents for stroke prevention, *Prescriber's Letter* 24:detail document 24010, 2008.

24. Goodney PP, et al: A regional quality improvement effort to increase beta blocker administration before vascular surgery, *J Vasc Surg* 17:1–13, 2011.

25. Stephens S: State of the science: beta-blockers and reduction of perioperative cardiac events, *Crit Care Nurs Clin N Am* 22:209–215, 2010.

26. Foex P, Sear JW: Challenges of beta-blockade in surgical patients, *Anesthesiology* 113:767–771, 2010.

27. Wallace A, et al: Atenolol is associated with reduced mortality when compared to metoprolol, *Anesthesiology*, 114:824–836, 2011.

28. Singh N, et al: The effects of the type of anesthesia on outcomes of lower extremity infrainguinal bypass, *J Vasc Surg* 44:964–969, 2006.

29. Matyal R, et al: Preoperative stress testing in high-risk vascular surgery and its association with gender, *Gender Med* 7:584–592, 2010.

30. Lumb A: Anaesthesia for vascular surgery on extremities, *Anaesth and Int Care Med* 8:255–259, 2007.

31. Society for vascular nursing 2009. clinical practice guideline for patients undergoing carotid endarterectomy (CEA), *J Vasc Nurs* 28:21–46, 2010.

32. Acetominophen, *Prescriber's Letter* 18:52, 2011.

33. Nicosia A, et al: Classification for carotid artery stenting complications: manifestation, management, and prevention, *J Endovasc Ther* 17:275–294, 2010.

34. Moulakakis K, et al: Hyperperfusion syndrome after carotid revascularization, *J Vasc Surg* 49:1060–1067, 2009.

35. Medel R, et al: Hyperperfusion syndrome following endovascular cerebral revascularization, *Neurosurg Focus* 26:1–5, 2009.

36. Tinkham M: The endovascular approach to abdominal aortic aneurysm repair, *AORN* 89:289–306, 2009.

37. Thompson J, Bertling G: Endovascular leaks: perioperative nursing implications, *AORN* 89:839–830, 2009.

38. Robbins D: Current modalities for abdominal aortic aneurysm repair: implications for nurses, *J Vasc Nurs* 28:136–145, 2010.

39. Dooner J, et al.: Laparoscopic aortic reconstruction: early experience, *Am J Surg* 191:691–695, 2006.

40. Gabrhelik T, et al: Percutaneous upper thoracic radiofrequency sympathectomy in raynaud phenomenon, *Reg Anesth and Pain Med* 34:425–429, 2009.

41. Murphy M, et al: Upper dorsal endoscopic thoracic sympathectomy: a comparison of one-and two-port ablation techniques, *Eur J Cardiothor Surg* 30:223–227, 2006.

42. Tellings SS, et al: Surgery and endovenous techniques for the treatment of small saphenous varicose veins: a review of the literature, *Phlebology*, 26:1–6, 2011.

43. Brar R, et al: Surgical management of varicose veins: meta-analysis, *Vascular* 18:205–220, 2010.

44. Word R: Medical and surgical therapy for advanced chronic venous insufficiency, *Surg Clin N Am* 90:1195–1214, 2010.

45. Mowatt-Larssen E: Management of secondary varicosities, *Semin Vasc Surg* 27:107–112, 2010.

46. Gaspard S, Gaspard DJ: Retrivable inferior vena cava filters are rarely removed, *Am Surg* 75:426–428, 2009.

47. Comerota A: Retrievable IVC filters: a decision matrix for appropriate utilization, *Pers Vasc Surg Endovasc Ther* 18:11–18, 2006.

48. Spencer F, et al: A population-based study of inferior vena cava filters in patients with acute venous thromboembolism, *Arch Intern Med* 170:1456–1462, 2010.

NURSING CARE IN THE PACU

37 Care of the Orthopedic Surgical Patient

Nancy M. Saufl, MS, RN, CPAN, CAPA, and
Jan Odom-Forren, PhD, RN, CPAN, FAAN

Orthopedics (or orthopaedics) is a specialty of health care that is concerned with the prevention, diagnosis, and correction of disorders of the musculoskeletal system of the body. Orthopedic surgery is concerned with the treatment of diseases and injuries of the musculoskeletal system, mainly with manipulative and operative methods. Perianesthesia nursing care of the orthopedic patient can be challenging and rigorous. In this highly technologic age, the care needed by the orthopedic patient requires both vigilant general perianesthesia care and a sound knowledge of orthopedic surgical procedures. Familiarity with orthopedic procedures and the anticipated patient outcomes helps the perianesthesia nurse provide high quality postoperative care. The perianesthesia nurse must possess astute nursing observation and assessment skills to ensure a low incidence rate of morbidity in this patient population. The psychosocial challenges are generally more evident within this group because, more commonly, the goal of the surgery is focused on restoring mobility and relieving pain and disability. The nurse must be sensitive to heightened anxieties and empathetic to individual needs.

DEFINITIONS

Anesthesia: Local or systemic loss of sensation.

Arthrodesis: Surgical fixation or fusion of a joint.

Arthroplasty: Reconstruction of joints for restoration of motion and stability.

Arthroscopy: Surgical examination of the interior of a joint with the insertion of an optic device (arthroscope) capable of providing an external view of an internal joint area.

Arthrotomy: Surgical exploration of a joint.

Articulation: The connection of bones at the joint.

Cineplastic (Kineplastic) Amputation: An amputation that includes a skin flap built into a muscle; a portion of the prosthetic mechanism is activated by the muscle.

Disarticulation: Amputation at a joint.

Diskectomy (Discectomy): Removal of herniated or extruded fragments of an intervertebral disk.

External Fixators: Equipment used in the management of open fractures with soft tissue damage (provides stabilization for the fracture while it permits treatment of soft tissue damage).

Fasciotomy: Surgical separation of the fascia (a fibrous membrane that covers, supports, or separates the muscles) for relief of muscle constriction or reduction of fascia contracture.

Harrington Rods: Equipment used in spinal fixation for scoliosis and for some spinal fractures.

Hemiarthroplasty: Replacement and resurfacing of the femoral head with a prosthesis.

Internal Fixation: The stabilization of a reduced fracture with the use of metal screws, plates, nails, and pins.

Joint Replacement: The substitution of joint surfaces with metal or plastic materials.

Laminectomy: Removal of the lamina for exposure of the neural elements in the spinal canal or relief of constriction.

Lordosis: Abnormal anterior convexity of the lower part of the back.

Luque Rods: Contoured metal rods that are fixed to each segment (vertebrae) in the affected part of the spine.

Meniscectomy: Surgical removal of the damaged knee joint fibrocartilage.

Open Reduction: The reduction and alignment of a fracture through surgical dissection and exposure of the fracture.

Osteoporosis: Diminished amount of calcium in the bone.

Osteotomy: Surgical cutting of the bone.

Paresthesia: Numbness and a tingling sensation.

Scoliosis: Lateral curvature of the spine.

Sequestrectomy: Surgical removal of necrotic bone.

Spinal Fusion: A fusion of the cervical, thoracic, or lumbar region of the spine with an iliac or other bone graft that primarily fuses the laminae and sometimes the joints, most often through the posterior approach.

Syme Amputation: Modified ankle disarticulation (below-the-ankle) amputation of the foot.

Volkmann Contracture: The final state of unrelieved forearm compartment syndrome; contractures of tendons to wrist and hand.

GENERAL PERIANESTHESIA CARE

Specific nursing care related to the patient for orthopedic surgery that begins in the postanesthesia care unit (PACU) includes positioning, neurovascular assessment, care of immobilization devices, wound care, range-of-motion exercises, and observation for complications.

Positioning

After the initial assessment of the patient is made, attention is turned to positioning. Proper body alignment is important for all these patients and requires a sound knowledge of operative procedure and body mechanics. Individual surgeons generally have specific directives for positioning, but general guidelines apply to all patients. The goal is optimal comfort and safety for the operated limb or area. The upper extremities should be held close to the body; elevation should be achieved without undue pressure on the elbow or shoulder. The lower extremities are in a neutral position, with support provided for the entire length, and heels are off the bed.

Elevation of operative limbs is usually indicated to increase venous return, reduce swelling, and promote comfort. In the elevation of a hand or arm, the hand must be higher than the heart and no pressure should be placed on the elbow. This position can be achieved with the use of a stockinette device for suspension on an intravenous (IV) pole. The stockinette is measured from the elbow to approximately 12 inches beyond the fingertips; a piece is cut double this length. That piece is then folded in half, with the elbow resting in the fold. With safety pins, the sides are closed around the limb to form a tube, while ensuring that the fingers are exposed (for assessment of neurovascular status). With the excess material, a knot is tied and suspended from the IV pole. The elbow should be properly supported. If a pillow is used for elevation, the arm should be allowed slight flexion for maximum comfort and provide additional support for the elbow and shoulder.

Lower extremity elevation is most effective if the toes are above the heart. If the limb is not in an immobilization device, it is kept in a position of extension. This position is achieved by elevating the foot of the bed rather than with the use of pillows. The entire length of the limb should be supported if pillows are used and the heels are kept off the bed.

Shoulder immobilization can be accomplished with a sling or shoulder immobilizer. An airplane splint (a padded and Velcro shoulder orthotic used to position the shoulder in various degrees of abduction; Fig. 37-1) may be applied for rotator cuff repairs and other involved humerus fractures and postoperative shoulder or arm surgery where shoulder position and elbow flexion control are desired. If a sling is used, the patient is instructed to keep the arm close to the chest, with the wrist and elbow supported. All shoulder immobilizers require special care and padding to areas where skin contacts skin.

The patient with a hip pinning is positioned with proper body alignment, and the legs are in a proper neutral position. Care is given to avoid

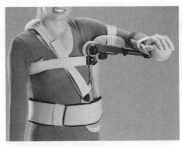

FIG. 37-1 Airplane splint. (From Coppard BM, Lohman H: *Introduction to splinting: a clinical-reasoning and problem solving approach*, ed 2, St. Louis, 2001, Mosby.)

stress to the operative area with exaggerated flexion or rotation. A pillow is placed between the knees during turning to prevent adduction and rotation.

For the patient with a posterior or lateral total hip replacement, proper body alignment is achieved with placement of an abduction pillow between the knees at all times (Box 37-1). Most important with these patients is to avoid flexion and adduction of the newly placed joint. There are four basic positions to be avoided after hip surgery: 1) no flexion of the hip past 90 degrees with respect to the axis of the body; 2) no abduction of the leg past the midline of the body; 3) no combined extension of the hip joint with external rotation of the lower extremity; and 4) no flexion with internal rotation. Use of the abduction pillow helps to prevent the patient from getting into positions that could cause dislocation. The patient who has had an anterior total hip replacement does not require dislocation precautions. Therefore there is no need for an abduction pillow, traction sling, or hip cushion to assist with positioning.[1]

The perianesthesia nurse should also be familiar with various types of orthopedic equipment that may be used and that can affect positioning. Often, patients with total knee replacement and those with more extensive knee arthrotomy are placed in a continuous passive motion (CPM) machine. The purpose of CPM is to enhance the healing process by providing CPM to the joint, thus increasing circulation and movement. Traction may also be used with various patients to immobilize and align a specific area. The perianesthesia nurse is not usually involved in setting up the traction, but should be aware of some basic principles for maintenance: (1) the traction must be continuous, (2) the patient is centered in bed in good alignment to maintain the line of pull in line with the long bone, (3) weights should hang freely and not resting on the floor or bed, and (4) the pulley ropes should be in alignment and free of knots. One type of traction is depicted in Fig. 37-2.

BOX 37-1   Surgical Approaches for Total Hip Arthroplasty

The approaches for total hip arthroplasty vary in the invasiveness of the hip musculature: (1) the posterior approach, (2) the lateral or transgluteal approach, (3) the anterolateral approach, and (4) the anterior approach.

1. The posterior approach (i.e., Kocher-Langenbeck approach) splits the gluteus maximus muscle and detaches the posterior external rotator muscles (i.e., the piriformis, obturator internus and externus, superior and inferior gemellus).
2. The lateral or transgluteal approach (i.e., Harding approach) splits the gluteus medius muscle and detaches the gluteus minimus and the anterior third of the gluteus medius muscles from the femur.
3. The anterolateral approach (i.e., Watson-Jones approach) is performed posterior to the tensor fascia lata and anterior to the gluteus medius and splits the hip deltoid muscle, which consists of the gluteus maximus and tensor fascia lata muscles.
4. The anterior approach (i.e., short Smith-Petersen and Hueter approach) does not split or detach muscles. This approach is performed over the tensor fascia lata, inside the tensor sheath, anterior and medial to the tensor fascia lata, and lateral to the sartorius and rectus femoris muscles.

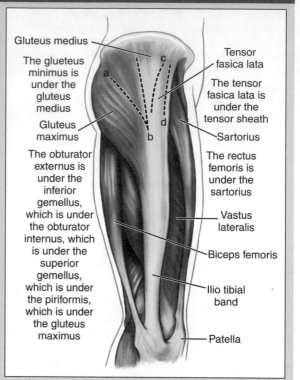

Gluteus medius

The glueteus minimus is under the gluteus medius

Gluteus maximus

The obturator externus is under the inferior gemellus, which is under the obturator internus, which is under the superior gemellus, which is under the piriformis, which is under the gluteus maximus

Tensor fasica lata

The tensor fasica lata is under the tensor sheath

Sartorius

The rectus femoris is under the sartorius

Vastus lateralis

Biceps femoris

Ilio tibial band

Patella

(From Munro CA: The perioperative nurse's role in table-enhanced anterior total hip arthroplasty, *AORN J* 90:54, 2009. Illustration by Kurt Jones.)

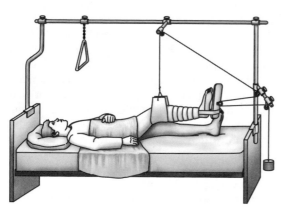

FIG. 37-2 Russell skin traction (single) with overhead frame and trapeze.

Neurovascular Assessment

Critical to the care of the patient for orthopedic surgery is assessment of the neurovascular status of the operative limb. Any alteration in blood flow to the extremity or nerve compression requires immediate intervention. Assessment is recommended every 30 minutes because problems can occur within 2 to 4 hours. Baseline neurovascular indicators should be noted in the admission nursing assessment. These indicators can be used to establish any deleterious effects from the surgery and to avoid the masking of potential complications. Both the affected and unaffected limbs are assessed.[2]

The hallmarks of neurovascular changes from constriction and circulatory embarrassment are pain, discoloration (skin that is pale or bluish), decreased mobility, coldness, diminished or absent pulses, altered capillary refilling, and swelling. Pain is common with patients for orthopedic surgery, and the approach to treatment must be individualized. Pain unrelieved with conventional methods, such as elevation and repositioning and the administration of opioids, must be assessed further. Color indicates circulatory compromise.[2] Cyanosis suggests venous obstruction; pallor suggests arterial obstruction. Mobility is assessed by determining the range of motion of the fingers or toes and strongly indicates neural compromise. Fingers are flexed, extended, spread, and wiggled. Toes should be dorsiflexed, plantarflexed, and wiggled. An inability to move the fingers or toes, pain on extension of the hand or foot, or coldness of the extremity is indicative of ischemia. Sensation is described as normal, hypesthetic (dulled), paresthetic, or anesthetic. Alteration in sensation suggests nerve compression or circulatory compromise. Limb perfusion is further assessed with the presence of peripheral pulses and capillary refilling. Capillary refilling is assessed with compression of the nail bed, which causes blanching; when the compression is released, color briskly returns. Compromise delays the filling time. With the development of pulse oximetry, a more reliable method of perfusion assessment is available. With placement of the oximeter sensor on a finger or toe of the affected limb, the pulsation is sensed and oxygen saturation is displayed. This method is more reflective of perfusion than capillary refilling and is valuable when pulses cannot be assessed because of the presence of a cast or dressing.

Care of Immobilization Devices (Cast Care)

Immediate assessment of the patient after orthopedic surgery in the PACU should include the type of immobilization device applied. The soft knee immobilizer should be checked for proper placement and closure, and the surgical dressing should be checked for drainage. For care that involves traction, refer to the previous section in this chapter on positioning.

The cast is a rigid immobilization device molded to the contours of the part to which it is applied. The cast has a dual purpose: immobilization in a specific position and provision of uniform pressure on the encased soft tissue. The cast should be inspected for visibility of fingers and toes for neurovascular assessment. If the cast is bivalved, the edges should be inspected for roughness to avoid discomfort and potential skin breakdown. When the patient arrives in the PACU, the cast is likely still wet, and special care must be taken to prevent indentations. A wet cast must be handled carefully with the palms of the hand to avoid pressure from fingertips. The cast should be supported on a pillow, and hard flat surfaces should be avoided. Improper handling and flat surfaces can cause indentations that can lead to the development of pressure sores. More frequently, a fiberglass cast is applied with quicker drying properties, but the same general principles still apply.[2] In general, a full cast may not be placed on a patient where wound drainage is expected (a temporary splint or cast would be used), but any drainage noted on the cast should be circled, and the time should be noted. This documentation can provide a guide for postoperative blood and fluid loss and can alert the nurse if the drainage appears to be excessive. Note that orthopedic wounds tend to ooze and may bleed more than other surgical wounds.

Wound Care

All surgical dressings should be checked for drainage and closure. Patients with orthopedic surgery are highly susceptible to infection; therefore strict asepsis is required when changing dressings or handling drains. Drains may be placed in the wound to minimize blood accumulation and the possibility of infection. Care must be taken to attend these drains and maintain suction.

A patient with total joint replacement may commonly have a large amount of blood loss in the immediate postoperative period. This loss can be as great as 250 to 300 mL in the first hour. With advances in technology and the implementation of minimally invasive techniques, blood loss of even 150 mL in the first hour could be significant and may require surgeon notification. The retrieval of this blood for reinfusion (autotransfusion), when coupled with preoperative autologous blood donation, has substantially reduced the need for homologous transfusions. Autotransfusion is accomplished with the use of self-contained disposable systems that are designed for easy setup and safe use.

Range-of-Motion Exercises

Range-of-motion exercises can be initiated in the PACU as soon as the patient is alert and cooperative. Flexion, extension, and rotation of joints distal to the operative area assist in stimulating circulation and strengthening muscles. Quad tightening exercises, if permitted by the physician, may also be helpful. Prevention of venous stasis decreases the incidence rate of thromboembolism, and early movement of joints promotes healing and stabilization.

Observation for Complications

Postoperative complications for the patient after orthopedic surgery include deep vein thrombosis, pulmonary embolism, fat embolism syndrome, compartment syndrome, shock, and urinary retention.

Deep Vein Thrombosis

Prevention of deep vein thrombosis (DVT) is a major concern for patients undergoing orthopedic surgery, especially total joint replacement.[3] Other contributing risk factors include age, previous history of DVT or pulmonary embolism (PE), metastatic malignancy, smoking, estrogen or current pregnancy, vein disease, obesity, and genetics (Box 37-2). Thrombosis is the formation of a blood clot associated with three conditions outlined by Virchow in 1846: venous stasis, altered clotting mechanism, and altered vessel wall integrity.[4] Immobilization and the insult of the surgical procedure

BOX 37-2 Risk Factors for Venous Thromboembolic Disease	
Clinical Risk Factors	**Hemostatic Abnormalities (Hypercoagulable States)**
Advanced age	Antithrombin III deficiency
Fracture of pelvis, hip, femur, or tibia	Protein C deficiency
Paralysis or prolonged immobility	Protein S deficiency
Prior venous thromboembolic disease	Dysfibrinogenemia
Operation involving abdomen, pelvis, or lower extremities	Lupus anticoagulant and antiphospholipid antibodies
Obesity	Myeloproliferative disorder
Congestive heart failure	Heparin-induced thrombocytopenia
Myocardial infarction	Disorders of plasminogen and plasminogen activation
Stroke	

Adapted from Anderson FA, Spencer FA: Risk factors for venous thromboembolism, *Circulation* 107:S19, 2003; Lieberman JR, Hsu WK: Current concepts review: prevention of venous thromboembolic disease after total hip and knee arthroplasty, *J Bone Joint Surg* 87A:2097, 2005.

place the orthopedic patient at high risk. DVT refers to the formation of a thrombus within the deep vein, typically the thigh or calf. In reports of total hip arthroplasty before routine prophylaxis, venous thrombosis occurred after total hip replacement in 50% of patients, and fatal pulmonary emboli occurred in 2%.[3] Immobilization impairs the leg muscle action needed to move the blood sufficiently, and the surgical procedure injures vessel walls that activate and alter clotting mechanisms. An inflammation process begins within the vessel wall and leads to deep vein thrombosis. The patient usually has pain and tenderness. Signs include swelling and sometimes localized redness. Palpation of the calf reveals firmness or tension of the muscle. A positive Homans sign may be seen, although a positive sign does not accurately diagnose a DVT alone.[5] DVT can be difficult to diagnose. Diagnostic tests such as venography, magnetic resonance imaging, or Doppler ultrasound may be indicated.

Prevention of DVT includes providing adequate hydration, early mobility, and exercise and applying compression elastic stockings and external compression devices to enhance venous flow. Rehabilitation beginning the first day after surgery will help to prevent venous complications. The pneumatic stockings (alternating–pressure gradient stockings) automatically provide a consistent compression-decompression system and are used in patients having many surgical procedures, including total hip replacement and spinal surgery. Surgeon's preference typically dictates the choice of postoperative anticoagulant therapy for patients at high risk, such as those with total joint replacements. The ideal agent for pharmacologic prevention of DVT has not been determined.[3] Most hospitals use a detailed DVT prophylaxis screening tool or protocol

to assess each patient's individual need for anticoagulation therapy and thromboprophylaxis. All health care facilities who are accredited by The Joint Commission must comply with National Patient Safety Goal 03.05.01 to "take extra care with patients who take medication to thin their blood."[6]

Pulmonary Embolism

The most serious sequela of deep vein thrombosis is PE. The severity of symptoms depends on the size and number of clots. Symptoms range from none if the clot is small to a myriad that may include, with increasing severity, anxiety, dyspnea, tachypnea, hemoptysis, substernal pain, stabbing pleuritic pain, tachycardia, cough, signs and symptoms of cerebral ischemia, fever, elevated sedimentation rate, shock, and sudden death. Immediate nursing care involves administration of oxygen and relief of pain. Medications usually include heparin-bolus doses with continuous infusion or other antithrombolytic agents. After hip surgery, thrombus formation may occur in the thigh, making it more likely that a PE may occur. After knee surgery most thrombi occur in the calf and are less likely to lead to PE,[3] but perianesthesia nurses must be vigilant for signs and symptoms of DVT and PE.

Fat Embolism Syndrome

Fat embolism syndrome is a condition that leads to respiratory insufficiency and is related to multiple fractures, especially of the long bones. It is caused by fat droplets released into the circulation from the bone marrow and local tissue trauma. Similar to pulmonary embolism, these fat globules migrate to the lungs, where they cause occlusions.

The fat globules break down into acids and irritate vascular walls and cause extrusion of fluids into the alveoli. The lung involvement alters ventilation and leads to hypoxemia. Fat embolism syndrome can lead to adult respiratory distress syndrome. The symptoms related to lung involvement include tachypnea, tachycardia, anxiety, chest discomfort, petechiae over the chest, PO_2 less than 60 mm Hg, fever, pallor, and confusion.[7] Brain involvement is evidenced by agitation, confusion, delirium, and coma. Immediate nursing care of this sometimes-fatal complication includes administering oxygen, keeping the patient quiet, and preventing motion at the fracture site. Prompt ventilation-perfusion scans may be warranted.

Compartment Syndrome

Compartment syndrome is a condition in which increased pressure within a muscle compartment causes circulatory compromise and leads to tissue necrosis and diminished function of the limb. Left undetected, the compression may cause permanent damage to the extremity. The compartment is described as a fascial sheath that encloses bone, muscle, nerves, blood vessels, and soft tissue. The two main causes of increased pressure to this space are: (1) constriction from the outside, such as a cast or bandage that decreases the size of the compartment, or (2) increased pressure within the compartment, such as swelling. The hallmark symptoms of compartment syndrome include intense pain unrelieved with conventional methods, paresthesia, and sharp pain on passive stretching of the middle finger of the affected arm or the large toe of the affected leg. The most significant sign is pain that is out of proportion to that expected with the injury or surgery.[3] Progressive symptoms include decreased strength, decreased sensation (numbness and tingling), and decreased capillary refilling; peripheral pulses are not generally compromised. Immediate intervention includes elevation of the extremity, application of ice, and release of restrictive dressings. Compartmental pressures may be determined by the surgeon. If compartmental pressures are greater than 30 mm Hg in the presence of clinical findings, immediate fasciotomy is indicated. Ambiguous readings require continuous monitoring and continued clinical examinations (Fig. 37-3).[3] Fasciotomy may be required within 4 to 6 hours of onset of symptoms if conservative measures are unsuccessful.

Shock

Because of the highly vascular composition of bone and secondary injury to the soft tissue, hemorrhage is always a potential risk after trauma and

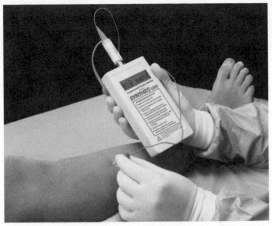

Fig 37-3 Synthes (West Chester, Penn.) hand-held compartment pressure monitor. (From Canale ST, Beaty JH: *Campbell's operative orthopaedics*, ed 11, Philadelphia, 2008, Mosby.)

orthopedic surgery. Vigilant observation of the operative area and blood pressure and pulse alerts the perianesthesia nurse to any impending danger. Immediate nursing measures include keeping the patient warm and flat in bed, monitoring vital signs, and replacing fluid volume. The surgeon is notified immediately, and more definitive treatment is initiated (see Chapter 54).

Urinary Retention

Urinary retention refers to the inability to void despite the urge or desire. This condition can occur in adult patients on whom hip or back surgery has been performed. The retention may be the result of spinal anesthesia or possibly the inability to void in the supine position. These patients should be monitored for bladder distention and pain in the lower abdomen. The surgeon should be notified if distention occurs or if the patient is unable to void within 8 hours after the surgery is completed. It is common practice in many perianesthesia units to use a bladder ultrasound to assess bladder volume, urinary retention, and postvoiding residual volume in postoperative patients.

PERIANESTHESIA CARE AFTER HAND SURGERY

Hand surgeries have become highly specialized, and there are numerous procedures including carpal tunnel release, excision of ganglions, fractures of carpal bones, or digit reimplantation.[8] There are several anesthesia options for patients undergoing hand surgery. Regional blocks to selectively block sensory functions of specific nerves are frequently used; these include digital blocks, wrist blocks, IV regional blocks, and axillary blocks. Therefore, many times patients with hand surgery bypass PACU Phase I and are admitted directly to PACU Phase II. Large bulky dressings may be in place on the hand and forearm. Ace wraps or elastic bandages for application of pressure may also be in place outside the dressing. The hand should be elevated above the level of the heart at all times to prevent edema and hemorrhage. The hand may be placed on pillows on the chest of the patient or suspended from the bed frame or IV pole with a stockinette. The elbow should be supported with a pillow. Support under the shoulder and wrist aids in decreasing pressure to the elbow. If a drain is present, it should be checked to ensure that it is activated, or it may be connected to a vacuum blood tube. The drain is placed to minimize the bleeding into the wound and to reduce the possibility of infection. Drains should be checked every 1 or 2 hours to maintain a proper vacuum, and the output should be recorded on the intake and output records. The tips of the fingers should be visible, and the neurovascular status should be assessed every 30 minutes for signs of change. If a regional block is used for anesthesia, the perianesthesia nurse must be aware that the patient's sensation and movement might not fully return for several hours after surgery and extremities must be protected from injury. Baseline neurovascular indicators should be noted in the admission nursing assessment and can be used to establish any deleterious effects from the surgery.

PERIANESTHESIA CARE AFTER ARM AND FOREARM SURGERY

Postanesthesia care of the patient who is recovering from arm and forearm surgery centers on elevating the extremity, observing for excessive bleeding, and monitoring for neurovascular changes. The radial pulse should be taken every 30 minutes and compared with that of the unaffected limb. If pulses cannot be assessed because of a dressing or cast, the pulse oximeter sensor should be placed on a finger of the affected arm; the pulsation reflects perfusion to the limb. Any decrease in intensity of the pulse or in bilateral strength of the hand, any excessive bleeding, and any changes in neurovascular status should be reported to the surgeon. Symptoms of excessive pain, weakness, or decreased sensation, especially on passive extension of the fingers, usually indicate compartment syndrome, which constitutes an orthopedic emergency. Patients should be encouraged to perform active range-of-motion

exercises with the wrists and hands. The perianesthesia nurse should keep in mind that peripheral nerve blocks are frequently used as primary anesthesia or for prolonged postoperative analgesia for these types of surgeries. Patients should be aware that they will have temporary loss of motor function and sensation from these blocks, and protective precautions must be taken.

PERIANESTHESIA CARE AFTER SHOULDER SURGERY

Shoulder surgery can include arthroscopy, arthrotomy, rotator cuff repair, or total shoulder joint replacement. The patient may be admitted to the PACU with a bulky pressure dressing in place along with a sling-style shoulder immobilizer. The immobilizer should not interfere with chest expansion, because this inhibits adequate respiratory exchange. The surgical dressing should be inspected for bleeding because the shoulder is a vascular area in which hemorrhage is difficult to manage.

Inspection should include checking to see whether any skin surface is in contact with another. If this situation occurs, a protective pad should be inserted between the two skin surfaces. The radial pulse should be monitored, because flexion of the arm in the immobilizer can reduce blood flow to the hand. The immobilizer should be checked for areas that might be causing pressure to the shoulder and arm. The elbow and wrist should be supported to prevent any undue pressure to the ulnar and radial nerves. Again, neurovascular observations are a critical part of the postanesthesia assessment of these patients. The patient should be encouraged to perform active range-of-motion exercises with the hand. Ice packs or cryotherapy may be ordered to decrease edema and pain. Management of pain can include intraoperative intraarticular injection of local anesthetic, interscalene block, opioids, and or nonsteroidal antiinflammatory drugs (NSAIDs).[2] Some surgery patients benefit greatly from peripheral nerve block for prolonged postoperative analgesia (see Chapter 25 for further information on regional anesthesia).

PERIANESTHESIA CARE AFTER HIP OR FEMORAL SURGERY

Total joint replacement or arthroplasty may be indicated in patients with painful debilitating arthritis that has failed to respond to conservative treatment over a period of time. It may also be indicated for patients with degenerative joint disease, rheumatoid arthritis, or avascular necrosis. A hip arthroplasty is a replacement of damaged or arthritic surfaces of the hip joint with materials to restore the integrity of the hip joint. The materials can be metal, plastic, or ceramic. The joint is replaced with a ball that is solidly fixed to a stem inserted into the femur and a cup that is fixed to the acetabulum, or socket. The implants are designed to create a new smoothly functioning joint that prevents painful bone-on-bone contact. A minimally invasive surgical technique is available for hip replacement. The minimally invasive technique reduces the incision from 6 to 8 inches to 3 to 4 inches and reduces the extent of soft tissue disruption in the hip. The decreased trauma to the muscles, ligaments, and tendons results in less postoperative pain. Other advantages of the minimally invasive hip replacement include shorter hospital stays, earlier mobilization, quicker rehabilitation, less blood loss, and a faster return to productivity and normal activities. The anterior approach is becoming more widely used for hip replacement because it does not split or detach muscles (see Box 37-1).[1] Advantages to the anterior approach include less postoperative pain, shorter length of stay, a single and small incision, no postoperative dislocation precautions because of decreased risk of dislocation, and immediate weight bearing on the leg.[1]

A hemiarthroplasty resurfaces the femoral head and is often used for displaced femoral fractures. Hip fractures include femoral neck fractures, intertrochanteric fractures, and subtrochanteric fractures. These types of fractures generally require open reduction with internal fixation. They occur in women more frequently than in men, mainly because of osteoporosis. Efforts should always be made to get these patients to surgery as soon as possible to avoid complications related to immobility, pressure, thrombophlebitis, or pulmonary compromise. Femur fractures are also frequently seen in trauma patients and will also require open reduction with internal fixation.

When the patient who has had hip or femoral surgery is admitted to the PACU, nursing assessment should include pulmonary and neurovascular function, body alignment, and the amount and type of bleeding from the surgical incision. Because of long bone trauma and the often advanced age of this group of patients, these patients represent the highest risk group for postoperative orthopedic complications. Many of these patients receive spinal anesthesia and the perianesthesia nurse must monitor the level of spinal blockade close and be alert for hypotension associated with spinal anesthesia (see Chapter 25 for further information on spinal anesthesia).

Preexisting medical conditions and the effects of anesthetic agents may compromise respiratory function. Coughing and deep breathing, sustained maximal inspirations, and position changes, when possible, are of utmost importance. The incentive spirometer can be used to facilitate good lung expansion. Any change in pulmonary dynamics should be reported to the anesthesia provider.

Because swelling at the operative site can reduce blood flow to the feet, neurologic signs along with pulses of the affected foot should be monitored and compared with those of the unaffected foot. The dorsalis pedis pulse can be palpated on the dorsum of the foot and lateral to the extensor tendon of the great toe. The posterior tibial pulse can be palpated just behind and slightly below the medial malleolus of the ankle. The extremity is elevated where indicated.

The body should be aligned as normally as possible. The legs and feet are maintained in a neutral position, elevated as indicated, and supported to avoid rotations of and pressure on the heels. Traction may be applied and has been discussed previously in this chapter. These patients may have antiembolism hose, sequential compression devices, or abduction pillows in place and should be observed for peroneal nerve compression. Compression can occur where the peroneal nerve crosses the knee at the head of the fibula. Decreased sensation over the dorsum of the foot, tingling, extremity weakness, and an inability to bring the foot up are indicative signs of this injury, which is a common cause of foot drop. The patient should be encouraged to perform active range-of-motion exercises of the ankle to enhance venous return.

The patient with posterior total hip replacement has an abduction pillow placed between the knees at all times. This position must be maintained to avoid adduction and internal rotation of the newly placed joint. The patient should not be allowed to flex the hips at a greater than 30- to 40-degree angle or to adduct the leg of the affected side. The muscle groups are weakened, and dislocation of the joint is a potential risk. If turning is necessary, the patient may be turned to the unoperated side no more than 45 degrees, with hip abduction maintained and total leg support provided. The head of the bed can be elevated no more than 45 degrees. The patient who has had an anterior total hip replacement does not require an abduction pillow, traction sling, or hip cushion to assist with positioning.[1] Many of these patients use a walker and begin ambulation the same day of surgery.

An autotransfusion system or other drain with suction, such as a Hemovac, may be inserted at the operative site to facilitate the removal of blood; the color and amount should be inspected frequently. Autotransfusion is a technique that salvages red blood cells lost by the patient at the wound site and re-infuses that blood into the same patient. Autotransfusion may be used if the patient is expected to lose enough blood during the perioperative period to require transfusion and can reduce or eliminate the need for allogeneic transfusion. The patient may also receive autologous blood that was provided by the patient before surgery.[9] The perianesthesia nurse should know how to operate any device that is used for drainage or autotransfusion and the hospital policies and procedures that apply (Fig. 37-4). If drainage systems are in use, the nurse should monitor the drainage and notify the surgeon for excessive volume or bright red blood.

PERIANESTHESIA CARE AFTER KNEE SURGERY

Total knee arthroplasty is a surgical procedure to replace the worn surfaces of the knee. This goal of this surgery is to relieve the patient's complaints of chronic knee pain and instability. The replacement implants are designed to create a new, smoothly functioning joint that prevents painful bone-on-bone contact. Many different types of designs and materials are currently used in total knee replacement surgery, nearly all of which consist of three components: the femoral component (made of a highly polished strong metal), the tibial component (made of a durable plastic often held in a metal tray), and the patellar component (also plastic). Surgeons may elect to replace all or part of the knee, depending on the patient's condition and the extent of the

arthritis affecting the knee (Fig. 37-5).[3] In patients with only limited knee arthritis, surgeons may choose to perform a unicompartmental or partial knee replacement. Unlike total knee replacement that involves removal of all the knee joint surfaces, a unicompartmental knee replacement replaces only one side of the knee joint. Usually knee osteoarthritis occurs first in the medial compartment of the knee, because this side of the knee bears the most weight. If the knee is otherwise healthy, a unicompartmental approach allows the outer compartment and the ligaments to remain intact, which may help the joint bend better and function more naturally. The partial knee replacement is done through a small incision, with minimal trauma to surrounding tissue. Many patients leave the hospital on the same day of or on the day after the surgery. Patients also have less postoperative pain,

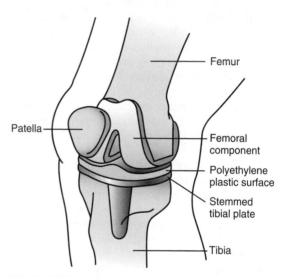

FIG. 37-5 Knee implant components. Up to three bone surfaces may be replaced in a total knee replacement: 1) The lower ends of the femur. The metal femoral component curves around the end of the femur (thighbone). It is grooved so the kneecap can move up and down smoothly against the bone as the knee bends and straightens. 2) The top surface of the tibia. The tibial component is typically a flat metal platform with a cushion of strong, durable plastic, called polyethylene. Some designs do not have the metal portion and attach the polyethylene directly to the bone. For additional stability, the metal portion of the component may have a stem that inserts into the center of the tibia bone. 3) The back surface of the patella. The patellar component is a dome-shaped piece of polyethylene that duplicates the shape of the patella (kneecap). (Modified with permission from OrthoInfo © American Academy of Orthopaedic Surgeons, available at http://orthoinfo.aaos.org.)

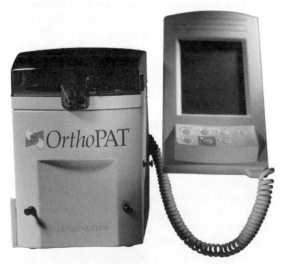

FIG. 37-4 OrthoPAT orthopedic perioperative autotransfusion system. (Used with permission of Haemonetics Corporation, Braintree, Mass.)

earlier mobilization, and less blood loss, which results in a faster return to activities of daily living. The total knee replacement is performed more frequently than the unicompartmental knee and involves replacing the opposing femorotibial joint and the patellofemoral joint.

Postanesthesia care of the patient who has had surgery of the knee involves observation for complications and proper knee positioning. After knee surgery, the patient may arrive in the PACU with a bulky compression dressing in place. Ice over the surgical site may be ordered to provide comfort and minimize swelling. The leg should be elevated and positioned in full extension, which can be facilitated by elevation at the ankle so that maximum extension of the leg can be accomplished. Assessments of neurovascular status should be performed frequently. Any decrease in sensation over the dorsum of the foot should be noted because it can represent compression of the peroneal nerve where it crosses the fibula at the knee. The surgeon should be notified if any neurologic or circulatory change is found, because early detection and correction prevent permanent nerve deficit or ischemic muscular injury. If the patient received a spinal anesthetic, the nurse cannot initially assess the patient's motor function. One of the most significant complications after total knee arthroplasty is the development of DVT, possibly resulting in a PE[3] (see the previous discussion of DVT and PE).

These patients should be encouraged to flex, extend, and rotate the ankles as soon as possible to improve circulation. Knee-strengthening exercises can also be started in the PACU. Isometric exercises and quadriceps sets aid in healing the muscle and providing stability to the joint. Isometrics involve a 6-second contraction of the entire leg followed by relaxation. The quadriceps sets require contraction of the quadriceps muscle while pressing the knee to the bed for 5 to 10 seconds and then relaxation.

The patient with total knee replacement and the patient who has undergone extensive arthrotomy knee repair are sometimes placed in a CPM machine (Fig. 37-6). This device provides a safe method of elevation, comfort, and continuous range-of-motion to the operative knee. The CPM promotes healing by increasing circulation and movement of the knee joint. The machine should be inspected to ensure proper positioning of the limb. The flexion and extension settings of the machine should be determined by the physician and are generally 0 to 30 degrees at slow speed initially.

Extensive knee procedures may have large amounts of drainage. An autotransfusion device or Hemovac drain may be present to facilitate removal of drainage from the wound.

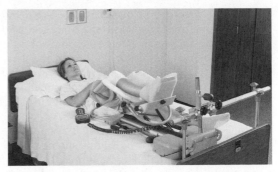

FIG. 37-6 OptiFlex Knee continuous passive motion machine with bed mount. (Courtesy Chattanooga Group, Hixson, Tenn.)

The Hemovac drain is emptied and reactivated as necessary. Drainage amounts of 250 to 300 mL in 1 to 2 hours are not uncommon. See the section on Hip Replacement Surgery for a discussion of autotransfusion.

Arthroscopic examination of the knee is done to facilitate minor repairs and the diagnosis of more extensive damage to the knee. In general, fewer postoperative complications occur because this procedure is less invasive. However, neurovascular assessment remains an important part of the postanesthesia care of these patients.

PERIANESTHESIA CARE AFTER FOOT SURGERY

The patient who has had a surgical procedure performed on the foot has either a cast or a bandage over the operative site. The amount and color of bleeding should be noted. Neurovascular signs should be monitored every 30 minutes. The extremity should be elevated above the level of the heart, with pillows supporting the entire length of the leg.

PERIANESTHESIA CARE AFTER SPINAL SURGERY

Several types of spinal procedures exist. The important features of the postoperative assessment relate mostly to the surgical area of the spine. Patients who have had a cervical procedure should be monitored for neurologic signs of the upper extremities. Symptoms such as weakness and radiating pain should be reported to the surgeon. Patients in halo traction should be monitored for any deficiency in the sixth cranial (abducent) nerve. Any decrease in the lateral movement of the eye is indicative of injury to the abducent nerve.

If the surgical procedure involves C3, C4, or C5, respiratory movements should be monitored because the diaphragm muscle is innervated by the spinal outflow from these vertebrae. The patient with this nerve deficit has a lack of diaphragmatic excursion and shortness of breath and uses the intercostal and accessory muscles in breathing. If these symptoms appear, oxygen should be administered and assistance in ventilation may be necessary.

An ileus can develop in patients who have had midthoracic or lower spinal surgery. This complication is signaled by abdominal distention, diminished or absent bowel sounds, and tympany on percussion of the abdomen. The usual treatment is to withhold oral food and fluids and to decompress the stomach with a nasogastric tube.

Patients who have had lumbar or sacral spinal surgery should be observed for loss of strength in the lower extremities and bladder distention. Bladder distention may be indicated by diaphoresis, hypertension, tachycardia, tachypnea, and a feeling of distress. If the patient has a catheter in place, it should be irrigated to remove any obstruction. If the patient has no urinary catheter and cannot urinate, the surgeon should be notified.

Patients with progressive curvature of the spine (scoliosis) may undergo a Harrington or Luque rod insertion for correction or stabilization of the spine. The procedure entails a spinal fusion followed by rod placement. The postanesthesia assessment entails those features included in the assessment of the patient after thoracic and lumbosacral spine surgery.

Patients who have surgery on the spine should also be observed for bleeding from the site of the operation. The patient should be turned from side to side to help reduce stasis of fluids in the lungs. The technique for turning the spinal patient is called *log rolling*.[2] All parts of the patient's body should move in unison. To facilitate this action, a pillow is placed between the patient's knees, and the knee opposite the side the patient is turned to should be flexed. The use of a draw sheet can also help to facilitate turning in one smooth motion. Pillows should be placed to support the length of the back and buttocks along with the pillow between the patient's knees. This method of turning the patient puts the least amount of pressure on the spine. With the advent of microdisk surgery, disturbance to the stability of the spine is minimal, and these patients are generally allowed activity as desired and often go home on the first postoperative day.

All spinal surgery patients with restricted movement should be wearing antiembolism or pneumatic stockings, and ankle pumping and rotation should be encouraged to decrease the stasis of blood in the lower extremities. The patient should be encouraged to use the incentive spirometer every hour to reduce the stasis of fluids in the lungs. Neurovascular evaluation is performed every 30 minutes to assess any improvements or deficiencies. Pain is a relative experience for the patient after spinal surgery. In many instances, the relief from nerve compression pain is so dramatic that the operative site pain is minimized. In other instances, the pain from spinal fusion is often difficult to manage. As discussed previously in this chapter, the pain experience must be individualized and treated appropriately. The perianesthesia nurse's goal is to help the patient perceive the pain as something that can be controlled rather than a fearful unrelenting burden.

PERIANESTHESIA CARE AFTER LIMB AMPUTATION

Patients who have had an amputation of the leg are admitted to the PACU with a dressing or a cast applied to the extremity. A cast is used to provide uniform pressure to the soft tissue, to control swelling, and to position the limb to avoid contracture (see cast care discussed previously in this chapter in the section on immobilization devices). To prevent hip contracture, elevation of the lower extremity with a soft compression dressing should be achieved by elevating the foot of the bed rather than using a pillow.[2] The patient with an amputation of the arm usually has a bulky compression dressing in place. The dressing should be assessed for drainage. The extremity should be elevated, and ice can be applied to reduce postoperative edema and discomfort. Opioids should be given for pain control. Phantom limb pain should be assessed and treated with appropriate pharmacologic agents. Adequate treatment is important to reduce the risk of chronic phantom pain syndrome.[2]

POSTOPERATIVE PAIN MANAGEMENT FOR THE PATIENT AFTER ORTHOPEDIC SURGERY

Orthopedic pain can be severe because of the significant muscle and skeletal tissue repair or reconstruction.[10] Pain management is vital in allowing the orthopedic patient to participate in early ambulation and physical therapy; both are key components of recovery.[10] Pain management for the orthopedic patient involves conventional pain protocols and can include the insertion of an epidural catheter or use of a patient-controlled analgesia pump (see Chapter 31). The patient-controlled analgesia pump administers a predetermined intravenous dose of the prescribed pain medication. The pump can be set to allow a continuous infusion of analgesic and bolus administration when the patient finds it necessary. Nonopioid analgesics such as acetaminophen, aspirin, and NSAIDs can also be used, with the possibility of gastrointestinal irritation, renal and hepatic toxic effects, and the inhibition of platelet aggregation kept in mind. Opioids such as hydromorphone, morphine, and fentanyl can be administered via IV drip, epidurally, or intrathecally to promote analgesia. Increasingly, orthopedic surgeons are using single-use systems that provide continuous delivery of local anesthetic through a small catheter inserted directly into the surgical site to decrease postoperative pain. The catheter is secured at the operative site with the dressing and with tape. Frequently, the patient is discharged home with this type of pain management. Also

of note is the increased use of peripheral nerve blocks for postoperative pain management. These blocks are well tolerated by the patient and greatly increase patient satisfaction. A multimodal approach to pain management allows the lowest effective dose of each medication (opioids, NSAIDs, local anesthetics) to be administered, resulting in less side effects.[10] Anticonvulsants can also be used and can produce an opioid dose-sparing effect and improve pain control.[10]

The perianesthesia nurse must collaborate with the surgeon and the anesthesia provider to determine an individualized plan of care to provide the patient with appropriate and effective pain management (Box 37-3).

Evidence-Based Practice

Wong and colleagues conducted a study to examine the effectiveness of pain management educational intervention on level of pain, anxiety, and self-efficacy among patients who had musculoskeletal trauma and subsequent orthopedic surgery. Patients were assigned to either a control group (usual care) or experimental group (usual care plus educational intervention). The educational intervention was 30 minutes long and included information about pain, coping strategies, and breathing relaxation exercises. The experimental group had significantly lower levels of pain, less anxiety, and better perceived self-efficacy during hospitalization. The experimental group requested significantly more analgesics on day 2 only. There were no significant differences on length

of hospitalization. When evaluated at 3 months, there were significantly lower anxiety levels among those in the experimental group.

IMPLICATIONS FOR PRACTICE

Patients may benefit from an educational intervention that focuses on relieving pain and anxiety and improving self-efficacy. Self-efficacy interventions such as seeking pain relief and practicing breathing relaxation techniques could result in decreased anxiety and pain. This educational intervention could be part of routine care for musculoskeletal trauma patients before surgery. Similar interventions could be applied to other patients who require orthopedic surgery.

Source: Wong EM, et al: Effectiveness of an educational intervention on levels of pain, anxiety, and self-efficacy for patients with musculoskeletal trauma, *J Adv Nurs* 66:1120–1121, 2010.

BOX 37-3   Management of Postoperative Orthopaedic Pain: Summary of Key Points

- Screen all patients preoperatively for underlying chronic (persistent) pain.
  - If present, assess pain control and medication use.
  - Contact primary care provider if pain is poorly controlled.
  - With the exception of nonselective NSAIDs, continue pain medications; switch from a nonselective NSAID to a COX-2 selective NSAID or a nonselective NSAID with minimal antiplatelet effect.
  - Anticipate higher opioid requirements in patients who are taking regular daily doses of opioids preoperatively.

- Establish comfort-function goals with patients preoperatively whenever possible.
- Teach the use of equipment that will be used postoperatively, such as IV PCA pumps, during the preoperative interview whenever possible.
- Ensure multimodal analgesia regardless of primary mode of therapy. The following applies to any treatment plan.
  - Unless they are contraindicated, acetaminophen (oral or rectal) and an NSAID (oral, rectal, or IV) should be administered preoperatively or as soon as possible in the PACU.

Continued

BOX 37-3   Management of Postoperative Orthopaedic Pain: Summary of Key Points—cont'd

- Consider a COX-2 selective NSAID after fracture or procedures requiring bone healing.
- Consider adding an anticonvulsant for neuropathic pain or difficult-to-control pain.
- Administer IV opioid doses to patients who have pain on admission to the PACU until a safe and satisfactory level of comfort is achieved.
- Opioid analgesics
  - Give scheduled, around-the-clock doses for continuous pain.
  - Consider a long-acting formulation for moderate-to-severe pain if an oral opioid is appropriate.
  - Establish a protocol for RN administration of IV opioid range orders.
  - Avoid IM administration of opioids because of unreliable and variable absorption; it is not recommended for any type of pain management.
- PCA
  - Patient must understand relationships between pain, taking pain medication, and pain relief and be cognitively and physically able to use the PCA equipment.
  - Ensure that the patient is relatively comfortable before initiating PCA therapy.
  - For IV PCA, use basal rates with caution in opioid-naive patients.
  - Oral PCA is appropriate for treatment of intermittent or breakthrough pain in patients who
- can take oral medications and are cognitively and physically able to use the PCA equipment.
  - Iontophoretic transdermal fentanyl PCA is indicated for pain that is expected to be moderate to severe for approximately 24 hours.
- Intrathecal anesthesia or analgesia is administered by single bolus dose technique; therefore it has short duration and is used most often as part of a multimodal plan.
- Epidural analgesia
  - Administered by single or intermittent bolus doses and continuous infusion only or with PCA capability (PCEA).
  - Cautious timing of epidural catheter placement and removal and anticoagulant dosing is crucial to prevent epidural hematoma.
- Continuous local anesthetic (block) infusions
  - Wound infusion: catheter inserted into or next to surgical site.
  - Perineural infusion: catheter inserted near peripheral nerves or nerve plexus.
  - May be administered with PCA capability.
  - Disposable pumps are used for administration in outpatient setting.
  - Provide opioid analgesic as needed for breakthrough pain.
  - Patient or family member may be taught to remove catheter at end of therapy.

Copyright © Chris Pasero and Margo McCaffery, 2006. Used with permission.
NSAID, Nonsteroidal antiinflammatory drug; *COX,* cyclooxygenase; *IV,* intravenous; *PCA,* patient-controlled analgesia; *PACU,* postanesthesia care unit; *PCEA,* patient-controlled epidural analgesia; *RN,* registered nurse; *IM,* intramuscular.

SUMMARY

Postanesthesia care unit nurses are highly skilled to assess, plan, and care for patients as they recover from surgery and anesthesia. When caring for the patient after orthopedic surgery in the PACU, the patient must be provided with appropriate care related to the surgical treatment received for a specific musculoskeletal disorder. These procedures can vary from outpatient hand and foot surgeries to more major joint and spine surgeries. Regardless of the complexity of the surgery, the patient is susceptible to joint stiffness and skin breakdown from impaired physical mobility, neurovascular compromise from pressure on major blood vessels or nerves caused by compartmental edema or immobilization devices, infection of the surgical site, and general discomfort and pain. The PACU nurse who has a basic understanding and knowledge of orthopedic procedures and associated nursing care is able to provide the patient with safe and efficient care in the immediate postoperative period.

REFERENCES

1. Munro CA: The perioperative nurse's role in table-enhanced anterior total hip arthroplasty, *AORN J* 90(1):53–72, 2009.
2. Saufl N: Orthopedic care. In Schick L, Windle PE: *Perianesthesia nursing core curriculum: preprocedure, phase I and phase II PACU nursing,* ed 2, St. Louis, 2010, Saunders.
3. Canale ST, Beaty JH: *Campbell's operative orthopaedics,* ed 11, Philadelphia, 2008, Mosby.
4. Townsend CM, et al: *Sabiston textbook of surgery: the biological basis of modern surgical practice,* ed 19, Philadelphia, 2012, Saunders.
5. Urbano FL: Homan's sign in the diagnosis of deep vein thrombosis, *Hospital Physician,* March 2001, available at www.turner-white.com/pdf/hp_mar01_homan.pdf. Accessed January 1, 2012.
6. The Joint Commission: *2012 Hospital national patient safety goals,* available at www.jointcommission.org/assets/1/6/2012_NPSG_HAP.pdf. Accessed January 1, 2012.
7. Kulik S: Orthopedic surgery. In Stannard D, Krenzischek D: *Perianesthsia nursing care: a bedside guide for safe recovery,* New York, 2012, Jones & Bartlett.
8. Bowen B: Orthopedic surgery. In Rothrock J: *Alexander's care of the patient in surgery,* ed 14, St. Louis, 2011, Mosby.

9. Joyce JA: Anesthesia for orthopedics and podiatry. In Nagelhout JJ, Plaus KL: *Nurse anesthesia*, ed 4, St. Louis, 2010, Saunders.
10. Pasero C: Orthopaedic postoperative pain management, *J Perianesth Nurs* 22:160–174, 2007.

RESOURCES

Altizer L: Compartment syndrome, *Orthopaedic Nurs* 23:391–396, 2004.

Altizer L: Neurovascular assessment, *Orthopaedic Nurs* 21(4):48–50, 2004.

American Academy of Orthopedic Surgery, available at www.orthoinfo.aaos.org. Accessed January 1, 2012.

American Society for Surgery of the Hand, available at www.assh.org. Accessed June 1, 2011.

American Society of Regional Anesthesia and Pain Medicine, available at www.asra.com. Accessed June 1, 2011.

Atlee J: *Complications in anesthesia*, ed 2, Philadelphia, 2007, Saunders.

Barrett K: *Ganong's review of medical physiology*, ed 23, New York, 2010, McGraw-Hill Professional.

Boezzart A: *Anesthesia and orthopaedic surgery*, New York, 2006, McGraw Hill.

Encyclopedia of Nursing & Allied Health: Bladder ultrasound, available at www.enotes.com/nursing-encyclopedia/bladder-ultrasound. Accessed January 1, 2012.

Fleisher LA: *Anesthesia and uncommon diseases*, ed 5, Philadelphia, 2007, Saunders.

Hall J: *Guyton & Hall's textbook of medical physiology*, ed 12, Philadelphia, 2010, Saunders.

Harvey CV: Complications, *Orthopaedic Nurs* 25:410–412, 2006.

Hohler SE: Looking into minimally invasive total hip arthroplasty, *OR Nurse* 1(1):32–37, 2007.

Mamaril M, et al: Care of the orthopaedic trauma patient, *J Perianesth Nurs* 22:184–194, 2007.

Miller R, et al: *Miller's anesthesia*, ed 7, Philadelphia, 2009, Churchill Livingstone.

Mulroy MF: *A practical approach to regional anesthesia*, ed 4, Philadelphia, 2009, Lippincott Williams & Wilkins.

Pasero C, McCaffery M: *Pain assessment and pharmacologic management*, St. Louis, 2011, Mosby.

Shugars RA, More RC: Arthroscopic hip surgery, *AORN J* 82(6):975–976, 978–984, 986–992, 2005.

Surgical Care Improvement Project Module 1: Infection prevention update, available at www.medscape.org/viewarticle/557689. Accessed July 31, 2011.

Swank ML, Lehnert IE: Orthopedic roles in the OR for computer-assisted total knee arthroplasty, *AORN* 82(4):631–640, 2005.

Warner C: The use of the orthopaedic perioperative autotransfusion (OrthoPAT™) system in total joint replacement surgery, *Orthopaedic Nurs* 20(6):29–32, 2001.

Watson DS: *Perioperative safety*, St. Louis, 2011, Mosby.

NURSING CARE IN THE PACU

38 Care of the Neurosurgical Patient

Melissa Thomas, BSN, RN, CAPA

As shown in Chapter 10, the physiology of the nervous system is extremely complex. Many neurologic care units have emerged because of the specific type of care needed in the perioperative period. Special education on the physiology, pharmacology, and nursing care is necessary to facilitate appropriate outcomes for the neurosurgical patient. Because nurses in the postanesthesia care unit (PACU) are able to render highly specialized nursing care to these patients, most facilities require that these patients first recover from anesthesia in the PACU before returning to the neurologic care unit or a routine care unit. Neurosurgical patients, or those with underlying neurologic conditions, present a challenge to the perianesthesia nurse. In addition to familiarity with routine perianesthesia care, the nurse must have a basic understanding of the nervous system and pathologic conditions or injuries that may affect this system and must be able to translate this knowledge into the skills necessary to assess, provide care for, and evaluate the neurosurgical patient. This chapter is divided into two sections: cranial surgery and spinal surgery. The division is made solely for this discussion because some aspects of care related to each topic are common to both areas. In addition, disease or injury in any portion of the nervous system may also affect other organs and systems of the body. In caring for the neurosurgical patient, the nurse must consider each structure of the nervous system (see Chapter 10) as it relates to the individual as a whole.

DEFINITIONS

Atony: Decreased or absent muscle tone.
Babinski Reflex: A reflex that is normal in newborns but abnormal in adults; in adults, it indicates a lesion in the pyramidal tract. The reflex is elicited with firm stroking of the lateral aspect of the sole of the foot, which normally elicits dorsiflexion of the big toe with extension and fanning of the other toes.
Baroreceptor: A sensory nerve cell aggregate present in the wall of a blood vessel that is stimulated by changes in blood pressure.
Compliance: The ability of the brain to yield when a pressure or force is applied.

Cranial Surgery: Surgery classified by infratentorial and supratentorial location.
Craniectomy: Removal of a portion of the skull without a replacement.
Cranioplasty: Repair of the skull with replacement of a part of the cranium with a synthetic material.
Craniotomy: A surgical opening of the skull.
Crepitus: A crackling sound produced by the rubbing together of fractured bone fragments or by the presence of subcutaneous emphysema.
Cushing Reflex: An elevated systolic blood pressure, bradycardia, and widening pulse pressure.
Decompensation: The inability of the heart to maintain adequate circulation because of an impairment in brain integrity.
Diabetes Insipidus: A metabolic disorder caused by injury or disease of the posterior lobe of the pituitary gland (the hypophysis).
Focal Deficit: Any sign or symptom that indicates a specific or localized area of pathologic alteration.
Infratentorial: The area below the tentorium that includes the brain stem, cerebellum, and posterior fossa. This approach is used for lesions in the brain stem and cerebellum region.
Laminectomy: Excision of the posterior arch of a vertebra to allow excision of a herniated nucleus pulposus.
Phrenic Nucleus: A group of nerve cells located in the spinal cord between the levels of C3 and C5. Damage to this area abolishes or alters the function of the phrenic nerve.
Pyramidal Signs: Symptoms of dysfunction of the pyramidal tract, including spastic paralysis, Babinski's reflex, and increased deep tendon reflexes.
Queckenstedt Test: The veins of the neck are compressed on one or both sides. In a healthy person, the cerebrospinal fluid (CSF) pressure rises rapidly and then quickly returns to normal when the pressure is taken off the neck. In a patient with spinal cord obstruction, little or no increase in pressure is found. This test is diagnostically accurate for most cord compressions; however, false-negative results may be obtained if the lesion is located high in the cervical spine area. This test is not performed in patients with known or suspected increased intracranial pressure (ICP).
Rhizotomy: Surgical interruption of the roots of the spinal nerves within the spinal canal.
Spinal Shock: A state that occurs after a spinal cord injury. All sensory, motor, and autonomic activities are lost below the level of the transection, and reflexes are absent. Paralysis is of a flaccid nature and includes the

urinary bladder. Autonomic activity gradually resumes as spinal shock subsides. When autonomic activity has returned, bladder and bowel training programs can be started. Flaccid paralysis may develop into varying degrees of spastic paralysis, as evidenced by spasms of flexor or extensor muscle groups. The presence of autonomic activity also allows for episodes of autonomic hyperreflexia.

Subarachnoid Block: The injection of a local anesthetic into the subarachnoid space around the spinal cord.

Subluxation: Partial or incomplete dislocation.

Supratentorial: The area above the tentorium that includes the cerebrum. The supratentorial approach is used for frontal, temporal, parietal, and occipital lobe lesions.

Tonoclonic Movements: Tense muscular contractions that alternate rapidly with muscular relaxation.

Valsalva Maneuver: Contraction of the thorax in forced expiration against the closed glottis; results in increases in intrathoracic and intraabdominal pressures.

CRANIAL SURGERY

Diagnostic Tools

Techniques used to ascertain the presence and extent of cranial injury or disease include invasive and noninvasive techniques. A brief discussion of invasive and noninvasive diagnostic procedures is included to familiarize the PACU nurse with the techniques and special considerations necessary in the care of these patients. Many interventional neuroradiology procedures with general anesthesia are now done; these patients go to the PACU after the procedure is completed. The specific PACU care is presented; if information on types of sedation (usually dexmedetomidine) for these patients is needed, please see Chapter 21.

Conventional Radiography

Skull radiographs are not ordered as often as computed tomographic (CT) scans and magnetic resonance imaging (MRI) scans. Radiographs are most often ordered to diagnose the presence of a skull fracture; information about the size, shape, and integrity of the skull and facial bones and any unusual calcification; and presence of air.

Computed Tomography

CT scanning creates a cross-sectional picture that separates various densities in the brain by means of an external x-ray beam. A computer-based apparatus allows the assessment of brain-emitted radiation and stores this information in the computer. The computer performs thousands of simultaneous equations on the radiation input and output data and delivers an accurate detailed picture of the brain and any abnormalities. The computer images correlate to tissue density. The dense structures, such as bone, appear white in color. Air and cerebrospinal fluid (CSF) appear as a black area because they have much less density. The radiologist looks at the structures, changes in density, and any abnormalities in shape, size, or location of structures.

Contrast material may be used to enhance images and explore the vasculature. An iodinated radiopaque material is injected intravenously. Scans are usually taken before and after the administration of the radiopaque material. The accuracy and rapidity of CT scanning render it advantageous in emergency situations. The entire procedure may last 15 to 20 minutes and may be difficult to use in an agitated, confused, or restless patient. The CT scan is most helpful in diagnosis of hematomas, subarachnoid hemorrhage, hydrocephalus, cerebral atrophy, and tumors.

Care before the CT scan should include an assessment of the patient's allergies, specifically allergies to shellfish, iodine, or contrast dye. Blood urea nitrogen and creatinine levels should be checked to assess kidney function. Some patients may have a headache, feeling of warmth, salty taste in the mouth, or nausea or vomiting when given contrast dye. After the procedure, the patient must be well hydrated to help excrete the contrast dye.

Magnetic Resonance Imaging

Also known as *nuclear magnetic resonance imaging,* MRI is a technique used for obtaining cross-sectional pictures of the human body without exposing the patient to ionizing radiation. MRI yields anatomic information that is comparable in many ways with the information supplied by a CT scan, but often more accurately discriminates between healthy and diseased tissues. MRI is excellent in detection of soft tissue changes. It can detect necrotic tissue, small malignant tumors, and degenerative diseases.

The patient is placed within a cylindric high-powered magnet. Body tissues are then subjected to a magnetic field, which causes some of the hydrogen ions to align themselves with the field. A burst of low-energy radio waves is then applied to knock atomic protons within the tissues out of alignment. When the radio waves are discontinued, these protons release tiny amounts of energy that are "read" by a computer. Next, the MRI generates an image based on this information, thus yielding a detailed picture of the structural content and contours of the internal organs. Contraindications for MRI include claustrophobic, agitated, or obese patients and patients with metallic devices or fragments present in the body.

Positron Emission Tomography

The positron emission tomography (PET) scan measures glucose uptake and metabolism, cerebral blood flow patterns, and oxygen uptake to ascertain the functioning of the tissues or organs. The patient is injected with a glucose analogue that is tagged with a radionuclide. As the radionuclide decays in the tissue, the protons emitted are recorded with detectors and a computerized picture is generated. PET scans have been helpful in identifying schizophrenia, Alzheimer disease, epilepsy, cardiovascular disease, head trauma, and other brain disorders.

Recent advances in technology have emerged combining the PET and CT scan together. The PET/CT imaging results in shorter imaging times than the PET scan alone. In addition, research indicates improved lesion localization in addition to more exact tumor staging.[1]

Cerebral Angiography

Arteriography, or angiography, is the diagnostic tool for aneurysms, arteriovenous malformations, and other cerebrovascular abnormalities. A cannulated needle[2] is introduced into the femoral or axillary artery and threaded to the level of the common carotid artery. Radiopaque dye is then injected, and radiographs record its path through the cerebral vasculature (Fig. 38-1). Irritation brought on by use of the dye may manifest itself in altered states of consciousness, hemiparesis, or speech difficulties that are usually transient. During and after arteriography, the patient may have an allergic reaction to the dye that can range from mild urticaria to anaphylaxis. Resuscitative equipment must be immediately available until the danger of allergic reaction has passed.

Postprocedure care includes proper hydration to prevent renal complications from the dye.[3] In addition, the patient will require close neurologic and cardiovascular monitoring. The proceduralist may have used a closure device at the arterial site. Manufacturer recommendations, institutional policies and proceduralist orders should all be maintained. These orders will consist of bedrest, puncture site checks for bleeding or hematoma and vascular check of the affected limb.[4] Intravenous fluids are maintained until the danger of untoward reaction has passed and the patient no longer has the transient nausea that occasionally occurs.

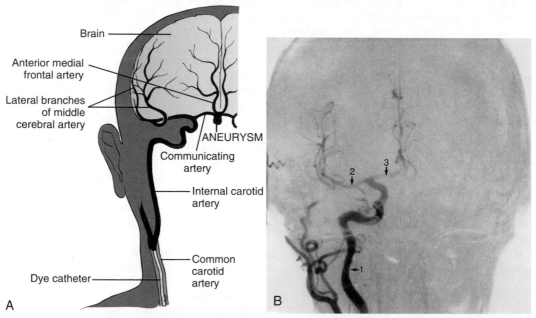

FIG. 38-1 Cerebral angiography allows x-ray visualization of the brain's vascular system when a contrast dye is injected arterially. **A,** Insertion of dye through a catheter in the common carotid artery, subsequently outlining vessels of the brain. **B,** An angiogram using the subtraction technique. *1,* Internal carotid artery. *2.* Middle cerebral artery. *3,* Anterior cerebral artery A1 segment. (From Black JM, Hokanson Hawks JH: *Medical-surgical nursing: clinical management for positive outcomes,* ed 7, St. Louis, 2005, Saunders.)

Injuries and Pathologic Conditions of the Brain

Types of Injuries

When a head injury occurs, the most crucial concern is the extent of injury to the brain itself. The injury becomes more severe when the fracture involves depression of fragments into the brain, penetration of a foreign object, leakage of CSF, expanding hematomas, or signs and symptoms of herniation. The primary goal is to protect the brain and facilitate the patient's return to an optimal level of functioning.

Skull fractures are categorized as linear, comminuted, depressed, or basilar. The linear skull fracture associated with mild brain injury[4] and do not require treatment. A comminuted fracture, also known as the *eggshell fracture,* is a culmination of multiple linear fractures.[5] A depressed skull fracture is an inward depression of the skull and is classified as open (compound) or simple (closed).[5] Infection is a primary concern, and surgery may be necessary to remove bony fragments, clean the wound, and elevate the depressed bone. Basilar skull fractures occur in the base of the skull and are difficult to diagnose with radiographs. Diagnosis is confirmed with clinical data. Patients often have "raccoon's eyes" (periorbital ecchymosis), Battle sign (ecchymosis around the mastoid process), or CSF otorrhea.

Concussion is caused by a violent jar or shock to the skull, such as rapid acceleration-deceleration. The patient may be dazed, "see stars," or have a period of impaired consciousness. When consciousness is regained, these patients may have posttraumatic amnesia and remember nothing of the injury itself or the events immediately preceding the injury.

Contusion is a bruising of the brain or hemorrhage on its surface. The extent of severity depends on the site and degree of brain injury. Consciousness may or may not be lost, but coma indicates diffuse injury. Laceration is the tearing of the brain. Laceration and contusions of the brain are usually found in the frontal and parietal lobes.

Consequences of Injury

Traumatic head injury can cause hemorrhage beneath a skull fracture or from a shearing of the veins or cortical arteries and results in epidural, subdural, subarachnoid, or intraventricular hemorrhage (Fig. 38-2). The signs and symptoms of brain ischemia and increased intracranial pressure (ICP) vary with the speed at which the functions of vital centers are altered. A small clot that accumulates rapidly may be fatal; however, the patient may survive a slowly developing, much larger hematoma through effective compensatory mechanisms.

An epidural hematoma, or extradural hematoma, accumulates in the epidural space, which is between the skull and the dura mater. The hematoma is most often arterial and caused from a rupture or laceration of the middle meningeal artery, which runs between the dura and the skull in the temporal region. Epidural hematomas may also be seen in the frontal, occipital, and posterior fossa regions. The patient usually loses consciousness and then has a lucid period after which a rapid deterioration occurs. The hemorrhage may be massive, and treatment consists of evacuation of the clot through burr holes made in the skull.

Subdural hematoma may result from trauma and the shearing of the bridging veins. Venous blood usually accumulates beneath the dura and spreads over the surface of the brain. A subdural hematoma may be acute, subacute, or chronic, depending on the size of the vessel involved and the amount of blood present. Patients with acute subdural hematomas have a rapid deterioration in condition and are critically ill.

Subacute subdural hematomas fail to show acute signs and symptoms at onset. Brain swelling is not great, but the hematoma may become large

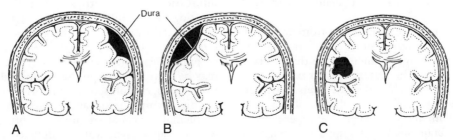

FIG. 38-2 Types of hematomas. **A,** Subdural hematoma. **B,** Epidural hematoma. **C,** Intracerebral hematoma. (From Black JM, Hokanson Hawks JH: *Medical-surgical nursing: clinical management for positive outcomes,* ed 8, St. Louis, 2009, Saunders.)

NURSING CARE IN THE PACU

enough to produce symptoms. Progressive hemiparesis, obtundation, and aphasia often appear 2 to 14 days after injury. The degree of ultimate recovery depends on the extent of damage produced at the time of injury.

Chronic subdural hematomas are seen most often in older adults. A history of head injury may be lacking because the causative injury is often minimal and long forgotten or deemed insignificant by the patient. The history is usually one of progressive mental or personality changes with or without focal symptoms as blood slowly accumulates and compresses the brain. The blood itself becomes thicker and darker within 2 to 4 days and within a few weeks resembles motor oil in character and color. Papilledema may be present. Chronic subdural hematomas can mimic any disease that affects the brain or its coverings. Treatment consists of evacuation of the defibrinated blood through multiple burr holes or a craniotomy incision.

Intracerebral hematomas are more commonly found in the elderly, often after a fall, but are also seen as a result of spontaneous rupture of a weakened blood vessel or aneurysm. Hemorrhage may be scattered or isolated and occurs in the brain parenchyma. Surgical evacuation of an isolated or well-defined clot may be attempted, but the mortality rate remains high.

Subarachnoid hemorrhage may occur as the result of traumatic brain injury. Bleeding into the subarachnoid space may result in a vasospasm. A vasospasm is the narrowing of the blood vessel lumen and places the patient at risk for a delayed ischemic event. The risk of development of vasospasms is greatest 3 to 7 days after the bleed.

Intraventricular hematoma, which is usually caused by a subarachnoid or intracerebral hemorrhage, is bleeding into the ventricles.[6] This can be caused by brain trauma such as penetrating wounds or from an anterior communicating and basilar tip aneurysm.[5] An intraventricular hematoma is associated with high mortality, and treatment includes a ventriculostomy with CSF drainage and ICP management.[6]

Herniation of the brain occurs from untreated, increased ICP. Supratentorial herniation is regarded as an emergency more severe than an epidural hematoma. The tentorium is an extension of the dura mater, which forms a transverse partition or shelf that divides the cerebral hemispheres from the cerebellum and brain stem. The superior portion of the brain stem passes upward through an aperture in the tentorium known as the *tentorial hiatus*. No space-occupying mass or lesion that expands within the cerebral hemispheres can escape upward or outward because of the confinement of the skull. Consequently, expansion within and compression of the hemispheres cause herniation of its contents (usually a portion of the temporal lobe known as the uncus) through the tentorial hiatus.

Uncal herniation is accompanied by compression of the lateral brain stem on the same side, which thus shuts off its blood supply and suppresses certain basic functions. The third cranial nerve (oculomotor) is in close proximity to the herniated uncus, and the pupil on the injured side becomes fixed and dilated. The reticular-activating system located in the brain stem that is responsible for waking and alertness becomes affected, and the patient rapidly becomes less and less responsive. Displacement of the midbrain causes compression of the pyramidal tract and results in contralateral hemiparesis or hemiplegia and plantar extensor responses (Babinski reflex). The respiratory center in the medulla may be affected, which results in changes in the respiratory pattern or cessation of respiration altogether.

In addition to these changes, the cerebellum itself may be so compressed that the cerebellar tonsil herniates inferiorly through the foramen magnum. This condition usually results in immediate death because the centers vital to life are compressed or sheared. The best treatment for supratentorial herniation is prevention through early detection and treatment of increased ICP and its causes. If efforts to minimize edema and increased ICP fail, surgical intervention, if possible, is necessary as a life-saving measure.

Types of Pathologic Conditions

Cerebral aneurysms are round dilations of the arterial wall that develop as a result of weakness of the wall from defects in the media layer of the artery. Most cerebral aneurysms occur at bifurcations close to the circle of Willis and usually involve the anterior portion. Common bifurcations include those with the internal carotid, the middle cerebral, and the basilar arteries and in relation to the anterior and posterior communicating arteries. The exact cause or precipitating factor is not well defined but may be related to congenital abnormality, arteriosclerosis, embolus, or trauma. Aneurysms are usually asymptomatic and present no clinical problem to the patient unless rupture occurs, which results in neurologic deficits. Ruptured cerebral aneurysm is the major cause of subarachnoid hemorrhage or hemorrhagic stroke. Depending on the severity of the cerebral bleed, the rupture of a cerebral aneurysm can often be fatal.[6] If treatable, surgical intervention usually involves clipping or coiling of the aneurysm after identification through angiography. Careful consideration is given to the complications that can occur after aneurismal rupture or bleeding, which are rebleeding, vasospasm, and hydrocephalus.[6]

An intracranial arteriovenous malformation (AVM) is a vascular network that appears as a tangled mass of dilated vessels that create an abnormal communication between the arterial and venous systems. The communication may be singular or multiple and resembles an arteriovenous fistula in that no connecting capillary system between the arteries and the veins exists. AVMs most commonly occur in the supratentorial structures and usually involve the vessels of the middle cerebral arteries. AVMs are usually present at birth as the result of congenital abnormalities, but may have a delayed age of onset. Patients may never experience symptoms until the AVM ruptures, causing an intracranial hemorrhage and increased ICP. If symptoms do occur, they most commonly appear between the ages of 10 and 20 years. These symptoms may include headache, seizures, and altered level of consciousness (LOC). The treatment of choice is complete surgical excision via dissection or obliteration with ligation of feeder vessels. Radiation is used to treat AVMs that are not surgically accessible. Although AVMs are rare, their impact can be enormous and cause serious neurologic problems or even death.

Intracranial tumors are space-occupying lesions. Through invasion, infiltration, and compression, they destroy brain tissue and nerve structures and produce an increased ICP.

Intracranial tumors can be primary or metastatic. Primary tumors are classified as primary intracerebral (intraaxial) tumors, which originate from glia cells, or primary extracerebral (extraaxial) tumors, which originate from supporting structures of the nervous system. Metastatic tumors most commonly arise from breast malignant disease in women and lung malignant disease in men. Clinical manifestations can be both localized and generalized in nature. Local pathophysiologic changes, such as focal neurologic deficits, seizures, visual disturbances, cranial nerve dysfunction, and hormonal changes, result from the tumor itself destroying tissue at a particular site in the brain. Generalized pathophysiologic changes result from the effects of increased ICP. The treatment for cerebral tumors is surgical excision or surgical decompression if total excision is not possible. Surgery is often performed before, during, or after radiation treatment and chemotherapy.

Hydrocephalus is not a disease entity, but is a clinical syndrome characterized by excess fluid within the cerebral ventricular system, the subarachnoid space, or both. Hydrocephalus occurs because of abnormalities in overproduction, circulation, or reabsorption of CSF. Hydrocephalus can be classified into two categories: noncommunicating (obstructive) or communicating (nonobstructive). Noncommunicating hydrocephalus is the result of an obstruction in the ventricular system or the subarachnoid space that prevents the flow of CSF to the location of the arachnoid villi, where reabsorption occurs. The obstruction can be caused by congenital abnormalities or space-occupying lesions. Communicating hydrocephalus occurs when the flow of CSF is normal, but absorption of the fluid at the arachnoid villi is impaired. Common causes of communicating hydrocephalus include inflammation of the meninges, subarachnoid hemorrhage, congenital malformation, and space-occupying lesions.

Intracranial Pressure Dynamics

ICP is pressure that is exerted against the skull by its contents: brain tissue, CSF, and blood. These contents are essentially not compressible, and a volume change in any compartment requires a reciprocal change to occur in one or both of the other compartments if the ICP is to remain constant (Monro-Kellie hypothesis). The contents of the skull allow for partial compensation when increased ICP occurs. These compensation capabilities are limited because of the small amount of CSF that the spinal subarachnoid space can hold, and total displacement of cerebral blood results in cerebral ischemia. Normal ICP is 0 to 15 mm Hg. Intracranial hypertension occurs when a sustained increased ICP at the level of the head occurs and exceeds 15 mm Hg.

Volume may be added to any of the cerebral compartments and results in increased ICP when the compensatory capacity is exceeded. Brain volume can be increased by a tumor, a hematoma, or edema. Blood volume can be increased through dilation of the vascular bed. CSF volume can be increased through obstruction in the ventricles, resistance to reabsorption, or, in rare instances, increased production of the CSF. Large brain tumors increase pressure by their mass, by blocking the rate of CSF reabsorption, or both. If the tumor is near the surface of the brain, it can cause inflamed meninges that may exude large quantities of fluid and protein into the CSF, thus increasing ICP. Hemorrhage or infection also causes increases in ICP. Large numbers of cells suddenly appear in the CSF and can almost totally block CSF absorption through the arachnoid villi. Regardless of the mechanism, when the volume added exceeds the volume that can be displaced, intracranial compliance is greatly reduced and ICP begins to increase.

Fig. 38-3 illustrates the relationship between intracranial volume and pressure. Phase I shows the success of compensatory mechanisms in maintenance of a constant ICP despite early increases in volume. In phase II, the limited capability of compensatory mechanisms has been exceeded and ICP begins to rise. In phase III, even a slight increase in volume causes a dramatic rise in ICP and thus results in complete decompensation and death. The shape of the curve may be altered by the rate at which the volume increases. Slowly developing increases in volume broaden the curve, whereas rapid increases narrow it.

Perianesthesia care for the patients with the potential for increased ICP requires an understanding of cerebral blood flow (CBF) and the factors that affect it; these factors become defective during increased ICP and are manipulated to reduce ICP. CBF is directly proportional to cerebral perfusion pressure (CPP) and inversely proportional to cerebrovascular resistance. CPP described as the pressure required to perfuse the brain.[7] CPP is typically expressed as the difference between the mean arterial pressure (MAP) and the ICP:

$$CPP = MAP - ICP$$

Consequently, any increase in ICP or reduction in MAP reduces CPP and resultant CBF. Average CBF is 50 mL per 100 g/min.[4] The CBF below which cerebral ischemia occurs has been termed the *critical CBF,* which is a flow rate of 16 or 17 mL per 100 g/min. Average CPP is 80 mm Hg.[4] CBF begins to fail at a CPP of 30 to 40 mm Hg.[6] Irreversible hypoxia occurs at a CPP less than 30 mm Hg. When ICP equals MAP, CPP equals zero and CBF ceases.

Factors that influence CBF regulation are partial pressure of oxygen in arterial blood (PaO_2) and partial pressure of carbon dioxide in arterial blood ($PaCO_2$; metabolic regulation), arterial blood pressure and autoregulation, and venous blood pressure. Metabolic regulation works in two ways. The first is regulation of blood flow based on the tissue needs for metabolic substrates: oxygen and glucose. As the activity of neuronal and glial cells in the brain increases, the demand for oxygen and glucose increases. The increased demand causes vasodilatation of arterioles, which increases CBF. Likewise, if the metabolic demand decreases, vasoconstriction occurs and CBF decreases.

The second, and most significant, way metabolic regulation affects CBF is the presence of metabolic byproducts, specifically carbon dioxide. Carbon dioxide is the most potent vasodilator of cerebral blood vessels. Normal cerebral vessels respond to changes in carbon dioxide by dilating when carbon dioxide increases and constricting when carbon dioxide decreases. The relationship between CBF and carbon dioxide is linear, and changes in CBF are in direct proportion to changes in carbon dioxide. A decrease of 1 mL per 100 g/min in CBF occurs for every 1 mm Hg decrease in carbon dioxide. In treatment of elevated ICP, carbon dioxide levels of 30 to 35 mm Hg are used to lower CBF.

Autoregulation is the ability of the cerebral vasculature in normal brain tissue to alter its resistance so that CBF remains relatively constant over a wide range of CPP. This mechanism causes vasoconstriction when perfusion pressure increases and vasodilation when perfusion pressure decreases. The limits of autoregulation are at a CPP of approximately 60 mm Hg at the lower end and 160 mm Hg at the upper end. Beyond the limits of autoregulation, CBF becomes passively dependent on CPP. When CPP increases to more than the upper limit of autoregulation, it exceeds the ability of the vasculature to constrict; CBF becomes directly related to and possibly dependent on CPP.

The lower limit of CBF autoregulation is the blood pressure below which vasodilatation becomes inadequate and CBF decreases. When CPP decreases to less than 60 mm Hg because of increases in ICP, autoregulation ceases to be beneficial or effective in regulation of CBF. Defective autoregulation aggravates pressure increases and creates critical or irreversible levels of ICP by increasing the blood volume within the cranium in an effort to maintain CBF. Defective autoregulation generally

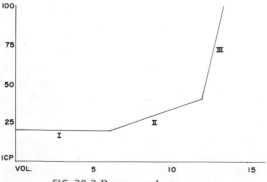

FIG. 38-3 Pressure-volume curve.

occurs when ICP exceeds 30 to 35 mm Hg. Eventually, autoregulation ceases altogether, and blood flow fluctuates passively with changes in arterial pressure, regardless of metabolic activity or regulation.

When ICP is increased, CPP and CBF are reduced, which renders the tissues ischemic. Ischemic cerebral tissue releases acid metabolites that cause a relatively fixed reduction in cerebrovascular tone. Autoregulation ceases and any increase in MAP causes further increase in cerebral blood volume and elicits further increase in ICP. CPP is reduced and thus causes ischemic areas to enlarge, such as those that surround an expanding intracranial mass. As can be seen in Fig. 38-4, a pathologic cycle ensues in which ICP and MAP eventually equilibrate, the CPP drops to zero, CBF stops, and death occurs.

Neurosurgical Procedures

With further developments in technology, neurosurgeons have more options in the treatment of patients. Surgical procedures that use instrumentation, lasers, and radiation therapy have increased the surgeon's ability to treat neurologic disorders.

Stereotaxis

Stereotaxis enables precise localization of a specified point. A stereotactic frame is applied to the patient's head, and the target tissue is located with the stereotactic frame's coordinates and CT scanning. Hemorrhage evacuation, catheter, shunt, or electrode placement and implantation of radioactive seeds are all procedures that may benefit from the use of stereotaxis. Additional uses include destruction of intracranial sensory pathways and the treatment of intractable chronic pain.[8]

Stereotactic Radiosurgery

The most common approaches to stereotactic radiosurgery (SR) are gamma knife and medical linear accelerator units. Stereotactic radiosurgery can destroy deep and surgically inaccessible areas. The goal of SR treatment is the delivery of high-dose radiation to a specific target area without delivery of the radiation to surrounding tissue. Regardless of the type of SR, a stereotactic frame is secured to the patient's head for accurate determination of target location. The placement of the stereotactic frame necessitates local anesthesia. Complications after SR may not appear for months to years later. Potential complications include permanent neurologic deficit, rebleeding, and worsening clinical symptoms.

Laser Surgery

The benefit of laser surgery is that it enables the neurosurgeon to access areas that were surgically inaccessible with conventional surgery. With laser surgery, the surgeon can dissect a structure without trauma to the surrounding tissue, shrink tumors, and coagulate blood vessels. See Chapter 47 for a complete discussion on laser surgery.

Anesthetic Agents and Intracranial Pressure

Although the brain represents only 2% of the body's total weight, it receives 12% to 15% of the total cardiac output because of the brain's high metabolic rate.[9] Anesthetic agents alter ICP by increasing or decreasing CBF and cerebral metabolic rate (CMR). In addition to the effects on ICP, some of these agents may also reduce systemic blood pressure and cause cerebral ischemia as a result of inadequate CPP.

Inhalation Anesthetics

The inhalation anesthetic agents generally decrease blood pressure and may increase ICP in the patient for cranial surgery. They produce a clinically significant degree of cerebrovascular vasodilation and metabolic depression and can modify autoregulation. In fact, high doses of volatile anesthetic agents can cause a total loss of autoregulation. The resulting increase in CBF ultimately leads to increased ICP. In patients with decreased intracranial compliance from neurologic disease, anesthetic agents that increase CBF may produce marked changes in ICP.

Isoflurane (Forane) at normocarbia has been shown to increase ICP. The initiation of hyperventilation simultaneously with the introduction of isoflurane prevents the increase in ICP that occurs at normocarbia. Isoflurane does not alter production of CSF and actually decreases resistance to absorption. It does not cause excitation of the central nervous system. Isoflurane produces

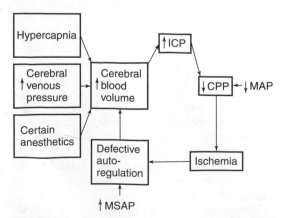

FIG. 38-4 Intracranial pressure dynamics with failed compensatory mechanisms.

NURSING CARE IN THE PACU

reductions in CMR, and autoregulation is not impaired to any degree. The greater decrease in CMR may explain why CBF increases are minimal at low concentrations.

Desflurane and sevoflurane have essentially the same characteristics as isoflurane. During normocarbia, desflurane and sevoflurane cause cerebral vasodilation with resultant increases in CBF and ICP. The cerebrovascular response to carbon dioxide is maintained; therefore the increase in CBF can be attenuated with hyperventilation. The CMR is reduced in a dose-dependent manner similar to that of isoflurane, and no neuronal excitation is seen. Both agents cause cardiovascular depression and can be used with caution for controlled hypotension to reduce CBF. Desflurane, unlike sevoflurane, can result in an increase in MAP and heart rate when used for induction or at initially high concentrations. This effect may be reduced with the use of opioids or beta blockers. Both desflurane and sevoflurane have relatively low blood–gas partition coefficients that allow for rapid elimination of the agent, which makes them desirable for use because of the more rapid recovery.

Nitrous oxide has become controversial for use during intracranial surgical procedures. When used alone, nitrous oxide can cause an increase in CBF, ICP, and CMR at normocarbia. These effects, however, are attenuated with the use of barbiturates, benzodiazepines, opioids, and hyperventilation. To a small extent, nitrous oxide is a cerebral vasodilator and does not interfere with autoregulation of the CBF. Nitrous oxide may be an acceptable choice when combined with other agents to benefit from its rapid onset and elimination for neurosurgical patients in whom increased ICP is not a problem; however, it should be used cautiously in patients with increased ICP.

Intravenous Anesthetics

A combination of inhalation and intravenous anesthetic agents are frequently used, but intravenous anesthetic agents (with the exception of ketamine) are usually the anesthetics of choice in cranial surgery.

Barbiturates, such as thiopental (Pentothal), are potent cerebral vasoconstrictors that can reduce CBF with subsequent reduction in elevated ICP. Cerebral vasoconstriction that is produced by barbiturates and the effect on CBF and ICP are dose related. The reduction in CBF produced by barbiturates is even greater if hypocarbia is also present and is maintained at a constant level. Deep thiopental anesthesia during normocarbia

results in an approximately 50% reduction in both CMR and CBF.

Benzodiazepines, such as diazepam (Valium) and midazolam (Versed), produce sedation and amnesia by stimulating specific receptors in the brain. The benzodiazepines produce dose-related reductions in CMR and CBF. When central benzodiazepine receptors are pharmacologically saturated, these drugs can decrease CMR by as much as 40%.

Opioids, such as fentanyl, morphine, and meperidine, are typically classified as cerebral vasoconstrictors, with resultant reductions in CBF. This effect is readily abolished by vasodilation that can accompany opioid-induced ventilatory depression and the resultant increase in $PaCO_2$. Inconsistencies do exist throughout the literature related to the actual effect CBF and CMR has on the unstimulated nervous system.[9] During normocarbia, the combination of nitrous oxide and morphine does not significantly alter CBF or autoregulation. Fentanyl causes a reduction in CBF and ICP in patients with normal CSF pathways. Alfentanil and sufentanil may in fact cause increased ICP in patients with compromised cerebral compliance.

Etomidate (Amidate) produces a maximum 45% decrease in cerebral metabolic rate and CBF; like the barbiturates, it can produce complete electroencephalographic suppression and appears to be comparable with lowering of ICP. Unlike the barbiturates, etomidate has less effect on MAP and offers greater stability in patients with hemodynamic compromise.

Propofol (Diprivan) reduces CMR, CBF, and ICP and increases cerebrovascular resistance in a dose-dependent manner. The use of propofol in patients with elevated ICP might not be appropriate because of the substantial decrease in MAP and resultant decrease in CPP. Although often used in rapid sequence intubation and continuous infusion during surgery, propofol has a short half-life and is therefore also used for sedation purposes in the neurosurgical patient; this facilitates the neurologic evaluation when needed.[10]

Dexmedetomidine (Precedex) is a sedative that allows for the patient to be easily aroused and often calm and cooperative while sedated; this enables the completion of the neurologic assessment. Although some precautions remain with this somewhat new drug, respiratory and hemodynamic stability are typically maintained with dexmedetomidine.[6,11]

Ketamine (Ketalar, Ketaject) can rapidly increase ICP and often reduce CPP, despite mild increases in blood pressure. Ketamine is

generally contraindicated for use in neurosurgical patients unless the fontanels are open, CSF aspiration is instituted, or ventilatory control is maintained.

The use of controlled ventilation to produce PCO_2 levels in the range of 30 to 38 mm Hg and administration of nitrous oxide and oxygen and possibly low concentrations of isoflurane, together with opioids and muscle relaxants, is a generally accepted anesthetic technique for the neurosurgical patient.[12]

Adjunctive Drugs and Interventions Used to Reduce Intracranial Pressure
Diuretics
Mannitol and furosemide (Lasix) are diuretics often used to control increased ICP. Mannitol, an osmotic diuretic, is the agent of choice for intracranial hypertension because it decreases intracellular edema.[6] Appropriate infusion of crystalloid and colloid solutions is often necessary to prevent adverse changes in plasma concentrations of electrolytes and intravascular fluid volume because of the rapidity of diuresis. Potential complications of the use of mannitol include hyperosmolarity, electrolyte loss, changes in blood viscosity and coagulation, transient intravascular hypervolemia, and rebound or secondary elevation of ICP.

Whereas mannitol reverses edema, furosemide is a loop diuretic and is more effective in decreasing circulating blood volume, thus reducing edema.[5] Furosemide is more effective than mannitol in reducing ICP and is the drug of choice in patients with congestive heart failure.

Furosemide, when combined with mannitol, has been shown to potentiate the ICP-reducing effects of mannitol at the cost of rapid loss of intravascular volume and electrolytes. The ICP effects of these drugs are lost after 1 or 2 hours.

Corticosteroids
The drugs most commonly used are dexamethasone and methylprednisolone. Steroids are effective in lowering increased ICP because of localized vasogenic cerebral edema associated with mass-type lesions, such as neoplasm, abscess, and intracerebral hematoma. Use is controversial with head trauma and cerebral infarctions with edema. The mechanism for the beneficial effect of corticosteroids is not known but may involve stabilization of capillary membranes, reduction in CSF production, blood-brain barrier repair, prevention of lysosomal activity, enhanced cerebral electrolyte transport, improved brain metabolism, and promotion of water and electrolyte excretion.

Evidence-Based Practice

A literature search by the Brain Trauma Foundation produced a Level I recommendation for the use of steroids. This was the only Level 1 recommendation contained in the Guidelines for the Management of Severe Traumatic Brain Injury. "Level I recommendations are based on the strongest evidence for effectiveness, and represent principles of patient management that reflect a high degree of clinical certainty." Guideline XV, *Steroids* states, "The use of steroids is not recommended for improving outcome or reducing intracranial pressure (ICP). In patients with moderate or severe traumatic brain injury (TBI), high-dose methylprednisolone is associated with increased mortality and is contraindicated." There are numerous patient trials related to this, mostly prospective and double-blind, as noted in the guideline. "The majority of available evidence indicates that steroids do not improve outcome or lower ICP in severe TBI. There is strong evidence that steroids are deleterious; thus their use is not recommended for TBI."

IMPLICATIONS FOR PRACTICE
Knowledge of perianesthesia nurses related to appropriate treatment options in traumatic brain injury is beneficial to the patient. Awareness of the difference between steroid use in patients with localized vasogenic cerebral edema and traumatic brain injury patients is imperative.

Source: Brain Trauma Foundation, et al: *Guidelines for the management of severe traumatic brain injury*, ed 3, New York, 2007, Brain Trauma Foundation.

Barbiturate Therapy
Initiation of barbiturate therapy is the last medication adjunct used in treatment of intracranial hypertension. The patient must have an intracranial pressure–monitoring device, usually started when ICP is more than 30 mm Hg for 30 minutes and CPP is less than 70 mm Hg. The most common barbiturate is pentobarbital, which lowers the ICP by inhibiting free radical–mediated lipid peroxidation, altering vascular tone, suppressing metabolism, and hopefully maintaining an ICP of 15 to 20 mm Hg.[5]

Temperature Management
Hyperthermia is a common crisis in neurocritical care, occurring in an estimated 70% of head-injured patients.[4,13] As the patient's temperature increases, so does CBF and CMR, which could therefore also increase ICP.[6] Temperature should be monitored closely, and the patient's body temperature should be

maintained at normothermia or even permissive hypothermia, which is becoming the current trend.[12] Other advanced cooling methods include cool saline intravenous infusion and surface-cooling pads or wraps.[4] Cooling measures such as antipyretics, hypothermia blankets, and other traditional cooling methods are used as needed.[4,5] Methods such as intravascular temperature management may be effective as well.[13]

Positioning

Body positioning, among many other factors described previously is yet another aspect in proper care of the neurology patient. Positioning can affect ICP, CPP, and MAP.[14] Although elevating the head of the bed to 30 degrees is preferred by most physicians, this is a topic of recent discussion.[6]

Intracranial Pressure Monitoring

The most precise indicator of the pressure state within the cranium is the CSF pressure, which is obtained through an ICP monitoring device. Trends in ICP, CPP measurement, and intracranial compliance are all functions of ICP monitoring.[8] Monitoring of ICP is the standard of care for patients at risk for intracranial hypertension.

A measurement of this pressure can be obtained from the lateral ventricles, subarachnoid space, epidural or subdural spaces, or the intraparenchymal. Values from these areas are meaningful indicators of ICP only if pressure is freely transmitted between these compartments. Because injury and disease of the brain often create obstruction in CSF flow, the most accurate values are those obtained from the ventricle.

Lumbar puncture values reflect only a relative index of the actual ICP. These values depend on the state of the spinal canal and all the factors that affect it. However, measuring the ventricular fluid pressure gives a direct and absolute value of the ICP, regardless of the influence or condition of the spinal canal. Lumbar puncture has other limitations; its use is limited to patients without suspected intracranial mass or to those whose ICP is not elevated or is elevated only slightly. In patients with these conditions, herniation of the brain tissue with the removal of CSF is a risk. ICP monitoring does not present this risk and can be used in a variety of conditions.

The ICP monitoring devices are categorized into two primary categories. The first category includes devices that use fluid or hydrostatic coupling to transmit to an external transducer. Ventricular catheters, subarachnoid bolts or screws, and subdural catheters fall into this group. The second group uses a transducer to directly monitor

ICP. These intracranial devices use fiberoptics to transmit ICP pressures and can be placed in the intraventricular, subarachnoid, intraparenchymal, epidural, or subdural spaces (Fig. 38-5).[6]

The subarachnoid bolt or screw was developed in 1973 and requires only a twist-drill hole in the skull and a nick in the dura for insertion. As the name implies, the sensor lies in the subarachnoid space. The advantages of this type of monitoring device are less risk of infection and use in patients with small ventricles. However, in the presence of moderately severe cerebral edema, a small piece of brain tissue may be driven into and occlude the proximal end of the screw, thus rendering it useless.

The intraventricular catheter (IVC) is the most common and least expensive ICP monitoring device, and it allows for drainage of CSF.[6] The tip is introduced into a CSF-containing ventricle via a twist-drill burr hole and is connected to an external transducer that converts the hydrostatic pressure force into a graph and numeric readout. The advantages of the IVC are that it provides a direct ICP reading and is easily kept patent. Another advantage is that CSF can be drained through the catheter for treatment of ICP elevations. In this way, the IVC may serve as a temporary artificial extension of the CSF-shunting compensatory mechanism. Intracranial compliance can also be tested with injecting fluid into the cranium and reading the responding pressure. If an abrupt and steep rise in ICP occurs, one can assume that compliance no longer exists and that the volume-pressure curve is a steep one. When the patient's arterial pressure is monitored simultaneously, exact CPP can be calculated at any time. The ventricular catheter also has the advantage of allowing instillation of contrast media or air for study of the size and patency of the ventricle. The principal disadvantage of the IVC is the risk of infection and hemorrhage.

The fiberoptic catheter uses the fiberoptic transducer-tipped probe and can be placed in the ventricles and in subarachnoid, subdural, and intraparenchymal sites. The advantages are its easy placement and lack of relation to ventricular size. The major disadvantages are its expense, its inability to allow for CSF sampling or drainage, its possible need for probe replacement, and the fragility of the fiberoptic cable, which breaks easily.

Intracranial pressure monitoring is a valuable tool in assessing the efficacy of nursing interventions that are intended to decrease ICP. Continuous monitoring of the pressure state within the cranium accelerates the treatment of elevations in ICP before the patient's condition deteriorates.

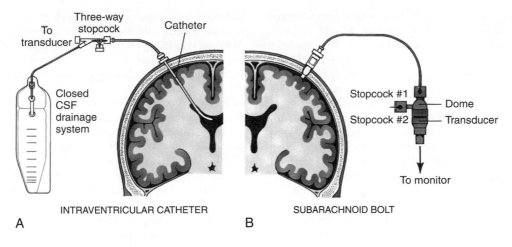

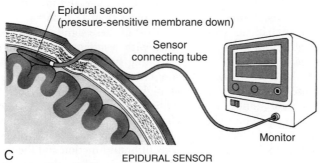

FIG. 38-5 Intracranial pressure monitoring devices. **A,** Intraventricular catheter monitoring system with a closed cerebrospinal fluid (CSF) drainage system. **B,** Subarachnoid bolt monitoring system. **C,** Epidural monitoring system. (From Barker E: *Neuroscience nursing,* ed 3, St. Louis, 2008, Mosby.)

Pressure Waves in Increased Intracranial Pressure

Pressures waves are discussed in two separate categories: the ICP waveform and the ICP waveform trends (Fig. 38-6).

The ICP waveform is valuable at the bedside as a means for the nurse to determine the adaptability of the patient.[5] The waves correlate with the patient's heart rate. Ideally there are three or more peaks in the wave, with the P1 (percussion) wave as the first and most prominent. P1 is thought to

be arterial in origin and consistent in its amplitude. P2, the tidal wave, is also arterial in origin and is related to the state of compliance. The last wave is the dicrotic wave or dicrotic notch and is venous in origin.[3-5] Decreased intracranial adaptive capability and impaired autoregulation are thought to be associated with an elevation in the P2 wave.[4]

Three patterns have been identified with the ICP waveform trends. The first and most significant type is the A wave, which is more commonly

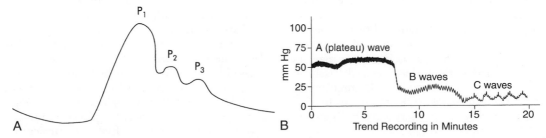

FIG. 38-6 **A,** ICP waveform. **B,** ICP waveform trends (From Barker E: *Neuroscience nursing,* ed 3, St. Louis, 2008, Mosby.)

called a *plateau wave*. These waves are associated with increases in ICP between 50 and 100 mm Hg that last for 5 to 20 minutes. They are seen only in advanced stages of increased ICP (the last phase of the volume-pressure curve) and superimpose themselves when the baseline ICP is elevated and exceeds 20 mm Hg. Early increases in mean systolic arterial pressure do not accompany plateau waves, and autoregulation is impaired. Thus, plateau waves signal hypoxia of brain cells and a decrease in CPP. They may cause both transient and irreversible damage to the brain and may be premonitory signs of acute incidents.

The second type of pressure wave pattern is called the *B wave*. These waves are sharp rhythmic oscillations with a sawtooth pattern that occurs every 30 seconds to 2 minutes. These waves can indicate increases in ICP as much as 50 mm Hg and are more commonly seen in patients with unstable increases in ICP usually from accelerations producing apneic episodes.[5]

The third type of pattern is the C wave. These waves are smaller rhythmic oscillations in ICP that occur 4 to 8 times per minute[4,6] and indicate increases in ICP by as much as 20 mm Hg. These waves are associated with respiratory influence on blood pressure, but their significance is questionable.

Intracranial Pressure Assessment

With the availability of high-resolution noninvasive imaging techniques such as CT scanning and MRI, these studies themselves may be the chief determining factor in the decision to initiate ICP monitoring. Some of the indications for ICP monitoring are expanding intracranial tumors, hydrocephalus, benign intracranial hypertension, trauma, vascular anomalies, certain cases of metabolic coma with cerebral edema, certain cases of viral hepatitis or fulminant hepatic encephalopathy, and patients in a controlled barbiturate coma for status epilepticus.

Continuous ICP monitoring is the only accurate method of assessing ICP at any given time. This method has two advantages: (1) it provides an ongoing record of the ICP and (2) it provides a means of assessment of intracranial dynamics. These advantages allow guided therapy and management of ICP through CSF drainage. The clinical signs of increased ICP are numerous. The early signs are often vague and overlooked, and research has shown the unreliability of these signs in determination or recognition of increased ICP. Regardless, frequent clinical assessment is necessary and often is the first sign of deterioration.

Early signs of increased ICP are change in LOC (restlessness, confusion, agitation, irritability,

lethargy), abnormal pupillary function, deterioration of motor function, and severe headache.[4,8] Nausea, vomiting, paralysis, visual field deficits, conjugate deviation of the eyes, sensory loss, and nuchal rigidity are also early signs. The presence of these signs may or may not confirm a diagnosis of increased ICP, but they can still inform treatment while treatment is effective.

The late signs of increased ICP are decreasing responsiveness and LOC; additional pupillary changes; increased systolic blood pressure; bradycardia; widening pulse pressure; alteration in respiratory pattern; decorticate or decerebrate posturing; and absence of or decrease in cough, gag, corneal, and deep tendon reflexes. A positive Babinski reflex is normal in infants younger than 18 months of age, but indicates increased ICP in those older than 18 months.

Most of these signs are manifestations of brain shift, with resultant dysfunction of the reticular-activating system, brain stem, and medulla. Pressure either has to elevate rapidly or be sustained at high levels to affect these structures so dramatically. Primary injury to these structures may elicit the same signs without appreciable increases in ICP. In this situation, they could indicate the level of brain function and the gravity of the situation, but not reflect the pressure dynamics that exist at that moment.

Just as these signs may be present without increase in ICP, ICP may be dangerously high with few signs, if any. Classic brainstem signs (reflecting changes in cardiac, respiratory, or vasomotor function) usually occur late, after the onset of intracranial hypertension, if at all. The most important factor in determining the degree of secondary brain damage incurred by elevated ICP is the effect of altered CPP on the brain. Clinical research has shown that the level of CPP is the best indicator of outcome from severe head injuries. CPP less than 40 mm Hg has been associated with poor outcomes. CPP needs to be maintained at no less than 50 to 60 mm Hg to provide a minimally adequate blood supply to the brain.

Most hospitals with the capacity for cranial surgery also have the capacity for continuous ICP monitoring. It is still important to be able to recognize signs and symptoms of intracranial hypertension without the assistance of an ICP monitor. Thus, the traditional signs and symptoms of increased ICP are discussed here, although they are not precise or infallible as indicators of increased ICP. At the least, they indicate that "something is not right" and that constant vigilance and further investigation are necessary. Even the transient appearances of these pressure signs are important; they indicate the development of a highly delicate and unstable intracranial situation, a sign that the patient may be having plateau waves.

Perianesthesia Nursing Management

The following four major areas of assessment are necessary in PACU care of the cranial surgical patient: (1) vital signs, (2) LOC, (3) motor and sensory functioning, and (4) pupillary signs. These areas should be assessed routinely at least every 15 minutes for the first 2 hours after surgery. Then, if results are within normal limits or unchanged since surgery, the areas should be assessed every 30 minutes. If the patient's condition is unstable or deteriorating or if the surgeon specifies, assessments should be made more frequently. If the patient's ICP is monitored, correct calibration of the monitor must be ensured, ICP value recorded, and waveform described. The same approach is used for arterial pressure recording.

Reports should be taken from both the anesthesia provider and the surgeon. Of particular importance are surgical procedure, pathologic findings, bone flap presence, allergies, preexisting medical problems, anesthetics, and any problems that occurred during surgery. Special positioning orders or restrictions, the presence of drains, and known CSF leaks must be noted. The Glasgow Coma Scale (GCS; Table 38-1) is a widely used neurologic assessment tool because of its simplicity, consistency, and reliability between raters who use it. However, the GCS cannot be used to assess subtle changes in the patient's neurologic status. When the GCS is used, the patient's responses are scored on a scale of 3 to 15. A score of 3 indicates coma, and a score of 15 indicates a fully alert oriented person with all neurologic functions intact.

Vital Signs

Assessment of vital signs includes blood pressure, pulse, respirations, and ICP (if monitored). Changes in vital signs may indicate increasing ICP, shock, hemorrhage, electrolyte imbalance, or other disturbances. The perianesthesia nurse should keep in mind that the injured patient may have other pathophysiologic processes unrelated to the head injury. Temperature is always monitored, and an elevation usually represents an infectious process, most often in the respiratory or urinary tract. Infrequently, elevations are attributable to direct damage to the temperature-regulating center in the hypothalamus. Temperature elevation also increases the metabolic rate of the brain, which may further increase ICP.

Airway patency is ensured, and the rate, depth, and rhythm are noted. If the rhythm is irregular, its pattern should be determined. Changes in the respiratory pattern may indicate injury to the respiratory center of the brain and the severity of the neurologic injury (Fig. 38-7). If the patient requires a ventilator, the machine should be checked for proper functioning and settings; however, mechanical ventilation can mask changes in the respiratory pattern.

For many years, the nursing literature has documented a relation between changes in blood pressure and pulse and increases in ICP. These changes are often referred to as *Cushing reflex, Cushing triad,* or *Cushing response.* Cushing reflex is described as elevated systolic blood pressure, bradycardia, and widening pulse pressure. Additional increases in ICP can lead to Cushing triad, which is described as bradycardia, hypertension,

Table 38-1	Glasgow Coma Scale	
CATEGORY	RESPONSE	SCORE
Eye opening	Spontaneous	4
	To speech	3
	To pain	2
	None	1
Best verbal response	Oriented to person, place, and time	5
	Confused	4
	Inappropriate words	3
	Incomprehensible sounds	2
	No response	1
Best motor response	Obeys commands	6
	Localizes to pain	5
	Withdrawal from pain	4
	Abnormal flexion	3
	Abnormal extension	2
	Flaccid	1

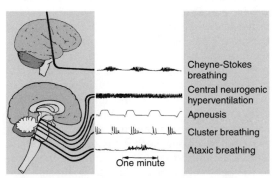

FIG. 38-7 Abnormal respiratory patterns with corresponding levels of central nervous system activity. (From Urden LD et al: *Critical care nursing,* ed 6, St. Louis, 2010, Mosby.)

and bradypnea. Cushing reflex and triad are late clinical signs of increased ICP and may indicate brain stem herniation. Patients with head injury often have a higher than normal blood pressure and heart rate that may be the result of pain, hypoxia, and agitation or the release of endogenous catecholamines.

Level of Consciousness

The most important indicator of brain function is the LOC, but it is not necessarily indicative of altered ICP. A decreased LOC in the PACU can be caused by the lingering effects of the anesthesia or by neuromuscular-blocking agents sometimes used with patients on positive-pressure ventilation. A change in LOC may also be the result of hypoxia, hypoglycemia, vitamin deficiency, or fluid and electrolyte imbalances. Other underlying pathologic changes can cause alterations in LOC. For assessment of LOC, a description of the patient's response is best instead of vague terms such as *stuporous, semiconscious,* or *unconscious.* A standard assessment form such as the GCS (see Table 38-1) should be available for assessment of the LOC. A change in LOC may also be indicative of deterioration or improvement in the patient's condition.

Motor and Sensory Functioning

Assessment of motor and sensory function is part of an ongoing neurologic assessment and is performed to note changes from the baseline assessment. It can also provide clues to extending hemorrhage or expanding edema. Focal changes, such as decreased hand strength unilaterally or an inability to move one side of the body, often accompany these events. Sensations may be decreased because of brain involvement, not just spinal cord injury (SCI). Observe whether the patient can move all four extremities. Check both hand grasps simultaneously. Are they weak or strong; equal or unequal? Foot strength can be tested by having the patient push or pull against the nurse's hands. (Be sure the patient uses only the foot and ankle, not the entire leg.) If the patient does not respond to simple commands, test to see whether a painful stimulus such as a pin prick or pinch induces movement. (Test both sides to determine sensory impairment.) If the patient does not respond to pain, test for motor function by raising both arms or both legs and letting them fall together. A paralyzed limb falls to the bed more quickly than an unaffected one. To further check leg motor ability, flex both of the patient's knees with the feet flat on the bed; release them at the same time. The healthy leg maintains its position momentarily and then resumes the original position. The affected limb abducts while falling and maintains knee flexion.

Facial muscle movement should also be tested. If possible, ask patients to wrinkle the forehead, shut the eyes tightly, smile, and show the teeth. Any asymmetry should be noted. If the patient is not responsive to verbal commands, noxious stimulation may elicit a grimace or other facial movement. The presence of a Babinski reflex is pathologic and indicates pyramidal tract dysfunction in any person older than 18 months. Starting at the heel and using a moderately sharp object, such as the rounded tip of a bandage scissors or the tip of a retracted pen, stroke the lateral sole and proceed to the ball of the foot. Firm pressure is necessary to elicit an accurate response. The Babinski reflex is present when the great toe dorsiflexes (bends toward the head) and the remaining toes "fan out." The Babinski reflex is not present when the stimulus elicits a plantar or downward flexion of the great toe.

Motor response to a painful stimulus may be one of decerebrate or decorticate rigidity, or these postures may exist in the absence of any stimulation. Decerebrate posturing is characterized by rigidity and contraction of all the extensor muscles. The legs are stiffly extended with the feet plantar flexed. The arms are extended and hyperpronated. Decerebrate rigidity is usually the result of upper brain stem damage, which means that the cerebral hemispheres are functionally cut off. Decorticate posturing indicates that function has been cut off at a lower level and that the entire cortex is physiologically cut off. In this instance, the legs are extended and internally rotated, and the feet are plantar flexed. The arms are flexed at all joints, and the hands are often held beneath the chin.

Pupillary Activity

Pupillary reactions are controlled by the third cranial nerve. In assessment of the pupils, the perianesthesia nurse should examine both simultaneously for shape, size, and equality. Normal pupils are round and, at a midpoint diameter, within the range of 1 to 9 mm. Instead of using terms such as *constricted* or *dilated,* measurement of the diameter directly with a pocket millimeter ruler is more precise. Test the direct light reflex of each pupil with a small bright flashlight. Normally the pupil constricts briskly. If it reacts sluggishly or not at all, the reaction is abnormal. To test the consensual light reflex, hold both eyelids open, shine the light in one eye, and observe the other pupil. The opposite pupil should constrict simultaneously with the lighted one, although perhaps not to the same degree.

Normal pupillary size and reactivity can be altered by some medical situations and by certain drugs. Previous surgery or direct injury to the eye may alter or abolish reactivity. Blindness abolishes reactivity to light because the sensory part of the reflex pathway is absent.

Unusual eye movements should be noted. Normal gaze in a person who is awake and alert is straight ahead, with no involuntary movements. This condition is generally true of unresponsive patients, although the eyes may rove slowly and in random fashion. (In detection of this movement, do not be misled into thinking that the patient is actually following you or your movements.) The eyes should move together in the same direction (conjugate gaze). If the eyes are disconjugate, they move in a jerky oscillatory fashion (nystagmus) or the gaze deviates from the midline. These ocular movements are abnormal and should be detailed in the nursing notes.

Nursing Care in the Postanesthesia Care Unit

The PACU nurse has three primary responsibilities in the care of the neurosurgical patient: (1) to institute measures of care to sustain optimal physiologic function in the perianesthesia patient, (2) to recognize and prevent conditions that increase ICP beyond normal limits, and (3) to detect and communicate signs and symptoms of the patient's condition to the physician (Box 38-1).

SPINAL SURGERY

In the United States there are approximately 200,000 people living with SCI, and 12,000-20,000 new cases are estimated to occur annually.[15] The goal of surgical intervention is minimization of complications related to SCIs, spinal cord tumors, or developmental abnormalities. Complete or incomplete SCI, bony fragments in the canal, unstable dislocation, and evidence of cord compression are some indications for immediate surgical intervention.

Diagnostic Tools

Several methods are used in the diagnosis of injury or disease involving the spine or spinal canal.

Conventional radiography and fluoroscopy are used to identify fractures and fracture-dislocations.

BOX 38-1   General Postoperative Considerations

AIRWAY, OXYGENATION STATUS
- Determine length of time to remain intubated, if applicable.
- Obtain respiratory vitals and arterial blood gases as needed before extubation.
  - Ensure that the patient is able to ventilate to maintain a $PaCO_2$ of 35 to 45 mm Hg.
- Before extubation, assess difficulty of maintaining airway and reintubation.

CARDIOVASCULAR AND HEMODYNAMIC STATUS
- Cardiac rhythm
- Fluid loss, replacement
- Electrolyte values
- Monitoring lines

NEUROLOGIC ASSESSMENT
- General considerations
  - The patient should be the same or better than during preoperative assessment.
  - Anesthetic agents may be reversed for more accurate assessment.
- Differential diagnosis for decreased level of consciousness
  - Anesthesia not fully reversed
  - Elevated ICP, decreased CPP

- Hypoxia
- Complications from surgery
  - Cerebral edema
  - Intracranial hematoma
- Differential diagnosis for respiratory depression
  - Anesthesia not reversed
  - Bronchospasm
  - Pneumothorax from central line placement, thoracic spine surgery
- ICP, CPP, and acceptable hemodynamic parameters
- Appropriate patient positioning
- Assess dressing and other sites of intervention (e.g., pin sites if the patient was placed in rigid skull fixation for posterior cervical spine surgery)

PAIN ASSESSMENT AND TREATMENT
- Measure intake and output
  - By shift and cumulative from first encounter
  - Drains, drainage

DOCUMENTATION
- Document critical information and the manufacturer lot number of any implantable device placed in the patient during surgery.

Adapted from Bitters L: Perioperative surgical considerations. In Bader MK, Littlejohns LR, editors: *AANN core curriculum for neuroscience nursing*, Glenview, Ill, 2010, American Association of Neuroscience Nursing.
PaCO₂, Partial pressure of carbon dioxide in arterial blood; *ICP*, intracranial pressure; *CPP*, cerebral perfusion pressure.

NURSING CARE IN THE PACU

Narrowing of an intervertebral space is sometimes evident as a result of a herniated nucleus pulposus (slipped disk). Fluoroscopy is used to show instability of the injured part on manipulation. Splintered or displaced bone fragments and radiopaque foreign bodies, such as bullets or other metal fragments, are also seen on radiographs. Radiographs also show abnormalities such as scoliosis and osteoporotic and arthritic changes. Tumors may be evidenced by erosion, calcium deposits within the mass, increased interpediculate distance, enlargement of an intervertebral foramen, or collapse of a vertebra.

CT scanning is used to delineate mass lesions that exist in the same plane as the spine and spinal cord and when conventional radiography is not adequate. Large blood clots may also be localized with this method.

MRI is being used increasingly for accurate detection and assessment of space-occupying lesions of the spine, such as herniated nucleus pulposus and tumors. In addition, MRI is appropriate to detect the degree of an SCI.

Myelography is one of the most valuable tools available in the diagnosis of compression of the spinal cord caused by tumor, fracture-dislocation, or herniated nucleus pulposus. A lumbar puncture is performed, at which time a Queckenstedt test may also be done. The myelogram consists of the injection of a radiopaque dye into the CSF canal and the fluoroscopic observation of its flow in the suspected area. Cord compression is evidenced by an interruption in the contour of the spinal cord. Disruption of the contours of the spinal nerve roots may also be found.

Injuries of the Spine

The spine protects the spinal cord and the terminal nerve roots. Injuries to the spine and spinal cord occur as a result of flexion, hyperextension, rotation with both flexion and extension, compression, and penetrating wounds (Fig. 38-8). Head injuries often accompany injuries to the spine and vice versa. The cervical spine is extremely mobile and therefore particularly susceptible to injuries that hyperflex or hyperextend the neck. Propulsion can occur anteroposteriorly or laterally. The spinal cord is relatively large in the cervical area and sustains damage fairly easily after injury. This area is unique in that the superior portion of C2 lacks a vertebral body. Instead, the neck has a dens, or projection, called the *odontoid*. Many injuries to the odontoid extend into C1, or atlas, which has no vertebral body at all.

The thoracic spine is fixed by the ribs, but the lumbar spine is not; therefore an increased incidence rate is seen of injury to the thoracic, lumbar, or sacral regions of the spine. Motor vehicle crashes are the leading cause of spinal cord injuries.[15]

Consequences of injury to the spine are the result of the mechanical insult or biochemical and hemodynamic changes. Mechanical insult includes the direct injury and changes to the cord structure, motion stress on the cord, and continuous compression to the cord. This physical injury to the cord results in the primary or initial spinal cord dysfunction. Edema of the cord, which causes cellular changes and ischemia, may occur in the hours after the initial injury. This process is called *secondary injury* and can last up to 5 days.

The primary goal in the early treatment of spinal cord injuries is prevention of further compromise of spinal cord tissue from secondary injury. If the damage to tissue as the result of the direct injury cannot be altered, an attempt is made to protect the remaining tissue by alleviating compression and movement of the spinal cord. Spinal cord immobilization, surgical intervention to alleviate cord compression, and pharmacologic therapies to reduce edema are used as immediate therapies.

Complete Spinal Cord Lesion

The extent of injury to the spinal cord is described as a *complete* or *incomplete lesion*. In a complete SCI, no motor or sensory function is seen more than three levels below the level of injury. When this type of injury lasts more than 24 hours, no recovery of distal function is indicated. Clinical findings during the acute phase after total cord transection include the following:

1. There is immediate loss of all sensory, motor, autonomic, and reflex functions below the level of the injury from spinal shock. Spinal shock can persist for days or weeks, depending on the injury and the patient's general state of health. It usually lasts 4 to 8 weeks.
2. Urinary retention as a result of bladder sphincter paralysis is present.
3. Paralytic ileus with progressive abdominal distention is present.
4. There is respiratory insult or cessation. Injury to the lower cervical or upper thoracic spine results in cessation of intercostal function. In this event, respiration is under the sole stimulus of the phrenic nerve, and breathing is diaphragmatic. Injury to the cord at the levels of C3 to C5 affects the phrenic nucleus and thus paralyzes the diaphragm and causes respiratory failure.

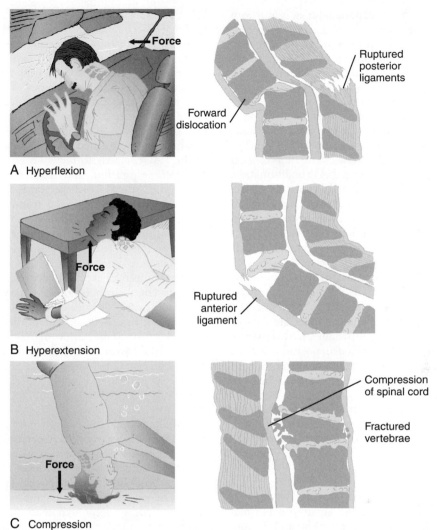

FIG. 38-8 Patterns of cervical spine injury. **A,** Hyperflexion injury of the cervical spine ruptures the posterior ligaments. **B,** Hyperextension injury of the cervical spine ruptures the anterior ligaments. **C,** Compression fractures crush the vertebrae and force bony fragments into the spinal canal. (From Black JM, Hokanson Hawks JH: *Medical-surgical nursing: clinical management for positive outcomes,* ed 8, St. Louis, 2009, Saunders.)

5. There is a loss of sweating below the level of the lesion.
6. Point tenderness over the injured part is present. Crepitus may or may not be present.

Initial therapeutic efforts are directed at the preservation of life. Mechanical stability, protection of nervous tissue, and freedom from pain are long-term therapeutic goals.

Incomplete Spinal Cord Lesion

Incomplete spinal cord lesion indicates residual motor or sensory function more than three segments below the level of injury. Indications of incomplete lesion are sensation, sense of position, or voluntary movement of the legs; sensation around the anus; voluntary rectal sphincter contraction; and voluntary toe flexion.

Various syndromes or types of incomplete lesions may result from the injury. Incomplete lesions include central cord syndrome, Brown-Séquard syndrome, anterior cord syndrome, and posterior cord syndrome.

Central cord syndrome (CCS) is the most common type of incomplete lesion. CCS occurs more commonly in older adults as a result of a hyperextension injury, such as a blow to the face or forehead. CCS from sports injuries is also seen in younger patients.

The center of the cord is contused and may hemorrhage, thus resulting in bilateral upper extremity weakness and a burning sensation. If CCS is caused by a contusion, lower extremity function usually returns first, then bladder function, upper extremities, and lastly finger movement.

Brown-Séquard syndrome may occur after injuries that transect the cord, such as knife or gunshot wounds, epidural hematoma, herniated cervical disc, spinal cord tumor, spinal AV malformation, and cervical spondylosis. Clinical signs are ipsilateral loss of motor, touch, pressure, and vibration below the lesion and contralateral loss of pain and temperature below the lesion. This type of lesion has the best functional recovery rate; many patients regain independent ambulation.

Anterior cord syndrome usually occurs as the result of compression of the anterior portion of the cord and loss of blood supply from the anterior spinal artery. Clinical signs are loss of motor function, pain, temperature, and sensation below the level of injury. Touch, position, and vibration sensation are still intact. Anterior cord syndrome is usually caused by flexion injuries in the cervical area.

Posterior cord syndrome is a rare disorder. Clinical signs are pain and paresthesias in the neck, upper arms, and torso. Mild paresis of the upper arms may occur.

Surgical Intervention for Spinal Cord Injuries

Surgeons differ in opinions about the optimal timing for surgical decompression and fusion. Early surgical intervention is indicated to decompress the spinal canal from bone or disk fragments, provide stabilization, and repair damage caused by penetrating objects.

Patients who need surgery may have exploration, insertion of Harrington rods or stabilization instruments, or decompression laminectomy procedures. Procedures can be performed through an anterior or posterior approach, depending on the cord lesion. Fusion is accomplished with the placement of a bone graft taken from tibial or iliac bone into the involved interspace or of a fixation device. External immobilization is often used after surgery until osseous union is complete.

General contraindications to surgery are the existence of associated life-threatening injuries, depressed respiratory function caused by high cervical injuries, lack of skilled personnel and necessary equipment, improved neurologic status, and need for stabilization.[6]

Perianesthesia Nursing Care for the Patient with Spinal Cord Injury

Permanent injuries of this nature are devastating to the patient and the patient's family. The nursing responsibilities are great during the acute, rehabilitative, and chronic phases. Patients with SCI may be sent to the PACU in any of these phases, and care requires special consideration and knowledge of SCI pathophysiology.

The initial assessment of the patient with SCI in the PACU needs to focus on airway patency, adequate respiration, and maintenance of systemic and spinal cord perfusion. Vital signs should be assessed every 15 minutes until the condition is stable. Baseline neurologic assessment including motor and sensory evaluation should be completed with the initial and ongoing assessments.

Immobilization is a primary intervention to help prevent the process of secondary injury. The standard of care for immobilization is placement of the neck in a neutral position and in a rigid cervical collar. Stabilization of fractures may be accomplished with several devices that promote alignment.

Complications Associated with Spinal Cord Injury
Spinal Shock
Spinal shock is a form of neurogenic shock characterized by a loss of motor, sensory, autonomic, and reflex activity below the level of the lesion and resulting in flaccid paralysis and paralytic ileus. The classic signs and symptoms of spinal shock include systemic hypotension, bradycardia, and hypothermia. Spinal shock is a condition that occurs immediately after injury or up to hours after an SCI that progressively worsens and may last hours to months, depending on severity of the injury.[6]

Hypotension
Hypotension is not uncommon because of vasodilation of the vessels below the level of the injury. The goal of treatment is maintenance of systemic and renal perfusion. Bradycardia may accompany the hypotension. Dopamine is indicated for the treatment of hypotension and bradycardia. Other causes of hypotension, such as a gastrointestinal hemorrhage, must be considered and ruled out. Hypotension is usually not caused by hemorrhagic shock; therefore the patient volume status should be monitored closely and not overloaded with intravenous fluids.

Bradycardia
Bradycardia is associated with spinal shock and nursing interventions such as manipulation of an endotracheal tube, suctioning, turning, and

insertion of a nasogastric tube, which may elicit a vasovagal response that leads to bradycardia. Nursing interventions should closely monitor for and provide prevention from a vasovagal response.

Thrombosis

Conditions are optimal for the development of deep vein thrombosis and pulmonary embolus because of venous pooling and loss of movement below the level of injury. Calf measurements, antiembolism stockings, compression devices, low-dose heparin, and low-molecular weight heparin are used to prevent these complications.

Autonomic Dysreflexia

Autonomic dysreflexia is a syndrome of massive imbalanced reflex sympathetic discharge.[16] It occurs in patients with SCI greater than the splanchnic sympathetic outflow (T5-T6)[16] and after the resolution of spinal shock and the return of reflex activity. Autonomic dysreflexia results from excessive reflex stimulation of the sympathetic nerves below the level of injury. Causes of the reflex stimulation include bladder distension, fecal impaction, and noxious stimuli. Symptoms of autonomic dysreflexia are pounding headache, excessively high hypertension, decreased heart rate, profuse sweating, and flushed skin above the level of injury, pallor and goose bumps below the level of the injury, anxiety, and visual disturbances. Treatment is aimed at removing the noxious stimulus and preventing complications from hypertension.

The PACU nursing care focuses on the routine prevention of known precipitants of autonomic dysreflexia. For example, the bladder must not become distended, and skin breakdown must be prevented. If signs and symptoms appear, the stimulus must be sought and removed as rapidly as possible. If the symptoms cannot be alleviated, the nurse should notify the physician, elevate the head of the bed (if not contraindicated), and monitor the blood pressure every 5 minutes. Severe cases can require treatment with spinal anesthesia and the administration of ganglionic-blocking agents. For chronic problems, subarachnoid blocks or rhizotomy may be necessary.

Pain Management

Patients may have pain in areas about the level of injury. The pain may be described as sharp, dull, or burning and often is associated with muscle spasms. Morphine for pain or diazepam, cyclobenzaprine, or other antispasmodic agents may be ordered. Intramuscular medications should never be administered below the level of the lesion, because they cause local inflammation and tissue breakdown and absorption is negligible.

Concomitant Head Injury

Every patient with acute injury to the spine must be observed for signs and symptoms that indicate head injury. Evaluation of cranial status should be done at the same intervals as the vital sign measurements. Abnormawl neurological signs should be reported to the physician immediately, because they may indicate injury to the brain or increased ICP that results from the upward expansion of cord edema.

Respiratory Complications

Respiratory insufficiency or failure is the most serious complication of SCI. Respiratory complications can be independent of the level of injury. C4 and higher injuries require mechanical ventilation because of the direct involvement of the phrenic nerves. Assessment of a patient's ventilation should include the following parameters: status, rate, depth, pattern, and oxygen saturation. Evaluation of pulmonary function should include tidal volume, inspiratory force, and vital capacity. Changes in pulmonary function are early indicators of deterioration in respiratory status and may necessitate ventilator support. Intubation of the patients may depend on the ability to clear secretions and to maintain adequate gas exchange. A program of chest physiotherapy and the use of pressure support ventilation and positive end-expiratory pressure assists with the prevention of atelectasis. Auscultation of lung sounds should also be performed routinely to assess the presence of abnormal lung sounds. Chest radiographic examinations and arterial blood gas determinations should be monitored routinely and ordered immediately if signs of deterioration occur. Potential respiratory complications that result from SCI include pneumonia, aspiration, pulmonary edema, and pulmonary embolism. Rotational beds before surgical stabilization facilitate the mobilization of secretions and help prevent respiratory complications. A team approach by nursing staff members, physicians, respiratory therapists, and physical therapists is necessary for the treatment of SCI. Because of the rapid onset of pulmonary complications, the PACU nurse must be aggressive in caring for the patient with SCI.

Skin Breakdown

As with the patient for cranial surgery, skin care for the patient with SCI is an important aspect of PACU nursing care. Skin breakdown is one of the most obvious, costly, and detrimental complications that a patient with SCI can have. The patient must be turned and repositioned at least every 2 hours to prevent skin breakdown and damage to underlying body tissues. A specialty surface such as an air mattress or alternating pressure mattress may be necessary to prevent skin breakdown.

Gastrointestinal Complications

Generalized atony and loss of motility render the stomach and intestine distended and highly susceptible to fecal impactions and obstructions. Distention is relieved with intermittent nasogastric suction. Programs of bowel training are initiated within 24 hours of admission.

A high incidence rate of stress ulcers is seen among these patients, especially in those with quadriplegia. Here, parasympathetic vagal action is unopposed because of sympathetic block from the ascending and descending visceral nerve paths, and gastric acid secretion by the parietal cells of the stomach is increased. This stressful situation can be further compounded by the administration of corticosteroids used to reduce cord edema. Corticosteroids alone are capable of inducing hyperacidity of gastric juices. Antacids or a histamine-2 antagonists, or both, are given prophylactically to prevent stress ulcers. If gastric juices are accessible through a nasogastric tube, gastric pH can be monitored as a guide to treatment. Serial hematocrit determinations establish a baseline and may be the first indication of "silent" gastrointestinal hemorrhage.

Urologic Complications

After transection of the spinal cord, the bladder sphincter becomes paralyzed and urinary stasis develops. Indwelling urinary catheterization is necessary to prevent bladder distention during the acute phase.

Long-term catheterization, osteoporosis, decreased muscle tone, fluid and electrolyte abnormalities, alterations in cardiovascular dynamics, anemia, and catabolism contribute to urologic complications. Stasis, calculi and fistula formation, and chronic urinary tract complications can lead to septicemia. Pneumonia and septicemia have the greatest effect on reduced life expectancy in patients with SCI.[17]

Anesthetic Considerations

The most influential factors in the anesthetic management of the patient with SCI are the duration of the injury (acute or chronic), fluid and electrolyte status, airway management, and autonomic hyperreflexia.

The use of a depolarizing muscle relaxant (succinylcholine) for intubation purposes in the patient with SCI is conservatively contraindicated because of the release of potassium. The succinylcholine-induced release of potassium is the result of proliferation of cholinergic receptors in muscle tissue below the level of transection. The resultant hyperkalemia, often as high as 14 mEq/L, can lead to ventricular fibrillation and cardiac arrest. The release of potassium caused by succinylcholine administration can be seen as early as 1 day after injury and as long as 9 months later. The degree of muscle involvement, not the dose of succinylcholine, is the determining factor in the amount of potassium released.

Patients with SCI may have some degree of hypotension because of a relative hypovolemia that results from sympathetic nervous system depression. The degree of the hypotension depends on the level of transection and the duration of the injury in regard to whether the patient still has spinal shock. The patient must be adequately resuscitated with fluids, and measures must be taken to monitor fluid status and ensure adequate organ perfusion.

Airway management is a significant problem in patients with SCI whose injuries involve the cervical spine. Endotracheal intubation must be performed without manipulation of the cervical spine to avoid further irreversible damage. Intubation may be accomplished with awake blind oral or nasal approach, fiberoptics, or retrograde intubation. When the airway obstruction is severe, tracheostomy or cricothyrotomy may be necessary. Patients may arrive in the PACU with the endotracheal tube in place and not undergo extubation until adequate management of the airway and ventilation are ensured.

Herniated Intervertebral Disk

Herniated intervertebral disk is also known as *herniated nucleus pulposus* (Fig. 38-9).[8] This condition can occur in any of the intervertebral disks, but is most commonly found in one of the last two lumbar interspaces. Pain and some degree of compromise in sensory or motor function along the distribution of the involved nerve are common preoperative findings. Before surgical intervention is undertaken, diagnostic confirmation is sought and the suspected herniated nucleus pulposus is differentiated from tumor, subluxation of the facets, or rheumatoid spondylitis.

Surgery consists of partial hemilaminectomy and removal of the diseased disk. If fusion is necessary to prevent recurrence of pain or deformity, a bone graft is removed from the iliac crest or tibia and placed as a bridge over the defective space. Spinal fusion lengthens the operative procedure and requires a second operative wound

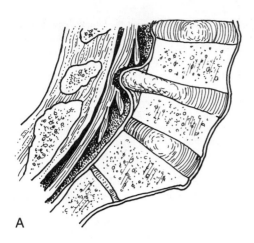

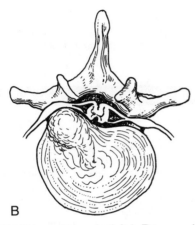

FIG. 38-9 Ruptured invetebral disk. Diagram shows herniation of the nucleus pulposus. **A,** Herniation presses on the structures of the spinal cord. **B,** Herniation may press on the exit of the spinal nerve and produce pain and other symptoms. (From Barker E: *Neuroscience nursing,* ed 3, St. Louis, 2008, Mosby.)

site; therefore a greater potential for postoperative complications exists, and the recuperative phase may be lengthened. The threat of shock is also greater because of increased blood loss and pain.

Movement restrictions in the PACU are determined by the surgeon and depend on the extent of the surgery and whether a fusion was done. If a fusion was not done, the patient is often allowed to stand at the bedside, and ambulation is allowed as soon as the effects of the anesthetic have subsided. If the spine is fused, mobility restrictions are more severe. Usually turning is allowed if done in the log-rolling fashion.

As in all spinal procedures, sensory function and motor strength of the extremities should be assessed along with the vital signs in the PACU. Evidence of CSF leaks must be sought on dressings and bed linens.

Intraspinal Neoplasms

Intraspinal neoplasms can occur at any level of the cord from the foramen magnum to the sacral canal. Most of the tumors are found in the thoracic region because this is the longest subdivision of the spine. Cord compression and neurologic deficit produce symptoms similar to those produced by displaced fracture of the spine, but they usually develop and progress at a slower pace. Neurologic examination, myelography, and tomography are used to determine the exact location of the lesion.

Intraspinal tumors may arise from the cord or its coverings, from fibrous tissue, or as a result of metastatic disease. For descriptive purposes, they are placed in the following subdivisions:

- *Intramedullary tumors:* those that arise solely from the substance of the cord
- *Extradural-extramedullary tumors:* those that arise outside the dura, either in the epidural space, vertebrae, or surrounding tissues
- *Intradural-extramedullary tumors:* those that arise within or under the dura but do not invade the cord

Early diagnosis and treatment are essential to prevent irreversible damage to the spinal cord. Most intraspinal neoplasms are benign and the remainders are usually caused by metastasis, although some are primarily malignant. The decision to intervene surgically is made after the patient's general condition and life expectancy are considered. Also considered are other metastases and the type and location of the primary tumor.

Treatment consists of laminectomy, surgical exploration, and excision of the mass. Most benign tumors can be excised completely. Prognosis depends on the location of the tumor, the severity and duration of the preoperative neurologic deficit, and whether the tumor is completely removable. Intramedullary tumors are associated with a more guarded prognosis because they can rarely be excised without increasing the neurologic deficit.

Postoperative Care for Spinal Cord Injury Surgical Interventions

Perianesthesia care of patients for lumbar surgery should include keeping the head of the bed flat and log-rolling the patient to help maintain proper body alignment, promote skin integrity, and minimize discomfort. The surgical site should be inspected for drainage and hematoma, and if spinal fusion was performed, the donor site should

NURSING CARE IN THE PACU

also be inspected. Assessment of the patient's comfort should be performed frequently because of muscle spasms that are often associated with lumbar surgery. The neurologic examination should include assessment of sensation in the lower extremities and notation of the presence of tingling, numbness, or paralysis. The pedal pulses, color, temperature, and capillary refill of the lower extremities should also be assessed.

SUMMARY

Perianesthesia care of the neurosurgical patient can be complex. However, modern pharmacology and technology in addition to our improved understanding of patient's physiology should facilitate the removal of many of the challenges in the care of these patients. Consequently, for a neurosurgical procedure or central nervous system trauma that necessitates radiologic studies with anesthesia, the anatomy and physiology (see Chapter 10) and pathophysiology have been described to include the monitoring equipment that can be used, all in an effort to ensure that outcomes are as favorable as possible. Besides the basic principles of PACU nursing management, which include airway management, ventilatory assistance, and hemodynamic support, the neurosurgical case entails unique preparation and management. This chapter has provided an in-depth discussion of the perianesthesia care of the neurosurgical patient in an effort to facilitate favorable outcomes.

REFERENCES

1. Czernin J, Schelbert H: PET/CT imaging: facts, opinions, hopes, and questions, The Journal of Nuclear Medicine 45:1S-3S, 2004.
2. Phillips N: Berry & Kohn's operating room technique, ed 11, St. Louis, 2007, Mosby.
3. Urden LD, et al: Critical care nursing, ed 6, St. Louis, 2010, Mosby.
4. Bader MK, Littlejohns LR: AANN core curriculum for neuroscience nursing, ed 5, Chicago, Ill, 2010, AANN.
5. Barker E: Neuroscience nursing, ed 3, St. Louis, 2008, Mosby.
6. Hickey J: The clinical practice of neurological and neurosurgical nursing, ed 6, Philadelphia, 2009, Lippincott Williams & Wilkins.
7. Noble KA: Traumatic brain injury and increased intracranial pressure, J Perianesth Nurs 25:242-247, 2010.
8. Schick L, Windle PE: Perianesthesia nursing core curriculum: preprocedure, phase I and phase II PACU nursing, ed 2, St. Louis, 2010, Saunders.
9. Miller RD, et al: Miller's anesthesia, ed 7, Philadelphia, 2005, Churchill Livingstone.
10. Souba WW, et al: ACS surgery: principles and practice, ed 6, New York, 2007, BC Decker.
11. Kemp KM: Precedex: Is it the future of cooperative sedation? Nursing 38 Suppl Critical: 7-8, 2008.
12. Yentis SM, et al: Anaesthesia and intensive care A-Z, ed 4, Edinburgh, 2009, Churchill Livingstone.
13. Fisher M, et al: Keep the brain cool – endovascular cooling in patients with severe traumatic brain injury: a case series study, Neurosurgery 68: 867-873, 2010.
14. Ledwith MB, et al: Effect of body position on cerebral oxygenation and physiologic parameters in patients with acute neurological conditions, J Neurosc Nurs 42: 280-286, 2010.
15. Centers for Disease Control and Prevention: Spinal cord injury (SCI): fact sheet, available at http://www.cdc.gov/TraumaticBrainInjury/scifacts.html. Accessed April 23, 2011.
16. Campagnolo DI: Autonomic dysreflexia in spinal cord injury, available at http://emedicine.medscape.com/article/322809-overview. Accessed April 27, 2011.
17. National Spinal Cord Injury Statistical Center: Spinal cord injury facts and figures at a glance, available at https://www.nscisc.uab.edu/PublicDocuments/nscisc_home/pdf/Facts%202011%20Feb%20Final.pdf. Accessed April 4, 2012.

RESOURCES

Aitkenhead A, et al: Textbook of anaesthesia, ed 5, Edinburgh, 2007, Churchill Livingstone.
Alspach J: Core curriculum for critical care nursing, ed 6, Philadelphia, 2005, Saunders.
Atlee J: Complications in anesthesia, ed 2, Philadelphia, 2007, Saunders.
Baird MS, Bethel S: Manual of critical care nursing, ed 6, St. Louis, 2011, Mosby.
Barash P, et al: Clinical anesthesia, ed 6, Philadelphia, 2009, Lippincott Williams & Wilkins.
Barrett KE et al: Ganong's review of medical physiology, ed 23, New York, 2009, McGraw-Hill Medical.
Brain Trauma Foundation, et al: Guidelines for the management of severe traumatic brain injury, ed 3, Guideline XV, Steroids S-91-S-95, 2007.
Brunton L, et al: Goodman and Gilman's the pharmacological basis of therapeutics, ed 11, New York, 2005, McGraw-Hill Professional.
Chulay M, Burns S: AACN essentials of critical care, St. Louis, 2005, AACN.
Fleisher LA: Anesthesia and uncommon diseases, ed 5, Philadelphia, 2007, Saunders.
Gallager C, Issenberg B: Simulation in anesthesia, Philadelphia, 2007, Saunders.
Hall J: Guyton & Hall's textbook of medical physiology, ed 12, Philadelphia, 2010, Saunders.
Lynn-McHale Wiegand DJ: AACN Procedure manual for critical care, ed 6, St. Louis, 2011, Saunders.
McCance K, Huether S: Pathophysiology: the biologic basis for disease in adults and children, ed 5, St. Louis, 2006, Mosby.
Nagelhout J, Plaus K: Nurse anesthesia, ed 4, St. Louis, 2009, Saunders.
Stoelting R, Miller R: Basics of anesthesia, ed 6, Philadelphia, 2011, Churchill Livingstone.
White P: Perioperative drug manual, ed 2, Philadelphia, 2005, Saunders.

39 Care of the Thyroid and Parathyroid Surgical Patient

Matthew D. Byrne, PhD, RN, CPAN, and
Joni M. Brady, MSN, RN, CAPA, CLC

Surgery of the thyroid gland was first performed around AD 500, and the first successful removal of a goiter occurred in AD 1000. By the 1800s, numerous thyroidectomies had been performed; however, nearly half of the patients died after surgery as a result of tetany. This morbidity rate was secondary to the removal of the parathyroid glands, whose function was not well understood at the time. In the early 1900s, a greater understanding of the role of the parathyroid glands promoted the subtotal thyroidectomy procedure which significantly reduced postoperative complications. In the late 1990s, endoscopic and minimally invasive techniques further reduced some postoperative complications and expanded the number of outpatient cases performed. The type of thyroid surgical procedure chosen depends on the patient's age, tumor cell type and size, presence of an encapsulated or extracapsular tumor, and any invasion of adjacent structures (Fig. 39-1).

DEFINITIONS

Bilateral Subtotal Thyroidectomy: Removal of most of the thyroid tissue in both lobes with a small remnant of thyroid tissue left at the back portion of the thyroid to protect the parathyroid glands and prevent recurrent laryngeal nerve damage (a potential complication associated with total thyroidectomy).

Parathyroidectomy: Excision of one or more diseased parathyroid glands.

Subtotal/Partial Thyroidectomy: Removal of the thyroid gland with the exception of a small portion retained on the opposite side of the thyroid.

Thyroidectomy: Total excision of the thyroid gland with the parathyroid glands left intact. Normally, a total thyroidectomy is only performed in patients with medullary malignant disease, because total thyroidectomy renders the patient immediately unable to produce any thyroid hormone, thus requiring thyroid hormone supplementation for the remainder of the patient's life. Patients who are not a candidate for radioablation may also be considered for thyroidectomy.

Thyroid Lobectomy with Isthmusectomy: Removal of one lobe of the thyroid and the isthmus that connects the two lobes.

ANESTHESIA

Surgery on the thyroid and parathyroid glands is commonly performed with general anesthesia. Regional and local techniques, such as a cervical plexus blockade, are growing in popularity as minimally invasive techniques and the number of outpatient cases grows.[1-3] Appropriate postoperative care for a patient receiving general anesthesia is instituted in the postanesthesia care unit. Minimally invasive techniques and those procedures performed with regional or local anesthesia may minimize the recovery requirements for this patient population.

PERIANESTHESIA NURSING CARE

Preoperative Considerations

A preoperative euthyroid state is considered the safest strategy for prevention of thyroid storm (see Thyroid Storm). Preoperative and postoperative calcium and vitamin D supplementation can be used to reduce the complications of hypocalcemia. Evaluation of a patient's voice quality provides the baseline to assess the presence of postoperative laryngeal nerve damage.

Positioning

The patient should be placed in the side-lying position to protect the airway when minimally responsive on arrival in the postanesthesia care unit. Once the patient is responsive, or if the patient is responsive on admission, a semi-Fowler position of at least 30 degrees elevation is used to promote venous return. The nurse must position the patient with specific attention given to head and neck support in order to prevent undue tension on the suture line.

Cardiopulmonary Assessment and Care

The nurse should carefully monitor the airway, respiratory rate, breath sounds, and pulse oximetry. Palpation to assess for crepitus should also be done, because a positive finding is an indication of

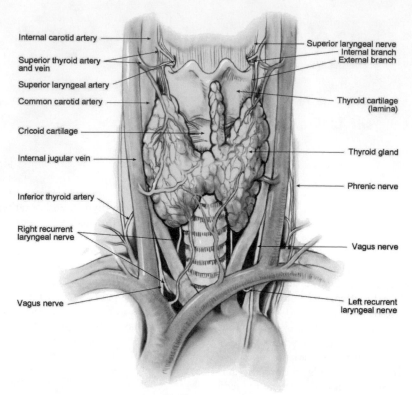

Internal carotid artery

Superior thyroid artery
and vein

Superior laryngeal artery

Common carotid artery

Cricoid cartilage

Internal jugular vein

Inferior thyroid artery

Right recurrent
laryngeal nerve

Vagus nerve

Superior laryngeal nerve
Internal branch
External branch

Thyroid cartilage
(lamina)

Thyroid gland

Phrenic nerve

Vagus nerve

Left recurrent
laryngeal nerve

FIG. 39-1 Thyroid gland and surrounding anatomic structures. (From Elisha S, et al: Anesthesia case management for thyroidectomy, *AANA J* 78(2):152, 2010.)

the presence of subcutaneous emphysema. Signs and symptoms of impending respiratory obstruction, such as tracheal deviation, stridor, air hunger, or falling oxygen saturations, should be reported immediately to the anesthesia provider and surgeon. In some situations, immediate reintubation or tracheostomy may be necessary; therefore the associated reintubation or tracheostomy equipment should be readily available for use. Hypertension and transient elevations of blood pressure should be avoided to decrease stress on suture lines and to avoid hematoma and hemorrhage. Prevention and management of heavy coughing, nausea, vomiting, or dry retching is essential.

Pain Management

Pain may be minimal after thyroidectomy and parathyroidectomy when performed on an outpatient basis. Postoperative analgesia requirements are greater in the open procedure population. Small doses of an opioid may be needed in the first 24 hours for patients admitted to a facility. Severe pain is an abnormal finding that can indicate unexpected bleeding or nerve damage, and it is a risk factor for unwanted hypertension.

Dressings and Drains

Postoperative dressings are small, and drains are generally not required. Postoperative drainage is minimal and should not visibly soak through the dressing. Some disagreement persists regarding the use of surgical drains. There are questions regarding whether the presence of a drain causes increased pain, scarring, cost, length of stay, and a drain's limited ability to identify and prevent hematoma.[4,5] Drains may be indicated in the presence of greater intraoperative blood loss or an extensive procedure or when a large space is left after removal of a tumor or goiter.

Intake and Output

As with any surgical patient, intake and output monitoring is important for the evaluation of cardiovascular stability. Because many thyroid surgeries are performed on an outpatient basis, it is important to ensure that the patient is capable of tolerating oral fluids before discharge. Routine phonation and swallowing evaluations serve to rule out laryngeal nerve damage, which could precipitate aspiration.

NURSING CARE IN THE PACU

Evidence-Based Practice

Debate about drain placement and the associated effects on scarring, infection, hematoma, and length of stay continues for the postthyroidectomy patient population. In a randomized prospective clinical trial, 55 patients requiring thyroidectomy were randomly assigned to drain and no-drain groups. The researchers found statistically significant results demonstrating that the no-drain group had a 1.12-day reduction in hospital stay, a cost savings of $2177 per patient, and no increase in postoperative complications.

IMPLICATIONS FOR PRACTICE

Although thyroidectomy patients can arrive with or without surgical wound drains, care outcomes appear to be equivalent or improved in the no-drain population. The presence of a surgical drain in the postthyroidectomy patient should not create a false sense of security regarding potential complications, particularly for the development of hematomas. Vigilance and routine hematoma assessment compose the cornerstone of care for this population.

Source: Morrissey AT, et al: Comparison of drain versus no drain thyroidectomy: randomized prospective clinical trial, *J Otolaryngol Head Neck Surg* 37:43-47, 2008.

Complications

As knowledge of thyroid and parathyroid function and interventional surgical techniques improved, postoperative complication rates decreased and now reportedly occur in less than 1% of patients. Complications are largely attributed to surgeon skill level, type and invasiveness of tumor, anatomic visualization during the procedure, and the patient's preoperative thyroid state.

Bleeding and Airway (Respiratory) Compromise

As surgical techniques became more refined and less invasive, the risk of postoperative bleeding was reduced significantly. Cardiopulmonary status compromise depends on the technique used and extent of the procedure. Techniques such as an endoscopic approach requiring insufflations can result in arterial or venous injury, hemorrhage, or pneumothorax. Open procedures used for large tumor removal may be more prone to cause hemorrhage and airway compromise. Excessive postoperative bleeding may cause tracheal compression and subsequent airway obstruction,

and this finding should be reported to the surgeon immediately.

Respiratory difficulties range from dropping oxygen saturations to stridor (a result of airway obstruction or compromise from bleeding). In cases that involve extensive dissection or insufflations, vocal cord and laryngeal nerve damage, laryngeal edema and pneumothorax can occur. Neck swelling, pain, pressure, fullness in the neck, dysphagia, and dysphonia (hoarse voice) can be specific indications of bleeding or nerve damage and indicate an existing potential for airway or respiratory compromise. Any excess bleeding requires the nurse to initiate immediate reporting to the surgeon.

Recurrent Laryngeal Nerve Injury

The recurrent laryngeal nerve may be injured during surgery because of clamping, compression, severing, or stretching. Unilateral recurrent laryngeal nerve injury can appear as a weak cough and change in voice. In some cases, although the damage actually occurred, no notable signs may be present. Aspiration is another potential risk with this type of injury. Symptoms of bilateral recurrent laryngeal nerve injury can result in life-threatening airway obstruction and may necessitate immediate intervention, including a potential for reintubation and tracheostomy. Nerve injury is generally transient and can be treated with corticosteroids.

Hypoparathyroidism and Hypocalcemia

Hypoparathyroidism is a complication that can occur after total thyroidectomy or total parathyroidectomy. The condition can be caused by intentional removal of the parathyroid glands or inadvertent or unavoidable damage during thyroidectomy. This complication manifests as hypocalcemia and is usually transient. Signs and symptoms of hypocalcemia, caused by neuromuscular irritability, rarely occur in the immediate postoperative period, but may appear 24 to 72 hours after surgery. Symptoms include numbness and tingling of the fingers, toes, and area around the mouth (perioral), muscle cramps (tetany), and spasm. If calcium levels are not restored, seizures and laryngeal stridor are imminent.

The assessment of any patient who verbalizes tingling symptoms includes testing for the presence of Chvostek sign (the development of a lip twitch or facial spasm when the cheek is tapped over the facial nerve) and Trousseau sign (carpal spasm development when a blood pressure cuff is applied and the circulation transiently occluded). Laboratory findings, Chvostek sign, and an evaluation of carpopedal spasms (clonus in the feet when dorsiflexed) are preferred over assessing for Trousseau sign, which can sometimes be painful. Definitive treatment involves intravenous administration of calcium. Although both calcium chloride and calcium gluconate may be used, calcium gluconate is preferred for its greater bioavailability and lesser arrhythmogenic potential. When intravenous calcium is administered, it is given via slow push with continuous electrocardiographic monitoring performed before, during, and after the infusion. Early and routine calcium and vitamin D supplementation have been indicated as a useful strategy in the reduction of hypocalcemic complications.[6-8]

Thyroid Storm

Thyroid storm, or thyrotoxic crisis, is a rare complication that can occur after surgical manipulation of a hyperactive thyroid. Rapid diagnosis of the underlying cause for an apparent postoperative hypermetabolic state is crucial for appropriate treatment of the problem. The presence of malignant hyperthermia (another potential cause for postanesthetic hyper-metabolic state) versus thyroid storm must be differentiated, because these disorders have significantly different treatment algorithms.

Ideally, an overactive thyroid is controlled with medication so that the patient arrives in the preoperative setting in a euthyroid state. Thyroid storm more commonly occurs when a patient with hyperthyroidism and thyrotoxicosis is involved in an emergent procedure or in circumstances when inadequate preoperative time is available to normalize thyroid levels. The patient can initially develop fever and tachycardia during surgery and subsequently appear in the postanesthesia setting in a hypermetabolic state that can include agitation, disorientation, hypertension, tachycardia, and heart failure proceeding to shock. Treatment should focus on thyroid level normalization, maintenance of cardiopulmonary integrity through reduction or management of sympathetic output, and reduction of the other signs and symptoms of hypermetabolism, most notably hyperthermia. Treatment generally includes administration of beta blockers, iodine, vasopressors, fluid support, oxygen, salicylates, steroids, and cooling measures.

Infection

Disagreement exists about the need for routine antibiotic administration, because the incidence of postoperative infection in patients who have undergone thyroid and parathyroid surgery is rare.[9] Any postoperative infection symptoms should be investigated and treated with appropriate antibiotic therapy and wound care.

SUMMARY

Increased knowledge of thyroid and parathyroid function, and improved and minimally invasive surgical techniques significantly decreased the length of stay and postoperative complication rates in the thyroid surgical population. Surgery on the thyroid and parathyroid glands is commonly performed with general anesthesia, and postoperative nursing care is focused on the recovery of the patient from general anesthesia. Selected minimally invasive procedures performed under local anesthesia minimize postoperative recovery requirements and length of stay, and they are becoming increasingly popular.

Postoperative nursing assessment should focus on the potential for cardiopulmonary compromise owing to sympathetic output related to a hyperthyroid state, hemorrhage, and venous oozing or laryngeal edema. The nurse should proactively address pain management, proper positioning to minimize suture line stress, ongoing assessment of the operative dressing and intake and output status. Although rare, thyroid surgery complications can include inferior or superior laryngeal nerve damage with possible vocal cord paralysis, laryngeal stridor, airway and respiratory compromise, bleeding that causes cervical or neck hematoma requiring surgical evacuation, hypocalcemia, tetany, seizures and mental disturbances, thyroid storm, and infection. Recognition of potential complications and implementation of appropriate and rapid treatment interventions are essential for an optimal postoperative outcome.

REFERENCES

1. Suri KB, et al: Postoperative recovery advantages in patients undergoing thyroid and parathyroid surgery under regional anesthesia, *Semin Cardiothorac Vasc Anesth* 14: 49-50, 2010.
2. Tuggle CT, et al: Same-day thyroidectomy: A review of practice patterns and outcomes for 1,168 procedures in New York State, *Ann Surg Oncol* 18:1035-40, 2011.
3. Elisha S, et al: Anesthesia case management for thyroidectomy, *AANA J* 78:151-160, 2010.
4. Dunlap WW, et al: Thyroid drains and postoperative drainage, *Otolaryngol Head Neck Surg* 143:235-238, 2010.
5. Morrissey AT, et al: Comparison of drain versus no drain thyroidectomy: Randomized prospective clinical trial, *J Otolaryngol Head Neck Surg* 37:43-47, 2008.
6. Roh JL, et al: Prevention of postoperative hypocalcemia with routine oral calcium and vitamin D supplements in patients with differentiated papillary thyroid carcinoma undergoing total thyroidectomy plus central neck dissection, *Cancer* 115:251-258, 2009.
7. Roh JL, Park CI: Routine oral calcium and vitamin D supplements for prevention of hypocalcemia after total thyroidectomy, *Am J Surg* 192:675-678, 2006.

8. Sabour S, et al: The role of rapid PACU parathyroid hormone in reducing post-thyroidectomy hypocalcemia, *Otolaryngol Head Neck Surg* 141:727-729, 2009.

9. Moalem J, et al: Patterns of antibiotic prophylaxis use for thyroidectomy and parathyroidectomy: Results of an international survey of endocrine surgeons, *J Am Coll Surg* 210:949-956, 2010.

RESOURCES

AACE/AME Task Force on Thyroid Nodules: American association of clinical endocrinologists and associazione medici endocrinologi medical guidelines for clinical practice for the diagnosis and management of thyroid nodules, 2010, available at https://www.aace.com/sites/default/files/ThyroidGuidelines.pdf. Accessed March 22, 2012.

Gal I, et al: Minimally invasive video-assisted thyroidectomy and conventional thyroidectomy: A prospective randomized study, *Surg Endosc* 22:2445-2449, 2008.

Hopkins B, Steward D: Outpatient thyroid surgery and the advances making it possible, *Curr Opin Otolaryngol Head Neck Surg* 17:95-99, 2009.

Johnson K: Laparoscopic or open removal of parathyroid? *Intern Med News* 38:28, 2005.

Lee KE, et al: Outcomes of 109 patients with papillary thyroid carcinoma who underwent robotic total thyroidectomy with central node dissection via the bilateral axillo-breast approach, *Surgery* 148:1207-1213, 2010.

Mazzaferri EL, et al: *Practical management of thyroid cancer: A multidisciplinary approach*, New York, 2010, Springer.

McKennis A, Waddington C: *Nursing interventions for potential complications after thyroidectomy*, available at www.sohnnurse.com/thyroidectomy.html.

Muenscher A, et al: The endoscopic approach to the neck: A review of the literature, and overview of the various techniques, *Surg Endosc* 25:1358-1363, 2011.

Noble KA: Thyroid storm, *J Perianesthesia Nurs* 21:119–125, 2006.

Oertli D, Udelsman R, editors: *Surgery of the thyroid and parathyroid glands*, New York, 2007, Springer.

Patel M, et al: Fibrin glue in thyroid and parathyroid surgery: Is under-flap suction still necessary? *Ear Nose Throat J* 85:530–532, 2006.

Takesuye D, et al: Practice analysis: Techniques of head and neck surgeons and general surgeons performing thyroidectomy for cancer, *Qual Manage Health Care* 15:257–262, 2006.

NURSING CARE IN THE PACU

40 Care of the Gastrointestinal, Abdominal, and Anorectal Surgical Patient

Denise O'Brien, DNP, RN, ACNS-BC, CPAN, CAPA, FAAN

Care of the patient after abdominal surgery or surgery on the gastrointestinal tract is an extremely broad subject. Surgical intervention within the abdominal cavity is generally directed toward restoring normal function and therefore involves repair of congenital abnormalities, reconstruction of deformities, removal of obstructions to restore patency of the gastrointestinal tract and the biliary tract, treatment of malignant disease, and maintenance of the integrity of related organs, such as the liver, pancreas, and spleen (Fig. 40-1).

DEFINITIONS

Antrectomy: Removal of the distal part of the stomach.

Appendectomy: Removal of the vermiform appendix, performed with an open or laparoscopic technique.

Cholecystectomy: Removal of the gallbladder; the procedure can be performed with an open or a laparoscopic approach.

Cholecystostomy: Placement of a tube or drain into the gallbladder to permit drainage of the organ, and rarely can be used to remove stones. This procedure is performed infrequently except to provide relief in a patient with cholecystitis who has prohibitive operative risk precluding cholecystectomy. This procedure is usually performed percutaneously in the radiology suite.

Colostomy: Colon brought through the abdominal wall to drain into a drainage device (bag); may be permanent or temporary, single or double lumen. May be performed with either an open procedure or a laparoscopic approach.

Diverticulum: A herniation of mucosa or submucosa through a weakness in a muscular wall of the colon, most commonly in the sigmoid colon, but may be found throughout the colon.

Endoscopic Retrograde Cholangiopancreatography (ERCP): A side-viewing fiberoptic endoscope is used to cannulate pancreatic and biliary ducts through the ampulla of Vater for cholangiography, pancreatography, stone removal, and invasive manipulation such as sphincterotomy.

Endoscopy: Visualization of a body cavity with a lighted tube or scope. Most commonly performed to visualize the inside of the esophagus, stomach, and duodenum or colon.

Esophagogastroduodenoscopy (EGD): Passage of a fiberoptic endoscope, usually with topical anesthesia and intravenous sedation, to view the esophagus, stomach, and duodenum. Biopsies or control of bleeding may also be performed with this procedure.

Esophagoscopy: Direct visualization of the esophagus and cardia of the stomach by means of a rigid or flexible lighted instrument (esophagoscope). Esophagoscopy can be used to obtain a tissue biopsy or secretions for study to aid in diagnosis.

Gastrectomy: Removal of the stomach. If less than a total gastrectomy is performed, in which only part of the stomach is removed, the procedure is typically described as distal gastrectomy, proximal gastrectomy, or subtotal gastrectomy, suggesting only a small proximal gastric remnant remains. Total gastrectomies are most commonly performed for cancers in the proximal part of the stomach.

Gastroscopy: Direct inspection of the stomach with possible removal of a tissue specimen by means of a lighted instrument (gastroscope); bleeding can also be controlled and biopsy specimens can be obtained with this procedure.

Hemorrhoidectomy: Surgical excision of dilated veins of the rectum.

Hernia: The displacement of any viscus (usually bowel) or tissue through a congenital or acquired opening or defect in the wall of its natural cavity, most commonly the muscular wall of the abdomen. Usually this term is applied to protrusion of abdominal viscera; however, it is actually the defect itself through which abdominal contents have protruded.

Herniorrhaphy: Repair of a hernia. Hernias are classified according to anatomic site and condition of the viscus that has protruded. Reducible hernias are those in which the bowel or contents of the hernia sac can be replaced into the normal cavity. An irreducible, or incarcerated, hernia is one in which the contents cannot be replaced. A strangulated hernia is one in which the blood supply to the protruding segment of bowel is obstructed. When a segment of bowel becomes strangulated, it rapidly becomes necrotic. A strangulated hernia constitutes a surgical emergency. Hernias can be repaired with an open or laparoscopic technique.

Herniorrhaphy, Diaphragmatic: Replacement of abdominal contents that have entered the thorax through a defect in the diaphragm and repair of the diaphragmatic defect.

Herniorrhaphy, Epigastric and Hypogastric: Repair and closure of the abdominal wall defect.

Herniorrhaphy, Femoral: A defect in the region of the femoral ring, which is located just below the Poupart (inguinal) ligament and medial to the femoral vein. Femoral hernias are seldom found in children and occur most often in women.

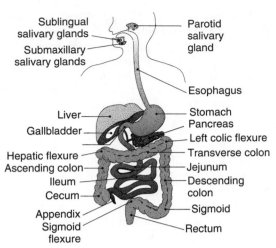

FIG. 40-1 Digestive system and its associated structures. (From Sole ML, et al: *Introduction to critical care nursing*, ed 5, Philadelphia, 2008, Saunders.)

Herniorrhaphy, Incisional: Repair of a defect in the abdominal wall that was a prior site of placement of a surgical incision. These types of repairs commonly involve placement of prosthetic (synthetic) mesh (e.g., Prolene, Gore-Tex, Parietex).

Herniorrhaphy, Inguinal: Repair of a defect in the inguinal region; may be direct (through Hesselbach triangle) or an indirect (through the internal ring) inguinal hernia. These repairs also commonly use some type of prosthetic mesh, most commonly Prolene or Parietex.

Herniorrhaphy, Umbilical: Reconstruction of the abdominal wall beneath the umbilicus (umbilical ring) can occur in pediatric patients and is most common in African American infants. In children, this hernia often closes spontaneously in infants before 2 years of age; therefore these repairs should generally not be performed until after the age of 2 years. Umbilical hernias in adults will never resolve spontaneously.

Ileostomy: Terminal ileum brought through the abdominal wall to empty into a drainage device (bag). Commonly used to treat inflammatory conditions of the bowel, such as ulcerative colitis and regional enteritis (Crohn disease), and to provide a permanent or temporary stoma after surgery for obstruction or cancer.

Intussusception: Telescoping of the bowel into itself.

Laparoscopy (Peritoneoscopy): Direct visualization of the peritoneal cavity by means of a lighted instrument (often connected to a color video monitor) inserted through the abdominal wall via a trocar placed through a small incision. An increasing number of abdominal procedures are performed assisted via laparoscopic techniques. Gastrointestinal or abdominal procedures commonly performed via laparoscopy include cholecystectomy, gastrojejunostomy, splenectomy, Nissen fundoplication, inguinal herniorrhaphy, appendectomy, jejunostomy, colostomy, colectomy, ileocolectomy, and pancreatectomy.

Laparotomy (Celiotomy): An opening made through the abdominal wall into the peritoneal cavity, to perform an operation in the abdomen in an open fashion (e.g., not laparoscopic).

Pancreaticoduodenectomy (Whipple Procedure): Removal of the head of the pancreas, the entire duodenum, the gallbladder, a portion of the jejunum, the distal third of the stomach, and the lower half of the common bile duct, with reestablishment of continuity of the biliary, pancreatic, and gastrointestinal systems. The procedure, which is used primarily for the treatment of malignant disease of the pancreas, duodenum, and ampulla, is associated with a less than 3% risk of perioperative mortality if performed in a high volume center. Sometimes a pylorus-sparing procedure is performed, which leaves the entire stomach intact.

Percutaneous Endoscopic Gastrostomy (PEG): Endoscopic procedure for the insertion of a tube into the stomach, either for the purpose of decompression or feeding, performed with local anesthesia and intravenous sedation.

Pyloromyotomy (Fredet-Ramstedt Operation): Enlargement of the lumen of the pylorus with longitudinal splitting of the hypertrophied circular muscle without severing of the mucosa; used as treatment for pyloric stenosis in infants. Pyloric stenosis is most common in firstborn male infants.

Pyloroplasty: A longitudinal incision made in the pylorus (full thickness) and closed transversely to permit the muscle to relax and establish an enlarged outlet. Heineke-Mikulicz is the most common type of procedure.

Splenectomy: Removal of the spleen; can be performed in an open or minimally invasive approach.

Transduodenal Sphincteroplasty: Partial division of the sphincter of Oddi and exploration of the common bile duct for treatment of recurrent attacks of acute pancreatitis caused by formation of calculi in the pancreatic duct or blockage of the sphincter of Oddi. Can also be used in treatment of biliary stones which cannot be removed by endoscopic or percutaneous means.

Volvulus: Intestinal obstruction as a result of twisting of the bowel, most commonly sigmoid colon or cecum.

GENERAL CARE AFTER ABDOMINAL SURGERY

Abdominal or gastrointestinal surgery can be performed with regional or general anesthesia. The choice of anesthesia varies with the type of procedure, the patient's cardiac and pulmonary status, and the surgeon's need for muscle relaxation. Usually only short, simple procedures are performed with regional (spinal or epidural) anesthesia. Diagnostic procedures such as endoscopy, biopsy, and percutaneous gastrostomy often are performed with sedation only. Inguinal or femoral herniorrhaphies are often performed with regional (spinal) or general anesthesia, and occasionally with only local anesthesia. Most other abdominal surgical and laparoscopic procedures are performed with general anesthesia. All laparoscopic procedures require general anesthesia because of the need for relaxation of the abdominal wall and the need to control the patient's respirations.

A number of abdominopelvic incisions have been developed and are commonly used (Fig. 40-2). An ideal incision ensures ease of entrance, maximal exposure of the operative site, and minimal trauma. It should also provide good primary wound healing with maximal wound strength.

The reader should review Chapters 26 through 31 for general care after surgery. See Chapter 45 for a discussion on bariatric surgical procedures and care.

Perianesthesia Care

As with any procedure, the surgeon and anesthesia care provider should give the perianesthesia nurse a full report on the anesthesia used

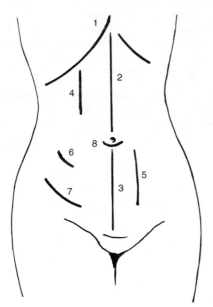

FIG. 40-2 Commonly used abdominal incisions. *1*, Kocher incision: *right side*, gallbladder and biliary tract surgery; *left side*, splenectomy. *2*, Upper abdominal midline incision: rapid entry to control bleeding ulcer. *3*, Lower abdominal midline incision: female reproductive system. *4*, Upper paramedian incision: *right side*, biliary tract surgery, cholecystectomy; *left side*, splenectomy, gastrectomy, vagotomy, hiatal hernia repair. *5*, Lower paramedian incision: *right side*, appendectomy, small bowel resection; *left side*, sigmoid colon resection. *6*, McBurney incision: appendectomy. *7*, Inguinal incision: inguinal herniorrhaphy. *8*, Infraumbilical: umbilical herniorrhaphy.

and the procedure performed. With every procedure, the surgeon will write an operative note, which describes the procedure performed, viscera removed, drains present, and any other relevant intraoperative findings or complications. This action assists those who are caring for the patient in an assessment of the wounds, dressings, and expected drainage.

Positioning

After abdominal surgery, patients are often positioned on the side until laryngeal reflexes have started to return. The patient is then placed in a semi-Fowler position to ease the tension on suture lines and to promote respiratory effort. After some procedures on the stomach or esophagus, strict aspiration precautions with the head of the bed elevated to 30 degrees may be required. After hemorrhoidectomy, the patient may assume any position of comfort, which is most likely on the right or left side.

Dressings and Drains

All dressings should be checked. The nurse must know what kind of incision was used and whether any drains are in place. Drains are discussed in more detail in the specific procedures. Drainage should be assessed for character, volume, and odor. The nurse should determine who can or should remove the dressing if needed. Some surgeons reinforce the abdominal incision and dressing with a binder; they believe that this gives the incision valuable support. Others, however, believe that binders restrict respiratory effort and that this disadvantage outweighs the limited advantage of incisional support.

Because drainage may be copious after gastrointestinal surgery, frequent reinforcement of dressings may be necessary. Ask the surgeon for anticipated or expected amounts of drainage for the patient and procedure. If drainage becomes excessive (more than expected from the particular procedure), the surgeon should be notified and the incision directly inspected.

All tubes should be connected to the appropriate drainage devices, usually straight-gravity or closed-bulb suction drainage, as the surgeon specifies. Nasogastric tubes will usually be attached to constant or low intermittent wall suction. Maintenance of the patency of these tubes is one of the most important nursing functions after gastrointestinal surgery. Irrigation of nasogastric tubes after esophageal or gastric surgery should be directed by the surgeon's orders.

Respiratory Function

The promotion of good respiratory function is a nursing priority for the patient who has had abdominal surgery. Painful abdominal incisions cause the patient to restrict chest expansion voluntarily, which is especially true with high abdominal incisions. The patient must be coached often in sustained maximal inspirations, coughing, and changing position to prevent respiratory complications. Assisting the patient with splinting of the incision and judicious use of pain medications aid in deep breathing and coughing and help to prevent the development of atelectasis. Coughing and incentive spirometry in the postanesthesia care unit (PACU) setting are valuable in promotion of respiratory function.

Frequent assessment of breath sounds during the postoperative period can alert the nurse to impending respiratory problems. An unrecognized injury to the diaphragm during upper abdominal surgery is possible and can result in respiratory distress. Positive pressure ventilation during anesthesia can also lead to respiratory problems. Breath sounds must be monitored closely to assess for pneumothorax and other respiratory complications.

Fluid and Electrolyte Balance

Fluid and electrolyte shifts or losses can be substantial during gastrointestinal surgery. Losses continue after surgery through gastrointestinal tubes or other drains, and through third-spacing of fluid into the abdomen. For this reason, accurate intake and output records are mandatory. This recording begins with the intake and output report from the anesthesia care provider, which should be the first PACU entry. All drainage from incisions should be included in the assessment of electrolyte balance. Frequent serum electrolyte determinations may be necessary if losses are great. Intravenous fluids are used for replacement for at least the first 24 hours after surgery and at least until the nasogastric tube is removed. See Chapter 14 for a discussion of the specific problems in electrolyte loss from the gastrointestinal tract.

For patients who do not arrive in the PACU with a urinary catheter in place, urinary retention can become a problem after abdominal surgery because of incisional pain, opioid analgesics, anesthetics, and physiologic splinting. Urine output should be checked frequently, and accurate records should be kept. The nurse should also check for bladder distention and document the findings; the patient might not recognize the need to void, particularly after spinal or epidural anesthesia. Ultrasound examination of the bladder with a bedside scanner can aid in assessment of bladder status. The patient should void within 6 to 8 hours after surgery. If the patient has not voided by the time of discharge from the PACU, the receiving unit should be notified to check specifically for urinary retention. If permissible, the male patient may benefit by standing to void. If urinary retention causes pain, distends the abdomen, or becomes prolonged, urinary catheterization may become necessary. Patients who have had extensive surgery will return to the PACU with a urinary catheter in place. Accurate output records should be maintained. For an adult with normal renal function, a minimum of 30 mL/hour of urine output is expected; if less than this, the surgeon should be notified.

Care of the Patient with Nasogastric or Intestinal Tubes

Anesthesia and manipulation of the viscera during surgery cause gastric and colonic peristalsis to diminish or disappear completely for up to 5 days after surgery. Nasogastrointestinal or nasogastric tubes can be used after surgery to prevent the sequelae of this hypomotility. Edema at the operative site also can result in temporary obstruction.

If gastric decompression is needed, short tubes are generally used; long intestinal tubes are no longer used. Short tubes used include the Levin and the plastic Salem sump, which is a double-lumen nasogastric tube and is the most commonly used tube. The double lumen prevents excessive negative pressure from developing when the tube is connected to suction. To benefit from the double-lumen tube, however, it is important that the lumen to air is not obstructed and is "sumping," or the tube will become obstructed by sucking on the gastric wall.[1]

When the patient returns from the operating suite with a nasogastric tube in place, the nurse must ascertain why the tube was placed, where it was placed, and whether it should be connected to suction or to straight-gravity drainage. The physician often orders the tube to be connected to low-pressure intermittent suction (20 to 80 mm Hg). Usually only low-pressure intermittent suction is used, because excessive negative pressure in either the stomach or the bowel pulls the mucosa into the lumen of the tube and can cause traumatic ulcers. For double-lumen nasogastric tubes, continuous suction at 40 to 60 mm Hg is usually ordered and is necessary for the tube to function properly. Keeping the open lumen above the midline improves functioning of the double-lumen tube.

Tube Patency

Patency of the tube must be ensured. The nurse should observe for drainage from the tube. All characteristics of the drainage must be noted: consistency, color, odor, quantity, and any deviations from the expected drainage. After gastrointestinal surgery, initial drainage may be bright red in small volumes but should become dark or thin, watery, cherry pink–colored liquid after 24 hours. Bloody drainage should not be expected from a nasogastric tube placed only for decompression of the stomach after biliary tract, liver, or spleen surgery. If no drainage is present, if the patient's abdomen becomes distended, or if the patient vomits around the nasogastric tube or has nausea, the tube may be clogged or the suction apparatus may be malfunctioning; check both. For maintenance of the patency of the nasogastric tube, irrigation with 20 to 30 mL of normal saline solution can be performed every hour, or more frequently if necessary. Before irrigating the tube, check with the surgeon regarding the permissibility of nasogastric tube irrigation. Plain water in 20-mL amounts can be used to irrigate the tube without creation of electrolyte abnormalities. Larger amounts of plain water should not be used when irrigating for gastric bleeding because of the large volume and the risk of electrolyte alterations. Frequent irrigations increase the loss of electrolytes from the gastrointestinal system. Some surgeons advocate the use of air to irrigate the nasogastric tube to maintain patency. Only air should ever be passed through the second ("sump") lumen of the double lumen tube.

Irrigation

The amount of irrigating solution instilled should be recorded as such, unless its equivalent is aspirated via syringe. All gastrointestinal drainage should be accurately measured and recorded. If irrigations do not clear the tube, the tubing should be checked for clogs by milking it toward the suction container to dislodge any obstruction. The suction apparatus is checked by disconnecting the nasogastric tube at the junction of the nasogastric tube and the drainage tube that leads to the container. With the suction turned on, the end of the drainage tube is placed in a glass of water; if the water is sucked up, the suction device is functioning. If these measures fail, gastric mucosa may be occluding the lumen of the tube or the tube may be kinked. In this instance, the patient or the tube may need to be repositioned. If the patient has had gastric, pancreatic, or esophageal surgery, the tube should not be manipulated. The

surgeon should be notified of the malfunctioning tube. In general, unless ordered by the surgeon, checking with the surgeon before manipulating or replacing a nasogastric tube is always prudent.

Patient Comfort

The presence of a nasogastric tube is an uncomfortable experience for the patient. However, appropriate nursing care can relieve sore throat, dry mouth, hoarseness, earache, sore nose, and dry lips. The tube should be taped securely and properly (hypoallergenic tape or a specially designed tube securing device) in a position to prevent pressure on the naris. The tube can be secured to the nose in the position it naturally assumes. The tube should not be taped to the patient's nose and then to the forehead; this causes pressure on the underside of the nostril and can cause tissue necrosis within minutes. To lessen the pressure and pull on the patient's nose, the tube can be taped or pinned to the gown.

Petrolatum ointment is applied to the tube where it enters the nose and around the nares. The outside portion of the tube is kept free of mucus or other drainage, which prevents encrustations from forming and reduces irritation of the nostril. Petrolatum ointment, cream, or lip balm is applied to the lips to keep them soft and to prevent cracking. Good and frequent mouth care is essential for the comfort of the patient and prevention of parotitis. Moistened swabs, mouthwash, or even a toothbrush can be used to provide mouth care for the patient. The nurse should ensure that the patient understands not to swallow any of the material used. This, of course, is not fatal but could make assessment of accurate nasogastric tube output difficult.

Gargling with warm tap water or warm saline solution (or with viscous lidocaine or applications of a local anesthetic spray) can relieve the patient's sore throat. A physician's order should be provided for these measures. Some surgeons allow patients to suck on isotonic ice chips or hard candy or to chew gum. Anesthetic throat lozenges, if allowed, may be comforting to the patient. All patients with a gastrointestinal tube in place are given essentially nothing by mouth until the tube is removed. The only exception may be certain medications, given orally or through the tube, or ice chips (less than 200 mL every 8 hours). Some surgeons believe that allowing patients to consume ice chips increases comfort and also helps to keep the tube patent by having the melted ice chips frequently sucked out of the stomach by the tube.

DIAGNOSTIC STUDIES

Invasive diagnostic procedures are occasionally performed at the patient's bedside on the nursing unit, but they are more commonly performed in a special procedures room, often located within the surgical suite. These procedures require local anesthesia and appropriate sedation or general anesthesia. Patients may be sent to the PACU for a brief observation period. Care after endoscopy includes all the general care afforded a perianesthesia patient. After esophagoscopy and gastroscopy, the nurse should be alert for the return of the gag reflex. When pharyngeal reflexes have returned, the patient can start consuming liquids and then progress to a regular diet as tolerated unless contraindicated by diagnosis or in anticipation of further surgery. Rest is the most important treatment for this patient. Bleeding, swelling, or dysfunction of the involved area may occur and are indications of complications from the procedure.

Patients who have had laparoscopy have only bandages or tape strip closures (Steri-Strips) or tissue glue over the small incisions used for entry of the scope and its accessories. These bandages should remain clean and dry. The patients are probably apprehensive regarding discovery about conditions during the diagnostic procedure; the surgeon should give accurate information after the procedure. The nurse should be familiar with what the patients have been told regarding findings of the diagnostic laparoscopy so that information can be interpreted or repeated for the patient, if necessary.

CARE AFTER SURGERY ON THE GASTROINTESTINAL TRACT

Esophagus

Surgery on the esophagus includes repair of hiatal hernia and various forms of tracheoesophageal fistulas, excision of esophageal diverticula, treatment of stenosis of the lower end of the esophagus, esophagomyotomy, esophagectomy, and antireflux procedures.

Postoperative care depends on the kind of incision used to expose the operative site: abdominal, thoracic, or laparoscopic. Surgery on the esophagus frequently involves a thoracic incision. Care for the patient after a thoracic incision is discussed in Chapter 34. Procedures involving the esophagus are performed with general anesthesia.

On arrival to the PACU, the patient should be placed in a semi-Fowler position. This position aids in the drainage of blood from the pleural space and prevents tension from impinging on the suture lines. The incision is generally long (from the tip of the scapula to the seventh or eighth rib area) and painful. Analgesics must be given in adequate doses to promote rest and adequate respiratory effort. An interpleural or epidural catheter often is in place for postoperative analgesia. Patient-controlled analgesia may be used.

A nasogastric tube is in place and should be cared for as previously discussed. The nurse should not manipulate the tube. Chest tubes should be managed as discussed in Chapter 34. A large, sterile dressing should be in place and should be checked frequently for drainage and reinforced as necessary. Excessive bloody drainage should be reported to the surgeon.

Stomach

Surgery on the stomach involves procedures to treat the complications of ulcers (e.g., pyloroplasty, gastric resection, gastrectomy), removal of portions of the stomach for malignant disease, and rerouting of the gastrointestinal system at this point to treat pyloric obstruction. In addition, gastric restrictive procedures for the treatment of clinically severe obesity (bariatric surgery) are also performed commonly (see Chapter 45). These procedures can be conducted as both open and laparoscopic procedures. All postoperative care of the patient is generally the same, and anesthesia is general.

After surgery, the patient should be placed in a semi-Fowler position to relieve tension on the abdominal wall suture line, to prevent aspiration, and to promote drainage. When the patient's condition is hemodynamically stable, the obese patient (e.g. a patient requiring bariatric surgery) may benefit from positioning in a reverse Trendelenburg position at 45 degrees to maximize respiratory effort and decrease the effects of the abdominal weight interfering with adequate ventilatory effort. For open procedures, the abdominal incisions are fairly high, long, and painful; particular attention must be paid to pulmonary toilet. This patient must be encouraged more often than any other to expand the lungs and to cough and must generally have assistance to change position. Assistance in splinting the wound with the hands or with a firm pillow is usually appreciated by the patient. These procedures generally produce considerable postoperative pain, and analgesics should be used generously but judiciously. Patient-controlled or continuous epidural analgesia may be effective for upper abdominal incisional and visceral pain. Patients who have diagnosed or may have obstructive sleep apnea or obesity hypoventilation syndrome are extremely sensitive to opioid analgesics.[2] Cautious administration and vigilant monitoring are essential, especially in these patients, to avoid respiratory depression and complications.

A nasogastric tube is in place and should be cared for as discussed previously. Small volumes of bloody drainage from the nasogastric tube can be expected for the first 2 to 3 hours, because bleeding at the anastomotic site is common in these procedures. However, bright red bleeding that does not decrease after this period or bleeding that becomes excessive (more than 75 mL/h) should be reported immediately to the surgeon. Observe the nasogastric tube and its drainage closely, because blood easily clots and clogs the tube. Notify the surgeon immediately if the tube stops draining or appears obstructed with blood. Because blood loss can be highly significant in this patient, cardiovascular status must receive careful scrutiny. Vital signs are checked frequently. If hypotension and tachycardia persist or maintain a downward trend, the surgeon should be notified.

Blood replacement may have to be instituted. Hemoglobin and hematocrit levels should be determined 4 to 6 hours after surgery, and the surgeon should be notified if the levels are significantly lower than previous determinations. Little or no drainage should be expected from the incision unless drains are in place. If drainage appears, the dressing should be reinforced and the surgeon notified. The nurse in the PACU should not replace the initial dressing unless so directed by the surgeon. Drains with copious output may need a drainage device applied over them to protect the patient's skin and to allow for accurate measurement of drainage, but the surgeon should be notified first.

Urinary retention may be a problem after abdominal surgery if an indwelling balloon-tipped catheter is not in place. Accurate measurements of output should be ascertained. If a urinary catheter is not in place, the patient should be checked frequently for bladder distention, which can indicate an overfull bladder and urinary retention. If the patient is unable to void, a catheterization order should be obtained.

Perforated Ulcer

Perforation of an ulcer is usually a surgical emergency, and neither the patient nor the family members are adequately prepared, either physically or emotionally, for the surgery. This situation concerns the perianesthesia nurse because complications, especially hypovolemia and shock, may more readily occur in this patient.

Pyloric Stenosis

Specific care for infants after surgery for pyloric stenosis is detailed in pediatric nursing or medical textbooks. However, the perianesthesia nurse should be aware of general care. Position is important. The infant should be kept either on the right side or on the abdomen until the danger of vomiting and aspiration has subsided and then should be placed in an upright position. Careful placement of the diaper is important to avoid contamination of the wound. Application of a pediatric urine collector may also be helpful to prevent contamination of the wound with urine and to determine accurate output. Feedings are usually begun for these infants 4 to 6 hours after surgery, but the surgeon's instructions should be strictly followed.

Bariatric Gastric Surgery

After bariatric procedures, the nurse should also be aware of the risk of leaks that occur with anastomoses or staple lines on the stomach. Leaks may occur and can be fatal if unrecognized. Symptoms of leaks range from abdominal tenderness, left shoulder pain, tachycardia, decreased urine output, fever, elevated white blood cell counts, oxygen desaturation, or a patient's anxiety (e.g., sense of impending doom). It is important to note that morbidly obese patients often do not manifest signs of intraabdominal catastrophe in expected ways; often tachycardia is the only sign. The surgeon should be notified immediately if any of these signs or symptoms occur. See Chapter 45 for a detailed discussion on bariatric surgical procedures and care.

Small Bowel

Operations on the small bowel include exploratory laparotomy with lysis of adhesions and resection for obstruction or perforation. Care after these procedures is essentially the same as that already mentioned. No excessive drainage from incisions should be noted unless drains have been placed. Fluid and electrolyte balance must be monitored carefully. Remember that the loss of sodium and bicarbonate ions is great, which results in imbalance, and that fluid losses during surgery may be significant, but fluid overload must be avoided.

The patient with an ileostomy enters the PACU with a bag in place over the stoma. The condition of the stoma should be pink and moist. Returns may be expected almost at once and should be recorded. Particular attention must be paid to this stoma, the drainage, and the collection device; no leakage onto the skin should be allowed because this causes significant skin irritation. Under the collection device, the peristomal skin is protected with a skin barrier that includes pectin-based and karaya-based wafers or paste.

Large Bowel

Surgery on the large bowel includes appendectomy, colostomy, various types of colonic resection for removal of tumors or correction of other problems, total proctocolectomy with ileostomy or ileoanal anastomosis (Fig. 40-3), and abdominoperineal resection with permanent colostomy (Fig. 40-4). Most of these surgical procedures are performed with general anesthesia. On return to

the PACU, patients are kept flat and on one side until the reflexes have returned; thcy may then assume a position of comfort unless otherwise specified by the surgeon. Specifically after abdominoperineal resection, patients should not have any direct pressure on their perineal wounds. Postoperative care is essentially the same as for small bowel surgery.

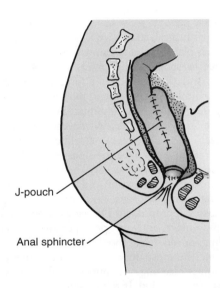

FIG. 40-3 Ileoanal anastomosis with J-pouch for treatment of ulcerative colitis. (From Black JM, Hokanson Hawks JH: *Medical-surgical nursing: clinical management for positive outcomes,* ed 8, St. Louis, 2008, Saunders.)

Evidence-Based Practice

Preoperative care for colorectal surgery has included mechanical bowel preparation and use of oral antibiotics to decrease the risk of septic complications. This review by the Cochrane Collaboration looked at all studies that compared any kind of mechanical bowel preparation with no preparation and mechanical bowel preparation with rectal enema. The review included 18 trials and determined that there were no statistically significant differences in the surgical outcomes of the three groups in leakage at surgical site of bowel, mortality rates, peritonitis, need for reoperation, wound infection, and other complications. They determined that there was no evidence that mechanical bowel preparation improves the outcome for patients and called for further research.

IMPLICATIONS FOR PRACTICE

When patients are undergoing colorectal surgery, there is no evidence to support the use of mechanical bowel preparation. The bowel cleaning can be omitted without compromising patient safety. Further study is warranted in these patients.

Source: Guenaga KF et al: Mechanical bowel preparation for elective colorectal surgery, *Cochrane Database Syst Rev* 1:CD001544, 2005.

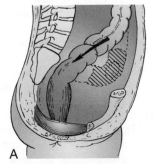 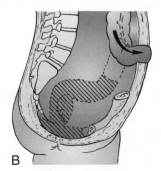 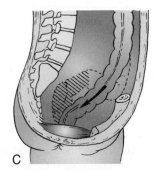

FIG. 40-4 Large bowel procedures for resection of malignant disease. **A,** Anterior resection with primary anastomosis. **B,** Abdominoperineal (anteroposterior) resection with permanent colostomy. **C,** Proctosigmoidectomy with "pull through." (From Black JM, Hokanson Hawks JH: *Medical-surgical nursing: clinical management for positive outcomes,* ed 8, St. Louis, 2008, Saunders.)

If the patient returns from surgery with a colostomy, some special care is required. The colostomy usually does not start functioning immediately after surgery; however, spillage must be prevented from contaminating the incision or excoriating the skin. A pouch or collection device will be in place over the colostomy. The skin around the stoma should be protected with an appropriate skin barrier if drainage is present. The color and appearance of the stoma (it should be pink and moist) should be assessed and documented in the nursing record.

Fluid and electrolyte balance must be monitored carefully. Some blood-tinged urine can be expected after colectomy, because retractors used in surgery may have caused contusions of the bladder; however, gross blood can indicate that the bladder was more severely injured. If ureteral catheters were used during surgery, this will also cause bloody urine. Dressings should remain dry unless drains were placed in the wound. If drains were placed, some bloody drainage may be expected, and dressings should be reinforced as necessary. Drainage that soaks through the dressings is considered excessive and must be reported to the surgeon.

Incisions may be left open to heal with delayed primary closure or secondary intent if there was significant contamination at the time of surgery. Abdominal wounds for bowel surgery may be contaminated (e.g., traumatic penetrating injuries, colostomies) with an increased risk of infection. For a delayed primary closure, the wound is left open, protected with moist gauze, and, when it is clean and red, closed with sutures that were placed during the original surgery and left slack. The cleanliness of the wound and the health of the granulation tissue in the wound generally determine the best time for closure.

Abdominoperineal Resection

Abdominoperineal resection for cancer of the rectum is a major procedure that results in permanent colostomy and two separate incisions (abdominal and perineal). Vital signs are monitored carefully, and any adverse trend is reported. Drains are usually left in place and should be noted on the patient's chart and nursing care plan. The perineal dressings often become saturated with bloody drainage and must be reinforced. If drainage remains bright and obviously new bleeding occurs, and if frequent dressing changes are necessary, the surgeon should be notified. If sump catheters are used to drain the perineal wound, they may be attached to a grenade or bulb drainage device and an accurate measurement of drainage may be obtained. The perineal drains may be brought out from the perineum directly or the abdomen, depending on surgeon preference.

The patient who has undergone abdominoperineal surgery has a colostomy. Check the blood supply to the stoma frequently because impaired blood supply is an early and serious complication. Pain may be severe and should be relieved with adequate doses of opioid analgesics or use of epidural analgesia to ensure comfort of the patient and promote respiratory sufficiency.

Appendectomy and Herniorrhaphy

Patients who have undergone surgery for appendectomy or herniorrhaphy usually return to the PACU almost fully awake and without serious postoperative complications. Generally, no nasogastric tube, indwelling urinary catheter, or drain is in place, and recovery is generally uneventful. However, patients who have large ventral hernia repairs with mesh may have nasogastric tubes and drains in place. Patients can assume a position of comfort as soon as pharyngeal reflexes have returned, and they can start a progressive diet as tolerated unless a nasogastric tube is in place. All the postoperative care outlined in Chapters 26 through 31 is applicable. When the laparoscopic approach is used, general anesthesia usually is given. Patients may have shoulder pain or bloating because of insufflation of air. They may also have sore throat from intubation and the neuromuscular blocking agents. Monitor fluid intake and replace fluid losses appropriately. Dressings should remain dry and intact, and any postoperative incisional bleeding or drainage should be reported to the surgeon. The most important postoperative complication is bleeding. The nurse should also watch for urinary retention. If the patient has undergone inguinal hernia repair, the nurse should watch for development of scrotal edema or hematoma, which may indicate slow bleeding from the operative site.

Lower Rectum and Anus

Surgery on the lower rectum and anus includes excision of pilonidal cysts, rectal fissures, fistulas, rectal abscesses, tumors, and hemorrhoids. Perianesthesia nursing care is the same as for any patient who undergoes local, regional, or general anesthesia. Dressings should be checked frequently for excessive drainage and bleeding. The incisions may be closed, but often are packed to facilitate drainage of infected material and aid in healing. Urinary retention can be a problem because the proximity of the bladder and operative site can make urination difficult. Pain can be severe, but patients are often embarrassed by the location of the operative site and might not ask for analgesia. The nurse should be alert to signs and symptoms of pain and discomfort and administer analgesia as necessary for relief.

SURGERY ON RELATED ORGANS WITHIN THE ABDOMINAL CAVITY

Liver

Surgery on the liver includes biopsy, excision of tumors, major resection, repair of traumatic lacerations, and liver transplant.

Percutaneous liver biopsy is a common procedure that is usually performed in the endoscopy suite, although the patient may be taken to the operating suite and may return to the PACU for a short period of observation. Postoperative care depends on the type of anesthesia used; anesthesia is usually local, but may involve other types if the patient cannot or will not cooperate. The patient should remain positioned on the right side for at least 2 hours after the procedure. Vital signs should be determined frequently: every 10 to 15 minutes for the first hour and every 30 minutes for the second hour. Complications include hemorrhage from penetration of a blood vessel and peritonitis from accidental puncture of the biliary tree. If the patient's vital signs begin a downward trend or if the patient reports severe abdominal pain or becomes febrile, the surgeon should be notified immediately.

Open or laparoscopic surgery on the liver for the excision of tumors or the repair of lacerations is done with general anesthesia and, if open, involves a fairly long upper abdominal vertical or bilateral subcostal oblique (chevron) incision. Liver transplantation may be indicated in patients with end-stage liver disease, fulminant acute liver failure, hepatocellular carcinoma, and pediatric metabolic liver diseases when a patient meets established criteria.[3] The transplanted liver may be from a living donor or cadaver. All care previously discussed for patients after general anesthesia and upper abdominal incisions applies. Respiratory care is of paramount importance. The liver is an extremely vascular organ. It is difficult to suture; gross bleeding is common and often involves large blood losses, especially when surgery is necessitated by traumatic injury or large resection. Large drains of the suction (grenade or bulb) type are placed in the region of the laceration or excision of the tumor and are brought through separate sites to the skin surface. For the first 8 hours, expect approximately 100 to 250 mL of serosanguineous drainage from the drains.

Coagulation studies must be performed frequently and monitored closely, because many patients have coagulation abnormalities that develop during and after liver surgery. Specific coagulation factors may be administered, according to the results of the coagulation tests. Phosphate levels must also be monitored closely after major liver resection.

Vital signs must be assessed frequently, and any downward trend should be reported to the surgeon at once. Blood replacement or hemostasis may be inadequate. Rapid infusions of fluid replacements may be needed, especially after extensive liver resection or transplant. Occasionally, this patient also has a T-tube in place in the common bile duct (Fig. 40-5). This tube should be attached to straight-gravity drainage, and accurate measurements of the output should be made. A nasogastric tube is often in place and should receive care as discussed previously. Pain may be severe, and opioid analgesics or epidural analgesia are necessary to promote rest and respiratory effort.

Spleen

Surgery on the spleen involves general anesthesia and removal of the organ, with either an open or laparoscopic technique. The spleen is removed because of rupture from trauma; accidental trauma from associated surgery; diseases that cause damage, such as mononucleosis and malaria; a variety of hematologic diseases; left-sided portal hypertension; and hypersplenism. If the procedure is done with an open technique, a midline or left subcostal incision is used. Postoperative care for

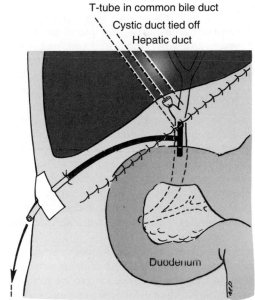

T-tube in common bile duct
Cystic duct tied off
Hepatic duct

Duodenum

To drainage collection

FIG. 40-5 T-tube placement in common bile duct. (From Black JM, Hokanson Hawks JH: *Medical-surgical nursing: clinical management for positive outcomes*, ed 7, St. Louis, 2005, Saunders.)

NURSING CARE IN THE PACU

the patient after splenectomy is the same as that for the patient after repair of a lacerated liver. Dressings should remain dry and intact. A drain may be placed in the subdiaphragmatic space to prevent the collection of blood under the diaphragm and to detect unrecognized injury to the pancreas that may have occurred.

The perianesthesia nurse should know the circumstances that lead to the patient's splenectomy. If it was necessitated by trauma, the nurse must be particularly alert for signs that indicate development of unrecognized complications from the accident. Vital signs should be determined frequently, and trends should be watched, especially those that indicate progressive bleeding. Neurologic signs should be checked, and the patient should be assessed carefully for any signs of injury to the extremities. Any dysrhythmia should be reported, because it can indicate cardiac injury.

Pancreas

Surgery on the pancreas is difficult and technically demanding. It involves general anesthesia, and care for these patients is the same as for other postoperative patients.

Postoperative care of the patient after a pancreaticoduodenectomy (Whipple procedure) requires particular attention to drains and catheters. All postoperative care for the abdominal surgery patient applies. Surgeons should augment their reports to the nurse by explaining exactly what procedure was performed, where drains or wound catheters were placed, and how to care for them. Surgeons should brief the nurse on expected drainage and what should be considered excessive. As with all abdominal surgeries, intravenous lines and intravenous therapy have already been initiated.

All respiratory, cardiac, and renal functioning must be monitored carefully, and the surgeon should be notified of any untoward signs. If frequent arterial blood gas analysis is needed for this patient, an arterial line should be in place for this purpose. Blood gas analysis yields valuable information about the patient's respiratory acid-base status. Urine output should be determined hourly, and at least 0.5 to 1 mL/kg/h should be expected.

Frequent assays of blood glucose levels should be ordered for all patients after pancreatic surgery. Most of these patients need to receive intravenous insulin during the postoperative period. Generally, insulin doses are titrated to maintain the blood glucose levels between 140 and 180 mg/dL in the critical care setting and at less than 140 mg/dL in the noncritical care setting.[4] The insulin aids in preventing hyperglycemia.

Large fluctuations in serum glucose levels or acid-base balance can precipitate electrolyte abnormalities in these patients. Potassium and calcium levels, in particular, should be monitored closely.

Biliary Tract

Surgery on the biliary tract includes exploration for removal of stones from the gallbladder and the ducts and removal of the gallbladder. It can also include repair of biliary tract injuries and resection for malignant disease or benign strictures. Anesthesia is general, regional, or a combined technique. For cholecystectomy, the procedure is performed with a laparoscope, the

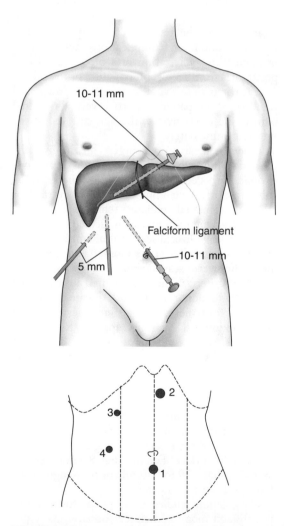

FIG. 40-6 Placement of laparoscope and instrument ports for laparoscopic cholecystectomy. (Redrawn from Malt RA: *The practice of surgery,* Philadelphia, 1993, Saunders.)

patient has an umbilical incision and three small subcostal incisions for instruments (Fig. 40-6); if performed open, the incision is either a right subcostal or a midline incision. On return to the PACU, the patient is placed in a semi-Fowler position. All tubes must be cared for appropriately. A nasogastric tube is typically placed during surgery and is often removed when the operative procedure ends. A T-tube is placed in the common bile duct if the common duct was opened during surgery. This tube is usually connected to straight-gravity drainage to a bile bag. Careful attention must be paid to maintaining the patency of this tube and its attachment to the patient; the surgeon needs to be called immediately if the tube is dislodged.

Bile drainage should be carefully measured and accurately reported. Between 200 and 500 mL of bile drainage can be expected within a 24-hour period. Dressings should remain dry and intact and should be reinforced as necessary to keep the surrounding skin dry.

As with all upper abdominal incisions, pain is a challenge, and analgesics (intermittent, continuous, or patient-controlled), epidural analgesia, and relaxation exercises should be used to promote rest and respiratory effort. Any downward trend in vital signs, excessive bleeding from the incision, or bleeding noted in the bile drainage from the T-tube should be reported to the surgeon. Bleeding from the cystic artery is a rare but serious complication and can lead to hemodynamic deterioration in the patient.

After laparoscopic cholecystectomy, the patient may have one of the most stable conditions of any seen in the PACU. Any patient with unexplained pain, oliguria, or hypotension should be immediately discussed with the surgeon. Complications of gas embolism, deep vein thrombophlebitis, subcutaneous emphysema, injuries to major vessels and intestine, and bile leakage all have been reported after laparoscopic procedures. Right shoulder pain is often experienced because of the referred pain from a nerve running up from the diaphragm; however, this resolves fully within 72 hours.

SUMMARY

This chapter discussed the care involved after surgery on the gastrointestinal tract, including the esophagus and the anus, and the accessory organs: the liver, gallbladder, pancreas, and spleen. Surgery on the female reproductive organs, which are also contained within the abdominal cavity, is reviewed in Chapter 42. The care common to all patients undergoing abdominal surgery was discussed, and only the most important variations related to specific procedures were included.

REFERENCES

1. Altman GB, et al: *Fundamental and advanced nursing skills*, ed 3, Clifton Park, NY, 2010, Delmar.
2. Gross JB, et al: Practice guidelines for the perioperative management of patients with obstructive sleep apnea: a report by the American Society of Anesthesiologists Task Force on Perioperative Management of patients with obstructive sleep apnea, *Anesthesiology*, 104(5):1081-1093; 2006.
3. DuBay DA, Sung RS: Liver transplantation. In Minter RM, Doherty GM: *Current procedures: surgery*, available at www.accesssurgery.com.proxy.lib.umich.edu/content.aspx?aID=6563318. Accessed January 5, 2012.
4. Moghissi ES, et al: American Association of Clinical Endocrinologists and American Diabetes Association consensus statement on inpatient glycemic control, *Endocr Prac* 15(4):353-369, 2009.

RESOURCES

Black JM, Hokanson Hawks JH: *Medical-surgical nursing: clinical management for positive outcomes*, ed 8, Philadelphia, 2009, Saunders.
O'Brien D: Gastrointestinal Care. In Schick L, Windle PE: *Perianesthesia nursing core curriculum: preprocedure phase I and phase II PACU nursing*, ed 2, St. Louis, 2010, Saunders.
Nagelhout J, Plaus K: *Handbook of nurse anesthesia*, ed 4, St. Louis, 2010, Saunders.
Rothrock JC: *Alexander's care of the patient in surgery*, ed 14, St. Louis, 2011, Mosby.
Townsend CM, et al: *Sabiston textbook of surgery: the biological basis of modern surgical practice*, ed 18, Philadelphia, 2008, Saunders.

NURSING CARE IN THE PACU

41 Care of the Genitourinary Surgical Patient

Candace N. Taylor, BSN, RN, CPAN

Genitourinary surgery involves procedures performed on the kidneys, ureters, bladder, urethra, and male genitalia. The genitourinary system can be the host of multiple problems, either congenital or acquired. In caring for patients undergoing genitourinary surgeries, the perianesthesia nurse should have an understanding of anatomic location and normal function of this system. Adrenalectomy is included in this chapter for convenience and because of the proximity of the adrenal glands to the kidneys.

DEFINITIONS

Adrenalectomy: Partial or total excision of one or both adrenal glands.

Bladder Neck Operation (Y-V Plasty): A plastic repair of the bladder neck for correction of stricture.

Chordee: Downward bowing of the penis as a result of congenital malformation or hypospadias with fibrous bands.

Circumcision: Excision of the foreskin (prepuce) of the glans penis.

Cystectomy: Excision of the bladder and adjacent structures; may be partial (excision of a lesion) or total (excision of a malignant tumor). This operation usually involves the additional procedure of ureterostomy.

Cystolithotomy: Opening of the bladder for removal of stones.

Cystoscopy: Direct visualization of the urethra, prostatic urethra, and bladder by means of a tubular lighted telescopic lens.

Cystotomy: An incision into the bladder.

Epididymectomy: Excision of the epididymis from the testis. This procedure is rarely done but may occasionally be indicated for treatment of persistent infection.

Epispadias: Urethral meatus situated in an abnormal position on the upper side of the penis. Surgical correction involves plastic repair.

Extracorporeal Shock Wave Lithotripsy: Use of shock waves through a liquid medium into the body to disintegrate stones.

Heminephrectomy: Partial excision of the kidney.

Hydrocelectomy: Excision of the tunica vaginalis of the testis for removal of a hydrocele (a fluid-filled sac).

Hypospadias: A deformity of the penis and malformation of the urethral wall in which the urinary meatus is located on the underside of the penis, either short of its normal position at the tip of the glans or on the perineum or scrotum. This condition

is often associated with chordee. Surgical correction involves plastic repair; penile straightening and urethral reconstruction (urethroplasty) are usually done in two or more stages.

Intravenous Pyelogram: A radiologic procedure in which intravenous dye is injected to assist in the visualization of renal structure. This procedure is used to diagnose abnormalities and look for blockages.

Kidney Transplant: Removal of a donor kidney with nephrectomy and ureterectomy, followed by transplantation of the donor kidney into the recipient's iliac fossa.

Nephrectomy: Removal of a kidney; used in treatment of some congenital unilateral abnormalities that cause renal obstruction or hydronephrosis; sometimes necessitated by the presence of tumors or severe injuries.

Nephrostomy: An opening into the kidney for temporary or permanent drainage.

Nephrotomy: An incision into the kidney.

Nephroureterectomy: Removal of a kidney and the entire ureter that drains it.

Orchiectomy: Removal of the testis or testes. This procedure renders the patient sterile.

Orchiopexy: Suspension of the testis within the scrotum. This procedure is used in the treatment of an undescended or cryptorchid testis to bring it into the normal intrascrotal position.

Penile Implant: A penile prosthesis implanted for treatment of organic sexual impotence.

Percutaneous Nephrolithotomy: Removal or disintegration of renal stones with passage of a nephroscope through a percutaneous nephrostomy tract.

Phimosis: Tightness of the foreskin so that it cannot be drawn back from over the glans; also, the analogous condition in the clitoris.

Prostatectomy: Enucleation of prostatic adenomas or hypertrophied masses.

Pyeloplasty: Revision or reconstruction of the renal pelvis.

Pyelostomy: An incision into the renal pelvis for drainage or for irrigation of the renal pelvis.

Pyelotomy: Incision into the renal pelvis.

Radical Prostatectomy: Common surgical treatment for prostate cancer in young men where the entire prostate is removed.

Spermatocelectomy: The removal of a spermatocele, which usually appears as a cystic mass within the scrotum, attached to the upper pole of the epididymis. A spermatocele is usually caused by an obstruction of the tubular system that conveys the sperm.

Transurethral Surgery: Piecemeal resection of the prostate gland and of tumors of the bladder and bladder neck and fulguration of bleeding vessels and of tumors with a resectoscope passed into the bladder via the urethra.

Urethral sling: Midurethral sling used as treatment for stress incontinence. A piece of mesh is introduced along the midurethral section using an introducer through either a retropubic approach or a vaginal approach.

Ureterectomy: Complete removal of one or both of the ureters.

Ureterolithotomy: Incision into the ureter and removal of stones.

Ureteroneocystostomy (Ureterovesical Anastomosis; Vesicopsoas Hitch Procedure): Division of the ureter from the urinary bladder and reimplantation of the ureter into the bladder at another site.

Ureteroplasty: Reconstruction of the ureter.

Ureteroscopy: Direct visualization of the ureters and upper urinary tract with the use of a lighted semirigid scope that passes through the urethra and bladder.

Ureterostomy, Cutaneous (Anastomosis of Transplant; Bricker Operation; Ureteroileostomy): Diversion of the urinary stream with anastomosis of the ureters into an isolated loop of ileum that is brought out through the abdominal wall as an ileostomy.

Urethral Dilatation and Internal Urethrotomy: Gradual dilation of the urethra and lysis of a urethral stricture.

Urethral Meatotomy: Incisional enlargement of the external urethral meatus for relief of stenosis or stricture.

Urethroplasty: Reconstructive surgery of the urethra.

Urethrovesical Suspension (Pubovaginal Slings): Suspension of the urethra with a permanent polypropylene mesh tape for the treatment of stress incontinence.

Varicocelectomy: Ligation and partial excision of dilated veins in the scrotum.

Vasectomy: Excision of a section of the vas deferens. This procedure is performed electively for birth control or before prostatectomy to prevent the spread of infection from the urethra to the epididymis.

Vasoepididymostomy: Anastomosis of the vas deferens to the epididymis.

Vasovasostomy: Anastomosis of two separate segments of the vas deferens for reversal of a vasectomy.

Vesicourethral Suspension: Suspension of the bladder neck to the posterior surface of the pubis in women for treatment of stress incontinence.

NURSING CARE AFTER DIAGNOSTIC PROCEDURES

Although there is an increase in the use of noninvasive diagnostic procedure, several invasive diagnostic procedures are performed on patients with genitourinary disease. If patients require monitored anesthesia care (MAC), spinal anesthesia, or general anesthesia, they are admitted to the postanesthesia care unit (PACU) for postanesthesia care.

Renal Angiography

For a renal angiographic examination, a small catheter is threaded through the femoral artery into the aorta or renal artery, radiopaque dye is instilled, and radiographs are made.[1] Local anesthesia is usually all that is needed; however, general anesthesia may be used for children or patients who cannot cooperate during the procedure. When the patient is admitted to the PACU, the groin area is inspected for bleeding at the site. A pressure-type dressing usually is present and can be replaced with a simple bandage after a few hours. Pedal pulses should be checked to ensure that no interruption of blood supply to the extremities has occurred. Urine output should be measured and closely monitored for hematuria. Special attention should be considered for the patient with renal insufficiency or renal failure. If possible, the leg should be kept straight. Fluids should be encouraged to facilitate excretion of the dye.[2]

Renal Biopsy

Renal biopsy is usually performed at the bedside with only local anesthesia, although general anesthesia may be used for children. The patient should maintain bed rest in a flat supine position for as long as 4 hours. Some physicians ask for the patients with a previous transplant to maintain a side lying or prone position. Pillows can be used for positioning for comfort and to decrease the risk of skin breakdown. Vital signs are monitored, and the site of the biopsy is checked for bleeding. Coughing and other activities that increase abdominal venous pressure should be avoided. Fluids should be increased to 3000 mL daily, and the urine should be observed for occult blood.[3]

Cystoscopy

Diagnostic cystoscopy can be performed in a special procedures room with only local anesthesia and appropriate sedation.[1] Children and patients who cannot or do not tolerate the procedure may need general anesthesia. This procedure can also be performed with spinal anesthesia.

On admission to the PACU, the patient is positioned to ensure airway patency if general anesthesia was used.[4] The patient may have to lie flat on the back if spinal anesthesia was used, with a gradual increase in the head of bed if tolerated and allowed by physician orders. After the effects of anesthesia have been eliminated, the patient may assume a position of comfort. The patient may have back pain, a feeling of bladder fullness, and bladder spasms. These symptoms may become severe enough to necessitate analgesia. Belladonna and opium suppositories or intravenous opioids may be administered to relieve patient discomfort as prescribed by the surgeon.[2,3]

Oral fluid administration should be encouraged and started as soon as the effects of anesthesia are gone. Urine output should be monitored carefully. The patient can expect frequency of urination and a burning sensation because of trauma to the mucous membranes from the procedure; this condition may inadvertently cause voluntary retention.[2,3] The urine may be pink tinged for several voidings, which is to be expected. Bright blood or clots in the urine, however, should be reported to the surgeon. Severe abdominal pain should be reported because it can indicate accidental urethral or bladder perforation or internal hemorrhage.[5]

The patient should be observed for signs of sepsis, because infection may spread throughout the urinary tract or into the blood stream after a cystoscopy. If symptoms of sepsis, such as chills, tachycardia, tachypnea, flushing, and temperature elevation, are noted, the surgeon should be notified.

GENERAL POSTOPERATIVE CARE

Assessment of the patient after genitourinary surgery involves particular attention to fluid and electrolyte balance. Intake and output records are especially important and must be accurately maintained. Postoperative care is directed primarily at urinary tract function, which is second in importance only to cardiorespiratory function. Maintenance of patency of the urinary tract often depends on the use of catheters, which come in a variety of shapes and sizes (Fig. 41-1).

Urethral catheters are used to drain urine from the bladder for decompression and accurate measurement of urine output. An indwelling catheter may be used after surgery and left in place until the patient's condition is stable and the surgeon orders its removal. The catheter is attached to a sterile, closed gravitational-drainage collection system. The urine collection reservoir may be a large (usually 2000 mL) container or a small calibrated chamber that can be emptied into a large reservoir after timed urine output volumes have been determined and recorded.

The catheter should be anchored securely to the patient's thigh with a leg strap and locking device with the tubing brought over the leg. The catheter should be secured to prevent undue tension on the urinary meatus. The connecting tubing should be attached to the bed linens so that no proximal loops of tubing lie below the distal tubing; this is a straight gravity drainage system. The tubing should never be under the patient, because compression of the tubing obstructs the flow of urine. The tubing should be checked frequently for kinks. The urine receptacle should

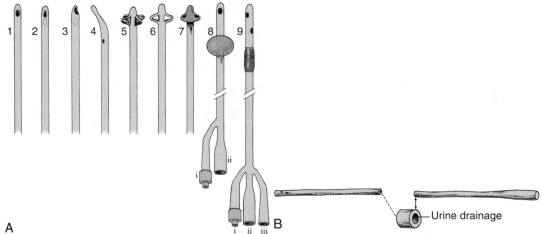

FIG. 41-1 **A,** Types of large-diameter catheters. *1,* Conical tip urethral catheter, one eye. *2,* Robinson urethral catheter. *3,* Whistle-tip urethral catheter. *4,* Coudé hollow olive-tip catheter. *5,* Malecot self-retaining, four-wing urethral catheter. *6,* Malecot self-retaining, two-wing catheter. *7,* Pezzer self-retaining drain, open-end head, used for cystotomy drainage. *8,* Foley-type balloon catheter, one limb of distal end for balloon inflation *(i),* one for drainage *(ii).* *9,* Foley-type, three-way balloon catheter, one limb of distal end for balloon inflation *(i),* one for drainage *(ii),* and one to infuse irrigating solution to prevent clot retention within the bladder *(iii).* **B,** Straight catheter. (**A,** From Canale ST, Beaty JH: *Campbell's operative orthopaedics,* ed 11, St. Louis, 2008, Mosby. **B,** From Potter PA, Perry AG: *Fundamentals of nursing,* ed 7, St. Louis, 2009, Mosby.)

always be kept below the bladder level to prevent urine reflux up the tubing. Particular attention must be paid to this principle during the transfer of patients.

For collection of a urine specimen from the closed system, a sterile syringe and needle are used. Some catheters have a small, specially constructed port from which to draw specimens. On those catheters that do not have such a port, the distal part of the catheter, close to the drainage tube, is used. The area is cleansed with alcohol or povidone-iodine (Betadine), the needle inserted, and a specimen withdrawn.

Mucus or blood, or both, can clog the tubing and prevent urine flow. Irrigations should be administered only according to the surgeon's orders. All irrigations are sterile procedures and can be either continuous or intermittent. For intermittent irrigation, a large sterile Toomey syringe and sterile irrigating solution (usually normal saline solution alone or with a selected antibiotic) are used. Care must be taken to keep all parts of the drainage system sterile. This action may be accomplished by placing a small sterile plastic cover on the drainage tubing while the irrigation is performed. Irrigations should never be given with pressure. When the bladder is irrigated, no more than 30 mL should be instilled at one time, unless ordered otherwise by the surgeon.[1]

After transurethral resection of the prostate (TURP), continuous irrigation is usually preferred. With continuous irrigation, normal saline solution is typically connected with a three-way urinary catheter. Nursing care should include vigilant monitoring of patients for hyponatremia and the development of TURP syndrome.[6] The report from the perioperative nurse should include the amount of intraoperative irrigation and the duration of the procedure. During the immediate postanesthesia phase, patient confusion should be monitored and differentiated from confusion as a result of amnesiacs, opioids, or hyponatremia (see also the Prostatic Surgery section in this chapter).

If hyponatremia is diagnosed, treatment may include the administration of hypertonic saline solution for a gradual increase in the patient's serum sodium level. Care includes monitoring for signs of intracellular to extracellular fluid shifts. As fluid moves back into the extracellular space, pulmonary edema and heart failure can occur quickly.[6]

Suprapubic Catheters

Suprapubic catheters are used to drain residual urine from the bladder. A temporary catheter can be placed into the urinary bladder via a stab

wound through the lower abdomen and into the anterior bladder wall. The catheter is sutured in place, and a dressing is applied (usually a type of dressing that allows direct observation of the puncture site). The catheter is connected to a straight gravitational drainage system. Care of the suprapubic catheter is similar to that of the urinary catheter. The catheter should be taped securely with a loop made to prevent tension on the bladder wall or the abdomen. The skin around the puncture site should be kept clean and dry. The catheter tubing should be checked periodically for kinks and to ensure that the stopcock valve is open to allow the urine to drain from the bladder.

A suprapubic catheter can also be placed into the urinary bladder via abdominal incision and cystostomy.[1] This procedure is typically done for more permanent or long-term use of the suprapubic catheter. The surgeon may choose this method if conventional methods of treatment for urinary incontinence fail, as with spinal cord injury or neurogenic bladder. The care of the catheter is the same as with the puncture wound, but the nurse should also apply nursing care that relates to the abdominal incision.

Ureteral Catheters

Ureteral catheters are used to drain urine or splint the ureters while they heal. The catheters can be placed through the urethra or through abdominal or flank incisions.[1] Care of these catheters is essentially the same as that for urethral catheters. Attention to patency must be especially meticulous because the renal pelvis can hold only 5 mL without overdistention and damage to the kidneys.[1,2]

Sterile irrigations are undertaken only as ordered by the physician. Only 5 mL of fluid should be used for the irrigation via gravitational flow. Irrigations should never be given with pressure, such as with a syringe and plunger. The nurse must be sure to avoid situations that can cause dislodgement or displacement of these catheters, which could be disastrous to the outcome of the surgery. Special care must be taken during patient transfer to ensure that these catheters stay in place. One person should be assigned this responsibility during the transfer. If the catheters should become dislodged despite all the precautions taken, the surgeon must be notified immediately.[1,5]

Intake

Optimal fluid intake is exceptionally important for the patient after surgery; increased fluids are the general rule. Fluids should be given orally if the patient can tolerate this preferred route, and intake should be increased to total of 3000 mL in a 24-hour period. Special consideration regarding type and amount of fluids should be taken with any patient with renal insufficiency. Parenteral fluid therapy is indicated for a short time until the effects of anesthesia have passed and is continued only if the oral route of intake is inadequate.[2,4]

Dressings

Care of dressings varies according to the procedure and can include anything from a bulky dressing to Steri-Strips or bandages. Dressings applied after urinary tract surgery often become soaked with blood and urine. They should be reinforced as necessary, and the surrounding skin should be kept clean and dry to prevent unnecessary excoriation and breakdown.[3] (Excessive staining that is unexpected for a particular procedure and indicates a complication is so indicated in the discussion of the specific procedure later in this chapter.) Excessive bleeding and hemorrhage are ever-present dangers of this surgery, because the kidneys and prostatic bed are extremely vascular. Vital signs must be monitored closely, and all avenues of output, especially the incisions and drainage tubes, should be evaluated frequently for bleeding.[2,3]

Abdominal Distention

All patients should be assessed for abdominal distention after surgery that involves abdominal and flank incisions (see Chapter 40 for care of the patient after an abdominal incision because the same care applies after genitourinary surgery). These patients often arrive with nasogastric tubes, the care for which is discussed in Chapter 40. In addition, the patient should be assessed for distention caused by overfilling of the bladder because of an inability to void or a malfunction of the catheters.

Bladder ultrasound scan is a noninvasive method to assess bladder volume for determining bladder distention or postvoid residual urine. This portable battery-operated device can be used at the bedside as a noninvasive replacement to intermittent catheterization (Fig. 41-2). This painless procedure eliminates discomfort, embarrassment, and risks associated with catheterization. Data from the bladder ultrasound scan can be printed and become part of the patient's chart. Depending on the volume and whether the patient is capable of voiding, straight catheterization should be performed to relieve urinary retention; this procedure is typically done with volumes greater that 300 mL. A bladder ultrasound scan can be repeated as necessary and has been shown to decrease the risk of urinary tract infections associated with intermittent catheterization.[7]

Evidence-Based Practice

In looking at urinary retention after spinal anesthesia, Feliciano and colleagues performed a retrospective, descriptive, exploratory study. This study evaluated incidence of postoperative urinary retention (POUR) and how it affects the length of stay (LOS) as well as the characteristics of POUR. A log of patients receiving spinal anesthesia was kept and reviewed for patient inclusion in the study. Of the 102 charts reviewed, complete data was available for 90 patients who met inclusion criteria that included 18 years of age or older, having spinal anesthesia only, and admission to the postanesthesia care unit (PACU) without an indwelling catheter. The incidence of POUR in the study facility was found to be 44.1%. Patients with POUR averaged a longer LOS by 26 minutes. POUR was defined as urine greater than 500 mL of bladder volume upon admission with inability to void for 30 minutes or longer. Complications of POUR include damage to the detrusor muscle and ischemia, increased vulnerability to urinary tract infections from high bladder pressures, tachycardia, and hypertension.

IMPLICATIONS FOR PRACTICE

Nursing assessment should include assessing for POUR. This can be accomplished with the use of a noninvasive bladder scan at the bedside. By instituting a protocol for assessment of POUR, the patient physically and psychologically benefits with a decrease in LOS in the PACU, patient comfort, and prevention of complications of bladder distention.

Source: Feliciano T, et al: A retrospective, descriptive, exploratory study evaluating incidence of postoperative urinary retention after spinal anesthesia and its effect of PACU discharge, *J Perianesth Nurs* 23(6):94-400, 2008.

Management of Discomfort and Pain

Discomfort after genitourinary surgery can be relieved with the administration of opioids, including intravenous morphine or fentanyl, belladonna, and opium suppositories. In the outpatient setting, the nurse may consider using oral medications such as oxycodone and hydrocodone. Nonsteroidal antiinflammatory drugs (NSAIDs) should also be considered.[8] The physiology of the need to void should be explained to the patient before surgery. The patient should be instructed not to attempt to void around the catheter, because exertion of pressure causes the bladder muscles to contract and results in painful bladder spasms. The avoidance of straining around the catheter and of intake of excessive fluids decreases bladder irritability and spasms. As the nerve endings become fatigued, the frequency and severity of the spasms diminish.

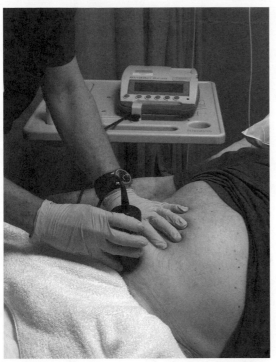

FIG. 41-2 Using a bladder scanner to determine amount of urine in the bladder. (From deWit S: *Fundamental concepts and skills for nursing,* ed 3, St. Louis, 2009, Saunders.)

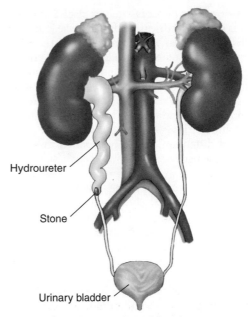

FIG. 41-3 Hydroureter is caused by obstruction in the lower part of the ureter. (From Leonard PC: *Building a medical vocabulary,* ed 8, St. Louis, 2012, Saunders.)

NURSING CARE AFTER SPECIFIC PROCEDURES

Renal and Ureteral Surgery

Procedures that involve the kidneys and ureters include excision of tumors and obstructions to urine flow (e.g., stones), reconstruction of urine outflow tracts, repair of lacerations, correction of deformities, excision of a kidney, and total organ transplant.

General anesthesia is commonly used for surgery on the kidneys and ureters. The kidneys are usually approached posteriorly through an incision that requires resection of the 11th or 12th rib. The surgical approach to the ureters is made through muscle-splitting flank incisions (Fig. 41-3).[1,5] The perianesthesia course for these patients is usually smooth and involves general care and maintenance of urinary tract function. The patient should be placed in a position that avoids tension on suture lines or as indicated by the surgeon.

All surgical patients are at risk for fluid volume deficit from the intake restrictions before surgery and from the decreased intake after surgery, possibly related to postoperative nausea or vomiting.[2,3] Maintenance of exceptionally accurate intake and output records is important. Low urine output should be reported to the surgeon.

Dressings should remain dry and intact unless drains are used, in which case dressings should be weighed when they are removed to determine output via this route. With the determination of output from the dressings, the dressings should be weighed before application and again at removal and the difference subtracted (1 g equals 1 mL of output). Patients with drains or stomas may need a small plastic bag over the area to collect drainage that consists primarily of urine. Drainage bags should be emptied frequently. If the bags are allowed to fill to capacity, the continual flow of urine is interrupted.

Skin care for these patients is important. Urine should not be allowed to remain on the skin. Plain water should be used to cleanse the skin, which should be carefully dried. No powders, lotions, or harsh skin preparations should be applied to the skin. If a ureteroileostomy has been performed, the stoma must be inspected frequently to ensure adequate vascularization. If skin turns a bluish hue, the surgeon should be notified immediately.[2]

NURSING CARE IN THE PACU

A urinary catheter is often in place and receives care as previously discussed. Fluid intake is increased both orally and parenterally to keep blood clots from forming in the ureters or bladder. Intestinal decompression may be necessary and is accomplished via nasogastric tube (see Chapter 40). Decompression is essential when an ileal conduit procedure (ureterostomy) is performed to allow healing of the intestinal anastomosis (Fig. 41-4).[3,5] Any evidence of abdominal distention should be reported to the surgeon immediately.

Extracorporeal Shock Wave Lithotripsy

After extracorporeal shock wave lithotripsy, the patient may be admitted to the PACU for a brief period of observation.[5] Vital signs should be monitored as with any renal or ureteral surgery. Fluids should be increased, and intake and output monitored carefully. Initially, the color of the urine may be cherry red to pink because of trauma from surgery; this condition may take several hours to clear. Petechiae, redness, and bruising may be seen on the skin at the site of lithotripsy. This petechiae should be documented by the perianesthesia nurse on assessment in the PACU. The patient may have pain from the force of the shock waves. This pain is usually localized to the skin and may be relieved with ice packs. Renal colic pain may also be experienced as the fragments of pulverized stones pass through the lower urinary tract.[2]

Ureteroscopy

Since the 1980s, rigid ureteroscopy has been used for the removal of distal ureteral calculi.[1] Today, flexible and rigid ureteroscopy are used for the diagnosis and treatment of stones, fulguration of epithelial tumors, analysis of gross hematuria, and management of ureteral strictures.[1] Complications are rare but include perforation of the ureter; therefore close observation of color and amount of urine output should be maintained. All urine should be strained, and any calculous fragments should be collected for inspection and identification. Ureteral stents are commonly placed during this procedure to facilitate urine flow and prevent obstruction or ureteral colic caused by edema.[1] If the surgeon has elected to externalize the stent suture, patients should be educated on its care.

Percutaneous Nephrolithotomy

Large stones that are not easily removed with ureteroscopy can be removed through a percutaneous tract into the renal collecting system. Local anesthesia or moderate sedation is used to establish the percutaneous nephrostomy tract with the guidance of fluoroscopy or ultrasound scan. A plastic sheath is left in place through which a rigid or flexible nephroscope can pass. Stones smaller than 1 cm can be removed manually with a grasping forceps. General anesthesia is used for the surgical procedure itself. For stones greater than 71 cm, lithotripsy is used according to the surgeon's preferred method and the location of the stone.[1]

Postoperative nursing care should include the consideration of surgical complications and all postanesthesia considerations.[2,3] Blood loss from damage to an intrarenal artery is the most significant complication of percutaneous nephrolithotomy. Extravasation of the irrigation solution used during surgery is another complication. Rare complications include damage to the surrounding organs caused by perforation with the placement of the percutaneous nephrostomy tube. The nephrostomy tube may be left in place for 1 to 5 days. Pain at the nephrostomy site may require management with opioids. As with all genitourinary surgeries, adequate fluid intake is encouraged.[2,3]

With each of the types of renal stone removal procedures, nursing care should include patient education on types of stones, diet for the prevention of stones, and fluid intake to improve the excretion of stones and prevention of new stone formation.[9] There are five types of renal stones:

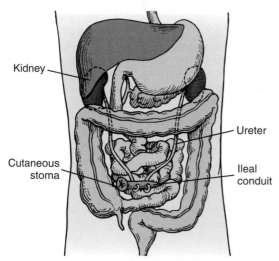

FIG. 41-4 Ileal conduit created from isolated segment of ileum with ureters anastomosed to segment between closed end and external stoma. Urinary collection device must be placed over incontinent stoma. Incontinent urinary diversion carries urine from kidneys through implanted ureters and ileal conduit to stoma. (From Phillips N: *Berry & Kohn's operating room technique*, ed 11, St. Louis, 2007, Mosby.)

Labels on figure: Kidney, Cutaneous stoma, Ureter, Ileal conduit

calcium oxalate, calcium phosphate, uric acid, struvite, and cysteine.[10,11] Of these the calcium oxalate stone is the most common. Each stone has different diet and fluid intake recommendations and restrictions. It is important to educate patients on the importance of follow-up with the surgeon in order to identify the type of renal stones they are producing. By knowing the chemical makeup of the stone, the surgeon is able to make specific recommendations to the patient (Box 41-1).

Kidney Transplantation

The kidney is the most commonly transplanted organ and the only one that can be preserved in a viable state for some time (Fig. 41-5). The kidney is relatively easy to remove and implant. Most people have two functioning kidneys and need only one to sustain life; therefore kidney transplantation is done only for patients who need the organ to replace a diseased or nonfunctioning solitary kidney. Transplantation can be accomplished two, three, or more times in the same patient, with the use of hemodialysis when a functioning kidney is not in place.[12]

Kidney grafts come from two sources: cadaver donors and living donors. Most living donors are a close blood relative of the recipient. Ideally, an identical twin is the best donor. The closer the recipient and donor in blood line, the better the chances for survival of the kidney graft. Although the living related donor is best, cadaver donors are the most common source for kidney graft.[1,5,12]

General anesthesia is the preferred method of anesthesia for both the donor and the recipient in renal transplantation.[4] After surgery, care of the living donor is essentially the same as that for the patient who has undergone nephrectomy.[12] All care considered previously for the urologic patient

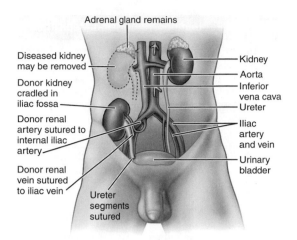

FIG. 41-5 Transplanted kidney in place. (From Black JM, Hokanson Hawks J: *Medical-surgical nursing: clinical management for positive outcomes,* ed 8, St. Louis, 2009, Saunders.)

applies, as does care for the patient after abdominal incision. If the laparoscopic approach was used for the living donor, four to five stab wounds are found from the trocars used during surgery.[1,12] Postoperative priorities include accurate intake and output, fluid volume and electrolyte replacement, adequate pulmonary perfusion, and pain and comfort measures.

Because postoperative care is routine, the donor patient often feels forgotten. Before surgery, the patient was considered heroic and received a generous helping of attention and glory. After surgery, attention is directed primarily to the organ recipient. The donor patient feels this even in the PACU. For this reason, the perianesthesia nurse must be aware of the needs of the postoperative donor and show concern for the patient's physical and psychologic well being. The care of these patients should be assigned to separate teams, if possible. In addition to normal self concern, the donor is concerned about the recipient and should receive factual information.[12]

For the renal transplant patient, the commonly used immunosuppressive agents are nonspecific and suppress the entire immune system. However, immunosuppressive therapy is vital to the treatment for the renal transplant patient to prevent rejection of the donor kidney. Calcineurin inhibitors, which block production of interluekin-2 in the T cell lymphocyte, purine inhibitors, and steroids are the first-line medications given for immunosuppression. A transplant patient receives one drug from each category. Sometimes, an antibody agent directed against T cells is given (Box 41-2).[8,12] PACU nurses should know the specific agents and transplant

---

BOX 41-1	Foods High in Oxalate

- Peanuts
- Tea
- Instant Coffee
- Rhubarb
- Beans
- Beets
- Berries (e.g., blackberries, cranberries, raspberries, strawberries, gooseberries)
- Chocolate
- Concord grapes
- Dark leafy greens
- Oranges
- Tofu
- Sweet potatoes

NURSING CARE IN THE PACU

BOX 41-2   Immunosuppression Medications

- Induction (administered in the first week after transplantation)
  - Antibody agents
  - Steroids
  - Purine inhibitors (azathioprine/mycophenolate mofetil)
  - Calcineurin inhibitors (cyclosporine/tacrolimus)
- Maintenance (administered during the first week and maintained throughout viability of transplant)
  - Steroids
  - Purine inhibitors (azathioprine/mycophenolate mofetil)
  - Calcineurin inhibitors (cyclosporine/tacrolimus)
- Rejection (administered when rejection is identified, often the first 2 to 4 weeks after transplant)
  - High-dose steroids
  - Antibody agents

From Barone CP, et al: The postanesthesia care of an adult renal transplant recipient, *J Perianesth Nurs* 18:32-41, 2003.

protocols used by their hospitals. Wound infections are among the common causes of death after kidney transplantation.[12] Meticulous aseptic technique is therefore imperative with these patients to prevent the introduction of infection.

On admission to the PACU, the recipient should be kept in a flat position for 12 hours, which allows the kidney to set. The head of the bed may be elevated 30 degrees to provide comfort and respiratory care. After 12 hours, the patient may turn to the side of the transplant. Turning to the opposite side may dislodge the graft. All vital signs are monitored continuously. Many renal transplant patients need antihypertensive medications after surgery. Blood pressures are more easily controlled as the fluid status becomes stable.[12]

A urinary catheter is in place, and all urine should be carefully monitored for volume and specific gravity. During the immediate postoperative period, the renal allograft is extremely sensitive to hypovolemia, and even a transient period of poor renal perfusion can result in oliguric renal failure. The kidney from a living donor may start to function almost immediately after transplantation, and diuresis occurs. The volume of urine output may be great enough to warrant measurement every 15 minutes. The cadaver kidney, however, reacts more slowly, depending on the cold ischemic time spent during transportation.[12]

Urine samples are generally collected hourly to ascertain electrolyte content, creatinine level, and osmolarity. Once daily, the total 24-hour urine collection (minus the small samples sent hourly) is sent to the laboratory for creatinine clearance test and culture. Urine output less than 1 mL/kg/h should be reported to the surgeon, because any decrease in urine output may be a sign of early rejection or complications of the anastomosis site.[12] Likewise, any gross hematuria should be reported immediately. A baseline postoperative weight should be ascertained as soon as feasible.

Other nursing considerations include care of the potential nasogastric tube that provides intestinal decompression and receives care as discussed previously. A central venous pressure line may be present for assessment of the patient's cardiovascular status. Monitoring of these systems is imperative to ensure adequate renal perfusion and prevent fluid overload. Skin integrity should be maintained, and the dressing over the incision site should exhibit a minimal amount of drainage. The recipient may have a stenting catheter from the renal pelvis out through the urethra along with the urinary catheter for the first 36 to 48 hours to ensure ureteral patency.[2,3]

Intravenous fluids provide most of the intake for these patients until the nasogastric tube can be removed. Intravenous replacement fluid composition is determined by the serum and urine electrolyte content, the hematocrit, and the clinical course of the patient. Volume is determined from necessary fluid requirements of the patient in normal status plus replacement on a volume-to-volume basis of drainage from the urinary catheter, nasogastric tube, ureterostomy, and cystostomy.[1,12] For the first 72 hours after operation, the major source of output is from the ureterostomy.[1] Meticulous handling of the closed urinary drainage system is mandatory to prevent the introduction of infection.

Vigorous pulmonary toilet should be instituted immediately to prevent atelectasis. The patient can be turned to the side of the kidney graft and back every 30 minutes to provide for change of position. The painful flank incision can be splinted either with the nurse's hands or with a firm pillow or a rolled blanket to assist the patient with coughing.

The threat of graft rejection is always present; therefore the health care professional must observe closely for signs of rejection.[2,12] Hyperacute allograft rejection can occur within minutes of the completion of the vascular anastomosis or in the first few postoperative hours.[1,12] Signs and symptoms of hyperacute rejection are noted in Box 41-3. To prevent irreversible damage to the kidney, treatment of a threatened rejection immediately is of the utmost importance.

BOX 41-3   Signs and Symptoms of Allograft Rejection

- Irritability
- Anxiousness
- Restlessness
- Lethargy
- Swollen tender kidney
- Decreased urine output
- Fever, may be low-grade
- Increased blood pressure
- Weight gain
- Anorexia
- Increased blood urea nitrogen and serum creatinine levels
- Decreased creatinine clearance
- Increased urine protein and lysozyme activity
- Lymphocytes in the urine

The patient may have a strong fear of rejection while still in the PACU. Many patients view this surgery as the last chance to live a normal life after facing numerous physical, psychologic, and socioeconomic stressors. The perianesthesia nurse may need to reassure the patient often that the kidney is functioning. After discharge from the PACU, the patient may be transferred to the surgical intensive care unit after surgery for close observation and intensive care.

Bladder Surgery

The bladder is a smooth muscle storage tank that holds urine until a reflex, normally with voluntary control, releases the urine to pass through the urethra to be eliminated.[1] Surgical procedures on the bladder include the removal of stones, foreign bodies, and tumors; the repair of strictures at the bladder neck and of injuries, such as lacerations; and the removal of the bladder itself.[1,5]

Anesthesia for these procedures may be either spinal or general.[1,4] On admission to the PACU, the patient is placed in a supine position. The head of the bed can be raised 30 degrees as soon as feasible. The removal of stones or foreign bodies and the resection of selected tumors can be accomplished via cystoscopy, which was discussed previously. After the repair of lacerations or after cystotomy for removal of stones, the patient is admitted to the PACU with a urinary catheter and a urinary diversion, such as a suprapubic cystostomy, usually in place. Urine from these drainage systems is pink tinged but should not become grossly bloody. Dressings should remain dry and intact, fluids should be increased, and oral fluids should be started as soon as the effects of anesthesia have passed.

Cystectomy

Lacerations or ruptures of the bladder are often the result of accidental trauma. They require emergency surgery, and the postoperative patient should be assessed carefully for any unrecognized associated injuries.[1] Pain should be minimal to moderate for these patients and easily controlled with analgesics. The presence of severe pain may represent a complication, such as internal hemorrhage and damage to a ureter, and should be reported to the surgeon.

Cystectomy may be performed as a result of trauma or underlying pathology, such as muscle-invasive bladder cancer. Whether the cystectomy is partial or radical (including hysterectomy and anterior vaginectomy in females and prostatectomy in males), urinary diversion is necessary.[1,5] Care for an ileal conduit was discussed in the section on ureteral surgery. Other forms of urinary diversion include Koch pouch, cutaneous continent ileocecal reservoir, and ileocolic neobladder and orthotopic bladder substitution. The type of urinary diversion is specific for each patient with consideration to age, height and weight, surgical history, and medical history.[13,14]

Postanesthesia care includes all the principles of surgical nursing along with special consideration to drains and catheters specific to type of diversion. The PACU nurse should observe the patient for potential complications that include stricture of the anastomosis site, rupture of the reservoir with neobladder or Koch pouch, infection, and any metabolic complications. Irrigation of the urethral catheter with 50 mL of saline solution 0.9% every 6 hours while the suprapubic catheter is freely draining is started immediately after surgery to prevent mucous from clotting the catheter.[13,14]

Patients may awaken in the PACU with questions regarding the surgeon's ability to remove the cancer in its entirety. Patients should be allowed to discuss fears and feelings. The nurse should pay close attention to patient concerns for changes in body image and fears for loss of intimacy with a partner.

Bladder Neck Suspensions

Quality of life challenges are significant in patients with incontinence. Bladder neck suspensions in a variety of techniques are performed to correct urinary stress incontinence.[1,5] Postoperative complications for all techniques include urinary retention, wound infection, urinary tract infection, continued incontinence, retroperitoneal hemorrhage, and organ perforation.[2]

Sling procedures including the Tension-Free Vaginal Tape (TVT Sling) are a recent development for the correction of urinary stress incontinence caused by pelvic floor relaxation in women and are considered a first-line surgical intervention. This procedure can be done with local anesthetic and MAC. Potential complications include postoperative voiding difficulties, bowel perforation, and erosion of the tape into the bladder, urethra, or vagina.[15]

Immediate postoperative care includes monitoring of patients, depending on the level of sedation after MAC. Pain medication should be administered as ordered. Close monitoring of voiding status ensures that bladder overdistention does not occur. When the patient is able to void, postvoid residual should be assessed with bladder ultrasound scan. If the patient is unable to void or postvoid residual is greater than 100 mL, an indwelling urinary catheter may be ordered. Nursing care then includes patient teaching on care of the catheter at home and instructions on follow-up with the surgeon for voiding trial.

Artificial Urinary Sphincter

Another treatment for urinary incontinence is the placement of an artificial urinary sphincter (AUS). This invasive procedure is a method to restore control over urinary function. AUS is a prosthetic device that consists of three parts: a balloon pressure reservoir, a control pump that is implanted in the scrotum or labia, and a cuff that occludes the urethra. This prosthetic device substitutes for the sphincteric mechanism and prevents the loss of urine. Indications for this procedure include post-prostatectomy urinary leakage, congenital disorders of the bladder, and unsuccessful reconstructive surgery of the urethra.[13,14]

Postanesthesia care includes principles of care for patients receiving general anesthesia. Specific assessment for this procedure includes observation for signs of hematoma along the plane of dissection for the pump in the scrotum or labia.[13] A bladder ultrasound scan can be used to assess for urinary retention that can result from edema around the cuff site.[1]

Along with the use of opioid analgesics to control pain, ice packs to the scrotum or labia and perineal areas provide comfort and prevent swelling. The patients arrive in the PACU with an indwelling catheter, and traction on the urethral catheter should be prevented to avoid increased pressure on the cuff of the sphincter.[13]

Prostatic Surgery

The prostate gland is a small, walnut-sized male reproductive organ. Its sole function is to manufacture a secretion that becomes part of the semen; the prostate gland is a nonessential organ. Surgical procedures performed on the prostate gland include the excision of tumors and the resection or total removal of the gland.[1]

The preferred anesthesia is spinal, although general anesthesia may be used. Several different approaches are common in surgery on the prostate.[6] The transurethral approach is the most common, especially if only minor obstructive lesions or small portions of the gland are to be removed. A resectoscope is introduced through the urethra, and the surgeon excises the tissue with a moveable tungsten wire that operates on high-frequency current controlled with a foot pedal.[1,5]

When the patient is admitted to the PACU after TURP, a three-way urinary catheter may be in place (see Fig. 41-1, *A*). One lumen allows filling of the retention balloon, one lumen allows outflow of the urine and irrigation fluid from the bladder, and one lumen is attached to the irrigation fluid system. Irrigation fluid, which is usually normal saline solution at room temperature, is available in 3000-mL plastic bags and may be regulated like intravenous solutions. To avoid creation of a hypothermic state with irrigation of the bladder with this solution, the saline solution should be warmed before administration, and the patient's body temperature should be monitored.[2] The triple-lumen catheter is advantageous in that blood clots do not regularly form and block the system when the flow is continuous. The irrigation rate should be regulated so that drainage remains a light-pink watermelon color. If drainage becomes bright red, speed up the irrigation; if the returning fluid is clear, slow down the irrigation. Some institutions use a Y-connecting system with one arm of the Y connected to the irrigating fluid and the other to straight-gravitational drainage from the bladder. In either instance, a fair amount of bleeding can be expected after TURP, because the prostatic bed is highly vascular. This bleeding may also increase as the spinal anesthesia wears off and may require frequent irrigation to prevent clogging of the drainage tube. If the catheter becomes clogged, the surgeon should be notified and may order irrigation with a piston syringe and the same normal saline irrigating solution. If patency of the catheter cannot be reestablished, the surgeon must be notified.[2,3]

The patient's vital signs should be monitored closely. Observe for signs and symptoms of post-TURP syndrome (hyponatremia) that can occur from venous absorption of the irrigation fluid through the venous sinuses. Serum sodium and potassium levels should be checked during the postoperative period, because changes in fluid balance may affect these electrolytes. Signs and symptoms of hyponatremia are a low serum sodium level, tachypnea, shortness of breath, nausea, vomiting, hypertension, bradycardia, increased pulse pressure, restlessness, apprehension, and mental disorientation.[6] If this syndrome occurs, the perianesthesia nurse should notify the anesthesia provider and surgeon, administer oxygen to the patient, monitor blood loss and electrocardiographic and fluid and electrolyte status, and administer intravenous fluid (hypertonic saline solution 3% or 5% in 100 mL/h increments until the serum sodium level is satisfactory) and diuretics to mobilize the edema.[2,6]

Oral fluids should be started and increased as tolerated as soon as possible. Diet may be progressed as tolerated in the absence of any postoperative nausea. Intravenous fluid replacement should be maintained until adequate oral fluids are maintained.

Pain should be minimal to mild and easily controlled with analgesics. Analgesics or tranquilizers can be administered to control the discomfort of bladder spasms and of the presence of the catheter, which makes the patient feel an urgency to void although the bladder is being emptied. Symptoms of abdominal pain, abdominal rigidity, increased pulse rate, and other signs of shock should alert the nurse to the possibility that the bladder wall or the capsule of the prostate was accidentally perforated during surgery; these symptoms should be reported to the surgeon immediately.[3,8]

Other approaches to prostatic surgery include retrograde or suprapubic, perineal, and retropubic incisions.[1,5] When the suprapubic approach is used, a midline vertical incision is made in the lowest part of the abdomen, the bladder is incised, and the tumors are removed.[1] This procedure is the choice when 60 g or more of tissue is to be removed. The patient is admitted to the PACU with a urinary catheter, which may or may not be attached to an irrigation system. If it is not connected to an irrigation system, the catheter has to be irrigated frequently via syringe to prevent clots from clogging the drainage system.[2,5] The patient also has a suprapubic catheter that should be connected to straight-gravitational drainage in place; output should be measured carefully (Fig. 41-6). In addition, a small Penrose drain is inserted in the suprapubic space and brought out through a separate stab wound. A dressing of several layers of 4 × 4 sponges should cover the incision and the drain. A moderate amount of serosanguineous drainage can be expected because of the presence of the drain. This dressing should be reinforced as necessary to keep the skin clean and dry. If excessive bright-red bleeding occurs, the surgeon must be notified.

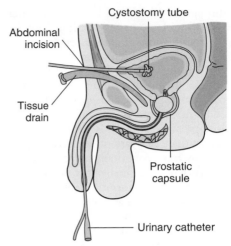

FIG. 41-6 Suprapubic prostatectomy. Note placement of inflated urinary catheter in prostatic fossa. (From Monahan FD, et al: *Phipps' medical surgical nursing: health and illness perspectives*, ed 8, St. Louis, 2007, Mosby.)

The surgeon can apply traction to the urinary catheter by taping the catheter to the inner thigh. Because the traction puts tension against the vesical outlet and promotes hemostasis, it can produce painful bladder spasms that may be relieved with the use of intravenous opioids or belladonna and opium suppositories as prescribed by the surgeon.[1,5] After the traction is removed, a small increase in bleeding can be expected for a short time.

The perineal approach, used for removal of large amounts of tissue, is the approach of choice for prostatic cancer.[1,5] A V-shaped incision is made above the rectum in this approach. The patient is admitted to the PACU with a urinary catheter and a perineal drain. Because of the perineal drain, a moderate amount of serosanguineous drainage can be expected, and the dressing should be reinforced as necessary. No instrumentation, including thermometers, should be placed in the rectum during the immediate postoperative period.

When a retropubic approach is used, a small incision is made above the pubis and a capsular incision is made into the upper surface of the prostate.[1] This approach is used in the nerve-sparing radical prostatectomy for patients whose carcinoma is confined within the prostate.[1] This approach is preferred because of the decreased risk of postoperative complications of long-term incontinence and impotence.

On the patient's arrival to the PACU, a urinary catheter is in place and a small drain may be present that was inserted in the incision or brought out through a stab wound lateral to the incision. As with all urologic patients, accurate intake and output records must be maintained after prostatic surgery. The perianesthesia nurse must be sure to indicate in the output data whether irrigation solution is included. Output should be documented hourly. Color and appearance of urine should be monitored closely and documented.

Most prostatic surgery is performed on adult men older than 50 years of age because prostatic hypertrophy most commonly occurs after 40 years of age.[10] As a result, assessment of cardiorespiratory status should be performed frequently. Oxygen should be administered and weaned with pulse oximetry. All patients should be connected to a cardiac monitor for assessment of changes. Astute observation of vital signs is imperative to monitor cardiovascular function, because postoperative bleeding may impair it. Observe carefully for decreasing blood pressure and increasing pulse rate, which may indicate impending shock.[2,3]

One of the most common postoperative complications after the nerve-sparing radical prostatectomy is pulmonary embolism. For this reason, the surgeon may order low-dose heparin. Care in the PACU should include deep-breathing exercises and position changes along with passive or active movement of the extremities.[2] As with other urologic procedures, some type of antiembolism stocking or sequential compression device should be used.[2,3]

Scrotal Surgery

The scrotum is a sac separated into two pouches: externally by the median raphe and internally by the dartos tunic. Each pouch contains a testis, an epididymis, and a spermatic cord. The vas deferens, which is continuous with the epididymis at the lower end of the testis, and the arteries, veins, nerves, and lymphatic vessels that are held together by spermatic fascia form the spermatic cord.[1] Operations on the scrotum include excision of masses and tumors, correction of deformities, and excision of diseased or abnormal structures that interfere with normal function.[1,5]

Anesthesia for scrotal surgery may be local, general, or spinal. Spinal anesthesia is commonly used for adult patients, whereas general anesthesia is usually preferred for children younger than 12 years. Local anesthesia is often used for simple procedures, such as vasectomy and epididymectomy.[1,4]

The PACU course after surgery on the scrotal structures is usually uneventful. Care is dictated primarily by anesthesia agent and its method of administration.[4] The patient may assume a position of comfort after surgery. Any dressings present should remain dry and intact. Oral food and

fluids may be reinstituted as soon as the patient tolerates them. An athletic supporter commonly is applied to provide scrotal support and elevation (Fig. 41-7). This device is suspended from thigh to thigh, with a tight sling across the expanse on which the scrotum is supported. A T-binder may also be used (Fig. 41-8).[2]

The application of a light crushed-ice bag helps to relieve scrotal edema, enhances hemostasis, and promotes comfort. Scrotal enlargement with apparent tension should be reported to the surgeon immediately. Progressive inguinal swelling may denote lymphatic obstruction after a varicocelectomy, and the surgeon must be notified. Pain should be minimal after these procedures and easily controlled with mild analgesics. Severe pain that is not controlled with mild analgesia should be reported to the surgeon.

As with any genital surgery, the patient's body image concerns and questions of fertility

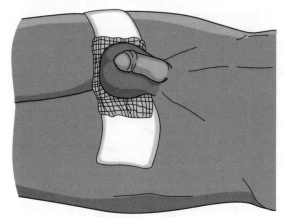

FIG. 41-7 A simple scrotal support. (From Monahan FD, et al: *Phipps' medical surgical nursing: health and illness perspectives,* ed 8, St. Louis, 2007, Mosby.)

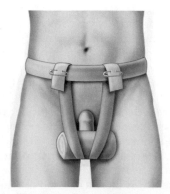

FIG. 41-8 T-binder for scrotal support. (From Harkreader H, et al: *Fundamentals of nursing: caring and clinical judgment,* ed 3, St. Louis, 2007, Saunders.)

in particular may be of paramount importance. These concerns are not usually addressed in the PACU, but the nurse must be sensitive to them and be prepared to assist the patient with factual information and reassurance. Often these patients feel an urgency to inspect the operative site and should be assisted to do so, if necessary.

The patient may be embarrassed by this type of surgery, may be reluctant to ask the nurse for assistance or to report pain, and may hesitate to allow the nurse to inspect the incision area. A matter-of-fact attitude on the part of the nurse and efficient care promote a sense of well being for the patient and may help to alleviate these feelings. The nurse should keep in mind that preadolescent and adolescent boys are especially sensitive about the genital area. If at all possible, a male nurse should be assigned to these patients to alleviate anxiety.

Penile and Urethral Surgery

Surgery on the penis and urethra involves removal of tumors or obstructions to urinary flow, plastic repair of deformities, and circumcision or excision of the foreskin.[1] Partial or total amputation of the penis is rarely necessary, but can be performed for malignant disease, which is essentially skin cancer. Laser technique is generally effective for the treatment of condyloma acuminata and squamous cell carcinoma of the penis.

Anesthesia for these procedures may be local, general, or spinal. The PACU course is usually smooth, and care is determined primarily by the type of anesthesia.[4] Physical care of the patient who has had a plastic repair of hypospadias or epispadias is dictated by the surgeon. Care after cystoscopy was discussed at the beginning of this chapter; the same care applies for patients who undergo cystoscopy for the resection of tumors.

After circumcision, which may be performed for correction of phimosis or for elective reasons, the nurse should check for bleeding. Usually, only a small band of petrolatum-impregnated gauze is applied as a dressing around the glans and is changed as directed. Bleeding that soaks this dressing is excessive and should be reported.

Patients who have undergone surgery on the penis should avoid erection during the PACU phase and for at least 1 week after surgery. Patients with penile prostheses should be admitted to the PACU with the penis in a flaccid state; the prosthesis should remain deflated. Inflation of the prosthesis should be avoided until after the first postoperative visit to the surgeon.[5]

Pain may be significant but should not be severe. Scrotal and penile support with a Bellevue bridge and the application of a light ice pack provide some relief; however, analgesia with small doses of opioids may be necessary.[2,5] Food and fluids may be restarted as soon as the patient tolerates them. Urine output should be checked and recorded. Low abdominal distention on palpation may be caused by voluntary retention, which is not uncommon because of fear that micturition creates pain. The patient should be reassured and informed that overdistention of the bladder causes an increase in discomfort and possible complications.[2]

Adrenalectomy

Adrenalectomy involves the removal of one or both of the adrenal glands, which are situated on top of the kidneys.[1,5] Adrenalectomy, an extensive and shock-producing procedure, may be performed for several reasons, including metastasized cancer from the reproductive organs, hyperfunction caused by hyperplasia of the organ, and adrenal tumors. The following two adrenal tumors are of major consequence: pheochromocytoma, a usually benign tumor that causes hyperfunction and results in severe symptoms, and neuroblastoma, a malignant tumor that is a leading cause of death in childhood.[1,11]

General anesthesia is used for adrenalectomy and can include the use of cortisone titrated to maintain catecholamine levels and blood pressure. Cortisone is usually necessary only when bilateral adrenalectomy is performed or when the uninvolved adrenal gland has poor function. The administration of cortisone, which is continued in the PACU, is an extremely important nursing procedure. The anesthesia provider and surgeon should give specific instructions for titration of the solution.[4] Failure to maintain postoperative levels of cortisone leads to hypovolemic and hyponatremic shock.[1] Perianesthesia care of these patients is a nursing challenge; observations must be especially astute.

The surgical approach for adrenalectomy may be lateral, anterior, or posterior.[1,5] On admission to the PACU, the patient is placed in the side-lying position until reactive from anesthesia, at which time the patient is placed in a semi-Fowler position. The surgeon may prefer the patient to be positioned on the operative side so that the perinephric space is obliterated to discourage bleeding. Assessment is aimed primarily at the cardiovascular status of the patient because hemorrhage and shock are the two most common and most disastrous complications. Profound shock may develop because of the reduction of circulating catecholamines that is precipitated by removal of the glands and the effects of the drugs used for preoperative control of hypertension.[1,2] The effects of these drugs usually last for a few hours after surgery. Because most of these drugs produce vasodilation, they are usually a factor in postoperative hypotension; therefore a fluid challenge usually is given in an attempt to treat hypotension. If fluid is not successful in increasing the blood pressure, then vasopressor drugs are used. Epinephrine or norepinephrine in an intravenous solution can be titrated to maintain blood pressure, according to the surgeon's instructions.

Shock can also result from hemorrhage because the adrenal glands are extremely vascular. Intravenous fluids, including hypertonic saline solutions, blood, plasma, dextran, and glucose in water can be used to maintain blood volume and prevent shock.[1,2] Dressings over the bilateral incisions should remain relatively dry, although drains are placed. If these dressings become soaked, the surgeon should be notified because this represents excessive bleeding. If the patient has abdominal pain, abdominal distention, nausea, or vomiting, development of an abdominal hematoma may be indicated; these signs should be reported to the surgeon.[2]

Other parameters of the patient's status that can give clues to the development of shock should also be assessed. Dehydration (increased urine specific gravity) and restlessness may indicate developing shock. Central venous pressure should be checked. A urinary catheter should be in place, and urine output should be monitored hourly. The development of oliguria or output of less than 1 mL/kg/h can indicate shock and subsequent renal shutdown.[2,3] Serum and urine electrolyte levels, especially sodium, should be determined hourly.

All care outlined for the patient after high abdominal incisions in Chapter 40 is applicable to this patient. Good pulmonary toilet should be instituted immediately in the PACU. A nasogastric tube often is necessary until normal intestinal peristalsis returns. Incisional pain may require the use of opioid analgesics. Because many opioids have a hypotensive effect, they should be titrated judiciously; blood pressure must be monitored continuously for at least 30 minutes after their administration.

The patient often is placed in protective isolation to avoid the introduction of infection. Meticulous sterile technique must be used when changing or reinforcing dressings. Because of extreme lability, which lasts for approximately 48 hours, these patients should be transferred to the surgical intensive care unit for continuous monitoring.

SUMMARY

This chapter has discussed the perianesthesia care of the patient who undergoes genitourinary surgery. The perianesthesia nurse should have an understanding of anatomic location and normal function of this system and the important postanesthesia nursing concerns for this type of patient. Adrenalectomy was included in this chapter because of the proximity of the adrenal glands to the kidneys.

REFERENCES

1. Tanagho E, McAninch: *Smith's general urology*, New York, 2007, McGraw-Hill.
2. Schick L, Windle PE: *Perianesthesia nursing core curriculum: preprocedure, phase I and phase II PACU nursing*, St. Louis, 2010, Saunders.
3. Stannard D, Krenzischek: *Perianesthesia nursing care: a bedside guide for safe recovery*, Sudbury, MA, 2012, Jones & Bartlett.
4. Stoelting R, Miller R: *Basics of anesthesia*, ed 6, Philadelphia, 2011, Churchill Livingstone.
5. Rothrock J: *Alexander's care of the patient in surgery*, ed 14, St. Louis, 2011, Mosby.
6. Eaton J: Detection of hyponatremia in the PACU, *J PeriAnesth Nurs* 18(6) 392-397, 2003.
7. Krapp K, Gale T: Bladder ultrasound, *Encyclopedia of Nursing & Allied Health*, 2002, eNotes.com 2006, available at http://www.enotes.com/bladder-ultrasound-reference/bladder-ultrasound. Accessed January 30, 2012.
8. Katzung B: *Basic and clinical pharmacology*, ed 10, Los Altos, CA, 2006, McGraw Hill.
9. National Kidney Foundation: *Diet and kidney stone fact sheet*, available at www.kidney.org/atoz/content/diet.cfm.
10. National Kidney and Urologic Diseases Information Clearinghouse: Kidney stones in adults, available at kidney.niddk.nih.gov/KUDiseases/pubs/stonesadults/index.aspx.
11. Litwin M, Saigal C: Uroligic diseases in America, Washington, DC, 2007, U.S. Government Printing Office: NIH pub No 07-5512.
12. Barone C, et al: The postanesthesia care of an adult renal transplant recipient, *J Perianesth Nurs* 18(1): 32-41, 2003.
13. Quallich S, Ohl D: Urinary sphincter, part I: overview. *Urol Nurs* 23(4): 259-268, 2003.
14. Quallich S, Ohl D: Artificial urinary sphincter, part II: patient teaching and perioperative care, *Urol Nurs* 23(4): 269-273, 2003.
15. Polt C: Taking the pressure off for women with stress incontinence, *Nursing* 36(2): 49-51, 2006.

RESOURCES

Alspach JG: *Core curriculum for critical care nursing*, ed 6, St. Louis, 2006, Saunders.
Atlee J: *Complications in anesthesia*, ed 2, Philadelphia, 2007, Saunders.
Barash PG, et al: *Clinical anesthesia*, ed 5, Philadelphia, 2005, Lippincott Williams & Wilkins.

Barrett K: *Ganong's review of medical physiology,* ed 23, New York, 2010, McGraw-Hill Professional.

Bickley LS, Szilagyi PG: *Bates' guide to physical examination and history taking,* ed 9, Philadelphia, 2005, Lippincott Williams & Wilkins.

Brunton L, et al: *Goodman and Gilman's the pharmacological basis of therapeutics,* ed 11, New York, 2005, McGraw-Hill Professional.

Canale ST, Beaty JH: *Campbell's operative orthopaedics,* ed 11, St. Louis, 2008, Mosby.

Cottrell J, Smith D: *Anesthesia and neurosurgery,* ed 4, St. Louis, 2001, Mosby.

Fleisher LA: *Anesthesia and uncommon diseases,* ed 5, Philadelphia, 2007, Saunders.

Hall J: *Guyton & Hall's textbook of medical physiology,* ed 12, Philadelphia, 2010, Saunders.

Hamlin L, et al: *Perioperative nursing: an introductory text,* Chatswood, Australia, 2009, Elsevier.

Hanson K: Minimally invasive and surgical management of urinary stones, *Urol Nurs.* 25:458–464, 2005.

Lake C, et al: *Clinical monitoring: practical applications for anesthesia and critical care,* St. Louis, 2001, Mosby.

Miller R, et al: *Miller's anesthesia,* ed 7, Philadelphia, 2009, Churchill Livingstone.

Nagelhout J, Plaus K: *Nurse anesthesia,* ed 4, St. Louis, 2009, Saunders.

Overstreet DL, Sims TW: Care of the patient undergoing radical cystectomy with a robotic approach, *Urol Nurs* 26(2):117–125, 2006.

Peliciano T, et al: A retrospective, descriptive, exploratory study evaluating incidence of postoperative urinary retention after spinal anesthesia and its effect on PACU discharge, *J Perianesth Nurs* 23(6):394-400, 2008.

Perimenis P, Koliopanou E: Postoperative management and rehabilitation of patients receiving an ileal orthotopic bladder substitution, *Urol Nurs* 24(5):383–386, 2004.

Stoelting R, Hillier SC, *Pharmacology and physiology in anesthetic practice,* ed 4, Philadelphia, 2005, Lippincott Williams & Wilkins.

Townsend CM, et al: *Sabiston textbook of surgery: the biological basis of modern surgical practice,* ed 19, Philadelphia, 2012, Saunders.

Wendy K. Winer, BSN, RN, CNOR

Traditionally, surgery on organs of reproduction usually involved an adult patient. However, in most recent years as girls reach puberty at earlier ages, it is becoming more frequent for young girls in their teens to have laparoscopic surgery for conditions such as endometriosis.[1] In addition, the perianesthesia nurse may encounter pediatric or adolescent female patients who undergo gynecologic surgery for repair or correction of congenital or traumatic deformities or incapacitating pelvic pain from causes such as endometriosis, ovarian cyst, or appendicitis. Surgery on the female genitalia may be conveniently divided into three major categories: obstetric, lower genital and vaginal, and abdominal gynecologic surgery. Abdominal surgery is then subdivided into either what used to be referred to as traditional surgery in the form of a laparotomy, mini-laparotomy (could include hand assisted surgery through a mini type laparotomy incision), or into the category of operative laparoscopy (typically two or three small incisions or robotic surgery, which may include four to seven incisions). The area of operative laparoscopy in gynecologic surgery has expanded and includes the majority of benign gynecologic surgery. However, there are still a great number of laparotomies currently performed. Many surgeons who previously have not felt comfortable performing laparoscopic procedures are now doing so with the aid of the robot. There is much debate among gynecologists as to whether the learning curve is shorter with the use of the robot. Whether or not that is the case, the bigger questions are "Is the cost of the robot warranted?" and "With proper training, can these same procedures be done just as effectively without the robot?" The perianesthesia nurse must be aware of how the care of the patient differs with these various approaches.

DEFINITIONS

OBSTETRIC SURGERY

Cerclage Procedure: Procedure for the treatment of incompetent cervix. The McDonald procedure involves the placement of a pursestring suture on the cervix at the level of the internal os. The Shirodkar's

procedure involves placement of a fascia lata (from the thigh) or a surgical band at the level of the internal os.

Cesarean Hysterectomy: Incision of the abdomen and the uterus, extraction of the infant and the placenta, and performance of a hysterectomy.

Cesarean Section (C-Section): Delivery of an infant through an incision made in the abdominal and uterine walls.

C-Section, Classic: A midline incision between the umbilicus and the symphysis pubis and an anterior incision through the uterine wall.

C-Section, Low Segment: An incision in the lower part of the uterus made after an abdominal incision.

Ectopic Pregnancy: Implantation of the fertilized ovum in any site other than the upper half of the uterus.

Uterine Aspiration (Suction Curettage): Dilation of the cervix and vacuum removal of the uterine contents.

LOWER GENITAL SURGERY, VAGINAL SURGERY, ABDOMINAL SURGERY (LAPAROTOMY AND LAPAROSCOPY)

Bartholin's Duct Cyst: A cyst that results from chronic inflammation of one of the major vestibular glands at the vaginal introitus.

Bartholinectomy: Removal of a Bartholin duct cyst.

Cervical Conization: Removal of abnormal cervical tissue via scalpel, electrosurgical current, or laser.

Colporrhaphy: Repair of the vaginal wall. May be anterior, as for cystocele repair, or posterior, as for rectocele repair or enterocele repair specifically for a vaginal prolapse.

Culdoscopy: An operative diagnostic procedure in which an incision is made into the posterior vaginal cul-de-sac, through which a tubular instrument similar to a cystoscope is inserted for the purpose of visualization of the pelvic structures, including the uterus, fallopian tubes, broad ligaments, uterosacral ligaments, rectal wall, sigmoid colon, and sometimes the small intestine. A newer technique for this procedure is transvaginal hydrolaparoscopy, which uses normal saline solution and a camera attached to a small-diameter rigid endoscope.

Cystocele: Prolapse of the bladder into the anterior vaginal wall.

Dilation of the Cervix and Curettage of the Uterus (D&C): Introduction of instruments (dilators) through the vagina into the cervical canal and scraping of the uterus with a curette for removal of substances, including blood. This procedure is used for diagnostic purposes and for treatment of conditions such as incomplete abortion, abnormal uterine bleeding, and primary dysmenorrhea.

Enterocele: Defect in the continuity of the endopelvic fascia most commonly seen after hysterectomy when the anterior pubic fascia is not attached to the Denonvilliers fascia.

Hysterectomy: Removal of the uterus; can be vaginal (with or without laparoscopic assistance) or abdominal (via laparotomy).

Hysteroscopy: Direct visualization of the canal of the uterine cervix and cavity of the uterus with an endoscope called a *hysteroscope*.

Procidentia: Herniation of the uterus beyond the introitus.

Prolapse of the Uterus: Downward displacement of the uterus. Vaginal hysterectomy is often recommended for a prolapsed uterus when childbearing is no longer desired or when marked prolapse is present.

Rectocele: Prolapse of the rectum into the posterior vaginal wall.

Trachelorrhaphy: Removal of torn surfaces of the anterior and posterior cervical lips and reconstruction of the cervical canal.

Urethrocele: Prolapse of the urethra into the anterior vaginal wall.

Vaginal Plastic Operation (Anterior and Posterior Repair): Reconstruction of the vaginal walls (colporrhaphy), the pelvic floor, and the muscles and fascia of the rectum, urethra, bladder, and perineum. Used to correct a cystocele or rectocele, restore the bladder to its normal position, and strengthen the vagina and the pelvic floor.

ABDOMINAL GYNECOLOGIC SURGERY (LAPAROTOMY, MINI LAPAROTOMY, OR HAND-ASSISTED AND LAPAROSCOPY WITH OR WITHOUT THE AID OF THE ROBOT)

Abdominal myomectomy: Removal of leiomyomas (fibroids) through a large or small incision; if this is done laparoscopically, then the abdominal cavity is visualized through a small incision, usually at the umbilicus after the establishment of a pneumoperitoneum. A video camera is attached to the eye piece of the laparoscope so that the surgeon and team can visualize the procedure while watching a video monitor; this provides a magnified view of the pelvis. If the robot is used, it is often set up after the umbilical trocar is in position.

Oophorectomy: Removal of an ovary.

Oophorocystectomy: Removal of an ovarian cyst.

Radical Hysterectomy: Removal of the uterus, the uterosacral and uterovesical ligaments, the upper third of the vagina, and all the peritoneum. This may or may not include removal of the fallopian tubes and ovaries.

Salpingectomy: Excision of the fallopian tube.

Salpingo-Oophorectomy: Removal of the fallopian tube and the associated ovary.

Salpingostomy (Tubal Plasty): Repair and opening of the fallopian tube to establish patency. This is often done in the case of a hydrosalpinx. Tubal plasty or tubal reanastomosis is used for removal of an obstructed portion of the tube and reconnection of each normal end of the tube after the obstruction has been removed to establish patency. Tubal reanastomosis increases the risk of ectopic pregnancy. Because the success rates of in vitro fertilization are so good, this procedure is seldom done anymore.

Total Abdominal Hysterectomy: Removal of the uterus, including the cervix (with or without the adnexa which refers to the tube and/or ovary), through an abdominal incision. Various types of hysterectomy include the following if done laparoscopically:

LTH or TLH: Laparoscopic total hysterectomy or total laparoscopic hysterectomy; the uterus is removed laparoscopically and the vaginal cuff is sutured laparoscopically.

LSH: Laparoscopic supracervical hysterectomy; the uterus is removed laparoscopically and the cervix remains. This is thought to be the hysterectomy with the least morbidity and the quickest recovery for the patient postoperatively.

LAVH: Laparoscopic assisted vaginal hysterectomy; the uterus is reached laparoscopically and removed vaginally. The vaginal cuff is sutured vaginally.

NOTE: If a robot is used, the robot must be disconnected for any tissue to be removed. One of the main reasons some physicians choose to use the robot is because they find suturing laparoscopically much easier with the robot.

Tubal Ligation: Interruption of fallopian tube continuity, which results in sterilization; this is most commonly done laparoscopically. The fallopian tube is cauterized or ligated, a clip is placed, or the tube is partially excised. Reversal procedures can be attempted with tubal reanastomosis using microsurgery; however, this is seldom done because the success rate of IVF is so high.

OBSTETRIC SURGERY

Obstetric surgery involves procedures on pregnant women to promote full-term pregnancy, to provide an alternative means of delivery when normal vaginal delivery is not feasible for reasons of fetal or maternal well being, and to interrupt pregnancy.

Care After Specific Procedures
Cesarean Section

Cesarean sections are performed on both an emergency and an elective basis. These patients have special physical and psychological needs. A selection of articles is included in the bibliography at the end of this chapter to assist the reader who provides care for families who experience cesarean birth.

Cesarean sections are indicated for dystocia (usually caused by cephalopelvic disproportion), antepartum bleeding; some toxemic conditions; certain medical complications, especially diabetes mellitus; and previous cesarean section. The low-segment cesarean section is usually the procedure of choice. Anesthesia may be general inhalation, spinal, or local infiltration of the operative field. Postoperative care after cesarean section includes all care rendered to a patient who undergoes abdominal surgery and postpartum care.

On admission to the postanesthesia care unit (PACU), a report is given by the circulating nurse who transports the patient with the anesthesia provider to the PACU area. The patient's vital signs should be monitored regularly in keeping with the PACU guidelines in the facility. As soon as condition permits, the patient can assume any position of comfort. Oxygen should be delivered and monitored with the use of pulse oximetry.[2]

Parenteral fluids are usually administered during the first 24 hours after surgery, but oral fluids can usually be resumed as soon as bowel sounds are audible and the patient desires. Intravenous fluids often contain oxytocin to increase uterine muscle tone and stop excessive blood flow. Usually 10 to 20 units of oxytocin are added to 1000 mL of lactated Ringer solution and infused at 125 mL/h. Side effects with oxytocin are not common. Serious side effects include an allergic reaction (shortness of breath; closing of the throat; hives; swelling of the lips, face, or tongue; rash; or fainting), difficulty in urination, chest pain or irregular heart beat, difficulty in breathing, confusion, sudden weight gain or excessive swelling, severe headache, rash, excessive vaginal bleeding, or seizures. Other, less serious, side effects may be more likely to occur and include redness or irritation at the injection site; loss of appetite; and nausea or vomiting. The physician should be notified if any side effects occur. Perianesthesia nurses should be familiar with potential side effects. Intake and output should always be monitored appropriately in the PACU regardless of what medications are given. A progressive diet is advised, pending the return of bowel sounds.

The patient has an abdominal dressing and a perineal pad; both should be inspected for drainage. The abdominal dressing should remain dry and intact. A moderate amount of lochia rubra is normal, but saturation of two or more perineal pads with blood during the first hour is considered excessive. The area underneath the buttocks should be checked for pooling of blood.

The fundus should be checked frequently to ensure that it is firmly contracted. Checking of the fundus is an uncomfortable procedure for the patient; therefore careful explanation should be provided before it is performed. The patient should be encouraged to relax the abdominal muscles as much as possible. Slow deep breathing with an open mouth facilitates relaxation of those muscles. If the uterus is firmly contracted, it need not be massaged, and in fact should not be massaged, because massage may cause uterine muscle fatigue and subsequent relaxation and bleeding. If the uterus is soft and "boggy," it should be gently but firmly massaged through the abdominal wall to stimulate contraction. The patient may be instructed to do this herself with supervision, which may allay anxiety and be more comfortable. Oxytocin often is administered intravenously and titrated to maintain the uterus in a state of contraction. If oxytocin is used, the uterus should be checked for firmness, but usually does not need frequent massage.

A full bladder is one cause of uterine atony. An indwelling urethral catheter commonly is left in place for the first 12 postoperative hours. A fundus palpated above the umbilicus or to the side of the abdomen (usually the right side) may indicate a nonfunctioning catheter. The catheter should be positioned for gravitational drainage and avoidance of kinks. The urine should be monitored for volume and color.

Many patients have transient trembling or shivering after delivery. Several theories have been proposed regarding this sense of chilling, although the actual cause remains unknown. This trembling is generally not associated with an elevation of temperature. Warmed blankets or warm-air therapy should be available as a comfort measure. Many hospitals have separate PACUs for postpartum patients; therefore the special considerations for the cesarean section patient pose no significant problems. The nurse who cares for the cesarean section patient within the general PACU must be judicious and often innovative to meet the needs of the mother and the new family. The mother, the neonate, and the father should be together as soon as possible to allow for the bonding experience. This experience can be accomplished using a quiet corner of the unit (if such a place exists), drawing curtains around the family, or expediting the discharge process to transfer the patient to the postpartum unit. The mother and father are anxious to review the details of the birth together, and the perianesthesia nurse should be prepared to answer questions. Consistent communication between the surgical nurse and the perianesthesia nursing staff makes answering these questions much easier.

Ectopic Pregnancy

Faulty implantation of the ovum can take place in the fallopian tube (in approximately 98% of all ectopic pregnancies), in the ovary, in any part of the abdominal cavity, or in the uterine cervix (Fig. 42-1). Until recently, the treatment of choice for an ectopic pregnancy in the fallopian tube was laparoscopy (or laparotomy) with removal of the ectopic pregnancy and most often with preservation of the fallopian tube. In cases in which bleeding cannot be controlled or the physician believes

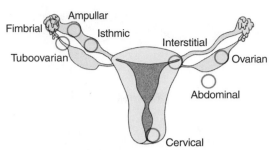

FIG. 42-1 Sites of implantation of ectopic pregnancies. Order of frequency of occurrence is ampulla, isthmus, interstitium, fimbria, tubo-ovarian ligament, ovary, abdominal cavity, and cervix (external os). (From Lowdermilk DL, et al: *Maternity and women's health care*, ed 10, St. Louis, 2012, Mosby.)

that the fallopian tube poses too much of a risk for the patient, removal of the fallopian tube at the time of surgery may be necessary. Obviously the patient must give proper consent before surgery, and all these possibilities are thoroughly discussed between the surgeon and the patient. More recently, however, patients with the early diagnosis of an unruptured ectopic pregnancy can receive intravenous methotrexate and not undergo surgery. Regardless of the treatment, these patients must have proper follow-up with their physicians to ensure successful treatment, which involves follow-up quantitative human chorionic gonadotropin studies and possibly ultrasound scans as well.

If laparoscopy is performed, the ovary preferably is not resected or removed; however, this procedure may be necessary if the ovary is involved with the ectopic pregnancy. If implantation occurs in the cervix, a hysterectomy is usually indicated to control hemorrhage. If abdominal implantation has occurred, the fetus is removed and the placenta often is left within the cavity to be reabsorbed.

Laparoscopy (or laparotomy) is performed with general anesthesia. The perianesthesia nurse should be especially observant for signs of intraabdominal hemorrhage and shock because these are not uncommon complications of ectopic pregnancy, especially one that has ruptured before surgery. All patients with ectopic pregnancy should have complete typing and cross-matching for whole blood, which should be kept available in the laboratory for 24 hours. Women who are Rh-negative should receive Rhogam to prevent sensitization. As mentioned previously, many ectopic pregnancies are being successfully treated without surgery and only with medications.

Cerclage Procedures

The McDonald or Shirodkar procedure is used to treat an incompetent cervix and is fairly successful in maintenance of pregnancy. The suture is usually placed between the fourteenth and eighteenth week of gestation. These procedures may be accomplished with general, spinal, or regional anesthesia.

On admission to the PACU, hospital guidelines are followed regarding patient admission to the PACU and care of the patient (see Chapters 27 and 28). Oxygen should be administered and weaned with pulse oximetry. Food and fluids can be resumed as soon as the patient is conscious and the laryngeal reflexes have returned. A perineal pad should be kept in place. Only a minimal amount of bloody spotting is normal. Pain should be minimal and easily controlled with a simple analgesic, such as acetaminophen. Any gross vaginal bleeding or abdominal cramping should be reported to the surgeon, because this procedure may induce labor and expulsion of the uterine contents. The surgeon may order an external fetal monitor to assess the presence of uterine contractions and fetal heart tones. If labor begins, the suture must be removed immediately.

Uterine Aspiration

Uterine aspiration is used in the termination of early pregnancy (i.e., first trimester) or in treatment of incomplete spontaneous abortion. The procedure is a type of dilation of the cervix and curettage of the uterus (D&C). A general anesthetic can be used, but the trend has been toward the use of paracervical block and sedation only. Nursing care in the PACU is essentially the same as after D&C by conventional means. The woman who is Rh negative should receive Rhogam to prevent sensitization. Complications from this procedure include incomplete evacuation and hemorrhage, which may be treated with oxytocin. Uterine perforation can occur and must be treated surgically.

GYNECOLOGIC SURGERY

Certain problems are inherent in gynecologic disease processes and the surgical procedures that deal with them. Because of prolonged or heavy menstrual periods, the patient may be more chronically anemic than even the peripheral blood indices indicate. Moreover, large amounts of blood may have accumulated within the pelvic organs at the time of the operation and may not be reflected in the external blood loss. Although the procedures are elective, many gynecologic operations are associated with significant blood loss, depending on the approach taken. This can be affected by the patient's age (more if she is premenopausal), a larger uterus, and large fibroids. One of the potential benefits of a well-trained laparoscopic team is a decrease in intraoperative complications and blood loss and a significant reduction in postoperative morbidity. For example, in the case of a hysterectomy or large fibroids in a premenopausal woman, the uterine vessels are large, vascular pedicles that need to be thoroughly coagulated to ensure hemostasis during surgery. For this reason, regardless of the approach (laparoscopy with or without a robot, vaginal, or laparotomy), these vessels must be identified and coagulated or ligated effectively. In addition, because of the proximity of the female organs to the urinary tract, great care must be taken during surgery to identify the ureters and bladder and provide proper follow-up during the observation period after surgery to ensure the integrity of this system. If there is any question of this, a cystoscopy should be done upon the conclusion of the surgery. In addition to overall assessment and general care of these patients, the perianesthesia nurse should direct specific attention toward the patient's cardiovascular status, renal function, and fluid balance.[3]

Laparoscopy

Operative laparoscopy commonly is performed as outpatient surgery for treatment of benign gynecologic problems and may involve advanced operative laparoscopic procedures for more significant problems that involve the pelvic organs. A small incision (approximately 1 cm) is made at the subumbilical site for insertion of the primary trocar (typically 10 to 12 mm in diameter), which houses the laparoscope with attached video camera for visualization of the pelvis (Fig. 42-2). The entry into the pelvic cavity can be done various ways; one of which includes open laparoscopy, particularly for patients who have had multiple previous surgeries to protect against injuring the bowel. When a patient has had multiple previous surgeries, the bowel is more likely to be adhered to the abdominal wall and oftentimes thought to be a safer way to enter. After pneumoperitoneum is established, the surgeon can visualize the organs within the peritoneum. The video camera enables the surgeon, first assistant, scrub technician, and entire team to view the procedure on the video monitor (Fig. 42-3). The video camera provides excellent resolution and visualization of the pelvis.

Advances in digital technology with high-definition (HD) cameras and monitors provide better resolution than ever before (Fig. 42-4). The

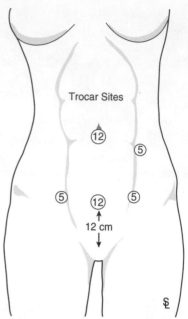

FIG. 42-2 Placement of trocars during advanced operative laparoscopy. Trocar in upper left quadrant is optional and only recommended in cases in which primary trocar is not sufficient because of severe adhesions. Laparoscope needs to be placed off to one side for taking down adhesions.

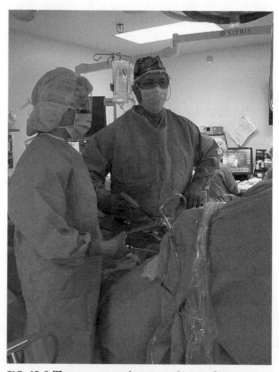

FIG. 42-3 The surgeon and registered nurse first assistant (RNFA) and the rest of the team are able to benefit from improved resolution attainable with high-definition cameras and monitors. (Courtesy Wendy Winer.)

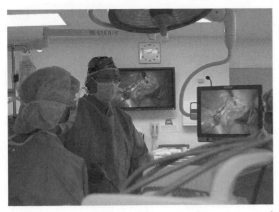

FIG. 42-4 High-definition cameras and monitors used for laparoscopic surgery at Northside Hospital in Atlanta, Georgia. (Courtesy Wendy Winer.)

surgeon is able to operate from HD monitors with instruments that are typically 5 mm in diameter (sometimes the instruments are as small as 3 mm in diameter or as large as 12 mm in diameter, depending on the procedure). In addition, an angled laparoscope can be used for improved visualization in the case of a large uterus. If the robot is to be used, it is connected after the trocars have been placed. The robot offers three-dimensional visualization that some find appealing. The surgeon sits at a console and is able to maneuver the instrumentation from that location while the surgical assistant is at the patient's side and using instrumentation such as suction and irrigation. In addition, a surgical technologist is typically present between the patient's legs (similar to laparoscopy without the robot) to manipulate the uterus with a uterine manipulator. In addition to the expense of the robot, there can be a significant amount of time required for the robot to be connected and disconnected. This includes the sterile draping of the arms of the robot. If an emergency arises with bleeding that cannot be controlled, the robot has to quickly be disengaged so that traditional surgery can quickly be initiated. For teaching purposes in particular, it is now possible to get a robot with two consoles so that the surgeon may have the student surgeon (resident or fellow) at the secondary console to work and receive instruction.

The surgeon examines the ovaries, fallopian tubes, pelvic side walls, uterosacral ligaments, bowel, appendix, peritoneum, anterior and posterior cul de sacs, and uterus after placement of the second and third incisions suprapubically in the right and left lower quadrants of the abdomen (this houses the ancillary instrumentation). If additional instrumentation is needed, a fourth incision may be made along the midsuprapubic area as well. During operative laparoscopy, the surgeon may differentially diagnose pelvic inflammatory disease or perform relatively simple procedures, such as aspiration of an ovarian cyst, lysis of adhesions, tissue biopsy, and tubal ligation. In addition, more advanced laparoscopic procedures may be done, including extensive lysis of adhesions, excision of mild, moderate or severe endometriosis, myomectomy, hysterectomy (laparoscopic total hysterectomy or laparoscopic supracervical hysterectomy), salpingectomy, salpingo-oophorectomy, removal of an ovarian remnant, ureterolysis, paravaginal repair or Burch procedures, repair of pelvic floor relaxation including laparoscopic sacral colpopexy with nonabsorbable mesh appendectomy, fibrinolysis, and tubal reanastomosis (Fig. 42-5). Various types of laparoscopic hysterectomy include laparoscopic supracervical hysterectomy, in which the cervix is preserved, laparoscopic-assisted vaginal hysterectomy (LAVH), and total laparoscopic hysterectomy. It is important to note that not all energy sources can be used with the robot, such as certain types of lasers and electrosurgery devices. In cases of severe endometriosis in which there is significant bowel involvement, a general surgeon may be called to do a laparoscopic bowel resection with the gynecologist. These surgeries may occur in patients with severe endometriosis and bowel symptoms and who have had a complete bowel preparation before surgery. The general surgeon, who is part of the endometriosis team, is on standby for that type of

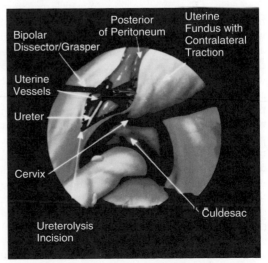

FIG. 42-5 Laparoscopic anatomy as seen through laparoscope. Figure shows bipolar instrument used for uterine occlusion. (Courtesy Center for Women's Care and Reproductive Surgery, Atlanta, Georgia.)

NURSING CARE IN THE PACU

procedure. PACU needs to be aware of any special needs postoperatively for patients undergoing either a laparoscopic bowel resection or a laparoscopic cystotomy and repair of the bladder for extensive invasion of these tissues with endometriosis. In regard to any type of bladder repair, it is common for the urinary catheter to be left in place for at least 7 to 10 days. With bowel surgery, the patients are generally kept inpatient for 3 to 4 days until bowel function returns. The diet generally is very limited, beginning with ice chips, followed by clear liquids, clear fluids, and then advance to a soft diet. In most cases, these patients no longer require a colostomy or a suprapubic urinary catheter. Always notify the surgeon if there is a significant amount of bleeding from any orifice. It is common for patients to have a pinkish urine output after cystoscopy. Often these patients have at least a mild form of interstitial cystitis. If there is any blood in the urine when the patient is brought to the PACU, the circulating nurse should communicate that information in the report.

Closure of the skin wound involves a few absorbable type sutures. It is important to close the fascia at the subumbilical site as well as any other incision sites that are 7 mm or larger to prevent the development of a hernia. Depending on the type of trocar used, some manufacturers recommend only closing the fascia for trocars 10 or 12 mm in size. The ancillary sites that are 5 mm can be sutured subcutaneously or a liquid glue can be used followed with liquid adhesive and Steri-Strips to approximate the edges of the skin incision. It is common for larger patients in whom the fascia of 7-mm trocar incisions or larger must be closed to be more tender the first couple of weeks postoperatively. If there is any oozing from an incision site, it is usually coagulated or an additional stitch is placed before the patient waking up. In addition, if there is any question about the amount of oozing, a pressure dressing can be place and the perianesthesia nurse can reinforce it with a 1-pound sandbag during the first hour postoperatively in the PACU. Dressings may include an eye pad or a 2 × 2-inch pad at the subumbilical site with clear adhesive type bandages over the other sites to allow the patients to shower. If patients have an allergy to adhesive, then use paper tape or Steri-Strips depending on the patient history. Initial pain in the PACU should be minimal to moderate and is generally successfully controlled with antiinflammatory agents or mild opioids. Severe pain may indicate a more severe condition, and the surgeon should be notified immediately. A firm abdomen could indicate abdominal bleeding that is not normal. Severe pain, nausea, or vomiting could indicate a bowel perforation. Generally these types of occurrences may show up in the first 24 hours, but also may not occur for 10 to 14 days postoperatively. For that reason, it is crucial that all this information is reinforced in writing to give the patient when they are discharged. If any of these conditions occur or anything is out of the ordinary, the surgeon should be notified immediately. Postoperative care instructions, including an explanation of the possibility of referred chest or shoulder pain, should be discussed with the patient and a significant other. Again, instructions should always be written and given to the patient preoperatively and reviewed prior to discharge.

A follow-up phone call to the patient within 24 to 48 hours is recommended. Special care for the patient who undergoes outpatient surgery is outlined in Chapter 46.

Lower Genital and Vaginal Surgery

The perianesthesia nurse may encounter pediatric or adolescent female patients who undergo gynecologic surgery for repair or correction of congenital or traumatic deformities or incapacitating pelvic pain (from causes such as endometriosis, ovarian cyst, or appendicitis). The conditions that require this type of surgery occur most often in women who have had multiple births, do frequent lifting in their occupation, are smokers, or frequently cough; they also occur as women age. Often this is seen in young women after they have had two or more children. These conditions are caused most commonly by exaggeration of the normal relaxation of the pelvic ligaments and support that occurs during childbirth and also after menopause. A number of specific procedures, named after their developers, may be encountered and include the following:

- Baldy-Webster procedure: Shortening of the round ligaments and changing of the direction of their pull by attaching them to the back of the uterus
- Fothergill-Hunter procedure: Complete repair of the vaginal wall (enterocele defect), from above downward toward the vulva, to correct faulty supportive structures of the pelvic floor; various defects commonly referred to as *vaginal defect* (enterocele repair), protrusion of the bladder (cystocele repair), or protrusion of the rectum (rectocele repair) and prolapse of the vaginal walls (paravaginal repair); generally a combination and not an isolated repair, which is why a urogynecologist is often the best person to most thoroughly make these

Evidence-Based Practice

A study was conducted to determine long-term outcomes after complete laparoscopic excision in a teenaged population, who were not specifically advised to take postoperative hormonal suppression. The design used was a prospective observational case series. All patients underwent diagnostic laparoscopy and complete excision of all areas of abnormal peritoneum with typical and atypical endometriosis. Patients were not specifically advised to take postoperative hormonal suppression. Complete laparoscopic excision of endometriosis in teenagers has the potential to eradicate the disease, and the results do not depend on postoperative hormonal suppression.

IMPLICATIONS FOR PRACTICE

Perianesthesia nurses can be actively involved in projects and studies that determine best practice for teenage patients following laparoscopic excision of endometriosis. Many of these patients have been suffering with severe dysmenorrhea since they began menarche. This is becoming more common in teenagers, particularly since the age of menarche is before they reach their teenage years. By the time they reach their teens, they have been taking a variety of pain medications, with the cause of their pain often diagnosed incorrectly, and taking numerous hormones in an attempt to alleviate their symptoms. As a result of short- and long-term follow-up, results show that thorough excision of endometriosis improves a patient's quality of life postoperatively. Additional studies postoperatively are being done to further evaluate the use of hormonal suppression in these patients.

From Yeung P, et al: Complete laparoscopic excision of endometriosis in teenagers: is postoperative hormonal suppression necessary? *Fertil Steril* 95:6:1909–1912, 2011.

repairs because there is so much overlap and it is important to evaluate the woman's entire pelvic floor for optimal success with the repairs
- Gilliam procedure: Shortening of the round ligaments by attaching them to the abdominal wall
- Le Fort operation (colpocleisis): Closure of the vagina with approximation of the anterior and posterior vaginal walls with or without attendant vaginal hysterectomy
- Radical vulvectomy: Abdominal and perineal dissection of the superficial and deep inguinal nodes and portions of the saphenous veins, reconstruction of the vaginal walls and pelvic floor, and closure of the abdominal wounds
- Vulvectomy: Removal of the labia majora, labia minora, and possibly the clitoris and perianal area, with a Z-plasty closure; used in treatment of leukoplakia vulva, carcinoma in situ of the vulva, and Paget disease of the vulva

The specialty of gynecologic oncologists typically perform procedures such as radical hysterectomy, vulvectomy, and lymphoidectomy, because they are usually performed on women with a form of gynecologic cancer.

Other vaginal surgical procedures include fistula repairs, correction of urinary stress incontinence (various sling procedures with nonabsorbable transobturator tape), and vaginal reconstruction to repair congenital or acquired defects developed during childbirth. Many of the pelvic floor repair procedures can be done laparoscopically if the surgeon is comfortable with laparoscopic suturing and is a well-trained laparoscopist. Currently there is a great amount of debate over the types of mesh being used in the body. In particular, mesh that is used for gynecologic pelvic organ prolapse procedures is under investigation because of infections and mesh erosion, which can cause subsequent pain months or years after surgery. In the past it was thought that the type of mesh and the pore size were the key factors; however, this is being discussed again. Patients with severe prolapse need some type of graft, and it is unclear what the eventual reality will be on this issue. Most importantly, patients must be sure to stay abreast of the research on this topic. Regardless of the type of graft that is used, a well-trained laparoscopist is required to do these procedures. Many gynecologists use the robot because they are not comfortable suturing laparoscopically. Other surgeons believe that the time and expense is unnecessary if the surgeon takes the time for proper training. In addition, many gynecologists believe that they can do the surgery more effectively and efficiently without the robot. Operative laparoscopy typically requires three to four incision sites, and the robotic laparoscopy may require four to seven incisions. In addition, there are single puncture devices that may be used at the umbilicus without the robot, and those are also being developed to be used with the robot. The debate continues about whether the surgery can be done effectively with one larger single site incision at the umbilicus. During a time when health costs are out of control, cost of instrumentation and equipment and length of surgery are important, and the

NURSING CARE IN THE PACU

question remains, does the robot offer advantages over advanced operative laparoscopy by a well trained, experienced laparoscopist and team?

There are several sides to this argument and debate. It appears that the robot is necessary for certain procedures in surgery, and there needs to be more follow-up and research to determine what procedures those will be and more specifically which ones those might include in the area of gynecology. It is important, however, to examine this data and to ascertain that comparisons of the robot are made to laparoscopy and that outcomes from robotic surgery are not compared to open surgeries.. The pelvic floor procedures are performed with nonabsorbable sutures and mesh for optimal long-term results. The role of the operative team in these procedures cannot be overemphasized in enabling the surgeon to focus on the surgery. The entire team can play an integral part in large part because of the video cameras and monitors being used during laparoscopic surgery.

General Perianesthesia Care

Anesthesia for lower genital and vaginal surgery can be local, general, or regional, depending on the amount of pelvic relaxation necessary to perform the procedures. Routine guidelines are followed when the patient is admitted to the PACU. When alert, the patient may assume a position of comfort and be encouraged to move about frequently as part of antiembolism care. After a general assessment of the patient's condition, all dressings should be checked carefully. Vaginal packing may be in place with some vaginal procedures, or a perineal pad only may be used vaginally in the case of laparoscopy. Intake and output is monitored as per routine. Saturation of the vaginal packing may be expected after any vaginal surgery; however, saturation of the perineal pad when vaginal packing is in place should be considered excessive bleeding and should be reported. Vaginal and groin wounds often have drains, and care must be exercised to avoid dislodgement. If drains are in place, a moderate amount of drainage may be expected.

Food and fluids can be resumed safely after the minor procedures, such as D&C and bartholinectomy, after the pharyngeal reflexes have returned. After more extensive procedures, the patient is usually not given anything by mouth until peristalsis is reestablished; intake is supplied with intravenous fluids. Urine output should be monitored carefully for amount and for the presence of blood. Often patients have a urinary catheter in place until they are ambulatory, and securing the catheter is important so

that no tugging or pulling causes irritation after its removal.

Pain must be carefully evaluated and may be alleviated with appropriate analgesics. Abdominal cramping is common after gynecologic surgery. For these patients, relaxation exercises are often helpful if they have been learned before surgery. Warm blankets over the abdomen can also aid in relaxation. Because the patient is often drowsy from the anesthesia, coaching is needed, especially during the first hour. If cramping is not relieved with relaxation exercises, analgesics, or other comfort measures, the surgeon should be notified because this may indicate a perforated uterus or more severe problem. After removal of tumors or cysts from the vaginal area, ice can be applied to reduce edema and provide comfort.[4]

ABDOMINAL GYNECOLOGIC SURGERY

Abdominal gynecologic surgery can be performed alone or in conjunction with vaginal surgery.

General Postoperative Care

Postoperative care after abdominal gynecologic surgery involves all the care and considerations rendered to the patient who undergoes any type of abdominal surgery. Anesthesia is most often general.[5] Overall assessment of the patient, with special emphasis on the cardiovascular status, should be undertaken as soon as the patient is admitted to the PACU.

The most common and dangerous complications of any obstetric or gynecologic surgery are excessive hemorrhage and shock; therefore the perianesthesia nurse should direct assessment to a complete evaluation of the patient's circulatory status at frequent intervals. All dressings should be checked for drainage. Pain should be evaluated, and appropriate comfort measures and analgesics should be administered.

After total abdominal hysterectomy or major abdominal procedures, the patient is usually not given anything orally until peristalsis has returned and nausea has subsided. Intake is supplied with intravenous fluids. Occasionally the patient is admitted to the PACU with a nasogastric tube to prevent abdominal distention. If abdominal distention develops, nasogastric and rectal tubes can be used to relieve it.[6]

A urinary catheter is often in place, and its patency must be ensured. The perianesthesia nurse should accurately document the amount of urinary output and the presence of blood. A possible complication of hysterectomy is accidental perforation or ligation of a ureter. Inadvertent injury to the bladder wall or the bowel may also occur.

To prevent vascular disorders, especially in the lower extremities, the patient's position should be changed frequently. A high Fowler position should be avoided, and active and passive range-of-motion exercises of the lower extremities should be instituted in the PACU as soon as possible.

If a hysterectomy is done laparoscopically and the uterus is removed vaginally (i.e., LAVH), vaginal packing typically is not used whether the vaginal cuff is repaired vaginally or laparoscopically. In addition, patients encounter some vaginal bleeding after LAVH and also after most laparoscopies, because a uterine manipulator is used during the procedure. Patients who have undergone a hysteroscopy likely have postoperative vaginal bleeding as well; however, in all these cases, the bleeding should not be heavier than that from a menstrual period. If heavier bleeding occurs, the surgeon should be notified immediately. After surgery, patients should be instructed to refrain from sexual intercourse and from vaginal insertion of foreign objects, including tampons for 2 weeks; these instructions may vary among physicians. On discharge, patients should be provided with written home instructions that outline specific guidelines to follow. These guidelines should include a telephone number for the patient to be able to contact the surgeon or the physician on call 24 hours a day. Many of the patients who undergo laparoscopic procedures are discharged within 24 hours after surgery; therefore they must know whom to call. Patients may have vaginal discharge in some form for several weeks after these procedures. After laparoscopic surgery, the surgeon typically has the patient return for a postoperative examination 2 weeks after surgery.

After laparoscopic surgery, patients should begin to feel significantly better within 48 to 72 hours. If they still have a great deal of discomfort or if they begin to feel better and then start to feel much worse a couple of days later, the surgeon should be notified immediately. This condition could indicate a postoperative complication that could involve the development of a hematoma, an infection, or an injury to the bowel, bladder, or ureter. A bowel injury often does not present itself until the patient has gone home. The injury could be serious, and the physician must identify and recognize it as soon as possible. All these criteria should be outlined in the written discharge instructions. Many facilities that discharge patients within 24 hours after surgery follow up by calling patients within 24 to 48 hours to see how they are doing. Usually this call is a courtesy call. If a problem is found, the patient is generally encouraged to contact the physician. If the patient ever has shortness of breath, severe pain, or bleeding heavier than a period, they should contact their physician immediately or go to the nearest emergency room.[7]

SUMMARY

This chapter discussed gynecologic surgery for repair or correction of congenital or traumatic deformities, incapacitating pelvic pain, abnormal bleeding, or potential abnormalities of the reproductive organs. The chapter discussed female surgery of three major categories: obstetric, lower genital and vaginal, and abdominal gynecologic surgery. Abdominal surgery can be what use to be referred to as *traditional surgery* in the form of a laparotomy, mini laparotomy (may include hand assisted surgery) or in the category of operative laparoscopy with or without the use of a robot. Robotics in the area of surgery continues to grow and seems to be increasing the number of minimally invasive procedures being done. Perianesthesia nurses must stay current to provide patients with optimal care before, during, and after surgery. Cost containment continues to be a focus as well as required guidelines that relate to the patient's temperature, administration of antibiotics, deep vein thrombosis prophylaxis, and other criteria that affect reimbursement. To provide optimal care for the patient, the perianesthesia nurse can combine knowledge about the procedures with knowledge of postanesthesia care of the patient undergoing gynecologic surgery.

REFERENCES

1. Yeung P, et al: Complete laparoscopic excision of endometriosis in teenagers: is postoperative hormonal suppression necessary? *Fertility and Sterility* 95(6):1909–1912, 2011.
2. McEwen DR: Gynecologic and obstetric surgery. In Rothrock J: *Alexander's care of the patient in surgery*, ed 13, St. Louis, 2007, Mosby.
3. Adolph A, et al: Laparoscopic supracervical hysterectomy for the large uterus, *J Am Assoc Gynecol Laparosc* 11(2):170–174, 2004.
4. Baughman VL, et al: *Anesthesiology and critical care drug handbook*, ed 9, Ohio, 2009, Lexicomp.
5. Lyons TL, et al: *Laparoscopic hysterectomy*, available at www.uptodate.com/contents/laparoscopic-approach-to-hysterectomy. Accessed August 28, 2011.
6. Winer WK: Core curriculum for the RN first assistant, section VIII: gynecology and obstetrics, *AORN* 197–212, 2005.
7. Winer WK, Seifert PC, editors: Advances in minimally invasive gynecology, *Perioperative Nursing Clinics* 1(4):305–380, 2006.

NURSING CARE IN THE PACU

43 Care of the Breast Surgical Patient

Nancy M. Saufl, MS, RN, CPAN, CAPA

Breast cancer, the most common cancer in women,[1] is a malignant tumor that develops from cells of the breast. Although breast cancer in men is rare, it does occur. With the newer forms of treatment of cancer of the breast, including improved forms of diagnosis, surgical procedures on the breast have increased. However, with earlier breast cancer diagnosis and with the advent of enhanced radiation and chemotherapy protocols, surgical procedures performed on the breast might not be as extensive as in years past. All women are at risk for breast cancer. The two most significant risk factors are female gender and older age.[2] Ninety-five percent of new cases and 97% of breast cancer deaths occurred in women older than 40 years.[2] Risk of breast cancer also increases if the woman's mother, sister, or daughter has had the disease. Breast surgery is most commonly performed on women; however, procedures are occasionally performed on men and children. In addition, nondisease breast procedures may be performed for cosmetic purposes. Breast cancer is the second leading cause of death for women after lung cancer.[1] The chances of a woman having breast cancer are one in eight. Chances of dying from breast cancer are approximately 1 in 33. Breast cancer is the most common cause of cancer in African American women and the second leading cause of death in African American women, exceeded only by lung cancer. Approximately 1 in 100 men is expected to develop breast cancer in a lifetime. As the patient's advocate, the perianesthesia nurse must be supportive, caring, and reassuring to the patient having breast surgery. Positive support is the start of the patient's rehabilitation process. Early detections, self examination, mammography, and an increased public awareness are all important factors in decreasing annual breast cancer mortality.[2] Breast cancer treatment today involves a combination of therapies, including surgical excision of the tumor, radiation therapy alone, or a combination of surgery, radiation and chemotherapy. New studies and treatment protocols are continuously being developed and subjected to trials, but early detection remains the best hope for cure.

DEFINITIONS

Adenocarcinoma: A general type of cancer that starts in glandular tissues anywhere in the body. Almost all breast cancers start in glandular tissue of the breast and therefore are adenocarcinomas. The two main types of breast adenocarcinomas are ductal carcinomas and lobular carcinomas. Benign breast lesions are the most commonly excised lesions (fibrocystic changes and fibroadenomas).

Augmentation Mammoplasty: Surgery to enlarge or augment the size of the female breast with a breast implant; the most popular cosmetic procedure.

Breast Biopsy: Excision of breast tissue. The specimen is sent to the pathology laboratory for frozen sectioning. In addition, a needle localization can be performed when a suspected lesion is identified with mammogram results. The procedure involves placing a thin needle or guide into the breast with mammographic visualization. The lesion is then excised and taken to the pathology laboratory for frozen sectioning to determine a diagnosis.

Breast Reconstruction (Mammoplasty): The breast is reconstructed after mastectomy.

Ductal Carcinoma In Situ (DCIS): Ductal carcinoma in situ (also known as *intraductal carcinoma*) is the most common type of noninvasive breast cancer. Cancer cells are inside the ducts, but have not spread through the walls of the ducts into the fatty tissue of the breast. Nearly all women diagnosed at this early stage of breast cancer can be cured. The best way to find DCIS is with a mammogram. With more women getting mammograms each year, diagnosis of DCIS is becoming more common. DCIS is sometimes subclassified based on its grade and type to help predict the risk of return of cancer after treatment and to help select the most appropriate treatment. *Grade* refers to how aggressive cancer cells appear with a microscope. Several types of DCIS exist, but the most important distinction among them is whether tumor cell necrosis (areas of dead or degenerating cancer cells) is present. The term *comedocarcinoma* is often used to describe a type of DCIS with necrosis.

Infiltrating (or Invasive) Ductal Carcinoma (IDC): With a start in a milk passage, or duct, of the breast, this cancer has broken through the wall of the duct and invaded the fatty tissue of the breast. At this point, it has the potential to metastasize, or spread, to other parts of the body through the lymphatic system and bloodstream. Infiltrating ductal carcinoma accounts for approximately 80% of invasive breast cancers.

Infiltrating (or Invasive) Lobular Carcinoma (ILC):
ILC starts in the milk-producing glands. Similar to IDC, this cancer has the potential to spread (metastasize) elsewhere in the body. Approximately 10% to 15% of invasive breast cancers are invasive lobular carcinomas. ILC may be more difficult to detect with mammogram than IDC.

Inflammatory Breast Cancer: This rare type of invasive breast cancer accounts for approximately 1% of all breast cancers. In inflammatory breast cancer, the skin of the breast appears red and feels warm, as though it were infected and inflamed. The skin has a thick, pitted appearance that doctors often describe as resembling an orange peel. Sometimes the skin develops ridges and small bumps that resemble hives. Doctors now know that these changes are not caused by inflammation or infection, but the name given long ago to this type of cancer still persists. Cancer cells that block lymph vessels or channels in the skin over the breast cause these symptoms.

In Situ: This term is used for an early stage of cancer in which it is confined to the immediate area at which it began. Specifically in breast cancer, *in situ* means that the cancer remains confined to ducts (ductal carcinoma in situ) or lobules (lobular carcinoma in situ). It has not invaded surrounding fatty tissues in the breast nor spread to other organs in the body.

Lobular Carcinoma In Situ (LCIS): Although not a true cancer, LCIS (also called *lobular neoplasia*) is sometimes classified as a type of noninvasive breast cancer. It begins in the milk-producing glands, but does not penetrate through the wall of the lobules. Most breast cancer specialists think that LCIS itself does not become an invasive cancer, but that women with this condition have a higher risk of developing an invasive breast cancer in the same or the opposite breast. For this reason, women with LCIS should have physical examinations two or three times per year and an annual mammogram.

Lumpectomy: Only the tumor and surrounding tissue of a "breast lump" are excised. The rest of the breast remains intact. The procedure includes dissection of the axillary lymph nodes. The lump is generally smaller than 4 cm in diameter.

Mastopexy (Breast Lift): Reshaping (uplifting) the sagging breasts with surgical tightening of the skin.

Medullary Carcinoma: This special type of infiltrating breast cancer has a relatively well-defined distinct boundary between tumor tissue and normal tissue. It also has some other special features, including the large size of the cancer cells and the presence of immune system cells at the edges of the tumor. Medullary carcinoma accounts for approximately 5% of breast cancers. The outlook, or prognosis, for this kind of breast cancer is better than for other types of invasive breast cancer.

Modified Radical Mastectomy: Removal of the entire breast and axillary lymph nodes; the pectoralis major muscle is left intact. In some instances, the pectoralis minor muscle is excised.

Mucinous Carcinoma: This rare type of invasive breast cancer is formed by mucus-producing cancer cells. The prognosis for mucinous carcinoma is better than for the more common types of invasive breast cancer. *Colloid*

carcinoma is another name for this type of breast cancer.

Paget Disease of the Nipple: This type of breast cancer starts in the breast ducts and spreads to the skin of the nipple and then to the areola, the dark circle around the nipple. It is a rare type of breast cancer and occurs in only 1% of all cases. The skin of the nipple and areola often appears crusted, scaly, and red with areas of bleeding or oozing. Women may notice burning or itching. Paget disease may be associated with in situ carcinoma or with infiltrating breast carcinoma. If no lump can be felt in the breast tissue and the biopsy shows DCIS but no invasive cancer, the prognosis is excellent.

Phyllodes Tumor: This rare type of breast tumor forms from the stroma (connective tissue) of the breast, in contrast to carcinomas, which develop in the ducts or lobules. Phyllodes (or hylloides) tumors are usually benign but rarely malignant, with the potential to metastasize. Benign phyllodes tumors are successfully treated by removing the mass and a narrow margin of normal breast tissue. A malignant phyllodes tumor is treated with removal along with a wider margin of normal tissue or with mastectomy. These cancers do not respond to hormonal therapy and are not so likely to respond to chemotherapy or radiation therapy. In the past, both benign and malignant phyllodes tumors were called *cystosarcoma phyllodes.*

Radical Mastectomy: Removal of the entire breast, skin, nipple, areolar complex, and pectoralis major and minor muscles with axillary node dissection.

Tubular Carcinoma: Tubular carcinomas are a special type of infiltrating breast carcinoma and account for approximately 2% of all breast cancers. They have a better prognosis than usual infiltrating ductal or lobular carcinomas.

SURGICAL INTERVENTIONS AND PERIANESTHESIA NURSING CARE

Breast Biopsy

Breast cancer is often first suspected when a lump is felt or an abnormal area is found on mammogram results. Lumps in the breast often are discovered during monthly self examination or with routine mammograms, breast ultrasound scans, or magnetic resonance imaging. A biopsy is done when the results of these other tests suggest breast cancer. The biopsy is the only way to know for certain. The lumps or masses are aspirated or excised and sent for definitive diagnoses.

For many of the female patients who undergo a biopsy, the diagnosis is fibrocystic disease. Fibro cystic disease describes a variety of benign and localized tumors or swelling within the breast tissues, including cysts, masses, and intraductal papillomas. Other nonfibrocystic conditions also may cause breast lumps. Inflammatory conditions, such as breast abscesses, fat necrosis, and lipomas of the skin (e.g., sebaceous cysts), can cause breast lumps.

A breast biopsy can be a one-step (biopsy and mastectomy, if needed) or two-step procedure. Two-step procedures are the most common practice. The two-step procedure allows the patient to be educated about the choices and given the opportunity to make an informed decision regarding the type of surgery to be performed in the event of a positive biopsy finding. The short delay between the biopsy and further treatment has not been shown to affect survival rates. If more extensive surgery is planned in the event of a positive biopsy result, the patient must have given preoperative informed consent for the definitive surgical procedure.

The patient is usually admitted as a same-day surgery patient. The patient may undergo needle biopsy, incisional biopsy, or excisional biopsy. A needle biopsy includes the introduction of a disposable cutting-type needle through the mass to entrap a core of tissue. The needle is withdrawn, and the specimen is sent to the pathology laboratory. In an incisional biopsy, a portion of the mass is surgically excised along a curved incision line. An excisional biopsy may be needed to remove the entire mass and some of the adjacent tissue around it for examination. A stereotactic procedure may be performed in which the patient lies face down on a special table. The breast protrudes through a hole in the table and is lightly compressed while the computer provides detailed diagnostic images. The biopsy area is located and a probe is inserted to remove the tissue specimens (Fig. 43-1).

Because of the patient's natural apprehension, the patient may receive intravenous moderate sedation along with local anesthesia. Monitored anesthesia care may also be indicated. If the patient meets phase I discharge criteria while still in the operating suite, the patient may bypass the phase I postanesthesia care unit (PACU). Otherwise, the patient is usually awake on arrival in the PACU but drowsy because of the sedation. Routine admission procedures are accomplished. The head of the bed may be elevated 45 degrees.

The dressing is usually a 4 × 4 sponge held in place with the patient's bra. It should be inspected for excessive drainage, which occurs only rarely. The patient can resume fluid and food intake as soon as the cough and gag reflexes have fully returned and nausea has subsided. Pain should be minimal, if any, and easily controlled with minor analgesics.

If midazolam has been administered, the patient may repeatedly ask the same questions. The perianesthesia nurse must patiently repeat the answers and also ensure that the person who accompanies the patient at discharge understands the home care instructions.

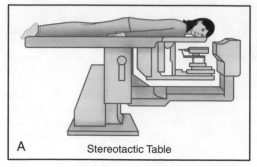

A   Stereotactic Table

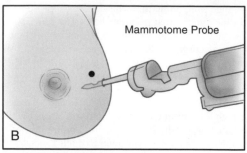

Mammotome Probe

B

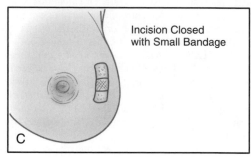

Incision Closed
with Small Bandage

C

FIG. 43-1 **A,** In stereotactic procedures, patients lie facedown on a special table. The woman's breast protrudes through a hole in the table's surface, where it is lightly compressed and immobilized while a computer produces detailed images of the abnormality. **B,** When the biopsy area has been located and mapped, the Mammotome probe is inserted through a ¼-inch incision in the breast, where it gently vacuums, cuts, and removes breast tissue samples. **C,** The incision is then closed with a small adhesive bandage. (From Rothrock J: *Alexander's care of the patient in surgery,* ed 14, St. Louis, 2011, Mosby.)

Surgical Choices for the Treatment of Cancer

Most women need some type of surgery to treat the breast tumor and remove as much of the cancer as possible. Surgical treatment choice depends on the stage of the disease, the size and site of the mass, and the patient's individual choice. Advances in early diagnosis and modifications in surgical techniques have increased the number of surgical choices in the treatment of breast cancer (Fig. 43-2). Surgical treatment may range from breast-conserving techniques (lumpectomy) to modified radical mastectomy that involves the breast and the axillary nodes.

Lumpectomy

Lumpectomy, also called *breast-conserving therapy*, is the surgical treatment of choice when the breast tumor is well defined and less than 5 cm in diameter. In landmark clinical trials reported in 1988, the National Surgical Adjuvant Breast Cancer Project reported that lumpectomy followed by radiation therapy produced 8-year disease-free survival rates equal to those of modified radical mastectomy.[3]

Lumpectomy is usually performed with general anesthesia. Only the breast tumor and a margin of 1 to 1.5mm of surrounding normal tissue are removed. Surgery may also be done to determine whether the cancer has spread to the lymph nodes. Lumpectomy with subsequent radiation therapy is frequently the treatment of choice for small tumors.

Sentinel Lymph Node Biopsy

A sentinel lymph node biopsy may be done to visually examine the lymph nodes without having to remove them first. Sentinel node biopsy was developed to reduce the morbidity associated with surgical staging of the axilla in patients with no palpable axillary nodes.[3] A blue dye alone or in combination

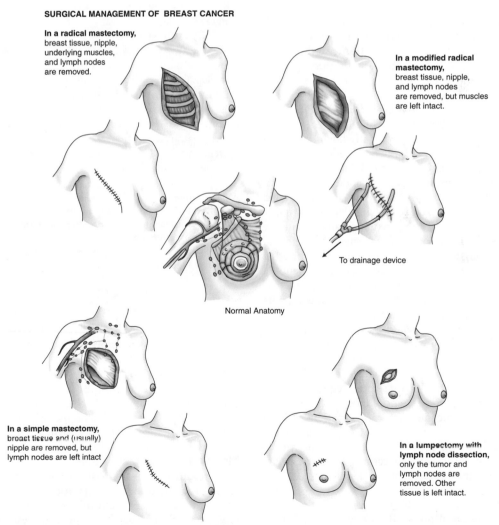

SURGICAL MANAGEMENT OF BREAST CANCER

In a radical mastectomy, breast tissue, nipple, underlying muscles, and lymph nodes are removed.

In a modified radical mastectomy, breast tissue, nipple, and lymph nodes are removed, but muscles are left intact.

To drainage device

Normal Anatomy

In a simple mastectomy, breast tissue and (usually) nipple are removed, but lymph nodes are left intact

In a lumpectomy with lymph node dissection, only the tumor and lymph nodes are removed. Other tissue is left intact.

FIG. 43-2 Surgical choices for treatment of breast cancer. (Redrawn from Ignatavicius DD, Workman ML: *Medical-surgical nursing: critical thinking for collaborative care*, ed 6, Philadelphia, 2010, Saunders.)

NURSING CARE IN THE PACU

with a radiolabeled colloid dye is injected near the tumor and is carried by the lymph system to the first (sentinel) node to receive lymph from the tumor. This lymph node is most likely to contain cancer cells if the cancer has spread. The sentinel node is not located in the same site in every patient. When this node is found, it is removed and examined. If it is free of cancer, further surgery may not be needed. If there is evidence of positive nodes and axillary node dissection and adjunct therapy may be required. It is done through a separate incision and involves a sample of 10 to 15 lymph nodes lateral and inferior to the pectoralis minor muscles for pathology. Removal and examination of the nodes allows for staging of the cancer and helps the patient and provider to choose adjuvant therapy and treatment options. A possible side effect from the removal of the lymph nodes is lymphedema or swelling of the arm (seen in 1 to 3 of 10 women; Box 43-1).

Patient complications from sentinel lymph node biopsy may include allergic reactions to the dye. Use of the dye in patients with known sensitivity is contraindicated and perianesthesia nurses should be alert for any signs of anaphylaxis.

When the patient is admitted to the PACU, all the initial assessment measures should be performed. The blood pressure cuff should be placed on the arm opposite the operative side. The arm on the operative side should be elevated on a pillow because the removal of lymph nodes increases the risk of lymphedema. The operative-side arm should be assessed frequently for circulatory adequacy with monitoring of color, temperature, capillary refill, and the presence and strength of the radial pulse. Venipunctures and injections should not be performed on the operative-side arm. Sentinel node biopsy is usually an outpatient procedure that allows rapid return to full mobility and permits return to work weeks sooner than after axillary dissection.[3] Dressings should be small, and bleeding or drainage should be minimal. A Hemovac or Jackson-Pratt closed-drainage system may be connected to drains placed at the incision site, but with a sentinel node biopsy are seldom required.

Nursing personnel should be aware that although this procedure allows the patient to keep the breast, it does not eliminate fear of the cancer diagnosis or concerns about whether the procedure was successful; therefore the nurse must provide factual reassurance and support.

Mastectomy
Partial (Segmental) Mastectomy
The partial mastectomy involves the removal of more of the breast tissue than in the lumpectomy

---

BOX 43-1   Lymphedema

Lymphedema may occur after breast surgery because of a build-up of fluid. This swelling often worsens the physical and emotional strain for patients as they deal with their diagnosis of breast cancer. Women who have multiple lymph nodes removed are more likely to develop lymphedema. Symptoms include swelling of the affected arm or upper chest, a heavy sensation in the arm, discomfort in the arm, difficulty moving the arm, stiffness, weakness, and numbness. Women with lymphedema should be instructed to avoid trauma or injury to the affected arm; avoid blood draws, intravenous catheters, and blood pressure monitoring in the affected arm; practice careful skin and nail hygiene to prevent infection; avoid heavy lifting; and avoid extreme temperature changes. Elevation of the arm and compression garments can help to promote lymph drainage. There is no cure for lymphedema, and the goal is to control the swelling and relieve the symptoms.

Clinical trials are underway to study the effectiveness of new treatments and therapies to reduce the incidence of lymphedema after breast cancer surgery. One current trial (CA:GB 70305) is investigating whether a combination of education, use of light arm weights with exercise, a light compression sleeve with vigorous activity, and regular breathing exercises can reduce the risk or severity of lymphedema after axillary lymph node dissection (www.cancer.gov/clinicaltrials/CALGB-70305).

Modified from Mohler III ER, Mondry TE: Patient information: lymphedema after breast cancer surgery, available at http://www.uptodate.com/contents/patient-information-lymphedema-after-breast-cancer-surgery?source=search_result&search=lymphedema&selectedTitle=5~109. Accessed December 11, 2011.

---

and is usually followed by radiation therapy. Some surgeons refer now to lumpectomy or partial mastectomy as a *wide local excision*.[3]

Simple Mastectomy
The simple mastectomy is the removal of the entire breast, but not the lymph nodes under the arm. Both breasts may be removed if the patient is at an increased risk for breast cancer. Most patients go home the next day.

Modified Radical Mastectomy
The modified radical mastectomy is the most commonly performed surgery for elimination of breast cancer. The entire involved breast and axillary, pectoral, and superior apical nodes are removed. The underlying pectoral muscles are not removed. The modified radical mastectomy is

performed with hopes of decreasing the chance of the malignancy spreading.

Radical Mastectomy

The radical mastectomy is rarely performed in the United States, because the modified radical mastectomy has been found to be just as effective for the patient and less disfiguring, with fewer side effects. The radical mastectomy involves the extensive removal of the entire breast, lymph nodes, and chest wall muscles under the breast. Refined techniques for diagnosis and surgery, radiation therapy, and chemotherapy have made it unnecessary in most instances.

Mastectomy is performed with general anesthesia. The patient is admitted to the Phase I PACU, with the head of the bed elevated 30 to 45 degrees. Admission assessments are performed per PACU protocol. Dressings may be bulky and should be checked frequently for excessive serosanguineous drainage and for constriction. Patients should be observed closely for signs of postoperative hematoma below the skin flaps. Attention to the drains and the maintenance of free drainage within the vacuum system prevent this potential complication. Drains are usually placed under the skin flaps to remove excess blood and serum that ordinarily collect under the wound site, thus causing edema, infection, and sloughing of the skin graft (Fig. 43-3).[4] The drains may be connected to Hemovac or Jackson-Pratt devices or some other closed suction device. Generally, additional vacuum is needed the first 8 postoperative hours, and the

Hemovac is connected to vacuum pressure of 20 to 30 mm Hg. These drains should be monitored for excessive bleeding, which must be reported to the surgeon. Dressings are necessarily snug, but should not impair respiration or circulation to the upper extremity. The arm on the operative side should be supported and elevated on a pillow; it must be checked frequently for cyanosis or pallor, and the pulse must be palpated for intensity. If signs of respiratory distress or impaired circulation arise, the surgeon should be notified to rearrange the dressing.

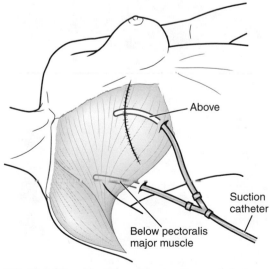

FIG. 43-3 Closed incision with closed wound drainage system in place.

Evidence-Based Practice

Thoracic paravertebral block (PVB) in breast surgery can provide regional anesthesia during and after surgery with the potential advantage of decreasing postoperative pain. In this study Boughey and colleagues report their institutional experience with PVB over the initial 8 months of use in their ambulatory care center. They reviewed 213 patients undergoing breast operations. Comparison was performed between a group of 178 patients who received PVB and the control group of 135 patients who did not. Pain scores were assessed immediately postoperatively, 4 hours postoperatively, 8 hours postoperatively, and again the morning after surgery. Immediately after surgery there was a statistically significant difference in the number of patients reporting pain between PVB patients and those without PVB. At all time points up until the morning after surgery, PVB patients were significantly less likely to report pain than controls. PVB in breast surgical patients provided improved postoperative pain control. Pain relief was improved immediately postoperatively, and this effect continued to the next day after surgery. PVB significantly decreased the proportion of patients who required overnight hospitalization after major breast operations and therefore may decrease cost associated with breast surgery.

IMPLICATIONS FOR PRACTICE

Paravertebral block greatly improves the quality of recovery and pain relief after breast cancer surgery. Most patients receiving a PVB have less postoperative pain, nausea, and vomiting. Perianesthesia nurses should be aware that these patients will have reduced opioid requirements and tolerate early ambulation or mobilization. Patients should be monitored for hypotension and signs and symptoms of pneumothorax.

Source: Boughey JC, et al: Improved postoperative pain control using thoracic paravertebral block for breast operations, *Breast J* 15(5):483-488, 2009.

Patients usually need intravenous fluid augmentation for the first 24 postoperative hours. Oral feeding is allowed after cough and gag reflexes have returned and if nausea is not present. Small sips of fluids may be offered and taken as desired, and diet resumed as tolerated. Postoperative pain can be moderate to severe and can usually be controlled with opioids such as meperidine and morphine. The incidence of persistent postsurgical pain in patients who received breast surgery has been identified as much as 65%.[5] With the increased preoperative use of paravertebral nerve blocks for breast surgery patients, pain management has been greatly enhanced, resulting in less need for opioids and improved patient satisfaction.[6] Hypothermia may be a problem because of prolonged exposure in the operating room, and rewarming should be accomplished with additional warmed blankets or a forced warm air device. Postoperative instructions for patients who have axillary node dissections should include hand and arm care instructions. Consistent education and support are necessary. Emotional support may be sought through support groups such as the Reach to Recovery program (American Cancer Society: web site, www.cancer.org/; or telephone, 800-ACS-2345).

Breast Reconstruction

The loss of a breast from cancer can be devastating to women, and the changes in body image may be difficult to manage. One of the advances made in breast surgery during recent years is the availability of effective means of reconstructing the breast after removal for cancer. Breast reconstruction can be accomplished in conjunction with mastectomy or at a later time, depending on each patient's individual decision and preference and the need for chemotherapy or radiation.

Breast reconstruction may be performed in a variety of methods in which the surgeon, in collaboration with a plastic surgeon, tailors the operation to the patient's individual irregularity. Reconstructive options can be divided into two main types: those that use autogenous tissue and those that require alloplastic material.[3] Breast reconstruction can be performed with three different techniques: available tissue with an implant, the use of tissue expanders, and the use of flaps. Use of the available tissue is the simplest procedure, but often sufficient tissue is not available after mastectomy. If enough tissue is available, an appropriately sized implant is placed under the remaining skin flap or muscle. The other breast may have its size adjusted with either a reduction mammoplasty or a mastopexy to achieve symmetry if necessary and the patient desires to do so. Autogenous methods of reconstruction give the best symmetry.[3]

Mastectomy can leave a shortage of enough skin tissue to create a breast mound. For these patients, a breast reconstruction technique with available tissue and implants is used to stretch the normal tissue to create extra tissue. A pocket is made under the remaining tissues into which a soft silicone bag is made to simulate the natural contour. The pocket can be made at the time of surgery or before the surgery with an inflatable tissue expander. The expander method requires the administration of several injections of gradually increasing volumes of saline solution over a period of weeks. When the desired amount of stretch has been reached, the temporary tissue expander is removed and replaced with a permanent breast implant.

Myocutaneous flap reconstruction (Figs. 43-4 and 43-5) involves moving nearby muscle and skin into the area of the mastectomy to replace the significant tissue deficiency after mastectomy. Commonly used muscle and skin flaps include the latissimus dorsi and rectus abdominis muscles with attached skin. Nipple-areola reconstruction can be accomplished with small portions of the labia and grafting to the selected location or

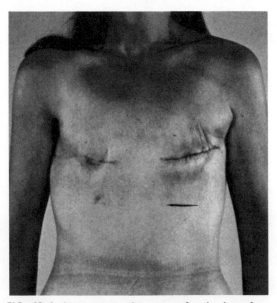

FIG. 43-4 Appearance of patient after healing from bilateral mastectomies for cancer.

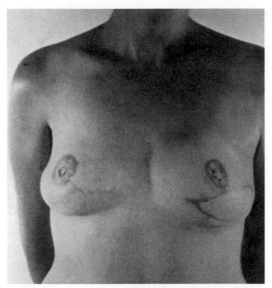

FIG. 43-5 Appearance of same patient in Fig. 43-4 after muscle-skin flap (latissimus) and nipple reconstructions. Patient has gained considerable weight, and later she delivered a healthy baby. She is free of disease 6 years after the mastectomy.

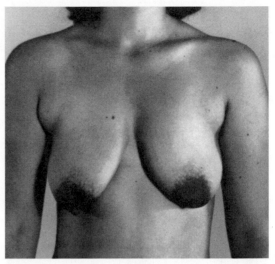

FIG. 43-6 Mastopexy (breast lift). Before surgery, this patient had sagging (ptosis) of the breasts.

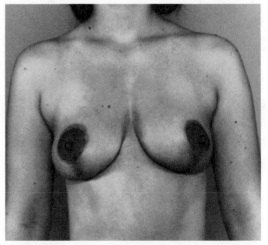

FIG. 43-7 Mastopexy, showing same patient in Fig. 43-6 several weeks after surgery. Scars are beginning to fade.

areola reconstruction with tattooed pigment.[3] Postoperative care is generally the same as for the patient who undergoes other types of breast surgery, with attention to graft and flap donor sites (see Chapter 44).

These operations have provided a measure of comfort to patients whose body image has been significantly disrupted by mastectomy. Patients report return of a sense of femininity and confidence. Many women do not choose to undergo additional surgery after mastectomy, but knowledge that the operation is available is reassuring.

Mastopexy (Breast Lift)

Breast ptosis (sagging) is defined by the position of the nipple areolar complex related to the inframammary crease. The reshaping process differs from reduction mammoplasty in the amount of tissue removed. There is usually minimal to no removal of breast tissue with use of a breast implant when needed.[7] Generally less than 300 g of tissue removed is considered a mastopexy procedure (Figs. 43-6 and 43-7).

Mastopexy is commonly performed as a same-day procedure, and postoperative care after mastopexy is generally not demanding. General anesthesia is most commonly used, and only minor adjustments in breast tissue are made.

The patient is positioned on the back after surgery and may assume a semi-Fowler to high-Fowler position for comfort as soon as she awakens. The motion of the arms is restricted to below shoulder level.

Postoperative dressings are minimal, and drains are rarely necessary because the entire procedure, with the exception of nipple release, is at the level of the dermis. Drainage should be minimal, and if frank bleeding occurs, the surgeon should be notified. Pain is usually not a problem, and discomfort can be controlled with mild anal-gesics. Food and fluids may be resumed as toler-ated after nausea has disappeared.

Augmentation Mammoplasty

Breast augmentation is done for hypomastia, to correct breast asymmetry, to recreate the breast af-ter mastectomy, or for the patient's desired en-hancement of breast size (Figs. 43-8 and 43-9).[7]

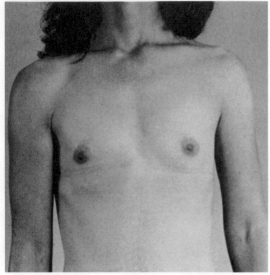

FIG. 43-8 Appearance of patient before breast aug-mentation.

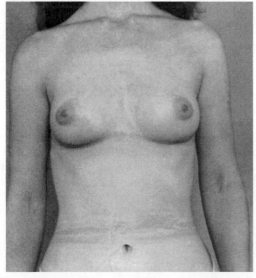

FIG. 43-9 Postoperative appearance of patient after breast augmentation with silicone bag prostheses.

Incisions may be inframammary, axillary, or semi-circular around the lower half of the areolar outline. The inframammary approach is the simplest, but the axillary incision provides the least visible scar after surgery. Breast implants can be placed be-neath the mammary tissue or under the muscle layer of the chest. Many surgeons believe that po-sitioning the implants beneath the muscle provides the patient with the most natural appearance. Breast augmentation can also be accomplished endoscopically with transluminal breast augmenta-tion in which a small incision is made inside the navel. These patients have self-adhesive wound strips over the umbilical incision and are fitted with an elastic bandage.

Breast augmentation patients usually receive general anesthesia, but local anesthesia with sedation is a viable consideration. The patients may have compression dressings in place on admission to the PACU, but some physicians have a brassiere placed on the patient immedi-ately after surgery. The patients usually go home the same day and see the physician in the office the following day to change the dressing. Inci-sional drains are rarely used with breast aug-mentation. Patients may need aggressive pain management in the initial phase I PACU, but generally can be comfortable with the use of oral analgesics. Patients should be encouraged to gently move their arms to prevent stiffness and discomfort.

Reduction Mammoplasty

Reduction mammoplasty is the surgical method to correct gigantomastia or macromastia in which patients have back pain, breast pain, postural changes, or shoulder strap discomfort from the weight of the breasts.[7] These women may also have an inability to participate in physical activi-ties such as jogging, aerobics, and horseback rid-ing. Breast reduction is performed with general anesthesia. Breast tissue and skin are excised; the nipple areolar complex is elevated superiorly on the new breast mound. Reduction mammoplasty is a lengthy procedure in which significant fluid and blood loss is anticipated. Because of the pro-longed anesthesia and surgery time, some provid-ers use a team approach to reduce the surgical time. Some patients donate autologous blood be-fore this surgery, but all patients should have a blood type and screen before surgery. Frequently, intravenous crystalloids are all that is necessary for fluid replacement.

A newer method in reduction mammoplasty is the laser deepithelialization technique. When the carbon dioxide laser is used to remove the epidermis from the inferior pedicle, reduction mammoplasty can be performed with little blood loss. The inferior pedicle technique is a commonly used approach to reduction mammoplasty. When the inferior pedicle technique is used, the laser simplifies skin removal. The laser is preferred for pedicle deepithelialization in all patients, especially patients who have large ptotic breasts, because rigid stabilization is not necessary.

On admission to the PACU, the patient is positioned on the back; as soon as the condition warrants, the patient is placed in a low Fowler position. Dressings may be of any variety, but most often wide strips of Elastoplast, which readily conforms to the patient's new skin contours, are used. A Velpeau bandage should be in place to restrain the patient from raising the arms, and the patient should be advised of this. Drains are rarely necessary, and drainage should be minimal. If drains are present, they should be connected to a vacuum source, such as the Hemovac. Because of the length of the surgery and the fluid volume loss, special attention should be paid to urine output, pulse rate, and blood pressure. Rewarming may be necessary to prevent or reduce hypothermia. Initially, parenteral opioids may be needed after surgery, followed by oral analgesics. Light ice packs may be used to relieve discomfort and minimize tissue swelling. Most patients spend one night in the hospital after surgery. As after mastectomy, the patient should be advised to not do anything that puts strain on the pectoral girdle.

Surgery in Gynecomastia

Gynecomastia, or benign hypertrophy of one or both breasts in boys and men, is relatively common (Fig. 43-10). The condition may be bilateral or unilateral. The causes may be hormonal, systemic disease-oriented, drug-related, or idiopathic.

In extreme instances or in cases in which gynecomastia causes problems in psychological adjustment, this excess tissue can be excised or removed with suction lipectomy. Suction lipectomy is useful when the gynecomastia is caused primarily by fat. Optimal cosmetic results can be obtained. The surgical procedure is similar to that of breast reduction in women. A peri-areolar incision is made, and tissue is removed. Suction drainage of the incision site is usually necessary and may be conveniently accomplished with a Hemovac or other closed drain system.

Postoperative care is essentially the same as that for women who undergo breast surgery. If no drains are necessary, the patient can be discharged the day of surgery after reflexes have returned, nausea has subsided, and food and fluids can be taken.

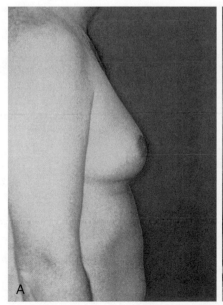 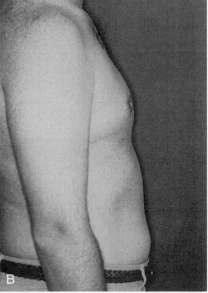

FIG. 43-10 **A,** Preoperative view of gynecomastia. **B,** Postoperative view after excision of gynecomastia. (From Rothrock J: *Alexander's care of the patient in surgery*, ed 14, St. Louis, 2011, Mosby.)

SUMMARY

Breast cancer is most commonly diagnosed in women, and the risk of development of breast cancer increases with age. All women are at risk for breast cancer, and one in eight women is predicted in the United States to have breast cancer develop at some point in life. Early detection with self examination or mammography is key and may be the reason for the slowly declining increase in breast cancer mortality rates. Surgical procedures on the breast are performed to establish a definitive diagnosis when cancer is a possibility or to treat a breast cancer. These surgeries range from biopsy to mastectomy. In addition, a sentinel node biopsy can be performed to help establish a diagnosis. Axillary node dissection may be necessary. Other breast surgeries include mastopexy, augmentation mammoplasty, and reduction mammoplasty.

A diagnosis of breast cancer can be overwhelming for both the patient and their family. Many facilities have hired breast care nurse navigators to offer support, answer questions, and "navigate" the patient through their journey.[8] After breast surgery, patients need emotional support and encouragement to express concerns and fears. Patients should be provided with accurate and complete information in a hopeful and positive manner, yet they should not be given unfounded or unreasonable hopes and promises. The nurse navigator, as an educator and patient advocate, can be a single point of contact for the patient and their family. In addition, perianesthesia nurses should encourage patients to discuss their fears and feelings regarding their diagnosis and treatment and provide patients with detailed postoperative instructions (see Chapter 28). The web site for the American Cancer Society (www.cancer.org) can provide the patient with an abundance of information regarding breast cancer after care and support groups.

REFERENCES

1. Centers for Disease Control and Prevention: *Cancer prevention and control,* available at www.cdc.gov/cancer/dcpc/data/women.htm. Accessed December 31, 2011.
2. American Cancer Society: *Breast cancer facts and figures 2011-2012,* available at www.cancer.org/acs/groups/content/@epidemiologysurveilance/documents/document/acspc-030975.pdf. Accessed December 31, 2011.
3. Townsend CM, et al: *Sabiston textbook of surgery,* ed 18, Philadelphia, 2008, Saunders.
4. Pearsall EB: Breast surgery. In Rothrock J, editor: *Alexander's care of the patient in surgery,* ed 14, St. Louis, 2011, Mosby.
5. Pasero C: Persistent postsurgical and posttrauma pain, *J Perianesth Nurs* 26:38–42, 2011.
6. Boughey JC, et al: Improved postoperative pain control using thoracic paravertebral block for breast operations, *Breast J* 15(5):483–488, 2009.
7. Dreger V: Plastic and reconstructive surgery. In Rothrock J, editor: *Alexander's care of the patient in surgery,* ed 14, St. Louis, 2011, Mosby.
8. Sein E, et al: Fox Chase Cancer Center partners develops orientation manual for breast care nurse navigators, *Oncology Nursing Forum* 36(3):45–6, 2009.

RESOURCES

Barash P, et al: *Clinical anesthesia,* ed 6, Philadelphia, 2009, Lippincott Williams & Wilkins.

Boughey JC, et al: Improved postoperative pain control using thoracic paravertebral block for breast operations, *Breast J* 15(5):483–488, 2009.

Elliott FL, et al: The scarless latissimus dorsi flap for full muscle coverage in device-based immediate breast reconstruction: an autologous alternative to acellular dermal matrix, *Plast Reconstr Surg* 128:71–79, 2011.

Fisher B, et al: Eight-year results of a randomized clinical trial comparing mastectomy and lumpectomy with or without radiation in the treatment of breast cancer, *N Engl J Med* 320:822–828, 1989.

Ganong W: *Review of medical physiology,* ed 23, New York, 2010, McGraw-Hill Professional.

Gutowski KA: Aesthetic and functional breast surgery, *Clin Obstet Gynecol* 49:337–345, 2006.

Hall J: *Guyton and Hall textbook of medical physiology,* ed 12, Philadelphia, 2011, Saunders.

Longnecker D, et al: *Principles and practice of anesthesiology,* ed 2, St. Louis, 1998, Mosby.

Mohler ER, Mondry TE: *Lymphedema after breast cancer surgery* (website). www.uptodate.com/contents/patient-information-lymphedema. Accessed July 26, 2011.

Miller R, et al: *Miller's anesthesia,* ed 7, Philadelphia, 2009, Churchill Livingstone.

Miller RD, Pardo M: *Basics of anesthesia,* ed 6, Philadelphia, 2011, Saunders.

Nagelhout J, Plaus K: *Nurse anesthesia,* ed 4, Philadelphia, 2011, Saunders.

National Comprehensive Cancer Network: NCCN Clinical Practice Guidelines in Oncology: *Breast Cancer, version 1.2011,* available at http://www.nccn.org/professionals/physician_gls/pdf/breast.pdf. Accessed July 31, 2011.

National Comprehensive Cancer Network: NCCN Guidelines for Patients: *version 2.2011,* available at http://www.nccn.com/files/cancer-guidelines/breast/index.html. Accessed July 31, 2011.

St. Francis Health: *Breast care nurse navigator,* available at www.stfrancishospitals.org/cancer. Accessed July 26, 2011.

Schick L, Windle PE: *Perianesthesia nursing core curriculum: preprocedure, phase I and phase II PACU nursing,* ed 2, Philadelphia, 2010, Saunders.

Susan G. Komen Breast Cancer Foundation: Breast cancer research, available at http://ww5.komen.org/BreastCancer/BreastCancerResearch.html. Accessed December 30, 2011.

44 Care of the Plastic and Reconstructive Surgical Patient

Joni M. Brady, MSN, RN, CAPA, CLC, and
Matthew D. Byrne, PhD, RN, CPAN

The field of plastic surgery encompasses cosmetic and reconstructive surgery, and related procedures and techniques have continuously evolved over time. This discipline is growing as consumer demand for cosmetic surgical procedures increases[1] and the ability to achieve aesthetic reconstructive surgical outcomes improves.

Plastic surgery derives its name from the Greek word *plastikos*, which means to mold or give shape. The first successful tissue transfers are said to have originated in India more than 2500 years ago. Modern grafting techniques were explored in nineteenth-century Germany. Today, reconstructive procedures involve much more than the correction of acquired and congenital deformities. They are also performed to correct defects related to tumors, trauma, infection, burns and postburn contractures, pressure ulcers, or disease.[2,3] Ideally, these procedures represent interconnected therapy[4] that strives to restore normal function and enhance appearance to maintain or improve body image and self-esteem.[5]

Few absolutes exist in plastic and reconstructive surgical techniques or in the associated preoperative or postoperative care. Perianesthesia nurses may encounter a wide variety of surgical techniques, from simple to complex, depending on the type of facility in which the procedures are performed. Only the basic aspects of postoperative plastic surgery patient care are presented in this discussion. Elements of nursing care related to the specific treatment of a specific body area affected during plastic or reconstructive surgical procedures are discussed in other chapters. The reader is advised to refer to the appropriate related chapter for more details.

DEFINITIONS

Abdominoplasty: Surgical removal of abdominal fat and skin.

Augmentation Mammoplasty: Surgical procedure performed to enhance the size and shape of a breast.

Blepharoplasty: Procedure done to correct deformities of the upper or lower eyelid with excision of redundant skin or protruding fat.

Dermabrasion: Surgical planing of the skin with removal of the epidermis and portions of the superficial dermis for elimination of high spots or other irregularities in an uneven skin surface.

Deep Inferior Epigastric Artery Perforator (DIEP) Flap: Autologous breast reconstruction performed using an abdominal wall flap. Less abdominal wall damage is incurred using this technique.

Gynecomastia: Benign hypertrophy of breast tissue in males.

Inosculation: Vessel anastomosis from host to graft that allows for graft revascularization.

Latissimus Dorsi Flap: Reconstructive procedure involving donor site muscle, adipose tissue, and skin blood supply that is left connected and then tunneled to the mastectomy site.

Lipectomy: Surgical removal of fatty tissue.

Otoplasty: Surgical procedure done to reduce prominence of the ears.

Pedicle Flap: A preferred flap for wound tissue that is somewhat avascular, such as cartilage, bone, and tendon, or in the presence of avascular scar tissue and radiation-affected tissue. This type of flap is used to provide soft tissue closure while allowing blood vessels to remain intact.

Reduction Mammoplasty: Surgical removal of glandular tissue, fat, and skin from the breasts to achieve lighter, smaller, and firmer breast proportions.

Rhinoplasty: Reshaping or reconstruction of the nose when its shape has been altered as a result of trauma or when the patient is unhappy with its form.

Rhytidectomy: Surgical tightening of facial and neck muscles with removal of excess skin; commonly called a *face lift procedure.*

Tissue Expansion: Insertion and positioning of a temporary inflatable balloon or implant device under the skin, which is periodically increased in size through instillation of normal saline solution to promote expansion of the skin for reconstructive purposes.

Transverse Rectus Abdominis Myocutaneous (TRAM) Flap: This procedure is performed after a mastectomy and involves the reconstruction of a breast with autografting of lower abdominal muscle, skin, and adipose tissue. A pedicle TRAM flap uses the entire rectus abdominal muscle, whereas the free flap technique only partially involves this muscle.

Tumescent Liposuction: A dilute solution of lidocaine, used in combination with epinephrine, is injected into the adipose tissue layer to facilitate the vacuum removal of fat cells via a small cannula.

PERIANESTHESIA NURSING CARE

Preanesthetic concerns for the patient undergoing skin grafting, flap repair, or any type of tissue grafting should include: evaluation of smoking status and smoking cessation education; assessment for vascular concerns that may threaten the healing process, such as diabetes; identification of peripheral vascular disease or hypertension; nutritional assessment of the patient; and patient education regarding the postoperative need for wound site immobilization, effective pain management, intensive care monitoring if necessary, and avoidance of straining or strenuous activities that may cause shearing of new grafts or increase the risk for hematoma development.

Basic plastic and reconstructive surgery techniques include excision of skin lesions, closure of skin wounds, and placement of skin grafts and skin flaps. Many minor plastic surgical procedures are performed with local anesthesia and require minimal postoperative nursing care, primarily involving close observation of the surgical site. When the patient receives general or regional anesthesia, postoperative nursing care includes all the appropriate considerations discussed for general care of the postoperative patient in addition to careful surgical site observation. Preoperative vital signs provide an important baseline for assessing possible postoperative complications.

SKIN GRAFTS

Skin grafting is the most common method for covering open areas that result from incomplete wound healing, trauma, burns, or large surgical incisions. Grafting involves the removal of a skin layer of varying thickness that is then transplanted to a host site. Transplanted skin layers can originate from the individual, be synthetic in origin, or be an expanded portion of the host's own skin. The lower abdomen supplies a good source for the full-thickness skin graft.[6]

The major types of skin grafts are outlined in Box 44-1. Revascularization generally takes 3 to 5 days and requires growth of vessels from the host or the recipient tissue via a process called *inosculation*. For cosmetically pleasing results, the color, texture, thickness, and hair-bearing nature of the skin used for grafting should be chosen to match the recipient site. As a rule, the closer the donor skin is located to the recipient area, the better the match.

Factors that influence graft survival include: adherence to the recipient tissue; adequate vascularity signs, which include color and capillary refill of site; close monitoring of graft tissue for early identification of complications; and strict management of oxygenation, hemodynamic stability, thermoregulation, pain control, and positioning. Postoperative monitoring and assessment for serum or blood in the graft site is important during the first 24 hours. Excess fluid can cause the graft to lift from its bed and must be removed. The donor site should be kept clean, and heals by forming a new layer of skin.[7] Many variations exist in the type of wound dressing used, use of pressure dressings, required positioning of the patient, use of ice or antibiotic ointments, and handling of donor sites.

Every effort should be made to keep the patient calm and still and to prevent touching, removing or shifting of dressings. Some dressings, such as

---

Box 44-1   Major Types of Skin Grafts

- A *full-thickness graft* includes all underlying dermis and epidermis and a small amount of subcutaneous tissue. These grafts, used to cover areas such as the nasal tip, dorsum, ala, and sidewall of the lower eyelid and ear, are more prone to necrosis.
- A *split-thickness graft* includes a portion of the underlying dermis and the entire epidermis. This graft is the least durable. It can be thin, medium, or thick, depending on the amount of dermis included.
- A *composite graft* comprises two or more tissue components and often includes skin and subcutaneous tissue, cartilage, or mucosa that can be used to reconstruct a patient's ear, nose, or eyelid.
- A *free cartilage graft* involves a portion of cartilage that is harvested and reimplanted to provide structure and support to the site. One example is the use of rib cartilage to create an ear structure in a patient with microtia.
- An *autograft* indicates that the donor and the recipient are the same person.
- An *isograft* signifies that the donor and the recipient are genetically identical.
- *Allograft* or *homograft* means that the donor and the recipient are of the same species; this procedure may entail the use of cadaver tissue.
- A *xenograft* indicates that the donor and the recipient are of different species (e.g., porcine or bovine sources).
- *Bioengineered skin* and *skin substitutes* contain cells that may be animal, human, or host hybrids which acclimatize to the wound and accelerate healing. The mechanism of action is unknown.

the bolster dressing shown in Fig. 44-1, may actually be sutured in place. Generally, the grafted area should be elevated and protected from both pressure and motion. The patient should be positioned to prevent any pressure on or other trauma to the graft or the donor site. The surgeon may order cold packs to reduce metabolic requirements of the graft and enhance its chances of survival. Dressings over grafts should be observed closely for drainage. The presence of excess drainage should be reported to the physician.

FLAPS

The term *flap* commonly refers to a skin flap; however, with recent advances in reconstructive surgery, flaps are not limited to skin tissue. Flaps are classified by anatomic composition: skin with muscle fascia or bone, or both; skin alone; omentum; or a composite of these tissues. The term *flap* implies maintenance of vascularity from the original location of harvest, unlike transplantation, which implies complete separation from original vascular site.

Pedicle flaps are the preferred surgical treatment method for covering of wounds with: inadequate vascularity to support a skin graft; reconstruction of full-thickness defects of specialized body parts such as ears, eyelids, nose, and lips; and concealment of gliding tendons. Reconstructions that require tissue bulk, such as decubitus ulcer closure, may also involve skin flap placement.

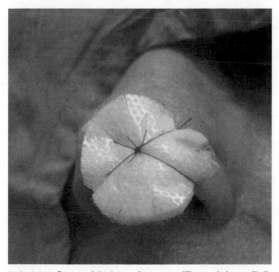

FIG. 44-1 Sutured bolster dressing. (From Adams DC, Ramsey ML: Grafts in dermatologic surgery: review and update on full- and split-thickness skin grafts, free cartilage grafts, and composite grafts, *Dermatol Surg* 31:1055–1067, 2005.)

Microvascular Tissue Transfer and Free Flaps

Microvascular tissue transfer represents an important advancement in the field of reconstructive surgery. This technique requires the use of a high-magnification operative microscope for reestablishment of vasculature. Regardless of the type of flap used, the newly positioned tissue is kept under constant observation by perianesthesia nursing personnel. Postanesthesia nursing management of the patient who has undergone microsurgery is consistent with established care requirements for the specific procedure performed with emphasis on notation of color changes in the skin at the operative site.

The most serious complication in a microvascular tissue transfer procedure is tissue necrosis. Tissue death occurs when the artery or the vein that supplies the flap develops a thrombus. Arterial thrombosis can result in complete flap failure within 4 hours of onset. Arterial occlusion is characterized by a pale cool flap that does not bleed when stuck with a needle. Hematomas can form at the recipient site and occur more commonly in the patient who preoperatively smokes or uses nonsteroidal antiinflammatory drugs or corticosteroids.[8]

Venous thrombosis is more commonly encountered, but it is not an immediate threat. Thrombosis is characterized by a congested warm mottled flap that continuously oozes dark blood. Objective assessment of the flap is possible with fluorometry, transcutaneous oxygen tension, thermometry, laser Doppler scan, temperature monitoring, buried Doppler probe, or photoplethysmograph disk for monitoring of blood flow. Any change in skin color from the normal baseline or monitoring findings that indicates imminent occlusion should be reported to the surgeon immediately. A donor site typically generates more painful stimuli than the transplanted skin graft or flap site.[9] Pain management should be individualized and based on the patient's self-reported pain levels. Nursing care should include administration of analgesics and selected nonopioid adjuvants with attention to comfort measures as needed.

Breast Reconstruction Flap Techniques

Breast cancer affects millions of women across the world each year, and reconstruction after mastectomy has become a routine part of breast cancer treatment. Breast reconstruction using autologous grafting is commonly accomplished in several ways, does not adversely affect cancer survival rates, and can serve to enhance the patient's psychologic state.

The transverse rectus abdominis musculocutaneous (TRAM) flap procedure involves the reconstruction of a breast with autografting of lower abdominal muscle, skin, and adipose tissue. The procedure can be performed using a pedicle TRAM flap or a free TRAM flap (Fig. 44-2). The pedicle TRAM procedure was first developed in the early 1980s. Through improved understanding of flap physiology and surgical techniques, common procedural options have evolved to include the use of a free TRAM

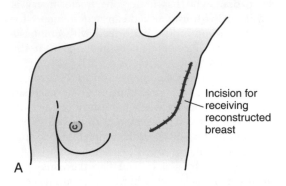

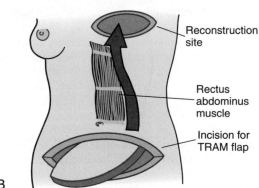

FIG. 44-2 Transverse rectus abdominis myocutaneous (TRAM) flap. **A,** After mastectomy of the involved breast, **(B)** a breast is reconstructed using the lower abdominal skin and fatty tissue. In a pedicled TRAM, the tissue's own blood supply remains attached, and the lower abdominal tissue is rotated into position on the chest. The tissue is tunneled under the skin to the chest area, where it is brought through the mastectomy incision. The reconstructed tissue is shaped to form a matching breast and placed in the mastectomy skin pocket. A *free TRAM flap* refers to using skin and tissue that are completely disconnected from their blood supply, moved from the abdomen to the new site, and reconnected to different blood vessels. A nipple and areola can be tattooed on later after healing has taken place. (From Goodman CC, Fuller KS: *Pathology: implications for the physical therapist*, ed 3, St. Louis, 2009, Saunders.)

flap, muscle sparing free TRAM flap, and deep inferior epigastric artery perforator (DIEP) flap. All these flap procedures use a segment of abdominal muscle mass to achieve the breast graft. This muscle resection has frequently resulted in an abdominal bulge, abdominal hernia, and some degree of permanent loss of the patient's abdominal strength. These findings occur at a lower incidence rate in the DIEP patient population. Surgeons performing the TRAM technique may choose to implant propylene mesh at the time of resection to better support the abdominal wall.[10]

Another procedure available for use in autologous breast reconstruction is the latissimus dorsi flap (LD) technique. The LD flap procedure is especially useful in the low body mass index patient who lacks the abdominal tissue reserves needed for flap harvest.[11] Although a functional option, this procedure has been associated with less overall patient satisfaction than with the abdominal graft options.[10] As with all postoperative flap procedures, nursing care of the postoperative breast reconstruction patient centers on observation of the graft site in addition to general perianesthetic breast surgery patient care (see Chapter 43).

Evidence-Based Practice

A comparison study evaluated patient satisfaction with four breast reconstruction techniques: transverse rectus abdominis musculocutaneous (TRAM), deep inferior epigastric artery perforator (DIEP), latissimus dorsi (LD) flap, and implants. A validated questionnaire was sent to 583 postreconstructive breast surgery patients with a 75% response rate obtained (119 pedicle TRAM, 117 DIEP, 116 LD, 87 tissue expander). Conclusive findings showed that the abdominal TRAM flap group had significantly greater aesthetic and general satisfaction with this procedure's results than did the LD flap population.

IMPLICATIONS FOR PRACTICE

Patients may have several options for the type of reconstructive breast flap procedure performed. Preoperative discussions surrounding the available breast surgery techniques and related patient satisfaction outcomes may better assist a patient in making an informed decision about the course of treatment pursued.

Source: Yeuh JH, et al: Patient satisfaction in postmastectomy breast reconstruction: a comparative evaluation of DIEP, TRAM, latissimus flap, and implant techniques, *Plast Reconstr Surg* 125:1585–1595, 2010.

BONE GRAFTS

After bone grafting has been performed, the graft site must be immobilized, and excessive movement of the patient should be avoided. The donor site is generally the greater source of postoperative discomfort over the graft site.[9] Pain should be anticipated and aggressively managed with opioid analgesics. If split-rib grafts are used, the patient should be placed in a low Fowler position. Respiratory status should be frequently assessed, and any signs of possible pneumothorax, such as tachycardia and tachypnea, should be reported immediately to the surgeon. Ice often is applied for reduction of swelling and pain management, and the graft site may necessitate elevation.

Surgical Repair of Facial Bone Injuries

The facial bones often are fractured during motor vehicle crashes, falls, fights, and sporting events because of their protrusion and prominence. Fractures differ in location and complexity, and repair can vary from closed reduction to internal fixation with plates and screws, interosseous wiring, and bone grafting. Repair of facial bones often requires general anesthesia. If the damage is extensive and airway obstruction or concomitant cranial or intrathoracic injury is present, a tracheostomy must be performed. All patients who have facial, jaw, or neck surgery need the placement of a tracheostomy tray at the postanesthesia care unit (PACU) bedside in the event an airway emergency should occur. When the patient is admitted, this equipment must also be available for immediate use on the inpatient nursing unit.

On admission to the PACU, the patient who has undergone repair of the facial bones is placed in a low Fowler position as soon as the condition warrants. The elevated position helps to minimize the development of head and neck edema. In the case of a patient with a wired jaw, treatment with antiemetics is essential to prevent vomiting and aspiration. Frequent suctioning of secretions may be necessary in the early postoperative period; therefore the nurse must maintain close airway monitoring with careful performance of oral and endotracheal tube suctioning as needed.

When interdental wire fixation is performed, opening of the jaws may become necessary if an airway emergency develops (see Chapter 32 for care of the patient with interdental fixation). A pair of wire clippers should be clearly visible and affixed to the head of the bed to facilitate rapid opening of the jaws if needed. Good oral hygiene is a priority for these patients, and petrolatum ointment should be applied to the lips to prevent drying and cracking.

Surgical Repair of Cleft Lip and Palate

Cleft lips and palates are among the more common congenital defects encountered in the U.S. population.[12] Children born with these defects may have associated problems, including facial growth abnormalities, dental irregularities, speech difficulties, ear diseases, psychological disorders, and cosmetic challenges. The infant with a cleft palate generally encounters difficulty nursing and swallowing. Repair of the cleft lip (Figs. 44-3 and 44-4) is usually accomplished when the "rule of 10" is met: 10 weeks of age, a body weight of at least 10 lbs, and a hemoglobin level of at least 10 g/dL. Repair is accomplished with general anesthesia, with palatal, maxillary regional nerve blocks available for use.[13,14]

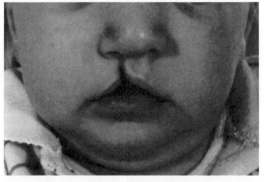

FIG. 44-3 Preoperative appearance of unilateral cleft lip.

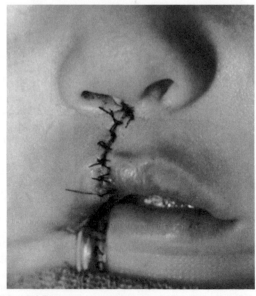

FIG. 44-4 Postoperative appearance of unilateral cleft lip. Incision is covered with antibiotic ointment to prevent crusting.

On PACU admission, the infant is placed in a semiprone position, and the arms should be guided away from the operative site to avoid disruption of the newly repaired lip. Postoperative complications can include acute airway obstruction, laryngospasm, bronchospasm, bleeding, and aspiration of secretions and blood.[15] Hemorrhage, although rare, is a possible complication. Because loss of even a few milliliters of blood in an infant can be significant, any bleeding requires rapid control intervention. Measures should be taken to minimize crying because it puts excessive tension on the newly repaired lip, and the parents should be present at the earliest possible time to facilitate soothing of the child. Depending on the type of anesthesia and intraoperative opioid dosing used, postoperative pain medication or sedation may be needed to comfort the infant. In addition to preventing lip trauma, the most important nursing activity is airway management. Humidified mist should be used to promote general respiratory well being and aid in clearing of secretions. In some cases, a nasal trumpet can be used to maximize oxygenation and may be sutured to the nostril to prevent dislodgement. When the child is fully awake from the anesthesia small sips of clear fluids may be given. Pain status, although difficult to assess in an infant, must be evaluated. Analgesia should be provided when indicated, and oral analgesics such as acetaminophen can be used. Iced normal saline solution–soaked gauze can be applied to the suture areas to reduce swelling and promote comfort.

Cleft Palate

Depending on the extent of the palate defect and accompanying lip defect, if present, repair may be completed when the child is 6 to 18 months of age. Optimization of speech and feeding is often a priority. The repair can be phased, requiring multiple procedures that include palatoplasty with bone grafts and orthodontic inserts.[16] Certain procedures, such as nasoseptal reconstructions, can be delayed until the child becomes a teenager. On admission to the PACU, the child is placed in the semiprone or "tonsil" position with careful attention given to airway maintenance. As in cleft lip repair, the child's arms should be guided away from the surgical site, and crying should be avoided. The head should not be flexed because this position tends to occlude the airway. Suctioning may be necessary but must be performed gently and only if the nurse's view is unobstructed. The catheter, plastic dental suction tip, or Yankauer suction tip should be passed over the dorsum of the tongue, and only minimal vacuum pressure should be used. A mist tent or cold-mist humidifier should be used

to aid in the elimination of secretions. Pain should be assessed and managed with opioids and adjuvants as indicated. Hemorrhage is a possible complication, and any active bleeding requiring control should be reported to the surgeon.

COSMETIC SURGERY

Men and women seek cosmetic surgery to enhance their physical appearance and emotional well being. Millions of cosmetic surgical procedures are performed each year in the United States, and many of these are performed in an outpatient surgery center or office-based practice setting. Most of these cosmetic procedures are performed on an outpatient basis. The anesthetic course depends on the selected procedure and the individual patient, and can involve straight local, local with sedation, or general anesthesia. Nursing assessments and nursing care should be adjusted to the type of anesthesia administered and then individualized for each patient's needs.

Blepharoplasty

Blepharoplasty is a procedure to correct deformities of the upper or lower eyelid with excision of redundant skin or protruding fat. The procedure may be performed for a cosmetic benefit or when eyelid drooping impedes vision.[17] The procedure is usually performed with local anesthesia with supplemental intravenous sedation. Iced compresses minimize swelling and bleeding. The patient may resume a regular diet after surgery; however, hot liquids are contraindicated for 24 hours to prevent vasodilation and bleeding. Activities such as bending and heavy lifting should be avoided. Pain should be assessed and managed with appropriate analgesics. Drugs that alter coagulation times should be avoided. Antibiotic ointment may be used for lubrication (see Chapter 33).

Dermabrasion

Dermabrasion is the surgical planing of the skin, with removal of the epidermis and portions of the superficial dermis, for removal of deep acne scarring, high spots, or other irregularities in an uneven skin surface. Enough of the dermal and epidermal elements are preserved to allow reepithelialization, and the result is smooth healing and blending of the scarred areas with the surrounding skin surface.

Usually the dermabraded areas are treated with the open method, and postanesthesia care includes protection of those areas from abrasion caused by rubbing on pillows or bed clothing. Facial edema, especially of the eyelids, may be expected, and the patient must be reassured that this subsides rapidly.

The dermabraded area should be observed closely for the development of moisture. If moisture develops, it should be dried with a heat lamp or a warm hair dryer. This procedure can produce an uncomfortable burning sensation for the patient and can be minimized by holding the lamp or dryer a considerable distance from the area to be dried. Appropriate analgesics should be administered to manage painful sensations.

Liposuction

Suction lipectomy (liposuction) removes subcutaneous fat to improve facial or body contours. It may be used in conjunction with other techniques. Liposuction is commonly performed on a same-day surgical basis, and anesthesia administration is local or general. However, if greater than 2500 mL of fat is removed, fluid replacement and an overnight admission may be required. In the tumescent liposuction approach, pain should be minimized because of local lidocaine infiltration, but the dose of tumescent lidocaine should not exceed 55 mg/kg.[18] However, if large areas are treated, an opioid analgesic could be required, and intravenous fluid replacement is needed. Postoperative bleeding and infection are possible complications. Drugs that alter coagulation times should be avoided. The patient can usually start oral fluids and a progressive diet as soon as pharyngeal reflexes have returned. Measures used to minimize discomfort, prevent fluid shifts, seroma or hematoma formation and ecchymosed areas include having the patient wear a binder, girdle, or elastic tape over the areas treated.[18]

Otoplasty

Otoplasty is performed to reduce prominence of the ears. The patient has a head dressing for support. Generally, patients have mild postoperative discomfort that lasts approximately 12 hours. Pain of a longer duration suggests a possible hematoma or other complication and should be reported to the surgeon.

Rhinoplasty

Rhinoplasty is performed to reshape or reconstruct the nose when its shape has been altered as a result of trauma or when the patient is unhappy with its form. Rhinoplasty can be performed with local anesthesia with supplemental opioids and intravenous sedation or general anesthesia. On admission to the PACU, the patient's head is elevated 30 to 45 degrees. Humidified oxygen is administered. In addition to routine assessment, the nasal area is assessed for swelling and bleeding. Nasal drip pads may be lightly taped under the nostrils.

Rhytidectomy

Rhytidectomy, commonly known as a *face lift*, is usually done with local anesthesia with supplementary sedation. It sometimes involves general anesthesia requiring PACU Phase I admission. The goal of the procedure is to lift and enhance facial soft tissue and skin, which gradually declines with age. The original procedure developed in the early 1970s involved repositioning of soft tissue and skin, but today include alloplastic implants and synthetic fillers.[19] Postoperatively, elevation of the head of the bed and promotion of a quiet atmosphere are indicated. Pain should be assessed and appropriately treated. Pain located on one side only is unusual and may indicate a potentially serious bleeding complication, which is more commonly found in patients with hypertension. Bleeding and hematoma formation can compromise the patient's airway and necessitate further surgical intervention; therefore the surgeon should be notified immediately when bleeding occurs.

SUMMARY

As the plastic and reconstructive surgery discipline and related surgical techniques continue to grow and evolve, the critical thinking, astute judgment, keen assessments, and targeted interventions of the perianesthesia nurse are paramount to quality patient outcomes. The perianesthesia nurse may encounter a variety of plastic surgical procedures, which can require simple local anesthetic outpatient education and treatment to technologically advanced surgical intensive care. Phase I and phase II perianesthesia nurses should become knowledgeable about the type and scope of plastic surgery care performed in the facility where care is delivered.

Primary postoperative concerns for this patient population include viability of flaps or transplanted tissue, minimization of and assessment for postoperative bleeding, conservative management of surgical sites and dressings, and aggressive pain control to facilitate healing and the patient recovery process. Psychosocial concerns and cosmetic outcomes are often a unique priority in this patient population. This personalized focus could significantly affect the course of care, the perianesthetic treatment and education performed, and the psychosocial integrity of the postoperative patient. Positive procedural outcomes, regardless of the surgical site, technique, or technology, require preparation, vigilance, and prompt intervention on the part of the perianesthesia nurse.

NURSING CARE IN THE PACU

REFERENCES

1. Hotta T: Plastic surgery on the rise, *Plast Surg Nurs* 31: 45-46, 2011.
2. Mahmoud SM, et al: Split-skin graft in the management of diabetic foot ulcers, *J Wound Care* 17:303-306, 2008.
3. Maillard GF, Garey L: Plastic surgery after ablative cancer surgery, *Aesthetic Plast Surg* 30:47–52, 2006.
4. Knobloch K, Vogt PM: The reconstructive clockwork as a 21st century concept in wound surgery, *EWMA J* 11: 25-27, 2011.
5. Borwick G: A holistic approach to meeting the needs of patients with conditions that affect their appearance, *Primary Health Care* 21:33-38, 2011.
6. Jabaiti SK: Use of lower abdominal full-thickness skin grafts for coverage of large skin defects, *Eur J Sci Res* 39:134-142, 2010.
7. Spear M, Bailey A: Treatment of skin graft donor sites with a unique transparent absorbent acrylic dressing, *Plast Surg Nurs* 29:194-200, 2009.
8. Kaplan ED: Preventing postoperative haematomas in microvascular reconstruction of the head and neck: lessons learnt from 126 consecutive cases, *ANZ J Surg* 78:383–388, 2008.
9. Davies SL, White RJ: Defining a holistic pain-relieving approach to wound care via a drug free polymeric membrane dressing, *J Wound Care* 20: 250-256, 2011.
10. Wan DC, et al: Inclusion of mesh in donor-site repair of free tram and muscle-sparing free tram flaps yields rates of abdominal complications comparable to those of DIEP flap reconstruction, *Plast Reconstr Surg* 126:367-374, 2010.
11. Elliott FL, et al: The scarless latissimus dorsi flap for full muscle coverage in device-based immediate breast reconstruction: an autologous alternative to acellular dermal matrix, *Plast Reconstr Surg* 128:71-79, 2011.
12. National Institute of Dental and Craniofacial Research: *Craniofacial birth defects*, available at http://www.nidcr.nih.gov/DataStatistics/FindDataByTopic/Craniofacial-BirthDefects/. Accessed August 22, 2011.
13. Jonnavithula N, et al: Efficacy of palatal block for analgesia following palatoplasty in children with cleft palate, *Pediatr Anesth* 20:727–733, 2010.
14. Mesnil M, et al: A new approach for peri-operative analgesia of cleft palate repair in infants: the bilateral suprazygomatic maxillary nerve block, *Pediatr Anesth* 20:343–349, 2010.
15. Kwari DY, et al: Cleft lip and palate surgery in children: anaesthetic considerations, *Afr J Paediatr Med* 7:174-177, 2010.
16. Eichhorn W: Influence of lip closure on alveolar cleft width in patients with cleft lip and palate, *Head Face Med* 7:3, 2011.
17. Perkins SW, Prischmann J: The art of blepharoplasty, *Facial Plast Surg* 27:58-66, 2011.
18. Coldiron B, et al: ASDS guidelines of care for tumescent liposuction, *Dermatol Surg* 32:709–716, 2006.
19. Hopping SB, et al: Volumetric facelift: evaluation of rhytidectomy with alloplastic augmentation, *Ann Otol Rhinol Laryng* 119:175-180, 2010.

RESOURCES

American Society of Plastic Surgeons: *Reconstructive procedures,* available at www.plasticsurgery.org/Reconstructive-Procedures.html. Accessed July 14, 2011.

Barlow JO: The placement of structural cartilage grafts under full-thickness skin grafts: a case series and strategies for successful outcomes, *Dermatol Surg* 36:1166–1170, 2010.

Bullocks J, et al: *Plastic surgery emergencies: principles and techniques,* New York, 2008, Thieme.

Habbema L: Safety of liposuction using exclusively tumescent local anesthesia in 3,240 consecutive cases, *Dermatol Surg* 35:1728–1735, 2009.

Hivelin M, et al: Ultrasound-guided bilateral transversus abdominis plane block for postoperative analgesia after breast reconstruction by DIEP flap, *Plast Reconstr Surg* 128:44–55, 2011.

Lazic T, Falanga V: Bioengineered skin constructs and their use in wound healing, *Plast Reconstr Surg* 127: 756S–90S, 2010.

Patel KM, et al: Management of massive mastectomy skin flap necrosis following autologous breast reconstruction, *Ann Plast Surg* 67, 2011. DOI:10.1097/SAP.0b013e3182250e23.

Stephan B, et al: The use of antithrombotic agents in microvascular surgery, *Clin Hemorheol Microcirc* 43:51–56, 2009.

Turgut G: Nipple reconstruction with bipedicled dermal flap: a new and easy technique, *Aesth Plast Surg* 33:770–773, 2009.

Wei FC, Mardini S: *Flaps and reconstructive surgery,* Philadelphia, 2009, Saunders.

45 Care of the Obese Patient Undergoing Bariatric Surgery

Theresa L. Clifford, MSN, RN, CPAN

Obesity is the most common nutritional disorder in the world today. Current estimates suggest that more than one third of the adult population in the United States is affected by excess weight. Approximately 33.3% of adult males, 35.3% of adult females, and 10% to 16.5% of teenagers and children are clinically obese.[1] Weight loss surgery is one treatment option for patients who are overweight. Bariatric surgeries increased during 1993 to 2005 from 9189 to more than 140,000 per year.[2] Caring for the patient with bariatric concerns presents a number of challenges for the perianesthesia nurse.

DEFINITIONS

Bariatrics: Branch of medicine dealing with the causes, prevention, and treatment of obesity.
Biliopancreatic Diversion (BD): Surgical procedure that involves reducing the size of the stomach and allowing food to bypass part of the small intestine to change the normal process of digestion.
Body Mass Index (BMI): A measure of body fat derived from a formula using a person's weight and height.
Laparoscopic Adjustable Gastric Banding (LAGB): One of the most common weight loss surgical procedures, it involves placing an adjustable silicone band around the upper portion of the stomach to restrict the size of the stomach. The band is tightened by adding saline through a port that is placed under the skin in the abdomen.
Malabsorptive Procedures: Weight loss surgeries combining the reduction of stomach size, with redirection of the digestive process causing poor absorption of nutrients and calories.
Metabolic Syndrome: A syndrome characterized by several common factors, including abdominal obesity and insulin resistance in which the body cannot use insulin efficiently.
Morbid Obesity: Generally involves a state of being 50% to 100% over normal weight, being more than 100 pounds (45.5 kg) over normal weight, having a BMI of 40 or higher, or being sufficiently overweight to severely interfere with health or normal function.
Obstructive Sleep Apnea (OSA): A sleep-disordered breathing; the risk increases with increased body weight.
Obesity: A condition involving an excess proportion of total body fat. A person is considered obese when his or her weight is 20% or more above normal weight.

Restrictive Procedures: Weight loss surgeries reducing the stomach size limiting the capacity of the stomach to hold food.
Roux-En-Y (RNY): Common gastric bypass surgery that divides the stomach into a small upper pouch leaving a much larger, lower remnant pouch and then rearranges the small intestine into a Y configuration to enable outflow of food from the small upper stomach pouch, via a Roux limb.
Sleeve Gastric Resection (SGR): A newer weight loss surgery that creates a thin, vertical sleeve of stomach using a stapling device, removing the rest of the stomach, thus limiting the amount of food eaten without causing any malabsorption.
Vertical Banded Gastroplasty (VBG): Weight loss surgery also known as *stomach stapling*, using both a band and staples create a small stomach pouch to restrict food volume.
Weight Loss Surgery (WLS): Procedures that either limit the amount of food a stomach can hold or restrict the amount of food digested.

DEFINING OBESITY

The most useful anthropometric index for determination of obesity is the body mass index (BMI). This measurement describes the relationship between height and weight using one of the following calculations:

$$BMI = \text{weight in kg} / \text{height in m}^2$$

or

$$BMI = \text{weight in lb} \times 703 / \text{height in in}^2$$

The higher the BMI, the greater the weight associated with a given height (Table 45-1). Recent studies have demonstrated that the patient who is considered overweight and one who is considered moderately obese usually experience minimal risks in the perioperative period.[3] Underweight patients, as well as patients with a BMI greater than 30, are found to have increased perioperative mortality rates. Although obesity is not equally distributed across gender or race, the incidence of obesity in a given community is relevant and clinically important. Patients in the obese and morbidly obese categories are seen in perianesthesia services for a wide variety of conditions for a wide variety of services, including surgery.

Table 45-1	Classification of Body Mass Index		
HEIGHT	WEIGHT RANGE	BODY MASS INDEX	CONSIDERED
5 ft, 9 in	≤124 lb	<18.5	Underweight
	125 to 168 lb	18.5 to 24.9	Healthy weight
	169 to 202 lb	25.0 to 29.9	Overweight
	≥203 lb	≥30	Obese

From Centers for Disease Control and Prevention: *Overweight and obesity*, available at www.cdc.gov/obesity/defining.html. Accessed September 12, 2011.

PHYSIOLOGIC CONSIDERATIONS IN OBESITY

Pulmonary

Preoperative evaluation of obese patients reveals that 85% have exertional dyspnea and some degree of orthopnea. Periodic breathing, especially when sleeping, may also be present.

Obese patients tend to develop some degree of thoracic kyphosis and lumbar lordosis because of a protuberant abdomen. In addition, the layers of fat on the chest and abdomen reduce the bellows action of the thoracic cage. The overall lung-thorax compliance is reduced and thus leads to increased elastic resistance of the system. Usually the diaphragm is elevated, and the total work of breathing is increased as a result of the deposition of abdominal fat. Because of these factors, the oxygen cost of breathing is threefold or greater than normal, even at rest.

The primary respiratory defect of obese patients is a marked reduction in the expiratory reserve volume. The reason for the decrease in expiratory reserve volume and other lung volumes is that the obese patient is unable to expand the chest in a normal fashion. As a result, diaphragmatic movement must account for the changes in lung volume to a much greater extent than thoracic expansion does. As discussed previously, the diaphragmatic movement is moderately limited by the anatomic changes of obesity, which account for the decreased lung volumes.

In the obese patient, the functional residual capacity may be less than the closing capacity in the sitting and supine positions; therefore the dependent lung zones may be effectively closed throughout the respiratory cycle. Consequently, inspired gas is distributed mainly to the upper or nondependent lung zones. The resulting mismatch of ventilation to perfusion produces systemic arterial hypoxemia. The hypoventilation and ventilation-perfusion abnormalities that contribute to systemic arterial hypoxemia also contribute to retention of carbon dioxide and thus lead to hypercarbia.

In the general population, undiagnosed obstructive sleep apnea (OSA) is common in obese patients despite awareness that increased abdominal girth is a significant risk factor. Reportedly more than 70% of patients undergoing weight loss surgery have been clinically diagnosed with sleep apnea.[4] OSA can occur in patients with redundant pharyngeal tissue. Obstructive sleep apnea is characterized by excessive episodes of apnea (approximately 10 seconds), apneic episodes occurring more than five times per hour, and a 50% reduction in airflow or a reduction sufficient to lead to a 4% decrease in oxygen saturation during sleep as a result of a partial or complete upper airway obstruction. Clinically significant apnea episodes of more than five episodes in 1 hour or 30 per night result in hypoxia, hypercapnia, systemic and pulmonary hypertension, and cardiac arrhythmias. In obese patients with OSA, there is an increased risk of difficult intubations as well as postextubation complications.[4]

Cardiovascular

Thirty pounds of fat are estimated to contain 25 miles of blood vessels, and the increased body mass in obesity leads to increased oxygen consumption and carbon dioxide production. It is not surprising that the cardiac output and the total blood volume are increased in the obese state. This increase in cardiac output is a result of an increase in stroke volume rather than an increase in heart rate; the latter usually remains normal.

The transverse cardiac diameter has been shown to be greater than normal in approximately two thirds of obese patients. A linear relationship seems to exist between cardiac diameter and body weight.

Obesity has been suggested to predispose one to electrocardiographic changes. The Q-T interval is often prolonged, and the QRS voltage is reduced because of the increased distance between the heart and the electrodes. Finally, the likelihood of ventricular arrhythmias is increased in the obese patient. These arrhythmias are believed to be a result of myocardial hypertrophy, hypoxemia, coronary artery disease, and fatty infiltration of the conducting and pacing systems.

A positive correlation exists between an increase in body weight and increased arterial pressure. Hypertension is a known risk factor for the development of coronary artery disease. A weight gain of 28 lb (12.75 kg) can increase the systolic and diastolic blood pressure by 10 and 7 torr, respectively. Systemic hypertension is tenfold more likely in the obese patient. The increase in blood pressure is probably caused by the increased cardiac output.

Chronic heart failure, although uncommon, can occur in persons with long-standing morbid obesity with or without hypertension. It is usually characterized by high output and biventricular dysfunction, with the left ventricle predominating. Clinically, heart failure can be difficult to diagnose because pedal edema may be chronically present.

Cerebral blood flow in obese persons does not differ significantly from that in persons of normal weight. Oxygen uptake of the brain remains normal in the obese person; however, the fraction of the total body oxygen represented in the cerebral metabolism is less than normal, because the total body oxygen requirement is increased. Although the kidneys of obese subjects weigh more than those of nonobese counterparts, renal blood flow is the same as or slightly lower than that of patients of normal weight.

Psychological

There are a number of contributing factors associated with obesity such as environment, genetics, highly processed and energy-dense foods, lack of exercise, ethnic culture, in addition to numerous psychological and social issues. Often eating has nothing to do with hunger. Many people eat in response to emotions such as boredom, sadness, or anger. Disordered eating may also be a symptom of depression and low self-esteem. Some individuals use food to fill emptiness, provide good feelings, and sooth job pressures and personal conflicts. Socially, obese people are perceived as lazy and lacking self-discipline and willpower, which can lead to a cycle of self-blame, guilt, shame, depression, and social withdrawal. Body image, along with the ability to interact with others, may be a problem for obese patients. Many bariatric patients have avoided routine medical care for fear of being judged and disrespected.

Integumentary

The presence of multiple skin folds can lead to impaired hygiene in the patient who may have difficulty seeing or reaching areas that need cleaning. Retained moisture on this redundant skin can lead to excoriations or rashes if not kept clean and dry. Problem areas tend to be found in the groin, perineum, or axilla, beneath the breasts, and in large skin folds. Wound infections can develop and commonly include yeast and fungi. Adipose tissue is poorly vascularized and can cause delayed wound healing.

Endocrine

Metabolic syndrome, also known as *insulin resistance,* is related to the effect of chronically high-normal serum blood sugars. The body has consistently high levels of glucose requiring the pancreas to secrete greater and greater amounts of insulin in order to keep blood sugar regulated. Eventually the cells no longer respond to insulin, and glucose begins to accumulate in the blood, leading to diabetes. Diabetes mellitus has been associated with obesity and metabolic resistance. It is the third most prevalent preoperative pathologic condition found in obese patients. Hypertension and dyslipidemia frequently occur concurrently and in association with resistance to insulin-stimulated glucose metabolism. When these risk factors cluster, the risks for CHD, stroke, diabetes, and cardiovascular disease mortality are further increased. This clustering of risk factors is frequent, but not invariably associated with obesity, particularly abdominal obesity. Insulin resistance is also associated with an unfavorable imbalance in the endothelial production of mediators that regulate platelet aggregation, coagulation, fibrinolysis, and vessel tone.

Other Disorders

Other problems associated with clinical obesity include abnormal liver function tests, fatty infiltration of the liver (nonalcoholic steatohepatitis), gallstones, hiatal hernia, stress incontinence, and varicose veins. Gastroesophageal reflux is prevalent among the obese. Overweight patients are at higher risk for deep vein thrombosis and pulmonary emboli because of the limited or lack of mobility, stasis, and polycythemia related to chronic respiratory insufficiency. Obese individuals will also have some degree of degenerative joint disease affecting mobility.

BARIATRIC PROCEDURES

For centuries, standard diet and exercise was the usual prescription for weight loss. With the increase in incidence of obesity and obesity-related health concerns, weight-related issues have become a priority in the health fields and the media. Multiple venues for managing weight have been established and newer, safer techniques in weight loss surgery are among the many treatment options for reducing excess body fat.

NURSING CARE IN THE PACU

Evidence-Based Practice

According to the extensive literature reviews conducted by Schumann and colleagues, safe pain management strategies for the patient undergoing weight loss surgery include a well-planned multimodal approach. Postoperative pain management options for the obese patient should include the use of preemptive agents including epidural or patient-controlled analgesia, surgical technique (open versus laparoscopic), the use of local anesthesia, and the use of nonopioid analgesics when indicated.

IMPLICATIONS FOR PRACTICE

Perianesthesia nurses caring for the bariatric patient can actively advocate for optimal pain management. This includes engaging multidisciplinary support for the development of appropriate order sets and policies and procedures for monitoring the postoperative bariatric patient, as well as soliciting active patient participation in postoperative pain management.

Source: Schumann R et al: Best practice recommendations for anesthetic perioperative care and pain management in weight loss surgery, *Obes Res* 13(2):254–266, 2005.

There are two basic types of bariatric surgery. Restrictive procedures are aimed at reducing the stomach size to limit the capacity of the stomach to hold food and to induce a state of satiation quickly. Malabsorptive procedures may include reducing the size of the stomach and redirecting the digestive process, causing an alteration in the body's ability to absorb and process nutrients and calories.

Two of the most common restrictive procedures include the laparoscopic adjustable gastric banding (LAGB; Fig. 45-1, *C*) and the vertical banded gastroplasty (VBG; see Fig. 45-1, *B*). The LAGB procedure involves the placement of an inflatable silicone band around the upper portion of the stomach. When in place, an access port is implanted just under the skin. This port allows for the injection or withdrawal of fluid into the band's lumen to either increase or decrease the diameter of the band. The end result is a smaller volume of food consumed with an early and longer sensation of fullness.

The second restrictive procedure is the VBG. In this procedure, the upper stomach near the esophagus is stapled vertically to create a small pouch (capable of holding approximately 30 mL) along the inner curve of the stomach. The outlet from the pouch to the rest of the stomach is restricted by a band, which delays the emptying of food from the pouch, causes an early feeling of fullness, and limits the volume of food consumed.

The most common malabsorptive weight loss procedure is known as the Roux-en-Y gastric bypass (see Fig. 45-1, *A*). Either open or laparoscopic, this procedure involves making the stomach smaller by creating a small pouch at the top of the stomach using surgical staples or a plastic band. The smaller stomach is then connected directly to the middle portion of the small intestine (jejunum), bypassing the rest of the stomach and the upper portion of the small intestine (duodenum). The smaller stomach reduces the amount of food taken in, and the bypass of the intestines result in fewer calories being absorbed.

The least commonly performed weight loss surgery is biliopancreatic diversion (BPD). BPD removes approximately three fourths of the stomach to produce both restriction of food intake and reduction of acid output. The small intestine is then divided with one end attached to the stomach pouch to create what is called an *alimentary limb*. All the food moves through this segment, but not much is absorbed. The bile and pancreatic juices move through the biliopancreatic limb, which is connected to the side of the intestine close to the end to supply digestive juice in the section of the intestine now called the *common limb*. The surgeon is able to vary the length of the common limb to regulate the amount of absorption of protein, fat, and fat-soluble vitamins.

PERIANESTHESIA CARE OF THE OBESE PATIENT

Equipment

Securing proper equipment throughout the continuum of care for the bariatric patient ensures patient comfort and safety. Properly sized blood pressure cuffs, gowns, bedside commodes, and transfer devices, such as wheelchairs and crutches, may be needed for the morbidly obese patient. In addition, special bariatric beds or stretchers for the operating room and postoperative care are also necessary. Adequate padding should be used to avoid pressure injuries that result in neurologic injury or rhabdomyolysis, a result of compartment syndrome and associated muscle necrosis. Because of problems associated with central lines in these patients, checking with the anesthesia care team to see what monitoring equipment is in use is important so that it can be continued in the postanesthesia phase.

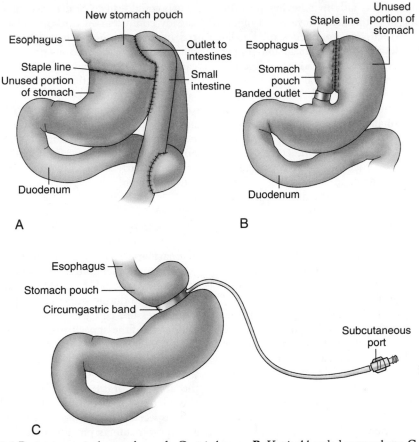

FIG. 45-1 Bariatric surgical procedures. **A,** Gastric bypass. **B,** Vertical banded gastroplasty. **C,** Laparoscopic adjustable gastric banding. (From Ignatavicius DD, Workman ML: *Medical-surgical nursing: critical thinking for collaborative care,* ed 5, St. Louis, 2006, Saunders.)

Respiratory

Significant problems arise in the PACU phase of the perioperative care of the obese patient. In fact, the problems associated with the rising incidence of obesity are becoming more apparent to all perianesthesia nurses, regardless of the reason for the surgical event. A direct correlation exists between the incidence rate of postoperative pulmonary complications and the degree of obesity. Expansion of the chest wall is restricted by the compression of weight. The mortality rate after upper abdominal operations in morbidly obese patients is 2.5 times that of the normal-weight counterparts.

Functional residual capacity (FRC) decreases with increasing BMI. The restriction of movement and crowding of structures within the chest because of weight contribute to this decreased FRC. In addition, expiratory reserve volume (ERV) decreases, and the residual volume (RV) stays the same. Thus, the FRC is reduced (ERV + RV = FRC) and the result is that the closing volume (CV) is increased, which leads to an increase in the alveolar-arterial oxygen (a-A PO$_2$) difference, resulting in hypoxemia. Therefore, the a-A PO$_2$ increases as the BMI increases. The bariatric patient is more susceptible to rapid desaturation and progressive hypercapnia. Vigilance to ventilation and oxygenation is crucial.

Positioning can be a valuable therapeutic tool for improving arterial oxygenation. Vigorous pulmonary toileting, including coughing, deep breathing, and the use of an incentive spirometer in the awake patient are also important nursing interventions. Position has been shown to significantly affect PaO$_2$ levels for 18 hours after surgery. The obese patient should be cared for in a semi-Fowler position unless cardiovascular instability exists. Routine use of the supine position should be avoided, because the functional residual capacity can decrease to less than the closing capacity and thus reduce the number of ventilated alveoli, which ultimately leads to hypoxemia.

Another position that aids in relieving pressure on the diaphragm is the head-elevated laryngoscopy position, which is a modified semi-Fowler position with elevation of the head and upper body with pillows to create a horizontal line between the sternum and ear that also improves the view for reintubation, if needed. Moreover, early ambulation and mobilization in the PACU is of great value in enhancement of lung volumes of the obese patient.

In the postanesthesia period, the position of the operative incision is a factor because obese patients with a vertical incision have been shown to have a more marked postoperative hypoxemia than obese patients who receive a transverse incision. Therefore supplemental inspired oxygen may be necessary after surgery for 3 to 4 days in patients with a vertical incision. Serial arterial blood gas determinations can serve as guides to supplemental oxygen administration. Moreover, after the patient's arterial line is in place, arterial blood gas determinations should be done to provide a baseline guide for proper ventilation. If the patient arrives in the PACU with the endotracheal tube in place, a ventilator should be started for the patient. The nurse should then auscultate for bilateral breath sounds to ensure proper placement of the endotracheal tube. Because of the many technical difficulties associated with tracheal intubation of the obese patient (e.g., size and mobility of the neck, increased tissue mass of the mouth and tongue), the perianesthesia nurse should constantly monitor the patient for proper placement of the tube. If the tube becomes displaced, the patient's lungs should be ventilated with a bag-mask system, and the anesthesia personnel should be summoned immediately.

Many patients will have a secondary diagnosis of OSA and may require the use of a continuous positive airway pressure device (CPAP) or bilevel positive airway pressure device (BiPAP) to maintain open airways. These devices may be contraindicated depending on the type of bariatric surgery performed, because CPAP and BiPAP devices have been linked to increased risk of anastomotic leaks. Morbidly obese adult patients with severe OSA may need a tracheostomy with local anesthesia before a general anesthetic is administered. If a patient with OSA arrives in the PACU and becomes obtunded, an emergency tracheostomy may be necessary to secure an airway.

Cardiovascular pathophysiology can reduce cardiac reserve, especially in the older obese patient. A reduction in arterial oxygen tension caused by incision site or postoperative position causes an increase in cardiac output to facilitate tissue oxygen delivery, which could lead to cardiac decompensation in an already compromised cardiovascular system. Arterial hypoxemia should be avoided because many obese patients cannot compensate for the increased cardiac output demand and the concomitant pulmonary vasoconstriction caused by the reduced arterial oxygen tension.

Early postoperative ambulation is important not only in enhancing lung volumes but also in helping to reduce the incidence of venous thrombosis. Indeed, relatively immobile obese persons are particularly susceptible to the development of pulmonary emboli.

Cardiovascular

The obese patient has a higher incidence rate of pulmonary hypertension, right-sided heart disease, coronary artery disease, myocardial infarction, and cardiomegaly; therefore careful electrocardiographic monitoring should be used. If an arterial line was not used during surgery, an appropriately sized blood pressure cuff that covers one third to half the length of the upper arm should be used. A baseline blood pressure measurement when the patient arrives in the PACU proves valuable in comparing the intraoperative measurements for assessment of the accuracy of the blood pressure reading. The PACU nurse may need a forearm blood pressure cuff, especially if used before and during surgery, and those readings provide a baseline blood pressure measurement.

Pain and Comfort Management

Bariatric patients are at higher risk for resedation and slower drug metabolism because many pharmacologic agents are lipophilic. Supplemental oxygen and pulse oximetry are often warranted depending on the extent of surgery or the length of anesthesia, or both. Respiratory sensitivity to the depressive effects of opioids should be assessed, and opioids should be used with caution and close monitoring. Multimodal treatments are encouraged using oral analgesics, nonsteroidal antiinflammatory drugs, opioids, patient-controlled analgesia, local anesthesia, and the epidural route of pain management.

Other comfort measures for the bariatric patient include the prevention of hypothermia. Lowered body temperatures will increase metabolic workload, increase oxygen demand, and ultimately increase the work of the cardiovascular system. Deep vein thrombosis prophylaxis requires attention to the proper fitting of compression devices, taking care to avoid a tourniquet effect that can impede blood flow and cause nerve or skin damage. Attention to skin integrity and condition is important for the bariatric patient. In addition to tension on skin during positioning and movement, care should be taken to keep skin clean and dry. Obesity-related stress incontinence is common and should be monitored. Last, close monitoring of serum glucose levels will help to minimize wide variations in blood sugars.

Fluid Dynamics

Subcutaneous fat often makes the process of initiating intravenous therapy a challenge. Careful monitoring of venous access sites should be a priority. Because fatty tissue is 6% to 10% water (compared with lean tissue, which is comprised of 70% to 80% water), fat contributes less fluid to total body water than does muscle mass. As a result, alterations in fluid requirements occur in the obese patient. In the healthy person, body water is 65%. In the obese person, the body water is approximately 40% of total weight. Calculations of fluid requirements must be adjusted to compensate for this reduction in total body water, and care taken to avoid rapid volume shifts will lessen cardiopulmonary compromise. Note that obese surgical patients have been found to have higher rates of postoperative nausea and vomiting, which will also affect fluid balance.

Psychological Aspects

Psychological support of the obese patient should not be overlooked when perianesthesia care is administered. The perianesthesia personnel should establish a positive rapport with the obese patient before surgery whenever possible. In addition, the perianesthesia staff must not express any negative feelings about the patient or about morbid obesity in general. Many obese patients have struggled with quality-of-life issues and clinical depression. Attention to psychological support serves to minimize fear and anxiety and ultimately improve outcomes of obese patients.

SUMMARY

The prevalence of obesity in patients seeking elective, bariatric, or emergency surgery has undoubtedly increased in recent years. Although patients with mild degrees of obesity pose few additional problems for perianesthesia and surgical management, those with a significant body mass index (BMI) require special consideration, equipment, and handling. Preoperative assessment is a key component of patient safety and preparation. Knowledge of the physiology of obesity is critical to understanding the implications of anesthesia and surgery on the overweight patient. In addition, the choice of anesthesia, patient positioning and handling, and postoperative care all require careful planning.

REFERENCES

1. Stewart M: Obesity and the perianesthesia patient, *J Perianesth Nurs* 24(5):332–334, 2009.
2. Tanner BD, Allen JW: Complications of bariatric surgery: implications for the covering physician, *The American Surgeon* 75:103–112, 2009.
3. Mullen JT, et al: The obesity paradox, *Annals of Surgery* 250(1):166–172, 2009.
4. Schumann R, et al: Best practice recommendations for anesthetic perioperative care and pain management in weight loss surgery, *Obesity Research* 13(2):254–266, 2005.

RESOURCES

Akinnusi ME, et al: Effect of obesity on intensive care morbidity and mortality: A meta-analysis, *Crit Care Med* 36(1): 151–158, 2008.

Boeka AG, et al: Psychosocial predictors of intentions to comply with bariatric surgery guidelines, *Psychology, Health & Medicine* 15(2):188–197, 2010.

Buchwald H, et al: *Surgical management of obesity*, Philadelphia, 2007, Saunders.

Flynn DR: Perioperative safety in the longitudinal assessment of bariatric surgery, *N Engl J Med* 361:445–454, 2009.

Houston DK, et al: Weighty concerns: the growing prevalence of obesity among older adults, *Journal of the American Dietetic Association* 109(11):1886–1895, 2009.

Ide P, et al: Perioperative nursing care of the bariatric surgical patient, *AORN* 88(1):30–54, 2008.

Jelic S, et al: Vascular inflammation in obesity and sleep apnea, *Circulation* 121:1014–1021, 2010.

Lotia S, Bellamy MC: Anaesthesia and morbid obesity, *Cont Edu Anesth Crit Care & Pain* 8(5):151–156, 2008.

Marley RA, et al: Perianesthesia respiratory care of the bariatric patient, *J Perianesth Nurs* 20(6):404–431, 2005.

McAtee M, Personett RJ: Obesity-related risks and prevention strategies for critically ill adults, *Crit Care Nurs Clin N Am* 21:391–401, 2009.

National Institutes of Health: Bariatric surgery for severe obesity, *NIH Publication* 08-4006:1–6, 2009. Available at: http://win.niddk.nih.gov/publications/PDFs/gasurg12.04bw.pdf. Accessed April 25, 2012.

Noble KA: The obesity epidemic: the impact of obesity on the perianesthesia patient, *J Perianesth Nurs* 23(6):418–425, 2008.

Pories WJ: Bariatric surgery: risks and rewards, *J Clin Endocrinol Metab* 93(11):S89 S96, 2008.

Reedy S: An evidence-based review of obesity and bariatric surgery, *The Journal for Nurse Practitioners* 5(1):22–29, 2009.

Schneider M: 11 Anesthesia safeguards for the obese, *Outpatient Surgery Magazine*, available at www.outpatientsurgery.net/guides/overweight-patients/2008/print&id=6960. Accessed August 18, 2011.

Sharkey KM, et al: Predicting obstructive sleep apnea among women candidates for bariatric surgery, *Journal of Women's Health* 19(10):1833–1838, 2010.

Silk AW, McTigue KM: Reexamining the physical examination for obese patients, *JAMA* 305(2):193–194, 2011.

Society of American Gastrointestinal and Endoscopic Surgeons: SAGES guideline for clinical application of laparoscopic bariatric surgery, *SAGES*, Los Angeles, CA: 2008. Available at http://www.sages.org/publication/id/30/. Accessed April 25, 2012.

Sood J, et al: Anaesthesia for laparoscopic bariatric surgery – our experience, *SAARC J Anaseth* 1(1):76–81, 2008.

Ward-Smith P: Obesity – America's health crisis, *Urologic Nursing* 30(4):242–245, 2010.

NURSING CARE IN THE PACU

Nancy Burden, MS, RN, CPAN, CAPA

Ambulatory surgery continues to grow, both in number of patients and in advancement of knowledge and technology. Providing quality nursing care in this setting requires a combination of many skills. The critical nature of surgery and anesthesia and potential complications demand critical thinking and advanced nursing skills. The short nature of the care cycle requires astute assessment skills and the ability to intervene rapidly and correctly. And the nature of more awake patients and family involvement places the nurse in the role of educator, counselor, and support system to help the patient experience correct preparation and safe aftercare in the home setting. Short-acting anesthetic agents and adjunctive drugs allow quick return to alertness and self care with fewer unpleasant side effects. In addition, consumers are more educated and sophisticated than in past generations, and current fast-paced lifestyles lend themselves to "in and out" care.

DEFINITIONS

Ambulatory Surgery Center (ASC): A facility that is separate from a hospital and may be on the same campus as or separate from other medical facilities.
Freestanding Ambulatory Surgery Center (FASC): Term used interchangeably with ASC.
Hospital Outpatient Department (HOPD): An area within a hospital that provides perioperative care for surgery patients who are discharged on the same day. These departments often function as a same-day admitting area for other surgical patients.
Joint Venture Surgery Center: An ambulatory surgery center that has more than one ownership entity, such as a corporation and physicians, a hospital and physicians, or a combination of all three.
Third-Party Payers: Payers that include insurance companies, health maintenance organizations, and the federal government; generally mandate that surgical procedures be performed in the appropriate lowest cost setting for payment eligibility. Thus, the trend has been to push procedures from hospitals to outpatient settings to physician offices. Ambulatory surgery and hospital industry organizations continually work with federal agencies to lobby for appropriate placement of procedures. Federal payment decisions often result in managed care companies following suit; therefore this is an important focus for administrators in all levels of health care settings.

AMBULATORY SURGERY ISSUES

A variety of factors drives the move toward outpatient surgery. Foremost, experience has shown the process to be successful and safe in both hospital outpatient departments and freestanding ambulatory surgery centers. Clinical outcomes have not suffered from shortened postoperative hospitalization in appropriate cases. In fact, avoidance of a hospital stay can reduce the opportunity for health care–associated infection and medical errors. However, the future growth of ambulatory surgery remains dependent on the effects of a variety of issues, including healthcare reform, the development of accountable care organizations (ACOs), Medicare and Medicare legislation, third party payer policies and other national influences. The great mobility of the population in the United States brings another challenge as families are scattered and the stronger family support systems of years past are reduced.

In addition to financial pressures to use the most cost-effective location for surgical procedures, other factors have contributed to the trend of same-day admission and early postoperative discharge. Technologic advances in instrumentation and equipment allow more complex procedures to be done with less invasiveness and physical trauma. Examples include advanced joint replacement procedures and laparoscopic gastric banding for weight loss, which has brought an increase in bariatric patients with their specific nursing care and environmental needs.

For patients who require nursing care in a much shortened time span, ambulatory perianesthesia nurses place emphasis on rapid yet comprehensive patient assessment along with complete understandable patient and family education. Ambulatory surgical nurses encourage the patient's self care and self responsibility for preadmission and postdischarge compliance with the planned medical and nursing care and then must assess the patient's ability, desire, and intentions to comply. In addition, nurses emphasize the patient's early ambulation and return to normal life activities, patient teaching, and family involvement in the patient's care.

Recognizing and addressing the social, emotional, and educational needs of patients as well as the physical needs are important. Unspoken questions may linger for patients and their families, such as relating to the final outcome of the procedure and concerns about health and well being, financial burdens, doubts about the availability and quality of postoperative support at home, vulnerability, and whether full preoperative life activities can resume and how quickly. Nurses should provide open doors for these types of questions and discussions.

Home support is essential because the patient returns there quickly after surgery. Involvement of the family or another responsible adult is integral to the overall plan of care. Postoperative complications such as nausea and vomiting might be considered minor or merely unpleasant for hospitalized patients who have nursing support. For ambulatory surgical patients, however, these problems become serious deterrents to discharge and can lead to a prolonged stay, costly unplanned hospitalization, or unpleasant home recuperation.

Assessment of the patient's medical, surgical, and social needs may lead to a physician's referral to a home health provider for general medical care, infusion therapy, pain management, physical therapy, or equipment-related needs. If needs are known before the day of the procedure, this referral can be in place, with equipment and supplies delivered to the patient's home to ensure its availability as soon as the patient arrives there.

Nursing care in this setting should promote wellness and self care to the degree possible. Patients should be continually encouraged to think positively and to provide self care as is appropriate and possible. Orem's general theory of nursing, a three part theory regarding self care, self care deficit, and nursing system, provides the basis for determining and using the patient's personal strengths relating to self care.[1] The Self-Care Deficit Nursing Theory describes nursing planning and intervention that is appropriate to the ambulatory surgical patient. The nurse calculates the patient's self-care demand and shares with the patient what must be done to regain or promote health in relation to postoperative recovery. Nursing actions revolve around teaching the patient and family, gaining acceptance of the prescribed actions, and then assessing the degree to which the nurse feels the patient can and will comply.

The concept of a self-fulfilling prophecy is a tool often used by managers to motivate a team. Nurses can use the concept to help patients expect success and comfort. According to the principles of a self-fulfilling prophecy, an outcome is more likely to happen just because the patient expects it. The outcome is preprogrammed by the patient's outlook; therefore the nurse's focus on wellness and uneventful recovery can be an important tool to shape the mindsets of the patient and caregiver in a positive direction.

Whether the patient has surgery in a hospital setting, a freestanding ASC, or a physician's office, the basic nursing needs remain the same. That care combines both critical assessment and monitoring during periods of high dependence, such as immediately after general anesthesia or sedation, with periods when the patient is encouraged and taught how to assume responsibility for self care. This care often is provided through a two-phase recovery process: the initial postanesthesia care unit (PACU) and a less care-intensive second phase unit from which the patient is eventually discharged.

More complex procedures are performed on sicker and older patients in the outpatient setting. Services such as 23-hour admission units, recovery care centers, and surgical specialty hospitals have provided a safety net of lengthier postoperative nursing care after more complex procedures. Early discharge after more complex procedures becomes more common as we gain more history of patient outcomes, the frequency and extent of complications, and the level of patient acceptance based on experience and research.

Without several shifts of nurses to prepare and educate patients and families before ambulatory surgery or to tend to the patient's postoperative needs, ambulatory surgical nurses must possess certain characteristics. Foremost, clinical assessment skills must be accurate and rapid. Nurses must be self motivated and able to communicate both in professional terms with peers and physicians and in lay terms with patients. Documentation skills and the forms used in the facility should allow for precise documentation of findings in minimal time. Probably most important from the patient's viewpoint, the nurse working in ambulatory surgery should present a positive, calm demeanor and show genuine concern for and interest in patients and their families.

ASSESSMENT AND PREPARATION OF THE PATIENT

Careful preoperative selection and preparation of patients for outpatient surgery help to reduce the risks of perioperative complications. Nonetheless, many patients may have significant physical, emotional or social challenges, yet they return home soon after surgery or other procedures because of insurance requirements. In addition to systemic illnesses that limit their ability to care for themselves and possibly increase the risk of perioperative complications, many people have limited social or family support. Nurses are especially challenged to prepare these more complex patients for an early transition to home.

The ultimate goals of complication-free recovery and early discharge are supported by what occurs before surgery. Proper patient selection, preparation, and education all contribute significantly to eventual patient outcome. Comprehensive physical assessment, history taking, and evaluation of the patient's social, emotional, and cognitive status are all essential to that care. The challenge for the ambulatory surgical nurse, however, is completing all those evaluations in a condensed time frame.

Nursing care also must reach beyond the facility into the patient's home setting, including preoperative education that helps to encourage preparation of a safe home setting for postoperative recuperation. Although nurses cannot be responsible for the actions of patients outside the facility, nurses do provide education, coaching, and suggestions for the patient's preoperative and postoperative care at home. The need to gain the patient's confidence and cooperation and to ensure the involvement of a responsible adult cannot be overstated. Support and education of the caregiver is another component of the nursing role.

Before the day of surgery, an on-site preadmission assessment is ideal for the nurse to establish a rapport with the patient, secure the patient's history, complete a physical assessment, help to reduce patient anxiety, provide comprehensive preoperative instructions, identify potential risk factors, and take steps to reduce those risk factors on or before the day of surgery. However, a telephone contact before the day of the patient's procedure is much more common today. The industry has come to this more streamlined approach for a number of reasons, including the busy lifestyles of the patient population, the economic restrictions of health care providers, the trend toward little or no diagnostic testing, and our current comfort with a telephone process borne out by history. Although a physical assessment or facility tour cannot occur via telephone, all other components of the preadmission care can be provided.

The Internet is another tool allowing patients and staff to share two-way information. Commercial and facility-developed assessment and educational tools allow patients to name their own time for providing preoperative health and demographic information. This does not preclude direct nursing interactions, but it provides a baseline from which to begin. Box 46-1 shows the

BOX 46-1 Quality Assessment and Performance Improvement in the Ambulatory Surgery Center

STUDY OBJECTIVE
To increase the use of an online system for gathering patient preoperative information.

BACKGROUND AND REASON FOR STUDY
The gathering of correct and comprehensive medical information is essential when providing surgical care. Anesthesia, physician, and nursing staff members all need and seek the most accurate and current information about medications, allergies, health, and past surgical or anesthesia experiences to be able to properly plan care for each patient.

The opportunity for an online option to allow patients and staff members to generate a clear document was available through a number of different commercial products. One Medical Passport System (Passport) created by Medical Web Technologies was chosen as an add-on to the software program used by the ambulatory surgery center (ASC). As with any new process, there was mixed response from staff members, ranging from excitement to refusal to use the new tool. Staff education, encouragement, and the positive leadership of management lent itself to improved use. However, we identified an opportunity to improve usage by staff members and patients.

It was difficult to get a true percentage of how many Passport records are completed compared with the patient load for that month, because Passport records are completed for future months as well as in the month of the patient's procedure. Thus, the percentages captured are of the ratio of Passport records completed in any month to the number of cases in that month. This number was not statistically accurate, but it gave us satisfactory data for trends upon which to make changes in the action planning and team education needed to improve.

Before implementation of the Passport system, we spoke with other ASCs using the system. We discussed the basis for the change in process to an electronic method of history retrieval. Those key reasons are:
1. To obtain more accurate information when the patient has quiet time at home to concentrate on the questions
2. To reduce illegibility of patient and nurse writing
3. To reduce potential for error in transferring information from a preadmission sheet onto other chart pages (The Passport system transfers essential information such as allergies onto the admitting, anesthesia, and admitting forms.)
4. To reduce nursing time for people who have completed their Passport records ahead of the preadmission testing (PAT) call. The nurse has the data available to review and only ask questions where gaps or concerns are found.

BOX 46-1   Quality Assessment and Performance Improvement in the Ambulatory Surgery Center—cont'd

5. To increase the ease of meeting CMS requirements for written and verbal notifications before the day of surgery

Current *Passport* usage was determined to be only 27%, whereas associated ASCs had 54% to 100% compliance. After discussion with the team, a stretch goal of 75% was set—just less than the 81% average of the other three ASCs. The team and leadership brainstormed ideas for improving the *Passport* usage and implemented actions throughout the year.

ACTION STEPS

ACTION	RESPONSIBLE PARTY	METHOD
Engage all staff	Administrator, manager	Educate team, encourage all team members go online to create personal *Passport* record, brainstorm ideas to encourage patient and nurse use
Improve physician office assistance	Administrator	Create new flier and deliver to offices; ask for more direction of patients to web site by office
Increase e-mail notifications to patients	Administrator, schedulers, physician advocate	Encourage physician offices to secure e-mails and provide those email addresses to the ASC
Increase e-mail notifications to patients	Registrars	Ask patients on all business calls about e-mail address and their use; consider common scripting
Improve ease of web site access	Physician advocate	Meet with corporate marketing to seek better linkage
Improve ease of tool	Director	Remove redundant or unnecessary questions from *Passport*
Provide more encouragement to patients to use site	Registrar or PAT	Telephone assistance to get into the site, positive communication to patients
Encourage nurse use	Administrator	Communicate necessity to all staff members; provide reward and recognition
Team education	Director, administrator	Provide ongoing modules to team for understanding success factors; use graphs and support documents
Data sharing	Information systems support	Provide information on usage; track improvements
Tracking and team education	Administrators, nurse managers	Ongoing review of processes and ways to encourage patients to use the online system
Assignment change	Manager	Change in process to move a specific nurse into PAT role on weekly basis

OUTCOME AND CONCLUSION OF STUDY

Over time, the level of *Passport* usage improved to 67.9%, ending the year with a December rate of 60.6%. Although the stretch goal of 75% was not met, the significant improvement in *Passport* usage was celebrated. Efforts continue to encourage patients to complete their own online *Passport* records. It is important to continue to focus on this effort and brainstorm further actions to meet a new goal of 85% of patients.

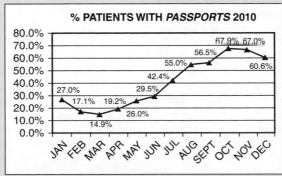

% PATIENTS WITH *PASSPORTS* 2010

27.0% 17.1% 19.2% 14.9% 26.0% 29.5% 42.4% 55.0% 56.5% 67.9% 67.0% 60.6%

JAN FEB MAR APR MAY JUN JUL AUG SEPT OCT NOV DEC

NURSING CARE IN THE PACU

work of one ambulatory surgery center to increase the use of such a tool using a quality improvement process.

Patients at high risk can be identified and may be asked to come to the facility for physical examination and anesthesia consultation. Early identification of significant risk factors allows time to correct any deficiencies or, if necessary, to reschedule the surgery to avoid day-of-surgery cancellations or unexpected postoperative complications and overnight admissions that are more costly to the institution, upsetting to the patient and physician, and generally time consuming.

A report by the American College of Cardiology (ACC) and American Heart Association (AHA)[2] has identified major, intermediate, and minor clinical predictors of increased perioperative risk.

- Unstable coronary syndromes, such as acute or recent myocardial infarction (MI) or unstable angina, decompensated congestive heart failure, and severe dysrhythmias or valvular disease, are major predictors of perioperative risk.
- Intermediate risk factors include mild angina, prior MI determined with history or Q waves, compensated or prior heart failure, diabetes mellitus, and renal insufficiency.
- Minor risks include advanced age, abnormal electrocardiogram results, dysrhythmias, low functional capacity, history of stroke, and uncontrolled hypertension.

These factors should be considered before any surgery, but especially before elective surgery that could wait until a more stable cardiac status can be attained. Active cardiac conditions for which the ACC and AHA recommend evaluation and treatment before elective surgery include: unstable coronary syndromes, decompensated heart failure, significant arrhythmias, and severe valvular disease, although these recommendations are not specific to ambulatory surgery. The same report identifies cardiac risk based on the type of procedure as low (less than 1%) for the following noncardiac surgeries: endoscopic and superficial procedures, cataract and breast surgery, and ambulatory surgery.[3] The physician will determine the need for adjunctive preoperative cardiac assessment.

Specific instructions necessary before the day of the procedure include arrangements for transportation and adult support, the projected length of stay, and general expectations on the day of surgery. The patient also should be instructed in the proper clothing to wear for ease of dressing after surgery, preparation of the home environment, physical restrictions after surgery, and any equipment or supplies to purchase or secure before arrival for surgery.

With the emphasis on safety in the perioperative period, involvement of the patient as fully as possible in safety practices is prudent. Boxes 46-2 and 46-3 provide information that can help to raise the patient's understanding and consciously set expectations that the patient and family will be part of the overall safety plan. With the proliferation of antibiotic-resistant microorganisms today, prevention of surgical site infection should be a key focus for all health care providers and the patient. Evidenced-based decisions are important to help reduce the potential for surgical site infection.

Evidence-Based Practice

In a randomized, double-blind study reported by Darouiche and colleagues, undertaken at six hospitals in the United States, researchers compared the difference in postoperative infection rates over 4 years in 813 surgical patients. Patients having clean-contaminated procedures were included in the study. Three hundred ninety-one patients were randomly assigned to the study group, in which a 2% chlorhexidine gluconate and 70% isopropyl alcohol combination was used as the preoperative skin scrub. The control group of 422 patients had preoperative skin preparation with an aqueous solution of 10% povidone-iodine. The study group showed a significantly lower rate of surgical site infection (9.5%) compared with the control group (16.1%).

IMPLICATIONS FOR PRACTICE

Ambulatory surgical nurses can be active in practice decisions by sharing insights from research studies that provide evidence of opportunities to reduce surgical site infections.

Source: Darouiche R, et al: Chlorhexidine-alcohol versus povidone-iodine for surgical-site antisepsis, *N Engl J Med* 362:18–26, 2010.

The Internet has become a common source of information. Nurses should be prepared to evaluate the value and accuracy of such information and advise the patient toward appropriate sites. Examples of sites providing information include the following:

- Agency for Healthcare Research and Quality (www.ahrq.gov)

BOX 46-2   Ten Tips to Keep You Safe in the Outpatient Setting

1. Be sure that everyone who cares for you identifies you by asking you to say your name and birth date and by checking your name band.
2. If you have any questions or concerns, ask a team member. Ask a family member or friend to speak for you if you are not able to do so.
3. If you believe that you are not steady on your feet, please ask us to help you. We do not want you to fall.
4. When you are asked about the medicines you take, please tell us about every medicine. Be sure to include creams, vitamins, herbs, diet supplements, and all prescription and over-the-counter medicines, including street drugs.
5. Tell us about all your allergies. Include allergies to medicines, tape, latex, shellfish, and anything else you may have reacted to in the past.
6. If you have a new prescription given to you while you are here, be sure you know what it is for, how to take it, and any possible side effects.
7. If you have any questions about a test or procedure, please ask your nurse or doctor.
8. Ask team members who have direct contact with you if they have washed their hands. It is the best way to prevent the spread of germs, and we will be glad you asked.
9. Be sure you know and understand how to take care of yourself when you go home.
10. If you notice any other safety concerns, please tell a team member so we can work to make our outpatient center a safer place for all.

BOX 46-3   Ten Things You Can Do to Help Prevent a Surgical Site Infection

BEFORE YOUR PROCEDURE

1. Shower or bathe with an antibacterial soap before your procedure.
2. Do not shave the skin near your incision area before surgery to prevent cuts in the skin that could harbor bacteria.
3. Do not apply creams or lotions near the incision area on the day of your procedure.

BEFORE AND AFTER YOUR PROCEDURE

4. Take care of yourself to enhance healing with adequate rest, plenty of fluids, and good nutrition: a diet high in protein and vitamin C, if not contraindicated by your health.
5. Avoid close contact with anyone who has an obvious infection, cold, or the flu.

AFTER YOUR PROCEDURE

6. If you do not see your health care workers wash their hands before caring for you, speak up and ask them to do so. Do not be embarrassed; we want to keep you safe.
7. Keep any dressing, bandage, or cast clean and dry. If it gets wet and you have been instructed not to remove or change it, tell your physician immediately.
8. If antibiotics are prescribed, take all the pills and take them according to directions.
9. Wash your hands before touching your bandage or caring for catheters and drains and ensure that any other people helping you also wash their hands.
10. Do not put anything on your incision area that is not prescribed.

- Accreditation Association for Ambulatory Health Care (www.aaahc.org)
- American Society of Anesthesiologists (www.asahq.org)
- American College of Surgeons (www.facs.org)
- Society for Ambulatory Anesthesia (www.sambahq.org)
- Institute for Healthcare Improvement (www.ihi.org)
- The Joint Commission (www.jointcommission.org)
- Society of Gastroenterology Nurses and Associates (www.sgna.org)
- American Association of Nurse Anesthetists (www.aana.com)
- Association of periOperative Registered Nurses (www.aorn.org)
- American Society of PeriAnesthesia Nurses (www.aspan.org)
- Leapfrog Group (www.leapfroggroup.org)
- Surgical Care Improvement Project (SCIP; www.jointcommission.org/surgical_care_improvement_project)
- National Quality Forum (www.qualityforum.org)
- ASC Quality Collaboration (www.ascquality.org)

NURSING CARE IN THE PACU

The American Society of PeriAnesthesia Nurses web site provides patient information on the following[3]:

- Preanesthetic interview and testing
- Expectations for the day of surgery
- What to expect in the preoperative holding area
- What to expect in the operating room
- What to expect in the postanesthesia care unit
- Admission to a facility
- Outpatient surgery
- What to expect if you are going home on the day of surgery
- Pain management
- Preverification checklist

Patients who take routine medications need instructions by the attending physician or anesthesiologist about which medications should be taken on the morning of surgery, usually with a small sip of water. Medications most often continued until the time of surgery include antihypertensives, cardiac antiarrhythmics, coronary artery dilators, bronchodilators, and respiratory inhalants (should be brought on the day of surgery).

Precise instructions regarding blood thinners should be provided by the patient's physician. Specific information about insulin and diet for patients with diabetes can help to avoid wide swings in glucose levels. Medication instructions are the responsibility of the physician; however they are often confirmed, reinforced, and clarified by nursing personnel.

Patients should be encouraged to fill prescriptions for postoperative medications before the day of surgery to avoid delays at home. If patients have not yet received any prescriptions, they should know to bring money or insurance cards to obtain medications if it is likely that prescriptions will be given on the day of surgery.

Parents of small children are asked to have two adults accompany the child—one to drive and one to attend to the child during transit home. In some institutions, supporting adults are instructed that they must remain at the facility throughout the patient's stay. In others, only parents of minors or special needs adults are required to remain on site. Patients and families should be told about such expectations ahead of time.

Freestanding ASCs have an additional requirement imposed by the Centers of Medicare and Medicare Services (CMS).[4] In ASCs that are Medicare certified, before surgery all patients, not just those covered by Medicare, must be provided with both verbal and written information about their rights and responsibilities, the ASC policy on advance directives, and

any physician financial interest in the ASC. Three informational items must be provided to the patient before signing the consent for treatment. For clarity, the nurse should document the time of the notification and the time the consent is signed to verify that standards were met.

Admission of the Patient

The preparation of patients immediately before surgery is essentially the same as for all surgical patients. Physical assessment includes at least vital signs, breath sounds, peripheral pulses as indicated, baseline oxygen saturation levels, skin condition at the site of surgery or regional anesthetic injection, and other appropriate assessments. Essential safety practices include a valid, correct, and signed informed consent; verification of the fasting period; home support and driver; and careful preoperative identification of the patient with two consistent identifiers, neither of which should be the patient's bed or room location. Meticulous operative site identification begins with the scheduling of the patient, but during the time of admission, the site, side, and procedure must be confirmed with the patient and any discrepancies should be immediately investigated and clarified before marking the site.

Current pressure from government, industry, consumer, and other groups to reduce medical errors and improve overall patient safety is demonstrated by a list of the most common sentinel events reviewed by The Joint Commission. Their sentinel event data compiled from 1995 through 2010 demonstrates that wrong site surgery remains one of the top three reviewed events in the last few years, ranking number one in 2008 and 2009 and ranking third in 2010.[5] Although these events represent both inpatient and outpatient surgeries in all types of settings, the lesson remains that this is a serious opportunity for error. Nurses must enforce strict policies regarding site marking and timeout procedures in all cases all of the time; this includes preoperative anesthesia blocks as well as surgical and endoscopic procedures.

Fasting Before Surgery

Fasting requirements as defined per facility by the department of anesthesia are decidedly more lenient that in the past. Traditional guidelines for "nothing after midnight" have been challenged and are now rarely used. The American Society of Anesthesiologists advocates the following fasting guidelines for elective procedures that involve anesthesia and sedation.[6]

INGESTED MATERIAL	MINIMUM FASTING HOURS
Clear liquids	2
Breast milk	4
Infant formula	6
Light meal (e.g., toast and clear liquid)	6
Nonhuman milk	6
Meal with fried or fatty foods or meat	8 or more

In the ambulatory surgical population, ensuring the required fasting period can be more challenging because the nurse has decidedly less opportunity to teach and less ability to control the patient who is not admitted to a hospital bed overnight. Adult patients and parents of pediatric patients must be thoroughly educated about the specifics of the fasting period. They should know that in addition to food and beverages, they are to avoid water, gum, candy, coffee, and cough drops immediately before surgery. It may be helpful to explain in lay terms that although gum and hard candy are not swallowed, they stimulate the stomach to produce acids that can be harmful if aspirated. Patients must be informed about the seriousness of breaking the fasting period and of accurate reporting of nonadherence.

Parents should carefully monitor children at home and in the automobile so that the child does not eat or drink without the parent's knowledge. Adolescents also may be at particular risk because of their tendency to resist authority and their misguided sense of immortality. On the day of surgery, the nurse must strive to elicit truthful and accurate verification of the patient's actual adherence and may need to alter the questions asked to secure a full picture of the fasting or lack thereof.

Diagnostic Testing

Required preoperative diagnostic tests vary widely from one institution to another and are a matter both of clinical judgment by individual physicians and the policies set by the medical board that administers the ambulatory surgical program. Current trends are toward performing no or only essential diagnostic tests that are aimed at providing the basic information necessary for safe anesthesia and surgical interventions. The American Society of Anesthesiologists supports that preoperative tests may be useful in the preanesthesia evaluation; however, no routine laboratory or diagnostic screening is necessary. *Routine* refers to tests performed without regard to clinical indications for an individual patient. *Screening* refers to efforts to detect disease in asymptomatic patients in unselected populations.[7]

The use of generic screenings without clinical evidence of patient appropriateness has a significant financial effect on health care. Institutional policies prevail; however, some facilities or physician groups continue to prefer some baseline laboratory data. Continued controversy exists regarding routine preoperative pregnancy testing in women of childbearing age. The medical oversight committee of a facility and individual physicians will make decisions based on clinical and practice issues.

Nurses responsible for preparing patients for surgery should carry out physicians' orders and the policies of the facility for all diagnostic testing and ensure that results of any tests are included in the medical record. Abnormal results should be provided to the physician before the patient is medicated or transferred to surgery. Test results should be secured and the physician should be notified of abnormal values before the day of surgery whenever possible.

Preoperative Medications

Some providers prefer to avoid all premedications in the ambulatory surgical patient and may even encourage patients to walk to surgery to promote a sense of normalcy and self control. Others believe that certain goals can be met pharmacologically to smooth the anesthetic course.

Preoperative medications can be given to decrease salivation; reduce anxiety; promote calmness before induction of general anesthesia; and, for children, reduce the fear and stress of separation from parents. Antiemetic and gastrokinetic medications can be used to reduce the risk of vomiting and subsequent aspiration. Opioids can be added to the regimen before painful procedures, although their penchant to promote nausea and vomiting may preclude their preoperative use.

When premedications are given, intravenous (IV) administration is certainly the trend. This rapidly effective route spares the patient from the pain of intramuscular injections and helps to avoid prolonged sedative effects that can delay eventual postoperative discharge.

After the administration of any preoperative medications, patients should be monitored for allergic, atypical, or untoward drug reactions, such as respiratory or cardiac depression. Appropriate interventions to correct such situations should be initiated immediately with concurrent notification of the physician.

Emotional Support

Emotional support also helps to reduce patient anxiety and potential associated complications such

NURSING CARE IN THE PACU

as hypertension, tachycardia, vomiting, aspiration, and increased postoperative pain related to fear. Conversations with the patient should be positive. Questions or statements should imply the positive aspects of recovery, particularly the ability to go to a familiar and comfortable home soon after the surgery. The nurse also teaches the family directly and by example to speak in similar positive terms to encourage the patient's confident attitude. This approach supports a climate of wellness and positive outcome.

PREOPERATIVE GOALS

The primary goals of patient preparation for ambulatory surgery are focused on identifying and reducing the potential risks related to surgery and anesthesia, reducing the potential for surgical site infections through strict adherence to standard precautions, verifying the patient's true understanding, and promoting each patient's quick return to self care. This preparation includes a significant shift of responsibility to the patient and family by educating them and then encouraging and evaluating their actions. Although patient preparations may not necessarily be identical for inpatients and outpatients, they should meet the same quality standards of care. Nurses who admit and prepare patients for surgery must be thorough in their assessments. They must be prepared professionally and have adequate equipment to intercede effectively in emergencies.

The essential outcome of patients remaining infection free begins in the preoperative area and continues throughout their stays. The opportunity for surgical site and other acquired infections can be reduced by basic cleanliness of the environment, strict adherence to medical asepsis and sterile process, meticulous hand hygiene, safe injection practices, proper skin preparation which avoids shaving, proper antibiotic selection and timing, and the good health of the providers within the unit.

An important way to provide a safe experience for the ambulatory patient is to consistently apply safety policies in the same manner for all patients. A surgical safety checklist like the one developed by the World Health Organization (WHO) provides a method to document all essential areas of care at three points in the continuum of patient care: before anesthesia induction, before the skin incision, and before the patient leaves the operating room.[8] The tool that can be downloaded from the WHO web site is intended as a baseline, and modifications are encouraged to fit the specific types of care provided in a surgical setting.

INTRAOPERATIVE PERIOD

Intraoperative care of the ambulatory surgical patient parallels that of all surgical patients. Specific nursing responsibilities include maintaining asepsis; properly preparing the operative site; providing for patient safety in identification, transfer, and positioning; assisting the anesthesia team; maintaining confidentiality; protecting the patient's dignity; maintaining a safe environment; correctly handling and labeling specimens in the presence of the patient; and documenting and reporting the intraoperative care and events. Before initiating the procedure, a time-out period must be enforced in which every participant in the operating room stops what they are doing and focuses on the identification of the correct operative site, side, procedure, patient, and implants.

Because of the trend to reduce or eliminate preoperative sedative medications and the common use of topical, regional, or local anesthesia, patients may be more awake and aware of their surroundings. As a result, monitoring and controlling the appropriateness of any discussions that occur near the patient is an important nursing role.

In addition, the increased use of registered nurse–administered sedation or analgesia demands competency of the perioperative nurse in monitoring, dysrhythmia detection, medication effects and side effects, and effective reversal agents. The nurse's knowledge base should also include related cardiac and respiratory anatomy and physiology, airway management, and resuscitative techniques. The availability of emergency supplies and support personnel must be ensured before the procedure begins. In particular, flumazenil and naloxone— specific reversal agents for benzodiazepines and opioids, respectively—should be immediately available for treatment of serious respiratory or cardiac depression related to the sedative drugs. Advanced Cardiac Life Support (ACLS) certification is appropriate for nurses monitoring and sedating patients for procedures. During each reappointment cycle, the procedural physician responsible for patient care during nurse-monitored sedation and analgesia should demonstrate competency in the appropriate physiologic and pharmacologic concerns, including rescue methods and drugs and the preprocedural assessment and documentation of the airway and anesthesia risk level.

Anesthesia Considerations

Anesthesia for the ambulatory surgical patient incorporates the traditional goals of adequate analgesia, muscle relaxation, amnesia, and, in the event of general anesthesia, loss of consciousness to accomplish the intended procedure. Because the ambulatory surgical patient is discharged soon after the procedure, the anesthesia plan should promote reduced postoperative hangover and complications. Topical, regional, and local techniques are favored by many clinicians because the patient does not lose consciousness, can usually be discharged sooner after the procedure, and often has prolonged pain relief at the operative site or extremity.

The ongoing development of new and shorter-acting general anesthetic agents has significantly reduced complications such as postoperative nausea and vomiting and has encouraged rapid return to alertness, thus making general anesthesia as likely to be used as other techniques.

POSTANESTHESIA PERIOD

Recovery of ambulatory surgical patients often occurs in several stages. After general or major regional anesthesia or after intraoperative complications in any patient, a two-phase recovery is typical. Phase I begins when the patient arrives in a fully equipped and staffed PACU. When the patient regains consciousness, lucidity, and physiologic stability and meets PACU discharge criteria, transfer to a less-intensive care unit is appropriate. Phase II of recovery is usually completed in a department equipped with lounge chairs and more homelike surroundings where families reunite and where the patient's self care is encouraged. After sedation or local or regional anesthesia, which has a limited effect on physiologic stability, the patient may be transferred from the procedure room directly to the phase II level of care as long as they meet predetermined criteria for care in that setting. This latter process is typically called *fasttracking*.

The American Society of Perianesthesia Nurses has published a position statement that any fasttracking plan should be a collaboration of the anesthesiology department and perianesthesia services. Guidelines should include appropriate patient selection, preoperative education of the patient and family, appropriate selection and management of anesthetic agents, assessment criteria used to determine readiness for bypassing PACU care, discharge criteria, and monitoring and reporting of patient outcomes.[9]

Phase I and phase II care are not necessarily based on a physical location, rather the intensity of nursing monitoring and interventions. As a result, some facilities keep a patient in one postoperative location, but alter the level of care to conform with phase I and phase II standards.

Postanesthesia Care Unit

After a handoff report from the operating room and anesthesia personnel that allows for questions and answers among the staff, the nurse applies all the usual parameters of PACU care to the ambulatory surgical patient. Airway and respiratory management are paramount. The patient is closely observed for untoward cardiac, respiratory, or other effects from anesthetic agents. The operative site and any related areas are monitored for bleeding, and any existing parenteral fluids are maintained. Further nursing duties include oxygen delivery, monitoring of vital signs and oxygen saturation, and periodic stir-up of the patient to move and deep breathe. Observation for any complications of surgery or anesthesia is coupled with rapid and appropriate nursing interventions if problems are identified.

These parameters are essential to the care of all patients in the PACU, but certain specific needs of ambulatory surgical patients must be met as well. Nursing care should be planned in a manner that not only identifies, reports, and treats complications in the early stages, but also reduces the risk of unpleasant complications that delay the patient's discharge to home. For example, the speed of progressive head elevation should be paced to the individual patient's responses. Faintness, lightheadedness, hypotension, pallor, nausea, or vomiting implies the need to lower the patient's head and begin the process again. Adequate parenteral hydration before the patient sits upright may reduce the patient's risk of development of gastrointestinal symptoms related to hypovolemia or hypotension. Oral fluids are given slowly, with adequate time between drinks, to assess the patient's tolerance.

Pain should be managed aggressively and immediately, not only because it is humane and the nurse's ethical responsibility to do so, but also because prevention of pain is easier than controlling escalating pain. Intramuscular injections are generally avoided and can interfere with the goal of imminent discharge. Patients who have more complex procedures may benefit from the long action of an intramuscular injection, but for most patients the IV route is the first choice because of its immediate effects and the shortened observation time for related complications such as respiratory depression. The provision of adequate analgesia and general comfort measures is usually attained before the patient is transferred to the phase II recovery area, where analgesia is more likely to be addressed with oral medications.

The goal of adequate patient comfort is supported when the patient knows before surgery that the nurse is concerned about and eager to provide adequate pain relief. Patients should be encouraged to discuss their usual tolerance for pain and should not be judged in that regard based on the attitudes and prior experiences of the staff. The use of an objective pain scale helps in determining the patient's need for intervention, and patients should be educated on that scale before procedures for comparison. They should also know that although total absence of postoperative discomfort may not be a realistic goal, acute pain should be reported and treated. Patient comfort, supported by positive thinking, general comfort measures, and oral analgesics, is one of the criteria with which eventual discharge readiness is measured, and this goal must be addressed in the early stages of recovery.

In pediatric patients, some potential postoperative problems include bleeding, croup, nausea and vomiting, and fever of unknown origin, any of which can result in unplanned hospitalization. Children need gentle care and strong emotional support. The presence of one or both parents in the PACU can be reassuring to both the child and the parents. On the other hand, emotional parents can precipitate anxiety and distress in the child; therefore support and guidance of the parents becomes an adjunctive nursing responsibility.

Emergence delirium is more common in children than in adults. The child who is agitated and thrashing should be gently restrained to prevent self injury. This behavior is uncommon, but parents who observe it need explanation and support. In children and adults, accurate differentiation is essential for the restlessness associated with emergence delirium from other physiologic complications, such as hypoxia, bladder distention, and pain that must be treated appropriately.

Progressive or Phase II Care

Patients who do not require the intensity of PACU care are transferred to the phase II unit of the ambulatory surgical facility. This area is generally furnished with lounge chairs, and the decor is more homelike than in the PACU to encourage a sense of wellness and normalcy. The phase II area includes a nourishment center, patient bathrooms and changing areas, and ready access to an outside door for patient discharge. As in all acute health care settings, emergency equipment and support personnel must be readily available.

The goals of nursing care in this setting address the patient's physical, emotional, social, educational, and spiritual needs. This care includes attention to ongoing surgical site and general assessment, comfort management, hydration, ambulation, urinary status, cardiovascular stability,

and home care needs. The comprehensive goals also include meeting the needs of the family or other responsible adult. Close nursing observation for potential complications is ongoing during the patient's stay. Expediting a safe discharge and complication-free recuperation is the ultimate objective of all nursing and medical interventions.

Specific areas of concern in the phase II unit include observation of cardiorespiratory status and other vital signs to ensure stability in relation to the patient's preoperative normal levels. Other goals are to ensure adequate nutrition and fluid status, provide effective pain management, avoid unpleasant gastrointestinal symptoms, observe the operative site and associated symptoms, and encourage ambulation. Observation of the patient sitting up and then walking without orthostatic hypotension, faintness, or dizziness provides some element of confidence that the patient will be able to maneuver in a similar manner at home. Patients should be able to show proper use and care of ambulatory aids such as walkers, crutches, and casts. Existing parenteral fluids or IV access ports should be maintained until the patient is able to ambulate without faintness and discharge readiness is attained.

The tradition of a certain level of oral intake before discharge has come under scrutiny. Certainly the patient's level of hydration must be considered, but forced oral intake on someone who has no desire or interest can be self defeating and result in poor tolerance. The patient's appetite and desire to eat or drink are often considered the best indicators of readiness. In the decision of whether to delay discharge until the patient can tolerate oral fluids, the physician considers the patient's overall condition. This decision includes gastrointestinal status, the amount of IV fluid replacement given, the level of home support, and the patient's likeliness to report and to handle any inability to tolerate food or fluids at home. Extensive nausea or vomiting should be effectively treated before the patient is discharged.

Most often, the phase II unit is where patients reunite with family members or the responsible adults who will accompany and care for them at home. Early reunion should be encouraged, and nurses in this setting must purposefully involve the patient's support people. The responsible adult may need to learn how to care for the patient's physical needs, such as changing a dressing, observing extremity circulation, or emptying drains. Encouraging a return demonstration of manual skills or having the caretaker repeat information is a good way to reinforce learning and to evaluate the person's ability to provide support. The nurse should focus on the information specifically needed to provide care and not divulge extraneous health information.

The nurse also helps the responsible adult to understand that the patient should perform self care to the extent of the patient's ability and that encouraging such behavior is in the best interest of the patient for a speedy recuperation and a positive mental outlook.

Discharge of patients to home after anesthesia and invasive procedures is a serious responsibility. Planning for that discharge should begin well before the actual time of discharge, hopefully at the time the patient is scheduled for surgery. Still, the discharging nurse is the one who ensures that all those plans come together. Ensuring patient safety at home and in transit may require the nurse to discuss problems with the physician and enlist the assistance of home health agencies or transportation sources. Whatever is necessary, the nurse is ethically obliged to intervene for the patient's safety before discharge.

One of the most difficult situations is the unexpected lack of a driver or responsible adult. Although all efforts are made to verify and ensure this before beginning the procedure, surprises do occur and present a dilemma for staff members. No magic answer addresses all scenarios, but in conjunction with the physician, the staff must use creativity and common sense to address the patient's safe discharge.

The physician is ultimately responsible for the decision to discharge each patient. The nurse's application of written discharge criteria that have been previously approved by the physician staff must meet the standards of regulatory bodies such as accreditation organizations and federal and state requirements.

Any special concern about the patient's actual condition or ability to safely recuperate at home should prompt the nurse to solicit direct physician involvement in the discharge process. Various areas of concern typically included in discharge criteria include vital signs; level of consciousness; comfort (pain, nausea, use of oral analgesics); activity level; surgical site; instructions; the support of a responsible adult and driver; and to a lesser degree, nourishment, hydration, and ability to urinate.

When a patient does not meet the facility's discharge criteria, a specific physician's order for discharge should be secured that addressed any deficiencies. The nurse's notes should reflect why or how the patient did not meet existing criteria and what was done about it. For example, the criteria may require that all patients void before discharge, but a patient who cannot void after several hours of recovery may be discharged by the physician without meeting the criterion. The nurse should document the involvement of the physician, notification of the responsible adult about the problem area, an assessment of the patient's abdomen, the specific guidelines and instructions given to the patient about what symptoms might indicate a full bladder, the importance of avoiding overdistention of the bladder, how long to wait at home without voiding before seeking care, telephone numbers given to the patient for obtaining medical assistance, and any other specific instructions given.

The eventual closure of documentation also should include a nursing notation regarding the patient's status related to unmet discharge criteria on the following day or later that day as ascertained via telephone contact. This last portion of comprehensive care and documentation is possible only if the person who makes the postdischarge telephone call is aware that an issue exists. A mechanism should be in place for communicating information from one nurse to the next, or discharging nurses should be personally responsible for the eventual postdischarge follow-up of patients in their care.

Before discharge, written and verbal instructions for home care should be provided. Anxiety, discomfort, and the amnesic effects of many medications given to patients can result in poor or absent recall of information from the day of surgery; therefore, whenever possible, instructions should be given both to the patient and to the adult responsible for the patient after discharge.

Most facilities have developed preprinted discharge instruction sheets with carbonless copies that remain on the chart after being signed by the patient, the accompanying adult, or both, as proof that the instructions were given. In addition to the usual instructions about eating, hygiene, wound care, ambulation, return physician visit, and telephone numbers for assistance, the patient should receive a description of what symptoms may be usual and what should be reported to the physician. For example, knowledge that a slight sore throat or generalized sore muscles may follow general anesthesia helps the patient avoid worry. When those same discharge instructions have been followed by suggestions for alleviating possible minor symptoms, the patient has an even greater chance of recuperating comfortably.

Medication reconciliation is a focus of the National Patient Safety Goals and is the responsibility of the physician. The patient's list of usual medications should be compared and reconciled with any medications given in the center that have a prolonged effect into the home recuperative period and with medication prescriptions given. Reconciliation is a review of the medications to identify contraindications, misunderstandings, and potential for duplication of medication. For example, consider the patient who routinely takes Percocet at home who is given a prescription for acetaminophen–oxycodone. Without review and reconciliation of the lists with the patient, a duplication could occur with serious ramifications.

The individual patient's specific needs must be addressed as well. The nurse should ensure that the physician's discharge instructions have included areas such as the following:

- When should oral medications be resumed?
- When should the diabetic patient resume taking insulin, and how much?
- When should blood thinners such as warfarin, clopidogrel, or dipyridamole be resumed?
- When can the patient drive, watch television, or have a glass of wine?

Many patients also wonder whether sexual intercourse should be avoided and for how long and why, although they might not verbalize this question. Inclusion of this information in the general instructions as appropriate to the patient and procedure avoids the need for the patient to ask. Comprehensive discharge instructions result in individualized information for each patient.

POSTDISCHARGE FOLLOW-UP

Mechanisms should exist for assessing and documenting patient outcomes and patient and family satisfaction with the care provided by the ambulatory surgical unit. Telephone calls and written surveys that can be returned by mail are two means of providing that follow-up. Written surveys most often address satisfaction issues, but evaluation of the patient's recuperation from anesthesia and surgery requires a more aggressive and timely approach.

In many communities, the standard of care is that patients are telephoned within the next few days after surgery to ascertain their clinical condition, safety, and comfort level. Such a contact can serve as a valuable resource for patients who may have symptoms that should be evaluated by their physicians or questions about which they are embarrassed or reluctant to telephone and ask their physicians. Not only is the patient's safety and medical condition supported, but the nursing staff also can identify the effectiveness of current modes of care. Other reasons for a postdischarge call include promotion of the facility's caring attitude, identification and reduction of medicolegal issues, marketing, the meeting of accrediting and regulatory standards, and closure and a sense of job satisfaction for the nurses.

In some instances, a second call may be made at a date several weeks after the patient's discharge for the goal of assessing a particular concern related to a quality improvement or risk management study, such as a study on postoperative infection or the satisfaction of vision changes after cataract surgery. Documentation of patient contacts via telephone should become a permanent part of the medical record. This level of follow-up after the patient's discharge closes the loop of the evaluation phase of the nursing process in the ambulatory surgery setting.

In addition, Joint Commission standards now require a 1-year follow-up to identify infections in patients who have had implantable devices placed during their procedures. This is another imposed regulation that must be met to help reduce the potential for surgical site infections by understanding and investigating events.[10]

SUMMARY

The number of patients who have surgery in the outpatient setting has continued to increase. Sicker patients and more complex procedures are performed in these settings. The ambulatory surgery nurse must be cognizant of special requirements for preparation and discharge of the ambulatory surgery patient and must also be prepared for any complications that can occur in the PACU setting. This chapter provided an overview of care of the ambulatory surgery patient. Details of the care of patients who are in the PACU, require care for complications, or are undergoing specific procedures may be found in the appropriate chapters in the book.

REFERENCES

1. *Dorothea Orem's Self Care Theory,* available at http://currentnursing.com/nursing_theory/self_care_deficit_theory.html. Accessed March 18, 2011.
2. Fleisher LA, et al: *ACC/AHA* 2007 *guidelines on perioperative cardiovascular evaluation and care for noncardiac surgery: a report of the American College of Cardiology/American Heart Association Task Force on Practice Guidelines,* available at http://www.circ.ahajournals.org/content/116/17/e418.full?sid=31fe5f4f-448a-48d3-b6bc-b9bd5ec2527e. Accessed March 17, 2011.
3. American Society of Perianesthesia Nurses: *ASPAN patient information,* available at www.aspan.org. Accessed March 10, 2011.
4. Department of Health and Human Services: Centers for Medicare and Medicaid Services: 42 CFR Part 416, Washington, DC, 2008.
5. The Joint Commission, Office of Quality Monitoring: *Most frequently reviewed sentinel event categories by year,* available at www.jointcommission.org. Accessed March 18, 2011.

6. American Society of Anesthesiologists, Inc: Practice guidelines for preoperative fasting and the use of pharmacologic agents to reduce the risk of pulmonary aspiration: application to healthy patients undergoing elective procedures. *Anesthesiology* 114:495–511, 2011.

7. American Society of Anesthesiologists: *Statement on routine preoperative laboratory and diagnostic screening: approved by House of Delegates October 15, 2003, last amended October 22, 2008,* available at www.ASAHQ.org. Accessed March 16, 2011.

8. World Health Organization: *The WHO surgical safety checklist,* available at http://www.who.int/patientsafety/safesurgery/tools_resources/en/index.html. Accessed March 18, 2011.

9. American Society of Perianesthesia Nurses: *Position statement of fast tracking,* available at https://www.aspan.org/Portals/6/docs/ClinicalPractice/PositionStatement/6-Fast_Tracking.pdf. Accessed March 18, 2011.

10. The Joint Commission: *Comprehensive accreditation manual for ambulatory care (CAMAC),* Oakbrook Terrace, Ill, 2009, The Joint Commission, available at http://www.jcrinc.com/Joint-Commission-Requirements/Ambulatory-Care/. Accessed April 2, 2012.

NURSING CARE IN THE PACU

47 Care of the Laser/Laparoscopic Surgical Patient

Kay Ball, BSN, MSA, PhD, RN, CNOR, FAAN

The evolution of laser and laparoscopic procedures over recent years has greatly changed the face and pace of perianesthesia nursing care. More procedures are conducted on an outpatient basis. Patients who undergo procedures that 15 years ago required lengthy hospitalizations are now discharged within 24 to 48 hours. Much of this increase in ambulatory surgery and rapid hospital discharge has been driven by reimbursement and insurance issues. Anesthetic innovations such as bispectral index monitoring, improved inhalational agents and muscle relaxants, advances in pain management, and regional anesthetic and analgesic techniques have also had positive effects. Technologic advances in surgical techniques, however, have had the greatest effect because these advances allow for the performance of more complex procedures with less trauma to the patient. Laser and laparoscopic techniques form the foundation for many of these surgeries.

This chapter provides an overview of laser and laparoscopic technologies and how the use of this technology affects perianesthesia patient care. Details of the care of patients who undergo specific procedures may be found in the appropriate systems chapters throughout this book.

DEFINITIONS

Absorption: The action of the tissue taking up the laser energy, which causes a reaction within the tissue. Thermal damage caused by laser absorption depends on the wavelength and fluence of the laser beam and the tissue consistency, color, and water content.
Coherence: A state in which all the waves travel in the same phase and direction and all the peaks and troughs of the waves are synchronized.
Collimation: A state in which light waves travel parallel to each other and do not diverge or spread, which reduces the loss of power and allows for better focus and precision.
Laparoscopic Surgery: A form of endoscopic surgery with a fiberoptic laparoscope inserted into the peritoneum for surgical assessment or treatment of a wide and continually expanding range of conditions.
Laser (Light Amplification by Stimulated Emission of Radiation): A process by which energy is converted into a light form or light energy.
Monochromatic: Light composed of one color or wavelength.

Pneumoperitoneum: Created when gas is delivered into the abdominal cavity through a Veress needle that is advanced through the abdominal wall. A mechanical insufflator with a pressure-limiting function is connected with tubing to the Veress needle to inflate the peritoneum. When a pneumoperitoneum is achieved, the surgical team is able to visualize the abdomen and perform the indicated procedure.
Reflection: Occurs when the direction of the laser beam is changed after it comes in contact with a surface.
Scattering: Process in which the laser beam is distributed in many different paths after entering the tissue.
Transmission: Occurs when the laser beam passes through or is transmitted through a medium, such as fluids or tissue, with little or no thermal effect.

LASER SURGERY

The term *laser* is actually an acronym for *light amplification by stimulated emission of radiation*. It describes a process by which energy is converted into a light form or light energy. The theory on which laser technology is based was developed by Albert Einstein in 1917. Schawlow and Townes further explored this theory while Gordon Gould also researched light technology. The principle of LASER was introduced in 1958 by these researchers, and the first true laser device was built by Theodore H. Maiman in 1960. Laser devices, although initially controversial, revolutionized surgical procedures; technology and use continue to expand.[1,2] The benefits of laser-assisted surgery are many (Box 47-1).[2,3]

Laser Light

Laser energy is measured by the wavelength of the light, which is the distance between two successive peaks of a wave. Laser wavelengths are often measured in nanometers. One nanometer is equal to 10^{-9} m.[3] Some of the lasers used in surgery today are longer (e.g., the CO_2 laser at 10,600 nm or the Nd:YAG laser at 1064 nm) and are within the infrared section of the electromagnetic spectrum. Other laser wavelengths are in the visible area of the electromagnetic spectrum (400 to 750 nm), whereas shorter wavelengths are found in the

---

BOX 47-1   Benefits of Laser Surgery

- Seals small blood vessels, possibly reducing intra-operative and postoperative blood loss
- Often decreases postoperative edema and the chance of the spread of malignant cells with sealing effects of lymphatic and vascular vessels
- Sometimes seals nerve endings, thus reducing postoperative pain in certain procedures
- Decreases scarring through the possible reduction of postoperative stenosis and decrease in collagen reformation
- Laser beam precision usually minimizes adjacent tissue damage
- Usually decreases operative and anesthesia time
- Allows for increased use of local anesthetic techniques as opposed to general anesthesia
- More procedures can be done on an ambulatory basis
- Often quickens recovery time and return to activities of daily living

Modified from Houck PM: Comparison of operating room lasers: uses, hazards, guidelines, *Nurs Clin North Am* 41(2):193-218, 2006; Ball KA: Surgical modalities. In Rothrock JC: *Alexander's care of the patient in surgery,* ed 14, St. Louis, 2011, Mosby; Babin-Ebell J: Transmyocardial laser revascularization combined with intramyocardial endothelial progenitor cell transplantation in patients with intractable ischemic heart disease ineligible for conventional revascularization: preliminary results, *Thorac Cardiovasc Surg* 58(1):11-16, 2010.

---

ultraviolet region of the electromagnetic spectrum (100 to 400 nm; Fig. 47-1).[1,3]

Laser light differs from ordinary light in three distinct ways that make it both unique and effective in the surgical setting.[1,3]

1. Laser light is monochromatic, which means one color or wavelength. This pure color can determine how it reacts with certain tissues. Ordinary light, in comparison, is polychromatic, which means that it comprises a multiple array of colors or wavelengths.
2. Laser light is collimated. The light waves travel parallel to each other and do not diverge or spread. Collimation reduces the loss of power and allows for better focus and precision. Ordinary light spreads out in space as it travels away from its source.
3. Laser light is coherent. All the waves travel in an orderly manner in the same phase and direction, and all the peaks and troughs of the waves are synchronized. This coherence gives the laser beam its power. Ordinary light, in comparison, is incoherent as its waves travel out in random directions.

Tissue Interaction

Four different interactions can occur when laser energy comes into contact with human tissue (Fig. 47-2). These interactions include reflection, scattering, transmission, and absorption.[3] The extent of this interaction is dependent on the wavelength of the laser, power settings, spot size, duration of exposure of the laser beam with the tissue, and the characteristics of the tissue. These interactions can have both positive and negative effects.[1-3]

- *Reflection.* Reflection occurs when the direction of the laser beam is changed after it comes into contact with a surface. This direction change can be intentional or accidental and thus can have both positive and negative effects. Mirrors can be used to intentionally reflect the laser beam to direct the beam to a hard-to-reach area. This action must be done carefully,

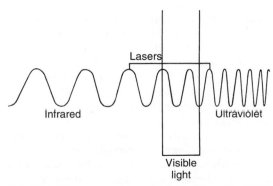

FIG. 47-1 Electromagnetic spectrum. (From Rothrock JC: *Alexander's care of the patient in surgery,* St. Louis, 2011, Mosby.)

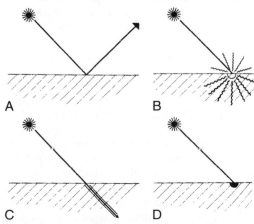

FIG. 47-2 Laser tissue interaction. **A,** Reflection. **B,** Scattering. **C,** Transmission. **D,** Absorption. (From Ball KA: *Endoscopic surgery,* St. Louis, 1997, Mosby.)

however, to prevent an inadvertent strike and possible damage to a nontargeted area. Reflection can also occur if the laser beam hits an obstacle (e.g., a surgical instrument) and then is inadvertently reflected to another area, thus causing a tissue burn. Reflection can be either specular (direct reflection) or diffuse (scattered reflection).

- *Scattering.* The laser beam can also scatter as it enters certain tissues. This scattering causes the beam to disperse over a large area and weakens its strength. Backscattering can also occur as the beam scatters backward up the endoscope, thus causing damage to the operator's eye, the endoscope optics, or the distal end of the scope.
- *Transmission.* Transmission occurs when the laser beam passes or is transmitted through fluids or tissue with little or no thermal effect. Transmission depends on the wavelength of the laser beam and the tissue with which it comes in contact. For example, an argon laser beam can be transmitted through the clear structures and solutions of the eye to coagulate a bleeding vessel on the retina. This action occurs because the argon energy is not absorbed by clear structures and solutions; therefore no thermal effect is noted on these tissues.
- *Absorption.* Thermal effects and tissue response occur only when tissue absorbs the energy of the laser that contacts it. The amount of absorption and penetration depends on the beam's wavelength and power, the characteristics of the contact tissue (color, consistency, and water content), the duration of the beam exposure, and the beam spot size. A thermal response can occur when tissue absorbs laser energy, thus heating the target cells. The degree of tissue change or thermal damage depends on the temperature to which the cells are heated. This temperature change is purposely regulated to affect the desired tissue response (Table 47-1).

Laser surgery can be categorized into three different types of tissue response, including thermal, mechanical, and chemical effects.[1] The thermal effect, as discussed previously, is the most common laser effect as tissue is vaporized, coagulated, ablated, cut, and welded depending upon the degree of thermal interaction. The mechanical (acoustical) effect from laser energy results when sound energy is created by the laser beam which disrupts tissue. The chemical effect is produced as the laser energy is used to activate a light-sensitive dye to disrupt and change tissue.

Table 47-1	Tissue Changes with Temperature Increases	
TEMPERATURE (°C)	VISUAL CHANGE	BIOLOGIC CHANGE
37-60	No visual change	Warming, welding
60-65	Blanching	Coagulation
65-90	White/gray	Protein denaturization
90-100	Puckering	Drying
>100	Smoke plume	Vaporization, carbonization

From Ball KA: *Lasers: the perioperative challenge*, ed 3, Denver, 2004, Association of periOperative Registered Nurses.

Types of Lasers

Lasers are classified by the four active mediums used to generate the laser energy: gas, solid, liquid, and semiconductor crystals. In a gas medium, electric energy is pumped through a gas, such as argon, to produce the laser energy. A solid medium uses a special rod doped with an element that is activated with exposure to flash lamps to create the laser energy. Liquid mediums are organic dyes that produce a wide range of wavelengths when activated with another laser beam. Semiconductor crystals are used in the medical field and in consumer products and fiberoptic communication systems. Experimental mediums that are currently being explored include free electron lasers. The actual laser name is usually derived from the active medium substance that is used to generate the laser energy.[1-3] A summary of the various lasers currently in use can be found in Table 47-2.

Preoperative Care

Preoperative care, as with any procedure, focuses on adequate preoperative assessment and preparation of the patient. Although procedure-specific issues are addressed in other chapters, certain issues unique to laser surgery must be addressed in this discussion. One of those issues is appropriate patient selection. Procedure-specific requirements and contraindications must be evaluated.

For example, transmyocardial revascularization with the laser is generally limited to patients with advanced cardiovascular disease who have hemodynamically stable conditions and are not candidates for traditional bypass surgery. This new laser treatment may offer a method to revascularize the heart muscle for patients with

Table 47–2   Summary of Laser Types and Uses

NAME	WAVELENGTH (NM)	ACTIVE MEDIUM	SPECIAL CHARACTERISTICS	USES
Ruby laser	694	Solid	First successful medical laser Has been replaced by newer technology	Tattoo and hair removal
Nd:YAG	1064–1318	Solid state	Transmitted through clear fluids and structures and more highly absorbed by darker tissue Can be focused to precise diameter for delicate procedures in confined areas such as middle ear Provides good penetration depth, although energy is not highly focused and laser light tends to scatter, thus causing thermal damage to approximately 2–6 mm Can be delivered in contact and noncontact modes	Primary function is coagulation Special pulsed mode also used in ophthalmology Used for skin rejuvenation and removal of pigmented lesions and tattoos in dermatology Interstitial laser prostatectomy Various applications also used in gastroenterology, pulmonary, oral surgery, and gynecology
Erbium:YAG	2900	Solid state	Highly absorbed by water Shallow depth of penetration	Used for oral surgery, ophthalmic surgery, dermatology Used with endoscopes
Holium:YAG	2100	Solid state	Produces vapor bubble to transmit beam to tissue in fluid environments Shallow depth of penetration Ablates tissue precisely Can be conducted through flexible fiber	Transmyocardial revascularization Oral surgery Fragmentation of stones Many other applications in surgical arena
Frequency-doubled (KTP) YAG	532	Solid state	Moderate depth of penetration Highly absorbed by pigmentation	Used with flexible or rigid endoscopes Used for general surgery, urology, gastroenterology, neurosurgery, otorhinolaryngology, dermatology, and cosmetic surgery
CO_2	10,600	Gas	Most versatile laser Can be operated in continuous or pulsed modes Different tissue and thermal effects can be created by varying duration of exposure and spot size Highly absorbed by water Requires articulating arm system or hollow core fiber for delivery	Performs coagulation, cutting, and vaporization functions Popular for use in cutaneous laser resurfacing Also used in following surgical specialties: general, gynecology, ENT, neurosurgery, plastic surgery, dermatology, and oral surgery

Continued

Table 47-2 Summary of Laser Types and Uses—cont'd

NAME	WAVELENGTH (NM)	ACTIVE MEDIUM	SPECIAL CHARACTERISTICS	USES
Argon	488 or 457 (blue), 514.5 or 528 (green)	Gas	Transmitted through clear structures and solutions Moderate depth of penetration Highly selective to pigmented tissue such as hemoglobin, melanin, and other similar tissues Because of high selectivity of beam to pigmented tissues, adjacent tissue injury significantly reduced	Used with rigid endoscopes Well suited for ophthalmic surgery Used in dermatology for ablation of vascular and pigmented lesions Also used in gastroenterology, gynecology, and otology
Krypton	531 (green), 568 (yellow), 647 (red)	Gas	Used in ophthalmology as alternative to argon laser	Effective for selective photocoagulation procedures Used primarily in ophthalmology Also used for removal of pigmented lesions
Dye	400-1000 (Variable with dyes)	Liquid	Can emit different wavelengths depending on dye used Can be used in continuous or pulsed modes	Used primarily in ophthalmology and dermatology Fragmentation of stones Limited applications such as photodynamic therapy and for vascular lesions Used with flexible or rigid endoscopes
Excimer	193-351	Excited dimmer	Complex delivery system Gases are extremely toxic and require appropriate laser housings and exhausts Larger units need more floor space	Excellent cutting capabilities with no significant damage to adjacent tissue Has been used successfully to sculpt corneas for refractive purposes and to ablate plaque in arteries Also used for phototherapeutic keratectomy procedures Other uses in orthopedics and dermatology also being explored
Diode	Varies	Semiconductor crystals	Extremely compact efficient crystals	Often used in consumer products such as video disc players and computers Now being used for surgical lasers primarily in ophthalmic and urologic applications such as interstitial laser prostatectomy Other applications are being explored, including pain management, oral surgery, and treatment of leg vein telangiectasia.
Free electron		Relativistic electron beam	Large experimental laser consisting of magnetic field Great versatility in emitting variety of wavelengths with high-precision capability	Currently under investigation

Modified from Ball KA: *Lasers: the perioperative challenge,* ed 3, Denver, 2004, Association of periOperative Registered Nurses; Houck PM: Comparison of operating room lasers: uses, hazards, guidelines, *Nurs Clin North Am* 41(2):193–218, 2006; Ball KA: Surgical modalities. In Rothrock JC: *Alexander's care of the patient in surgery,* ed 14, St. Louis, 2011, Mosby. *ENT,* Ear, nose, and throat; *YAG,* yttrium-aluminum-garnet; *Nd,* neodymium; *KTP,* potassium titanyl phosphate.

intractable ischemic heart disease.[1,4] Dermatologic procedures may require extensive skin preparation at home, preoperative administration of prophylactic antibiotics or antivirals, multiple treatments, and extensive postoperative skin care regimens that may last up to 1 month or more.[1,2,5] Preoperative care must include education concerning these issues and must be used to determine whether the patient will be able to comply with the treatment regimen.

The patient must also be prepared for expectations both during and after surgery. Many of these procedures are conducted without any anesthesia or with moderate sedation. The patient must be prepared for the sights, smells, and other sensations that will be experienced. Eye protection must be provided. Odors can include the smell of tissue burning or being vaporized. The patient may also have burning or stinging types of painful sensations with certain procedures.[1,6]

Intraoperative Issues

Intraoperative issues with laser procedures primarily concern safety. Lasers are considered a class III medical device and, as such, are subject to U.S. Food and Drug Administration jurisdiction.[3] Many other regulatory, industry, and professional bodies also address the safe use of lasers. Regulations addressed include the registration of laser devices, training requirements, laser safety officer responsibilities, and safety rules.[1,3]

Lasers must be further classified by the manufacturer according to their potential to cause biologic harm and their inherent level of hazard. The classification system is based on the laser output power, wavelength, exposure duration, and emergent beam exposure. The classification system ranges from I to IV; the higher the class, the greater the potential hazard. Most lasers used in surgery are classified as a class IV and can damage eyes and skin and present a fire hazard.[1,3] Because of the many provider and patient risks associated with laser use, a laser safety program should be in place in any facility in which laser procedures are conducted. This includes freestanding ambulatory facilities and physician's offices. A laser safety committee complete with a laser safety officer should be established and responsible for guiding and overseeing all laser use in the facility. Issues that should be addressed include staff education, physician credentialing, and the monitoring of quality and safety issues. All staff involved in laser use must receive appropriate education before using or being involved in laser procedures. Topics included in these special training classes include laser biophysics,

laser equipment, laser-tissue interaction, safety procedures, and clinical applications. Knowledge and skills should be verified through a competency-based credentialing program, and the skills should be reassessed and updated on a regular basis.[1-3] The three most important areas of safe laser use include eye protection, smoke evacuation, and fire safety.

The eyes are susceptible to damage from laser radiation. The damage may occur acutely or may go unnoticed and develop gradually over time. The type of damage also varies with the type of laser being used. Anyone who enters an operating room or treatment area where a laser is in use (including the patient) is at risk for eye damage and therefore should wear protective eyewear specific to the laser in use. Filtering devices should also be placed on operative microscopes and endoscopes. The patient's eyes should be protected with either the appropriate eyewear or moist gauze pads.[1-3] The protective eyewear should have inscribed on the side of the frame the laser wavelength that the lenses are protecting against along with the optical density (i.e., the lenses' filtering capabilities).[1-3]

Another major safety concern with the use of laser technology is the control of the smoke that the laser energy produces as it impacts tissue. This surgical smoke is also called *laser plume* or *surgical plume*. Surgical smoke contains extremely small particles of vaporized tissues, toxins, and steam. If inhaled, this particulate can end up in the alveoli of surgical team members or can coat the inside lumen of unprotected suction lines if used for smoke evacuation. Even short exposure to smoke particulate and odor from toxic gases may be related to headaches, nausea, myalgia, rhinitis, conjunctivitis, and respiratory conditions and complications.[1-3] In one study, perioperative nurses were shown to have twice the incidence of targeted respiratory problems, probably because of the repeated inhalation of surgical smoke.[7-9] In addition, there is a high chance that surgical smoke can transmit viable pathogenic material within the plume.[1-3,7]

Patients are also exposed to hazards when surgical smoke is not evacuated appropriately. One study demonstrated that laparoscopic surgery patients can absorb the byproducts of laser tissue interaction (surgical smoke), thus increasing the level of the patient's methemoglobin and carboxyhemoglobin. This in turn, will decrease the oxygen-carrying capabilities of the red blood cells. The patient is absorbing the toxins produced within surgical smoke and then exhibits symptoms of headache, double vision, or nausea in the postanesthesia care area.[10] When surgical smoke is properly evacuated during laparoscopy, vision of the surgical site is maintained, smoke is not absorbed by the patient, and these untoward symptoms are not routinely present in the recovering patient.

A smoke evacuation system with an ultra low penetration air filter (to remove small particles) and charcoal filters (to absorb toxic gases) must be used whenever surgical smoke is generated. The smoke collection device should be positioned as close to the laser–tissue impact site as possible. All persons in the room should also wear high-filtration masks to protect against any residual plume that may have escaped capture. Surgical masks are never to be the first line of defense to protect against plume inhalation. There are smoke evacuators available today that sense surgical smoke is being generated and automatically activate the system to gently evacuate the plume without destroying the pneumoperitoneum. There also are other different types of plume removal products that can be attached to the trocar sleeve to help clear the abdominal cavity of smoke without impacting the pneumoperitoneum. If any of these products require a suction line, then an in-line suction filter must be used so that plume particulate will not be drawn into the suction system. The in-line filter must be placed between the wall outlet and the suction canister to avoid pulling fluids through the filter, which would destroy it. Although smoke evacuation devices and supplies are available on the market today, compliance with smoke evacuation recommendations continues to be lacking.

Whenever a laser is in use, the risk of fire is also increased. A fire can be triggered anytime that a reflected laser beam or a direct beam comes in contact with a dry combustible item. The oxygen, anesthetic gases, and vapors from alcohol-based preparation solutions also contribute to the possible danger. All members of the laser team must be trained in fire safety and be able to respond quickly should a fire occur. All combustibles near the laser–tissue impact site should be kept wet to prevent ignition. Use of flammable draping materials and skin preparation solutions should be avoided. Sterile water or saline solution should be immediately available to douse any small fires that may occur.

Postoperative Care

A laser procedure does not require any technique-specific postoperative care. The laser is merely a tool that provides energy to cut, coagulate, and ablate during laparoscopic procedures. Patient management should include routine postanesthesia care unit (PACU) and phase II care that is geared to the type of anesthesia administered and the given procedure. Specific surgical procedure issues are addressed in the systems-appropriate chapters throughout this book.

Only one type of laser procedure requires special nursing care in the postanesthesia care unit. If the patient has undergone photodynamic therapy for selective destruction of a malignancy, the laser is used to activate a special light-sensitive dye that has been injected into the patient approximately

Evidence-Based Practice

Surgical smoke creates a serious workplace hazard for more than 500,000 health care workers as the gases within smoke create an offensive and harmful odor, the small particulate matter causes respiratory problems, and pathogens may be transmitted within surgical smoke. Patients can even absorb dangerous gases when smoke is generated during laparoscopy. Research has demonstrated the many hazards of surgical smoke, but compliance with smoke evacuation recommendations continues to be lacking. A descriptive exploratory study was conducted using a validated and piloted survey that was completed by a random sampling of perioperative nurses working with electrosurgery devices. Major findings revealed that specific key indicators influencing compliance include increased knowledge and training, positive perceptions about the complexity

of the recommendations, and larger facilities with increased specializations, interconnectedness, and leadership support. The barriers to compliance include a lack of availability of smoke evacuation equipment, physicians' negative attitudes about smoke evacuation, noisy smoke evacuation equipment, and staff complacency.

IMPLICATIONS FOR PRACTICE

For smoke evacuation recommendations to be followed, a comprehensive educational program on smoke hazards along with smoke evacuation equipment training needs to be implemented. Leadership support and active communication among health care providers need to be fostered. Barriers to compliance must be addressed to minimize any obstacles preventing the achievement of a 100% smoke-free surgical environment.

Source: Ball K: Surgical smoke evacuation guidelines: compliance among perioperative nurses, *AORN J* 92(8):e1–e23, 2010.

2 days before the procedure. The laser is introduced intraoperatively, which may be during a laparoscopic procedure, to activate the dye that in turn causes singlet oxygen to be formed, thus destroying a malignancy. Because some of the light-sensitive dye is retained for approximately 6 weeks in the skin cells, the patient cannot be exposed to bright lights or sunlight. Precautions to avoid this exposure must be followed in the postanesthesia phase and especially if the patient is discharged. Sometimes these procedures are performed later in the day so that the patient can be discharged during the evening hours when it becomes dark outside.[1]

LAPAROSCOPIC SURGERY

Laparoscopic surgery is a form of endoscopic surgery with a fiberoptic laparoscope inserted into the peritoneum for surgical assessment or treatment of a wide and continually expanding range of conditions.[11] This surgical approach affords many benefits to the patient and surgeon, including smaller incisions, decreased hospital stays and recovery time, and better visualization and magnification of surgical anatomy and pathology.[12] To understand the history of laparoscopy, one must first examine the origins of endoscopy, which began in ancient times and were driven by the innate human curiosity to peer inside body cavities. Speculums were first developed and used to examine various areas of the body, such as the rectum and vagina, as early as 400 BC. An Arabian physician first used a mirror to reflect light and examine the cervix in AD 1012. The first crude endoscope was developed in 1585 and used the sun as a light source for examination of the nasal cavity.[3,13,14]

The 1800s saw the addition of more reliable, but crude, light sources to these endoscopic examinations. The Italian physician Phillip Bozinni developed a device that used a candle for illumination to examine the urethra of a living patient. Later devices used alcohol lamps and a wick. Thomas Edison's development of the incandescent light bulb in 1880 truly spurred the evolution of modern endoscopy and laparoscopy as we know it today.[3,13,14]

True laparoscopy was first accomplished by George Kelling in 1901 when he viewed the abdominal viscera of a living dog with a cystoscope. Kelling is also credited with creating the first pneumoperitoneum with this procedure. Equipment and techniques continued to evolve, and the first laparoscopic tubal ligation was performed in 1941. By 1973, more than 500,000 gynecologic laparoscopic procedures had been performed. Laparoscopic cholecystectomy procedures all but replaced open procedures within 3 years of its introduction in 1987. The technology continues to expand today into multiple therapeutic and diagnostic procedures across most surgical specialties.[3,14]

Preoperative Issues

Preoperative care should be focused on the adequate assessment and preparation of the patient. Routine diagnostics and assessments that are conducted for all general anesthesia or surgical patients should be completed. Special attention should be paid to establishing the appropriateness of a laparoscopic procedure for this patient because laparoscopy, and the creation of a pneumoperitoneum, brings its own inherent risks and problems. A recommended preoperative checklist should include the following[14]:

- History and physical examination
- Evaluation of medical problems
- Thorough evaluation of the cardiac and respiratory systems
- Normalization of fluids and electrolytes
- Antibiotics, if needed
- Deep vein thrombosis prophylaxis
- Genitourinary system evaluation
- Appropriate laboratory and radiologic studies
- Informed consent

Numerous relative and absolute contraindications to laparoscopic procedures are well established (Box 47-2), and the patient should be closely evaluated in regard to these issues. Previous abdominal surgery should be thoroughly evaluated, because possible scarring or adhesions can affect the performance of the laparoscope or limit the surgeon's view of the surgical field. A comprehensive evaluation of the cardiovascular and pulmonary systems is mandated before any laparoscopic procedure, because a pneumoperitoneum can greatly stress these systems. Patients with significant pulmonary disease are at particular risk for developing respiratory acidosis from the accumulation of insufflation carbon dioxide in the abdomen. Large abdominal wall hernias, diaphragmatic defects, and previous scars can affect trocar placement. Pregnancy was once considered an absolute contraindication to laparoscopic surgery; however, these procedures have now been shown to be safe and effective well into the second trimester. Obese patients should also be closely evaluated with specific attention to cardiac and pulmonary status.[12,15,16]

Intraoperative Issues

The primary difference between laparoscopic surgeries and their open counterparts are the creation of a pneumoperitoneum and patient

BOX 47-2	Contraindications to Laparoscopic Surgery

RELATIVE	ABSOLUTE
Prior abdominal or pelvic surgery	Hypovolemic shock
Previous peritonitis or pelvic fibrosis	Large pelvic or abdominal mass
Obesity	Severe cardiac decompensation
Diaphragmatic or abdominal wall hernia	Hemodynamic instability
Umbilical abnormality	Massive bleeding
Abdominal or iliac aneurysm	Inability to tolerate laparotomy
Severe pulmonary disease	Inexperienced surgeon
Bowel obstruction	Condition unfit for general anesthesia
Intolerance to positioning	
Acute pancreatitis	
Uncorrected coagulopathies	
Portal hypertension	
Late pregnancy	
Severe acute cholecystis	
Ductal calculi	
Sepsis	
Thickened gallbladder (> 4 mm)	
Jaundice	

Modified from Wadlund DL: Laparoscopy: risks, benefits and complications, *Nurs Clin North Am* 41(2):219−229, 2006; Gerges FJ, et al: Anesthesia or laparoscopy: a review, *J Clin Anesthesia* 18(1):67−78, 2006; Jobe BA, Hunter JG: Minimally invasive surgery. In Brunicardi FC, et al, editors: *Schwartz's principles of surgery,* ed 8, New York, 2005, McGraw Hill; Soper NJ, et al, editors: *Mastery of endoscopic and laparoscopic surgery,* ed 2, Philadelphia, 2004, Lippincott Williams & Wilkins.

positioning, both of which can create patient management challenges during the operative and recovery phases.

Pneumoperitoneum

The creation of a pneumoperitoneum involves the insufflation of the abdomen with a gas. The most commonly used gas for insufflation is CO_2 because of its relatively low risk of venous gas embolism (rapidly dissolves) and noncombustibility. Other gases that have been evaluated in clinical and experimental settings include nitrous oxide, helium, and argon, but CO_2 gas has been chosen as the preferred insufflation gas for laparoscopic procedures.[12,17]

A pneumoperitoneum is created during laparoscopic surgery to allow the surgical team to visualize the abdomen and perform the indicated procedure. Unfortunately, the creation and maintenance of this pneumoperitoneum can have varying effects on the patient and is associated with many of the complications generally associated with laparoscopic surgery. The patient's position during surgery can exacerbate these adverse affects.[3,12,15]

The pneumoperitoneum is created when gas is insufflated into the abdominal cavity after the Veress needle is inserted through the abdominal wall. A mechanical insufflator with a pressure-limiting function is connected to the Veress needle with tubing to deliver the insufflations gas into the peritoneum. Normal insufflation pressures are maintained at 14 to 16 mm Hg.[3] Insufficient pressure produces an inadequate pneumoperitoneum and impairs surgical visualization of the target site. Excessive pressure creates even greater cardiovascular and respiratory compromise than that commonly associated with the procedure.[3,12] Insufflation control panels should monitor and display the rate of flow of the insufflations gas, volume of gas delivered, and the intraabdominal pressure.[3] High-flow insufflators that deliver 15 to 20 L/min are more effective than those delivering gas at slower rates.[3] When higher pressures are achieved in the abdomen, the insufflator must immediately stop the insufflation and release some of the gas if overpressurization is sensed.[3]

Cardiovascular Changes

A wide variety of hemodynamic effects have been reported with the insufflation of a CO_2 pneumoperitoneum. The increased abdominal pressure compresses veins within the abdominal cavity and results in an initial increase in cardiac preload; however, true preload is ultimately decreased because of impaired venous return. Cardiac afterload is also increased as a result of the increased abdominal pressure and the resultant neurohumoral reflexes. The most common net effects from these changes include increases in heart rate, systemic vascular resistance, and central venous pressure. Cardiac output drops, and mean arterial pressure may increase, decrease, or remain unchanged, depending on the relative changes in cardiac output and systemic vascular resistance. Hemodynamic monitoring can be used to monitor for pressure changes and myocardial compromise in patients at extremely high risk. Pneumoperitoneum can cause dysrhythmias to include sinus tachycardia, bigeminy, and premature ventricular contractions. When pneumoperitoneum has been established, a resultant increase in the abdominal pressure causes vagal stimulation that can lead to severe bradycardia and possible asystole.[12,15] As stated previously, automatic sensors are available within insufflators that provide continual monitoring and adjustment of the abdominal pressure so that cardiac problems are minimized.

Respiratory Changes

The creation of a CO_2 pneumoperitoneum also has several adverse effects on the respiratory system. Oxygenation may be impaired because of reductions in lung volume and the associated atelectasis that results from an elevated diaphragm. Ventilation may also be impaired and result in CO_2 retention and hypercarbia. Other untoward effects include reduced pulmonary compliance, increased airway resistance, and reduced vital capacity. All these effects are exacerbated by the commonly used Trendelenburg position.[3] These respiratory changes are also further aggravated by the following conditions: surgery that lasts more than 4 hours, a history of chronic obstructive pulmonary disease, age, obesity, and an American Society of Anesthesiologists physical status of III or greater.[3,12,15] A summary of these effects can be found in Table 47-3.

Other System Effects

In addition to the extensive cardiopulmonary changes affected by the creation of a pneumoperitoneum, various other body systems may be affected as well. The patient should be closely monitored for the development of hypothermia, and preventive measures should be taken to avoid this complication.[3] Hypercarbia can lead to increased cerebral blood flow with a net result of increased intracranial blood pressure, possible cerebral edema, and potential brain stem herniation. Renal failure can result from the impaired renal blood flow caused by the increased abdominal pressure[18] or hypercarbia. Increased abdominal pressure also compromises venous return and puts the patient at risk for development of deep vein thrombosis. Stress hormones are also elevated because of peritoneal distention, which can increase anesthetic time, pain, and acidosis, and decrease venous return.

Table 47-3	Cardiopulmonary Effects of a Pneumoperitoneum	
	ELEVATED	**REDUCED**
Respiratory	Respiratory rate	pH
	$PaCO_2$, mixed venous CO_2 tension, alveolar volume	Forced expiratory
	CO_2 tension	Forced vital capacity
	Arterial-venous CO_2 difference	Functional residual capacity
	Peak airway pressure	Total lung capacity
	Plateau airway pressure	Compliance
	Intrathoracic pressure	
	Airway resistance	
	Atelectasis	
Cardiovascular	Heart rate with initial insufflation	Stroke volume
	Systemic blood pressure	Cardiac output
	Mean arterial pressure	Venous return unchanged or reduced
	Central venous pressure	Bradycardia with maintenance of pneumoperitoneum
	Pulmonary artery pressure	
	Systemic vascular resistance	
	Myocardial oxygen demand	

Modified from Wadlund DL: Laparoscopy: risks, benefits and complications, *Nurs Clin North Am* 41(2):219–229, 2006; Gerges FJ, et al: Anesthesia or laparoscopy: a review, *J Clin Anesthesia* 18(1):67–78, 2006; Soper NJ, et al, editors: *Mastery of endoscopic and laparoscopic surgery*, ed 2, Philadelphia, 2004, Lippincott Williams & Wilkins.

NURSING CARE IN THE PACU

Concerns about the effect of a pneumoperitoneum on the implantation and spread of tumor cells also arise. The role of laparoscopic surgery for the treatment of cancer remains controversial with questions still being posed about the possibility of the CO_2 gas used to establish the pneumoperitoneum being the vehicle for dissemination of malignant cells causing port site metastasis.[19,20] More research needs to be conducted before a conclusive answer can be determined.

Gasless Laparoscopy

Several systems are currently being evaluated for use in gasless laparoscopy. These systems work with various slings and retractors to lift the abdominal wall away from the intraabdominal contents and create a surgical space in which the procedure can be performed. The primary advantage of this technique, of course, is the elimination of the need for a pneumoperitoneum. Disadvantages center around the inability to establish adequate surgical field exposure. Patient indications for gasless laparoscopy essentially parallel those for similar open and laparoscopic (with insufflation) cases. The gasless approach is better suited to lower abdominal procedures, because greater abdominal distension can be accomplished in this area, particularly with women.[21]

Patient Positioning

Exaggerated surgical positions are often necessary with laparoscopic surgery to affect adequate organ exposure. The two most commonly used positions are the Trendelenburg, or head-down, position for bowel surgery and the reverse Trendelenburg, or head-up tilt, position for upper abdominal procedures. Both positions result in changes in cardiac filling pressures and lung volumes that affect ventilation, oxygenation, and

lower extremity venous stasis. These changes are exacerbated with the addition of a pneumoperitoneum (Table 47-4).[3,12,21]

Postoperative Issues

Care of the patient immediately after any laparoscopic procedure should include basic PACU care and monitoring specific to the procedure and type of anesthesia administered. Postoperative pain management is typically easier after laparoscopic procedures than after open procedures and can often be accomplished with a small amount of opioids in combination with nonsteroidal agents and local anesthetics. Visceral discomfort is often more difficult to treat and more unpredictable. This pain is triggered by the retained gas in the peritoneal cavity and the resulting irritation of peritoneal surfaces; it commonly manifests as shoulder pain and may persist for several days after surgery. The patient should be prepared for this discomfort as a part of the preoperative education. The pain can generally be managed with oral analgesics.[15,21]

Postoperative nausea and vomiting can pose a significant problem with any intraabdominal surgery. Routine drainage of the stomach at the end of the case before removal of the nasogastric tube helps to reduce the incidence but does not completely eliminate it. Prophylactic treatment with an antiemetic is not indicated for all laparoscopic cases, although it may be appropriate when multiple risk factors for postoperative nausea and vomiting are present.[15]

If a recovering laser laparoscopic surgery patient complains of headaches, nausea, or double vision, these symptoms may be from the lack of smoke evacuation when the plume is created. A study by Ott[10] demonstrates that the patient may absorb surgical smoke toxic gases, such as carbon monoxide, when plume is not removed.[10]

Table 47-4	Physiologic Effects of Patient Position During Laparoscopic Surgery	
SYSTEM	**TRENDELENBURG**	**REVERSE TRENDELENBURG**
Cardiovascular	Increased central filling pressures Increased MAP No change in CO	Decreased central filling pressures Decreased MAP Decreased CO
Pulmonary	No change in oxygenation No change in ventilation	No change in oxygenation No change in ventilation
Venous stasis	No change in lower extremity venous blood flow	No change in lower extremity venous blood flow

Modified from Wadlund DL: Laparoscopy: risks, benefits and complications, *Nurs Clin North Am* 41(2):219–229, 2006; Gerges FJ, et al: Anesthesia or laparoscopy: a review, *J Clin Anesthesia* 18(1):67–78, 2006; Soper NJ, et al, editors: *Mastery of endoscopic and laparoscopic surgery,* ed 2, Philadelphia, 2004, Lippincott Williams & Wilkins; Henny CP, et al: Laparoscopic surgery: pitfalls due to anesthesia, positioning, and pneumoperitoneum, *Surg Endosc* 19(9):1163–1171, 2005.
MAP, Mean arterial pressure; *CO,* cardiac output.

Untoward symptoms, such as methemoglobin and carboxyhemoglobin, can be avoided through appropriate smoke evacuation during laparoscopic procedures.[10]

In addition to basic PACU care, careful attention should be paid to monitoring the patient for any complications associated with laparoscopic intervention. Laparoscopic procedures are remarkably safe when correctly performed; their major complication rate is less than 1%, and the overall mortality rate is 4 to 8 deaths per 1000 procedures.[21] Complications can occur, however, and are divided into two categories: those associated with the pneumoperitoneum and those associated with the procedure.

Pneumoperitoneum Complications

The complications associated with the creation of the surgical pneumoperitoneum are directly related to the physiologic changes associated with this procedure. Most complications occur during the initiation and maintenance of the pneumoperitoneum; however, the perianesthesia nurse may be the one who identifies the complication or is responsible for the continued care and management of the patient. Table 47-5 provides a summary of pneumoperitoneum complications and their causes. Nursing care should be based on the complication presented.

Laparoscopy Complications

Complications associated with the laparoscopic technique are usually trocar-related injuries and involve the bowel, vasculature, or bladder.[3,12,15,21] Early recognition and treatment in the operating room, of course, results in the best outcome; however, many injuries may go unrecognized at the time of surgery. As a result, vigilant PACU assessment, care, and thorough discharge teaching are essential to a positive patient outcome.

Bowel Injuries

Bowel injuries are most troubling because they tend to go unrecognized at the time of surgery. The most common bowel injury involves perforation of the small intestine. Injury to the colon, duodenum, and stomach can also occur. Almost 50% of these injuries go unrecognized for at least 24 hours.[12] Perforations that go unrecognized in the operating room can develop into peritonitis sometime after discharge. Delayed onset of sepsis is also common with these injuries. The mortality rate associated with unrecognized bowel injuries can be as high as 5%.[12,21] These injuries may go unrecognized in the PACU because the patient may be asymptomatic at that time. Discharge teaching that emphasizes reporting of unrelieved pain, nausea and vomiting, and unresolved fever is particularly important in the recognition and resolution of this complication.

Table 47-5	Pneumoperitoneum Complications	
SYSTEM	**COMPLICATION**	**POSSIBLE MECHANISM**
Cardiovascular	Tension pneumothorax	Diaphragm injury
		Dissection near esophageal hiatus
		Barotrauma
	Myocardial infarction	Inadequate perfusion to meet increased demand
	Metabolic acidosis	Inadequate tissue perfusion from reduced cardiac output
	Visceral organ ischemia	Hypercarbia
	Venous stasis, thromboembolism	Impaired visceral blood flow, impaired lower extremity venous return, endothelial damage from IAP
Pulmonary	Hypoxia	Atelectasis and reduced lung volume
	Hypercarbia	CO_2 retention
	Respiratory acidosis	Hypercarbia
	Aspiration	Increased risk of regurgitation of gastric contents from IAP
Other	CO_2 gas embolus	Entry of CO_2 bubbles through injured blood vessels

Modified from Wadlund DL: Laparoscopy: risks, benefits and complications, *Nurs Clin North Am* 41(2):219–229, 2006; Gerges FJ, et al: Anesthesia or laparoscopy: a review, *J Clin Anesthesia* 18(1):67–78, 2006; Soper NJ, et al, editors: *Mastery of endoscopic and laparoscopic surgery*, ed 2, Philadelphia, 2004, Lippincott Williams & Wilkins.
IAP, Increased abdominal pressure.

NURSING CARE IN THE PACU

Vascular Injuries

Although rare (occurring 0.02% to 0.03% of the time), vascular injuries carry a significant mortality rate of 15%.[12] Vascular injuries are most commonly associated with pelvic procedures and tend to occur near the distal aorta and its branches, the inferior vena cava, or iliac veins. Abdominal wall hemorrhage can also occur from inadvertent trocar insertion. Major vascular injury during laparoscopic procedures is rare. Most injuries are usually recognized quickly and repaired in the operating room with direct suture ligation, although a patch or synthetic graft may be necessary for more extensive damage.[12,21] Injuries that go unrecognized in the operating room again pose the greatest challenge to the perianesthesia nurse. Unresolved tachycardia and hypotension must be closely evaluated as possible signs and symptoms of hemorrhage. Unresolved or extremely severe postoperative pain and abdominal distension are also possible signs and symptoms of unexpected bleeding. Recognition of surgical hemorrhage and immediate evaluation is critical to a positive patient outcome.

Bladder Injuries

The risk of bladder injury can be decreased during laparoscopic procedures with the routine insertion of a urinary catheter to decompress the bladder; however, occasional bladder perforation still occurs. The risk of perforation is greatest in patients with previous abdominal or bladder surgery; risks are also elevated in patients with congenital anomalies. The most common signs and symptoms of bladder perforation are the appearance of air in the urinary drainage bag or unexplained urinary tract bleeding during the procedure. Diagnosis can be confirmed with a retrograde cystogram, and surgical repair can be performed.[12,21]

Other Complications

Other complications of interest include postoperative infection and laparoscopic electrosurgery complications. Antibiotic medications may be used for laparoscopic procedures and other types of surgical procedures as prophylaxis. Studies show that wound infection rates range from 0.1% for diagnostic laparoscopy to as high as 1% for laparoscopic cholecystectomies.[12] Electrosurgery has replaced laser energy as the preferred power supply during laparoscopic surgery because it is less expensive and more convenient. This energy, however, has been associated with secondary thermal injuries that may go unrecognized (direct coupling, insulation failure, or capacitive coupling) because they occur outside the surgeon's view through the laparoscope.[3] As with bowel perforations, these injuries often are seen days to weeks after surgery as peritonitis or sepsis, which again highlights the importance of thorough discharge instructions regarding the signs, symptoms, and management of postoperative infections.[1,3]

SUMMARY

Technologic advances in surgical techniques have had a significant effect on surgical procedures and perianesthesia care as more complex procedures can be conducted with less trauma to the patient. Laser and laparoscopic techniques form the foundation for many of these surgeries. Laser devices, which create a collimated beam of light energy, have revolutionized surgical procedures as technology and acceptance continue to expand. Laparoscopic surgery, a form of endoscopic surgery with a fiberoptic laparoscope inserted into the peritoneum for surgical assessment or treatment of a wide range of conditions, also continues to expand into multiple therapeutic and diagnostic procedures across most surgical specialties. This chapter provided an overview of laser and laparoscopic technologies and how the use of these surgical tools affects perianesthesia patient care. Details of the care of patients who undergo specific procedures may be found in the appropriate systems chapters throughout this book.

REFERENCES

1. Ball KA: *Lasers: the perioperative challenge*, ed 3, Denver, 2004, AORN.
2. Houck PM: Comparison of operating room lasers: uses, hazards, guidelines, *Nurs Clin North Am* 41(2):193–218, 2006.
3. Ball KA: Surgical modalities. In Rothrock JC: *Alexander's care of the patient in surgery*, ed 14, St. Louis, 2011, Mosby.
4. Babin-Ebell J: Transmyocardial laser revascularization combined with intramyocardial endothelial progenitor cell transplantation in patients with intractable ischemic heart disease ineligible for conventional revascularization: preliminary results, *Thoracic & Cardiovascular Surgeon* 58(1):11–16, 2010.
5. Tiffany J, et al: Patient compliance as a major determinant of laser tattoo removal success rates: A 10-year retrospective study, *Journal of Cosmetic & Laser Therapy* 12(4):166–169, 2010.
6. Kono T, et al: Split-face comparison study of cryogen spray cooling versus pneumatic skin flattening in skin tightening treatments using a long-pulsed Nd:YAG laser, *Journal of Cosmetic & Laser Therapy* 12(2):87–91, 2010.
7. Ball K: Surgical smoke evacuation guidelines: compliance among perioperative nurses, *AORN Journal* 92(8):e1-e23, 2010.
8. Ball K: Compliance with surgical smoke evacuation guidelines: implications for practice, *AORN Journal* 92(2):142–149, 2010.

9. Ball K: Stamping out electrosurgery smoke, *Outpatient Surgery* 11(12), 2010, available at http://www.outpatientsurgery.net/issues/2010/12/stamping-out-electrosurgery-smoke. Accessed February 28, 2012.

10. Ott DE: Smoke and particulate hazards during laparoscopic procedures, *Surgical Services Management* 3(3):11–13, 1997.

11. Venes D, editor: *Taber's cyclopedic medical dictionary*, ed 20, Philadelphia, 2005, F.A. Davis.

12. Wadlund DL: Laparoscopy: risks, benefits and complications, *Nurs Clin North Am* 41(2):219–229, 2006.

13. Ball KA: *Endoscopic surgery*, St. Louis, 1997, Mosby.

14. Soper NJ, et al, editors: *Mastery of endoscopic and laparoscopic surgery*, ed 2, Philadelphia, 2004, Lippincott Williams & Wilkins.

15. Gerges FJ, et al: Anesthesia or laparoscopy: a review, *J Clin Anesthesia* 18(1):67–78, 2006.

16. Jobe BA, Hunter JG: Minimally invasive surgery. In Brunicardi FC, et al, editors: *Schwartz's principles of surgery*, ed 8, New York, 2005, McGraw Hill.

17. Menes T, Spivak H: Laparoscopy: searching for the proper insufflations gas, *Surgical Endoscopy* 14(11):1050–8, 2000.

18. Abassi Z, et al: Adverse effects of pneumoperitoneum on renal function: involvement of the endothelin and nitric oxide systems, *American Journal of Physiology: Regulatory, Integrative, & Comparative Physiology* 63(3):R842–R850, 2007.

19. Chandrakanth A, Talamini M: Laparoscopy and malignancy, *Journal of Laparoendoscopic & Advanced Surgical Techniques*, 15(1):38–47, 2005.

20. Fletcher J, et al: Dissemination of melanoma cells within electrosurgery plume, *The American Journal of Surgery* 178(7):57–59, 1999.

21. Soper NJ, et al, editors: *Mastery of endoscopic and laparoscopic surgery*, ed 2, Philadelphia, 2004, Lippincott Williams & Wilkins.

22. Henny CP, et al: Laparoscopic surgery: pitfalls due to anesthesia, positioning, and pneumoperitoneum, *Surg Endosc* 19(9):1163–1171, 2005.

NURSING CARE IN THE PACU

48 Care of the Patient with Chronic Disorders

*Cecil B. Drain, PhD, RN, CRNA, FAAN, FASAHP and
Beverly Breyette, MSN, RN, CDE*

Patients in the perioperative phase of their hospitalization usually require a significant degree of advanced practice nursing care. If the patient's health can be enhanced before surgery, the patient's ability to have a positive perioperative experience will increase. Patients suffering from a chronic disorder are at greater risk of developing postoperative complications.

In this chapter, selected chronic disorders will be presented to enhance the use of appropriate and informed perianesthesia care. For example, patients with chronic obstructive pulmonary disease (COPD) can have significant preoperative respiratory dysfunction, of which some improvement can be accomplished with intense and knowledgeable nursing care. COPD is a serious condition that starts to develop up to 30 years before significant symptoms; it affects more than 25 million Americans and is responsible for about 80,000 deaths per year.[1] These patients have significant risks for anesthesia and surgery. The COPD disease process can be generalized to many pulmonary dysfunctions, as are the other chronic disorders described in this chapter. Therefore patients suffering from some of the other chronic disorders described in this chapter present a significant challenge to the perianesthesia nurse. In an effort to reduce the incidence of postoperative complications in patients suffering from chronic disorders, a complete understanding of the pathophysiology of the disease process will facilitate the appropriate evidence-based nursing interventions will lead to a positive outcome for the perianesthesia patient.

DEFINITIONS

Acetylcholine (ACh) Receptors: Cholinergic neurotransmitter receptors.

Anticholinesterases: Drugs that act to block the cholinesterase enzyme.

Asthma: A lung disease characterized by constriction and spasms of the muscles of the small airways; a component of COPD.

Atelectasis: Collapse of a lung or portion of the lung.

Bronchospasm: Muscle spasm in the bronchi that causes constriction and a reduction in airflow; a component of COPD.

Cardiomegaly: Enlargement of the heart.

Chronic Bronchitis: Lung disease usually caused by chronic infections in the lungs characterized by increased pulmonary secretions.

Cor Pulmonale: Right heart failure as a result of primary lung disease.

Diplopia: Double vision.

Dynamic Compliance: Elasticity of the lungs over the tidal volume range.

Emphysema: A disease of the lungs characterized by a physical breakdown of the pulmonary tissue and a disease component of COPD.

FEV$_1$: Forced expiratory volume in the first second.

Glycosuria: Glucose in the urine.

Hemolyze: Breakdown of red blood cells that causes a release of hemoglobin.

Hypercarbia: Abnormally high levels of carbon dioxide in the blood.

Hypervolemia: An increase in the volume of circulating blood.

Hypoglycemic Agent: A synthetic drug that lowers the blood glucose level for treatment of type 2 diabetes.

Immunosuppressants: Agents that significantly interfere with the ability of the immune system to respond to antigenic stimulation with inhibiting cellular and humoral immunity.

Microangiopathy: A disease of the small blood vessels.

Miosis: Contraction of the sphincter muscle of the iris that causes the pupil to become smaller.

Myasthenic Syndrome: Called the *Eaton-Lambert syndrome;* chronic fatigability and muscle weakness, especially in the face and throat.

Plasmapheresis: Removal of plasma from previously withdrawn blood via centrifugation, reconstitution of the cellular elements in an isotonic solution, and reinfusion of this solution into the donor or another person who needs red blood cells rather than whole blood.

Polycythemia: Increased number of red blood cells.

Ptosis: Abnormal condition in which the upper eyelids droop because of muscle weakness.

Rales: Crackling sound made inside the lungs during auscultation.

Rhabdomyolysis: A disease of the skeletal muscle characterized by the presence of myoglobin in the urine.

Rhonchi: Sound made inside the lungs during auscultation.

Thalassemia: Microcytic, hypochromic, and short-lived red blood cells caused by deficient synthesis of hemoglobin.

Thymectomy: Surgical removal of the thymus gland.

CHRONIC OBSTRUCTIVE PULMONARY DISEASE

Chronic obstructive pulmonary disease (COPD) describes bronchial obstructive respiratory diseases. It is characterized by dyspnea with or without cough and sputum. The two major clinical manifestations of COPD are airway obstruction and airway destruction. The magnitude of the various disease entities that the term *COPD* includes is great; therefore individual elaboration on the diseases is difficult because each deserves separate attention. This chapter briefly describes the overall characteristics of COPD and general care required in the postanesthesia care unit (PACU). Variations between patients with COPD exist. The perianesthesia nurse must consult with the physician about the specific nursing care to be administered to the patient with COPD. For discussion of specific COPD diseases, see the bibliography at the end of this chapter.

Description of COPD

The hallmark of COPD is the evidence of a productive cough and a progressive decrease in the patient's exercise tolerance. Three major diseases are part of COPD: asthma, emphysema, and chronic bronchitis.[2] All are characterized by airway obstruction. These diseases may have medically reversible components, such as bronchospasm, or they may have irreversible components, such as alveolar septal destruction. Some of the reversible components of asthma, such as retained secretions, bronchospasms, and infections, can be corrected with the interaction of the physician, nurse, physical therapist, and respiratory therapist. The treatment of asthma can include oxygen therapy, bronchodilators, chest physiotherapy, and proper hydration.

Chronic bronchitis is associated with chronic cigarette smoking. The nurse can contribute greatly to the patient's future health with strong influences to refrain from smoking.[3] Other therapy for the reversible components can include the use of bronchodilators, chest physiotherapy, and oxygen.

The patient with emphysema usually has airway destruction that is irreversible. As the alveolar septa are destroyed, insufficient alveolar ventilation ensues and eventually leads to hypercarbia. As the disease progresses, carbon dioxide cannot be expelled from the lungs and is retained there. The patient usually increases minute ventilation to try to compensate for the hypercarbia. Respiratory acidosis develops slowly as the various acid-base buffer systems try to neutralize the accumulated acid. In this compensated state, the patient usually has a near-normal pH, high plasma bicarbonate, low chloride concentration, and high total carbon dioxide levels. The $PaCO_2$ usually is low because some inspired oxygen is unable to cross into the blood from the lungs because of the decreased respiratory diffusion membrane surface area in the lungs. Pulmonary hypertension usually appears as the disease progresses. Cor pulmonale may develop, and because of the pulmonary venous engorgement, the right heart may begin to fail. The patient with emphysema who has irreversible destruction can be treated with chest physiotherapy, bronchodilators, and steroids.

Cigarette Smoking as a Precursor to the Development of COPD

Cigarette smoking has been well established as one of the major precursors to chronic bronchitis and emphysema—two of the three disease components of COPD. Cigarette smoking affects the manner in which a patient recovers from an anesthetic.[4,5] The perianesthesia nurse should be aware of the diverse reactions that smoking can have on the patient who is emerging from an inhalation anesthetic. Studies on the relationship between smoking and its effects on anesthesia indicate an increase in the risk factor in the patient who smokes. Although the incidence rate of smoking is decreasing slowly, it continues to rise in the teenage population.

Respiratory Effects of Smoking

A growing body of convincing scientific literature suggests that almost all pulmonary disease is related in some way to the inhalation of infectious or irritant particulate material. Cigarette smoke in its gaseous phase contains nitrogen, oxygen, carbon dioxide, carbon monoxide, hydrogen, argon, methane, hydrogen cyanide, ammonia, nitrogen dioxide, and acetone. In the particulate phase, cigarette smoke contains nicotine, tar, acids, alcohol, phenols, and hydrocarbons. The bottom line is that cigarette smoke contains oxidants, and the oxidants can damage cells and the extracellular matrix components of the lung, leading to significant damage to the tissue in the lungs. Smokers who inhale nicotine from a cigarette into the lungs actually receive 25% to 30% of the nicotine contained in the cigarette. Thirty percent is destroyed with combustion, and 40% is lost in the side stream. Therefore, if a person inhales the smoke from a cigarette that contains 2.5 mg of nicotine, 1 mg of nicotine is actually absorbed by the lungs. In addition, filters are known to make little difference in this absorption. Contrary to some opinions, the smoking of cigars and pipes also presents a risk for pulmonary disease.[6] Carbon monoxide combines with the hemoglobin molecule at the same point as oxygen does. It has an affinity for this receptor point that is 210-fold greater than that of oxygen[7]; therefore the oxygen-carrying capacity of hemoglobin is reduced, and the end result is that less oxygen is relinquished to the tissues by the hemoglobin. When carbon monoxide combines with hemoglobin, a compound called *carboxyhemoglobin* is formed. The amount of carboxyhemoglobin in the blood is especially important in the patient who has a diseased myocardium, because myocardial oxygenation is limited by the flow of the blood through the coronary arteries. During stress, such as in surgery and anesthesia, the amount of carboxyhemoglobin saturation could lead to severe myocardial hypoxia in patients who smoke heavily and have coronary artery disease because the diseased coronary arteries cannot increase the flow significantly. The only means of prevention of hypoxia is an increase in the extraction of oxygen from the hemoglobin. Small amounts of carboxyhemoglobin can hinder the uncoupling of the oxygen and thus result in yet more oxygen retention at any given tension. This effect clearly is greater when the oxygen tension is further reduced by local ischemia and any additional vasoconstriction associated with smoking.

Smoking is an important causative factor in chronic pulmonary disease, especially the obstructive type.[8] The characteristic pulmonary function alterations in smokers usually include a reduction in vital capacity, an increase in residual volume to total lung capacity, an uneven distribution of inspired gas, a decrease in dynamic compliance, and an increase in nonelastic resistance. Most critically, chronic cigarette smoking ultimately causes the forced expiratory volume in the first second (FEV_1) to be less that 80% of normal, a critical sign of COPD.

Chronic bronchitis is the disease most often associated with smoking and is seen often by the perianesthesia nurse. Hypertrophy of bronchial mucous glands with production of excessive mucus is the hallmark of this disease. A vicious cycle develops as this failure to remove the mucus leads to retention of pathogenic organisms and irritants. The resulting distorted alveolar septa and the increased pressure on the alveoli from chronic bronchitis can lead to emphysema.

Cigarette smoke can cause a progression from hyperplasia to metaplasia to neoplasia in the lungs. Eaton-Lambert syndrome is sometimes associated with bronchial carcinoma and is often called the *myasthenic syndrome* because its symptoms resemble those of myasthenia gravis (MG). This syndrome in some way affects neuromuscular transmission, and patients have the classic symptoms of muscle weakness. These patients are especially sensitive to the skeletal neuromuscular blocking agents used in clinical anesthesia. If the anesthetist is unaware of this syndrome and administers the normal dose of skeletal muscle relaxants, the patient will probably be unable to breathe spontaneously on emergence from anesthesia, even when pharmacologic reversal of the muscle relaxant is attempted. In this situation, postoperative mechanical ventilation is necessary.

Cardiovascular Effects of Smoking

The correlation between vascular disease and smoking is strong. Smoking can influence thrombosis, and because thrombi and platelets contribute to the development of arteriosclerosis, smoking can contribute to arteriosclerosis and its complications.

Inhalation of nicotine produces a release of catecholamines, activates the carotid and aortic chemoreceptor bodies, and directly stimulates the muscles of the vessel walls. As a result, the immediate effects of smoking even a small number of cigarettes can be fairly marked, with production of increases in heart rate, peripheral resistance, cardiac workload, and blood pressure. Each of these actions causes a greater myocardial oxygen demand. Furthermore, because the smoker's hemoglobin can provide less oxygen to the myocardium, smoking can cause cardiac arrhythmias, either through myocardial anoxia or epinephrine release.

Surgical Considerations

The incidence rate of pulmonary complications in patients who have undergone abdominal or thoracic surgery is high. Changes occur in the pulmonary status of the patient who undergoes anesthesia and surgery. In the postoperative phase, these changes are characterized by gradual or abrupt alveolar collapse. The patient with COPD, when subjected to surgery, then represents an even higher risk for postoperative complications. These patients must be given meticulous preoperative care so that they are in the best possible health when they enter surgery. This preoperative medical treatment usually includes hydration, nutrition, chest physiotherapy, bronchodilators, and prophylactic antibiotics if an infection is present. Serial pulmonary function tests and arterial blood gas determinations are used to monitor the progression of the preoperative treatment.[7]

When the patient's pulmonary function reaches a peak before surgery (i.e., when the pulmonary function test and arterial blood gas test results no longer show continued improvement), surgery is considered because the patient has reached optimal pulmonary status.

Care of the COPD Patient

Perianesthesia care focuses on prevention of complications. The modified stir-up regimen should include frequent cascade coughing, sustained maximal inspirations (SMIs), and repositioning of the patient (see Chapters 12 and 28). An appropriately implemented modified stir-up regimen is of great importance, especially in patients who are recovering from upper abdominal or thoracic operations. Surgery at these sites can cause decreased ventilatory effort and a complete absence of sighs by the patient. Given that the patient already has compromised respiratory function, the possibility of retained secretions and atelectasis is magnified. As a result, these patients represent a significant challenge to the perianesthesia nurse (Box 48-1).

When the patient is completely reactive from anesthesia, the use of the incentive spirometer may be helpful in reducing the incidence of atelectasis. Consequently, the perianesthesia nurse who is responsible for supportive measures should assist and encourage the patient in using the SMI with or without the incentive spirometer. On the basis of subjective research findings, if the perianesthesia nurse explains the rationale of the SMI maneuver and properly instructs the patient in the use of the technique before surgery, the patient is more likely to correctly use the SMI maneuver after surgery with or without coaching. The performance of the SMI maneuver, with or without mechanical devices, should be monitored by the nurse to ensure proper production of a sustained inspiration with a 3-second inspiratory hold. The perianesthesia nurse should also encourage and monitor the patient's performance of the cascade cough to facilitate early secretion clearance.

Patients with COPD have some component of reactive airways disease. Consequently, the airway becomes compliant and can become compressed during a forced expiratory maneuver. This dynamic compression of the airways is a function of the equal pressure point theory, as discussed in Chapter 12. To reduce the amount of dynamic compression

---

BOX 48-1 Risk Reduction Strategies to Decrease the Incidence of Postoperative Complications in Patients with COPD

PREOPERATIVE

- Encourage cessation of smoking for at least 8 weeks.
- Treat evidence of expiratory airflow obstruction (e.g., bronchodilator therapy).
- Treat respiratory infection with appropriate antibiotics.
- Initiate patient education regarding lung volume expansion maneuvers.

INTRAOPERATIVE

- Use minimally invasive surgical (laparoscopic) techniques when possible.
- Consider using regional anesthesia.
- Avoid the use of long-acting neuromuscular blocking drugs.
- Avoid surgical procedures longer than 3 hours.

POSTOPERATIVE

- Continue tracheal intubation and mechanical ventilation (likely after abdominal or intrathoracic surgery and a preoperative $PaCO_2 > 50$ mm Hg and $FEV_1/FVC < 0.5$; maintain PaO_2 at 60 to 100 mm Hg and $PaCO_2$ in a range that maintains the pH at 7.35 to 7.45).
- Institute lung-volume expansion maneuvers (voluntary deep breathing, incentive spirometry, continuous positive airway pressure).
- Use chest physiotherapy.
- Maximize analgesia (neuraxial opioids, intercostals nerve blocks, patient-controlled analgesia).

From Stoelting RK, Dierdoff SF: *Handbook for anesthesia and co-existing disease,* ed 2, New York, 2002, Churchill Livingstone; Data from Smetana GW: Preoperative pulmonary evalution, *N Engl J Med* 340:93–944, 1999.
FEV_1, Forced expiratory volume in the first second; *FVC,* forced vital capacity.

---

of the airway during exhalation, the patient should be encouraged to use pursed-lip breathing. Breathing through pursed lips during exhalation can be the same as adding 5 to 10 cm H_2O of positive end-expiratory pressure. Increasing the pressure inside the airway during exhalation reduces the amount of dynamic compression of the airways and decreases the amount of air trapping that commonly occurs in patients with COPD.

Audible wheezing will require the use of a fast-acting bronchodilator such as albuterol. Arterial blood gases may be ordered, and capnography may be used to monitor end-tidal CO_2.[9]

The cardiac status should be monitored meticulously because of the frequent involvement of the heart in the pathologic disorders of these patients. Kidney function should also be monitored because it may be altered, especially in patients with fluid retention and edema of the extremities.

The patient with severe COPD who has marked hypercarbia can present difficulties in the PACU. Patients who have severe emphysema usually fit into this category. Ventilatory effort in these patients is stimulated by the hypoxic drive, in which lack of oxygen stimulates ventilation. Hypoxia indirectly stimulates the respiratory center by means of chemoreceptors in the carotid bodies located at the bifurcation of the carotid artery. When the patient receives 100% oxygen to breathe in the PACU, oxygen tensions rise in the inspired gas; the carotid and aortic chemoreceptors cease to function; and the patient quickly becomes apneic. The patient's respiratory status should be assessed carefully and the physician consulted before 100% oxygen is administered. Mist therapy after surgery aids in liquefying the secretions and helps in the all-important maintenance of a patent tracheobronchial tree. If excessive bronchial drainage is not removed, it provides a convenient avenue for bacteria and might also obstruct the airways, thus leading to insufficient alveolar ventilation and hypoxia.

The patient with COPD should be under constant surveillance for signs of cardiopulmonary decompensation, including shallow rapid gasping respirations, severe dyspnea, substernal retraction, and disorientation. Blood pressure may be elevated or low, but the patient usually has tachycardia, fever, and muscle rigidity. Cyanosis may be present.

Patients who are cigarette smokers have significant postanesthesia risks.[6] Cigarette smokers who have smoked for a long period of time and have an FEV_1 less than 80% usually have an increased risk of pulmonary complications in comparison with nonsmokers. Patients who smoke more than two packs of cigarettes per day are especially prone to perianesthetic complications. In addition, patients who have had a long history of smoking (>20 pack years) and are presently in a nonsmoking situation still can have pulmonary complications. Many of these complications develop when cigarette smokers have a preexisting chronic respiratory disease, usually bronchitis. The major postoperative complications associated with smoking are infection, atelectasis, pleural effusion, pulmonary infarction, and bronchitis.

Complications associated with chronic cigarette smoking revolve around the inability of the patient to clear secretions. The goal of nursing care in the PACU centers on clearing the tracheobronchial tree, which necessitates frequent suctioning, cascade coughing, and the SMI maneuver. If rales and rhonchi are heard on auscultation, percussion and postural drainage should be initiated.

Because cardiovascular disease is associated with a long history of cigarette smoking, the patient should have continuous electrocardiographic monitoring. Arrhythmias, such as premature ventricular contractions, should be addressed because they may be the first signs of decreased myocardial oxygenation in the cigarette smoker.

Respiratory depressant drugs, such as opioids, should be given in low doses, or they should be avoided completely if the COPD is severe. Repositioning of the patient and splinting of the incision site, in addition to reducing the anxiety usually seen in these patients, reduces the need for opioids. Some form of regional analgesia may be beneficial for these patients.[8]

MYASTHENIA GRAVIS

The patient with MG deserves special consideration in the PACU because of the respiratory dysfunction and possible pharmacologic ramifications of the disease. The incidence rate of MG has been estimated to be between 1 in 7500 and 1 in 10,000.[1] MG occurs twice as often in females than in males and at earlier ages, and it occurs most often between the ages of 30 and 40 years.[7] The main symptoms are weakness in one or more of the muscle groups, fatigability on effort, and at least some partial restoration of muscle function after rest.[7]

MG is the prototype autoimmune disease because its pathophysiology involves the postsynaptic acetylcholine (ACh) receptors at the myoneural junction. The causative factor is an immune-mediated destruction or blockage that leads to an inactivation of the postsynaptic ACh receptors. Interestingly enough, the presynaptic ACh receptors continue to be normal. More specifically, patients with MG have developed antibodies to muscle acetylcholine receptors. The antibody does not bind exactly on the site that binds the ACh, but it does bind close to it. The ACh receptors are steadily destroyed, with a resulting reduction in the binding of acetylcholine at the postsynaptic myoneural junction. The patient with MG sometimes has a lesion in the myocardium that is a spotty focal necrosis accompanied by an inflammatory reaction. An alteration in the S-T segment and T wave is sometimes seen in these patients.

Ptosis of the eyelid is the most common sign of the disease. Ptosis is usually accompanied by diplopia, blurred vision, or nystagmus. Ocular signs and symptoms often are worsened by bright light. The patient may also have myasthenic facies, which is caused by weakness of the facial muscles and can progress to dysphagia and difficulties in speech.

Respiration is often affected in the patient with myasthenia. Dyspnea can be either inspiratory if the diaphragm is involved or expiratory if the intercostal and abdominal muscles are affected. The patient may also have emotional disturbances caused by anxiety and depression.

Diagnosis of MG is made on the clinical symptoms and the characteristic electromyographic results. The clinical symptoms can be assessed with the neostigmine test or the edrophonium test, both of which involve anticholinesterases that increase the strength of the myasthenic muscle. Should these tests show that MG may be present, serum levels of anti-AChR antibodies can be drawn. These antibodies are usually present in 85% to 90% of patients with myasthenia.

Treatment for this disease consists of various pharmacologic interventions designed to enhance neuromuscular transmission and slow the progression of the disease. Therefore the treatment may include cholinesterase inhibitors, corticosteroids, specific immunosuppressants, plasmapheresis, intravenous immunoglobulin, and thymectomy.[1]

Anticholinesterase drugs, which slow down the enzymatic destruction of acetylcholine at the neuromuscular junction, are commonly used. Oral pyridostigmine is the anticholinesterase of choice. Patients with MG seem to favor pyridostigmine over other anticholinesterases because its length of action is 3 to 4 hours when administered orally. Steroids and other immunosuppressive agents may be used in some patients to reduce antibody production responsible for the disease. Plasmapheresis, a plasma exchange, arrests severe refractive MG by reducing the concentration of circulating antibodies. Like the use of intravenous immunoglobulin, plasmapheresis is a short-term treatment.

Thymectomy seems to be an appropriate therapeutic mode because the thymus gland appears to be intimately involved in the disease process. Approximately 75% of the patients with myasthenia who do not have thymoma have improvement after thymectomy. Alternatively, approximately 20% of the patients with MG with thymoma show improvement in the disease process after thymectomy.

Because thymectomy has been used as a therapeutic intervention in the treatment of MG, the perianesthesia nurse will probably render nursing care to many patients with MG. Because of the location of the incision, the myasthenic patient does not usually receive any intraoperative skeletal muscle relaxants. Patients with myasthenia can have an exacerbation of symptoms in the PACU; therefore critical monitoring of the patient's ventilatory status should be the primary focus of the perianesthesia

nursing care. Patients with MG who are recovering from any type of surgical procedure and who have been administered any form of anesthesia (general, inhalation, or regional) can have exacerbated symptoms and myasthenic crisis develop in the PACU. Consequently, respiratory support should always be available for these patients.

Care of the Patient with Myasthenia Gravis

If a muscle relaxant is given during surgery, the patient has the neuromuscular blockade reversed. After reversal in the operating room, the patient must have a complete sustained return of skeletal muscle strength before extubation. If the patient does not meet the criteria for extubation, the endotracheal tube remains in place and the patient is taken to the PACU for ventilatory support. In patients with MG, the skeletal muscle strength may appear to be appropriate immediately after surgery, but may deteriorate a few hours thereafter.[7]

The patient with MG can have various difficulties because of an impaired respiratory system, possible poor nutrition, susceptibility to infection, altered psychiatric status, and possible altered response to drugs used during anesthesia. The patient should be placed in a quiet area, where no direct light shines in the eyes. The patient's respiratory effort and exchange should be monitored continuously. Oxygen should be administered with humidification, and secretions should be removed with frequent suctioning and postural drainage. Oxygen saturation levels for these patients should be maintained at more than 96%. Any change in respiratory status should be reported to the physician immediately.

Because cardiac mechanisms may be responsible for some sudden deaths in this patient population, cardiac monitoring should be instituted for every patient with myasthenia in the PACU. Monitoring of the fluids administered to patients with MG is also important. Hypovolemia and hypervolemia must be avoided because of their deleterious effects on the already compromised heart and lungs.

The patient should be kept as pain free as possible to facilitate good respiratory exchange. Morphine and other opioids are often potentiated by anticholinesterases; therefore the initial opioid dose should be reduced to half the normal dose and then increased if necessary. If the patient is receiving continuous mechanical ventilation, the normal amount of medication can be given without compromising the patient's respiratory status.

The PACU nurse should monitor for a myasthenic crisis, which is a severe exacerbation of the symptoms associated with MG. It can occur when an anticholinesterase is underdosed and does not reduce the amount of muscle weakness sufficiently. Alternatively, a cholinergic crisis can occur when too much anticholinesterase is administered, resulting in a surplus of acetylcholine at the myoneural junction and causing a depolarizing type block that leads to skeletal muscle weakness, which could be severe. For all the previous reasons, during PACU care of the patient with MG in the immediate postoperative phase, airway equipment must be kept at the patient's bedside. Along with the skeletal muscle weakness, muscarinic side effects occur, such as abdominal cramping, miosis, bradycardia, salivation, and diarrhea. See Chapters 10, 11, and 23, which provide the reader an in-depth discussion of the myoneural junction and nicotinic and muscarinic effects.

The emotional status of the patient with myasthenia is of considerable importance. As few clinicians as possible should be responsible for this patient throughout the emergent phase, because the patient is likely to be distrustful of anyone he or she does not know. Communication is important, and the patient should be informed about any nursing procedure to be performed. If the patient with myasthenia has a tracheostomy, paper and pencil should be used to facilitate communication between nurse and patient.

DIABETES MELLITUS

Diabetes mellitus (DM) affects approximately 29 million people in the United States and is the seventh leading cause of death. It is also believed that DM as a comorbidity is underreported.[10] However, it is what transpires between the diagnosis and death that determines the level of health, the health care needed, and the number of surgical interventions of the patient with DM.

Diabetes is a chronic, progressive disease characterized by the body's inability to metabolize carbohydrates, fats, and proteins leading to hyperglycemia.[11] The degree of hyperglycemia and the incidence of acute or long-term diabetes complications depend on the type of diabetes and the level of DM control over the lifetime of the person with diabetes.

The two forms of diabetes are insulin dependent and non–insulin dependent. Insulin-dependent diabetes, now called type 1, was formerly called *juvenile onset diabetes*. Type 1 diabetes may be genetic in predisposition, but the majority of those diagnosed with type 1 DM have no first-degree relatives with DM.[11] It is characterized by complete dependence on exogenous insulin therapy. Type 1 DM is caused by a vigorous autoimmune destruction of the beta cells in the islets of Langerhans in the pancreas. The onset of DM is usually before the age of 40 years; however, it can develop at any age. By the time of diagnosis, approximately 80% to 90% of the beta cells have been destroyed. Approximately 10% of the people with DM have type 1.[11] Treatment centers on meal planning, exercise, and insulin administration (Table 48-1).

The other main form of DM is non-insulin dependent diabetes, or type 2 diabetes. Formerly

Table 48-1   Insulin Formulations Used in the Treatment of Diabetes

TYPE OF INSULIN	GENERIC NAME (BRAND NAME)	ONSET	PEAK	DURATION
Rapid-acting analogs	Lispro (Humalog), aspart (Novolog), glulisine (Apidra)	5-15 min	1-2 hours	3-4 hours
Short-acting	Regular (Humulin R, Novolin R)	30-60 min	2-4 hours	6-8 hours
Intermediate-acting	NPH (Humulin N, Novolin N)	1-2 hours	4-8 hours	10-20 hours
Long-acting	Glargine analog (Lantus),	4-6 hours	Peakless	24-48 hours
	Detemire analog (Levemir)	4-6 hours	Peak with higher doses	24-48 hours
Mixed insulin: 75% intermediate and 30% short acting regular	Humulin 70/30 (Novolin 70/30)	30-60 min	2-8 hours	10-20 hours
Mixed insulin: 75% intermediate and 25% lispro insulin	Humalog mix 75/25	5-15 min	1-4 hours	10-20 hours
Mixed insulin: 70% intermediate and 30% aspart insulin	Novolog mix 70/30	5-15 min	1-4 hours	15-18 hours

Adapted from Furlong K, et al: Perioperative management of endocrine disorders. In Merli G, Weitz H, editors: *Medical management of the surgical patient*, ed 3, St. Louis, 2008, Saunders.

called *adult onset diabetes*, type 2 affects approximately 90% of people with DM. This type of DM is characterized by impaired insulin secretion or peripheral resistance to one's own insulin, resulting in a degree of endogenous insulin production, but not at a level sufficient to produce normal carbohydrate homeostasis. Most people with type 2 DM are older than 40 years and have a family history of diabetes, and 85% are obese.[11] As the U.S. population ages, becomes more obese, and is less active, a continued rise in the number of persons with DM is to be expected. Treatment focuses on meal planning, exercise, and weight loss with the possible inclusion of oral hypoglycemics, injectable noninsulin products, and treatment with insulin (Table 48-2).

The Centers for Disease Control and Prevention estimates that 25.8 million persons in the United States have DM, comprising 8.3% of the total population.[10] Of these, 18.8 million have been diagnosed, whereas 7 million remain undiagnosed. As the U.S. youth become more sedentary and obese, the incidence of type 2 DM in children is skyrocketing. In 2010, approximately 215,000 people younger than 20 years old had a diagnosis of type 1 or type 2 DM (Table 48-3).[10]

The diagnosis of DM has traditionally been determined by the fasting blood glucose (FBG) level. FBG greater than 126 mg/dL (7.0 mmol/L) indicates DM. An oral glucose tolerance test (OGTT) with a 75-g sugar load may also be used, with a resultant blood glucose (BG) of greater than 200 mg/dL (11.1 mmol/L) indicating DM. The glycosylated hemoglobin (HbA1c), now referred to as the *A1C level*, is a newer determinant of a diagnosis of DM. The A1C level was used for

Table 48-3	Diagnosed Persons with Diabetes Aged 20 Years or Older – U.S. 2010
GROUP	**NUMBER WITH DIABETES (%)**
Age ≥20 years	25.6 million (11.3)
Age ≥65 years	10.9 million (26.9)
Men	13.0 million (11.8)
Women	12.6 million (10.8)
Non-Hispanic whites	15.7 million (10.2)
Non-Hispanic blacks	4.9 million (18.7)

From Centers for Disease Control, U.S. Department of Health and Human Services. *National Diabetes Fact Sheet* 2011, available at http://www.cdc.gov/diabetes/pubs/pdf/ndfs_2011.pdf. Accessed May 5, 2012.

two decades to determine diabetes control, and in 2010 the American Diabetes Association allowed a laboratory-based standardized A1C to be used for diagnosis.[12] As the red blood cell travels throughout the body on its approximately 6-week life cycle, glucose molecules attach to the hemoglobin molecule in the red blood cell. The A1C test reports a percentage, correlating to the average BG level over the last 2 to 3 months (Table 48-4).

Although hyperglycemia is most often cited as the primary problem with diabetes, it is usually the resultant long-term physiologic changes that cause the person with DM to require surgery. It is estimated that people with diabetes have a 50% chance of requiring surgery in their lifetime and that approximately 20% of all surgical patients will have DM.[13] DM is the leading cause of nontraumatic lower limb amputations, increasing the likelihood of intervention in any surgical setting.

Table 48-2	Oral Medication or Non-Insulin Injectable Medications for Persons with Diabetes	
CHEMICAL CLASS	**AGENTS**	**ACTION**
Biguanides	Metformin	Decreases endogenous hepatic glucose production and increases peripheral glucose uptake
Sulfonylureas	Glipizide, glyburide, glimepiride	Increases the secretion of insulin from B cells
Meglitinides	Repaglinide, nateglinide	Increases the secretion of insulin from B cells
Thiazolidinediones	Pioglitazone, rosiglitazone	Improves insulin action in the periphery and the liver
α-Gglycosidase inhibitors	Acarbose, miglitol	Inhibits intestinal α-glucosidase, delaying glucose absorption
GLP-1 receptor agonist	Exenatide (injectable)	Stimulates insulin secretion and facilitates homeostasis follow food ingestion
Amylinomimetic	Pramlintide (injectable)	Regulates glucose concentration after a meal, increases satiety, slows gastric emptying, suppresses glucagon secretion

Adapted from Fain J: Management of clients with diabetes mellitus. In Black J, Hawks J, editors: *Medical surgical nursing; clinical management for positive outcomes*, ed 8, St. Louis, Saunders.

SPECIAL CONSIDERATIONS

Table 48-4	Criteria for the Diagnosis of Diabetes		
	PLASMA GLUCOSE VALUES		
DIAGNOSIS	FBG (mg/dL)	OGTT (mg/dL)	A1C (%)
Normal	<100	<140	4–5.7
Pre-diabetes	100-125	140-199	5.8-6.5
Diabetes	>125	>200	>6.5

From Fisher L: *Anesthesia and uncommon diseases*, ed 5, Philadelphia, 2007, Saunders.
FBG, Fasting blood glucose; *OGTT*, oral glucose tolerance test; *A1C*, glycosylated hemoglobin.

Determination of any long-term diabetes complications should be made in the preoperative period, hopefully weeks before the scheduled surgery (Box 48-2). Input from the primary care physician or diabetes specialist should be sought. Patient information from the medical record can also provide a thorough assessment for the emergent surgical patient with diabetes. Results of a current A1C provide an overview of the glucose control over the last 2 to 3 months; A1C values under 7% help to ensure fewer postoperative infections.[13] None of these complications are unique to people with diabetes, but the incidence of these complications is higher in those with diabetes. Macrovascular disease reflects an increase in atherosclerosis with deposits of lipids within the inner layer of vessel walls. Increased levels of BG over time cause a thickening of the cell basement membrane and intracellular edema

BOX 48-2	Chronic Complications of Diabetes Mellitus

MACROVASCULAR COMPLICATIONS
• Coronary artery disease
• Cerebrovascular disease
• Hypertension
• Peripheral vascular disease
• Infection

MICROVASCULAR COMPLICATIONS
• Retinopathy
• Nephropathy
• Leg and foot ulcers
• Sensorimotor neuropathy
• Autonomic neuropathy
  • Pupillary
  • Cardiovascular
  • Gastrointestinal
  • Genitourinary

and altered cell function. The resulting thickness causes a greater distance of travel for nutrients and cellular waste decreasing the oxygen and nutrition entering the cell and causing cellular waste buildup.[11]

Anesthesia and Diabetes

Preoperative guidelines for medications depend on the person's home regimen and should be discussed with the person's primary care physician and diabetes specialist before the surgical intervention. Varied combinations of medications make it unlikely to find a standardized preoperative plan that works for all patients with type 1 or type 2 DM. If possible, the person with diabetes should be scheduled for an early morning surgery to reduce the time without oral intake.[11] Ongoing preoperative monitoring of BG levels helps to prevent acute complications during the perioperative and postoperative periods.

In general, people with DM who take oral medications or non-insulin injectables should be advised to hold those medications the evening before or the day of surgery, primarily for prevention of hypoglycemia. Sulfonylureas can interfere with ischemic myocardial preconditioning and theoretically increase the risk of perioperative myocardial ischemia and infarction.[14] Metformin is withheld to prevent the possibility of lactic acidosis.

Persons with type 1 DM may be advised to reduce the bedtime insulin to prevent hypoglycemia while NPO before surgery; however, some form of maintenance insulin must be continued to prevent hyperglycemia from the lack of basal insulin. Basal insulin is the amount of exogenous insulin per unit of time necessary to prevent hepatic gluconeogenesis and ketogenesis. People with type 1 DM are usually maintained on a basal dose of one or two injections of a long-acting insulin or multiple injections of an intermediate insulin or continuous subcutaneous insulin infusion (i.e., insulin pump with a rapid acting analog).[15] Nutritional insulin is the amount of exogenous insulin necessary to prevent hyperglycemia associated with any type of nutritional supplement, such as discrete meals, total parenteral nutrition, and enteral feedings. Correctional or supplemental insulin is used to correct unexpected hyperglycemia that occurs before or between meals.[15] Nutritional and correctional insulin is usually a rapid-acting insulin or a short-acting insulin may be chosen. Each hospital tends to adopt different procedures for the person with diabetes using an insulin pump. Refer to individual hospital policies for details. In general, the pump may be set to the "suspend" mode for minor or short-duration surgeries. Longer procedures

Table 48-5 Acute Complications of Diabetes

	DKA	HHNS	HYPOGLYCEMIA
Type of diabetes	Usually type 1, but can occur with type 2	Type 2	Type 1 or 2
Clinical manifestations	Warm or dry skin, nausea, vomiting, flushed, dry mucosa, soft eyeballs, Kussmaul respirations, tachypnea, hypotension, tachycardia, abdominal pain, acetone breath, decreased LOC	Same as for DKA without Kussmaul respirations and acetone breath, altered LOC, severe dehydration, tachycardia, shallow respirations	Mild reaction: Tremors, palpitations, sweating, hunger Moderate reaction: Headache, irritability, drowsiness, weakness, visual disturbances, decreased mental acuity Severe reaction: Loss of consciousness, seizures
Preoperative precipitating factors	Undiagnosed DM, omission of insulin dose, infection, cardiovascular disorder, trauma	Undiagnosed DM, infection, some medications, dialysis, gastrointestinal bleeding, acute pancreatitis, central nervous system disorders	Delay or omission of meal, insulin overdose, improper timing of insulin and food
Overview of interventions	IV regular insulin; rehydration; potassium, phosphate, electrocardiogram; correct the underlying problem	Correct underlying problem; IV regular insulin, rehydration, potassium	Treat mild with 15 g simple carbohydrate (CHO); treat moderate with one or more simple CHO or glucagon; treat severe with glucagon IV or intramuscular or IV glucose

Fain J: Management of clients with diabetes mellitus. In Black J, Hawks J, editors: *Medical surgical nursing; clinical management for positive outcomes*, ed 8, St. Louis, 2009, Saunders.

LOC, Level of consciousness; *DKA*, diabetic ketoacidosis; *DM*, diabetes mellitus; *HHNS*, hyperosmolar hyperglycemic nonketotic syndrome; *IV*, intravenous; *CHO*, carbohydrate.

from which the person will have a longer period of sedation necessitate the removal of the pump and implementation of an IV insulin drip. The bagged and labeled pump and equipment should be sent home with the family and that action documented.

Care of the Patient with Diabetes

Perioperative goals for glycemic control include: the maintenance of fluid and electrolyte balance, prevention of ketoacidosis, avoidance of marked hyperglycemia, and avoidance of hypoglycemia.[13] If any of these problems occur, immediate treatment is imperative and diligent investigation is required to determine the underlying cause. Surgery induces a stress response mediated by the neuroendocrine system through the release of catecholamines, glucagon, and cortisol. Surgery and possibly anesthesia cause an elevation of sympathetic tone with a release of cortisol and catecholamines. The relative insulin deficiency (type 2) and the absolute insulin deficiency (type 1) limit

the body's ability to compensate for this deficiency, requiring supplemental insulin during the perioperative period. This stress response of hyperglycemia may also occur with surgical patients without DM, demonstrating a need for glucose control for all surgical patients. Multiple studies have shown that control of the perioperative serum glucose level has a positive effect on the outcomes of all patients (Table 48-5).[14]

The nature and duration of the surgical procedure affects the glucose levels and the insulin interventions needed. In patients who require minor surgical procedures of short duration or limited general, local, epidural, or spinal anesthesia might need only minimal changes in their diabetes regimen. Procedures of longer than 2 hours under general anesthesia will have greater glucose variations and require more frequent monitoring and treatment.[15] Intravenous regular insulin is used for glucose control during surgery. Doses and frequency may be determined by hospital or surgical center protocols. Subcutaneous insulin is not used

Evidence-Based Practice

Smith and colleagues conducted a retrospective study to explore the effect of hyperglycemia in the postanesthesia care unit (PACU) on postoperative complications, length of stay (LOS), and mortality in patients with diabetes undergoing spine, colon, or joint surgery. Results of the study determined that patients with blood glucose (BG) > 200 mg/dL in the PACU had a significantly longer LOS than patients with a maximum BG of 140 to 200 mg/dL. They also found that the rate of total complications significantly increased as the BG levels increased. There was a 70% increase in complications when the PACU BG was > 200 mg/dL.

IMPLICATIONS FOR PRACTICE

To establish consistent best practices in BG management in the PACU, perianesthesia nurses should advocate for consistent and clear parameters for BG for the perianesthesia patient. Prospective, controlled studies on the management of hyperglycemic patients in the PACU are needed and could be conducted by perianesthesia nurses. In the meantime, the PACU nurse should be aware of the latest research indications for care.

Source: Smith DK, et al: A study of perioperative hyperglycemia in patients with diabetes having colon, spine, and joint surgery, *J Perianesth Nurs* 24:362–369, 2009.

because the absorption is affected by the person's body temperature, circulating blood volumes, and certain anesthetics.[11]

Postoperative goals for the patient with DM include the universal outcomes of stabilizing vital signs, correcting fluid and electrolyte imbalances, preventing wound infection and promoting wound healing. Prevention of hypoglycemia depends on BG monitoring and physical indicators such as a decrease in blood pressure or an increased heart rate in the still unresponsive patient. Patients with peripheral vascular disease, neuropathy, or both require frequent skin inspection for signs of breakdown, pressure spots, or shearing injuries to the skin.[11] However, for the person with diabetes, reestablishing control of their DM is imperative.

What is considered to be the optimal BG levels for the postoperative period has been one of debate for several years. However, statistics demonstrate that infection accounts for 66% of postoperative complications for those with DM. Mortality rates in people in diabetes have been estimated at fivefold greater than for those without DM. Both infection and mortality are thought to be caused by impaired leukocyte function, altered chemotaxis, and phagocytic activity.[14]

Furnary and colleagues[16] and Van den Berghe et al[17] determined that tight glycemic control decreased the incidence of deep sternal wound infections and decreased mortality, respectively. A postoperative BG level between 80 mg/dl (4.4 mmol/L) and 110 mg/dl (6.1 mmol/L) was designated as the standard for cardiac surgical or critical care patients. The basic goal of balancing the BG levels while still preventing hypoglycemia remains paramount in the medical and surgical efforts to decrease mortality and morbidity. Current studies have shown that although tight glycemic control may still be beneficial for the postcardiac surgical patient, others benefit from less stringent goals of between 80 (4.4 mmol/L) and 150 mg/dL (8.3 mmol/L). Other guidelines propose "reasonable" normoglycemia with the majority of BG levels less than 180 to 200 mg/dL (<10 to 11 mmol/L).[13] The American Diabetes Association Standards of Medical Care has endorsed an FBG level of less than 140 mg/dL (7.8 mmol/L) for general hospitalized patients with random BG readings less than 180 mg/dL (10 mmol/L).[12,18]

Diabetes and BG control throughout the perianesthesia period determines the success of the procedure, the adverse or positive outcomes, and the overall health of the person with diabetes. DM remains the leading cause of kidney failure and is a major cause of heart disease and stroke; all of these are risks that may have an impact on the outcome of any surgical case. Minimizing BG variability during the perianesthesia period should be part of any glycemic control strategy.[18] Nursing consideration of the preoperative DM status, the perioperative BG levels, and the postoperative outcomes influence the person with DM for months beyond the surgical intervention portion of their health care.

RHEUMATOID ARTHRITIS

Rheumatoid arthritis (RA) is a relatively common disease that affects the connective tissue of the body. The clinical course varies, but it tends to be progressive and lead to characteristic deformities. Many patients become incapacitated over time. The disease affects more women than men, and its incidence rate in temperate climates is approximately 3%. The cause is not completely understood, but the disease is thought to be an autoimmune phenomenon. The outstanding clinical feature of this disease is proliferative inflammation. The patient often appears chronically ill, undernourished, and anemic.[19]

These patients often undergo surgery to correct restrictive deformities caused by the disease process (Table 48-6). On arrival in the PACU, they require comprehensive nursing management. Some of the hazards to be aware of in patients with rheumatoid arthritis are listed in Table 48-7.

Care of the Patient with Rheumatoid Arthritis

Airway

Extubation is often deferred in these patients until they are unquestionably able to maintain their own airways. This deference is of prime importance because these patients are often extremely difficult to intubate and are prone to airway obstruction.

Lungs

The patient with RA usually has pulmonary dysfunction, such as diffuse interstitial fibrosis, granulomatous lesions, or large silicotic nodules. These pulmonary dysfunctions lead to stiff lungs, and these patients are prone to atelectasis, hypoxemia, and hypercarbia in the PACU (see Chapter 12). Postoperative blood gas analysis and good pulmonary support are therefore important. Respiratory depressant opioids should be given with caution, if at all. Deaths in patients with RA have resulted from drug-induced respiratory failure during this period.[20]

Table 48-6 Corrective Surgery for Rheumatoid Arthritis

OPERATIVE SITE	COMMON OPERATIVE PROCEDURE
Neck	Atlantoaxial arthrodesis
Shoulder	Synovectomy and partial excision of acromion
Elbow	Synovectomy and radial head excision, resection arthroplasty
Wrist	Synovectomy and excision of distal ulna
Hand	Metacarpal phalangeal arthroplasty and flexor and extensor tenosynovectomy
Hip	Cup or total replacement, arthroplasty
Knee	Synovectomy (often bilateral), arthroplasty
Foot	Resection arthroplasty (often bilateral)

From Nagelhout J, Plaus K: *Nurse anesthesia,* ed 4, St. Louis, 2010, Saunders.

Table 48-7 Perianesthesia Hazards in Patients with Rheumatoid Arthritis

AREA OF CONCERN	COMPLICATION
Respiratory System	
Airway	Hypoplastic mandible restriction, cervical spine motion, atlantoaxial subluxation, laryngeal tissue damage
Ventilation	Rheumatoid nodules in lung, chronic diffuse interstitial fibrosis, costovertebral joint disorder that inhibits ventilation, thoracic vertebrae flexion deformity that inhibits ventilation, tuberculous lung
Cardiovascular System	Pericardial, myocardial, coronary artery disorders, aortic valve regurgitation, arrhythmias
Hemopoietic, Hepatic, and Renal Systems	Anemia, leukopenia, bleeding tendency (decreased platelets), renal amyloidosis
Miscellaneous	Skin fragility; postoperative chest complications, such as atelectasis, hypercarbia, and hypoxia; multiple joint disease

Modified from Bready L, et al: *Decision making in anesthesiology,* ed 4, St. Louis, 2007, Mosby.

Heart

Disease of the pericardium, myocardium, endocardium, and coronary vessels is usually associated with rheumatoid arthritis; therefore cardiovascular status should be monitored continuously in the PACU. Hypotension should be avoided because it can lead to left ventricular decompensation and acute heart failure.

Blood

The patient with RA usually has anemia, most commonly of the hypochromic microcytic variety. In most instances, this type of anemia can be treated with blood transfusion. Postoperative hematocrit and hemoglobin levels should be determined when the patient arrives in the PACU.

Blood loss should be extensively monitored, including observation of the stools for blood. The contents recovered from the nasogastric tube (if present) should be checked for blood, because these patients may have a bleeding peptic ulcer from long-term aspirin and steroid therapy.

Fluid Balance

Renal function is usually impaired in the patient with chronic rheumatoid arthritis; therefore drugs that are primarily excreted by the kidneys should be avoided, and urinary output should be monitored at regular, perhaps hourly, intervals.

SICKLE CELL DISEASE

Sickle cell disease is an inherited type of hemolytic anemia. It is a chronic disease marked by exacerbations. The clinical manifestations are based entirely on sickling of the red blood cells and its consequences.

More than 100 abnormal hemoglobins have been described in humans. When these hemoglobins are exposed to low oxygen tensions, this particular form of hemoglobin causes the red blood cell to distort its shape (sickle) and cause infarction and other complications. Normal hemoglobin is labeled *hemoglobin A,* whereas this sickling hemoglobin is labeled *hemoglobin S.*[7]

Hemoglobin S is thought to have arisen in Arabia in Neolithic times and from there to have spread eastward and westward; it is found today in parts of India, east and west Africa, the West Indies and among African Americans.

The common sickle cell disorders are sickle cell trait (SA), homozygous sickle cell disease (SS), sickle cell-hemoglobin C disease, and sickle cell-thalassemia. A combination of thalassemia and sickle cell anemia occurs in sickle cell-beta thalassemia.

Sickle cell trait is found in about 8% to 12% of the African-American population[21], which is heterozygous for sickling, and represents a combination of sickle hemoglobin (SA) and normal hemoglobin (AA). The red blood cells of such persons contain 20% to 40% hemoglobin S, but are not misshapen in normal living conditions. The person may have sickling with exposure to any conditions that cause hypoxia, such as depressed respiratory function from anesthetics in the PACU.

The most common form of sickle cell disease is the homozygous sickle cell disease. It occurs in 1 in 400 to 500 African Americans. These persons have inherited sickling genes from both parents, and they usually have 80% to 100% hemoglobin

S. Sickling is present all the time, and minor reductions in oxygen tension can cause a sickle cell crisis. The onset of symptoms occurs around the age of 2 years; rarely do these persons live past the age of 40 years.[21]

Sickle cell-hemoglobin C disease is caused by the presence of the gene for sickle hemoglobin and the gene for hemoglobin C. The course of the disease is usually milder than that of the homozygous sickle cell disease, although the person has discomfort and occasional sickle cell crises.

Sickle cell thalassemia, which occurs in persons who have traits for sickle cell thalassemia and beta thalassemia, has a less severe course and symptoms in comparison with the other forms of these diseases. The sickle cell crises are not seen as commonly in this disease.

Pathogenesis of Sickle Cell Disease

To understand the pathogenesis of this disease, knowledge of what happens to the red blood cell when sickling occurs is helpful. If oxygen tension is lowered, long crystals called *tactoids* are formed within the red blood cells because of rearrangement of the amino acid chains or polymers. The cell membrane becomes distorted by the twisting of the polymers. The result is the sickle cell shape for which the disease is named. The process can be reversed if the oxygen tension is increased.

The actual pathologic action of sickling occurs in the microcirculation. Because of increased viscosity and the distortion of the red blood cells with the formation of tactoids, which prevents the cells from molding to the size and structure of the capillaries, the sickled cells are wedged in the capillary bed and thus occlude normal flow. As the cells aggregate, a thrombus is formed. Symptoms depend on whether the thrombus becomes an embolus and, if so, on where it becomes lodged; infarctive episodes are caused in that tissue. Areas of infarctive crisis are the spleen, myocardium, kidney, liver, mesentery, bone marrow, and brain.

Oxygen tension causes sickling, but several other precipitating factors are also involved, such as acidosis, hypotension, regional vasodilation, dehydration, hemoconcentration, stasis of blood, hypothermia, sepsis, decreased cardiac output, and respiratory impairment.

Sickle Cell Anemia and Anesthesia

Anesthesia is not generally believed to be hazardous to patients with sickle cell trait. Nevertheless, sufficiently adverse hypoxic conditions can precipitate a sickling crisis. Definite hazards arise with anesthesia in patients with sickle cell and sickle cell–hemoglobin C disease. Because of its ability to cause the intravascular sickling syndrome, general anesthesia has been the subject of much research. The most important factor in this syndrome is hypoxemia, which generally occurs during the emergent period rather than during surgery. Local anesthesia or nerve block is the technique of choice. Epidural and spinal techniques should be avoided because of the possibility of hypotension with these two methods.

Care of the Patient with Sickle Cell Disease

Prevention of sickle cell crisis is the main objective in the PACU phase. A general guideline for preoperative preparation is a hemoglobin A level of at least 50% and a hematocrit value of 35%. A recent study indicated that a conservative transfusion regimen is effective as an aggressive regimen in preventing postoperative complications. The tendencies to administer preoperative intravenous fluid and to transfuse blood to patients with sickle cell increased with disease severity and extensiveness of the surgical procedure. Although 89% of respondents to a recent survey felt comfortable managing patients with sickle cell disease, 73% thought an advisory statement on optimal perioperative management was needed. Ultimately, there is a wide variation in the management of children with sickle cell disease, and clinicians determine management based on disease severity and procedure type.[22]

If diagnostic procedures are not available or if emergency surgery prevents testing for the sickling trait, all African American patients should be treated as possible carriers of the trait because the incidence rate of this disease is relatively high among African Americans.

In the patient with sickle cell disease, the postoperative period is critically important because incisional pain, analgesics, pulmonary infections, and low arterial oxygen partial pressures all are predisposing factors to the formation of sickle cells. In the PACU, supplemental humidified oxygen, along with appropriate monitoring of intravascular volume and core temperature, is of utmost importance for ensuring positive outcomes.

Temperature regulation is important for the patient with sickle cell disease. Although cold reduces tactoid formation, it also reduces body metabolism, which can lead to crisis. Hyperthermia causes excess sweating, however, and can lead to dehydration, which can also cause sickling. Temperature monitoring and the use of hypothermia and hyperthermia blankets can allow maintenance of body temperature in the optimal range of 36° to 37° C.

Cardiac monitoring is important because the occurrence of arrhythmias, such as extrasystole and prolonged P-R interval, in patients with sickling is high. Vasodilators or vasoconstrictors should be avoided, if possible, because the dilators can cause hypotension and the vasoconstrictors can cause circulatory stasis.

Respiratory rate and volume should be monitored closely so that hypoxia can be avoided. Oxygen saturation or arterial blood gas monitoring can aid in assessing respiratory status, and postoperative pain should be managed with drugs that do not depress respiratory function.

Kidney function should be monitored because the renal tubules become blocked by the hemolyzed red blood cells if crisis occurs and infarcts may occur in some areas of the kidney. Insertion of a urinary catheter to monitor urinary output at regular intervals has proved useful.

Sickle Cell Crisis

The types of crisis seen in sickle cell anemia are vasoocclusive, aplastic, sequestration, and hemolytic. The vasoocclusive crisis is the most common type and is characterized by tissue ischemia, infarction, and necrosis. The bones, tendons, synovia, spleen, liver, and intestine are common sites of occlusion. Infections, dehydration, high altitudes, extreme physical exertion, and emotional upsets can trigger this type of crisis.[23]

The aplastic crisis is most grave and constitutes a medical emergency. It is characterized by a sudden drastic decrease in red blood cell production. The patient initially appears weak and has signs of cardiac decompensation.[24]

The spleen is involved in sequestration crisis. A large amount of blood becomes trapped in the spleen and thus causes hypovolemia and shock, which constitutes a medical emergency. Clinically, the patient's blood pressure decreases and the pulse rate increases. Palpation and percussion reveal an enlarged mass in the right upper quadrant of the abdomen.

Bacterial infections, poisons, and medications, such as phenothiazines and sulfonamides, aspirin in large quantities, and quinine, can produce hemolysis of the red blood cell. The patient also has an enzyme deficiency (glucose-6-phosphodehydrogenase) in this type of sickle cell anemia.

If crisis occurs, the following modes of treatment are recommended: keep the patient warm; treat infections; and maintain oxygenation, hydration, and alkalinization. Heparin may be administered to reduce the risks of embolus formation, and magnesium sulfate may also be indicated for its vasodilator and anticoagulant properties.

SUMMARY

Patients with various chronic disorders present the perianesthesia nurse with significant challenges throughout the perianesthesia phase of hospitalization. The number of patients with COPD is increasing exponentially. These patients have altered lung mechanics; with the appropriate knowledge base for reversal of the altered lung mechanics, these patients have an excellent outcome during recovery from anesthesia. In addition, patients who have a history of cigarette smoking present significant challenges to the perianesthesia nurse. These patients often have COPD and usually need enhanced evidence-based care in the PACU because of the chronic bronchitis that is associated with cigarette smoking. Perianesthesia nursing care was presented with a focus on the maintenance of a patent airway and enhanced use of the modified stir-up regimen.

Another chronic disease that is becoming a national health issue is diabetes. As described in this chapter, these patients usually need enhanced care in regard to fluid and electrolytes and glucose management. Another chronic disease, sickle cell disease, was presented with a focus on identification of possible clinical problems and appropriate nursing interventions during the perianesthesia phase.

In many cases, the chronic disorders presented in this chapter have a pathophysiologic process that can be generalized to other patients. It is certainly important to acquire specific information on the disease process for a patient who is suffering from chronic diseases not specifically discussed in this chapter.

REFERENCES

1. Atlee J: *Complications in anesthesia*, ed 2, Philadelphia, 2007, Saunders.
2. Fisher L: *Anesthesia and uncommon diseases*, ed 5, Philadelphia, 2007, Saunders.
3. Warner D: Helping surgical patients quit smoking: who, when, and how, *Anesth Analg* 101:481–487, 2005.
4. O'Rourke J, et al: The effects of exposure to environmental tobacco smoke on pulmonary function in children undergoing anesthesia for minor surgery, *Ped Anesth* 16:560–567, 2006.
5. Theadom A, Cropley M: Effects of preoperative smoking cessation on the incidence and risk of intraoperative and postoperative complications in adult smokers: a systematic review, *Tob Control* 15:352–358, 2006.
6. Moores L: Smoking and postoperative pulmonary complications: an evidence-based review of the recent literature, *Clin Chest Med* 21:139–146, 2000.
7. Nagelhout J, Plaus K: *Nurse anesthesia*, ed 4, St. Louis, 2010, Saunders.
8. Marley R, Hoyle BL: Respiratory care. In Schick L, Windle PE: *Perianesthesia nursing core curriculum: preprocedure, phase I and phase II PACU nursing*, ed 2, St. Louis, 2010, Saunders.
9. Daley K: Patients with chronic diseases. In Stannard D, Krenzischek DA: *Perianesthesia nursing care*, Sudbury, Mass, 2012, Jones & Bartlett.
10. Centers for Disease Control, US Department of Health and Human Services: *National diabetes fact sheet*, 2011, available at www.cdc.gov/diabetes/pubs/factsheet11.htm. Accessed November 27, 2011.
11. Fain J: Management of clients with diabetes mellitus. In Black J, Hawks J, editors: *Medical surgical nursing; clinical management for positive outcomes*, ed 8, St. Louis, 2009, Saunders.
12. American Diabetes Association: Diagnosis and classification of diabetes, *Diabetes Care* 34(suppl 1):S1–2, S62–S69, 2011.
13. Khan N, et al: Perioperative management of diabetes mellitus, *UpToDate*, available at www.uptodate.com/contents/perioperative-management-of-diabetes-mellitus?source=search_result&search=perioperative+management+of+diabetes+mellitus&selectedTitle=1%7E150. Accessed December 30, 2011.
14. Loh-Trivedi M: Perioperative management of the diabetic patient, available at http://emedicine.medscape.com/article/284451-overview. Accessed May 5, 2012.
15. Furlong K, et al: Perioperative management of endocrine disorders. In Merli G, Weitz H, editors: *Medical management of the surgical patient*, ed 3, St. Louis, 2008, Saunders.
16. Furnary A, et al: Continuous intravenous insulin infusion reduces the incidence of deep sternal wound infection in diabetic patients after cardiac surgical procedures, *Annals of Thoracic Surgery* 67(2):352–60, 1999.
17. Van den Berghe G, et al: Intensive insulin therapy in the critically ill patients, *New England Journal of Medicine* 345:1359, 2001.
18. Raju TA, et al: Perioperative blood glucose monitoring in the general surgical population, *Journal of Diabetes Science and Technology*, 3(6):1282–1287, 2009.
19. MacKenzie C, Sharrock N: Perioperative medical considerations in patients with rheumatoid arthritis, *Rheum Dis Clin North Am* 24:1–17, 1998.
20. Longnecker D, et al: *Anesthesiology*, New York, 2007, McGraw Hill Medical.
21. Davis P, et al: *Smith's anesthesia for infants and children*, ed 8, St. Louis, 2011, Mosby.
22. Firth PG, et al: A survey of perioperative management of sickle cell disease in North America, *Pediatric Anesthesia* 21:43–49, 2011.
23. Miller R, Pardo M: *Basics of anesthesia*, ed 6, Philadelphia, 2011, Saunders.
24. Stoelting R: *Pharmacology and physiology in anesthetic practice*, ed 4, Philadelphia, 2005, Lippincott Williams & Wilkins.

RESOURCES

AACN: *Core curriculum for progressive care nursing*, Philadelphia, 2010, Saunders.
Aguilar D: Glycated hemoglobin as a prognostic marker in nondiabetic patients after acute myocardial infarction: what now? *Circulation* 124:666–668, 2011.

Barash P, et al: *Clinical anesthesia*, ed 6, Philadelphia, 2009, Lippincott Williams & Wilkins.

Barrett K, et al: *Ganong's review of medical physiology*, ed 23, New York, 2009, McGraw-Hill Medical.

Brunton L, et al: *Goodman and Gilman's the pharmacological basis of therapeutics*, ed 12, New York, 2010, McGraw-Hill Professional.

Drake R, et al: *Gray's anatomy for students*, ed 2, Philadelphia, 2009, Churchill Livingstone.

Deutschman C, Netigan P: *Evidence-based practice of critical care*, Philadelphia, 2010, Saunders.

Hall J: *Guyton and Hall textbook of medical physiology*, ed 12, Philadelphia, 2011, Saunders.

Hemmerling T, et al: Comparison of a continuous glucose-insulin-potassium infusion versus intermittent bolus application of insulin on perioperative glucose control and hormone status in insulin-treated type 2 diabetics, *J Clin Anesth* 13:293–300, 2001.

Hines R, Marschall K: *Handbook for Stoelting's anesthesia and co-existing disease*, ed 3, Philadelphia, 2009, Saunders.

Mason R: *Murray and Nadel's textbook of respiratory medicine*, ed 5, Philadelphia, 2011, Saunders.

Michaelian N, et al: Perioperative glycemic control: use of a hospital-wide protocol to safely improve hyperglycemia, *J Perianesth Nurs* 26:242–251, 2011.

Miller R, et al: *Miller's anesthesia*, ed 7, Philadelphia, 2009, Churchill Livingstone.

Pasero C, McCaffery M: *Pain assessment and pharmacologic management*, St. Louis, 2011, Mosby.

Pasero C, McCaffery M: Orthopaedic postoperative pain management, *J Perianesth Nurs* 22(3):160–174, 2007.

Townsend C, et al: *Sabiston's textbook of surgery*, ed 18, Philadelphia, 2008, Saunders.

Vincent J, et al: *Textbook of critical care*, ed 6, Philadelphia, 2011, Saunders.

49 Care of the Pediatric Patient

Elizabeth Howell, BS, BSN, CRNA

Delivery of optimal perianesthesia nursing care to pediatric patients requires an appreciation of the uniqueness of this population of individuals. Pediatric patients are not merely small adults; they are individuals with numerous unique anatomic, physiologic, and psychological characteristics. Because this population represents a wide range of ages and developmental stages, meeting the needs of this diverse group can present a multitude of challenges to the perianesthesia nurse. The goals of this chapter are to simplify approaches to managing and caring for our pediatric population in a safe environment and to promote a rewarding and enjoyable experience for both the nurse and patient. To meet these goals this chapter will provide an overview of the unique characteristics of pediatric patients and discuss the perioperative management of pediatric patients.

DEFINITIONS

Analgesia: Absence of pain.
Anesthetic: An agent used to produce anesthesia.
Anesthesia: Partial or complete loss of sensation, with or without loss of consciousness; referred to in this chapter as the administration of an anesthetic agent via injection or inhalation.
Antagonist: To counteract the action of something else, such as a drug that binds to a receptor site and prevents receptor stimulation.
Anticholinergic: A parasympatholytic; blocks the parasympathetic nerve fibers and parasympathetic nerve impulse conduction.
Anxiolytic: Medication used to reduce, relieve, or counteract anxiety.
Apnea/Apneic: Suspension of breathing.
Aspiration: The general use of this term is to draw in or out via suction; however, specifically referred to in this chapter are situations in which an individual is at risk for entry of gastric secretions, oropharyngeal secretions, or exogenous food or fluids into tracheobronchial passages, because of loss of the normal protective mechanisms as occurs with induction of general anesthesia.
Atelectasis: A collapse, lack of expansion, or airless condition of the lungs.
Barotrauma: An injury caused by a change in atmospheric pressure relative to a potentially closed space within a surrounding area.

Child: Younger than 13 years of age; before puberty.
Conception: Onset of pregnancy with implantation of a fertilized ovum in the uterine wall; fertilization.
Delirium: An acute and reversible condition characterized by agitation, confusion, disorientation, hallucinations or delusions, difficulty focusing attention, and inability to rest.
Desaturation: When oxygen is dissociated from hemoglobin.
Dissociative: A type of anesthesia with marked catalepsy, amnesia, and analgesia.
Dysphoria: A mood disorder of restlessness without apparent cause, anxiety, dissatisfaction, and discomfort.
Emergence: To evolve or rise out of anesthesia to a level of consciousness and status of protective reflexes, motor activity, and orientation.
Emergence Delirium: Occurs during initial cessation from general anesthesia to an awake state and initial transfer into the postanesthesia care unit.
Erythropoiesis: Forming red blood cells.
Gestation: Period of intrauterine fetal development from conception to birth.
Hemostasis: To stop bleeding; stasis refers to standing still.
Hypercarbia, Hypercapnia: Elevated above normal levels of carbon dioxide in the blood (>45 mm Hg).
Hyperflexion: Increased flexion of a joint; in this text, refers to the neck.
Hyperoxia: Increased levels of oxygen in the blood.
Hyperthermia, Hyperpyrexia: An elevated body temperature greater than the normal range.
Hypervolemia: An abnormal increase in circulating blood volume.
Hypothermia: A lower body temperature below normal range.
Hypovolemia: An abnormal decrease in circulating blood volume.
Hypoxemia: Decreased levels of oxygen in the blood.
Induction: Anesthetization, onset of general anesthesia.
Infant: Includes the neonatal period and extends through 12 months of age.
Inhalation: To draw a breath, vapor, or gas into the lungs.
Inspiratory Pressure: An active positive pressure ventilatory maneuver in which a delivered volume of gas is given to a set peak level of pressure before passive expiration.
Isotonic: In this chapter, pertains to an intravenous solution with the same osmotic pressure as normal body fluid.

Laryngospasm: A spasm of the laryngeal muscles.

Larynx: The musculocartilaginous organ at the upper end of the trachea, below the root of the tongue, and part of the airway and vocal apparatus.

Macroglossia: An abnormally small tongue.

Maintenance: Stage of anesthesia in which relaxation of muscles and loss of sensation and consciousness are adequate for the performance of surgery.

Micrognathia: Refers to the jaw; abnormal smallness, particularly of the lower jaw.

Neonatal Period: The first 28 days of life.

Newborn ("Newly Born"): Younger than 72 hours.

Occiput: The back part of the skull.

Parenteral: Any route of administration for a medication other than alimentary; such as intravenous, subcutaneous, intramuscular, or mucosal.

Pediatrics: The medical science specific to the care of children and treatment of diseases that occur in childhood.

Pharynx: Refers to the passageway from the nasal and oral cavity to the larynx and esophagus.

Postconceptual Age: Postgestational age (number of weeks since birth) plus conceptual age (number of weeks at delivery).

Premature Newborn: Birth before 37 weeks' gestation.

Rebreathing: Inhalation of a gas or gases previously exhaled.

Retrognathia: When the mandible lies behind the frontal plane of the maxilla.

Thermogenesis: Heat production. Nonshivering thermogenesis is a physiologic response of the newborn infant during periods of hypothermia with stimulation of the sympathetic catabolism of brown fat with release of energy in the form of heat. Brown fat is primarily located in the neck and chest of the infant.

ANATOMIC AND PHYSIOLOGIC CONSIDERATIONS

Respiratory System

Understanding the differences between the adult and pediatric respiratory systems is essential to properly manage the pediatric airway. There are several distinctions of the pediatric airway that make these patients more susceptible to airway obstruction and hypoxemia.[1,2-5] Respiratory distress will occur quickly in the pediatric patient if respiratory complications are not managed quickly and properly.[2]

The newborn has small nares, a large tongue, a small mandible, a short neck, and a large amount of upper airway lymphoid tissue.[2-6] Newborns are considered obligate or preferential nose breathers[4-6]; therefore anything that partially or fully blocks the nares can result in respiratory compromise. In the neonate, the epiglottis is at the level of the first cervical vertebra (C1); however, the epiglottis usually moves down to the level of C3 by 6 months of age (this makes oral breathing more feasible).[3] The epiglottis of the newborn is U shaped versus being flatter in the adult. A straight laryngoscope blade may be more maneuverable in the pediatric airway and is most commonly used for intubation in pediatric patients. The tracheal length is relatively short in children, which makes proper placement and securing of the endotracheal tube critical to avoid bronchial intubation (or accidental extubation).[7] When the endotracheal tube is secured (and anytime the patient is repositioned), the presence of bilateral breath sounds and end-tidal carbon dioxide ($ETCO_2$) should be reconfirmed.

The vocal cords of the newborn are more anterior (C4) than in adults (C6)[3-5]; this makes it more difficult to properly align the airway for ventilation and intubation.[5,6] Historically, the shape of the child's larynx has been thought to resemble that of an inverted cone with the narrowest portion of the trachea residing at the cricoid cartilage.[1,3,4,6] Recent research suggests that the narrowest portion of the pediatric trachea may actually be the glottis.[5] No matter where the smallest diameter lies, the diameter of the endotracheal tube that can be used is limited. In addition, because the diameter of the pediatric airway is small, airway edema may lead to significant narrowing (and potential occlusion) of the airway.

Newborns are diaphragmatic breathers.[5,6] The ribs of newborns are situated horizontally in a cylindrical thorax, which limits thorax expansion. Consequently, ventilatory efforts are the result almost entirely of the movement of the diaphragm. Newborns are susceptible to ventilator problems when excursion of the diaphragm is impeded. As a result, gastric distention caused by faulty bag and mask ventilation, improper positioning, or bowel obstruction can produce inadequate ventilation.[5] In the pediatric patient, the sternum and anterior rib cage are compliant, and the intercostal and accessory muscles of respiration are poorly developed. The respiratory rates of infants and young children (Table 49-1) are faster than those of adults.[5] This faster rate is a result of (1) the lung volumes in infants being extremely small in relation to their body size and (2) the higher metabolic rates in infants (oxygen consumption per unit body weight is double that of adults). This is the main reason that pediatric patients rapidly desaturate during short periods of hypoventilation or apnea.

The control of breathing in infants during the first several weeks of life differs significantly from that of the adult patient. As in the adult, the newborn's primary drive to ventilation is carbon dioxide;

Table 49-1	Respiratory and Cardiovascular Age-Related Changes in Children					
AGE	RESPIRATORY RATE (BREATHS/MIN)	HEART RATE AWAKE (BEATS/MIN)	HEART RATE ASLEEP (BEATS/MIN)	HEART RATE EXERCISE/FEVER (BEATS/MIN)	SYSTOLIC BLOOD PRESSURE (MM HG)	DIASTOLIC BLOOD PRESSURE (MM HG)
Newborn	45-60	100-180 (140)	80-160	<220	65	40
12 mo	40	80-160 (120)	70-120	<200	95	65
3 yr	30	80-120 (100)	60-90	<200	100	70
6 yr	25	70-115 (100)	60-90	<200	90	60
12 yr	20	65-90 (80)	50-90	<200	110	60

Modified from Davis PJ, et al: *Smith's anesthesia for infants and children,* ed 8, Philadelphia, 2011, Mosby.

however, hypoxemia depresses rather than stimulates respiration in the newborn.[5] This secondary response is potentiated further by hypothermia, a condition that can occur at any point in the perioperative period.

The respiratory control center in both full-term and premature infants can fatigue easily; therefore ventilatory reaction to high carbon dioxide tensions or to low percentage of oxygen is not as rapid in the newborn.[5] As a result, the newborn might not be able to compensate for rapid changes in arterial blood gas levels. By 3 weeks of age, hypoxemia induces sustained hyperventilation, as in older children and adults.[5] In addition, newborns and infants may breathe irregularly because of the lack of a mature respiratory center. Periodic breathing is often seen in this age group.[5]

Endotracheal intubation is more widely used in pediatric anesthesia today and is considered the preferable airway management technique for general anesthesia in premature infants and most neonates. The reason for this change is that the premature infant and neonate can prove difficult to ventilate by mask, which increases the risk of filling the stomach with air during mask ventilation.[1] Both endotracheal tube and laryngeal mask airways have been used safely in children of all ages (Table 49-2). The advantages of endotracheal intubation include decreased dead space, avoidance of laryngospasm and gastric distention, and prevention of aspiration; however, the incidence rate of post intubation edema from trauma and infection may be increased.

Cardiovascular System

As the pediatric patient matures, the cardiovascular system undergoes substantial changes. Normally the respiratory rate and heart rate decreases with increasing age.[5] Advancing age and increasing body size result in increases in the systolic and diastolic

blood pressure. The cardiovascular age-related changes for newborns, infants, and children are summarized in Table 49-1. The newborn heart functions near its peak ventricular function and therefore has little cardiac reserve. Thus, in the newborn, heart rate plays a major role in determination of cardiac function.[5] The newborn is relatively unable to compensate for suboptimal conditions such as hypoxemia, acidosis, or myocardial depression.[5] With the advent of more sophisticated blood pressure monitoring devices, measurements in infants can be taken with greater accuracy. The pediatric patient ordinarily has the usual signs of impending shock or airway obstruction, but physiologic status deteriorates rapidly if the problem is not rectified quickly.[1-3,5,6] The perianesthesia nurse should closely observe children for subtle changes in cardiovascular status. If abnormalities arise, prompt intervention is essential.

At birth, fetal hemoglobin levels are high compared with those in the adult patient; however, the fetal hemoglobin does not readily release the oxygen it carries to tissues. Hemoglobin values decrease progressively and reach their lowest values by 2 to 3 months of age.[5] By 4 to 6 months of age, the amount of oxygen available to tissues begins to increase and reaches the highest value usually by 10 months of age. This increase remains steady during the first decade of life. Research regarding the physiologic anemia of childhood suggests that, although children's hemoglobin levels are lower than adults, oxygen unloading at the tissue level is increased in children.[5] This allows a lower level of hemoglobin in infants and children to be as efficient in tissue oxygenation as a higher hemoglobin in adult patients (Table 49-3).

Composition and Regulation of Body Fluids

Maturation of the kidneys in newborns occurs rapidly. In the neonate, renal function is characterized

Table 49-2   Pediatric Airway Equipment

AGE	WEIGHT (KG)	INTERNAL DIAMETER (MM)	LENGTH ORAL (CM)	LENGTH NASAL (CM)	SUCTION CATHETER	LMA SIZE (NO.)	LMA CUFF VOLUME (mL)	ORAL AIRWAY SIZE*
Premature	0.7-1.0	2.5 uncuffed	7-8	9	5F	—	—	000-00
Premature	1.0-2.5	3.0 uncuffed	8-9	9-10	5F	—	—	000 (30 mm)
Newborn	2.5-3.0	3.5 uncuffed	9-10	11-12	6F	1	2-5	00 (40 mm)
3 mo	3.5-5.0	3.5 uncuffed	10-11	12	6F	1	2-5	0 (50 mm)
3-9 mo	5.0-8.0	3.5-4.0 uncuffed	11-12	13-14	6F	1.5	7	0 (50 mm)
9-18 mo	8.0-11	4.0-4.5 cuffed	12-13	14-15	8F	1.5	7	1 (60 mm)
1.5-3 yr	11-15	4.5-5.0 uncuffed	12-14	16-17	8F	2	10	1 (60 mm)
4-5 yr	15-18	5.0-5.5 uncuffed	14-16	18-19	10F	2	10	2 (70 mm)
6-7 yr	19-23	5.5-6.0 uncuffed	16-18	19-20	10F	2.5	14	2 (70 mm)
8-10 yr	24-30	6.0-6.5 cuffed	17-19	24-25	10F	2.5	14	3 (80 mm)
10-11 yr	30-35	6.0-6.5 cuffed	18-20	22-24	12F	3.0	15-20	3 (80 mm)
12-13 yr	35-40	6.5-7.0 cuffed	19-21	23-25	12F	3.0	15-20	3 (80 mm)
14-16 yr	45-55	7.0-7.5 uncuffed	20-22	24-25	12F	3.0	15-20	3 (80 mm)

Adapted from Davis PJ, et al: *Smith's anesthesia for infants and children*, ed 8, Philadelphia, 2011, Mosby.
LMA, Laryngeal mask airway; *ML*, milliliters of air for inflation of cuff.
*Oral airway size as a guide. A quick method of determining oral airway size is by placing the airway along the side of the face. The oral airway length should extend from the lips to the angle of the mandible.

Table 49-3   Equivalent Hemoglobin Values for Adults, Infants, and Neonates

	HEMOGLOBIN FOR EQUIVALENT OXYGEN DELIVERY TO TISSUES						
AGE	HEMOGLOBIN (g/dL)						
Adult	7	8	9	10	11	12	13
Infant (>6 mo)	5.7	6.5	7.3	8.2	9.0	9.8	10.6
Neonate (<2 mo)	10.3	11.7	13.2	14.7	16.1	17.6	19.1

From Davis PJ, et al: *Smith's anesthesia for infants and children*, ed 8, Philadelphia, 2011, Mosby.

with obligate salt loss, slow clearance of fluid overload, and an inability to conserve fluid.[8] Consequently, newborns are intolerant of both dehydration and fluid overload. The newborn can conserve sodium to some degree despite a low glomerular filtration rate and limited tubular function[5]; however, premature infants are prone to hyponatremia and water overloading. Dehydration in the neonate of any gestational age has harmful effects on renal function.[5] Moreover, decreased renal function can delay the excretion of drugs primarily eliminated by renal clearance. At 20 weeks after birth, maturation of glomerular filtration and tubular function is nearly complete.[4,5]

The blood volume of the newborn younger than 1 month of age is approximately 80 to 90 mL/kg[3]; however, the blood volume of the premature newborn is as high as 100 mL/kg. The estimated blood volume of an infant from 3 months until 3 years of age is 75 to 80 mL/kg. In children older than 6 years, the estimated blood volume approximates that of an adult (65 mL/kg in the adult female; 70 mL/kg in the adult male).[3]

Water distribution in the various body compartments is markedly different among the premature newborn, the full-term newborn, the child, and the adult. Water distribution is significant because body water composition affects the volume of distribution of drugs. Premature infants have the highest percentage of fluid in the extracellular fluid compartment. A progressive decrease in total body water and distribution to the extracellular fluid compartment is seen during the first year of life. Complete maturation of renal function occurs when the child reaches 2 to 3 years of age. The fluid requirements for infants and children are reviewed in Table 49-4.

It is important to assess the hydration status of the pediatric patient to formulate an appropriate therapeutic strategy. Guidelines for

SPECIAL CONSIDERATIONS

Table 49-4	Formula for Hourly Maintenance Fluid Requirements in Infants and Children
BODY WEIGHT (KG)	**HOURLY FLUID REQUIREMENT***
0-10	4 mL/kg/h for each 1 kg body weight
10-20	40 mL + 2 mL/kg/h for each 1 kg >10 kg
>20	60 mL + 1 mL/kg/h for each 1 kg >20 kg

From Davis PJ, et al: *Smith's anesthesia for infants and children,* ed 8, Philadelphia, 2011, Mosby.
*Based on 1 mL of fluid per 1 kcal of caloric expenditure.

assessing dehydration in children are provided in Table 49-5. Laboratory data, history and physical, and assessment of fluid input and output should be used to aid in the diagnosis of dehydration and guide therapy.

Thermal Regulation

Newborns and infants are sensitive to heat loss because they have a relatively large body surface area, a relatively small amount of subcutaneous fat, poor vasomotor control, and a decreased ability to produce heat.[9] The primary mechanism of heat production in a neonate is nonshivering thermogenesis mediated by brown fat.[1,5,10] Shivering is of little significance to thermal regulation. When ambient temperature falls (<33° C), epinephrine is released by the sympathetic nervous system to activate thermogenesis. The preterm newborn needs a higher ambient temperature (at least 35° C) to minimize oxygen consumption.[5] Ordinarily, to maintain a body temperature within normal limits, infants metabolize brown fat, cry, and move about vigorously. Newborns and infants respond to a cold environment by increasing their metabolism, which ultimately leads to an increase in oxygen consumption and the production of organic acids.

PREMATURITY

A premature newborn is defined as birth before 37 weeks' gestation.[3,5,6,8] The often labile condition of a premature neonate demands meticulous and vigilant perianesthesia care. Careful attention must be given to airway maintenance, medication dosage, fluid management, and temperature regulation. Premature infants and infants younger than 6 months are prone to airway obstruction and apneic episodes.[3,5] Most infants in whom postanesthesia apnea develops are less than 46 weeks of postconceptual age; however, apnea has been

Table 49-5	Assessment and Evaluation of Dehydration in Children		
CRITERIA	**MILD DEHYDRATION**	**MODERATE DEHYDRATION**	**SEVERE DEHYDRATION**
Signs and Symptoms			
Weight loss (%)	5	10	15
Fluid deficit (mL/kg)	50	100	150
Vital Signs			
Pulse	Normal	Increase; weak	Greatly increased; feeble
Blood pressure	Normal	Normal to low	Reduced and orthostatic
Respiration	Normal	Deep	Deep and rapid
General Appearance			
Infants	Thirsty, restless, alert	Thirsty, restless or lethargic, but able to be aroused	Drowsy to comatose, limp, cold, sweaty, gray color
Older children	Thirsty, restless, alert	Thirsty, alert, postural hypotension	Usually comatose, apprehensive, cyanotic, cold
Skin turgor	Normal	Decreased	Greatly decreased
Anterior fontanel	Normal	Sunken	Markedly depressed
Eyes	Normal	Sunken	Markedly sunken
Mucous membranes	Moist	Dry	Very dry
Urine			
Flow (mL/kg/h)	<2	<1	<0.5
Specific gravity	1.020	1.020-1.030	>1.030

From Davis PJ, et al: *Smith's anesthesia for infants and children,* ed 8, Philadelphia, 2011, Mosby.

reported in infants up to 60 weeks of postconceptual age.[2] In addition to apneic spells, pulmonary complications include hyaline membrane disease and bronchopulmonary dysplasia. In addition, the premature neonate is immunocompromised and at greater risk for postoperative infection. In the sick premature neonate, the likelihood of blood transfusions, artificial ventilation, and the need for parenteral nutrition is greater.[2] The risk of apnea in the postanesthesia care unit (PACU) may be decreased with intravenous (IV) administration of caffeine (10 mg/kg).[5] In neonates, the half-life of caffeine is 37 to 231 hours.[5] By 4 months of age, the half-life of caffeine decreases dramatically to approximately 6 hours and is similar to that in an adult. In addition, several authors cite the initial discovery of xanthine derivatives, such as theophylline or aminophylline, as a respiratory stimulant that can be used to decrease the frequency of apneic episodes in the newborn.[2,5,8]

Retinopathy of Prematurity

Retrolental fibroplasia is a fibrovascularization and scarring of the retina. Although this disease is associated with hyperoxia (too much oxygen), a multitude of other risk factors may be involved, and the role of oxygen therapy is controversial.[5,8] The risk of this retinal disorder is to newborns, especially premature infants who are born before 36 weeks' gestation and weigh less than 1000 to 1500 g.[5] Vascularization of the retina is complete at approximately 44 weeks' gestation.[8] The extreme prematurity may be the single most important factor in the development of retinopathy of prematurity. The normal PaO_2 in neonates is between 60 and 80 mm Hg. Oxygenation is recommended to be continuously monitored with pulse oximetry, and hyperoxia should be avoided; therefore a saturation of 90% to 95% results in a PaO_2 in the range of 60 to 80 mm Hg.[5,6,8] In addition, the pulse oximeter probe must be placed on the right upper extremity or ear lobe, in case of a patent ductus arteriosus. Placement of two pulse oximeter probes on the premature infant may be helpful. Moreover, when an arterial catheter is indicated, it also should be placed in the right upper extremity.

In susceptible patients who are exposed to a hyperoxic environment, blood gas tension should be measured and an oxygen analyzer used to confirm the oxygen concentration. It is not known what level of oxygenation, or what exact length of exposure time, might lead to the development of retinopathy of prematurity.[8] One must consider that attempts to prevent arterial hyperoxia and

visual impairment must be tempered with the realization that unrecognized arterial hypoxemia can result in irreversible brain damage.

Infant Respiratory Distress Syndrome

Infant respiratory distress syndrome (IRDS), once called *hyaline membrane disease,* is a severe disorder of the lungs of the newborn.[11] The incidence rate of IRDS increases in premature infants. The basis of the pathogenesis of IRDS is insufficient surfactant levels.[8] Surfactant is beneficial for the following two functions: (1) reduction of surface tension so that less pressure is required to hold the alveoli open and (2) maintenance of alveolar stability with adjustment of surface tension to changes in alveolar size. Insufficient surfactant levels increase surface tension at the alveolar air-liquid interface, resulting in alveolar collapse, an inordinate increase in the work of breathing, and impaired gas exchange. This impaired gas exchange results in hypoxemia and hypercarbia. In addition, the pulmonary vascular resistance is increased and leads to hypoperfusion of pulmonary and systemic circulation. This hypoperfusion, along with hypoxemia, causes tissue hypoxia and metabolic acidosis. An increase in survival with a decrease in serious complications is associated with administration of surfactant into the lungs at birth.[5] As lung compliance improves, a progressive decrease in tidal volume and positive inspiratory pressure helps to prevent further lung injury.

Treatment for neonates with severe IRDS includes oxygen therapy, maintenance of intravenous fluids and nutritional support, temperature regulation, arterial blood gas monitoring, and laboratory sampling.[8,11,12] Extremely preterm infants and those with severe disease often need intubation during delivery room resuscitation or shortly after birth.[8] In addition, intermittent positive-pressure mechanical ventilation with positive end-expiratory pressure may be necessary to ventilate the exceptionally stiff lungs of these neonates. Chronic air trapping in preterm infants can occur, and excessive inflation pressures must be avoided.[5]

PEDIATRIC PERIANESTHESIA CONSIDERATIONS AND TECHNIQUES

Preoperative Period

The preoperative meeting with the pediatric patient and his or her guardians begins the foundation of the perioperative care for this child. A thorough preoperative examination of the pediatric patient and the child's medical record enable the nurse to assess the patient's general state of health and identify chronic or acute disease processes. The preoperative evaluation includes (1) reviewing the patient's chart; (2) reviewing current and past medical history of the patient with the patient and guardian(s); (3) determining medication, latex, and food allergies; (4) determining the fasting (nothing by mouth [NPO]) status of the patient; (5) formulating a list of the patient's current medications (including herbal medications); and (6) reviewing any lab tests. Most importantly, the preoperative interview gives the nurse the opportunity to gain the confidence of the patient and caregiver which can help to alleviate anxiety. Depending on the age of the child, after the interview the nurse may be responsible for starting the intravenous catheter for the pediatric patient. If the child is healthy, this task may be postponed until the operating room, after mask induction with general anesthesia has been initiated.

Before initiating any preoperative interventions, the NPO status of the patient must be confirmed. NPO guidelines have been formulated to help prevent the aspiration of stomach contents into the lungs during surgery. The most current guidelines suggest the following: (1) solids are prohibited within 6 to 8 hours of surgery, (2) formula is prohibited within 6 hours of surgery, (3) breast milk is prohibited within 4 hours of surgery, and (4) clear liquids are prohibited within 2 hours of surgery.[1]

Even if the nurse gains the trust of the child and guardians, this may not be enough to alleviate all of the pediatric patient's anxiety. Premedication with various anxiolytic medications might aid in these situations. It must be remembered, however, that the most common fear for children concerning hospitalization is the pain from needles or venopuncture; therefore the route of administration should be considered carefully. Children 1 year of age and older benefit from anxiolytic premedication to decrease preoperative anxiety and modify behavioral changes after discharge.[13] Many anesthesia practitioners use oral midazolam premedication in pediatric patients 1 year of age and older, in whom a greater likelihood of uncontrollable separation anxiety exists. In addition, midazolam can be given intramuscularly, intravenously, rectally, or intranasally as an alternative route of administration for pediatric premedicant.[13] However, the oral route is generally preferred unless preoperative intravenous access is available. The effect of premedication

in children varies from sedation to extreme excitation. Flumazenil is a competitive antagonist at the benzodiazepine receptor and is used as a reversal agent for midazolam.[5,8,14] An initial dose has been recommended of 0.2 mg of flumazenil IV (8 to 15 mcg/kg IV) given over 15 seconds[14]; this usually reverses the central nervous system effects of midazolam within 2 minutes. If need, additional doses of 0.1 mg IV to a total of 1 mg IV can be administered at 60-second intervals.[14]

An anticholinergic drug, such as glycopyrrolate or atropine, may be given preoperatively to protect against bradycardia, which can occur with the induction of general anesthesia.[5,8,14] The most popular inhalation anesthetic agents used for pediatric anesthesia are halothane, sevoflurane, isoflurane, and desflurane. Halothane and sevoflurane are the most common induction inhalation agents, although halothane is no longer available for use in the United States. Sevoflurane may be superior to halothane for mask induction of general anesthesia because of (1) a quicker induction of anesthesia, (2) less incidence of cardiac arrhythmias, (3) more rapid psychomotor recovery postoperatively, and (4) less nausea and vomiting.[15] After induction of general anesthesia with either sevoflurane or halothane, and when the child reaches the maintenance phase of general anesthesia, the anesthesia provider may switch to either isoflurane or desflurane. To help prevent emergence delirium, an analgesic should be administered before emergence from general anesthesia and transfer to the PACU.

Ketamine, a dissociative anesthetic, is sometimes used in pediatrics as an induction agent or for short procedures, such as painful dressing changes that do not require muscle relaxation. Emergence time depends on route of administration and whether the drug was repeated during the operation. The most serious disadvantage to ketamine is a high incidence rate of emergence delirium, hallucinations, and possible psychosis.[14] Nystagmus can also occur. After the use of ketamine, the postanesthesia recovery area should be quiet and conducive to a slow peaceful emergence and recovery. A premedicant with a sedative, such as midazolam, can significantly reduce these side effects.[8] It is suggested that, if possible, ketamine should always be administered with a drug such as midazolam[1,8,14]; this helps to reduce the emergence delirium. Ketamine has the advantage of providing analgesia and supporting spontaneous respirations.[14] Caution should be used when additional opioids are given in the PACU. For uncooperative children or patients with Down syndrome or mental retardation, an intramuscular injection of midazolam combined with ketamine may be helpful.[2]

Evidence-Based Practice

In a retrospective study, Dahmani and colleagues investigated the utility of ketamine for postoperative pain management in children. The authors performed a comprehensive literature review and identified clinical trials that used ketamine as a perioperative analgesic medication for infants and children. The outcome measures for this study were postoperative analgesic requirements, pain intensity and duration, and duration of sensory block. The study revealed an association between ketamine use and decreased PACU postoperative pain intensity and decreased nonopioid analgesic requirements.

IMPLICATIONS FOR PRACTICE

Perianesthesia nurses can be actively involved in studies that evaluate the efficacy of pain management techniques. A prospective study evaluating these findings and investigating the effects of ketamine on the opioid consumption in pediatric patients postoperatively would be interesting. The use of ketamine as an adjunct to pain management techniques is increasing in all areas, including pediatrics. A perianesthesia nurse should have an understanding of the basic pharmacology of ketamine and how it affects patients to most effectively manage pain. The dissociative state induced by ketamine often results in an odd demeanor in patients (e.g., blank stare, nystagmus, difficulty verbalizing or odd verbalizations, hallucinations). When caring for a patient who has received ketamine, the nurse must remember that a calm, quiet environment will yield the best results.

Source: Dahmani S, et al: Ketamine for perioperative pain management in children: a meta-analysis of published studies, *Paediatr Anaesth* 21(6):636, 2011.

The opioid fentanyl can be given as a premedicant either IV or in the form of a lollipop called an *Oralet* (5 to 15 mcg/kg).[4] When using the Oralet, when the child becomes sedate, the Oralet naturally falls away from the child's mouth. With the Oralet, fentanyl levels continue to rise during surgery and contribute to postoperative analgesia. The fentanyl Oralet has fallen out of favor because of the potential for children to associate the medication with candy.

The introduction of the intravenous agent propofol has had a dramatic effect on pediatric anesthesia. Propofol can be used for sedation or general anesthesia and has minimal recovery time with few side effects.[8,14,16] Propofol can be used when administering anesthesia in remote locations and provides deep sedation for painful or frightening procedures.[1-3,5,8,14,17] This drug has advanced anesthesia care for children in remote locations such as magnetic resonance imaging or during procedures or therapy for hematology and oncology.[17,18] Propofol provides rapid onset of action and quick emergence from anesthesia with minimal residual effects.[19] Earlier discharge and decreased recovery time are particularly notable when propofol is the only anesthetic agent used.[20] Maintenance of anesthesia can be accomplished through repeated dosing or continuous infusion.[18] In addition, propofol has an antiemetic effect which has demonstrated usefulness in preventing postoperative nausea and vomiting in susceptible patients.[1,8,14]

POSTOPERATIVE CARE OF THE PEDIATRIC PATIENT

The pediatric patient is at high risk for complications in the postoperative period. Preparation for the pediatric patient's arrival from the operating room should begin well before the patient enters the PACU. If possible, the procedure, history, and physical examination for the patient should be reviewed before to the patient's arrival in the PACU. With computerized charting used more widely, the patient's history, antibiotics, and intake and output may be available before the patient's arrival. Information gained before the patient's arrival can help to prepare and anticipate potential complications.

A large percentage of children become hypoxic during the transfer from the operating room to the PACU. In addition, the primary organ dysfunction seen in children involves the respiratory system.[8] For these reasons, it is prudent to always transport the pediatric patient with supplemental oxygen. Furthermore, upon the patient's arrival to the PACU, the first task of the nurse is to administer humidified oxygen and then connect the pulse oximeter. While sufficient oxygenation is being confirmed, the blood pressure cuff and electrocardiogram (ECG) leads can be applied. Always remember airway, breathing, and circulation (ABCs). The initial assessment should include identification of a patent airway and confirmation of stable vital signs, including temperature. A humidified air-oxygen mixture (high-flow) should be administered, and a safe environment secured before report from the anesthetist is given. In a restless child or in one with a history of seizure disorder, side rail pads may be used. The pediatric patient is usually placed in the lateral position on the stretcher in the operating room for transport to PACU (Fig. 49-1). However, after an intraoral surgical procedure, the patient may be placed in the three-fourths prone position, more commonly

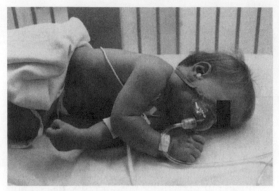

FIG. 49-1 An infant is transported to the postanesthesia care unit in lateral position. (From Motoyama E, Davis P: *Smith's anesthesia for infants and children,* ed 7, St. Louis, 2006, Mosby.)

known as the *tonsillar position,* to facilitate adequate drainage of secretions and blood.

During the report from the anesthesia provider and operating room circulating nurse, dressings should be checked for drainage and the intravenous infusion line should be checked for patency and that it is secured well to the patient. Children's teeth should be checked routinely on admission to the PACU and again before discharge. In the event of tooth loss, all teeth should be saved and given to the parents, if possible.

Over the years, anesthesia techniques have improved. With combined rapid-acting anesthetic agents, the pediatric patient usually arrives in the PACU awake and responsive, with good abdominal muscle tone. These patients are usually quickly responsive to verbal and tactile stimulation. However, it has been reported that as many as 30% of pediatric patients experience some type of agitation or delirium during their PACU stay.[8] Pediatric patients, especially those experiencing agitation, need constant nursing care to prevent injury to themselves. These patients can be extremely restless, vocal, and difficult to manage.

It must always be remembered that this agitation or excitement could be related to hypoxemia, the pharmacologic side effects of certain drugs, pain, or awakening in strange surroundings. Therefore, if a pediatric patient has hyperactive behavior, the perianesthesia nurse should assess the patient in the aforementioned areas to provide the appropriate interventions.

Psychosocial Considerations

The nurse must address issues of parental and child anxiety, which helps to lessen the stress on the child.[21] The parents should be allowed to be with the child as soon as is practical and preferably before the child awakens.[5,21] Remember that all surgical procedures and hospitalizations are extremely stressful for a family. When the pediatric patient emerges from anesthesia, the perianesthesia nurse should meet certain emotional needs of all children to facilitate positive outcomes of the perioperative experience. Explanations must be provided to the child in terms that can be understood. In addition, the nurse should always be completely honest with the child. The developmental age of the child determines which areas are of greatest concern (Table 49-6). For example, infants can become distressed when physical needs are not met. With the type of surgery and the degree of emergence from anesthesia taken into consideration, the primary caregiver should hold or rock the patient, if it is age-appropriate, or do both. This action usually relaxes the patient, and infants especially enjoy being swaddled in a warm blanket, cuddling, rocking, having the head or back rubbed, and hearing the voice of the nurse. In the infant younger than 6 months, the nurse is "mom."[7] Because the infant mimics facial expressions, the nurse should smile and use facial expressions of happiness when caring for all children. Another consideration is that the PACU is a strange environment for the child. Often, dolls, teddy bears, and other familiar objects from home are taken to surgery and arrive with the patient in

Table 49-6	Classic Stages of Development Theories for Children		
THEORY BASED ON AGE (YR)	FREUD PSYCHOSEXUAL	ERIKSON PSYCHOSOCIAL	PIAGET COGNITIVE
Infant (0-1)	Oral	Basic trust	Sensorimotor (stages 1-5)
Toddler (2-3)	Anal	Autonomy versus shame and doubt	Sensorimotor (stages 5, 6)
Preschool age (3-6)	Oedipal	Initiative versus guilt	Preoperational
School age (6-12)	Latency	Industry versus inferiority	Concrete operations
Adolescent (12-20)	Adolescence	Identity versus identity diffusion	Formal operations

From Kliegman RM, et al: *Nelson's textbook of pediatrics,* ed 19, Philadelphia, 2011, Saunders.

the PACU. These special toys should remain with the child, especially during emergence, to help the child cope with the environmental change.

In the older infant and preschool child, stranger anxiety remains the greatest fear. This stage is a particularly vulnerable one in childhood development. Children at 2 to 3 years of age are at the stage of autonomy versus self doubt. They may exhibit independence that alternates with sudden dependence and the need for periodic cuddling and reassurance. Their greatest fears include separation from parents, pain, physical harm, strange environments, and the unknown.[5] Often the only mechanism of self expression is crying. Negativism may be the child's means of demonstrating control; thus, "no" may actually mean "yes." Children of this age are prone to temper tantrums, ritualistic behavior, and breath-holding spells. The perianesthesia nurse should be sure to differentiate apnea from breath-holding spells when assessing the respiratory status of the patient. Three-year-old children are too young to use their own reason and can become impatient at times; therefore the perianesthesia nurse must avoid criticism and provide acceptable behavior alternatives to the patient.

Between 3 and 6 years of age, the child begins to become independent; however, in the PACU, dependency can occur because of pain, course of disease, or immobilization. Guilt can occur when the child desires to remain dependent.[8] Consequently, the perianesthesia nurse should provide as much opportunity for independence as possible. The nurse can foster independence by allowing the child to select alternatives in care.

The ages of 6 to 12 years coincide with entering school. These children are striving for approval when tasks are completed and usually do not tolerate failure because it promotes their sense of inferiority and inadequacy. The hospital environment is new to them, and the child may be unprepared to handle the situation and thus have difficulty with impulse control. The nurse should allow children as much individualization and self-care as possible, because children lose control when they are immobilized or ill. The nurse should also encourage self expression and compliment the child on accomplishments during recovery from anesthesia. Remember that a child of this age has a vivid imagination and could easily distort reality.[8]

The adolescent years of ages 12 to 20 are a transitory time characterized by vacillations between dependence and independence, idealism and realism, and confidence and uncertainty. The adolescent may experience anxiety over issues related to privacy, loss of control, autonomy, and competence. Privacy is of utmost importance to these patients; therefore the adolescent's body should be covered as much as possible to prevent exposure and resulting embarrassment.

The individual perioperative experience of each child greatly affects the success of future medical encounters. Addressing the developmental needs of the child and support of parental involvement can go a long way to meet the needs of the child and lead to a positive experience for the whole family. A preoperative program for elective surgical procedures that includes a tour of the PACU can help to reduce preoperative anxiety and minimize postoperative negative behaviors.

Monitoring

Initially, monitoring in the PACU includes respiratory rate, blood pressure, pulse oximetry, ECG, fluid balance, and temperature control.[1,5,8] When the vital signs are obtained, the PACU values should be first compared with the preoperative and intraoperative recordings of vital signs. After the initial blood pressure is ascertained, particularly for outpatients, pulse oximetry monitoring may be all that is needed. The pulse oximeter is superior to clinical judgment in providing the earliest warning of a desaturation event.[5,8] The frequency in measurement of other physiologic parameters depends on the status of the patient and the surgical procedure.

The rate and depth of ventilation should be monitored in the PACU. Respiratory depression occurs with greater frequency if muscle relaxants are used during general anesthesia. Because of the rapid ventilatory changes that can occur in the PACU, an oxygen saturation monitor should be used on all pediatric patients. A variable rate of fraction of inspired oxygen content delivery with supplemental oxygen can occur and is the result of delivery technique and patient depth of ventilation.

The most likely causes of respiratory failure in children with surgical disease include extrathoracic airway swelling and injury, thoracic dystrophy consistent with congenital disease or intraabdominal swelling, respiratory control abnormality such as occurs with congenital anomalies or drug induced, and loss of functional residual capacity that results in atelectasis.[8] The most common etiology involves the extrathoracic airway with swelling of the pharynx, larynx, or trachea. Infants and small children usually have a low incidence rate of postoperative atelectasis, because crying from pain or awakening in an unfamiliar environment stimulates ventilation. Older children tend to remain in one position and not move. They must be encouraged to cough and to perform the sustained maximal inspiration (SMI) maneuver to prevent atelectasis. If the pediatric patient is unable to perform the SMI maneuver, deep breathing should be encouraged.[5,8]

A change in heart rate of the pediatric patient is one of the first clues of impending physiologic dysfunction.[5] The PACU provider should initially consider hypoxia as the most likely cause of bradycardia. In the PACU, the heart rate of infants and children is influenced by physical activity, fluid volume replacement, and the administration of atropine, glycopyrrolate, and anesthetic agents. Glycopyrrolate (Robinul), an anticholinergic atropine-like drug, may elevate

the heart rate mildly, and not to the same degree as atropine.[14] Crying, struggling, or pain can also increase the heart rate.

In the event of respiratory dysfunction, the designated PACU attending anesthesia provider should be notified immediately. An ongoing airway assessment should be performed, and emergency airway management may be necessary. An oral airway must be of proper size and correct placement to relieve airway obstruction (Fig. 49-2). In addition, correct positioning of the patient assists with ventilation and intubation if necessary; however, correct positioning varies depending on the age of the child. For example, children 6 years of age and older benefit

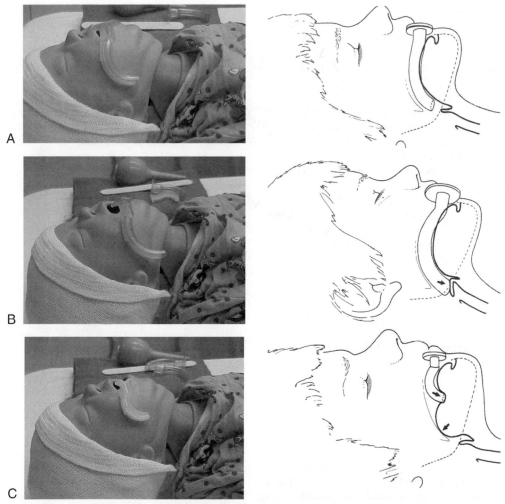

FIG. 49-2 Identification of correct oral airway selection. **A,** Correct oral airway size can be estimated when tip of airway ends just cephalad to angle of mandible. **B,** If oral airway is too large, tip of oral airway may obstruct glottic opening by pushing down on epiglottis. **C,** If oral airway is too small, tip of airway can lead to obstruction by pushing down on base of tongue. (From Cote CJ, et al: *A practice of anesthesia for infants and children*, ed 4, Philadelphia, 2009, Saunders; Courtesy Department of Nurse Anesthesia, Virginia Commonwealth University, Richmond, Va.)

from a folded towel or small pillow placed under the occiput in combination with extension of the head (Fig. 49-3). This position has often been referred to as the *sniffing position*. In infants and younger children, usually the size of the head is large relative to the trunk and hyperflexion of the neck occurs with lying flat on a bed. Further elevation of the occiput with a folded towel most likely hinders airway management. Mild flexion of the neck, with slight extension of the head, can be accomplished with the placement of a shoulder roll. Optimal positioning of the head and neck should assist in maintaining a patent airway and helping to ensure successful bag-mask ventilation when indicated. Excessive elevation of the

occiput or exaggerated extension of the head and neck should be avoided.

Reversal agents such as flumazenil (0.1 mg/kg IV) and naloxone (1 to 10 mcg/kg IV) should be readily available in the event of hypoventilation that is unresponsive to stimulation and to improve or reverse respiratory depression secondary to benzodiazepine (midazolam) or narcotic overdose respectively.[2,8,14] In addition, the anesthesia care team providers should be notified to offer additional assistance and follow-up care. Pressure-cycled ventilators are used in the neonatal intensive care unit to prevent barotrauma.[3] With a pressure-cycled ventilator, the risk of pressure trauma to the lungs is reduced by allowing the

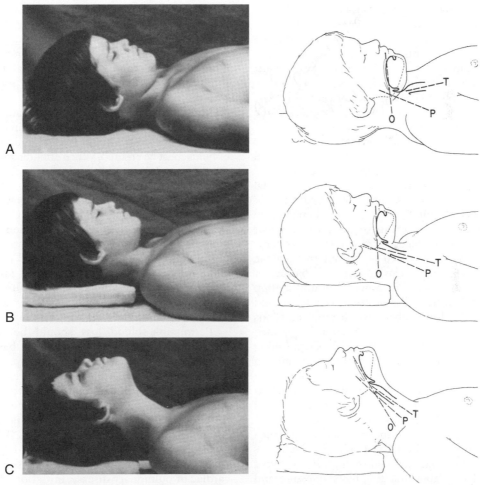

FIG. 49-3 Correct positioning for ventilation and tracheal intubation. **A,** When patient is lying flat on bed or stretcher, oral (O), pharyngeal (P), and tracheal (T) axes pass through three divergent planes. **B,** When folded sheet or towel is placed under occiput of head, pharyngeal (P) and tracheal axes align. **C,** With added extension of atlantooccipital joint, all three planes align to correct positioning for ventilation and tracheal intubation. (From Cote CJ, et al: *A practice of anesthesia for infants and children*, ed 4, Philadelphia, 2009, Saunders; Courtesy Department of Nurse Anesthesia, Virginia Commonwealth University, Richmond, Va.)

peak airway pressure to be varied to support optimum ventilation. However, a peak airway pressure alarm and limit must be maintained to decrease the risk of trauma to the lungs. Therefore, in the event of necessary postoperative mechanical ventilation of an infant, the setting is most likely an intermittent mandatory ventilation rate of 20 to 40 breaths/min, with a peak positive inspiratory airway pressure set at approximately 20 to 24 cm H_2O.[3]

A patent IV catheter should be maintained in the postoperative care unit. In ambulatory surgery with short-stay postanesthesia rooms, additional IV fluids may not be necessary if the intraoperative total fluid volume is sufficient to cover the initial postoperative recovery. However, in most instances, a patent IV catheter should be maintained throughout recovery. In the event of postoperative vomiting, additional fluids may be necessary. Initially, the care provider should administer an isotonic maintenance hourly fluid rate based on the kilogram weight of the patient. If the pediatric patient is moderately to severely ill, monitors for central venous pressure, ECG status, urine output, specific gravity, and an arterial line may be used.

The most likely indications for a central venous catheter include the need to monitor central venous pressure, cardiac surgery, inotropic drug administration, neurosurgery (with the potential risk of air embolism), major orthopedic procedures (such as spinal fusion), and abdominal surgical procedures when massive fluid shifting or blood loss is expected.[5] The central venous pressure line can be inserted via the internal jugular, external jugular, subclavian, femoral, basilic, or axillary veins.[5,8] This line provides for information on blood volume and serves as an avenue for fluid replacement. Remember that all rapid infusions of blood products or fluids should be warmed before administration. A fluid or blood warming device should have a visible thermometer and an audible warning that indicates excessive heating greater than 42° C.[3] The arterial line, which is inserted through the umbilical (neonate) or radial artery, can measure blood pressure and heart rate and provide for instantaneous blood gas or laboratory sampling. The ECG results provide information on cardiac rate and rhythm. In the event of circulatory abnormalities, blood pressure and pulse should be ascertained and recorded frequently. Any deviation in the cardiac or pulmonary physiologic parameters should be reported immediately to the attending physician.

Newborns and infants expend a great amount of energy maintaining alveolar ventilation, cardiac output, muscular activity, and an appropriate temperature. Because of these high-energy metabolic processes, glycogen and fat stores may be mobilized and depleted rapidly.[5,8] Consequently, cold, stress, pain, and increased muscle activity compound the need for adequate caloric intake in the PACU. In high-risk situations, plasma glucose concentrations should be monitored.[12] The patient's clinical condition dictates the final fluid and electrolyte requirements incurred as a result of trauma or complications from surgery. A glucose-containing infusion can be used for postoperative maintenance fluid replacement for children in high-risk circumstances[2,3,5,6,8]; however, rapid infusion of glucose-containing solutions should be avoided. During the administration of fluids, the perianesthesia nurse should ensure that the indwelling catheter is patent and not infiltrated and should use a constant infusion pump to facilitate the proper administration of the correct volume and rate of fluids. To prevent inadvertent overhydration, not more than one third of the day's maintenance intravenous fluid volume should be measured into the intravenous bag at any time.

Important considerations for fluid management of the pediatric patient include monitoring for hypervolemia or hypovolemia. Proper administration of fluids must be ensured. When attending to issues related to hydration, additional areas of assessment and monitoring can be helpful and include the following: (1) urine output, specific gravity, and osmolality; (2) body temperature; (3) ECG status, pulse, and blood pressure; (4) hydration of the mucosa; (5) assessment of the fontanel, in the newborn, for bulging or depression; and (6) blood loss.[5] An accurate assessment of blood loss must be made during and after surgery, because a small miscalculation of a few milliliters can have a serious effect on the total blood volume of an infant.

Permissible blood loss should be defined individually for each patient and is based on the patient's current medical condition, surgical procedure, and cardiovascular and respiratory function.[3,5,8] In healthy children with normal cardiovascular function, a lower hematocrit should be tolerated by increasing cardiac output when ventilation is not compromised. A higher inspired oxygen concentration should be provided. In the neonate or child with significant cardiac or pulmonary disease, initiation of blood loss replacement occurs earlier because of the patient's inability to compensate and because of a greater association with increased morbidity. Initially, ongoing blood loss is replaced with isotonic crystalloid at a ratio of 1:3; for every 1 mL of blood lost, 3 mL of isotonic fluid, such as lactated Ringer solution, is given. When losses are high, the usual blood replacement is such that for each 1 mL lost, 1 mL of packed red blood cells is administered (1:1) to the patient. Alternatively, if a colloid solution is used, it is replaced at the same ratio (1:1) as that for blood products, 1 mL of 5% albumin per 1 mL of blood lost, until the patient's hematocrit level reaches a predetermined critical level that requires packed red blood cells.[5]

Dressings should be watched for excessive bleeding. Such bleeding should be reported at once to the attending physician, because infants and small children have a narrower time span in which to compensate for loss. The leading cause of circulatory abnormalities in the postoperative pediatric patient is hemorrhage. The second most common cause of circulatory abnormality is plasma redistribution. Rarely is the cause cardiogenic in nature. Urine output and specific gravity may yield additional information on kidney function and volume expansion.

Thermal Regulation in the Postanesthesia Care Unit

Hypothermia can delay emergence from anesthesia and prolong the stay in the postoperative care unit (see Chapter 53). Hypothermia can have a detrimental affect on termination of neuromuscular blockade, metabolic balance, coagulation, and ventilatory control.[1-3,5,8] If an infant or small child arrives in the PACU with inadvertent hypothermia, the nurse should assess the patient for (1) vital signs (core temperature, pulse, and respiratory rate), (2) pulse oximetry waveform and saturation, and (3) the degree of emergence from anesthesia. If the patient has a delayed emergence from anesthesia, the nurse should protect the patient from aspiration of gastric contents and from hypoventilation with positioning (see Fig. 49-1) and stimulation. Dysrhythmias and cardiovascular depression are associated with profound hypothermia. Hypothermia can also lead to a detrimental effect on coagulation, ventilatory control, and metabolism.[1,3,5,8] Children with profound hypothermia should remain intubated and sedated. Continuous ECG monitoring is necessary until the core temperature reaches at least 35° C.[5] Finally, to avoid excess oxygen demand and acidosis associated with hypothermia, newborns and infants should be maintained in a neutral thermal environment in the PACU with the use of incubators, warm blankets, infrared heating lamps, warm-air heating blankets, or elevated room temperature when possible. Care should be taken to minimize environmental exposure during physical assessment, and the head should remain covered.

A word of warning is needed. If a water mattress is used to rewarm the patient, the temperature setting should be no greater than 37° C and a layer of sheets between the mattress, and the skin should be used as a barrier to prevent burns. When a forced warm-air heating device is used, it is imperative to follow the manufacturer's guidelines for proper use. Only the manufacturer's recommended blanket should be attached to the warm-air tube. Never place the warm-air heating tube between two blankets or directly blowing onto the infant or child, because these actions have resulted in burns. Whichever rewarming method is used, the temperature of the device should be monitored frequently to prevent overwarming or injury to the patient. Records should be kept of core body temperature (rectal, esophageal, or tympanic), room temperature, and device temperature.

Postoperative Pain Management and Regional Anesthesia

Analgesia is a right of all patients, including pediatric patients.[22] Inadequate management of a pediatric patient's pain can have severe negative consequences both acutely and chronically.[23] Therefore the management of postoperative pain in the pediatric patient must be a priority for the perioperative nurse. Numerous patient and situational factors must be considered when selecting and administering pain medications to children. If the postoperative plan of care includes hospital admission, then the analgesic regimen can be more flexible because the patient will have skilled nursing care available. Conversely, an alternate regimen may need to be selected for the outpatient.

The issues related to pain management for children have received increased attention in recent years.[5,23-28] Depending on the age and maturity of the child, various choices for pain management are available. Choices for pain management include parenteral or oral opioids, nonsteroidal antiinflammatory drugs (NSAIDs), regional anesthesia, and even patient-controlled analgesia (PCA). Medications such as NSAIDs, and oral or rectal acetaminophen in combination with parenteral opioids have been shown to be effective for pain control in the postoperative period. The use of this type of multimodal technique also has the advantage of decreasing opioid requirements, which may be beneficial in the outpatient setting. The overall opioid dose and incidence rate of opioid side effects is decreased when combined with NSAIDs.[22,25]

Acetaminophen and NSAIDs can treat minor to moderate pain and have been shown to be effective at reducing postoperative pain in pediatric patients.[22-30] Ketorolac is approved by the U.S. Food and Drug Administration for parenteral use (0.5 mg/kg, IV or intramuscular [IM], q6h).[25] The recommended dosing of ibuprofen is 8 to 10 mg/kg, orally, every 6 hours. Acetaminophen is a nonopioid analgesic and antipyretic that can be given via the oral (10 to 15 mg/kg q6h) or rectal (20 mg/kg q4h) route.[14] OFIRMEV (acetaminophen), the first IV formulation of acetaminophen in the United States, is indicated for the management of mild to moderate pain, management of moderate to severe pain with adjunctive opioid analgesics, and reduction of fever. It can be used in children who are 2 years old or older.[29]

Opioids are administered for moderate to severe pain. Routes of administration for opioids include oral, rectal, oral transmucosal (under the tongue), intramuscular, intravenous, transdermal, epidural, subarachnoid, and subcutaneous.[1-3,5,8,10,28-30] The most common postoperative parenteral opioids used in the pediatric population include fentanyl (0.5 to 1.0 mcg/kg, IV/IM), meperidine (0.5 to 1 mg/kg, IV/IM,) and morphine (0.05 to 0.1 mg/kg, IV/IM).[5] However, meperidine use is limited because its metabolite normeperidine can cause dysphoria, agitation, and seizures.[5,8] In low doses, meperidine can be used for the treatment of rigors and shivering in the PACU. The most common side effects that occur with opioid administration are sedation, pruritus, nausea, vomiting, constipation, and respiratory depression.[1-3,5,8] These side effects are dose dependent. Respiratory depression is of great concern in the pediatric patient; therefore vigilant monitoring of the patient's respiratory status after administration of opioids is imperative. Supplemental oxygen may be required when administering these medications. Fentanyl and its analogs can produce chest wall rigidity when administered as a bolus, which makes mask ventilation extremely difficult.

Ketamine is a sedative, hypnotic medication that produces dissociative anesthesia.[14] Ketamine is one of the only sedative, hypnotic drugs that also has analgesic properties. The preoperative or intraoperative use of ketamine has been shown to lower postoperative opioid requirements.[1,8,31] A benefit of ketamine is that it promotes spontaneous respirations.[1-3,8,14] This drug has been shown to be a highly effective adjunct to the management of postoperative pain in pediatric patients.[31] When used in small (subanesthetic) doses (0.1 to 0.5 mg/kg), the common side effects (i.e., tachycardia, delirium, hallucinations, nightmares) are minimal.[2,3] It has been suggested that ketamine always be administered with a benzodiazepine (midazolam) to help reduce the incidence of delirium, hallucinations, and nightmares.[1,8] For more information regarding ketamine, refer to the Evidence-Based Practice box.

PCA has been used successfully in children as young as 6 years of age, but requires the understanding and cooperation of the patient.[6,7,10,20] The inherent safety of PCA is based on the idea that a child who becomes too sleepy is not able to push the button to self-administer another dose of pain medication. Family members and nurses must not push the button for the child or medication overdose may result. By pushing a button, the child is able to deliver a precise opioid dose preprogrammed into the infusion pump. A minimum interval between dosing (a lock-out mechanism) and a maximum dose delivered over a set period of time are also preprogrammed to prevent overdose. A basal metabolic rate can be preprogrammed into the infusion pump to prevent severe breakthrough pain. In some cases, a basal infusion rate is not suggested for fear of additive sedation and for prevention of respiratory depression. Research has shown that the overall total drug consumption with PCA use is less.[5,22,30] The potential complications associated with PCA include overdose from incorrect programming of parameters or mechanical malfunction of the device. The perianesthesia care provider should assess the child for side effects associated with opioids (nausea, vomiting, itching, and ileus). An order should be written to discontinue all previous pain medications. Children should be instructed on the use of a pain score method, such as the visual analogue scale, and a record for assessment of pain should be included on the vital sign sheet (Table 49-7). Morphine is most often the opioid of choice for postoperative PCA use in children.[5] During orientation, all nurses should be trained in PCA use.

Regional anesthesia in children can dramatically improve pain management and lower general anesthesia requirements.[5] The most common regional blocks in children include a penile block for circumcision, ilioinguinal block for hernia repair, spinal anesthesia (most often in the neonate who is very ill), and caudal epidural. Caudal blocks have been used for a variety of surgical procedures, including circumcision, inguinal herniorrhaphy, hypospadias repair, clubfoot repair, anal surgery, and other procedures below the umbilicus and of the lower extremities.[8] A caudal catheter can be threaded to the thoracic epidural space and can provide a thoracic-level block for pain relief in small children; this is particularly useful for control of pain after open heart surgery.

Table 49-7 Age-Specific Pain Measurement Tools for Children

NAME	FEATURES	AGE RANGE	ADVANTAGES	LIMITATIONS
VAS	Horizontal 10-cm ruler; subject marks between "no pain" and "worst pain imaginable"	≥8 yr	Good psychometric properties; gold standard	Cannot be used in younger children or those with cognitive limitations
Faces scales (e.g., Wong, Baker, Oucher, Bieri, McGrath)	Subjects compare pain with line drawings of faces or photos of children	≥ 4 yr	More useful than VAS for younger children	Choice of anchors affects responses (neutral versus smiling)
Color analog scales	Horizontal or vertical ruler, on which increasing intensity of red signifies more pain	≥ 4 yr	Useful for younger ages; converges to VAS at older ages	Cannot be used in toddlers or those with cognitive limitations
Behavioral or combined behavioral-physiologic scales (e.g., CHEOPS, OPS, FACS, MIPS)	Scoring of observed behaviors (e.g., facial expression, limb movement) and heart rate and blood pressure	Some work for any age; other tests are age-specific	Can be used even for infants and nonverbal children	Overrates fear in toddlers and preschool children; underrates persistent pain; some inconvenient measures that require videotaping and complex processing
Autonomic measures (e.g., heart rate, blood pressure, heart rate spectral analyses)	Scores changes in heart rate, blood pressure, or measures of heart rate variability (e.g., vagal tone)	All ages	All ages; useful for patients with mechanical ventilation	Nonspecific; changes can occur unrelated to pain
Hormonal-metabolic measures	Plasma or salivary sampling of hormones (e.g., cortisol, epinephrine)	All ages	Can be used at all ages	Nonspecific; changes can occur unrelated to pain; inconvenient; cannot provide real-time information

From Kliegman RM, et al: *Nelson's textbook of pediatrics*, ed 19, Philadelphia, 2011, Saunders.
VAS, Visual analog scale

SELECTED POSTOPERATIVE CONCERNS IN PEDIATRICS

The most common reasons for postdischarge readmission to the hospital are protracted vomiting and surgery-related complications.[5,8] PACU nursing care of children must include constant assessment of airway patency, ventilation, and circulatory stability.[5] In addition, common postoperative concerns in children include the potential for a postanesthetic excitement phase commonly referred to as emergence delirium, and pain management.[1-3,5,8,30] Because the pediatric patient does not have the physiologic reserves of the adult patient, when complications occur, serious untoward sequelae take place. The perianesthesia nurse must monitor for and react to any complication in a timely fashion.

Laryngospasm

The larynx is the musculocartilaginous organ located at the upper end of the trachea. It is part of the airway and vocal apparatus.[1-3,8] Laryngospasm (closure of the larynx) is caused by sensory stimulation of the superior laryngeal nerve.[5,8] When this nerve is stimulated, a forceful involuntary spasm of the laryngeal musculature occurs.

In the PACU, laryngospasm can occur as the child awakens. Laryngospasm is usually caused by blood or pharyngeal secretions draining toward the vocal cords.[1,5,8,31] For this reason, children are placed in the three-fourths prone position to promote drainage of oral secretions away from the vocal cords. Posterior oral pharyngeal suctioning can cause additional trauma and should be avoided (or performed very carefully) after the child has been extubated.

Initial treatment of laryngospasm includes positive-pressure ventilation with a bag-mask device (Fig. 49-4). The two-person bag-mask ventilation technique provides superior ventilation in the event of significant airway obstruction or poor lung compliance. Intravenous lidocaine (1 to 1.5 mg/kg) also can be helpful.[1-3,8] If hypoxia develops and the laryngospasm is not relieved from positive-pressure ventilation via mask, then succinylcholine (0.25 to 1 mg/kg) should be given to allow control of ventilation with paralysis of the laryngeal muscles.[5,31] Succinylcholine is a rapid-acting and ultra-short–duration depolarizing muscle relaxant and is useful in situations that necessitate rapid endotracheal intubation and securing of the airway.[1,14] A word of caution is needed because succinylcholine use is associated

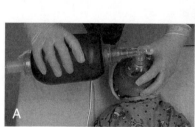
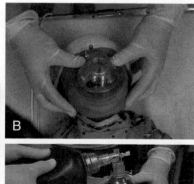
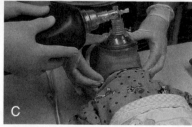

FIG. 49-4 **A,** One-person bag-mask ventilation. **B,** Two-handed technique for mask ventilation may be useful to improve mask fit and ventilation when one-person bag-mask ventilation is difficult or inadequate. Modified jaw-thrust–chin-lift maneuver is shown. Tips of index and ring fingers are applied to ascending ramus of mandible behind pinnae of ear. Thumbs apply downward pressure to facemask to ensure tight seal. Mouth should open, which helps to maintain airway patency. Soft structures of airway should be avoided. **C,** One person uses both hands to open airway and maintain tight mask-to-face seal while assistant compresses ventilation bag. (Courtesy Department of Nurse Anesthesia, Virginia Commonwealth University, Richmond, Va.)

with many profound side effects such as cardiovascular complications, severe hyperkalemia, increased intraocular pressure, increased intracranial pressure, prolonged apnea, and injured muscle membranes with associated hyperkalemia and can be a trigger for myotonia, masseter spasm, and malignant hyperthermia. The U.S. Food and Drug Administration issued a "box" warning against the elective use of succinylcholine outside of the operating room. Because of the combination of a box warning and an increased availability of alternative agents, succinylcholine use is limited outside the operating room, except when clearly indicated such as in emergency airway situations.

A perianesthesia care provider should have airway equipment and drugs readily available to facilitate re-intubation if necessary. When laryngospasm develops, large intrathoracic pressures are generated. A negative-pressure pulmonary edema can result even in healthy children, and close attention should be given to further respiratory compromise after the laryngospasm has resolved.[1-3,5,8] Positive-pressure ventilation is used to treat pulmonary edema after a laryngospasm. If the pulmonary edema is severe and the patient begins to show signs and symptoms of inadequate respiration (labored breathing, decreasing oxygen saturation even with supplemental oxygenation), then more aggressive measures should be used. These measures include the use of diuretics and possibly intubation of the patient.

Airway Obstruction

In the PACU, every pediatric patient, particularly children who have been intubated during anesthesia, should be monitored for signs of airway obstruction. Postintubation croup is caused by glottic or tracheal edema. When laryngeal swelling occurs, the diameter of the airway of the infant or small child can become significantly reduced; in fact, 1 mm of edema in the infant's trachea at the cricoid level decreases the diameter of the airway by 75%. The symptoms of laryngeal obstruction, in order of appearance, are croupy cough, hoarseness, inspiratory stridor, and aphonia. These symptoms are accompanied by increasing restlessness, tachypnea, use of accessory muscles of respiration, retraction of the suprasternal notch and intercostal spaces, and drawing in of the upper abdomen.[5] If these symptoms appear, the perianesthesia nurse should act immediately to relieve the obstruction, administer supplemental oxygen, and send someone to notify the PACU anesthesia provider. The progression of these symptoms can be rapid.

Treatment of postintubation croup involves use of a high-humidity atmosphere that is oxygen-enriched. Nebulized racemic epinephrine (0.5 mL of a 2.25% solution in 2.5 mL of normal saline solution) has been useful in the treatment of postintubation croup. In addition, corticosteroids such as dexamethasone (Decadron, 0.2 mg/kg, IV) have been useful to decrease the laryngeal inflammation associated with other causes of croup[5,8,14]; however, corticosteroid use for postintubation croup remains controversial.[6] If laryngeal edema is allowed to progress, the patient may need reintubation, although this rarely occurs.

Nausea and Vomiting

Nausea and vomiting (see Chapter 29) is a leading cause of delayed discharge from the PACU. Children who are undergoing tonsillectomy, strabismus, or orchiopexy surgery are at greater risk.[5] The incidence rate of postoperative nausea and vomiting (PONV) varies; anything that can be done to minimize PONV wins the approval of the patient, the parents, and the staff members. Early or forced administration of liquids before the child is ready can cause vomiting. If a greater likelihood of PONV exists, administration of prophylactic antiemetics is best whenever possible.[5] In most cases, vomiting can be treated successfully with the use of phenothiazines (rectal promethazine, 0.5 mg/kg), metoclopramide (0.15 mg/kg, IV), or the serotonin-3 antagonist ondansetron (0.05 to 0.15 mg/kg, IV; maximum dose, 4 mg). Phenothiazines and metoclopramide can cause dystonic reactions that can be treated with diphenhydramine (0.5 to 1 mg/kg, IV).[14] Ondansetron (Zofran) is safe to use without significant side effects, is approved for use in patients 1 month of age and older, and has been shown to be the most effective drug for treating PONV.[5] In the absence of an IV catheter, ondansetron can be given under the tongue for quick absorption without the need for swallowing. Propofol used alone for sedation has antiemetic properties, and it may decrease PONV when it is combined with other drugs for maintaining anesthesia.[1]

Malignant Hyperthermia

Although a detailed discussion on malignant hyperthermia (MH) is presented in an alternate chapter of this text (Chapter 53), a brief description of the condition is given here. The incidence rate of MH is approximately 1:3000 to 1:15,000 in children, compared with 1:40,000 to 1:100,000 in adults.[1-3,5,8] Halogenated inhalation anesthetic agents and the depolarizing muscle relaxant succinylcholine trigger this genetically determined condition. The pathophysiology of this condition centers on the enhanced release and diminished reuptake of calcium in the skeletal muscle. This decreased uptake of calcium causes sustained skeletal muscle contraction which results in profound hyperthermia. The muscle cells convert to anaerobic metabolism, and lactic acidosis ensues. Ultimately, muscle cell breakdown occurs. The drug dantrolene sodium effectively treats MH with inhibition of further release of calcium in the skeletal muscle. In most instances, MH occurs in the operating room; however, a patient may first be seen with the disorder in the PACU, or the patient with successfully treated MH may have an exacerbation of MH symptoms later in the recovery process.

The earliest clinical feature of MH is a rising $ETCO_2$ level; however, this feature is not readily apparent in the PACU unless the patient is intubated and an $ETCO_2$ level is being monitored. Therefore, in most cases of MH in the PACU, the first clinical sign is tachycardia with or without other dysrhythmias; tachypnea and a profound increase in tidal volume are then observed in the patient with spontaneous breathing. Generalized muscle rigidity may or may not occur. Hyperthermia is often a late sign. Additional signs include arrhythmias, hypertension, sweating, and mottled skin. Diagnosis of MH in the PACU may be difficult because this syndrome has a variable presentation. For example, fever is often an inconsistent and late sign.

Blood chemistry studies reveal an elevated potassium level and an initially elevated calcium level before it falls. Arterial blood gas levels show a severe fall in bicarbonate and pH and an elevated $PaCO_2$. The PaO_2 may be normal, depending on the use of controlled ventilation and the fraction of inspired oxygen content (FiO_2). Serum myoglobin, creatine kinase, lactic dehydrogenase, and aldolase levels usually rise.

To facilitate a reversal of this condition, the perianesthesia nurse must understand the pathophysiology of MH and should know exactly where the MH emergency cart is located. If a patient seems to be exhibiting signs and symptoms of MH, the nurse should send for help immediately. The nurse should start to assist ventilation of the patient with high-flow 100% oxygen and ensure that the IV catheter is patent. When the appropriate personnel arrive, more than one person should mix the dantrolene sodium (20 mg per 60 mL of sterile water). A note of warning is needed to ensure that the sterile water does not contain preservatives and that much sterile water will be used. The usual starting dose of dantrolene sodium is 2.5 mg/kg IV. This dose can be repeated up to 10 mg/kg over 45 minutes or until the patient's condition stabilizes and temperature is reduced.

When the protocol is initiated, the need for endotracheal intubation and active cooling with frequent temperature monitoring begins. Recognition and treatment of arrhythmias along with correction of the associated acidosis and electrolyte imbalance (hyperkalemia) should be anticipated. Most likely an arterial line, nasogastric tube, and three-way urinary catheter is placed. The most successful outcome occurs when the syndrome is identified and treated early.[6,26] The child is transferred to a pediatric intensive care unit usually for at least 24 hours for close monitoring and continued therapy.

SPECIAL CONSIDERATIONS

Otolaryngologic Surgery

The most common surgical procedures performed in pediatrics involve the ear, nose, and throat. The leading cause of obstructive sleep apnea (OSA) and hypoventilation in children is adenotonsillar hypertrophy.[5] Other anatomic factors that lead to OSA include micrognathia, retrognathia, or macroglossia. In addition, morbid obesity in children or a congenitally small airway narrows the nasopharynx. Chronic OSA can disrupt sleep and breathing patterns and lead to impaired daytime performance and more serious complications such as polycythemia, growth failure, heart failure, pulmonary hypertension, and arrhythmias.[5,8]

Pediatric patients who have tonsillectomies and other operations on the pharynx, larynx, and esophagus need intensive PACU care because the airway can become obstructed after surgery as a result of surgical manipulation and bleeding. When the patient is admitted to the PACU, the laryngeal and pharyngeal reflexes should be present. The patient should be placed in the tonsillar position, three-fourths prone, with the arm and leg flexed and the head turned to the side. This position improves drainage of secretions and blood from the mouth and is helpful in prevention of possible aspiration or laryngospasm. The patient should be kept in this position until the gag reflex has returned completely.

Nausea with vomiting can lead to bleeding and airway compromise in the PACU. During report, the nurse should note whether a perioperative antiemetic was given. The combination of propofol and ondansetron effectively reduces the incidence of vomiting in children after tonsillectomy. Before emergence and extubation in the operating room, common practice is for the surgeon to suction gastric content and the oral pharynx and to assess for hemostasis. After the child has been extubated, avoidance of deep oral pharyngeal suctioning is best to prevent trauma and bleeding.

Trauma Victim

Special consideration should be considered with airway management for the child with head or cervical spine injury. When assisted airway support is needed to relieve airway obstruction in the PACU, the jaw-thrust maneuver is indicated to open the airway (see Figs. 49-3 to 49-5).[5,8,30] An anesthesia provider should be notified at once to offer assistance and airway management. If a second care provider is available, assistance should be placed with emphasis on immobilization of the cervical spine with maintenance of a neutral alignment. The head tilt–chin lift is contraindicated in the presence of cervical spine injury.[1,5,8] When the airway is controlled, a semirigid cervical collar, spine board, linen rolls, and tape can be used to immobilize the child. To support oxygenation and ventilation, intubation may be indicated. Inline traction and spine immobilization are necessary during mask ventilation, laryngoscopy, intubation, and transport.

DISCHARGE FROM THE POSTANESTHESIA CARE UNIT

With the advancement in pharmacologic drugs and inhalational agents for general anesthesia, rapid recovery with decreased side effects has led to earlier discharge from the PACU for children. Certain criteria must be met for safe transition from the PACU to a short-stay recovery unit or hospital ward; however, the goals of recovery vary depending on the discharge location planned for the patient.[5] In the evaluation of a child for possible discharge from the PACU, the perianesthesia nurse should observe for each of the following: (1) an alert and easily aroused child; (2) protective airway reflexes; (3) strong muscle strength; (4) oxygen saturation maintained above 95% on room air or at the baseline preoperative level; (5) normothermia; (6) pain under control; (7) absence of vomiting; (8) no sign of active bleeding; and (9) stable vital signs. Children continue to recover in an ambulatory or short-stay recovery unit after outpatient procedures.

Discharge of the pediatric patient depends on the overall functional status of the child. However, after procedures involving the airway, such as tonsillectomies, the child may stay in the hospital for a longer period of time, such as the 23-hour admission for observation.

Factors that delay postoperative recovery in children include residual anesthetic or neuromuscular blockade, hypothermia, hypoxemia, acid-base imbalance, hypocarbia, hypercarbia, hypovolemia, and elevated intracranial pressure.[5] Forcing fluids by mouth to facilitate discharge is never advisable, and one should wait until the child vocalizes a desire to decrease the likelihood of vomiting. A delay of discharge until the child has voided is not necessary. The anesthesia provider should be notified to assess the child; write the discharge notes, including any findings or recommendations for postoperative care; and sign for discharge from the PACU. The parents or guardian must be instructed concerning discharge care. A phone number should be included with written information on what to do in case of an emergency for further clarification of post discharge questions or concerns.

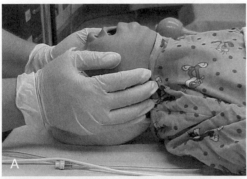
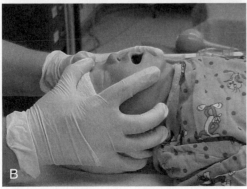

FIG. 49-5 **A,** Jaw thrust maneuver. Elevate the jaw by placing the tips of the index and ring fingers along the ramus of the mandible (on the bony prominences), while avoiding the soft structures overlying the larynx and glottic opening, which potentially can lead to airway obstruction. **B,** Spine immobilization with airway opening in infant with potential head and neck trauma. Combined jaw thrust and spinal stabilization maneuver. (Courtesy Department of Nurse Anesthesia, Virginia Commonwealth University, Richmond, VA.)

SUMMARY

Successful transition of the pediatric patient through the perioperative period requires careful coordination by skilled perioperative nurses. The pediatric patient's journey begins with a thorough assessment and proper preparation by the preoperative nurse. The care is then transitioned to the intraoperative nurse and anesthetist. In the PACU, the nurse must be constantly vigilant and aware of any minor changes in the pediatric patient that may be early signs and symptoms of problems. The perioperative nurse must be skilled in airway assessment and the provision of basic airway support and management, in the use of oral and nasal airways, bag-mask ventilation, and assistance with intubation and extubation. The nurse must be prepared to manage emergence delirium and postoperative pain and potentially assist with basic and advanced life support measures. All these tasks must be performed while providing an age-appropriate level of comfort and reassurance to a frightened child.

REFERENCES

1. Barash PG, et al: *Clinical anesthesia*, ed 6, Philadelphia, 2009, Lippincott Williams & Wilkins.
2. Morgan GE, et al: *Clinical anesthesiology*, ed 4, New York, 2006, Lange Medical Books/McGraw Hill Publishing Division.
3. Nagelhout J, Plaus K: *Nurse anesthesia*, ed 4, St. Louis, 2010, Saunders.
4. Moore KL, et al: *Clinically oriented anatomy*, ed 6, Philadelphia, 2010, Lippincott Williams & Wilkins.
5. Davis PJ, et al: *Smith's anesthesia for infants and children*, ed 7, St. Louis, 2011, Mosby.
6. Holzman RS, et al: *A practical approach to pediatric anesthesia*, Philadelphia, 2008, Lippincott Williams & Wilkins.
7. Galbusera V, et al: The assistance of the ventilated infant: role of the nurse in the management of the endotracheal tube, *Minerva Pediatrica* 62(3 Suppl 1):169, 2010.
8. Miller R: *Anesthesia*, ed 7, New York, 2009, Churchill Livingstone.
9. Hines RL, Marschall KL: *Stoelting's anesthesia and coexisting disease*, ed 5, Philadelphia, 2008, Saunders.
10. Cousins MJ, et al: *Cousins & Bridenbaugh's neural blockade in clinical anesthesia and pain medicine*, ed 4, Philadelphia, 2009, Lippincott Williams & Wilkins.
11. Townsend GM, et al: *Sabiston textbook of surgery*, ed 18, New York, 2008, Saunders.
12. Mason RJ, et al: *Murray and Nadel's textbook of respiratory medicine*, ed 5, New York, 2010, Saunders.
13. Eckhenhoff J: Relationship of anesthesia to postoperative personality changes in children, *Am J Dis Childhood* 86:587–591, 1953.
14. Stoelting RK: *Pharmacology and physiology in anesthetic practice*, ed 3, Philadelphia, 1999, Lippincott Williams & Wilkins.
15. Redhu S, et al: A comparative study of induction, maintenance and recovery characteristics of sevoflurane and halothane anaesthesia in pediatric patients (6 months to 6 years), *Journal of Anaesthesiology-Clinical Pharmacology* 26(4):484, 2010.
16. Cravero J, et al: The incidence and nature of adverse events during pediatric sedation/anesthesia with propofol for procedures outside the operating room: a report from the pediatric sedation research consortium, *Anesthesia and Analgesia* 108(3):795, 2009.
17. Weiss M, et al: Deep propofol sedation for vacuum-assisted bite-block immobilization in children undergoing proton radiation therapy of cranial tumors, *Paediatric Anaesthesia* 17(9):867, 2007.
18. Martin L, et al: Total intravenous anesthesia with propofol in pediatric patients outside the operating room, *Anesth Analg* 74:609–612, 1992.
19. Westrin P: The induction dose of propofol in infants 1–6 months and children 10–16 years of age, *Anesthesiology* 74(3):455–459, 1991.
20. Hannallah R: Propofol: effective dose and induction characteristics in unpremedicated children, *Anesthesiology* 74(2):217–219, 1991.
21. Bevin J, et al: Preoperative parental anxiety predicts behavioral and emotional responses to induction of anaesthesia in children, *Can J Anaesth* (37):177–182, 1990.
22. Savoia G, et al: Postoperative pain treatment SIAARTI recommendations 2010, (short version), *Minerva Anestesiologica* 76(8):657, 2010.
23. Ali S, et al: Pain management of musculoskeletal injuries in children: current state and future directions, *Pediatric Emergency Care* 26(7):518, 2010.
24. Mubroy J: Safety and efficacy of alfentanil and halothane in paediatric surgical patients, *Can J Anaesth* 38(4):445–449, 1991.
25. Sutters K, et al: Comparison of morphine patient-controlled analgesia with and without ketorolac for postoperative analgesia in pediatric orthopedic surgery, *Am J Orthop* 28(6):351–358, 1999.
26. Vesely C: Pediatric-patient-controlled analgesia: enhancing the self-care construct, *Pediatr Nurs Rev* 21(2):124–128, 1995.
27. Migita R, et al: Sedation and analgesia for pediatric fracture reduction in the emergency department: a systematic review, *Archives of Pediatrics Adolescent Medicine* 160(1):46, 2006.
28. Neuhuser, et al: Analgesia and sedation for painful interventions in children and adolescents, *Deutsches International* 107(14):241, 2010.
29. Groudine S, Fossum S: Use of intravenous acetaminophen in the treatment of postoperative pain, *J Perianesth Nurs* 26(2):74–80, 2011.
30. Macintyre PE, et al: *Acute pain management: scientific evidence*, ed 3, 2010, Australian and New Zealand College of Anaesthetist and Faculty of Pain Medicine, Melbourne, Australia.
31. Dahmani S, et al: Ketamine for perioperative pain management in children: a meta-analysis of published studies, *Paediatric Anaesthesia* 21(6):636, 2011.

RESOURCES

Costanza LS: *Physiology*, ed 3, Philadelphia, 2006, Saunders.
Kliegman R, et al: *Nelson textbook of pediatrics*, ed 19, Philadelphia, 2011, Saunders.
Walbergh E: Plasma concentrations of midazolam in children following intranasal administration, *Anesthesiology* 74(2):233–236, 1991.

50 Care of the Older Patient

Tracey Gendron, MSG, and E. Ayn Welleford, MSG, PhD, AGHEF

The world's population is aging at a rapid pace. The current population of adults older than 65 years constitutes 34 million people, or approximately 13% of the population. Projections suggest that by 2030, 69 million individuals will be older than 65 years, or approximately 19% of the population.[1] This trend represents two important phenomena: the increase in life expectancy and the aging of the baby boomers (those born between 1946 and 1964) who began to turn 65 in 2011. Older adults are not only living longer; they are doing so free of disease and disability. According to "compression of morbidity theory," the limit to life span may be stretched significantly with a concurrent delay in the onset of chronic conditions.[2] This stretching of the lifespan would result in a population living longer and healthier than any generation to date.

DEFINITIONS

Activities of Daily Living: Daily self-care activities, including bathing, eating, dressing, toileting, and grooming.

Cognitive Impairment: Reduction in mental functioning that results in cognitive changes, including short-term memory loss and impaired judgment and thinking.

Cultural Competence: The ability to provide culturally relevant and appropriate care to persons with diverse values, beliefs, and behaviors.

Dementia: A loss of brain function that occurs with certain a group of diseases. It affects memory, thinking, language, judgment, and behavior. The most common form of dementia is Alzheimer disease.

Geriatrics: Medical aspect of gerontology in the treatment of acute and chronic conditions in older adults (i.e., a person 65 years of age or older).

Gerontology: The scientific study of age, aging, and the aged using a lifespan, biopsychosocial approach.

Health: A state of physical, mental, and social well-being.

Instrumental Activities of Daily Living: The activities performed by people living independently, including meal preparation, money management, shopping, and taking medications.

Person-Centered Care: Focuses on individual care needs by understanding how the individual experiences his or her situation in order to most effectively address needs and desired outcomes.

Presbycusis: Age-associated hearing changes or the slow loss of hearing as people get older.

Presbyopia: Age-associated visual changes of diminished ability to focus on near objects.

The World Health Organization defines health as a state of complete physical, mental, and social well-being and not merely the absence of disease or infirmity.[3] In this view, older adults may then perceive themselves as healthy despite physical limitations or disease. It is essential in caring for the older patient to recognize overall health from physiologic, psychological, and social perspectives. In assessing an older adult's health, an appropriate delineation is between an individual's chronological age versus their functional age. Some individuals who are more judicious in using preventive health measures and who maintain more active lifestyles may have little decline or age-related comorbidities, reflecting greater functioning relative to chronologic age, whereas others may have multiple comorbidities, perhaps at an even earlier age, reflecting functional limitations relative to age. Gerontologists often use the distinctions *young-old, old-old,* and *oldest-old* to differentiate between older adults. In terms of functional capacity, gerontologists also describe aging in terms of primary, secondary, and tertiary aging.[4] Primary aging represents aging free of disability and disease. Secondary aging encompasses developmental changes affected by lifestyle, disease, or factors that are not inevitable processes of biologic aging. Tertiary aging is rapid loss and decline experienced at the end of life. Differentiation of age and functional capacity is essential to focus attention on the diversity of this population and establish some markers that are helpful in meeting the individual needs of older adults.

Many different chronologic markers are used for governmental determinations and legal purposes (i.e., 40 years of age for age discrimination determination, 50 years of age for AARP membership, and 65 plus years of age for Social Security). As a result, no one definition of old-age, elderly, or older adult is accepted. Because no biomarkers exist, a definition of when old age begins is difficult because individuals age at different rates than is reflected simply by chronologic age. The growing complexity and diversity of the aging population mandates a holistic interprofessional biopsychosocial approach to care to move beyond a simplistic chronologic marker of age toward a more accurate functional assessment.

Care of the older adult patient is particularly important in the postanesthesia care unit because of the normal physiologic changes that occur with aging and may be compounded by multiple comorbid conditions. With advancing age, the potential risks of complications from surgical procedures increases, because of the potential for multiple comorbidity. Morbidity and mortality are at least fourfold more likely in older adults and twentyfold more likely in emergency procedures.[5] These conditions include congestive heart failure, insufficient oxygenation of the blood, improper elimination of carbon dioxide, fluid and electrolyte imbalance, diabetes and the associated complications, and drug toxicity.

Advances in anesthetic care have resulted in a substantial reduction in perioperative morbidity and mortality in the aging population.[6] Successful anesthesia care of the older adult patient is highly dependent on the knowledge of the changes associated with aging and the effects of anesthesia on the older patient. Therefore, the focus of this chapter is primarily on the normal aging changes that take place in addition to the disease states associated with aging and their translation to functional status, especially of the cardiovascular system. It is essential to keep in mind throughout this chapter that the rate at which each individual and organ system age is highly individualistic. This phenomenon is referred to as the *individuation of aging.*[7] Individual genes, hormonal balance, diet, medications, environmental exposure, and emotional stress and burden are all factors that influence individual biological aging.

THE AGING BODY: AN OVERVIEW

Cardiovascular System

Cardiovascular health is essential to the overall well-being of the older adult. Healthy cardiovascular functioning can be maintained across the lifespan, and disease can be prevented through healthy lifestyle choices and preventive care; however, heart disease remains the leading cause of death for both males and females.[8] Of all of the body systems, the cardiovascular system exerts the most influence on anesthesia and general health outcomes.[8] Annually, more than 1 million surgeries are complicated by adverse cardiac outcomes,

such as postsurgical myocardial infarction or death from cardiac disease.[9] This risk can be reduced with a thorough preoperative interview and assessment that examines functional capacity and existing comorbidities and the current treatment regime.[8]

Functional Capacity

The assessment of functional capacity reflects the ability to perform activities of daily living that require sustained aerobic metabolism.[10] Exercise tolerance in daily life is the best indicator of the quality of biologic age. It is also one of the most important predictors of perioperative outcomes in older adult patients.[11,12] Poor exercise tolerance reflects low functional capacity and greater severity of disease. Functional status is usually reflected in metabolic equivalent (MET) levels. One MET corresponds to a resting oxygen consumption of 3.5 mL/kg/min. MET scores are multiples of resting metabolism, which are used as a point of reference to describe the oxygen demands of any activity.[13] Box 50-1 provides examples of MET ratings of activities. Functional status can be ascertained during the preoperative screening. Questions addressing daily activities and assessing lifestyle habits, such as house cleaning, vacuuming, walking, and stair climbing,

BOX 50-1	Estimated Energy Requirements for Various Activities
1 MET	Take care of yourself Eat, dress, or use the toilet Walk around the house Walk a block or two on level ground (2-3 mph)
4 METs	Perform light housework, such as dusting or dishes Climb a flight of stairs or walk up a hill Walk on level ground at 4 mph Do heavy housework such as scrubbing floors and lifting or moving furniture Engage in recreational activities such as bowling, golf, or dancing
>10 METs	Participate in strenuous sports such as swimming, singles tennis, basketball, or skiing?

Adapted from Hlatky MA, et al: A brief self-administered questionnaire to determine functional capacity, *Am J Cardiol* 64:651–654, 1989; Fletcher GF, et al: Exercise standards: a statement for healthcare professionals from the American Heart Association, *Circulation* 104:1694–1740, 2001.
MET, Metabolic equivalent.

and any participation in regular exercise should provide adequate information for a subjective assessment of the patient's functional status.[14] Objective assessment can be made via exercise testing. Patients who are unable to regularly meet a 4 MET demand have an increased perioperative cardiac risk.[15]

Structural Changes

There are several structural changes frequently seen with advancing or older age that occur within the cardiovascular system. Changes of the arteries include dilation of the large arteries accompanied by thickening of the arterial walls and changes in wall matrix. An increase in elastin and collagen tissues in the heart and arteries can cause arterial wall thickening and an increase in smooth muscle tone.[16-19] Increased vascular stiffness leads to elevated systolic arterial pressure and pulse wave velocity, early reflected pulse pressure waves, and late peak systolic pressure, which trigger a series of cardiac adjustments. A resultant augmenting of aortic impedance and cardiac mechanical load may be seen.

Clinically elevated left ventricular afterload causes an increase in myocyte size and thickening of the left ventricular wall.[18] When combined with augmentation of aortic impedance, elevated afterload prolongs myocardial contraction. This adaptive measure preserves cardiac function by lengthening the amount of time available for the heart to eject blood into stiffened vasculature. The resultant prolonged myocardial contraction delays ventricular relaxation time, which manifests as a decrease in early ventricular filling.[19-23]

Between the ages of 20 and 80 years, the rate of early diastolic filling decreases by 50%.[24] This decrease may be the result of a prolonged isovolumetric relaxation time between aortic valve closure and mitral valve opening. With aging, alterations in calcium release from the myoplasm to the sarcoplasmic reticulum may contribute to the changes in early diastolic filling.[16,23]

For maintenance of stroke volume, end diastolic filling is increased.[16] The effectiveness of this strategy is dependent on the atrial contribution to end diastolic filling; therefore left atrial size increases.[20] Enlargement of the atria raises the likelihood of atrial fibrillation among elders, thus underscoring the importance of stable hemodynamics to ensure normal sinus rhythm.

Gender differences may be found in certain age-related changes in cardiac function.[16] Men seem to have different compensatory mechanisms than women. To maintain stroke volume in the presence of the age-associated decrease in heart rate, men have an increase in left ventricle end-systolic volume and left ventricle end-diastolic volume. This mechanism preserves cardiac output in aging men, whereas a 15% decrease is seen in cardiac output in women. Table 50-1 summarizes cardiac changes in response to exercise that occur with age.[25]

The most clinically relevant age-related changes in cardiovascular function are increased myocardial stiffness and all of the subsequent compensatory actions and blunted beta-adrenergic responses. During increased oxygen demand, the most relevant changes in the older patient are autonomic reflex dysfunction and beta-adrenoreceptor responsiveness.

Table 50-1	Changes in Cardiovascular Response to Exercise with Comparison of 20 and 80 Years of Age	
CARDIOVASCULAR PHYSIOLOGY	**PEAK RESPONSE AT AGE 20 YEARS**	**CHANGE IN PEAK RESPONSE BETWEEN 20 AND 80 YEARS**
LV end-diastolic volume	↔,↓	↑30% males; ↔ females
LV end-systolic volume	↓	↓100%
Ejection fraction	↑	↓15%
Stroke volume	↑	↔
Heart rate	↑	↓25%
Cardiac output	↑	↓25%
Stroke work	↑	↑15% males; ↔ females
SVR	↓	↑30%
Oxygen consumption	↑	↑50%
Plasma catecholamines	↑	↑
Myocardial contractility	↑	↓60%
Beta-adrenergic stimulation	Fully functional	↓

Adapted from Eagle KA: Perioperative cardiac assessment for noncardiac surgery: eight steps to the best possible outcome, *Circulation* 107:2771–2774, 2003.

LV, Left ventricular; ↔, no change; ↑, increase; ↓, decrease; *SVR*, systemic vascular resistance.

See Table 50-1 for cardiovascular age-related changes to upright peak exercise.

Cardiovascular Risk Assessment

Preoperative risk assessment is an important component in minimizing perioperative morbidity and mortality. This assessment is best achieved through the work of an interdisciplinary team that consists of the patient, the primary care physician, the surgeon, and the anesthesia professional. In addition, training and expertise are essential to the quality care of older adult patients. This assessment relies on the evaluation of the interaction of clinical markers, functional capacity, type of surgical procedure, and age. When risks are identified, measures should be used to minimize the risks before surgery and to improve immediate periprocedural outcomes and long-term clinical outcomes. Some clinical markers act as predictors of perioperative cardiovascular risk. These markers can be categorized by the perioperative risk associated with them (Box 50-2) as major, intermediate, and minor perioperative risk.[11]

In addition, the type of surgery coupled with the degree of hemodynamic stress incurred during the surgery are the major determining factors of perioperative risk.[11,12] Emergency surgeries are particularly high risk, especially in older patients. Other high-risk surgeries include vascular, cardiac, abdominal, and thoracic surgeries.[26] Box 50-3 categorizes surgery-specific risk according to the incidence rate of cardiac death and nonfatal myocardial infarction for noncardiac surgical procedures.

Heart

It is difficult to determine which changes in the cardiovascular and circulatory systems represent

BOX 50-2	Clinical Predictors of Perioperative Cardiovascular Risk
Major	Unstable coronary syndromes, decompensated CHF, significant arrhythmias, severe valvular disease
Intermediate	Mild angina pectoris, myocardial infarction (>30 d old), compensated or previous CHF, diabetes mellitus
Minor	Advanced age, abnormal ECG results, rhythm other than sinus, low functional capacity, history of stroke, uncontrolled systemic hypertension

CHF, Congestive heart failure; *ECG,* electrocardiogram.

BOX 50-3   Cardiac Risk Stratification for Noncardiac Surgical Procedures*

HIGH (REPORTED RISK, ≥ 5%)
- Emergency major operations
- Aortic, major, and peripheral vascular surgery
- Extensive surgical procedures with large volume shifts or blood loss

INTERMEDIATE (REPORTED RISK, ≥1% AND <5%)
- Intraperitoneal and intrathoracic surgery
- Carotid endarterectomy
- Head and neck surgery
- Orthopedic surgery
- Prostate surgery

LOW (REPORTED RISK, <1%)
- Endoscopic procedures
- Superficial biopsy
- Cataract surgery
- Breast surgery

Adapted from Mukherjee D, Eagle KA: Perioperative cardiac assessment for noncardiac surgery: eight steps to the best possible outcome, *Circulation* 107:2771–2774, 2003.
*Combined incidence rate of cardiac death and nonfatal myocardial infarction.

---

normal aging and which are disease states. Current research suggests that overall heart size in healthy older adults does not change significantly with age.[27] However, there are many cellular and biochemical changes associated with older age.[16,24,28] These changes include altered growth-controlling factors, impaired excitation-contraction coupling, impaired calcium homeostasis, increased myocyte apoptosis, and an increase in atrial natriuretic peptide secretion.

As a result of these age-related biochemical and molecular changes, a number of morphologic changes manifest as changes in cardiac function (Table 50-2). It is important to note that cardiac senescence can result in a number of functional impairments. These impairments can include decreased mechanical and contractile efficiency, prolongation of the contraction phase, stiffening of myocardial cells, stiffening of valves and mural connective tissue, decreased number of myocytes, increased myocyte size, increased rate of myocyte apoptosis, and a blunted beta-adrenoceptor–mediated inotropic response.[29-31]

There is tremendous variability in both the level and intensity of age-related changes to the heart. In nonstressful conditions, the normal aging heart functions appropriately. Under stress or with damage from disease, the effects of age become more profound and can lead to functional limitations and reduced quality of life for the patient.

Table 50-2	Changes in Cardiovascular Physiology in Healthy Individuals Between Ages 20 and 80 Years*
LV end-diastolic volume	↑20% males; ↔ females
LV end-systolic volume	↑20% males; ↔ females
Ejection fraction	↔
Stroke volume	↑20% males; ↔ females
Heart rate	↓10%
Cardiac output	↔ males; ↓ 15% females
Stroke work	↑15%
Early diastolic filling rate	↓50%
Systolic arterial pressure	↑15%
Systemic vascular resistance	↔ males; ↓ 45% females

Adapted from Eagle KA: Perioperative cardiac assessment for noncardiac surgery: eight steps to the best possible outcome, *Circulation* 107:2771–2774, 2003.
LV, Left ventricular; ↔, no change; ↑, increase; ↓, decrease.

Respiratory System

The structural and age-related changes that can occur in the respiratory system are clinically influential to the perioperative care of the older adult patient. Structurally, an increase in chest wall rigidity increases the work of breathing. By the time an individual is 70 years of age, an approximately 20% decrease in respiratory muscle strength and endurance and a 15% decrease in alveolar surface area are seen. Older patients have an attenuated response to hypoxemia and hypercapnia. Changes in lung volume include a 20 to 40 mL/yr decrease in vital capacity, a 30% increase in residual volume by the age of 70 years, increased closing volume, and a 0.05% annual decrease in gas exchange.[32]

These changes in the older adult patient may hinder the ability of the patient to meet additional postoperative workloads, thus increasing the risk for acute respiratory failure. The older adult patient is more likely to develop apnea in response to opioids and benzodiazepines. The blunted response to hypoxia and lower baseline arterial oxygen tension increases the risk of postoperative hypoxemia, which can contribute to myocardial ischemia and infarction.[25]

Renal System

The kidneys have a crucial role in fluid and electrolyte balance. As with other body systems, the aging process affects the efficiency of the kidneys and the urinary and renal systems. Age-related changes in renal function can elevate cardiovascular risk in

older adults and make them more prone to hypervolemia and hypovolemia, hypertension or hypotension, and heart failure. By the age of 70 years, glomerular filtration rate decreases at least 30% and as much as 50%; cortical nephrons are decreased; decreases are seen in renal blood flow, ability to concentrate urine, ability to conserve sodium, and tubular secretion; thirst perception is lowered; and a 10% to 15% reduction in total body water is seen.[33]

Attention to fluid and electrolyte balance is of the utmost importance in the perianesthesia care of the older patient. Altered thirst, rennin response, and ability to concentrate urine are likely to facilitate sodium and volume depletion, which may disrupt the Starling mechanism and challenge the older patient's ability to maintain cardiac output and arterial pressure during periods of increased demand.

Hepatic Function

By the time an individual is 80 years old, an approximate 40% reduction in hepatic mass and a 40% decrease in hepatic and splanchnic blood flow are seen. Decrease in the activity of hepatic cholinesterase and microsomal demethylation pathway may also accompany increasing age.[34,35] These changes lead to an impaired ability to meet the increased demands of metabolism, biotransformation, and protein synthesis after surgery. Drugs that rely on hepatic metabolism have a prolonged effect for older adults. For prevention of hepatic injury from medication, hypoxia, or transfusion, careful attention to appropriate drug dosage and adequate oxygenation should be made.

Thermoregulation

Temperature regulation is slower with advanced age, with the shivering and sweating responses showing marked reductions.[17] As a result, advanced age is considered a predisposing factor for perioperative hypothermia,[36-39] which can impose increased demands on the cardiovascular system. Specifically, perioperative hypothermia exerts a number of adverse effects, including prolonged drug action,[40] negative postoperative oxygen balance,[41] immune dysfunction,[42] and subsequent increased incidence of wound infection.[43] Cardiac changes include a leftward shift of the hemoglobin-oxygen saturation curve, increased vascular resistance, cardiac arrhythmias, and up to a fourfold increase in cardiac output and oxygen consumption associated with rewarming and shivering.[42] Special care to maintain normothermia can minimize the risk of postoperative ischemia and angina in older patients.

Sensory System

Although sensory changes are significantly affected by lifestyle, by midlife most individuals experience presbyopia (age-associated vision change) and presbycusis (age-associated hearing change). Being mindful of sensory changes improves the care for patients.

Communication with a person with age-associated hearing loss, or presbycusis, can be improved by:

- Identifying yourself.
- Assuming the person understands everything you are saying. Include the patient in the conversation unless they tell you otherwise.
- Addressing the person by last name unless asked to do otherwise. Avoid pet names such as "honey" and "sweetie."
- Always approaching the patient from the front. Face the patient when you speak. This action enhances the patient's ability to hear you and demonstrates interest and respect.
- Using good eye contact. Use a positive friendly facial expression. Elders are much better at interpreting social cues and notice on negative messages much easier than younger people.
- Using expanded speech and speaking in a lower pitch, rather than raising the voice. This action is helpful because presbycusis is marked by loss of high pitches, and raising your voice also raises your pitch. Also, a lower pitch is more calming.
- Using proper enunciation. Loss of hearing "S" and "F" sounds is most frequent.
- Encouraging the patient to wear a hearing aid, if the patient uses one.
- Being certain that the environment is "elder friendly" or is a low-distraction and low-noise environment. Presbycusis specifically affects a person's ability to filter ambient sound.
- Using written instructions if hearing loss is significant.

Communication with a person with age-associated vision loss, or presbyopia, can be improved by:

- Approaching the person face to face.
- Identifying yourself when you approach and avoiding startling the patient.
- Telling the person your intentions before you begin.
- Using large-print (sans serif, high-contrast print is best) or recorded material when available.
- Encouraging the patient to wear glasses and keep them clean, if he or she uses glasses.
- Being certain that older patients have sufficient time to adjust to light changes and that stairs and walkways are clutter free and clearly marked. Presbyopia specifically affects the ability to adjust between light and dark surroundings and depth perception.

A person-centered approach and respectful language is foundational to providing quality care and assisting patients to maintain a sense of self. Frequently, ageist stereotypes lead to inaccurate assumptions regarding compliance and performance. Poor cognitive performance once thought to be the result of age-related cognitive decline is now understood to be the result of extraneous variables such as sensory changes, fatigue, low education levels, hypermotivation, and polypharmacy.

THE AGING MIND: AN OVERVIEW

Memory and Cognition

The majority of older adults perform well cognitively in day-to-day lives throughout late life. Although cognitive changes do not significantly affect day-to-day functioning, older adults in a vulnerable state (e.g., hospitalization, illness, injury) may show poor concentration, confusion, and disorganized thought patterns. Long-term memory is not altered as a part of normal aging, but attentional abilities and working memory are often affected as part of normal aging by 80 years of age.

Compared with younger cohorts, older adults do not encode new information as deeply, causing greater difficulty with new information retrieval. This difference is the result of many factors: anatomic changes in the brain, poor sensory encoding, cohort differences in the use of memory strategies, and difficulty filtering irrelevant environmental stimuli and noise. Recent research indicates that older adults trained in memory strategies can improve performance on cognitive tasks. Although these changes do not typically affect day-to-day functioning, they can affect understanding and compliance to the care plan particularly in high-stress situations in which cognitive and physical reserve and challenged. Therefore, avoidance of inaccurate assumptions from ageist attitudes and careful communication are essential to quality care. Implementing adult learning techniques and providing care plan information in multiple formats (verbal and print) can be helpful.

Dementia and Delirium

Differentiating dementia, cognitive impairment, and delirium is essential for the anesthesia provider. Whereas true dementias are inherently irreversible, delirium and cognitive decline are potentially reversible if properly diagnosed and treated.

It is well established that dementia is not a normal or inevitable part of the aging process. Although Alzheimer disease (AD) is the most common type of dementia and accounts for 60% to 70% of all dementia, other forms of dementia also affect older adults. For example, vascular dementia, Lewy body dementia, and frontotemporal dementia are also prevalent forms.

The dementias are characterized by a global decline in cognitive function resulting in significant social or functional impairment.[44] Dementia seriously affects a person's ability to perform activities of daily living, including feeding, bathing, and dressing. Initial involvement is in parts of the brain that control thought, memory, and language. Although the exact cause of AD is unknown, autopsies reveal three different types of lesions on patients' brains: senile plaques, neurofibrillary tangles, and vascular lesions. Senile plaques and vascular lesions contain high levels of beta-amyloid protein. The important consideration from an anesthesia perspective is that the presence of dementia also indicates that the patient has increased metabolic risk and comorbidities that need to be addressed during preanesthesia and perianesthesia phases.

Cognitive impairment refers to cognitive changes including short-term memory loss, confusion, and decreased performance on neuropsychological tests. Symptoms of cognitive impairment are greater than changes caused by normal aging, but are insufficient to meet the criteria for a dementia diagnosis. Delirium is a disorder that disrupts brain functionality. Delirium clinically presents with major behavioral changes not explained by a preexisting dementia.[27]

Postoperative cognitive decline and delirium are adverse events that occur frequently in older adults.[45] One study of delirium in older adult patients found a prevalence of 31.4% at initial assessment and an incidence of 31.1% during the course of hospitalization.[44] Postoperative deliriums can be particularly prevalent and problematic for older patients. Preexisting patient factors, medications, and various intraoperative and postoperative causes have been implicated in the development of postoperative delirium.[45]

There are a number of tools available for assessing and screening for delirium, including the confusion assessment method (CAM), and the delirium rating scale (DRS).[46,47] A physical examination, history assessment, and laboratory study are all important tools for identifying possible causes of delirium.

WORKING WITH THE AGING POPULATION: ESSENTIAL CONCEPTS

Geropharmacology

Older adults living in the community take an average of 2.7 to 4.2 prescription and nonprescription medications.[48] Nonprescription medications include both over-the-counter (OTC) drugs as well as dietary supplements. Among prescription medication users, approximately 46% concurrently use OTC drugs and 52% concurrently use dietary supplements.[49] Concurrent use of prescription medications, OTCs, and dietary supplements can lead to medication-related adverse events. Medication-related problems have many forms, often as a result of polypharmacy: overuse of medications, inappropriate prescribing, and drug interactions. Hanlon and colleagues[48] found that 55% of outpatients were taking drugs with no indication, 33% were taking ineffective drugs, and 17% were taking drugs with therapeutic duplications.[50,51] Thirty percent of hospital admissions are linked to medication-related problems; furthermore, medication-related problems are the fifth leading cause of death in the United States.[52]

Almost one quarter of community-dwelling older adults use medications that should be avoided. The Beers criteria, a list of medications that are usually considered inappropriate when given to elderly people, were created to measure inappropriate prescribing and highlight common drug interactions.[53] These criteria are updated regularly and should be a companion when working with older adult patients. For example, long-acting benzodiazepines, dipyridamole, propoxyphene, and amitriptyline were the most frequently inappropriately prescribed medications.[51] Table 50-3 illustrates some possible adverse effects or drug interactions that can take place in older patients during the perioperative period. Age-related changes to organ systems affect a drug's pharmacokinetic and pharmacodynamic properties.

Pharmacokinetics refers to the time it takes for the drug to be liberated, absorbed, distributed, metabolized, and excreted. Drug distribution is altered by the age-related decrease in total body water and lean mass, increase in total body fat, decrease in serum albumin, decrease in cardiac output, reduction in blood volume, and increase in α_1-acid glycoprotein.[54] Injection of medication into a contracted blood volume produces a higher plasma concentration of drug. High protein–bound drugs may have an exaggerated clinical effect (e.g., lidocaine,

Table 50-3	Adverse Effects or Drug Interactions Associated with the Older Adult Patient
DRUG	**ADVERSE EFFECT OR DRUG INTERACTION**
Antibiotic	Prolongation of muscle relaxants
Antidysrhythmic	Prolongation of muscle relaxants
Benzodiazepine	
Diazepam	Decreased metabolism
Chlordiazepoxide	Increased CNS effects
Flurazepam	Prolonged drowsiness
Digoxin	Decreased renal excretion with increased CNS disorientation, anorexia, nausea, and cardiotoxicity; blood levels twofold to threefold higher in older adult with any given dose
Diuretic	Hypokalemia, hypovolemia
Halothane	Decreased anesthetic requirement
Lithium	Clearance decreased by 65% and effective dose by 30% in comparison with patients at 25 years of age; increased side effects of tremor, diarrhea, and edema
Meperidine	Markedly elevated plasma levels and decreased red blood cell and plasma binding of drug; increased incidence rate of nausea, respiratory distress, and hypotension
Methyldopa	Enhanced hypotensive effects
Pancuronium	Decreased clearance from plasma
Propranolol	Plasma level approximately threefold to fourfold higher in elderly because of decreased metabolism; bradycardia, congestive heart failure, bronchospasm, mental confusion, and attenuation of autonomic nervous system activity
Tricyclic antidepressant	Increased anticholinergic effects: confusion, agitation, and disorientation; cardiac conduction disturbances; increased anesthetic requirements
Warfarin	Enhanced sensitivity

Adapted from Krechel S, editor: *Anesthesia and the geriatric patient,* New York, 1984, Grune & Stratton; Miller R, editor: *Anesthesia,* ed 5, New York, 2000, Churchill Livingstone.
CNS, Central nervous system.

propranolol, thiopental, etomidate, profol, alfentanil) because of a higher level of unbound (free) drug. Decreased distribution of water-soluble drugs can cause an adverse reaction because of the initial high plasma concentrations. Conversely, increased distribution of fat-soluble drugs can prolong the action of that medication (e.g., diazepam, midazolam).[54]

Pharmacodynamics is the ability of the drug to react with a specific receptor and to translate that effect on the receptor into a physiologic response. This reaction can render older adults more sensitive to a given concentration of most drugs; however, the opposite is true in regard to beta-adrenoreceptor antagonist and agonist and to digoxin. A higher incidence rate of hyperkalemia, renal failure, and death from gastrointestinal bleeding is associated with the use of nonsteroidal antiinflammatory drugs.[18,54]

In the assessment of the older adult patient, the informed clinician must consider changes in cardiovascular, renal, hepatic, and respiratory function; the compensatory mechanisms; and coexisting comorbid conditions. As a result of marked heterogeneity of drug response in older adult patients, no strict age rules can be applied across the entire older adult population.[25]

Person-Centered Care and Cultural Competence

Adults 65 years of age and older compose a culturally diverse and heterogeneous population. Although cohort effects (e.g., being raised during the Great Depression) result in some similarities in terms of preferences from living within one historic time period, many years of lived experience lead to enormous interindividual diversity.

Person-centered care necessitates taking the time to know the patient's personal preferences, goals, and priorities to provide the highest quality care. A person-centered approach views the patient as the center of defining what is most important to effective delivery of his or her care and care outcomes. An individuals' life experience affects their personal health beliefs, which results in a wide variety of understanding, preferences, and knowledge regarding care provision and medical practice. Assurance of understanding is essential to quality patient care and is at the foundation of person-centered care. Contrary to popular belief, older adults are among the most compliant in regard to care planning. Most frequently, poor compliance is the result of external barriers (e.g., income restrictions) and lack of understanding from poor communication.

Evidence-Based Practice

Gerontological content was infused within three core graduate nursing courses for advanced practice nurses: Theoretical Foundations in Advanced Nursing Practice; Critique and Utilization of Research in Nursing; and Law, Policy, and Economics of Health Care. Gerontological content in core courses provides a foundation for core competencies, which are addressed in the support and specialty of nurse anesthesia as well as other nursing disciplines. Introducing advanced practice nursing students to gerontological content early in their program can encourage students to seek further training and education in a gerontological nursing specialty.

IMPLICATIONS FOR PRACTICE

Perianesthesia nurses can be engaged learners of gerontological content during their training and education, adequately preparing them to deliver quality care to older adults. Gerontological education is paramount to preparing nursing professionals serving the aging community.

Source: Kohlenberg E, et al: Infusing gerontological nursing content into advanced practice nursing education, *Nurs Outlook* 55:38–43, 2007.

The population of older adults includes increasing numbers of individuals from diverse ethnic groups and backgrounds. This diversity presents practitioners with both opportunities and challenges in providing culturally relevant care to the individual. Cultural competency challenges us to understand how people of different cultural backgrounds might approach health, health care, and treatment options. Cultural competence also means having the ability to provide care to persons with diverse values, beliefs, and behaviors and to tailor care delivery to their social, cultural, and linguistic needs. Being culturally competent entails being aware and accepting of differences, thinking about how one's own culture influences oneself, and being aware of when cultures interact, what stereotypes are at play, and what patterns of communication are necessary to avoid misinterpretations or misjudgments.

SUMMARY

Perianesthesia nursing care of older patients requires a thorough understand of physiologic and psychological changes that occur with aging. An accurate assessment of the individual is necessary based on personal functioning, the presence of co-morbidities, medication regimen, and psychological

outlook of the older adult patient. When caring for older adults, keep in mind that age is just a marker of years lived and does not accurately represent the totality of the older patient.

REFERENCES

1. U.S. Census Bureau of Census: *Current population survey*, Washington, DC, 2003, U.S. Government Printing Office.
2. Fries JF: Aging, natural death and the compression of morbidity, *N Engl J Med* 303:130−135, 1980.
3. World Health Organization: *Preamble to the Constitution of the World Health Organization as adopted by the International Health Conference*, available at www.who.int/about/definition/en/print.html. Accessed August 13, 2011.
4. Birren JE, Cunningham WR: Research on the psychology of aging: principles, concepts, and theory. In Birren JE, Schaie KW, editors: *The handbook of the psychology of aging*, New York, 1985, Van Nostrand Reinhold Co, Inc.
5. Bailes BK: Perioperative care of the elderly surgical patient, *AORN J* 72(2): 186−206, 2000.
6. Bekker A, et al: Does mild cognitive impairment increase the risk of developing postoperative cognitive dysfunction? *Am J Surgery* 199:782−788, 2010.
7. Henderson JL: *Thresholds of initiation*, Middletown, Connecticut, 1967, Wesleyan University Press.
8. Centers for Disease Control: *Trends in health and aging: aging and chronic disease statistics branch* (website). www.cdc.gov/index.htm. Accessed August 2, 2011.
9. Maddox TM: Preoperative cardiac evaluation for noncardiac surgery, *Mt Sinai J Med* 72(3): 185−192, 2005.
10. Arena R, et al: Assessment of functional capacity in clinical and research settings, *Circulation* 116(3):329−343, 2007.
11. Eagle KA, et al: ACC/AHA guideline update for perioperative cardiovascular evaluation for non-cardiac surgery: executive summary: a report of the American College of Cardiology/American Heart Association Task Force on Practice Guidelines (Committee to update the 1996 Guidelines on Perioperative Cardiovascular Evaluation for Noncardiac Surgery), *Circulation* 94:1052–1064, 2002.
12. Fleisher LA: Preoperative cardiac evaluation, *Anesthesiol Clin North Am* 22: 59−75, 2004.
13. McArdle WD, et al: *Exercise physiology: energy, nutrition and human performance*, ed 3, Philadelphia, 1991, Lea & Febiger.
14. Hlatky MA, et al: A brief self-administered questionnaire to determine functional capacity, *Am J Cardiol* 64:651–654, 1989.
15. Fletcher GF, et al: Exercise standards: a statement for healthcare professionals from the American Heart Association, *Circulation* 104:1694–1740, 2001.
16. Lakatta EG: Cardiovascular aging research: the next horizons, *J Am Geriatic Soc* 47: 613–667, 1999.
17. Lakatta EG: Aging effects on the vasculature in health: risk factors for cardiovascular disease, *Am J Geriatr Cardiol* 3:11–17, 1994.
18. Lakatta EG, et al: *Heart disease: a textbook of cardiovascular medicine*, ed 5, Philadelphia, 1997, Saunders.
19. Wei JY: Age and the cardiovascular system, *N Engl J Med* 327:1735–1739, 1992.

20. Klein AL, et al: Effects of age and physiologic variables on right ventricular filling dynamics in normal subjects, *Am J Cardiol* 84:440–448, 1999.
21. Gardin JM, et al: Left ventricular diastolic filling in the elderly: the cardiovascular health study, *Am J Cardiol* 82:345–351, 1998.
22. Palka P, et al: The effect of long-term training on age-related left ventricular changes by Doppler myocardial velocity gradient, *Am J Cardiol* 84:1061–1067, 1999.
23. Schulman SP, et al: Age-related decline in left ventricular filling at rest and exercise, *Am J Physiol* 263: H1932–H1938, 1992.
24. Lakatta EG: Changes in cardiovascular function with aging, *Eur Heart J* II (suppl C):22–29, 1990.
25. Priebe HJ: The aged cardiovascular risk patient, *Br J Anesth* 85:763–778, 2000.
26. Eagle KA: Perioperative cardiac assessment for noncardiac surgery: eight steps to the best possible outcome, *Circulation* 107:2771–2774, 2003.
27. Saxon SV, et al: Physical change and aging: a guide for the helping professions, ed 5, New York, 2010, Springer.
28. Folkow B, Svanborg A: Physiology of cardiovascular aging, *Physiol Rev* 73:725–764, 1993.
29. Lakatta EG: Cardiovascular mechanisms in advanced age, *Physiol Rev* 73:413–467, 1993.
30. Olivetti G, et al: Cardiomyopathy of the aging human heart: myocyte loss and reactive cellular hypertrophy, *Circ Res* 68:1560–1568, 1991.
31. Yang B, et al: Age-related left ventricular function in the mouse: analysis based on in vivo pressure-volume relationships, *Am J Physiol* 46:HI906–HI913, 1999.
32. Carpo RO, Campbell EJ: Aging of the respiratory system. In Fishman AP, editor: *Pulmonary diseases and disorders*, New York, 1998, McGraw-Hill.
33. Shannon RP, et al: The influence of age on water balance in man, *Semin Nephrol* 4:346–352, 1984.
34. Shannon RP, et al: The effect of age and sodium depletion on cardiovascular response to orthostasis, *Hypertension* 8: 438–443, 1986.
35. Kampnann JP, et al: Effect of age on liver function, *Geriatrics* 30:91–95, 1975.
36. Woodhouse KW, et al: The effect of age on pathways of drug metabolism in human liver, *Age Ageing* 13:328–334, 1984.
37. Freidl LP, et al: Risk factors for 5-year mortality in older adults: the cardiovascular health study, *JAMA* 279:585–592, 1998.
38. Kurz A, et al: The threshold for thermoregulatory vasoconstriction during nitrous oxide/isoflurane anesthesia is lower in the elderly than in young patients, *Anesthesiology* 79:465–469, 1993.
39. Vaughan MS, et al: Postoperative hypothermia in adults: relationship with age anesthesia, and shivering to re-warming, *Anesth Ana* 60:746–751, 1981.
40. Heier T, et al: Mild intraoperative hypothermia increases duration of action and spontaneous recovery of verconium blockade during nitrous oxide-isoflurane anesthesia in humans, *Anesthesiology* 74:815–819, 1991.
41. Carli R, et al: Effect of preoperative normothermia on post operative protein metabolism in elderly patients undergoing hip arthroplasty, *Br J Anesth* 63:276–282, 1989.
42. Valeri RC, et al: Hypothermia-induced reversible platelet dysfunction, *Ann Surg* 205:175–181, 1987.
43. Kurz A, et al: The study of wound infection and temperature group: perioperative normothermia to reduce the incidence of surgical wound infection and shorten hospitalization, *N Engl J Med* 334: 1029–1035, 1996.
44. Ajilore OA, Kumar A: Delirum and dementia, *Journal of Lifelong Learning in Psychiatry* 2: 211–220, 2004.
45. Fong HK, et al: The role of postoperative analgesia in delirium and cognitive decline in elderly patients: A systematic review, *Anesth Analg* 102:1255–1266, 2006.
46. Trzepacz PT, et al: A symptom scale for delirium, *Psychiatry Res* 23:89–97, 1988.
47. Inouye SK, et al: Clarifying confusion: the confusion assessment method, *Ann Intern Med* 113:941–948, 1990.
48. Hanlon JT, et al: Suboptimal prescribing in older inpatients and older outpatients, *JAGS* 4: 200–209, 2001.
49. Qato DM, et al: Use of prescription and over-the-counter medications and dietary supplements among older adults in the United States, *JAMA* 300(24):2867–2878, 2008.
50. Fick DM, et al: Updating the Beers criteria for potentially inappropriate medications in older adults: results of a U.S. consensus panel of experts, *Arch Intern Med* 163:2716–2724, 2003.
51. Aparasu RR, Mort JR: Inappropriate prescribing for the elderly: Beers criteria-based review, *Ann Pharomacother* 34:338–346, 2000.
52. Simon SR, Gurwitz JH: Drug therapy in the elderly: improving quality and access, *Clinical Pharmacol* 73:387–393, 2003.
53. Beers MH: Explicit criteria for determining potentially inappropriate medication use by the elderly: an update, *Arch Intern Med* 157:1531–1536, 1997.
54. Montamat SC, et al: Management of drug therapy in the elderly, *N Engl J Med* 304:405–412, 1989.

RESOURCES

Allen J: Geriatric education and competence a nursing necessity, *J Perianesth Nurs* 24(3):185, 2009.
Asher M: Surgical considerations in the elderly, *J Perianesth Nurs* 19(6):406–414, 2004.
Doerflinger DMC: Older adult surgical patients: Presentation and challenges, *AORN* 90(2):223–244, 2009
Frank SM, et al: The perioperative ischemia randomized anesthesia trial study group: unintentional hypothermia is associated with post-operative myocardial ischemia, *Anesthesiology* 78:468–476, 1993.
Kuchta A, Golembiewski J: Medication use in the elderly patient: focus on the perioperative/perianesthesia setting, *J Perianesth Nurs* 19(6):415–427, 2004.
Monarch S, Wren K: Geriatric anesthesia implications, *J Perianesth Nurs* 19(6):379–384, 2004.
Paynter D, Mamaril M: Perianesthesia challenges in geriatric pain management, *J Perianesth Nurs* 19(6):385–391, 2004.
Saufl N: Preparing the older adult for surgery and anesthesia, *J Perianesth Nurs* 19(6):372–378, 2004.

51 Care of the Pregnant Patient

Mallorie Croal, BS, MSN, CLE,
and Joseph F. Burkard, DNSc, CRNA

The incidence rate of surgery performed on pregnant women for reasons unrelated to the pregnancy itself has been reported to be as high as 50,000 to 75,000 cases per year, with a frequency range of 0.75% to 2%.[1] The most common conditions that require surgical intervention are acute appendicitis, ovarian cysts, and breast tumors, with laparoscopy being the most common first-trimester procedure. However, more complicated procedures have been reported and include craniotomy, open-heart surgery, and aneurysm repair that have been performed successfully in pregnant patients.[1,2]

In care of the pregnant patient after surgery, one must remember that two patients require nursing care and assessment: the mother and the fetus. Perianesthesia nursing care should be directed toward emotional support for the mother and avoidance of uterine stimulation that could produce preterm labor. Also of prime importance are prevention of respiratory depression in the mother and maintenance of normal uterine placental blood flow to ensure adequate fetal supply of oxygen and nutrients.[1-3]

DEFINITIONS

Aortocaval Compression (Scott Syndrome): Obstruction of the inferior vena cava and the pelvic veins by the enlarging uterus.

Aspiration Pneumonitis: An inflammatory condition of the lungs and bronchi caused by material in the stomach regurgitated into the pharynx and inhaled through the epiglottis into the lungs and bronchi.

Cesarean Section: A surgical procedure in which the abdomen and pregnant uterus are incised and the baby is delivered transabdominally.

Cricoid Pressure (Sellick Maneuver): Used in rapid sequence intubation of the trachea in which the cricoid cartilage is pushed against the body of the sixth cervical vertebra in an effort to compress the esophagus to prevent passive regurgitation.

Defasciculation: Administration of a nondepolarizing muscle relaxant 1 to 3 minutes before the administration of succinylcholine to prevent the muscle twitches that usually occur after the administration of a depolarizing muscle relaxant with the intended outcome of reducing the amount of gastric pressure created by the muscle twitches or fasciculations.

Esophagitis: The inflammation of the mucosal lining of the esophagus.

Gastric Motility: The spontaneous peristaltic movements of the stomach that move the stomach contents through the pyloric sphincter into the duodenum.

Gastroesophageal Reflux: Often referred to as *heartburn;* a result of a backflow of stomach contents as a result of an incompetent lower esophageal sphincter muscle.

Hypovolemia: A reduction from normal in blood volume.

Physiologic Anemia of Pregnancy: A normal reduction in hemoglobin in the blood as a result of the normal physiologic process of pregnancy.

Plasma Cholinesterase: An enzyme in the plasma that is responsible for the metabolic breakdown of acetylcholine to choline and acetate.

Pruritus: The symptom of itching of the skin.

Retained Placenta: After the birth of the infant, the placenta is usually delivered within 30 minutes; if it is expelled after 30 minutes, it is considered to be a retained placenta.

Sepsis: Infection or contamination.

Thromboembolism: A situation in which a blood vessel becomes obstructed by a clot or thrombus that had been carried by the bloodstream from its site of formation.

PHYSIOLOGIC CHANGES OF PREGNANCY

Almost every system in the body is affected in some way during pregnancy, either from hormonal changes or from the increasing size of the uterus. The changes that affect perianesthesia nursing care are outlined in Box 51-1 and are discussed in the following sections.

Cardiovascular Changes
Hemodynamic Alterations

The cardiovascular system undergoes significant change as pregnancy advances. Cardiac output and heart rate increase progressively during pregnancy until, at 30 to 34 weeks' gestation, the cardiac output is 30% to 50% higher than normal and the heart rate is approximately 15% greater than the nonpregnant

BOX 51-1   Physiologic Changes in Pregnancy

CARDIOVASCULAR SYSTEM
- Flow and pressure changes
  - Cardiac output increases from 20% at the end of the first trimester to 40% at term
  - Heart rate at more than 15% of nonpregnant level
  - Stroke volume increases
  - Ejection fraction increases
  - Pulmonary capillary wedge pressure has no significant change
  - Central venous pressure has no significant change
  - Systolic blood pressure decreases to approximately 10 mm Hg below nonpregnant level at term
  - Diastolic blood pressure decreases by 15 to 20 mm Hg in early gestation through 30 weeks and then returns to pregestation levels at term
- Blood volume and constituents
  - Total blood volume increases to approximately 45% above nonpregnant levels
  - Total plasma volume increases to approximately 55% above nonpregnant levels
  - Red blood cell mass increases to approximately 30% above nonpregnant levels
  - Hematocrit levels decrease to approximately 36 mg/dL during gestation
  - Hemoglobin levels decrease to approximately 11.6 g/dL
  - Plasma cholinesterase levels decrease as much as 80% of nonpregnant levels
- Coagulation
  - Prothrombin time and partial thromboplastin time decreases 20%; platelet count decreases 15%; bleeding time decreases 10%

RESPIRATORY SYSTEM
- Anatomic changes
  - Capillary engorgement of the nasal and oropharyngeal mucosa and larynx
  - Increased circumference of the thoracic cage
  - Elevated diaphragm

- Respiratory system flow, volume, and ventilation changes
  - No change in FEV_1
  - No change in flow-volume loop
  - Total pulmonary resistance decreases
  - Tidal volume increases from 20% to 45% above nonpregnant levels
  - Functional residual capacity decreases by 20% to 60% below nonpregnant level
  - Alveolar ventilation increases by 30% to 45% above nonpregnant level
  - Minute ventilation increases by 45% above nonpregnant level
- Changes in blood gases
  - $PaCO_2$ decreases to approximately 30 mm Hg
  - PaO_2 increases to approximately 103 to 105 mm Hg
  - Arterial pH from 10 weeks' gestation until delivery is approximately 7.44
- Metabolic rate and acid-base status
  - Metabolic rate is depressed during first 12 to 16 weeks
  - Metabolic rate is 15% above nonpregnant level at term
  - Oxygen consumption is 35% above nonpregnant level at term
  - Oxygen consumption is 40% above nonpregnant level during first stage of labor
  - Oxygen consumption is 75% above nonpregnant level during second stage of labor
  - Respiratory alkalosis with some metabolic compensation is present

GASTROINTESTINAL SYSTEM
- Gastric emptying delays after 34 weeks' gestation
- Gastric volume increases
- Gastric pH decreases
- Pyrosis (heartburn) is present in approximately 50% of pregnant women
- Intragastric pressure increases
- Hepatic blood flow and function not altered

RENAL SYSTEM
- Glomerular filtration rate increases
- Urine output increases

FEV_1, Forced expiratory volume in 1 second, $PaCO_2$, Partial pressure of carbon dioxide in arterial blood, PaO_2, Partial pressure of oxygen in arterial blood.

normal level, with electrocardiographic changes and heart sounds possibly developing (Box 51-2). The systolic blood pressure is minimally affected by pregnancy, with a maximum decline of approximately 8% during early to middle gestation and a return to the pregnant level at term. Diastolic blood pressure falls to a greater degree than does systolic pressure, with early to middle gestational decreases of approximately 20%. It also returns to a prepregnancy level at term.[4]

Perhaps the most significant effect on the cardiovascular system for the nurse to consider in routine postanesthesia management is obstruction of the inferior vena cava and the pelvic veins by the enlarging uterus (Figs. 51-1 and 51-2). This condition, known as *aortocaval compression* or *Scott syndrome,* can develop by the second trimester and cause supine hypotension. Avoidance of the supine position becomes mandatory after surgery, because it can significantly aggravate the

BOX 51-2   Possible Alterations in Cardiovascular Parameters

- Heart sounds are louder with the development of a split S_2
- Short systolic murmur
- More forceful apical impulse
- Inverted T waves in leads III, V_1, and V_2
- Left axis deviation in months 2 to 6
- Flattened T waves
- Depressed ST segments
- If findings develop during pregnancy, they usually disappear after delivery

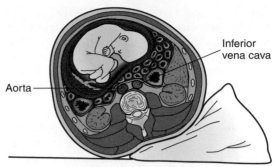

FIG. 51-3 Uterine displacement with wedge under hip to relieve aortocaval compression. (From Lowdermilk DL, et al: *Maternity and women's health care*, ed 10, St. Louis, 2012, Mosby.)

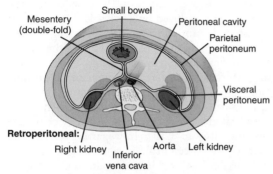

FIG. 51-1 Cross section of lower abdomen (nonpregnant). (From Bontrager KL, Lampignano JP: *Textbook of radiographic positioning and related anatomy*, ed 7, St. Louis, 2010, Mosby.)

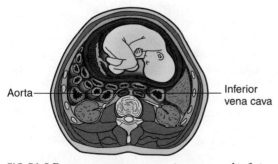

FIG. 51-2 Pregnant uterus compressing aorta and inferior vena cava (aortocaval compression). Patient is in supine position. (From Lowdermilk DL, et al: *Maternity and women's health care*, ed 10, St. Louis, 2012, Mosby.)

obstruction. Treatment includes the administration of additional intravenous crystalloid, the placement of the mother in the side-lying position, and the administration of supplemental oxygen (Fig. 51-3).[5,6]

Collateral circulation for venous return develops through the intervertebral venous plexus and the azygos vein. This condition reduces the volume of the epidural and subarachnoid spaces; therefore the amount of drug during regional anesthesia should be decreased. With this in mind, the perianesthesia nurse should assess the patient on admission for a high block and monitor dermatome levels frequently thereafter (see Chapter 25).[5,6]

In the nonpregnant patient, the sympathetic nervous system plays a role in promoting venous return to the heart from the lower extremities. This sympathetic stimulation of vasomotor tone is enhanced during pregnancy in an effort to counteract the negative effects of uterine compression of the vena cava. Clinically, this protective mechanism is abolished with spinal or epidural anesthesia because it acts as a pharmacologic sympathectomy. Without an appropriate preload of fluids (500 to 1000 mL intravenous lactated Ringer solution), the pregnant patient could have a 30% to 50% decrease in blood pressure during the anesthesia. The pregnant patient must receive an appropriate preload of fluids before epidural or spinal anesthesia. Hemodynamic stability can be secured with the infusion of 15 mL/kg of colloid solution or 30 mL/kg of crystalloid solution. If the patient is to receive an inhalation anesthetic agent such as isoflurane or sevoflurane, similar fluid preloading is given because the inhalation anesthetic agents produce peripheral vasodilation.[7]

This increased fluid requirement has significant implications for the perianesthesia care of the pregnant patient. Consequently, the patient's cardiac and hydration status must be monitored closely throughout the emergence phase of regional anesthesia (see Chapter 25).[7,8]

Hematologic Alterations

Blood volume along with the number of platelets, fibrinogen levels, and the level of activity of several clotting factors (VII, VIII, IX, X, and XII) increases by 15% during the first trimester, rises rapidly during the second trimester to 50% above the pregnant levels, and changes little during the remainder of the pregnancy.[7,8] However, a smaller rise in the number of circulating red blood cells occurs. This difference results in lower hematocrit and hemoglobin levels (see Box 51-1), although red blood cell mass actually increases. This condition is known as *physiologic anemia of pregnancy*.[7,8]

The plasma concentration of the enzyme cholinesterase is decreased during pregnancy. Because plasma cholinesterase is involved in the mechanisms of clotting, the perianesthesia nurse should monitor the pregnant patient for thromboembolism. Plasma cholinesterase is also involved in the destruction of the depolarizing muscle relaxant succinylcholine. The recovery time from succinylcholine is unaltered and in fact may be somewhat faster in pregnant women, which is explained by the fact that the volume distribution of succinylcholine increases during pregnancy because of an elevation in the plasma volume. In the immediate postpartum period, the plasma cholinesterase concentration and the plasma volume distribution are further reduced.[7-10]

Respiratory Changes
Upper Airway Anatomy
During pregnancy, capillary engorgement of the upper respiratory tract includes the nasal and oropharyngeal mucosa and larynx, and pregnant women may have nasal stuffiness. In addition, nose breathing is difficult, and nosebleeds can occur. This capillary engorgement of the respiratory mucosa during pregnancy predisposes the upper airways to trauma, bleeding, and obstruction. Gentle laryngoscopy and the use of small endotracheal tubes (6 to 6.5 mm) should be used during general anesthesia.[7-10]

Lung Mechanics and Ventilation
The diaphragm elevates, and the rib cage flares; therefore at term, 85% of respiratory effort is intercostal and 15% diaphragmatic (normally, approximately 70% is intercostal, and 30% is diaphragmatic). Because of the mechanical changes in the lungs and chest wall, the lung volumes and capacities change during pregnancy. Overall, the inspiratory lung volumes and capacities moderately increase, and the expiratory lung volumes and capacities decrease. The inspiratory reserve volume and the inspiratory capacity increase by 5% to 15%. The functional residual capacity (FRC) decreases by approximately 20% to 60%. The residual volume and expiratory reserve volume,

which compose the FRC, are decreased. The combination of decreased FRC and increased oxygen consumption promotes rapid oxygen desaturation during periods of apnea.[7-10]

The tidal volume also increases 20% to 45%, and the respiratory rate does not change, which leads to a 30% to 45% increase in the alveolar ventilation and the minute ventilation. Therefore, during pregnancy, the arterial oxygen level ranges from 95 to 105 mm Hg and the arterial carbon dioxide level is approximately 30 mm Hg, with an arterial pH of 7.44. Consequently, the pregnant patient has some respiratory alkalosis for which the renal excretion of bicarbonate compensates. As a result, the normal bicarbonate level during pregnancy is approximately 19 mEq/L, and the base excess is reduced by 2 mEq/L.[7-10]

Limited information exists regarding the effects of pregnancy on characteristics of the central chemoreflex control of breathing. Some studies suggest that the increased circulation of hormones, particularly progesterone and estradiol, significantly lowers the threshold and increases the sensitivity of the central ventilatory chemoreflex response to CO_2. In regard to flow rate changes, the forced expiratory volume in 1 second and the flow-volume loop remain unchanged. In addition, the closing capacity (see Chapter 12) does not change during gestation.[7-10] Consequently, the conductance and resistance of the small and large airways do not change during pregnancy.

Gastrointestinal Changes
Motility and Secretions
Gastric emptying slows during pregnancy because the stomach is displaced as the uterus enlarges, which leads to gastroesophageal reflux and esophagitis during pregnancy. All parturients have a gastric pH less than 2.5, and more than 60% have gastric volumes greater than 25 mL. The gastric volume also increases during hours 1 to 8 in the postpartum period; therefore the perianesthesia nurse must be cognizant of the potential for vomiting and aspiration, particularly in patients who have had general anesthesia. Muscle relaxants may have been used and can result in the patient's normal protective mechanisms being obtunded. Again, the side-lying position becomes of significant importance.[7-10]

Hepatic System
Liver function test results are abnormal, but no evidence suggests alteration in liver function. Hepatic blood flow remains constant; therefore anesthetic agents that are metabolized in the liver should have the same duration of effect.[7-10]

Renal Changes

Early in pregnancy, the kidneys receive an increased blood flow because of renal vasodilation, and glomerular filtration and urine formation rates increase. This increase is necessary to handle the increased amount of waste products produced. Monitoring of output should reflect this expected increase in volume. Intervention may be necessary for hypovolemia even though the urine output is within ranges acceptable in a nonpregnant patient.[7-10]

Loss of glucose in the urine is not uncommon or necessarily pathogenic during pregnancy, but is merely a reflection of the kidney's inability to reabsorb all of the glucose filtered by the glomeruli. This observation, combined with anatomic changes leading to ureteral atonia and stasis of urine in the ureters, increases the risk for urinary tract infection in the pregnant patient.

Increased water retention is a basic chemical alteration of pregnancy. This alteration leads to a decrease in plasma sodium concentration from 140 to 136 mmol/L and a decrease in plasma osmolality from 290 to 280 mOsmol/kg. Serum potassium levels decrease by an average of 0.2 to 0.3 mEq/L.[7-10]

CARE OF THE OBSTETRIC PATIENT

Because the effects of anesthesia have such a profound effect on the emergence of the pregnant patient, a complete review of the techniques and procedures of general and regional anesthesia is presented.

Positioning

The supine position causes a reduction in uterine blood flow in the pregnant patient; therefore the semi-Fowler position is used when possible. To prevent aortocaval compression, the patient is placed in the lateral decubitus position, and the right hip is elevated with a pillow, or the uterus is displaced to the left with devices on the operating table.[11,12]

Gastrointestinal Considerations

The pregnant patient has a reduced gastric emptying time and a reduced gastric pH. Research has shown that gastric volume and acidity in the pregnant patient do not differ significantly from those in the nonpregnant patient. However, many anesthesia clinicians believe strongly that the pregnant patient, especially the patient with pyrosis (heartburn), is at risk of developing aspiration pneumonitis. Consequently, preoperative pharmacologic interventions are usually taken. Drugs that can be administered include a nonparticulate antacid such as 30 mL of 0.3 mmol/L sodium citrate (Bicitra) to increase the gastric pH; cimetidine (Tagamet) or 50 mg ranitidine (Zantac) or granisetron (Kytril), which are histamine-2 receptor blockers that reduce gastric acid secretion; and 10 mg metoclopramide (Reglan), which accelerates gastric emptying time and elevates lower esophageal tone.[13-15]

General Anesthesia
Induction

Because of the strong full-stomach considerations, the pregnant patient is intubated with a rapid-sequence endotracheal intubation technique (see Chapter 30) that includes intravenous (IV) propofol, etomidate, or ketamine followed by succinylcholine. A defasciculation dose of a nondepolarizing muscle relaxant can be given before the administration of the succinylcholine to avoid the increase in intragastric pressure. Some clinicians do not administer a defasciculating dose of a nondepolarizing muscle relaxant, because most pregnant patients do not have fasciculation after succinylcholine. Cricoid pressure (Sellick maneuver) is applied with an assistant's thumb and index fingers exerting downward pressure on the cricoid cartilage to displace the cartilaginous cricothyroid ring posteriorly and thus compress the underlying esophagus against the cervical vertebrae.[16-19]

The endotracheal tube should be a small tube, usually 6.0 to 6.5 mm in diameter or smaller, because of increased mucosal engorgement in the nasal and oropharyngeal areas. Nasotracheal intubation is not used because of the high risk of tissue trauma.[16-19]

Maintenance

Nitrous oxide in 50% concentration with oxygen is usually administered. Inhalation agents such as sevoflurane, isoflurane, and desflurane can be used. Analgesic concentrations of 0.5 minimum alveolar concentration (see Chapter 20) or less to avoid significant uterine relaxation can be used safely for these inhalation drugs. However, these inhalation agents, particularly sevoflurane, may be used in high concentrations for a short period to produce uterine relaxation for intrauterine manipulation of the fetus or removal of a retained placenta. The clinical implication in the postanesthesia care unit (PACU) for the patient who received a high concentration of an inhalation agent, even for a short period (less than 2 minutes) is monitoring for postpartum hemorrhage and maternal hypotension. The uterine response to oxytocic drugs is reduced when high concentrations of these inhalation agents are used.[16-19]

SPECIAL CONSIDERATIONS

Evidence-Based Practice

In recent history, 0.45% of deliveries developed severe hemorrhage, resulting in the second leading cause of maternal mortality with a rate of 0.66 deaths per 100,000 deliveries. Obstetric hemorrhagic emergencies can be subdivided into antepartum and postpartum. The more common causes of postpartum hemorrhage are uterine atony, uterine inversion, and placenta accreta. Knowledge of the latest preventive or rescue management strategies applicable to massive blood loss in obstetric cases is important.

The American Society of Anesthesiologists taskforce guidelines suggest red blood cell (RBC) transfusion is often needed when hemoglobin is 6 gm/dL and not needed for hemoglobin concentration greater than 10 g/dL in the absence of uncontrolled ongoing bleeding. Borgman and colleagues state that in nonobstetric hemorrhagic trauma patients, there are several cohort studies suggesting improved outcome or survival with early administration of fresh frozen plasma (1 unit of fresh frozen plasma for every 2 units of packed RBCs) and platelets (1 six-pack of pooled platelets for every 6 to 7 units of packed RBCs).

IMPLICATIONS FOR PRACTICE

Perianesthesia nurses can be actively involved in the early diagnosis and multidisciplinary planning for the postpartum hemorrhaging parturient. It is important to have availability of blood and blood products, rapid fluid infusing devices, venous accesses, and consideration for prophylactic internal iliac artery balloon placement for occlusion and embolization, and appropriate availability of obstetric, radiologic, surgical, and anesthesia personnel.

Source: American Society of Anesthesiologists Task Force on Perioperative Blood Transfusion and Adjuvant Therapies: Practice guidelines for perioperative blood transfusion and adjuvant therapies, *Anesthesiology* 105:198–208, 2006; Borgman MA, et al: The ratio of blood products transfused affects mortality in patients receiving massive transfusions at a combat support hospital, *J Trauma* 63:805–813, 2007.

In regard to skeletal muscle relaxation, succinylcholine infusion or short-acting nondepolarizing muscle relaxants such as rocuronium and vecuronium can be used safely, because they lack autonomic side effects and have a low degree of placental transfer. In the immediate postpartum period, the neuromuscular-blocking effects of vecuronium are prolonged.[16-19]

Emergence

At the end of the surgical procedure, the residual effects of the nondepolarizing muscle relaxants are reversed and the inhalation anesthetic agents are discontinued. When the patient is awake, responsive, and able to ventilate without assistance, she is extubated.[16-19]

Regional Anesthesia

Regional anesthesia, primarily spinal and epidural, is used extensively for anesthesia in the pregnant patient because it produces analgesia without causing neonatal depression. This technique also reduces the risk of maternal hypoventilation and the need for opioids and sedatives. Regional anesthesia does not require airway management, preserves airway reflexes, and allows the mother to remain awake during birth. It is contraindicated in patients with severe coagulation problems, severe hypovolemia, sepsis, and infection at the needle insertion site; in situations in which immediate delivery is crucial, such as in fetal distress; and when the patient refuses the procedure.[16,20,21]

The level of sensory blockade for either spinal or epidural anesthesia for cesarean section is from T4 to S4. The commonly used local anesthetic drugs for spinal anesthesia are lidocaine and bupivacaine (see Chapter 24). For epidural anesthesia, the commonly used local anesthetic agents are 2-chloroprocaine (Nesacaine), lidocaine with epinephrine, bupivacaine, and ropivacaine, which may be preferable because of possibly less motor blockade and reduced potential for cardiotoxicity.[16,20,21]

In comparison with the spinal approach, the epidural approach is the preferred technique because drugs can be administered throughout the surgical procedure via a continuous epidural catheter. The anesthesia clinician then has the ability to control the onset, distribution, and duration of anesthesia. In addition, the incidence rate of postdural puncture is much lower in comparison with the spinal technique.[16,20-21]

PERIANESTHESIA CARE OF THE MOTHER AND THE FETUS

Studies have not shown one anesthetic technique to be better than another in the gravid patient. As with nonpregnant patients, the choice of technique is determined by the following:
1. Surgery to be performed
2. American Society of Anesthesiologists classification of the patient
3. Anesthetist preference
4. Patient preference
5. Underlying disease entities

The care of the pregnant patient after surgery should be the same as for any patient who undergoes that procedure or for one who recovers from that particular anesthetic. However, additions to the routine nursing care must be instituted for all pregnant patients.[22-24]

Positioning

To alleviate compression of the vena cava, the uterus should be displaced to the left, either by positioning the patient on her left side or by tilting the pelvis with a folded sheet or bath towel under the woman's right iliac crest. Slight elevation of the legs and the use of thigh-high elastic stockings should be standard.

Psychologic and Emotional Support

The mother's concern for her unborn child is paramount. Constant reassurance is mandatory. If possible, allow the mother to listen to the fetal heartbeat frequently during the recovery phase. Explain all procedures and why they are being done before they are followed. If the PACU allows visitors, involvement of the father should also be considered.[25-27]

Fetal Monitoring

The fetal heart rate must be monitored every 15 minutes if the fetus has reached viability (Table 51-1). If available, an indirect fetal monitoring system should be used for constant assessment of fetal stability (Fig. 51-4). If the fetus is considered previable, it is generally sufficient to ascertain the fetal heart rate by Doppler before and after the procedure.[25,28]

The second type of monitoring required is close observation of the patient for signs of premature labor. These signs include spontaneous rupture of membranes, increased fetal heart rate, presenting of vaginal mucus plug, uterine palpitations, uterine contractions, and restlessness of the mother.[25,28]

Initially, the patient might not feel the contractions or be aware of membrane rupture; therefore palpation of the abdomen and assessment of vaginal discharge must be performed by the nurse. If premature labor begins, transfer of the patient to the labor and delivery area as soon as possible is recommended. A drug may be necessary to stop

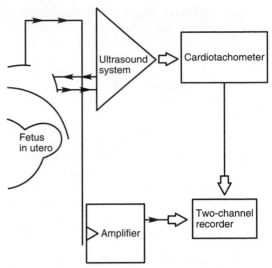

FIG. 51-4 Indirect fetal monitoring system. Doppler ultrasound scan device transmits a beam for determination of fetal heart rate. When the beam strikes a moving object within the fetus, such as mitral valve leaflet, the frequency of transmitted beam is shifted up or down, depending on which way leaflet is moving. This valve movement is counted and displayed as heart rate on the recorder.

labor. These drugs should be administered by personnel familiar with proper protocols for administration and side effects.[25,28]

Pain Management
The Patient After Cesarean Section

The patient after cesarean section presents unique challenges in regard to pain management. More specifically, more women desire to care for their newborns within the first 24 hours. Heavy sedation with opioids and IV or epidural catheters inhibits the mother's ability to care for the infant. In addition, the infant can be affected through the transfer of the drug in breast milk.[20,23,29]

Patient-controlled analgesia (PCA) is becoming popular in pain management of the patient after cesarean section (see Chapters 22, 27, and 31). PCA interrupts the pain cycle, gives the patient a feeling of control, hastens the time to ambulation, and reduces the length of stay in the hospital. Morphine is the preferred drug to be administered via PCA. The usual dose is 1 to 1.5 mg, with a lockout of 10 minutes and an hourly limit of 10 to 12 mg.[16,29]

Epidural administration of opioids is another option that can be used for the control of pain in the PACU. Morphine is the preferred drug because of its demonstrated safety and prolonged duration of action after a single dose of 5 mg. The primary side effects of epidural morphine are

Table 51-1	Fetal Heart Rates
DESCRIPTION	RATE (BEATS/MIN)
Normal fetal heart rate	120-160
Moderate tachycardia	160-180
Marked tachycardia	>180
Moderate bradycardia	100-120
Marked bradycardia	<100

SPECIAL CONSIDERATIONS

pruritus and nausea. Some clinicians have advocated the use of the opioid antagonist naloxone (5 to 10 mcg/kg/h) to treat these side effects; however, problems arise with some reversal of the analgesia. Most clinicians treat the nausea with 2 to 4 mg of ondansetron (Zofran) IV and the pruritus with 12.5 mg of IV diphenhydramine (Benadryl).[16,29]

Fentanyl is an alternative to morphine for epidural analgesia. The difficulty with fentanyl is that its duration of action is less than 5 hours and that it must be administered via continuous infusion or intermittent boluses. The epidural fentanyl technique provides excellent analgesia; however, most women desire to be ambulatory as soon as possible and do not like to be encumbered with the catheter, tape, and pump.[16,29,30]

When administered epidurally with opioids, 2-chloroprocaine inhibits the analgesic effects of the opioids. This inhibitory action of 2-chloroprocaine is probably caused by the ethylenediaminetetraacetic acid (EDTA) that is used in the solution of the drug. EDTA is an antioxidant that has analgesic antagonism properties because it is a strong chelator of calcium. Clinically epidural opioids should be avoided for at least 6 to 8 hours after 2-chloroprocaine has been administered.[16,29,30]

A variety of receptor-specific drugs to include opioids, alpha$_2$-adrenergic agonists, and local anesthetics are being evaluated for use via the intraspinal approach. With the refining of the spinal technique to include the use of small needles, this technique is gaining in popularity for post–cesarean section pain relief. Morphine, 0.3 mg administered intrathecally, has a longer duration of action than 4 mg of morphine administered via the epidural route. Some anesthesia clinicians are now adding morphine to bupivacaine during surgery, with the outcome of excellent analgesia that lasts well into the postanesthesia period.[16,29,30]

Along with the various opioid analgesics, the patient after cesarean section should be administered supplemental oxygen during anesthesia and for the first 2 hours after surgery, not only to enhance pulmonary function but also to potentially help in the prevention of postoperative nausea and vomiting. More research is needed to evaluate the effectiveness during the immediate postanesthesia period.[16,29,30]

The Pregnant Patient

Because of the growth in consumer awareness, the administration of medication during pregnancy has become a controversial issue that must be addressed on an individual basis. For pain management in the PACU, when the pregnant patient is in a hypersuggestive state, distraction techniques such as guided imagery and breathing exercises have had favorable results in place of drugs.[31,32]

If a mild analgesic is needed, the drug of choice is acetaminophen (Tylenol). For moderate pain management, oral or sublingual opioids (morphine, methadone, codeine, and in some countries oxycodone, buprenorphine, and fentanyl) can be used safely for short periods during pregnancy. If prolonged administration is expected, drugs without active metabolites are preferable, such as methadone rather than morphine for short-term pain management. Opioid analgesia may be warranted for severe pain but must be used judiciously, with the respiratory depressive effects kept in mind.[31-33] Ketorolac (Toradol), a prostaglandin synthetase inhibitor, is becoming popular in postoperative pain therapy. However, nonsteroidal antiinflammatory agents, such as ketorolac, are not recommended in the parturient, because they suppress uterine contractions and promote closure of the fetal ductus arteriosus.[31-34]

The gravid patient in the PACU is a rare occurrence that requires the nurse to have a great deal of knowledge and the ability to provide continual support during this stressful situation. The nurse must be able to provide a quiet calm reassuring atmosphere for the patient. The objective of the care delivered is an optimal environment for both the mother and the fetus.[31-34]

SUMMARY

The perianesthesia nursing care of the obstetric patient who is undergoing a nonobstetric surgical procedure is both challenging and rewarding. Statistics indicate that approximately 1 in 500 pregnancies are complicated by nonobstetric surgical conditions. The intent of this chapter is to provide information on the pregnant patient and fetus undergoing nonobstetric surgery. The physiologic changes, types of surgery, and perianesthesia nursing care were highlighted and should provide the perianesthesia nurse with valuable knowledge to facilitate the appropriate outcomes for the mother and fetus.[35]

REFERENCES

1. Abboud T: Nonobstetric surgery during pregnancy, *Semin Anesth* 11(1):51–54, 1992.
2. ACOG Committee Opinion Number 474: Nonobstetric surgery during pregnancy, *Obstetrics and Gynecology* 117(2):420–421, 2011.
3. Alspach J: *Core curriculum for critical care nursing*, ed 6, Philadelphia, 2005, Saunders.

4. Barash P, et al: *Clinical anesthesia*, ed 6, Philadelphia, 2009, Lippincott Williams & Wilkins.
5. Benumof J, Saidman L: *Anesthesia and perioperative complications*, ed 2, St. Louis, 1999, Mosby.
6. Belfort M, et al: *Critical care obstetrics*, ed 5, Oxford, 2010, Wiley-Blackwell.
7. Chestnut D: *Obstetrical anesthesia: principles and practice*, ed 4, Philadelphia, 2009, Mosby.
8. Chichester M: When your patient is from the obstetric department: postpartum hemorrhage and massive transfusion, *J Perianesth Nurs* 20(3):167–176, 2005.
9. Conklin K: Maternal physiological adaptations during gestation, labor, and the puerperium, *Semin Anesth* 10(4):221–234, 2005.
10. Hall J: *Guyton and Hall textbook of medical physiology*, ed 12, Philadelphia, 2011, Saunders.
11. Bowdle T, et al: *The pharmacologic basis of anesthesiology*, New York, 1994, Churchill Livingstone.
12. Martin J: *Positioning in anesthesia and surgery*, ed 3, St. Louis, 1997, Mosby.
13. Miller R, et al: *Miller's anesthesia*, ed 7, Philadelphia, 2009, Churchill Livingstone.
14. Moran D, Dewan D: Anesthesia for cesarean delivery, *Semin Anesth* 10(4):286–294, 1991.
15. Morgan E, et al: *Clinical anesthesiology*, ed 4, New York, 2006, McGraw-Hill.
16. Nagelhout J, Plaus K: *Nurse anesthesia*, ed 4, Philadelphia, 2010, Saunders.
17. Shnider S, Levinson G: *Anesthesia for obstetrics*, ed 4, Philadelphia, 2002, Lippincott Williams & Wilkins.
18. Stoelting R: *Pharmacology and physiology in anesthetic practice*, ed 4, Philadelphia, 2005, Lippincott Williams & Wilkins.
19. Miller R, Pardo Jr. MC: *Basics of anesthesia*, ed 6, New York, 2011, Saunders.
20. Eisenach J: Pain management in the parturient: theoretical and practical aspects, *Semin Anesth* 11(1):55–65, 1992.
21. Estafanous F, et al: *Cardiac anesthesia*, ed 2, Philadelphia, 2001, Lippincott Williams & Wilkins.
22. Coté C, et al: *A practice of anesthesia for infants and children*, ed 4, Philadelphia, 2008, Saunders.
23. Gbods A, Set al: Effect of postoperative supplemental oxygen on nausea and vomiting after cesarean birth, *J Perianesth Nurs* 20(3):200–205, 2005.
24. Torgersen K: Communication to facilitate care of the obstetric surgical patient in a postanesthesia care setting, *J Perianesth Nurs* 20(3):177–183, 2005.
25. Lake C, et al: *Clinical monitoring: practical applications for anesthesia and critical care*, St. Louis, 2001, Mosby.
26. Davidson M, et al: *Maternal-newborn nursing and women's health across the lifespan*, ed 9, Upper Saddle River, NJ, 2011, Pearson Education.
27. Curran C: Perianesthesia care following obstetric emergencies at risk for multisystem organ dysfunction, *J Perianesth Nurs* 20(3):185–199, 2005.
28. Motoyama E: *Smith's anesthesia for infants and children*, ed 8, St. Louis, 2011, Mosby.
29. Schick L, Windle PE: *Perianesthesia nursing core curriculum: preprocedure, phase I and phase II PACU nursing*, St. Louis, 2010, Saunders.
30. Hardman J, Limbird L: *Goodman and Gilman's the pharmacological basis of therapeutics*, ed 12, New York, 2010, McGraw-Hill.
31. Chestnut DH, et al: *Chestnut's obstetric anesthesia*, ed 4, Philadelphia, 2009, Mosby.
32. Shaver S, Shaver D: Preoperative assessment of the obstetric patient undergoing abdominal surgery, *J Perianesth Nurs* 20:160–166, 2005.
33. Fleisher LA: *Anesthesia and uncommon diseases*, ed 5, Philadelphia, 2007, Saunders.
34. Katzung B, editor: *Basic and clinical pharmacology*, ed 11, Los Altos, CA, 2009, Appleton & Lange.
35. Ziadlourad F, Conklin K: Anesthesia for obstetric emergencies, *Semin Anesth* 8(3):222–231, 1989.

SPECIAL CONSIDERATIONS

52 Care of the Substance-Using Patient

Cecil B. Drain, PhD, RN, CRNA, FAAN, FASAHP

Substance abuse is the major public health issue in America. More than 25 million Americans have used illicit drugs on a monthly basis, and more than 80% of all the opioids in the world are probably used primarily in the United States.[1-5] Add to this the fact that the abuse of prescription drugs has become a major contributing factor to the increase in the use of illicit drugs. Consequently, the significant increase in the number of persons who use opioids, amphetamines, cocaine, hallucinogens, barbiturates, and date rape drugs has created new problems in today's perianesthesia nursing care. One in five patients in the perioperative area has an alcohol use disorder, one in three patients has a nicotine use disorder, and one in 10 patients has a drug use disorder.[6]

Drug dependence is the nonmedical use of a drug and consists of the self administration of any drug in a manner that deviates from the approved medical or social practices within a given culture.[5] Physical dependence is an altered physiologic state caused by repeated administration of a drug that necessitates the continued administration of the drug to prevent the appearance of withdrawal or abstinence syndromes characteristic for that drug. Psychologic dependence is habituation-compulsive drug use. In this type of dependence, a drug is used to alter mood and feeling. Eventually, dependent people come to believe that the effects of the drug are necessary to maintain an optimal state of well being. Another term that should be defined in discussions of substance dependence is tolerance. Drug tolerance is a state in which, after repeated administration of a drug, a given dose produces a decreased effect or in which increasingly larger doses are needed to obtain the same effect as that of the original dose.

The pharmacologic agents that are most commonly seen in dependence can be grouped as follows: (1) opioid analgesics; (2) general central nervous system (CNS) depressants, such as alcohol and barbiturates; (3) CNS sympathomimetics, such as amphetamines and cocaine; (4) cannabinoids, such as marijuana; and (5) psychedelics (of which lysergic acid diethylamide (LSD) and phencyclidine are the prototypic drugs; Table 52-1), inhalants, club drugs, and date rape drugs.

DEFINITIONS

Alcoholic: A person who is excessively dependent on alcohol and who has a noticeable degree of mental, physical, psychologic, or pathologic disorders.

Alcoholic Cirrhosis (Laënnec's Cirrhosis): A fibrotic form of cirrhosis precipitated by alcohol abuse.

Anterograde Amnesia: The inability to form new memories or recall events that occur after the onset of the amnesia.

Delirium Tremens: An acute and sometimes fatal psychotic reaction caused by cessation of excessive intake of alcoholic beverages over a long period of time.

Endocarditis: Inflammation of the endocardium and heart valves.

Hallucinations: A sensory perception that does not result from an external stimulus and that occurs in the waking state.

Plasma Cholinesterase: An enzyme in the blood plasma that acts as a catalyst in the hydrolysis of acetylcholine to choline and acetate.

Potentiated: A synergistic action in which the effect of two drugs given simultaneously is greater than the sum of the effects of each drug given separately.

Sensorium: The part of the consciousness that includes the special sensory perceptive powers and their central correlation and integration in the brain. A clear sensorium conveys the presence of a reasonably accurate memory together with spacial orientation.

Substance Abuse: The overuse of stimulant, depressant, or other chemicals or drugs that is detrimental to the patient's physical or mental health.

Substance Dependence: The total psychophysical state of one addicted to drugs or alcohol who must receive an increasing amount of the substance to prevent the onset of withdrawal symptoms.

Substance Use: A maladaptive pattern of the use of a drug, chemical, or biologic entity that is capable of being abused because of its physiologic or psychologic effects.

Tremulousness: Involuntary muscle contraction.

OPIOID ANALGESICS

Opioid analgesics cause strong psychological dependence. Physical dependence is manifested by the withdrawal syndrome of autonomic storm and CNS irritability. A strong tolerance for these drugs and a cross tolerance with other drugs of the same classification of opioid analgesics develop. Studies indicate that in people who are

Table 52-1	Categories of Substance Dependence: Effects and Signs of Dependence and Withdrawal		
CATEGORY	**POSSIBLE EFFECTS**	**SIGNS OF DEPENDENCE**	**SIGNS OF WITHDRAWAL**
Opioid Analgesics			
Opium Morphine Codeine Heroin Meperidine (Demerol) Sublimaze (Fentanyl) Methadone (Dolophine)	Euphoria, "rush" with IV injection, feeling of detachment, drowsiness, miosis, nausea, respiratory depression Tolerance and physical and psychologic dependence	Injection scars or needle marks, usually on inner surfaces of arms Thrombophlebitis at injection sites, cellulitis Pinpoint pupils Uncoordinated movements Confusion, disorientation Heavy smoking	Watery eyes, runny nose, scratching, yawning, anorexia, irritability, tremors, panic, chills and sweating, muscle pains and cramps, nausea, vomiting, diarrhea
General CNS Depressants			
Alcohol	Loss of inhibitions Impaired judgment Carefree mood Impaired motor coordination, concentration, memory Ataxia, incoherence Stupor, coma Tolerance and physical dependence	Reported intake: Heavy drinker* Alcohol-addicted† GI disturbances Malnutrition Heavy smoking Trauma Psychologic problems Social maladjustment	*8 hours after abstinence:* Tremors, GI disturbances, anxiety, jittery feeling, and headache *24–72 hours or longer of withdrawal:* Increased tremors, hyperactivity, irritability, nervousness, insomnia, delusions, hallucinations, seizures, DTs, high fever, profuse sweating, tachycardia, hyperventilation, nausea and vomiting
Barbiturates			
Amytal Butisol Nembutal Seconal Tuinal Phenobarbital	Euphoria, reduced anxiety, dry intoxication (drunken behavior without odor of alcohol) Tolerance and physical and psychologic dependence	Drowsiness, lack of interest, fatigue, irritability Changes in personality and behavior Possession of pills of varying colors and shapes	Range from anxiety, weakness, confusion, anorexia, and mild tremors to delirium, disorientation, hallucinations, and convulsions
Benzodiazepines			
Valium Librium Serax Ativan Versed	Same as barbiturates	Same as barbiturates	Same as barbiturates

Continued

Table 52-1   Categories of Substance Dependence: Effects and Signs of Dependence and Withdrawal—cont'd

CATEGORY	POSSIBLE EFFECTS	SIGNS OF DEPENDENCE	SIGNS OF WITHDRAWAL
CNS Sympathomimetics			
Amphetamines	Increased alertness, euphoria, anorexia, insomnia, elevated blood pressure, tachycardia, anxiety Tolerance, psychologic dependence	Possession of pills of varying color Injection scars, needle marks Compulsion to talk, extreme activity, chain smoking Frequent nose rubbing or scratching, licking of dry lips, bad breath Changed eating and sleeping habits Projected sense of prowess or capability Possible aggressive or antisocial behavior	"Crashing" (response produced when stimulant effect ends); hunger, extreme lethargy, profound depression, and sleep disturbance
Cocaine	Same as amphetamines Possible tolerance, no physical dependence, high psychologic dependence	Same as amphetamines Inflamed nasal mucosa	Same as amphetamines "Crashing" may be profound
Cannabinoids			
Marijuana (hashish)	Sense of relaxation and well being Distorted orientation to time and space Altered sensory perception Occasional excitement and spontaneous (often uncontrolled) laughter Increased appetite Tolerance and psychologic dependence, degree of physical dependence unknown	Possession of off-white or brown cigarette papers and coarse brownish-green tobacco Conjunctival congestion, dilated pupils Wearing of dark glasses because of light sensitivity	*Reported abstinence symptoms:* Hyperexcitability, insomnia, decreased appetite
Psychedelics			
Lysergic acid diethylamide (LSD) Phencyclidine (PCP)	Illusions Distorted perceptions of time, distance, body image, mood, affect Depersonalization and ego dissociation Psychotic behavior Tolerance, degree of psychologic dependence unknown	Possession of perforated small squares of blotter paper with colored designs, ampules of clear liquid, or capsules of white or colored powder, or tablets Unusual body odor Marked mood changes Dreamlike or trancelike state	None reported

From Bready L, et al: *Decision making in anesthesiology*, ed 4, St. Louis, 2007, Mosby.
IV, Intravenous; *CNS*, central nervous system; *GI*, gastrointestinal; *DT*, delirium tremens.
*A person who consumes five or more drinks on some occasions and at least 45 drinks a month.
†A person who consumes approximately 20 drinks of beer, wine, or liquor per day and has developed physiologic tolerance.

chronically addicted to opioid analgesics such as morphine, the minimum alveolar concentration of inhalation anesthetics (see Chapter 20) is increased, which indicates that a cross tolerance with general inhalation anesthetics may exist.[7,8]

Heroin, an opioid analgesic that is derived from morphine, is degraded in the body to morphine approximately 30 minutes after injection. The most common problem associated with the use of heroin and other opioid analgesics is pulmonary edema; other dysfunctions include superficial bacterial infections, adrenal insufficiency, bacterial endocarditis, liver disease, urinary abnormalities (proteinuria and glycosuria), and false-positive serology. In addition, approximately 30% of the persons dependent on opiates have positive results on the Venereal Disease Research Laboratory test for syphilis, but approximately 25% of these results are true positive when checked with the *Treponema* immobilization test.

Perianesthesia nursing care of a patient who is dependent on an opiate, such as heroin dependency, focuses on monitoring the patient for complications.[3] Monitoring for the withdrawal (abstinence) syndrome is the foremost concern. The abstinence syndrome after dependence on an opiate occurs in two phases. The acute phase occurs during the first few days. The protracted phase, which is not readily treatable, can persist for as long as 2 to 6 months. The acute opiate abstinence phase is not dangerous to life because it usually is not associated with convulsions and delirium. Instead, the symptoms are anxiety, nervousness, jittery behavior, anorexia, rhinorrhea, hypotension, muscle twitching, insomnia, sweating, pupillary dilation, gooseflesh, nausea, and vomiting. Symptoms during the protracted phase include those of the acute phase, along with convulsions and delirium. Treatment for the acute opiate abstinence phase is accomplished with any opioid analgesic; reports indicate that clonidine has proved to be most effective in attenuating the symptoms. New research indicates that dexmedetomidine may also be effective in attenuating the symptoms. Treatment for the protracted phase focuses on protection of the patient and abatement of the symptoms shown by the patient. If a patient is suspected of dependence on an opiate, opioid antagonists such as naloxone (Narcan) should not be administered because the withdrawal syndrome can be precipitated. No attempt should be made at withdrawal of the patient who is actively dependent on an opiate during the postanesthesia care unit (PACU) period. Liberal use of morphine or methadone in the PACU appears to be satisfactory. Patients who are formerly dependent on opioids should not receive opioids;

analgesics such as pentazocine (Talwin) and butorphanol (Stadol) should be used in their place. Nonsteroidal antiinflammatory drugs may also be considered in a multimodal approach for these patients.[6]

GENERAL CENTRAL NERVOUS SYSTEM DEPRESSANTS

The patient dependent on a barbiturate may appear only nervous and anxious before surgery; however, the patient should be monitored after surgery for anxiety, tremors, and hallucinations. These symptoms usually develop on the second or third postoperative day and can be treated with a barbiturate until acute illness has passed. These patients also appear to have an increased tolerance to anesthesia and therefore have an increased chance of anesthetic toxicity.

The dependency rate of persons taking benzodiazepine compounds has increased significantly during the last decade. The benzodiazepine drug is usually taken in combination with marijuana or alcohol to obtain a high. Chronic intoxication has been reported with the use of these compounds. The benzodiazepine that produces the most dependency is diazepam (Valium); however, midazolam (Versed) will soon rank at the same level as diazepam. These drugs are becoming popular because of their rapid onset of action coupled with their pleasure-giving effects. The pharmacologic effects of the benzodiazepines are similar to those of the barbiturates.[9] This classification of drugs is somewhat addictive and includes withdrawal syndromes.

For treatment of mild to moderate overdoses of benzodiazepines, the drug physostigmine in an adult dosage of 1 to 2 mg given intravenously can be used. Flumazenil (Romazicon), is a true benzodiazepine receptor antagonist with longer action and fewer side effects. The usual adult dose is 0.1 to 0.2 mg given intravenously. As with naloxone for patient dependence on an opioid, flumazenil must be used with caution with patients who are benzodiazepine dependent. More specifically, reversal of benzodiazepine dependence is associated with precipitating the withdrawal syndrome, including seizures (see Chapter 21).

Alcoholism has long been widespread, but it is difficult to define. An alcoholic, for the purposes of this discussion, is a person who is excessively dependent on alcohol and who has developed a noticeable degree of mental, physical, psychologic, or pathologic disorders. Alcohol was the first anesthetic; it can produce anesthesia, respiratory depression, and hypotension. Alcoholic dependency has been linked to complications during the perianesthesia phase including alcohol withdrawal syndrome, increased infections, acute respiratory distress syndrome, cardiovascular complications, and secondary hemorrhage.[6]

Alcohol affects many of the body's major systems.[10] Cirrhosis of the liver is common in the later stages of alcoholism. This knowledge is of importance to the perianesthesia nurse because the liver detoxifies many drugs administered during the perioperative period (see Chapter 16). Hepatic cirrhosis can produce significant alterations in pulmonary and cardiovascular functions. Hyperventilation and arterial oxygen desaturation are common findings caused by an increase in shunting of blood away from areas in the lung where diffusion of oxygen occurs. Concomitant with this is an increase in blood volume that can lead to cardiac hypertrophy and eventually to congestive heart failure. Fluid balance is affected by the presence of alcohol, because alcohol exhibits antidiuretic effects by inhibiting the release of antidiuretic hormone. Alcoholic cirrhosis (Laënnec's cirrhosis) is also associated with portal vein hypertension, renal failure, hypoglycemia, duodenal ulcer, esophageal varices, and hepatic encephalopathy.

The alcoholic, in comparison with the nonalcoholic, usually requires a larger amount of sodium thiopental for induction and a higher concentration of anesthetic agents during surgery. Prediction of the time or the character of emergence from anesthesia is difficult in the alcoholic patient. This patient may be anxious and may have a stormy emergence and postoperative phase.

During the PACU phase, the alcoholic patient should be monitored for withdrawal symptoms. The minor alcohol withdrawal syndrome is characterized by symptoms such as tremulousness, insomnia, and irritability. Because of autonomic nervous system imbalance, signs such as tachycardia, hypertension, and cardiac dysrhythmias are often observed. The minor alcohol withdrawal syndrome can occur within 6 to 8 hours after abstinence by the alcoholic patient. The signs and symptoms of this syndrome usually disappear within 48 hours without treatment.

In approximately 5% of the alcoholic population, the severe alcohol withdrawal syndrome, or delirium tremens, occurs with abrupt cessation of alcohol ingestion. The mortality rate from this syndrome is approximately 15%; it is considered a medical emergency. The time of onset of delirium tremens is 48 to 72 hours after the abrupt discontinuation of alcohol ingestion.[11]

The patient is difficult to manage if withdrawal symptoms are allowed to develop. The severe withdrawal syndrome should be suspected if symptoms occur, such as restlessness, disorientation, tremulousness, and hallucinations. In addition, because of activation of the sympathetic nervous system, symptoms such as diaphoresis, hyperpyrexia, tachycardia, and hypertension are seen. When any of these symptoms are observed, hypoxia should first be ruled out because the symptoms of withdrawal can be confused with those of hypoxia. The treatment used to control the withdrawal symptoms is sedation with diazepam, along with intravenous fluids and electrolytes, vitamin replacement (i.e., thiamine), and glucose. If deemed necessary by the attending physician, propranolol may be given to suppress the clinical manifestations of the increased sympathetic nervous system activity. If cardiac dysrhythmias occur, lidocaine can be administered intravenously.

CENTRAL NERVOUS SYSTEM SYMPATHOMIMETICS

Cocaine has a two-pronged effect—vasoconstriction and mood alteration—because it inhibits the reuptake of catecholamines.[9,12] The mood-altering effect is similar to the psychological effect produced by amphetamines. Cocaine is steadily becoming one of the most popular drugs among persons dependent on a substance. Patients who are known to be dependent on cocaine should be closely monitored in the PACU for hypertension and cardiac arrhythmias. These patients are prone to nosebleeds, and care should be taken in giving nursing care near or directly to the nose and nasal cavity.

CNS stimulants, which include amphetamines, are becoming extremely popular with the teenage population; they tend to have the pharmacologic effect of long-acting vasopressors. The patient has dilated pupils, tachycardia, palpitations, cardiac arrhythmias, and changes in temperature regulation and appears to be extremely anxious. If the stimulant is wearing off, the patient is lethargic and depressed. Continuous electrocardiographic monitoring for cardiac arrhythmias is necessary and is coupled with frequent blood pressure and pulse measurements. The mental sensorium should also be monitored throughout the patient's stay in the PACU.

CANNABINOIDS

The hemp plants, for which *cannabis* is the generic name, contain approximately 30 active substances that are called *cannabinoids*. Of these, tetrahydrocannabinol (THC) is the most active. *Marijuana* is the generic term applied to the hemp plants.

The marijuana cigarette contains rolled or crushed dried leaves from the hemp plant. Each marijuana cigarette contains approximately 0.005 g of THC. The cannabinoids are threefold more potent when inhaled than when ingested orally. Psychological changes occur minutes after inhalation of marijuana, and the effects peak in 1 hour for as long as 3 hours.[3]

The peripheral effects of THC on the autonomic nervous system include vagal blockade and beta-adrenergic stimulation. The person dependent on marijuana has tachycardia, peripheral vascular dilation, bronchodilation, conjunctival congestion, and a dry mouth. The actual effects of THC on the CNS are not known.[13]

Because of the rapid effects of the drug, along with the short duration of action and the absence of physiologic dysfunction or changes, patients dependent on marijuana do not seem to present any added problems in the PACU. Because of the chronic irritation produced by the inhalation of smoke from the marijuana cigarette, chronic dependence should be monitored for chronic bronchitis.

PSYCHEDELICS

Phencyclidine is the hallucinogen most commonly used today. This drug is a popular veterinary anesthetic agent (Sernylan) and is related pharmacologically to the drug ketamine. It can be ingested, taken parenterally, or inhaled. The sensory effects have a rapid onset and last approximately 1 to 2 hours, and the CNS effects can last for 1 or more days. The CNS activation usually produces sympathetic nervous system activation.[14]

The perianesthesia nurse is unlikely to have much contact with a patient under the influence of this drug. If a patient who is dependent on this drug should require perianesthesia care, the nurse must monitor this patient for sympathetic activation; symptoms such as dilated pupils, increased pulse, and elevated blood pressure should be reported immediately to the attending physician.

LSD is a hallucinogen that reached its peak of use in the late 1960s and remained popular through in the 1990s. This drug is ingested orally, and its major effects occur in a dose-related manner. Moderate doses of the drug cause euphoria, marked sensory distortion (including heightened awareness of sensory stimuli), and occasional visual hallucinations. Large doses of LSD usually lead to frightening hallucinations and a distorted body image, commonly known as a *bad trip*. This drug also produces some hypertension, dilated pupils, and increased temperature, by virtue of its stimulation of the central hypothalamic area of the brain. The onset of the psychologic effects of LSD is after approximately 40 minutes, and the duration is approximately 2 hours. Some of the milder effects of LSD have been reported to last as long as 8 hours after ingestion.

The primary focus of perianesthesia nursing care for the patient who is in the hallucinogenic state is to prevent self injury and sedation. The bad trip effects can be managed with a phenothiazine or benzodiazepine such as diazepam. Other considerations in regard to the patient who has ingested LSD are that the analgesic effects of opioids are potentiated by LSD and that the plasma cholinesterases are somewhat inhibited by LSD. Opioid dosage may need to be reduced in these patients, and if succinylcholine is to be administered to the patient, the possibility of prolonged apnea exists (see Chapter 23).

INHALANTS

Inhalants can make a person extremely dependent and consist of breathable chemical vapors that produce mind-altering effects. Persons who use inhalants can have significant dependence; they are likely to be teenage people because the drugs are easily accessible and inexpensive.[14,15] Inhalants are classified into three categories: solvents, gases, and nitrates.

The solvents consist of paint thinners or solvents, electronic contact cleaners, and felt-tip marker fluid. The gases consist of such household products and commercial products as butane lighters and propane tanks, whipping cream aerosols, spray paints, hair or deodorant sprays, and fabric protector sprays. Gases used for anesthetic medical purposes, such as isoflurane, sevoflurane, desflurane, and nitrous oxide (see Chapter 20), are now being used illicitly and can cause dependency.[16] The nitrates—such as cyclohexyl nitrite and butyl nitrite, which are available to the public, and amyl nitrite, which is only available by prescription—are now used as substances that can produce dependency.

The inhalants that cause dependency produce effects that are similar to the inhalational anesthetics as described in Chapter 20. Basically, these inhalants cause an intoxicating effect when they are inhaled through the nose or mouth into the lungs. When inhaled in high concentrations, these inhalants can induce heart failure and even death. Some of the irreversible effects of these inhalants can include hearing loss, peripheral neuropathies or limb spasms, central nervous system damage, and bone marrow damage. Some of the serious yet potentially reversible effects include hemoglobin oxygen depletion and liver or kidney damage.[17]

The implications in the perianesthesia care of a patient who is using inhalants can be great. Given the fact that these substances can cause reversible and irreversible effects, each patient should be evaluated individually for use of these drugs. Health care professionals who care for these patients should remember that these inhalants are mainly used by children, with the highest usage between grades 6 and 12, and that usage continues to be a significant problem among youths. For perianesthesia nursing, the deliberate misuse of these volatile substances poses a significant risk or considerable morbidity and mortality in the adolescent population in the PACU. All these inhalants basically cause severe dysfunction to the liver and cause it to be unable to detoxify most drugs used in anesthesia. Consequently, even small doses of opioid or nonopioid drugs have a prolonged length of action. Should the perianesthesia nurse suspect that a patient is dependent on inhalants, the anesthesia care provider must be advised because an entirely new regime of pain relief care has to be developed. Certainly, the lowest dose of any opioid or nonopioid should be considered, and the perianesthesia nurse should monitor for signs of cardiovascular and respiratory depression.

CLUB DRUGS

Club drugs are most popular in the teenage and young adult population who are part of the nightclub, bar, rave, or trance scenes. Raves and trance parties are usually nightlong events that include adolescents who might not use the specific drugs; however, those who do are attracted to the use of these rather low-cost agents that appear to produce increased stamina and intoxicating highs. Research now shows that these drugs can change critical parts of the brain. Because of the different effects on the E-C coupling mechanisms of muscles as opposed to skeletal muscle relaxants (see Chapter 23), these agents are not implicated in malignant hyperthermia (see Chapter 53).

3,4-Methylenedioxymethamphetamine (MDMA, or ecstasy) is a psychoactive drug that has both stimulant (amphetamine-like) and hallucinogenic (LSD-like) properties. This drug has many street names such as *ecstasy*, *Adam*, *XTC*, *hug*, *beans*, and *love drug*. MDMA has many routes of administration, including oral, rectal, intravenous, or inhalation.[18]

The problems associated with MDMA are similar to those found with the use of amphetamines and cocaine, which were discussed previously. The psychological difficulties may include such phenomena as confusion, depression, sleep problems, severe anxiety, and paranoia. The physical difficulties include such things as muscle tension, involuntary teeth clenching, nausea, blurred vision, faintness, and chills or sweating. Physiologic concerns are that this category of drugs can cause hypertension and tachycardia, and long-term use can result in damage to the brain in the parts that focus on thought, memory, and pleasure.

Research on the effects of MDMA on the patient recovering from anesthesia continues to be desperately needed. The reader is encouraged to review the effects of cocaine because the pharmacologic actions are similar, and consequently the effects of the MDMA category of drugs on emergence from anesthesia could be significant, resembling the emergence of the patient with cocaine dependence.

DATE RAPE DRUGS

Gamma hydroxybutyrate (GHB) is a euphoric, sedative, and anabolic. It is a widely used drug that was obtained over the counter in health food stores until 1992. It has street names of *liquid ecstasy*, *soap*, *easy lay*, and *Georgia home boy*. Coma and seizures can occur after the use of GHB. Combined with alcohol, GHB can cause nausea and dyspnea. GHB has been associated with poisonings, overdoses, date rapes, and deaths. This drug has a short duration of action and is not easily detectable on routine hospital toxicology screening tests. Research needs to be conducted on this drug to determine its long-term effects, and actual dependency has not been established.

Flunitrazepam (Rohypnol) is a benzodiazepine that when mixed with alcohol incapacitates victims and prevents them from resisting sexual assault. This drug, like midazolam, produces anterograde amnesia. This drug is not approved for use in the United States and its importation is illegal. The street names for this drug include *rophies*, *roofies*, *roach*, and *rope*, and its illegal use continues to be a problem in the border states, particularly Texas and Arizona.

Ketamine is an intravenous anesthetic drug (see Chapter 21) that is used illegally in the club and rave scenes and has been used as a date rape drug. It can be injected or snorted and is known on the street as *special K* or *vitamin K*. This drug produces a dreamlike state and hallucinations.[18] In high doses, ketamine causes delirium, amnesia, impaired motor function, high blood pressure, depression, and apnea. The veterinary form of this drug appears to create the most dependency; its frequency of use is steadily increasing.

CARE OF THE SUBSTANCE ABUSE PATIENT IN THE POSTANESTHESIA CARE UNIT

The use of illicit drugs has become a national issue, particularly in the health care arena. It is even a greater issue for the health care providers in the perianesthesia nursing setting. The recreational drugs, such as alcohol, along with the many other illicit drugs such as cannabis, "crack," LSD, cocaine, and amphetamines present a significant challenge to the PACU nurse. Many of these patients that abuse drugs can have a "normal" anesthetic experience and then experience acute drug withdrawal in the PACU. If a patient exhibits increased blood pressure, tachycardia, abdominal cramping, irritability, tremors, diarrhea, or sweating, acute drug withdrawal should be suspected. The patient should be examined for the signs and symptoms as described in Table 52-2. After the evaluation is performed, the PACU nurse should notify the attending physician or anesthetist to facilitate the appropriate intervention. The treatment should be symptom oriented, and use of scoring systems to determine treatment approach is becoming more prevalent.[6] In addition, the emergency drugs and equipment should be placed at the patient's bedside. Other interventions will probably include a blood sample and a urine sample to aid in the identification of the specific drug in question.

Evidence-Based Practice

Kleinwächter and colleagues conducted a study to compare the anesthesia provider detection rate of illicit substance use (ISU) during routine preoperative assessment with a self-assessment questionnaire completed by the patients. The questionnaire asked patients about ISU, alcohol use disorder, nicotine use, and socioeconomic information. Findings after 2938 patients had completed the questionnaire were that 7.5% of patients reported ISU within the past year. ISU was associated with 18 to 30 years old, men, smokers, and positive for alcohol use disorder. Anesthesia providers detected ISU in 1 of 43 patients, whereas the patients self-reported on the computerized questionnaire as 1 in 13 patients with ISU.

IMPLICATIONS FOR PRACTICE

If anesthesia providers underestimate the prevalence of ISU, we can assume that perianesthesia nurses in the preoperative assessment areas also underestimate use. Preoperative assessment clinics provide an appropriate setting for interventions regarding ISU, determining high-risk behavior, and effective strategies to institute lifestyle changes. Perianesthesia nurses in the preoperative setting should consider the use of a structured computerized self-assessment questionnaire about ISU with the goal of increased recognition and decreased perioperative risks for the patient.

Source: Kleinwächter R, et al: Improving the detection of illicit substance use in preoperative anesthesiological assessment, *Minerva Anestesiol* 76:29–37, 2010.

Table 53-2   Initial Patient Evaluation for Suspected Substance Abuse

EVALUATION FOCUS	EVIDENCE OF SUBSTANCE ABUSE
Evidence of drug injection	Track marks or scaring, thrombotic veins, phlebitis, tattoos used to mask the injection site, subcutaneous skin abscesses, poor venous return in effected arm or hand
Ophthalmologic changes	Pupillary constriction (from opioid use), papillary dilation (from amphetamine use), nystagmus (from phencyclidine use)
Nourishment	Malnourishment (from amphetamine use and/or alcohol use), normal nourishment (opioid users)
Nasal	Nasal perforation from cocaine abuse
Teeth	Poor dental care, bruxism from involuntary grinding and clenching of teeth from amphetamine use
Lymphatic system	Lymphadenopathy that can be caused by the chronic use of injections with impurities resulting in activation of the immune system

Adapted from Nagelhout J, Plaus K: *Nurse anesthesia*, ed 4, St. Louis, 2010, Saunders.

SPECIAL CONSIDERATIONS

SUMMARY

Substance dependence in the United States is increasing at an alarming rate. All ages and people from all walks of life are affected by this problem. This chapter provides evidence that a person can become dependent on a variety of formulations. Even more serious is the number of practitioners on the anesthesia care team who are becoming dependent on drugs that may be readily available.

Health care practitioners must recognize the severity of the addiction trends among subsets of health care professions.[4] It is important to learn to recognize, report, and prevent this continued escalation of drug dependence. The key feature is that all must agree that early intervention may save the lives of colleagues and fellow practitioners. Probably the most difficult abuse issue that has become of national epidemic is the abuse of prescription drugs. This problem presents the PACU nurse with a variety of signs and symptoms that are difficult to explain or justify. However, if the patient demonstrates abnormal physiologic function, prescription drug abuse should be considered.

The intent of this chapter was to provide the reader with an overview of the many drugs and substances that can be used by a person to become dependent. Not all the drugs and substances were identified or discussed because this area is ever changing. The key point presented was the overview of how the perianesthesia practitioner should modify the PACU nursing care with regard to patients who are dependent on a drug or substance category presented. Armed with this knowledge, the outcomes of the perianesthesia patient are enhanced. Certainly the use of illicit drugs is an ever increasing public health issue. In the PACU, drug withdrawal can and does occur. Identification of the specific abused drug is essential, and rapid intervention can be life saving for this type of patient.

REFERENCES

1. Conlay L, et al: *Case files anesthesiology,* New York, 2011, McGraw Hill Medical.
2. Frost E, Seidel M: Preanesthetic assessment of the drug dependent patient, *Anesthesiol Clin North Am* 8(4):829–842, 1990.
3. Kaye A, et al: Perioperative anesthesia clinical considerations of alternative medicines, *Anesthesiol Clin North America,* 22:125–139, 2004.
4. Luck S, Hedrick J: The alarming trend of substance abuse in anesthesia providers, *J Perianesth Nurs* 19(5):308–311, 2004.
5. Manchikanti L: National drug control policy and prescription drug abuse: facts and fallacies, *Pain Physician* 10:399–424, 2007.
6. Kork F, et al: Perioperative management of patients with alcohol, tobacco and drug dependency, *Current Opinion in Anaesthesiology* 23:384–390, 2010.
7. Mitra S, Sinatra R: Perioperative management of acute pain in the opioid-dependent patient, *Anesthesiology* 101:212–227, 2004.
8. Miller R, Pardo M: *Basics of anesthesia,* ed 6, Philadelphia, 2011, Saunders.
9. Fisher L: *Anesthesia and uncommon diseases,* ed 5, Philadelphia, 2007, Saunders.
10. Atlee J: *Complications in anesthesia,* ed 2, Philadelphia, 2007, Saunders.
11. Huckabee M: Perioperative care of the active substance dependent, *J Post Anesth Nurs* 3(4):254–259, 1988.
12. Longnecker D, et al: *Anesthesiology,* New York, 2007, McGraw Hill Medical.
13. Kurtzman T, Otsuka K: Inhalant dependent by adolescents, *J Adolesc Health* 28(3):170–180, 2000.
14. Nagelhout J, Plaus K: *Nurse anesthesia,* ed 4, St. Louis, 2010, Saunders.
15. Davis P, et al: *Smith's anesthesia for infants and children,* ed 8, St. Louis, 2011, Mosby.
16. Stoelting R: *Pharmacology and physiology in anesthetic practice,* ed 4, Philadelphia, 2005, Lippincott Williams and Wilkins.
17. Brouette T, Anton R: Clinical review of inhalants, *Am J Addict* 10(1):79–94, 2001.
18. Morgan M: Ecstasy (MDMA): a review of its possible persistent psychologic effects, *Psychopharmacology (Berl)* 152(3):230–248, 2000.

RESOURCES

AACN: *Core curriculum for progressive care nursing,* Philadelphia, 2010, Saunders.
Aitkenhead A, et al: *Textbook of anesthesia,* ed 5, Philadelphia, 2007, Churchill Livingstone.
Alspach J: *Core curriculum for critical care nursing,* ed 6, Philadelphia, 2005, Saunders.
Barash P, et al: *Clinical anesthesia,* ed 6, Philadelphia, 2009, Lippincott Williams & Wilkins.
Barrett K, et al: *Ganong's review of medical physiology,* ed 23, New York, 2009, McGraw-Hill Medical.
Bready L, et al: *Decision making in anesthesiology,* ed 4, St. Louis, 2007, Mosby.
Brunton L, et al: *Goodman and Gilman's the pharmacological basis of therapeutics,* ed 12, New York, 2010, McGraw-Hill Professional.
Drake R, et al: *Gray's anatomy for students,* ed 2, Philadelphia, 2009, Churchill Livingstone.
Deutschman C, Netigan P: *Evidence-based practice of critical care,* Philadelphia, 2010, Saunders.
Hall J: *Guyton and Hall textbook of medical physiology,* ed 12, Philadelphia, 2011, Saunders.
Hines R, Marschall K: *Handbook for Stoelting's anesthesia and co-existing disease,* ed 3, Philadelphia, 2009, Saunders.
Kaplan J, et al: *Cardiac anesthesia,* New York, 2011, Churchill Livingstone.
Miller R, et al: *Miller's anesthesia,* ed 7, Philadelphia, 2009, Churchill Livingstone.
Pasero C, McCaffery M: *Pain assessment and pharmacologic management,* St. Louis, 2011, Mosby.

Rogers E: Postanesthesia care of the cocaine dependent, *J Post Anesth Nurs* 6(2):102–107, 1991.

Sandberg W, et al: *The MGH textbook of anesthetic equipment,* New York, 2011, Churchill Livingstone.

Schick L, Windle PE: *Perianesthesia nursing core curriculum: perianesthesia nursing core curriculum,* ed 2, Philadelphia, 2010, Saunders.

Schirle L: Polyuria with sevoflurane administration: a case report, *AANA J* 79(1):47–50, 2011.

Shorten G, et al: *Postoperative pain management: an evidence-based guide to practice,* Philadelphia, 2006, Saunders.

Teter C, Guthrie S: A comprehensive review of MDMA and GHB: two common club drugs, *Pharmacotherapy* 21(12): 1486–1513, 2001.

Townsend C, et al: *Sabiston's textbook of surgery,* ed 18, Philadelphia, 2008, Saunders.

Vincent J, et al: *Textbook of critical care,* ed 6, Philadelphia, 2011, Saunders.

White P: *Perioperative drug manual,* ed 2, Philadelphia, 2005, Saunders.

Weiss S: Anesthesia for the alcoholic and addict, *AANA J* 47(3):309–312, 1979.

SPECIAL CONSIDERATIONS

53 Care of the Patient with Thermal Imbalance

Vallire D. Hooper, PhD, RN, CPAN, FAAN

Patients admitted to the postanesthesia care unit (PACU) usually have some form of thermal imbalance. Thermal imbalance is defined as body core temperature that is outside the normothermic rage of 36° to 38° C.[1,2] This chapter reviews the physiology of thermoregulation, the concepts of perioperative thermoregulation and hypothermia, malignant hyperthermia, and the effect of these issues on the care of the patient in the PACU.

DEFINITIONS

Active Warming Measures: Include the application of forced air convective warming, circulating-water mattresses, resistive heating blankets, radiant warmers, negative-pressure warming systems, and warmed humidified oxygen.

Core Thermal Compartment: Consists of the organs of the trunk and head, which compose 50% to 60% of the body mass. Tissues are well perfused and maintain a relatively uniform temperature.

Malignant Hyperthermia: A hereditary abnormality of muscle metabolism caused by certain triggering agents and resulting in a life-threatening pharmacogenetic disorder.

Normothermia: A core temperature range of 36° to 38° C.

Passive Insulation: Warmed cotton blankets, reflective blankets, socks, head covering, and limited skin exposure.

Perioperative Hypothermia: A core body temperature less than 36° C.

Peripheral Thermal Compartment: Consists of the arms and legs. Temperature is not homogenous and varies over time.

Preventative Warming: Initiation of passive insulation or active warming measures to maintain normothermia.

Thermal Comfort: A patient's subjective description of temperature comfort level.

OVERVIEW OF THERMOREGULATION

The body maintains its temperature between the narrow range of 36° to 38° C.[1-3] Although the peripheral thermal compartment (consisting of the arms and legs) temperatures can vary with environmental and thermoregulatory responses, temperature in the core body compartment is controlled within a 0.2° C range by a balance of heat production and heat loss typically regulated by thermoregulatory mechanisms in the central nervous system (CNS). These mechanisms receive input from various thermoreceptors located in the skin, nose, oral cavity, thoracic viscera, and spinal cord. These thermoreceptors send sensory information in hierarchical order: spinal cord, reticular formation, and primary control in the preoptic hypothalamic region of the brain.[3-6]

The central temperature controls maintain body temperature with two primary responses: physiologic and behavioral. The physiologic thermoregulatory response consists of sweating, shivering, and alterations in the peripheral vasomotor tone. These responses control the regulatory process of body temperature; consequently, heat loss is reduced with vasoconstriction and increased with vasodilation and sweating. The responses also work by reducing heat production, lowering the metabolic rate, and increasing muscle tone and shivering to enhance heat production. Behavioral thermoregulation is triggered by subjective feelings of discomfort or comfort. For example, in a hot environment, a person seeks air conditioning; in a cold environment, the person seeks heat. The response mechanism is stronger, but does not exhibit fine motor control as in the physiologic thermoregulatory response system.[3,4,6]

Body heat is produced by metabolism and has a circadian cycle, with the core temperature lower in the morning than in the afternoon.[7] Body heat is removed with four methods of heat transfer: radiation, conduction, convection, and evaporation, all of which play a significant role in the development of perioperative hypothermia (Fig. 53-1).

Radiation

Radiation involves the loss of energy, in this case heat, through the radiant electromagnetic waves in the infrared spectrum. It involves no direct contact between the objects involved, but simply occurs as heat radiates from a warmer object to a cooler one. Radiation heat loss accounts for 40% to 60% of all heat loss and occurs in the operating room (OR) as the uncovered skin of the surgical patient radiates energy away from the patient,

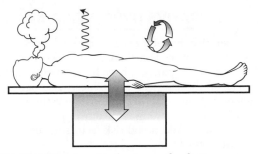

FIG. 53-1 Heat loss mechanisms of radiation, convection, conduction, and evaporation in patients under anesthesia. (From Nagelhout J, Plaus K: *Nurse anesthesia*, ed 4, St. Louis, 2010, Saunders.)

resulting in a drop in body temperature. Neonates and older adults are particularly prone to heat loss via this mechanism.[2-6]

Conduction

Conduction involves the transfer of heat energy through direct contact between objects. Conduction loss accounts for as much as 10% of heat loss in the OR and can occur via several mechanisms, including patient contact with a cold OR table, skin preparation solutions, intravenous (IV) fluids, irrigants, and cold sheets and drapes.[2-6]

Convection

Convection involves the loss of body heat via transfer to the surrounding cooler air and occurs with a temperature gradient between the body and surrounding air. It accounts for 25% to 50% of heat loss in the OR. This transfer can occur in two ways. Passive movement occurs as a loss of body heat from basic skin exposure as warm air rises. Active movement, which can be facilitated by the laminar flow systems in an OR, occurs as a loss of body heat from a fan or wind blowing across the body surface.[2-6]

Evaporation

Evaporation results in a loss of body heat from the transfer of heat that occurs when a liquid is changed into a gas. Evaporation accounts for up to 25% of heat loss in the OR and can occur via perspiration, evaporation, and exposed viscera during surgery or trauma.[2-6]

TEMPERATURE MEASUREMENT

Patients have rapid core temperature changes during the perioperative period. During such periods of rapid temperature fluctuation, a core temperature measurement provides the most accurate indication of body temperature.

Temperature measurement during this period must be accurate and consistent and provide a true reflection of the core temperature. The relationship between temperatures measured at various body sites during this period, however, may differ significantly from a true core reading. Consideration of the best method for obtaining a temperature must also account for accessibility of the measurement site, patient comfort and safety, and the practitioner's ability to consistently use the device correctly.[1,2,4,6,8] The same route of temperature measurement should be used throughout the perianesthesia period to allow for accurate temperature comparisons across the surgical continuum, and any extreme temperature (hypothermic or hyperthermic) detected with a noncore measurement instrument should be interpreted with caution.[1]

The most accurate core temperature measurement is obtained via use of a pulmonary artery (PA) catheter, because the artery bathes the catheter with blood from the core compartment and its surroundings. Temperature readings at the site can be affected by the rapid infusion of large amounts of warmed or cold IV fluids, by respiratory cycles, and by lower limb pneumatic compression devices. Readings from the distal esophagus and nasopharynx provide accurate alternatives to the PA catheter and are commonly used during surgery; however, like the PA catheter, these methods are invasive in nature and are not appropriate outside the operative setting after the patient has been extubated.[2,4,6,8]

Oral temperature measurement with electronic digital thermometers is a popular method of temperature measurement that is easily accessible, is less prone to operator error, and quickly reflects changes in core body temperature. Oral temperature readings vary based on placement in the oral cavity (Fig. 53-2).[9] Oral temperature measurement taken in the right or left posterior sublingual (buccal) pocket provides an accurate reflection of core temperature, even in the presence of oxygen therapy, warmed and cooled inspired gases, and varied respiratory rates.[1,8,10]

Temporal artery thermometry is a noninvasive radiation thermometer used with a scanner probe to scan the forehead and capture the infrared heat from the arterial blood supply and record the highest temperature sensed. Current evidence supports the accuracy of temporal artery readings as a core temperature measurement at normothermic temperatures; however, the accuracy of temporal artery measures at temperature extremes has not been established.[1,11-13]

Infrared tympanic thermometry, previously considered a preferred method for noninvasive

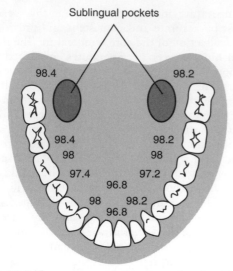

Sublingual pockets

FIG. 53-2 Temperature variations in oral cavity. (From Nicoll LH: Heat in motion: evaluating and managing temperature, *Nursing* 32:s12, 2002; Schick L, Windle PE, editors: *Perianesthesia nursing core curriculum: preprocedure, phase I and phase II PACU nursing*, ed 2, St. Louis, 2010, Saunders.)

core temperature measurement, can be adversely affected by common sources of instrument error, including poor operator technique, patient anatomy (site), and the calibration, accuracy, and inherent instrument error of the thermometer used.[8] Given the issues surrounding temperature measurement with this instrument, it is no longer recommended as an accurate means of temperature measurement during the perianesthesia period.[1]

PERIOPERATIVE HYPOTHERMIA

Perioperative hypothermia is defined as a core body temperature less than 36° C.[1] As many as 70% of surgical patients have hypothermia in the course of the surgical experience.[5] All patients undergoing general or regional anesthesia are at risk for developing unplanned perioperative hypothermia. Additional risk factors include[1]:

• Extremes of ages
• Female gender
• Systolic blood pressure less than 140 mm Hg
• Level of spinal blockade
• Length and type of surgical procedure
• Normal or below normal body mass index
• Body surface or wound area uncovered
• History of diabetes with autonomic dysfunction
• Use of cold irrigants
• Use of general or regional anesthesia

Adverse effects associated with perioperative hypothermia include[1,2]:

• Patient discomfort
• Increased adrenergic stimulation
• Untoward cardiac events
• Coagulopathy
• Altered drug metabolism
• Impaired wound healing
• Surgical site infection
• Increased PACU and hospital length of stay
• Increased hospital costs

The typical temperature drop associated with perioperative hypothermia is between 1° and 3° C and depends on the type and dose of anesthesia, amount of surgical exposure, and ambient room temperature. This temperature drop

Evidence-Based Practice

In a descriptive correlational study, Fetzer and Lawrence evaluated the correlation between tympanic and temporal artery temperature measurements in adult perianesthesia patients. Tympanic and temporal artery temperatures were consecutively taken in 222 patients both preoperatively and postoperatively. Mean temperature differences and temperature correlations were evaluated. Results indicated that the two thermometers did not obtain comparable temperatures on the same patient.

IMPLICATIONS FOR PRACTICE

Consistent temperature measurement is critical to the diagnosis and subsequent management of

thermoregulatory disturbances in the perianesthesia patient. Invasive core temperature measurement is preferred because it yields the most accurate temperatures; however, such methods are generally not plausible in the preoperative and postoperative periods. Noninvasive core temperature measurement methods vary in their relationship to invasive core temperature measurements. As such, nurses should use the same temperature measurement approach throughout a patient's perianesthesia experience to establish accurate temperature trends.

Source: Fetzer SJ, Lawrence A: Tympanic membrane versus temporal artery temperatures of adult perianesthesia patients, *J Perianesth Nurs* 23(4):230–236, 2008.

occurs from a loss of normal physiologic thermoregulatory mechanisms that are impaired by anesthetic drugs. As a result, the patient becomes poikilothermic and, without intervention, takes on the cooler temperature of the operative environment.[3,14]

Intraoperative temperature loss typically occurs in a characteristic pattern as a result of core-to-peripheral redistribution (Fig. 53-3). Redistribution occurs as a result of a reduction in the vasoconstriction threshold from the inhibitory impact of general anesthesia, resulting in a drop in core temperature, and peripheral vasodilation triggered by both general and regional anesthesia, which causes an increase in the blood flow to the skin and a resulting loss in core body heat. An initial heat loss of 1° to 1.5° C occurs during the first hour of surgery, followed by a slower more linear drop over the next 2 to 3 hours. Core temperature loss generally does not stabilize until 2 to 4 hours into the surgical procedure (Fig. 53-4). Postoperative return to normothermia occurs when the brain anesthetic concentration decreases enough to allow a normal thermoregulatory response. This response can take as long as 2 to 5 hours to occur and may be inhibited by residual anesthetics and postoperative opioids.[2-4,6,14]

Every patient should be assessed for hypothermia on arrival in the PACU, and postoperative care should be provided per the multidisciplinary American Society of PeriAnesthesia Nurses (ASPAN) *Clinical Guideline for the Maintenance*

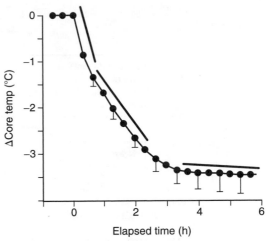

FIG. 53-4 Perioperative heat loss over time. (From Sessler DI: Perioperative heat balance, *Anesthesiology* 92:583, 2000. In Schick L, Windle PE, editors: *Perianesthesia nursing core curriculum: preprocedure, phase I and phase II PACU nursing*, ed 2, St. Louis, 2010, Saunders.)

of Perioperative Normothermia (Fig. 53-5).[1] In the case of normothermia, preventative warming measures and passive insulation should be instituted. The ambient room temperature should be maintained at or greater than 24° C, and the patient's thermal comfort level should be assessed at least on admission and discharge. In addition to constant observation for the signs and symptoms of hypothermia, the patient's temperature should be reassessed when the thermal comfort level decreases, with any emerging signs or symptoms of hypothermia, and on discharge from the PACU. In addition to the previous measures, active warming should be initiated for any patient with hypothermia who is admitted. In addition, IV fluids should be warmed; all gases (oxygen) should be humidified and warmed; and temperature should be monitored at least every 15 minutes until normothermia is achieved. The expected outcomes for all patients in PACU Phase I include a return to normothermia (minimum discharge temperature of 36° C), resolution of the signs and symptoms of hypothermia, and patient verbalization of an acceptable level of warmth. Preventative warming measures and continued assessment for hypothermia should continue at whatever location to which the patient is discharged.[1]

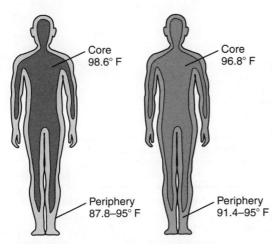

Vasoconstricted — Anesthesia → Vasodilated

FIG. 53-3 Core-to-peripheral redistribution after administration of anesthesia. (From Sessler DI: Perioperative heat balance, *Anesthesiology* 92:583, 2000. In Schick L, Windle PE, editors: *Perianesthesia nursing core curriculum: preprocedure, phase I and phase II PACU nursing*, ed 2, St. Louis, 2010, Saunders.)

MALIGNANT HYPERTHERMIA

Malignant hyperthermia (MH) is a genetic abnormality of muscle metabolism initiated by certain

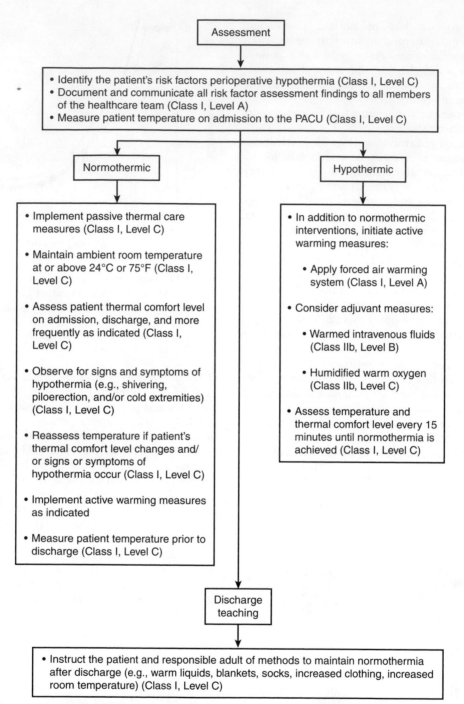

FIG. 53-5 Phase I/II PACU postoperative patient management recommendations. (From Hooper VD et al: ASPAN's evidence-based clinical practice guideline for the promotion of perioperative normothermia: second edition, *J Perianesth Nurs* 25(6):346–365, 2010.)

triggering agents resulting in a hypermetabolic state. MH is precipitated by certain general inhalation anesthetics, depolarizing skeletal muscle relaxants, and stress.[4,15-17] The incidence of MH ranges from 1 in 5000 to 1 in 100,000 anesthetics. MH averages approximately 600 cases per year in the United States, with hot spots including Wisconsin, Michigan, and West Virginia.[17] A study of the clinical manifestations of MH in North America from 1987 to 2006 noted that almost 75% of MH cases occurred in males, with almost 70% of those incidences in whites.[18] The study showed that the most commonly presenting clinical symptom was hypercarbia, followed by sinus tachycardia and masseter spasm.[18] Additional signs and symptoms include generalized muscle rigidity, unstable blood pressure, tachypnea, mixed respiratory and metabolic acidosis, myoglobinuria, hyperkalemia, and body temperature that may exceed 110° F (43° C).[4,16-20] Research shows that time from induction to first sign of MH was less than 30 minutes in the majority of cases.[18] After the acute episode is treated in the OR, the patient may be admitted to the PACU. Because successful management of MH depends on early assessment and prompt intervention, the perianesthesia nurse must be knowledgeable of the pathophysiology and treatment of this syndrome.

Identification of Patients with Malignant Hyperthermia Susceptibility

Genetics

Humans probably inherit susceptibility to MH with more than one gene or more than one group of possible mutational forms of a gene. The pattern of inheritance can range from recessive to dominant, with graded variations in between. The ease of initiation of an episode of MH seems to depend on the degree of genetic susceptibility and on environmental factors, which explains why some patients who are known to be susceptible show no signs of MH when exposed to confirmed MH-triggering agents. A patient with MH susceptibility (MHS) could be given an anesthetic in the presence of trigger agents, and this patient might not experience an acute MH reaction during surgery, but could have MH develop in the PACU instead.[6,15-17,20]

Evaluation of Susceptibility

Before anesthesia is administered, identification of patients who may be susceptible to MH is of major therapeutic importance. On history and physical examination, patients with MHS usually show some subclinical muscle weakness or abnormality, such as deficient fine motor control. Many patients with MHS have muscle cramps that occur spontaneously, during an infectious illness, or during or after exercise. When these cramps are present, they can be so severe that they are almost incapacitating. The patient may also describe heat prostration during physical exertion that is associated with environmental heat stress. In addition, a positive patient history or a positive genealogy may go back two generations (i.e., the patient or immediate relatives may show MH symptoms during an anesthetic experience). Physical examination of the person with MHS

may reveal myopathies such as wasting of the distal ends of the vastus muscles and hypertrophy of the proximal femoral muscles of the thigh. Other myopathies that are associated with MH susceptibility are cryptorchidism, pectus carinatum, kyphosis, lordosis, ptosis, and hypoplastic mandible. Electromyographic changes are seen in fewer than half of patients with MHS. Electrocardiographic results of patients with MHS may reveal ventricular or atrial hypertrophy (or both), bundle branch block, myocardial ischemia, and ventricular dysrhythmias. Measurements of blood creatine phosphokinase are usually approximately 70% reliable in estimating to MHS. The most definitive test for detection of MH susceptibility is the biopsy of skeletal muscle. Samples are obtained from the quadriceps muscle and are subjected to isometric contracture testing. The skeletal muscle of the patient with MHS has an increased isometric tension when exposed to caffeine or halothane.[16,17,20]

A new molecular genetic screening test has recently been developed that detects anywhere from 30% to 50% of those patients at risk for development of MH. A genetic test and DNA analysis is performed with a simply obtained blood sample. Although this method does not detect all people susceptible to development of MH and thus cannot be used to replace the more definitive muscle biopsy testing, the procedure is less costly, does not require the patient to travel to one of the few muscle biopsy testing centers, and shows great promise for future development.[16,17,20]

Patients at high risk for development of an acute MH crisis have been classified as follows: (1) patients who have an MH-positive muscle biopsy or who have survived an acute MH crisis; (2) patients who have a first-degree relative known to have MHS or to have had a positive muscle biopsy; (3) patients whose family members have a clinically demonstrated muscle abnormality; and (4) patients who are members of a family whose plasma creatine phosphokinase measurements have been found to be elevated in one or more samples (taken on at least three occasions).[17,20]

Normal Skeletal Muscle Physiology

Although a complete discussion of skeletal muscle contraction can be found in Chapter 23, a brief synopsis is presented here. The events that lead to the contraction of a skeletal muscle begin with an electric impulse that is transmitted down the axon to the motor nerve terminal, where vesicles that contain acetylcholine are located. On stimulation, the contents of the vesicles are released. This quantum of acetylcholine crosses the myoneural junction and interacts with its receptor on the postsynaptic membrane. This receptor activation causes a transient increase in the permeability for sodium and potassium ions, which ultimately creates an electric action potential (nerve impulse) that is propagated along the muscle membrane. This action potential electrically excites the sarcolemma and releases into the myoplasm calcium ions that are stored in the sarcoplasmic reticulum. These calcium ions then attach to troponin C, an inhibitory muscle protein that, when stimulated by the calcium, permits the actin and myosin protein filaments to interact and cause muscle contraction. The calcium ions in the myoplasm are then taken up via a reuptake mechanism into the sarcoplasmic reticulum. The process by which the electrically excited sarcolemma is coupled to the calcium released from the sarcoplasmic reticulum is known as *excitation-contraction* (E-C) *coupling*.[20,21]

Pathophysiology of Malignant Hyperthermia

When a susceptible patient is exposed to a trigger agent, such as halothane, that causes MH to occur, the clinical features are produced by an excess of calcium ions in the myoplasm. Although the exact pathophysiology of MH is not known, in MH the reuptake of calcium from the myoplasm by the sarcoplasmic reticulum appears to be decreased. It has also been suggested that the E-C coupling mechanism is defective. With an elevated calcium ion concentration in the myoplasm, the skeletal muscle contraction is intense and prolonged, finally leading to a hypermetabolic state of acid and heat production. More specifically, heat is produced by the accelerated and continued synthesis and use of adenosine triphosphate during glycolysis. The metabolic byproduct of glycolysis, lactic acid, is transported to the liver, where part of it is oxidized to provide the adenosine triphosphate necessary to help make glucose. This glucose, along with glycogen, is released from the liver and transported back to the metabolically active muscle, where the entire cycle repeats. This revolving process liberates much heat and produces a significant amount of metabolic acid. Respiratory and metabolic acidosis develop because of this hypermetabolic state, and symptoms such as tachycardia, tachypnea, ventricular dysrhythmias, and unstable blood pressure appear. Because of intense vasoconstriction, the skin is mottled and cyanotic (Box 53-1). Elevated body temperature can actually be a late sign of MH; for this reason, the nurse should not prolong the assessment of the patient on the assumption that

---

> **BOX 53-1   Signs and Symptoms of Malignant Hyperthermia**
>
> - The most consistent indicator of potential MH in the OR is an unanticipated increase (e.g., doubling or tripling) of end-tidal CO_2 when minute ventilation is kept constant.
> - Unexpected tachycardia, tachypnea, and jaw muscle rigidity (masseter spasm) are often common signs of MH that follow the significant CO_2 increase.
> - Respiratory and metabolic acidosis usually indicate fulminant MH. However, metabolic acidosis is not always present before severe temperature increase.
> - A specific sign of the MH syndrome is body rigidity (i.e., limbs, abdomen, and chest).
> - Temperature elevation is often a late sign of MH. Temperature change during MH is best detected with core temperature measurement (nasopharyngeal or oropharyngeal, esophageal, or pulmonary artery). Forehead skin temperature is less acceptable; it is slower in reflecting changes in core temperature and could be influenced by peripheral vasoconstriction.
> - Although most commonly presenting within the first 30 minutes of anesthesia induction, malignant hyperthermia can occur at any time during anesthesia or on emergence from anesthesia, including in the immediate postoperative period.

MH, Malignant hyperthermia; *OR*, operating room.

---

the patient's body temperature must be significantly elevated before intervention is attempted. When the patient's body temperature begins to rise, it may increase at a rate of 0.5° C every 15 minutes and may approach levels as high as 46° C.[15,20-22]

Muscle rigidity occurs in approximately 75% of patients with MH, especially after the administration of succinylcholine. In fact, the spasm of the masseter muscles after the injection of succinylcholine may be so severe that the anesthesia provider cannot open the patient's mouth to insert an airway. The onset of skeletal muscle rigidity after the administration of succinylcholine could be a sign of the impending development of MH.[15,17,18,20-22]

Triggering of Malignant Hyperthermia

Various environmental stimuli and pharmacologic agents can stimulate an acute episode of MH (Box 53-2). The symptoms of heat exertion and heat stroke are similar to MH. However, most patients with heat-related illness are not MH

repeated every 5 to 10 minutes, with a maximal dose of 10 mg/kg. If the acute episode of MH occurs in the OR and the patient is treated successfully, dantrolene therapy is continued into the recovery period in the PACU to prevent recurrence of MH. After the acute period in the PACU has passed, the patient is given oral dantrolene in four divided doses. Because dantrolene is poorly soluble, it is supplied in vials in the form of a lyophilized powder. To reconstitute a vial of lyophilized powder, 60 mL of sterile water for injection is added to the vial and is shaken until the solution is clear; many compatibility problems arise when dantrolene is mixed with solutions other than sterile water for injection. In addition, the sterile water for injection, used to reconstitute the dantrolene, should not contain any bacteriostatic agents because it is not unusual to use more than 2000 mL of diluent during the treatment of acute MH in an adult who weighs 70 kg.[4,16,17,19-21]

Perioperative Management of the Patient with Malignant Hyperthermia Susceptibility

Although pretreatment with dantrolene was previously recommended for the patient with MHS, current evidence indicates that pretreatment is ineffective and not indicated.[16,23] Premedication with anticholinergics, such as atropine, should be avoided because they interfere with the normal heat loss mechanisms and, in the case of atropine, can cause tachycardia that may cause confusion in the diagnosis of acute MH. Phenothiazine should also be avoided in the perioperative period because it can cause a release of calcium from the sarcoplasmic reticulum. Intraoperative anesthesia requires the use of agents that do not trigger an episode of MH (Box 53-3). Although regional anesthesia avoids the use of the general inhalation anesthetic agents and skeletal muscle relaxants, elevated temperatures in patients with MHS have been reported with its use.[16,17,21,23]

Intraoperative monitoring of the patient with MHS includes electrocardiogram, temperature, arterial blood gas (including acid-base), and precordial stethoscope determinations. These monitoring parameters should be continued into the PACU period (Box 53-4). Because some patients with MHS have had MH triggered in the postoperative period, patients should be followed for a minimum of 24 hours after surgery and should not be subjected to anxiety or stress. These patients should be reassured that physicians and nurses have reliable instruments to monitor for MH and that prompt and effective treatment will be provided if it develops.[16,17,20-23]

susceptible. In a few cases, MH susceptibility has been diagnosed with muscle biopsy in patients who had heat stroke (nonfatal), and some experts believe that heat stroke may occur more often in individuals with MH susceptibility. This area is an area of intense interest and investigation.[15,17,18,20-22]

The anesthetic agents that trigger MH seem to affect the sarcoplasmic reticulum or the E-C coupling mechanism, or both. Because of their wide use, halothane and succinylcholine are the most common trigger agents, although all inhalation agents are triggering agents. In patients with MHS or in patients who have had an episode of acute MH in the OR, all possible trigger agents should be stringently avoided.[15,17,18,20-22]

Dantrolene Sodium (Dantrium)

Dantrolene, the primary pharmacologic agent used in the treatment of MH, is a muscle relaxant that is chemically and pharmacologically unrelated to other muscle relaxants. It is the only known pharmacologic agent that is effective in the treatment of MH. The site of action of this drug is distal to the end plate within the muscle fiber. The main pharmacologic action of dantrolene reduces the release of calcium by the sarcoplasmic reticulum without affecting reuptake. Consequently, the concentration of calcium in the myoplasm is reduced, thus inhibiting the E-C coupling mechanism and causing muscle contraction to cease. When administered orally, dantrolene has a half-life of 8 hours; with IV administration, the half-life is 5 hours. When it is used in the treatment of acute MH, the intravenous dosage is 1 to 2 mg/kg, which can be

BOX 53-3   Drugs that Are Considered Safe to Administer to a Patient with MHS

BARBITURATES AND INTRAVENOUS ANESTHETICS
Diazepam
Etomidate (Amidate)
Hexobarbital
Ketamine (Ketalar)
Methohexital (Brevital)
Midazolam
Pentobarbital
Propofol (Diprivan)
Thiopental (Pentothal)

OPIOIDS
Alfentanil (Alfenta)
Anileridine
Codeine (Methyl Morphine)
Diamorphine
Fentanyl (Sublimaze)
Hydromorphone (Dilaudid)
Meperidine (Demerol)
Methadone
Morphine
Naloxone
Oxycodone
Phenoperidine
Remifentanil
Sufentanil (Sufenta)

ANXIETY-RELIEVING MEDICATIONS
Centrax
Chlordiazepoxide (Librium)
Clorazepate (Tranxene)
Diazepam (Valium)
Flurazepam (Dalmane)
Halazepam (Paxipam)
Klonopin
Librax
Lorazepam (Ativan)
Midazolam (Versed)
Oxazepam (Serax)
Temazepam (Restoril)
Triazolam (Halcion)

INHALED NONVOLATILE GENERAL ANESTHETIC
Nitrous oxide

SAFE MUSCLE RELAXANTS
Arduan (Pipecuronium)
Atracurium (Tracrium)
Cisatracurium (Nimbex)
Curare (active ingredient is tubocurarine)
Doxacurium (Neuromax)
Gallamine
Metocurine
Mivacurium (Mivacron)
Pancuronium (Pavulon)
Rocuronium (Zemuron)
Vecuronium (Norcuron)

LOCAL ANESTHETICS
Amethocaine
Articaine
Bupivicaine
Dibucaine
Etidocaine
Eucaine
Lidocaine (Xylocaine)
Levobupivacaine
Mepivacaine (Carbocaine)
Procaine (Novocain)
Prilocaine (Citanest)
Ropivacaine
Stovaine

MHS, Malignant hyperthermia susceptibility.

BOX 53-4   Suggested Components of Monitoring of Patient with Acute Malignant Hyperthermia

- Continuous ECG (consider 12-lead ECG and EEG after acute phase)
- Core temperature
- Urine output
- Arterial pressure line
- Pulse and blood pressure
- Central venous pressure*
- Pulmonary artery catheters*

ECG, Electrocardiogram; *EEG*, electroencephalogram.
*Should be considered; however, do not delay treatment if insertion of these monitors is physically or technically difficult.

Treatment of Acute Malignant Hyperthermia in the Postanesthesia Care Unit

The cornerstone of the successful treatment of MH is early detection (see Box 53-1). Box 53-5 lists the suggested equipment and drugs that should be kept in the PACU to be used in the treatment of acute MH. Chapter 1 also provides information on equipment and drugs that should be available for the treatment of acute MH. If assessment indicates that the patient is developing acute MH, the following steps should be taken[4,6,19,20,22]:

1. Discontinue the use of any trigger agent (see Box 53-3) and send for help.
2. Rapidly ventilate the patient's lungs with large tidal volumes with a bag-mask system and oxygen (total oxygen flow should exceed 15 L/min). Oral endotracheal intubation should be performed if the patient's airway is compromised.
3. Insert arterial and central venous lines and send venous and arterial blood samples to the

---

BOX 53-5   Suggested Equipment and Drugs to Be Used in Treatment of Acute Malignant Hyperthermia

EQUIPMENT NEEDED

- Intravenous lines with assorted cannula gauges
- Central venous pressure sets (2)
- Transducer kits for arterial and central venous cannulation
- Esophageal or other core temperature probes
- Pulmonary artery catheter
- Laboratory test tubes for blood chemistry analysis
- Syringes (60 mL × 5) to dilute dantrolene
- Crystalloid solution (ten 1000-mL bottles), labeled *for hyperthermia only* and stored in PACU refrigerator
- Bucket of cracked ice, labeled *for hyperthermia only* and stored in freezer of PACU refrigerator
- Cooling blanket
- Nasogastric tubes
- Urine meter (1)
- Irrigation tray with piston syringe
- Fan
- Large clear plastic bags for ice

DRUGS NEEDED

- Sodium bicarbonate (8.4%): 50 mL × 5
- Furosemide: 40 mg/ampule × 4 ampules
- Calcium chloride (10%): 10-mL vial (2)
- Glucose (two bottles of 50% strength)
- Iced intravenous saline solution (ten 1000-mL bottles in refrigerator)
- Lidocaine for injection: 100 mg per 5 mL or 100 mg per 10 mL in preloaded syringes (3)
- Amiodarone is also acceptable (ACLS protocol for treatment of cardiac dysrhythmias)
- Regular insulin (1 ampule of 100 units; refrigerated)
- Dantrolene (Dantrium) intravenous: 36 vials of lyophilized powder with at least 2200 mL of sterile water for injection, USP (without a bacteriostatic agent), to reconstitute dantrolene

Note: All the equipment and drugs listed in the box should be stored in a box or cart in the PACU. The box or cart should be labeled *hyperthermia*.
PACU, Postanesthesia care unit; *ACLS*, advanced cardiac life support.

---

laboratory for immediate results on electrolyte and arterial blood gas analysis. Also obtain creatine kinase (CK), myoglobin, comprehensive metabolic panel, prothrombin time/partial thromboplastin time (PT/PTT), fibrinogen, fibrin split products, complete blood count (CBC), and platelets.

4. Start reconstituting the dantrolene as soon as possible.

5. Administer the intravenous dantrolene, 1 to 2 mg/kg over 1 to 2 minutes, up to 10 mg/kg or until the patient's temperature starts to decrease.

6. Cool the patient. Cover all exposed surfaces with towels soaked in water. Cover the wet towels with ice. Use cooling blankets and fans if possible. Use cold gastric lavage and hydrate with iced intravenous fluids. To avoid hypothermia, discontinue all the cooling interventions when body temperature decreases to 38° C.

7. Administer sodium bicarbonate IV at a dose of 1 to 2 mEq/kg. When results of the arterial blood gas analysis are available, correct the base deficit with sodium bicarbonate according to the following formula:

$$\text{Base deficit} = 0.3 \times \text{weight (kg)} \times \text{base excess (mEq/L)}$$

If the $PaCO_2$ is elevated, increase the tidal ventilation of the patient. Do not administer sodium bicarbonate to correct respiratory acidosis, because the $PaCO_2$ only increases, which may lead to ventricular fibrillation.

8. Constantly monitor the patient's core temperature, blood pressure, pulse, cardiac rhythm, and pupil size and reactivity and watch for cyanosis (see Box 53-4).

9. Hyperkalemia should be treated with intravenous insulin and glucose (0.25 to 0.5 U/kg of insulin to 0.25 to 0.5 g/kg of glucose) or calcium.

10. If possible, catheterize the bladder and monitor urinary output and appearance. To secure a high urinary output, furosemide (1 mg/kg) or mannitol (1 g/kg) can be given.

11. Avoid calcium channel blockers. Dysrhythmias usually subside with resolution of the hypermetabolic phase of MH. They can be treated with amiodarone, lidocaine, procainamide, adenosine, or other drugs according to the advanced cardiac life support protocol.

12. Hypotension can be treated with the infusion of cold crystalloid solution.

13. Continue to send arterial and venous blood samples to the laboratory for prompt determination of arterial blood gases and electrolytes.

14. Look for such hopeful prognostic signs as lessening coma, hyperactive tendon reflexes, and stabilization of the temperature. When the temperature returns to normal, continue constant observation of the patient.

Complications After Acute Malignant Hyperthermia

Renal failure can occur because of myoglobinuria or hypotension. Consumption coagulopathies, such as disseminated intravascular coagulation, have been reported along with acute heart failure and pulmonary edema. Because the brain is the organ most sensitive to hyperthermia (permanent brain damage at ≥41° C), brain deterioration can occur in patients who are not promptly diagnosed and treated for MH.[4,6,18]

SUMMARY

Thermal imbalance issues encompass one of the most common, and one of the rarest, complications experienced by the patient in the PACU. Perioperative hypothermia, a commonly occurring yet easily preventable complication, can precipitate many adverse patient events, resulting in increases in both morbidity and mortality. Malignant hyperthermia, although rare, requires rapid diagnosis and treatment to avoid certain death. This chapter has provided an overview of the physiology of thermoregulation, the basic concepts of perioperative thermoregulation and hypothermia, malignant hyperthermia, and the effects of these issues on the care of the patient in the PACU. Astute assessment, appropriate prophylaxis, and aggressive patient management by the PACU nurse are critical to assuring safe quality patient outcomes in the patient with thermal alterations.

REFERENCES

1. Hooper VD, et al: ASPAN's evidence-based clinical practice guideline for the promotion of perioperative normothermia: second edition, J Perianesth Nurs 25(6):346–365, 2010.
2. Kurz A: When is forced-air warming cost-effective? In Fleisher LA, editor: Evidence-based practice of anesthesiology, ed 2, Philadelphia, 2009, Saunders.
3. Sessler DI: Perioperative heat balance, Anesthesiology 92:578–596, 2000.
4. Hooper VD: Thermoregulation issues. In Stannard D, Krenzischek DA, editors: Perianesthesia nursing care: a bedside guide for safe recovery, Sudbury, Mass, 2012, Jones & Bartlett Learning.
5. Welch TC: AANA journal course, AANA Journal 70(3):227, 2002.
6. Hooper VD: Thermoregulation. In Schick L, Windle PE, eds: Perianesthesia nursing core curriculum: preprocedure, phase I and phase II PACU nursing, ed 2, St. Louis, 2010, Saunders.
7. Holtzclaw BJ: Circadian rhythmicity and homeostatic stability in thermoregulation, Biol Res Nurs 2:221–235, 2001.
8. Hooper VD, Andrews JO: Accuracy of noninvasive core temperature measurement in acutely ill adults: the state of the science, Biol Res Nurs 8(1):24–34, 2006.
9. Nicoll LH: Heat in motion: evaluating and managing temperature, Nursing 32(5):s1–s12, 2002.
10. Lawson L, et al: Accuracy and precision of noninvasive core temperature measurement in adult intensive care patients, American Journal of Critical Care 16:485–496, 2007.
11. Calonder EM, et al: Temperature measurement in patients undergoing colorectal surgery and gynecology surgery: a comparison of esophageal core, temporal artery, and oral methods, J Perianesth Nurs 25(2):71–78, 2010.
12. Fetzer SJ, Lawrence A: tympanic membrane versus temporal artery temperatures of adult perianesthesia patients, J Perianesth Nurs 23(4):230–236, 2008.
13. Washington GT, Matney JL: Comparison of temperature measurement devices in post anesthesia patients, J Perianesth Nurs 23(1):36–48, 2008.
14. Sessler DI, Akca O: Nonpharmacological prevention of surgical wound infections, Helathcare Epidemiology 35: 1397–1404, 2002.
15. Hernandez JF, et al: Scientific advances in the genetic understanding and diagnosis of malignant hyperthermia, J Perianesth Nurs 24(1):19–34, 2009.
16. Watson CB: Is there an ideal approach to the malignant hyperthermia-susceptible patient? In Fleisher LA, editor: Evidence-based practice of anesthesiology, ed 2, Philadelphia, 2009, Saunders.
17. Rosenburg H: Malignant hyperthermia syndrome, available at www.mhaus.org/NonFB/Slideshow_eng/SlideShow_ENG_files/frame.htm. Accessed May 29, 2011.
18. Larach MG, et al: Clinical presentation, treatment, and complications of malignant hyperthermia in North America from 1987 to 2006, Analgesia & Anesthesia 110(2):498–507, 2010.
19. Glahn KPE, et al: Recognizing and managing a malignant hyperthermia crisis: guidelines from the european malignant hyperthermia group, British Journal of Anaesthesia 105(4):417–420, 2010.
20. Hommertzheim R, Steinke EE: Malignant hyperthermia-the perioperative nurse's role, AORN J 83(1):149–167, 2006. [erratum appears in AORN J, 83(3):601, 2006].
21. Gurunluoglu R, et al: Evidence-based patient safety advisory: malignant hyperthermia, Plastic and Reconstructive Surgery 124(4S):68S–81S, 2009.
22. Naecsu A: Malignant hyperthermia, Nurs Stand 20(28): 51–57, 2006.
23. Wappler F: Anesthesia for patients with a history of malignant hyperthermia, Current Opinion in Anesthesiology 23:417–422, 2010.

RESOURCES

Malignant Hyperthermia Association of the United States (MHAUS), available at www.mhaus.org. Accessed May 30, 2011.
North America MH Registry of MHAUS, available at www.mhreg.org. Accessed May 30, 2011.

54 Care of the Shock Trauma Patient

Myrna E. Mamaril, MS, RN, CPAN, CAPA, FAAN

Shock trauma care continues to change dramatically in response to innovative surgical technologies, advancements in anesthesia agents, and trauma research. Likewise, the medical advances continue to be driven by the state of the trauma science directly resulting from military medicine's evolving combat casualty management from the wars in Iraq and Afghanistan. In peacetime, the civilian trauma centers take the lead in timely research and evidence-based medicine to establish new trauma protocols and to translate the trauma research to the practice at the bedside. However, in wartime, it is military medicine's combat medical research and scientific data outcomes that guide the cutting edge benefiting civilian trauma centers.[1] The history of advancements in shock trauma care is directly linked to wars and the military's battlefield medicine.[1] Trauma care continues to advance in the twenty-first century with the wars in Afghanistan and Iraq. Permissive hypotension and damage control hemorrhage bring new dimensions in treating severe hemorrhagic shock. Consequently, the treatment of shock is now focused on rapid transport and guided resuscitation within the "golden hour."[2] Advances in vascular surgery have led to better patient outcomes. Today, the battlefields in Iraq and Afghanistan have continued to advance shock trauma nursing care that directly correlates with enhance trauma patient outcomes.

This chapter will focus on the epidemiology of traumatic injuries, mechanism of injury (MOI), pattern of injury, anatomy, physiology, and the patient's presenting symptoms that guide the postanesthesia nurse in the delivery of care for the adult, pediatric, and obstetric patient.

The postanesthesia nurse's focus includes primary and secondary assessments for systematic prioritization of nursing interventions and outcomes of care. The mechanism of injury is vital to understanding the pathogenesis of injury and anticipated complications, including shock during the patient's recovery from anesthesia and surgery. The emphasis of the trauma patient's postanesthesia care is on ensuring vital life functions, promoting safety, and supporting the psychosocial and spiritual needs. Preparedness for emergence delirium from posttraumatic stress disorder (PTSD) assists the nurse in understanding and effectively managing emergence from anesthesia. Finally, the use of evidence-based practice brings the best available science to the practice arena and advances trauma care.

DEFINITIONS

Compartment Syndrome: A pathologic condition caused by the progressive development of arterial compression and consequent reduction of blood supply.

Damage Control Resuscitation: A systematic approach to control bleeding at the point of injury by definitive treatment interventions of minimizing blood loss and maximizing tissue oxygenation.

Injury: A state in which a patient experiences a change in physiologic or psychological systems.

Microvascular: Pertaining to the portion of the circulatory system that is composed of the capillary network.

Motor Vehicle Crash (MVC): Occurs when a vehicle collides with another vehicle or object and can result in injuries or death.

Pattern of Injury: The circumstance in which an injury occurs, such as causation from sudden deceleration, wounding with a projectile, or crushing with a heavy object.

Permissive Hypotension: A guided intervention that limits fluid resuscitation until hemorrhage is controlled.

Primary Assessment: The first in order of importance in the evaluation or appraisal of a disease or condition.

Resuscitation: Use of emergency measures in an effort to sustain life.

Secondary Assessment: Evaluation of a disease or condition with previously compiled data.

Shock: An abnormal condition of inadequate blood flow and nutrients to the body's tissues, with life-threatening cellular dysfunction.

Shock Trauma: A sudden disturbance that causes a wound or injury and results in acute circulatory failure.

Systemic Inflammatory Response Syndrome (SIRS): Inflammatory disturbance that affects multiple organ systems of the body.

Trauma: Tissue injury, such as a wound, burn, or fracture, or psychological injury in which personality damage can be traced to an unpleasant experience related to tissue injury, such as a wound, burn, amputation, or fracture.

EPIDEMIOLOGY OF TRAUMA

In the United States, trauma injuries continue to be the fourth leading cause of death, affecting the lives of more than 70 million people each year.[3-7] Furthermore, trauma accounts for more deaths in the United States during the first four decades of life than any other disease. Surprisingly, fatality rates for older adults are now higher than rates for younger adults.[5,6] Mortality from trauma is the tip of the iceberg, a small indication of a much bigger problem; many patients survive trauma, need surgical intervention, and require lengthy rehabilitation.

Although 50% of all deaths attributed to trauma occur within minutes to hours after the injury, 30% of patients die within 2 days of neurologic injury; the remaining 20% of deaths occur as a result of complications.[3] Overwhelming infection and sepsis result from these traumatic injuries, and trauma patients are at risk for multiple complications, including respiratory, circulatory, neurologic, and renal failure. Numerous pathologic conditions and inflammatory derangements can contribute to this high incidence rate of late mortality from sepsis. Trauma patients who need surgery and anesthesia have greater vulnerability to life-threatening conditions and mandate vigilant, astute postanesthesia nursing care.

PREHOSPITAL PHASE

During the prehospital phase, vital information regarding the trauma patient's condition at the scene and MOI reveals important clues in the clinical finding of how the patient presents in the resuscitation area or later in the postanesthesia care unit (PACU). If the patient had a prolonged extrication period at the scene, the airway may have been compromised; the patient may have active or uncontrolled bleeding; or the patient may have been exposed to environmental elements (e.g., decreasing core temperature).

Other conditions at the scene that can influence the trauma patient's outcome include such considerations as: (1) whether restraint devices were used; (2) whether airbags were deployed during impact; (3) whether the passenger was ejected from the car; (4) in what position the patient was found; (5) whether the car rolled over; (6) whether the windshield was broken; (7) the speed at which the vehicle was traveling; (8) where the impact was on the car; (9) whether the patient sustained an impaled object; (10) whether the patient wore a motorcycle helmet; (11) whether other fatalities occurred at the scene; and (12) what, if anything, bystanders did to assist the victim. All these observations by the first providers help to piece each part of the trauma puzzle together to ensure a comprehensive approach to the management of the trauma patient.

Mechanism of Injury

The pattern or MOI simply refers to the manner in which the trauma patient was injured.[8] For accurate assessment of the trauma patient in the PACU, the nurse needs a basic understanding of the different types of MOI. Patterns of injury are related to the categories of the injuring force and the subsequent tissue response. A thorough understanding of these aspects of injury helps in determining the extent and nature of the potential injuries. Damage occurs when the force deforms tissues beyond failure limits.[8] Injuries result from different kinds of energy (kinetic forces, such as motor vehicle crashes [MVCs], falls, or bullets) or acute exposure (thermal, chemical, electrical, radiation, or high-yield explosives) to the tissues and underlying structures. Some of the major factors that influence the severity of the injury are the velocity of the objects and the force in terms of physical motion to moving or stationary bodies. The force is the mass of an object multiplied by the acceleration. Numerous studies conclude that the MOI helps identify common injury combinations, predict eventual outcomes, and explain the type of injury sustained.[8] Although a certain pattern of injury may be predictable for specific injuries, trauma patients may sustain other injuries. A thorough assessment for identification of all actual and potential injuries is needed.[8,9]

Various forms of traumatic injuries are: blunt force (high-velocity); penetrating, such as those that cut or pierce; falls from great heights; firearms; and chemical, electric, radiant, and thermal burns. MVCs create impressive forces that can fracture extremities, crush organs, and lead to massive blood loss and soft tissue damage. At the time of a crash, three impacts occur: (1) vehicle to object; (2) body to vehicle; and (3) organs within body. Forces are exerted in relation to acceleration, deceleration, shearing, and compression.[8,9] Acceleration-deceleration injuries occur when the head is thrown rapidly forward or backward, resulting in sudden alterations. The semisolid brain tissue moves slower than the solid skull and collides with the skull, causing injury. The injury where the brain makes contact with the skull is called a *coup*. The brain injury can also occur as the brain tissue is thrown in the opposite direction, causing damage in the contralateral skull surface, which is known as *contrecoup injury*. Ever-changing MOIs also create the need for new nursing educational programs and competencies for postanesthesia nurses to stay up to date and to advance practice.

Blunt Trauma

Blunt trauma is one of the major types of trauma injuries that is best described as a wounding force that does not communicate to the outside of the body. Blunt forces produce crushing, shearing, or tearing of the tissues, both internally and externally.[8-10] High-velocity MVCs and falls from great heights cause blunt-trauma injuries that are associated with direct impact, deceleration, continuous pressure, and shearing and rotary forces.[8-10] These blunt-trauma injuries are usually more serious and life threatening than other types of trauma because the extent of the injuries is less obvious and diagnosis is more difficult. Because blunt-trauma injuries can leave little outward evidence of the extent of internal damage, the nurse must be extremely vigilant and astute in making observations and ongoing assessments.

When the body decelerates, the organs continue to move forward at the original speed. As the body's organs move in the forward direction, they are torn from their attachments by rotary and shearing forces.[8-10] Furthermore, blunt forces disrupt blood vessels and nerves. This MOI to the microcirculation causes widespread epithelial and endothelial damage and thus stimulates cells to release their constituents and further activates the complement, the arachidonic acid, and the coagulation cascade that activated the systemic inflammatory response syndrome. This unique inflammatory response is covered later in this chapter. Finally, blunt trauma may mask more serious complications related to the pathophysiology of the injury.

Penetrating Trauma

Penetrating trauma refers to an injury produced by a foreign object, such as stab wounds and firearms. The severity of the injury produced by a foreign body is related to the underlying structures that are damaged. The MOI causes the penetration and crushing of underlying tissues and the depth and the diameter of the wound that results from penetrating trauma. Tissue damage inflicted by bullets depends on the bullet's size, velocity, range, mass, and trajectory. Knives often cause stab wounds, but other impaling objects can cause damage. Tissue injury depends on length of the object, the force applied, and the angle of entry. These penetrating wounds cause disruption of tissues and cellular function and thus result in the introduction of debris and foreign bodies into the wound.[8,10]

Impaled objects are left in place until definitive surgical extraction is available because of the tamponade effect of vascular injuries. Finally, the insult to the body may occur as local ischemia or extend to a fulminant hemorrhage from these penetrating injuries.[10]

Contusion of Tissues

When blunt trauma is significant enough to produce capillary injury and destruction, contusion of tissues occurs. Consequently, the extravasation of blood causes discoloration, pain, and swelling.[8-10] If a large vessel ruptures, a hematoma may produce a distinct palpable lesion. With a massive contusion or hematoma, an increase in myofascial pressures often results in sequelae known as *compartment syndrome*.[9,10] A compartment is a section of muscle enclosed in a confined supportive membrane called *fascia;* compartment syndrome is a condition in which increased pressure inside an osteofascial compartment impedes circulation and impairs capillary blood flow and cellular ischemia, resulting in an alteration in neurovascular function.[9,10] This syndrome occurs more frequently in the lower leg or forearm but can occur in any fascial compartment. Damaged vessels in the ischemic muscle dilate in response to histamine and other vasoactive chemical substances, such as the arachidonic cascade and oxygen-free radicals. This dilation, with resultant leakage of fluid from capillary membrane permeability, results in increased edema and tissue pressure.[9] The increased edema and pressure compress capillaries distal to the injury, impeding microvascular perfusion. These pathologic changes cause a repetitive cycle within the confined tissues, which increases swelling and leads to increased compartment pressures. Fascial compartment syndrome can be measured if indicated. Normal pressure is more than 10 mm Hg, but a reading of more than 35 mm Hg suggests possible anoxia.[11,12] A fasciotomy may be indicated to prevent muscle or neurovascular damage.

SCORING SYSTEMS

Numerous scoring mechanisms have been designed to assist in measuring the severity of injuries and attempt to forecast morbidities, mortalities, and the likelihood of functional outcomes. Each scoring system is unique and measures the physiologic status of the patient. Some scoring systems work better for penetrating versus blunt trauma.[11,12] The PACU nurse may record the injury scoring measurement as initial baseline severity indices; however, accuracy can be limited despite the score.

STABILIZATION PHASE

The initial assessment, resuscitation, and stabilization processes that are initiated in the emergency department and trauma center extend into the operating room (OR), the PACU, and the critical care unit. Temperature of the trauma rooms may be increased to prevent hypothermia during resuscitation. Because the most common cause of shock (Table 54-1) in the trauma patient

Table 54-1	Types of Shock			
TYPES	**DEFINITION**	**CAUSES**	**SIGNS**	**TREATMENT**
Hypovolemic	Decrease in intravascular volume	Internal or external hemorrhage, third spacing of fluids, plasma volume loss	Increased HR Decreased BP Decreased CVP Decreased PCWP Increased respirations Visible signs of bleeding or fluid loss Pallor Diaphoresis Anxiety Decreased urine output	Fluids or blood administration
Cardiogenic	Circulatory failure from impairment of contractility	Blunt chest trauma Cardiac contusion Injury to heart muscle Myocardial infarction	Decreased BP Cardiac ischemia Anxiety Confusion Tachypnea Decreased pulse pressure Cool and clammy skin Elevated CVP Elevated PCWP	Support cardiac rhythm Increase cardiac output Inotropics Vasoactive drugs Decrease afterload
Obstructive	Decreased cardiac output from compression to aorta or great vessels that prevents atria from filling and decrease in stroke volume	Cardiac tamponade Tension pneumothorax	Decreased BP Increased HR JVD Tracheal shift Muffled heart sounds Diminished or absent lung sounds Tachypnea	Treat cause Needle decompression and chest tube Pericardial centesis and surgical intervention
Distributive	*Neurogenic:* Vasodilation from decreased neurogenic tone to vessels *Anaphylactic:* Histamine release into bloodstream after allergic reaction, increased capillary permeability and vasodilation *Septic:* Massive infection resulting in vasodilation and inadequate tissue perfusion	Bacteria Allergens Spinal cord injury Spinal anesthesia	Warm skin Flushed color Increased HR Decreased HR (if neurologic in origin) Increased temperature Decreased BP Increased cardiac output Laryngeal edema with bronchospasm (anaphylaxis)	Treat cause Fluids Antibiotics Vasopressors Steroids Epinephrine Antihistamines

HR, Heart rate; *BP*, blood pressure; *CVP*, central venous pressure; *PCWP*, pulmonary capillary edge pressure; *JVD*, jugular venous distension.

is hypovolemia from acute blood loss, the ultimate goal in fluid resuscitation is prompt restoration of circulatory blood volume through replacement of fluids so that tissue perfusion and delivery of oxygen and nutrients to the tissues should be maintained.[10-13] Rapid identification and ensuing implementation of correct aggressive treatment are vital for the trauma patient's survival. Although hypovolemia is the most common form of shock in the trauma patient, cardiogenic shock, obstructive shock (tension pneumothorax, cardiac tamponade), and distributive shock (neurogenic shock, burn shock, anaphylactic shock, and septic shock) can occur. Rapid-volume infusers deliver warmed intravenous fluids at a rate of 950 mL/min with large-bore intravenous catheters.[10] Many trauma centers initially infuse 2 to 3 L of lactated Ringer or normal saline solutions and then consider blood products. The fluids should be warmed to prevent or minimize hypothermia. Crystalloids, colloids, or blood products can be used for effective reversal of hypovolemia.

Crystalloids are electrolyte solutions that diffuse through the capillary endothelium and can be distributed evenly throughout the extracellular compartment. Examples of crystalloid solutions are lactated Ringer solution, Plasma-Lyte, and normal saline solution. Although controversy exists regarding crystalloid versus colloid fluid resuscitation in multiple trauma, the American College of Surgeons Committee on Trauma recommends that isotonic crystalloid solutions of lactated Ringer or normal saline solution be used for that purpose.[11] Furthermore, crystalloids are much cheaper than colloids. Administration of crystalloids should be threefold to fourfold the blood loss.[11]

Colloid solutions contain protein or starch molecules or aggregates of molecules that remain uniformly distributed in fluid and fail to form a true solution.[13-16] When colloid solutions are administered, the molecules remain in the intravascular space, thereby increasing the osmotic pressure gradient within the vascular compartment. Volume for volume, the half-life of colloids is much longer than that of crystalloids. Colloid solutions commonly used are plasma protein fraction, dextran, normal human serum albumin, and hetastarch.

Researchers in several new randomized control trials have used hypertonic solutions to resuscitate patients in shock.[14-18] According to Beekley,[18] hypertonic saline solution (3% sodium chloride) can be used in resuscitation of the child with a severe head injury because it maintains blood pressure and cerebral oxygen delivery, decreases overall fluid requirements, and results in

improved overall survival rates.[16] In addition, patients with low Glasgow Coma Scale (GCS) scores from head injuries have improved survival rates in the hospital.[16]

Although crystalloid and colloid solutions serve as primary resuscitation fluids for volume depletion, blood transfusions are necessary to restore the capacity of the blood to carry adequate amounts of oxygen. Furthermore, blood component therapy is considered after the trauma patient's response to the initial resuscitative fluids has been evaluated.[11] In an emergency, universal donor blood (type O negative for women in childbearing years) packed red blood cells can be administered for patients with exsanguinating hemorrhage. Untyped O negative whole blood can also be given to patients with an exsanguinating hemorrhage. Other blood products, such as platelets and fresh frozen plasma, may need to be given to the trauma patient because of a consumption coagulopathy. Most notable are the leukemic trauma patients with low platelet counts. With fluid resuscitation of these patients with immunosuppression, colloids are contraindicated because of the antiplatelet activity that exacerbates hemorrhaging.[17] Type-specific blood often times is available within 10 minutes and is preferred over universal donor blood. Fully cross-matched blood is preferred in situations that can warrant awaiting type and cross match, which often takes up to 1 hour.[10-12] Finally, the therapeutic goal of all blood component therapy is to restore the circulating blood volume and to give back other needed blood with red blood cells and clotting factors to correct coagulation deficiencies.[19-22]

New evidence recognizes "permissive hypotension" by keeping the patient's systolic blood pressure at approximately 90 mm Hg correlates with better outcomes owing to conservation of important clotting factors.[21] In addition, there also seems to be a protective mechanism of myocardial suppressive factors that conserve homeostasis of fluid shifts. The intent of this protective response is to prevent further hemorrhaging or bleeding out of the red blood cells and clotting factors. By sustaining the hypotension, the blood pressure supports basic perfusion until the patient is in the OR and surgically resuscitated.[19,21] Damage control resuscitation and warm, fresh whole blood are now associated with better survival rates in combat-related massive hemorrhage injuries. Restoration of blood volume before homeostasis is achieved may have adverse complications of exacerbation of blood loss from increase in blood pressure.[18-22]

In summary, fluid resuscitation of the trauma patient is essential to ensure that adequate circulating volume and vital oxygen and nutrients are delivered to the tissues. However, new studies recommend permissive hypotension with the use of damage control resuscitation to decrease mortality and morbidity and optimize the patient's survival.[18-22] These combat-related studies are now influencing the management of civilian resuscitation of massive hemorrhage injuries in trauma centers throughout the United States.

Diagnostic Studies and Protocols

Diagnostic tests and laboratory studies have a vital role in establishing the patient's baseline and current status. The results of these tests predicate the treatment protocols that are initiated. Comprehensive diagnostic studies are required to establish an accurate diagnosis and to plan effective treatment of the patient with multiple injuries. The initial routine studies may be arterial blood gas determinations, urinalysis (myoglobinuria), complete blood count, electrolyte levels, lactate, prothrombin and partial thromboplastin times, and type and cross match. Other diagnostic studies that can be ordered for suspected injuries include lateral cervical spine, upright anteroposterior chest, and anteroposterior pelvic radiographs; computed tomographic scan; 12-lead electrocardiogram; ultrasound scan; and toxicology laboratory studies. Diagnostic peritoneal lavage is performed only on the severely injured patient with hypotension, especially if the result of an abdominal examination is suggestive of injury or is unreliable. Pregnancy tests should be performed on all women of childbearing age, but should not delay treatment of life-threatening injuries.

Collaborative Approach

Collaborative practice is essential in the care of the trauma patient. During the prehospital phase, vital communication with the trauma team is initiated at the trauma center. Subsequently, when the patient is first admitted to the PACU, the approach to patient care is comprehensive. Together, the postanesthesia nurse, anesthesia provider, respiratory therapist, surgeon, and radiology technician create a collaborative environment so that care becomes focused and directed. This collaborative practice continues through the intraoperative and postanesthesia periods.

The anesthesia provider or OR nurse communicates a comprehensive systems report to the perianesthesia nurse and verbally reviews any definitive findings of the computed tomographic scan, including whether generalized edema or lesions are found. Vital nursing information is communicated to the appropriate OR and postanesthesia nurses caring for the trauma patient. The anesthesia provider and trauma surgeon should communicate the significant findings during the intraoperative period that may be problematic during the recovery phase, what the PACU nurse should look for and report promptly to these physicians, and what the PACU nurse should do to prevent harm during the postanesthesia phase of care.[23]

POSTANESTHESIA PHASE I

Before the shock trauma patient is admitted to the PACU, the postanesthesia nurse begins preparing for the PACU admission. When the OR nurse calls the PACU to notify the admitting nurse that the trauma surgeon is beginning to close the patient's surgical site, important prehospital and intraoperative information is communicated. The transfer of care, or hand-off, communication from the OR nurse to PACU nurse consists of a detailed yet succinct report of all pertinent findings, such as surgical operation, type of anesthesia including opioids, vital signs, oxygen saturation, ventilation settings, hemodynamic monitoring, drains, vasoactive drugs, intravenous sites with type of solutions, and other pertinent findings so that the PACU nurse can begin to prepare for the patient's needs.

Primary Assessment

The nursing assessment of the shock trauma patient in the PACU begins with evaluation of the ABCDs (airway, breathing, circulation, and disability). Foremost in this vital primary survey is the patency of the airway. This assessment begins with proper positioning of the patient's head, with cervical spine protection always maintained if injury is suspected. Cervical collars should not be removed unless specifically directed by the trauma or neurosurgeon after confirmation of the absence of spinal cord injury. The patient may need to have the airway cleared with suctioning and removal of secretions or blood. In addition, airway adjuncts may be needed, such as oropharyngeal and nasopharyngeal airways. If the patient is intubated via endotracheal tube or nasotracheal tube, ventilatory support should be provided with the proper settings to achieve optimal oxygenation and ventilation.

Next, the postanesthesia nurse evaluates the patient's work of breathing. While recalling the MOI, such as blunt or penetrating trauma to the chest, the nurse should be highly suspicious of pulmonary contusions, fractured ribs, or injuries from shearing forces. The nurse assesses spontaneous respirations, respiratory excursion, chest wall integrity, symmetry, depth, respiratory rate, use of accessory muscles, and the work of breathing. With palpation, the nurse should evaluate for the presence of subcutaneous emphysema, hyperresonance or dullness over the lung fields, and tracheal deviation. With auscultation, the nurse assesses the lungs for bilateral breath sounds and evaluates for adventitious breath sounds. In addition, pulse oximetry and end-tidal CO_2 monitoring augment the complete respiratory assessment of the trauma patient.

After a thorough evaluation of the airway and breathing, the nurse begins the circulatory assessment. With the use of palpation, the nurse evaluates the circulation, checks the quality, location, and rate of the pulses, and compares the right with the left and the upper extremities with the lower. If the nurse can palpate a radial pulse, the arterial pressure is at least 80 mm Hg. If no radial pulse is palpable, the nurse then palpates the femoral pulse (a situation that indicates a pressure of 70 mm Hg). If only a carotid pulse is palpable, the arterial pressure is approximately 60 mm Hg. The patient's blood pressure and pulse (rate and rhythm) should be monitored via the cardiac monitor. Any changes in the patient's appearance should be investigated and prompt the nurse to reassess the patient. Pulseless electric activity may show as electric impulses on the cardiac monitor without the presence of a palpable pulse. Pulseless electric activity may be seen in the trauma patient related to a variety of causes, such as pneumothorax, cardiac tamponade, hypovolemia, or hypothermia.

Simultaneously during the palpation of pulses, the nurse assesses the patient's skin temperature, color, and capillary refill. Capillary refill is a good indicator of tissue perfusion, especially in children. Another aspect of circulatory assessment is observation of the patient for any significant or uncontrollable bleeding from the operative site. The nurse should inspect the peripheral, central, and arterial lines to ensure the patency of the lines and integrity of the sites. Each line should be identified and labeled with the date and time to distinguish the type of parenteral fluid and medication administration in use.

The final component of the primary survey is the disability or neurologic examination. The patient's mental status should be assessed with the AVPU (Alert, Voice, Pain, Unresponsive) scale or the GCS. The AVPU is described as follows: *A* for awake and responding to nurse's questions; *V* for verbal response to nurse's questions, *P* for responding to pain; and *U* for unresponsive.[10,11] The GCS is used in many PACUs

for evaluating neurologic status and predicting outcomes of severe trauma. This neurologic scoring system allows for constant evaluation from field to emergency room to PACU. One must remember that anesthesia blunts the neurologic response; therefore the response is not as useful in the immediate postanesthesia period. Next, bilateral pupil response is evaluated for equality, roundness, and reactivity: brisk, slow, sluggish, or no response to light and accommodation. Before the primary assessment is complete, the PACU nurse quickly reassesses the ABCDs for stability and then is ready to receive a report from the anesthesiologist.

Anesthesia Report

The anesthesia provider's report provides valuable information concerning the trauma patient's presenting status to the perianesthesia nurse. This report includes significant facts that pertain to the MOI, prehospital phase, admitting and stabilization period, operative report, intubation, anesthetic agents, estimated blood loss, fluid resuscitation, cardiopulmonary status, and treatment abnormalities.

In the review of the anesthesia report, the nurse should note any difficulty in intubation of the patient. The nurse should take note if the oral secretions are tinged pink or bloody, which can indicate an infectious process, pulmonary edema, trauma, or uncontrolled hemorrhage.

Another important aspect of the anesthesia report is estimated blood loss and fluid replacement, which are carefully monitored through the hemodynamic status of the trauma patient. With the use of arterial lines and pulmonary artery catheters, the anesthesiologist can closely monitor the patient's hemodynamic status. In severe chest injuries, closed chest drainage units and auto transfusions or Cell Saver blood recovery systems can be used to conserve the vital life-sustaining resource blood. Because the goal of treatment is to keep the patient in a hyperdynamic state, the intraoperative trending should reveal that the patient is volume supported, because the body responds hypermetabolically to trauma and achieving that state ensures the delivery of oxygen and other nutrients to essential tissues in the body. End-organ perfusion is monitored and measured with the urinary output and hemodynamic monitoring. Urinary catheters are essential in management of fluids in the trauma patient and assessment of kidney function. Hemodynamic monitoring reflects the body's hydration status and reveals the work of the heart. A detailed operative report reveals the surgical insult to the patient. It also presents a comprehensive review of all anesthetic agents that reflects a rapid sequence of induction, balanced analgesia, and heavy use of opioids, including the time these agents were given and the amount and type of muscle relaxants and reversal agents used. The anesthesia report should reveal any untoward events that occurred during surgery, such as hypothermic or hypotensive events and significant dysrhythmias, including ischemic changes.

Secondary Assessment

After the anesthesia report is received, a brief initial primary survey is completed, and the postanesthesia nurse begins the secondary comprehensive survey with a high degree of suspicion concerning the trauma patient's MOI for specific perianesthesia problems. The initial surgery often is directed at repair of the major life-threatening injuries, such as a ruptured aorta. Consequently, additional injuries may manifest themselves during this later time in the PACU, after swelling or bruising are allowed to develop. During the comprehensive secondary survey, head-to-toe assessment is performed as the trauma patient is emerging from anesthesia. The perianesthesia nurse may discover other injuries, such as pulmonary, cardiac, or renal contusions and compartment syndrome of different extremities.

The head-to-toe assessment begins with a neurologic assessment, including the patient's level of consciousness; the appropriateness of verbal response; pupillary reactivity, size, and shape; equality of pupillary response to light and accommodation; movement; sensation; and pain response in the extremities. Each aspect is carefully evaluated and documented. Next, the head and face are inspected for abrasions, lacerations, puncture wounds, ecchymosis, and edema. These structures are palpated for subcutaneous emphysema or tenderness. The eyes are assessed for gross vision by asking the patient to identify the number of fingers the nurse is holding up. Furthermore, the eyes are evaluated for ecchymosis, "raccoon eyes," and possible conjunctival hemorrhage. Extraocular movements are also evaluated by asking the patient to follow the nurse's finger in six directions. The presence of maxillofacial injuries can be of great concern because of the potential to compromise the patient's airway.

The ears are inspected for Battle sign (ecchymosis behind the ears). The nose is examined for drainage of blood or clear fluid. Clear fluid draining from the nose or ears should be checked for the presence of cerebrospinal fluid (CSF). A draining nose or ears should never be packed. If CSF is suspected or Battle sign is seen, a nasogastric tube should never be inserted through the patient's nose. An orogastric tube is the placement of choice. Finally, the nurse should

immediately report a positive CSF finding to the trauma surgeons.

The neck should be evaluated for edema, ecchymosis, tracheal deviation, pulsating or distended neck veins, and subcutaneous emphysema. As the perianesthesia nurse continues the assessment of the chest, the anterior and the lateral thorax and axilla are inspected for lacerations, abrasions, contusions, puncture wounds, ecchymosis, and edema. The nurse carefully palpates the chest for tenderness and subcutaneous emphysema. The chest wall is observed for symmetry, depth, and equality of expansion and excursion. If the trauma patient has a flail chest from the injury sustained, astute monitoring for effective oxygenation and ventilation are essential. Breathing is observed for rate, degree of effort, use of accessory muscles, or paradoxic chest wall movements. Breath and heart sounds are auscultated, noting adventitious lung sounds (e.g., wheezing, rales, friction rubs) or murmurs, bruits, and muffled heart sounds. The perianesthesia nurse carefully notes facial expressions or body reactions that may suggest possible cardiac contusions or rib fractures. The operative site and all dressings and drains should be assessed and described. Furthermore, all drains should be labeled, drainage of fluid is measured, and color and consistency are described. Precise documentation of all fluid output is essential for accurate fluid replacement.

The next areas to be inspected are the abdomen, pelvis, and genitalia. All abrasions, contusions, edema, and ecchymoses are noted. The abdomen is auscultated for bowel sounds before palpation for tenderness and rigidity. The nasogastric tube, jejunostomy, or tube drainage is examined for color, consistency, and amount of fluid. In suspected internal abdominal or retroperitoneal hemorrhage, abdominal compartment measurements should be assessed. Some common causes of abdominal compartment syndrome are pelvic fractures, hemorrhagic pancreatitis, ruptured abdominal aortic aneurysm, blunt and penetrating abdominal trauma, bowel edema from injury, septic shock, and perihepatic or retroperitoneal packing for diffuse nonsurgical bleeding. If intraabdominal hypertension or abdominal compartment syndrome are suspected or considered, the standard of care is measurement of bladder pressures.[24] A catheter or similar device is connected to a pressure transducer that is connected to the urinary catheter. The urinary catheter is clamped near the connection, 50 mL of saline solution is instilled to the bladder, the transducer is leveled at the symphysis pubis, and the pressure is measured at end expiration. If the pressure is elevated, a decompression laparotomy should be performed to release the pressure that develops from bowel edema.[24] The abdomen is then left open and covered with a sterile wound vacuum until the swelling has resolved and the abdomen can be closed.

The pelvis is palpated for stability and tenderness, especially over the crests and the pubis. Priapism, which is persistent abnormal erection, may be noted.[10,11] In addition, preexisting genital herpes may also be present. The urinary catheter is inspected for color and amount of drainage. Urinary output should be at least 0.5 to 1.0 mL/kg/h in adults and 1 to 2 mL/kg/h in children.[8] Hematuria can indicate kidney or bladder trauma. Furthermore, urinary output must be vigilantly monitored to ensure a minimum of 30 mL/h in adults so that the patient does not develop acute renal failure from rhabdomyolysis, which can occur after traumatic injuries. The vagina and rectum are checked carefully for neurologic function and bloody drainage.

All extremities are examined for circulatory, sensory, and motor functions with range of motion. Because the trauma patient is rushed to the OR to correct life-threatening injuries, minor soft tissue injuries often may be missed. Later in the PACU, these soft tissue and musculoskeletal injuries can develop into compartment syndrome. Each extremity must be thoroughly examined for abrasions, contusions, puncture wounds, ecchymosis, and edema. If neurovascular compromise is found, an arteriogram or venogram can be performed as a conclusive diagnostic study.

The patient is then log-rolled onto the side, with maintenance of cervical spine integrity, for assessment of the back, flanks, and buttocks for abrasions, contusions, and tenderness. Rectal tone is noted if spinal cord injury is suspected. Posterior chest assessment is completed as a last step in the head-to-toe assessment. Finally, a detailed yet succinct description of the primary and secondary assessment is documented.

Pain

Assessment and management of pain are important parts of the scope of care provided to the trauma patient in the PACU. The trauma patient may have musculoskeletal injuries or ruptured organs that cause severe pain, which may include more than the surgical site. Identification of alcohol or opioid withdrawal requires a specialized management approach and may be difficult to assess in the patient with multiple traumas during the postanesthesia period. Substance abuse pain assessment scales, such as the Clinical Institute Narcotic Assessment Scale and Clinical Institute Withdrawal Assessment Scale, are more appropriate.[25] The perianesthesia nurse needs to recognize that because pain is subjective, verbal, nonverbal, and hemodynamic, changes that indicate the patient may be exhibiting signs of pain should be noted. Pain can manifest itself with increased heart rate, increased blood pressure, pallor, tachypnea, guarding or splinting, and nausea and vomiting. Pain scales should be used to augment the nursing assessment of pain.

Optimal management of acute pain may use the following techniques: (1) patient-controlled analgesia with intravenous or epidural infusions; (2) intravenous intermittent doses for pain or sedation; and (3) major plexus blocks. Guidance for medications should be based on choosing drugs that minimize cardiovascular depression and intracranial hypertension. A higher incidence rate of substance abuse, both alcohol and recreational or addictive mind-altering drugs, in the trauma patient population may require higher doses of opioids or analgesics.[25,26] Other complementary techniques, such as music therapy and guided imagery, may be initiated and used as adjuncts when the trauma patient returns for subsequent surgical procedures or wound debridement. Finally, continual pain assessment is vital to the patient's optimal care.

Nausea

Nausea can be a concern for the trauma patient. Trauma patients rarely fast before the traumatic event; therefore patients enter anesthesia with a potentially full stomach. Vomiting can lead to aspiration and a host of issues. Extubation of trauma patients should be delayed until the gag reflex returns to avoid aspiration. Many times, nasogastric tubes are present, but if the patient has consumed food before the event, particles may be too large to be evacuated. Nausea needs to be treated after surgery and is seen with a higher incidence rate in the traumatized patient.

Psychologic Assessment

Often, the psychological and emotional condition of the trauma patient is not considered a priority because the initial events are life threatening. However, when the patient regains consciousness in the PACU, this aspect of the patient's care may prove to be the most challenging.

Posttraumatic Stress Disorder

Trauma patients can emerge from anesthesia in a confused or combative state because of pain, disorientation, or PTSD. Emergence delirium or emergence excitement is a recognized complication of patients recovering from anesthesia. Trauma patients are at increased risk for emergence delirium because of PTSD that occurs after

SPECIAL CONSIDERATIONS

the experience or witnessing of life-threatening events, such as military combat, a terrorist incident, a natural disaster, or sexual assault.[27] The PACU nurse should be prepared to critically assess the patient on emergence from anesthesia for restlessness, agitation, "thousand-mile stare," or sudden outbursts when the patient experiences flashbacks from the traumatic event.[27] The nurse must provide a calm, soft, but directive communication, always remembering to orient the recovering patient from anesthesia. Family or friends may be appropriate visitors in PACU Phase I to help orient the patient to an unfamiliar hospital environment. In severe cases of PTSD, the PACU nurse should consider collaborating with an anesthesia provider to resedate the emerging patient.[27] As the patient emerges from anesthesia, the perianesthesia nurse orients the patient to place and time. Because the patient might not remember or recall the event that caused the accident, the nurse orients the patient to the hospital. Fear of death, mutilation, or change in body image can increase the patient's anxiety. The trauma patient may regain consciousness only to find that the extremities are immobilized or amputated. Because a high incidence rate of injuries is related to alcohol or substance abuse, the patient may have no memory of events before, during, or after the injury. The patient may have alterations in visual and auditory functions. If the patient was alert at the scene and remembers that loved ones were severely injured or killed, the patient may become upset or hysterical, often reliving the tragic event. Consequently, the patient not only experiences loss of body integrity and control, but also the loss of loved ones.

The perianesthesia nurse needs to be supportive yet focused on maintaining the patient's integrity and coping skills. The nurse needs to speak to the patient calmly, slowly, and clearly, with simple language that is easily understood. Often the same information has to be repeated as the patient emerges from anesthesia. The clinician should be honest with the patient. Psychologic aspects of trauma care include the following three concepts, according to the Emergency Nurses Association: (1) need for information, (2) need for compassionate care, and (3) need for hope.[10]

NURSING CARE

The focus of the nursing care of the trauma patient is on vigilant continuous reassessments. Consequently, treatment priorities are established on the basis of vital signs, presenting signs and symptoms, clinical findings, abnormal laboratory values, and diagnostic studies. The perianesthesia

nurse must be cognizant of the subtle cues— complex pathophysiologic responses to the traumatic injury—and always anticipate that the trauma patient might exhibit subtle or overt signs of shock. Furthermore, if shock progresses, the perianesthesia nurse should be aware of other complications, such as systemic inflammatory response syndrome, which causes a myriad of cascading pathophysiologic etiologies: adult respiratory distress syndrome, clotting derangements (coagulopathies), acute renal failure, and ultimately multisystem organ failure. Nursing care of the trauma patient provides a special challenge because of the unique physiologic responses.

Infection Control

Infection is the predominant complication that delays recovery and threatens the life of the trauma patient. Wound infections are related to disruption of the skin that compromises the integrity of the skin and consequently results in an infection. At highest risk are massive open soft tissue injuries, such as traumatic amputations, high-energy fractures, burns, and degloving and avulsion injuries. During surgery, the surgeon classifies the wound contamination, which is determined according to the degree of expected bacterial contamination relative to the surgical procedure. The PACU nurse must be diligent in the timing and documentation of postoperative antibiotics. In addition, the type of antibiotic and the time the antibiotic was given should be communicated during the transfer of care.

SHOCK AS A COMPLICATION IN THE PATIENT WITH MULTIPLE TRAUMAS

The most common complication associated with traumatic injuries is shock. Although different types of shock exist, all types exhibit a profound problem with inadequate delivery or utilization of oxygen and nutrients to the cells. Consequently, this anaerobic state results in inadequate tissue perfusion.[28-35] A measure of the body's overall metabolism is expressed as oxygen consumption (VO_2) and oxygen delivery to the cells (DaO_2).[28] When VO_2 is inadequate, cellular hypoxia evolves. The magnitude of oxygen debt correlates with the lactic acid levels, and this measurement quantifies the severity and prognosis in different shock states.[28] Consequently, this complex syndrome of disequilibrium between oxygen supply and demand causes a functional impairment (oxygen debt) in cells, tissues, organs, and eventually body systems.[28] Vital tissues such as the brain, heart, and lungs require large amounts of oxygen to support their specialized functions. Other important tissues, such as the liver, kidney, and gut, need essential amounts of oxygen to support their specialized functions. Furthermore, these functions can be maintained only with energy derived from aerobic metabolism, and they cease when oxygen is in short supply.

Unfortunately, ischemia rapidly initiates a complex series of events that affect every organelle and subcellular system in the body. As cells become anoxic, adenosine triphosphate stores are depleted and virtually all energy-dependent functions cease. Protein synthesis is depleted. Changes in ion transport and glycolysis result in the loss of intracellular potassium and the production of lactic acid, which can result in lethal complications for the ischemic heart. Finally, irreversible anoxic cellular injury kills vital tissues.

Clinical manifestations of shock include signs and symptoms of decreased end-organ perfusion: cool, clammy skin; cyanosis; restlessness; altered level of consciousness; altered skin temperature; tachycardia; dysrhythmias; tachypnea; pulmonary edema; decreased urinary output; increased platelet, leukocyte, and erythrocyte counts; sludging of blood; and metabolic acidosis.[34]

TYPES OF SHOCK

The four major types of shock are hypovolemic, cardiogenic, obstructive, and distributed (see Table 54-1). The first and most common type of shock, hypovolemic, results from an acute hemorrhagic loss in circulating blood volume that decreases vascular filling pressure.[32,33] Cardiogenic

shock results from an inadequate contractility of the cardiac muscle; it is rare in the trauma patient, but can be caused by blunt cardiac injury or myocardial infarction (MI). In obstructive shock, obstruction or compression of the great vessels or the heart itself is the cause. Both tension pneumothorax and cardiac tamponade can cause obstructive shock.[10,11] Distributive shock causes an abnormality in the vascular system and activation of systemic inflammatory response syndrome and produces a maldistribution of blood volume.[29,30] Distributive shock includes neurogenic, anaphylactic, and septic types. The most common type among trauma patients is neurogenic shock from spinal cord injuries.

Hypovolemic Shock

Hypovolemic shock is the decrease in intravascular volume that results in the fluid volume ineffectively filling the intravascular compartment.[29] Consequently, hypovolemic shock can evolve from many causes, such as internal and external hemorrhage, plasma volume loss in burns, third spacing of fluids, and decreased venous return.[32,33]

Classifications of Hemorrhage

As hemorrhage progresses, the cardiovascular system produces characteristic clinical manifestations that are classified according to approximate blood loss (Table 54-2).[11] The following hemorrhagic classifications are described in the conceptual framework of the Committee on Trauma of the American College of Surgeons Advanced Trauma Life Support Course.[11]

Class I hemorrhage, or the early phase, is the loss of as much as 750 mL of blood, or 1% to 15%

Table 54-2	Identification of Hemorrhagic Shock			
	CLASS I	**CLASS II**	**CLASS III**	**CLASS IV**
Blood loss	Up to 15%; 750 mL	15%-30%; 750-1500 mL	30%-40%; 1500-2000 mL	>40%; >2000 mL
Pulse rate (beats/min)	>90	100	120	>140
Capillary refill	Normal	Positive	Positive	Positive
Pulse pressure	Normal or increased	Decreased	Decreased	Decreased
Blood pressure	Normal; 90-100 SBP	Normal	Decreased	Decreased
Respirations (breaths/min)	14-20	20-30	30-40	>35
Urine output (mL/h)	>30	20-30	5-15	Negligible
Mental status	Slightly restless or anxious	Mildly restless and anxious	Anxious and confused	Confused, lethargic to unresponsive
Treatments				
Fluid replacement	Possibly	Always	Always	Always
Blood replacement	No	Possibly	Almost always	Always

From American College of Surgeons, Committee on Trauma: *Advanced trauma life support for doctors*, Chicago, 2009, ACS.
SBP, Systolic blood pressure.

of the body's total blood volume. Minimal physiologic changes occur in heart rate, blood pressure, capillary refill, respiratory rate, and urinary output. However, the patient may have mild anxiety in response to the sympathetic nervous system.

Class II hemorrhage, or the moderate phase, is the loss of 750 to 1500 mL of blood, or 15% to 30% of blood volume. In this phase, multiple incremental physiologic changes occur. The patient may have increased anxiety and restlessness as a result of cerebral stimulation by the sympathetic nervous system and subsequent catecholamine release. The heart rate may be greater than 100 beats/min. Although minimal changes in blood pressure occur, peripheral vasoconstriction does develop, and a rise in diastolic blood pressure results, decreasing pulse pressure. Capillary refill is delayed slightly, and the skin is cool and pale. Finally, urinary output may be slightly depressed.

Class III hemorrhage, or the progressive phase, is the loss of 1500 to 2000 mL of blood, or 30% to 40% loss of blood volume. These patients have signs of cerebral hypoperfusion, hypoxia, and acidosis that create a progressive reduction in the level of consciousness. The patient may be confused, agitated, and anxious, and the heart rate may be greater than 120 beats/min. The patient may have systolic and diastolic hypotension. Capillary refill time may be delayed more than 2 seconds. Deep rapid respirations result from the ensuing metabolic acidosis. As renal perfusion decreases, urinary output may be 5 to 15 mL/h.

Class IV hemorrhage is the loss of more than 2000 mL of blood, or approximately 40% of the body's blood volume. This significant blood loss profoundly affects the trauma patient. The patient's level of consciousness may be lethargic, stuporous, or unresponsive. The heart rate may be 140 beats/min or greater, and the peripheral pulses may be weak and difficult to palpate. The capillary refill time may be more than 10 seconds. The patient may have severe hypotension, and blood pressure may be difficult to obtain. The skin may be cold, clammy, diaphoretic, or cyanotic. The respiratory rate is shallow, irregular, and greater than 35 breaths/min. Finally, no renal end-organ perfusion occurs, which results in anuria.[11]

According to the American College of Surgeons Advanced Trauma Life Support Course[11], the treatment of patients with blood loss hemorrhage is infusion of crystalloids and possibly blood. A rough guideline for the total volume of replacement fluid is 3 mL of crystalloid for each 1 mL of blood loss.[10,11] This guideline is referred to as the *3:1 rule*.[11] When the blood loss results in a class III hemorrhage, administration of blood should be considered; the patient with a

class IV hemorrhage needs blood administration and without aggressive measures dies within minutes. The goal is assessment of the patient's response to fluid resuscitation and evidence of adequate end-organ perfusion and oxygenation (e.g., urinary output, level of consciousness, tissue perfusion). The same signs and symptoms that alert the presence of shock must be reassessed to determine the patient's response.[11] The first hour after injury is termed the *golden hour*, in which successful treatment of shock is associated with lower mortality.[34,35]

Treatment

The primary treatment goal for patients with hypovolemic shock is fluid replacement. By filling the vascular "tank," the heart is able to generate adequate cardiac output and produce enough hydrostatic pressure to allow perfusion of the tissues.

Cardiogenic Shock

Cardiogenic shock induced by inadequate cardiac output usually occurs in the trauma patient as a result of blunt injury to the heart muscle (e.g., contusions and ruptured heart or injury to heart valves or septa) or occasionally MI.[10,11,30] MIs, however, may either precipitate or precede the traumatic event. Consequently, the patient with a history of heart disease or age-related cardiac reserve limitations or who needs myocardial depressants, such as anesthesia, has a high propensity for cardiogenic shock.[34] Finally, this trauma patient population is also at greater risk for developing cardiac failure because of the rapid fluid resuscitation.

Cardiogenic shock is circulatory failure caused by a consequence of impairment of cardiac contractility, not by a loss of intravascular fluid volume. This impaired pumping ability of the heart can result from destruction of contractility of the ventricles, as in MI. Another cause of pump failure occurs from the disruption of normal conduction sequence, as in heart blocks or dysrhythmias. Myocardial depression that results from the release of vasoactive substances like myocardial depressant factor during septic shock causes dysfunction and decreased myocardial contractility.

Another method to classify causes of cardiogenic shock is identification of the shock as either coronary or noncoronary. Rice[32] described coronary cardiogenic shock as an obstructive coronary artery disease process that interrupts blood flow and oxygen delivery to heart muscle cells, resulting in ischemia and death. The infarcted area of heart muscle is necrotic and dead and thus provides no function. Because the area of infarction and the surrounding area of ischemic heart muscle do not contract normally, the heart is unable to maintain forward blood flow or cardiac output.

Patients with acute MIs are at greatest risk of developing cardiogenic shock, especially when a significant portion (myocardial injury, >40%) of the left ventricle is involved. This loss of contractility reveals a low cardiac output, elevated left-ventricular filling pressure, peripheral vasoconstriction, and arterial hypotension. Another problem involves the volume of blood that accumulates in the left ventricle after systolic ejection and increases the left-ventricular filling pressure. This back-pressure mechanism causes the following sequence of events: (1) an increased left-atrial pressure; (2) an increased pulmonary venous pressure; and (3) an increased pulmonary capillary pressure that results in pulmonary interstitial edema and intraalveolar edema.[34] A small percentage of MIs, however, involve the damaged right ventricle, which does not propel sufficient blood forward through the lungs into the left heart.[34] Cardiac output decreases, and systemic circulation is insufficient to maintain the body's needs.

As discussed previously, noncoronary cardiogenic shock can develop in the absence of coronary artery disease and heart muscle damage, such as with cardiomyopathies, valvular heart abnormalities, cardiac tamponade, and dysrhythmias.[34]

Cardiogenic shock is defined as shock from acute myocardial dysfunction, including the following clinical and diagnostic criteria: systolic blood pressure less than 80 mm Hg, or less than 30 mm Hg of baseline in the patient with hypertension; cardiac index less than 2.1 L/min/m²; urinary output less than 20 mL/h; diminished cerebral perfusion evidenced by confusion or obtundation; and cold, clammy, cyanotic skin characteristic of a low cardiac output state. However, classic signs and symptoms of cardiogenic shock, such as pulmonary congestion, edema, neck vein distention, and hepatic congestion, may not be seen in the trauma patient with coexisting acute hypovolemia.

Other clinical indicators can be obtained through hemodynamic monitoring. Cardiac, stroke, and left-ventricular stroke work indexes are decreased because of pump failure. Pulmonary artery and pulmonary capillary wedge pressures are increased, which indicates an increased left-ventricular end-diastolic pressure. Systemic vascular resistance is increased and reflects vasoconstriction. Systemic venous oxygen saturation is decreased because of decreased cardiac output and increased oxygen extraction from the capillary bed. Arterial blood gas determinations reveal respiratory and metabolic acidosis that is associated with hypoxemia. Consequently, cardiogenic shock is the most lethal and results in mortality rates that range from 80% to 100%.

Treatment

The importance of early recognition and treatment of cardiogenic shock cannot be overemphasized. Prompt improvement of myocardial oxygen supply and tissue perfusion, with a decrease in myocardial oxygen demand, is vital not only to minimization of heart damage but also to the trauma patient's chance of survival. The goals of treatment for cardiogenic shock are to establish an airway, maintain ventilation and oxygenation, provide proper positioning, relieve pain, correct acidosis, monitor urinary output, and deliver pharmacologic support to improve or correct cardiac rhythm. Furthermore, increasing cardiac output can may be achieved by judiciously increasing intravascular volume to improve preload. The heart rate and myocardial contractility may be increased with the inotropic and vasoactive drugs such as epinephrine, dopamine, and dobutamine. Another goal of therapy is to decrease afterload, which may be accomplished by lowering peripheral vascular resistance. Other important pharmacologic agents that may be used in cardiogenic shock are vasopressors, vasodilators, adrenergic blocking agents, corticosteroids, digitalis, and thrombolytic agents.

When pharmacologic support fails to improve the oxygen supply-and-demand balance, alternative methods such as the intraaortic balloon pump and the right-ventricular and left-ventricular assist devices help to increase myocardial oxygen supply, decrease myocardial VO_2, relieve pulmonary congestion, and improve organ perfusion.[34,35]

Distributive Shock

Distributive, or vasogenic, shock is an abnormal placement or a maldistribution of the vascular volume. The heart's ability to pump blood and the body's blood volume are normal. Therefore this category of shock describes a unique pathologic condition that exists within the vascular circulatory network and causes an alteration in blood vessels. The three types of distributive shock are neurogenic, anaphylactic, and septic.

Neurogenic Shock

Neurogenic shock reflects the domination of the parasympathetic nervous system and results in venous pooling and bradycardia. Neurogenic shock can occur from acute spinal cord injury or in patients who are paraplegic or quadriplegic and have a full bladder. Decreasing bladder pressure with catheterization helps to resolve symptoms in the patient with nonacute spinal cord injury. Likewise, neurogenic shock is described as a tremendous increase in the vascular capacity such that even the normal amount of blood becomes incapable of adequately filling the circulatory system.[35] When the body has an increase in vascular capacity, the mean systemic pressure decreases, which causes a decreased venous return to the heart. 'Because the sympathetic nervous system causes vasoconstriction to maintain vascular tone, the loss of sympathetic enervation results in domination of the parasympathetic nerves, causing vascular dilation (or venous pooling). This massive vasodilation of veins occurs as a result of the loss of sympathetic vasomotor tone. Neurogenic shock, however, often is transitory and does not commonly occur.

Although neurogenic shock can be caused by deep general or spinal anesthesia, loss of sympathetic vasomotor tone in the trauma patient can occur directly from a brain concussion or contusion of the basal regions of the brain or from spinal cord injury above the level of T6.

Because massive unopposed vasodilation induces arterioles to dilate, decreasing peripheral vascular resistance, venules and veins also dilate and thus cause blood to pool in the venous vasculature and decrease venous return to the right heart.[30,31] Consequently, the following series of events occurs: (1) decreased ventricular filling pressure, (2) decreased stroke volume, (3) decreased cardiac output, (4) decreased blood pressure, (5) decreased peripheral vascular resistance, and (6) decreased tissue perfusion.

The clinical presentation in neurogenic shock is different from that in hypovolemic shock, even though the blood pressure is low. The patient is frequently bradycardic, and the skin is warm, dry, and flushed. Hemodynamic monitoring reveals a decrease in cardiac output, as a result of a decrease in resistance in arteriolar vasculature, and also a decrease in venous tone.

Treatment

The treatment of neurogenic shock may require extensive volume expansion and the use of vasopressors, such as ephedrine. In the case of spinal anesthesia, the perianesthesia nurse should place the patient in a supine position and, if possible, decrease the head of the bed elevation and elevate the legs. Finally, the goal of treatment in neurogenic shock is to balance volume expansion with the titration of vasopressor administration.[32,33,34,35]

Anaphylactic Shock

Anaphylactic shock results from a severe antigen-antibody reaction. Although this type of shock is not commonly seen in trauma patients, the condition can occur as an iatrogenic complication during resuscitation.[29-32] Other causes of anaphylactic shock are reactions to antibiotics, contrast media, and blood transfusions.

The pathophysiologic response of anaphylaxis relates to the systemic inflammatory response syndrome process and the activation of the complement and arachidonic cascades. The sequence of events involved in the development of anaphylactic shock are divided into three phases[32,33,34,35]:
1. The sensitization phase, in which immunoglobulin E antibody is produced in response to an antigen and binds to mast cells and basophils
2. The activation phase, in which reexposure to the specific antigen triggers mast cells to release their vasoactive contents
3. The effector phase, in which the complex response of anaphylaxis occurs as a result of the histamine and vasoactive mediators released by the mast cells and basophils

These vasoactive mediators act on blood vessels and cause massive vasodilation and increased capillary permeability, which allows fluid to leak from the intravascular space to the interstitial space.[30]

Clinical symptoms of anaphylactic shock include conjunctivitis, angioedema, hypotension, laryngeal edema, urticaria, bronchoconstriction, dysrhythmias, and cardiac arrest. One or all of these symptoms may occur; therefore immediate and effective life-saving treatment must be initiated.

Treatment

The initial treatment of the patient in anaphylactic shock is identification and removal of the specific antigen that has caused the allergic reaction. Furthermore, if the patient is receiving an infusion of blood or blood products, the perianesthesia nurse should immediately discontinue the transfusion and initiate an intravenous infusion with normal saline solution. Administration of oxygen via facemask should be started. The initial pharmacologic agent of choice is epinephrine, a bronchodilator that helps restore vascular tone and increase arterial blood pressure.

Aminophylline can be administered to reduce bronchial constriction and wheezing and to minimize respiratory distress.[35] Diphenhydramine, an antihistamine, is another drug of choice. Corticosteroids can be used to decrease the inflammatory response. Finally, gastric acid blockers such as the histamine 2 (H_2) blockers (famotidine, ranitidine) are given.

Septic Shock

Septic shock is the most common type of distributive shock and results from an acute systemic response (systemic inflammatory response syndrome) to invading bloodborne microorganisms. The sepsis can be caused by gram-positive bacteria; however, the most common cause is gram-negative bacteria. Other pathogens that can cause septic shock are viruses, fungi, parasites, or rickettsiae. The trauma patient is predisposed to the following determinants that affect the outcome of septic shock: infection as a result of contaminated wounds, poor nutritional status, preexisting disease state, and altered integrity of the body's defense mechanisms.[32,33,35] Furthermore, sepsis-associated tissue damage is a major complication and remains the principal cause of death in trauma patients who survive the first 3 days after injury.[34]

Septic shock is a clinical syndrome that, on a continuum, begins with sepsis and ends with multisystem organ dysfunction or failure. Septic shock is primarily a complex cellular disease that results in a loss of autoregulation and in tissue dysfunction that occurs early and persists despite increased cardiac output. Interactions between bacterial toxins and the body's cellular, humoral, and immunologic systems are considered to activate the kinins and complement, arachidonic, and coagulation cascades, which generate other endogenous mediators that only intensify regional malperfusion.[12,28-35]

The profound hemodynamic instability of septic shock is revealed in the body's biphasic response. The first phase, or the hyperdynamic response, is characterized by a high cardiac output and a low systemic vascular resistance; the second phase, the hypodynamic response, reflects the classic shock picture with a low cardiac output and an extremely high systemic vascular resistance.[28-31] These phases are also referred to as *early shock,* or a warm hyperdynamic phase, and *late shock,* or a cold hypodynamic phase. During early shock, the patient's skin is pink, warm, and dry because of the increased cardiac output and peripheral vasodilation. With progressing shock, fluid leaks from the vascular compartment, and the patient develops relative hypovolemia, with decreasing cardiac output and increasing peripheral vasoconstriction.[33,34] The clinical manifestations of late shock are cold and clammy skin, decreased cardiac output, severe hypotension, and extreme vasoconstriction.[35]

In septic shock, the degree of myocardial depression is directly related to the severity of sepsis. Decreased force of contractions may be the result of the release of vasoactive chemical mediators, such as myocardial depressant factor, endotoxins, tumor necrosis factor, complement, leukotrienes, and endorphins.[32-35] Furthermore, decreased ventricular preload from increased capillary permeability augments the myocardial depression.

Rice[32,33] describes alterations in peripheral circulation as massive vasodilation that occur as a result of mediator activation of the bradykinins, histamines, endorphins, complement split products, platelet-activating factor, and prostaglandins.[32-35] Another aspect of altered circulation is observed in the maldistribution of blood volume that occurs when some tissues receive more blood flow than is needed and other tissues are deprived of needed oxygen and nutrients. Finally, increased capillary permeability causes reduced circulating blood volume, increased blood viscosity, hypoalbuminemia, and interstitial edema.[35]

One of the first target organs to be affected in septic shock is the lung.[28,33,34] Endotoxin stimulates the production of complement split products, producing bronchoconstriction, and the release of other vasoactive mediators that cause neutrophil and platelet aggregation to the lungs increases capillary permeability. Consequently, fluid collects in the interstitium and increases diffusion distance, decreases compliance, and thereby causes hypoxemia. Pulmonary vasoconstriction may be caused by thromboxane A_2, which augments capillary permeability and leads to acute respiratory distress syndrome or acute lung injury.[30,33]

Septic shock also causes a profound alteration in metabolism. This metabolic dysfunction is attributed to the following: (1) increasing oxygen debt and rising blood lactate levels, (2) sustained proteolysis, (3) altered gluconeogenesis with concurrent insulin resistance, and (4) liberation of free fatty acids.[34]

Treatment

The treatment of septic shock consists of identifying and eliminating the focus of infection. With culturing of the blood, urine, sputum, wound drainage, and invasive lines, the organism can be identified, and the proper definitive antimicrobial therapy can be initiated. Hemodynamic monitoring ensures an accurate means to assess the patient's circulatory status and the patient's response to therapeutic interventions. Initially, the perianesthesia nurse may elect to use supplemental oxygen and encourage the patient to breathe deeply. However, as the shock state progresses, the patient's respiratory status becomes compromised. Aggressive ventilator support must be established to maintain adequate oxygenation and tissue perfusion. Proper selection of parenteral fluid administration is important in correcting the cause of shock and supporting tissue perfusion.[32-33,35-36]

Pharmacologic support, including the use of positive inotropes (primarily dopamine, dobutamine, norepinephrine) and vasodilators (primarily nitroprusside and nitroglycerin), may be indicated to augment contractility, preload, and afterload. New evidence supports glycemic control to assist in control of the stress response.[36] Finally, promising research suggests that the use of arginine vasopressin in refractory septic shock, despite adequate fluid volume resuscitation and high-dose vasopressor therapy, helps to restore mean arterial pressure and is catecholamine sparing in septic shock.[36]

Obstructive Shock

Obstructive shock is caused by an obstructive source such as acute pulmonary embolism, dissecting aortic aneurysm, vena cava obstruction, cardiac tamponade, or tension pneumothorax. The result of all these pathologic mechanisms is decreased cardiac output from compression to the atria, which prevents the atrium from filling and thus leads to decreased stroke volume. Cardiac tamponade can compress the atria during diastole so that the atria cannot fill completely, resulting in decrease in stroke volume results.[10] Displacement of the inferior vena cava can obstruct return of venous blood to the heart, building up pressure as in a tension pneumothorax. Clinical manifestations are in alignment with causative mechanisms.

Treatment

Interventions should be aimed toward correction of the cause. Tension pneumothorax may need a needle decompression and chest tube. Cardiac tamponade may need pericardiocentesis and surgical intervention. Without prompt and appropriate treatment, obstructive shock is fatal.

PEDIATRIC TRAUMA

Pediatric trauma continues to be the leading cause of death in children older than 1 year.[37,38] These injuries significantly affect not only the children, but also the parents and the entire family unit. Furthermore, their health care problems lead to complex psychological trauma, increased financial burden, and the long-term medical costs for rehabilitation. Foremost, the postanesthesia nurse needs to understand the epidemiology of pediatric trauma, the risk factors related to the developmental ages (Table 54-3), and the unique pediatric anatomic and physiologic differences that directly affect the optimal management of the patient. Likewise, the PACU nurse should recognize the symptoms of families in crisis as well as signs of psychological posttraumatic stress in order to effectively intervene and promote coping techniques with the child and parents. Finally, the postanesthesia nurse should facilitate family visitation during invasive or resuscitative events in

the PACU as an advocate for the preservation of the family unit.

Epidemiology

Millions of children are seriously injured each year in the United States. Unintentional injuries are the leading cause of pediatric deaths of more than 21,000 children, adolescents, and young adults.[38] Interestingly, unintentional deaths peak during the toddler–preschool period and then again during adolescence and young adulthood. Although the most common injuries are open wounds, superficial injuries, contusions, dislocations, sprains, and strains, the more significant trauma injuries are blunt trauma, intracranial injuries, and burns.[10,11,39] Key predictive risk factors related to age group and types of injuries are the following: infants sustain suffocation, motor vehicle crashes (MVCs), burns and falls; toddlers and preschool-age children who sustain MVCs, drowning, fires, burns, suffocations, and falls; school-age children start to engage in more risk-taking behaviors that are linked to pedestrian injuries, bicycle injuries, drowning, and firearms; and finally MVCs lead the category in adolescent trauma injuries.[40-42] Overall age and gender are important characteristics and reflect that male children have higher injury and mortality rates than females.[40] Likewise, children with attention deficit disorders have a 1.5-fold greater risk of injury.[38] Effective injury prevention education and research continue to promote keeping children safe and decreasing the risk of traumatic injuries.[41]

Pediatric Pathophysiology

It is important to understand the differences between a pediatric and adult anatomy and physiology. The pediatric airway has several inherent differences. First, the pediatric head-to-body ratio is approximately 1:5, whereas the ratio for adults is 1:8. Head injuries are the leading cause of death in children and adults. Children are predisposed to head injuries because their heads are large and heavy in relation to their bodies. The risk of injury is increased because the child's balance and coordination are immature.

Airway

The child's mouth is relatively small compared with the child's large tongue, which can easily obstruct the airway. Furthermore, neonates and infants are obligate nose breathers and may become distressed if their nose becomes obstructed by mucus, blood, or foreign bodies. Likewise, the pediatric epiglottis is omega-shaped and floppy, the larynx is higher and more anterior, the

Table 54-3 Developmental Considerations for Pediatric Trauma Patients

	INFANT (0-1 YR)	TODDLER (1-3 YR)	PRESCHOOL CHILD (3-6 YR)	SCHOOL-AGE CHILD (6-12 YR)	ADOLESCENT (12-18 YR)
Developmental task (Erikson)	Trust vs. mistrust	Autonomy vs. doubt and shame	Initiative vs. guilt	Industry vs. inferiority	Identity vs. role confusion
Cognitive development (Piaget)	Sensorimotor knowing	Preoperational thought	Preoperational thought (late phase)	Concrete operations	Formal operations
Communication	Cries, facial expression, motor activity	Simple phrases, cries, physical activity	Sentences, crying, physical activity; Very literal; Does not comprehend cause and effect	Well-developed vocabulary	Abstract thinker; Generally seeks information
Stresses, fears	Disruptions in routine	Separation, pain	Separation, abandonment, pain, mutilation	Loss of control, bodily injury, death, separation, pain	Disfigurement, separation from peers, loss of control
Illness concept	None	None	Illness as feeling state	Understands various aspects of illness, some basic anatomy	Understands anatomy and physiology
Preparation		Simple, honest explanation just before event, using sensory information; Medical play with equipment	Simple, honest explanation just before event, using sensory information; Medical play with equipment	Explanation before procedure, using concrete and specific information; Medical play with equipment; Encourage questions; Allow child to have some control if possible	Explanation before procedure; Provide enough time for the adolescent to formulate questions; Explain why the procedure is necessary

From Moloney-Harmon PA, Czerwinski SJ, editors: *Nursing care of the pediatric trauma patient*, Philadelphia, 2003, Saunders.

tracheal length is only 4 to 5 cm in infants, and the cricoid ring is the narrowest part of the airway, making it more difficult to intubate the infant and young child.[43] It is vital to ensure that the child's airway is patent.

Breathing

Another critical assessment is breathing to ensure adequacy of the respirations. The postanesthesia nurse carefully evaluates the work of breathing by assessing the rise and fall of the chest, respiratory effort (use of accessory muscles), efficacy, quality of the bilateral breath sounds, and oxygenation.[44] When the child is intubated, end-tidal CO_2 may be monitored continuously. The PACU nurse needs to be vigilant in continually assessing the rate and work of breathing. Signs and symptoms of impending respiratory distress or failure are the following: respiratory rate greater than 60 breaths/min, nasal flaring, noisy, stridor, coarse rales, cyanosis, altered mental status, and irregular breathing patterns. It is important that the nurse be ready to intervene and be able to provide ventilatory support and oxygenation via the bag-mask device.

Circulation

The most common cause of shock in the pediatric trauma patient is hypovolemia through blood loss. One of the important circulation assessments for adequate end-organ perfusion is through palpating the central versus distal pulses and counting the pulse for 1 minute because of irregularities in an anxious or injured child. Pediatric patients are volume sensitive and in low-perfusion states will shunt their circulating blood to their vital organs. In hypotensive or low-flow states, the child's extremities will be cool to the touch, and distal pulses will be weak to nonexistent. One may find tachycardia in children with conditions such as a fever, anxiety, or early shock. However, bradycardia is an ominous sign that may reflect hypoxia, hypoglycemia, hypothermia, spinal cord injury, or increased intracranial pressure. In infants, it is essential to keep in mind that they have not yet developed the ability to compensate for hypovolemia by increasing heart rate; therefore bradycardia is especially concerning. Children maintain such strong circulatory compensatory mechanisms that even with a loss of 25% to 30% circulating blood volume loss, their bodies can maintain blood pressures through peripheral and superficial vasoconstriction (Table 54-4). Therefore hypotension is a late sign of hypovolemia. Accurate blood pressures should be assessed with the correctly sized cuff. It is important to assess for sources of external bleeding and, if found, apply direct pressure. Foremost to ensuring effective volume resuscitation is the need to assess the intravenous site for patency and that the fluid infuses properly.

Neurologic

Head injuries are the leading cause of death in children because of their large head size, proportionally larger cranial blood volume, malleable skull, and

Table 54-4	Classes of Hemorrhage for Children		
CLASS	**BLOOD LOSS**	**SIGNS**	**TREATMENT**
Class I	15% or less 40-kg child = 500 mL blood	Pulse: slight increase BP: normal Respiration: normal Capillary refill: normal Tilt test: normal*	Crystalloids
Class II	20%-30% 40-kg child = 800 mL blood	Pulse: tachycardia >150 BP: decreased systolic; decreased pulse pressure Respiration: tachypnea >35-40 Capillary refill: delayed Tilt test: positive Urine output: normal (1 mL/kg/h)	Crystalloids
Class III	30%-35% 40-kg child = 1200 mL blood	BP: decreased Narrow pulse pressure Urine output: decreased	Crystalloids Packed red blood cells
Class IV	40%-50% 40-kg child = 1600 mL blood	Pulse: nonpalpable BP: nonpalpable No response to verbal or painful stimuli	Crystalloids Packed red blood cells

BP, Blood pressure.
*A tilt test is performed by sitting the child upright. The test result is normal if the child can stay up for more than 90 seconds and maintain blood pressure.

incomplete myelinization of brain tissues that renders the brain vulnerable to shearing forces. A careful, thorough neurologic examination begins with assessing the level of consciousness, motor response, pupil size, and reactivity. The AVPU method of assessment determines the child's response to external stimulation.[10,11] The child whose level of consciousness changes, such as failure to recognize parents and failure to response to painful procedures (e.g., drawing blood, insertion of intravenous catheter), or becomes sleepy or lethargic should be reassessed frequently and monitored closely. Vomiting and irritability are early signs of increased intracranial pressure. The effects of elevated increased intracranial pressure may be revealed in Cushing triad: hypertension, bradycardia, and abnormal breathing patterns. Consequently, this severe compromise of blood flow to the brainstem indicates impending herniation that requires immediate emergency interventions. The goal of caring for the child with head trauma is to prevent or limit the secondary reperfusion injury to the brain.[44]

Exposure

Infants and children have a larger body surface area. As a result, pediatric trauma patients may experience hypothermia that can be life threatening because of the clotting cascade that is temperature dependent. Hypothermia can develop quickly and complicate recovery. The PACU nurse may use different methods to preserve body heat and warm their patients, such as warm thermal blankets, forced air warmers, and heat lamps. Close temperature monitoring during the postanesthesia recovery is essential.

Urinary Output

Urinary output is a measure of end organ perfusion in the kidneys. Urine output can vary with age. Output for the following ages groups should be expected: 2 mL/kg/h for infants (1-12 months), 1.5 mL/kg/h for younger children, and 0.5 mL/h for older children.[10,11]

Pain Management

The management of pain is an important aspect in the care of pediatric patients. The management of acute pain in pediatric patients includes both pharmacologic and nonpharmacologic modalities. Common pharmacologic interventions most often used in the PACU include nonopioid (e.g., acetaminophen, salicylates, nonsteroidal antiinflammatory drugs) and opioid medications (e.g., fentanyl, morphine, hydromorphone), dissociative medications (e.g., ketamine), anxiolytics medications (e.g., midazolam), and local nerve blocks.[45] Nonpharmacologic techniques that are often used include guided

imagery, music therapy, videos, toys, massage, cold, and warmth therapy.[45] Optimally, the combination of nonpharmacologic and nonpharmacologic interventions provide the best methods to decrease the traumatic pain experience in children and promote the healing process.[25]

OBSTETRIC TRAUMA

Acute traumatic injury during pregnancy is the leading cause of maternal death in the United States.[46-51]. Major causes of injury-related maternal deaths are from blunt trauma (e.g., MVCs, abdominal), penetrating trauma (e.g., gunshot wounds, stab wounds), burns, falls, and assaults.[46-51] Even more alarming is the significant rise in the incidence of domestic violence during pregnancy.[52,53] Tragically, these lethal injuries affect not only the pregnant woman, but also the unborn fetus she is carrying. Likewise, the risk of trauma to the mother and fetus increases as the pregnancy progresses, mainly because of the increasing size of the developing fetus and uterus.[51] Consequently the rapid, effective resuscitation of the mother is of paramount importance, because fetal survival is directly related to the maternal well-being.[49] Because there is a high maternal and fetal morbidity and mortality associated with these injuries, a multidisciplinary team approach to the acute management of their injuries is essential for optimal outcomes for both the mother and her baby.[46]

Epidemiology

According to Muench and Canterino,[54] although trauma complicates 6% to 7% of all pregnancies, it is the leading cause of nonobstetric maternal morbidity and mortality. As the size of the developing uterus and fetus expand, the risk to the mother and unborn baby also increases. Furthermore, there is direct correlation between the multiple anatomic and physiologic changes that occur during pregnancy and the movement of abdominal organs from the lower abdominal or pelvic regions to the upper abdominal and thoracic cavities,[55] thus exposing the pregnant patient to increased risk of traumatic injury.

Placental Abruption

The mechanism for placental abruption is related to the difference between the tissue properties of the elastic myometrium and the inelastic placenta.[55] Placental abruption is caused by shearing forces at the placental-uterine interface. Because amniotic fluid is not compressible, impact against the uterine wall results in amniotic fluid displacement and uterine distention.[55] Abruption can occur immediately after abdominal trauma impact or be delayed for several hours after the trauma episode.

Uterine Rupture

Blunt trauma to the abdomen of the pregnant patient can be so severe that it causes the uterus to rupture. Adding to the severity of injury is the increased vascularity that could result in severe hemorrhage. The greater the hemorrhage the more rapid the need for replacement of blood and clotting factors required to prevent disseminated intravascular coagulopathy.[46]

Obstetric Pathophysiology

During pregnancy, anatomic and physiologic changes occur in almost all maternal organs and complicate the anesthetic care and postanesthesia management of the trauma patient.[55-60] Anatomically, as pregnancy advances, there is compression and displacement of the pelvic, abdominal and thoracic organs.[56] The diaphragm rises, causing the heart to rotate on its axis while moving upward to the left; the small bowel is also displaced upward, increasing its vulnerability to penetrating traumatic injuries.[56,57] Another important phenomenon that occurs after 20 weeks' gestation is the enlarged uterus compressing the aorta and vena cava when the pregnant woman is lying supine, causing decreased venous return and uterine perfusion. Furthermore, as the uterus increases in size, it displaces the bladder upward and out of the pelvis, making it more vulnerable to rupture.[58,60] The physiologic changes involve the hematologic, cardiovascular, respiratory, gastrointestinal, and renal systems.

Airway

There are several airways considerations when caring for the pregnant patient. The airway may become more difficult to visualize during intubation because of: weight gain, especially in the breast tissue; the position of the larynx being pushed upward more anteriorly; the mucosa of the larynx and pharynx becoming edematous and friable from the increase in extracellular fluid and vascular engorgement; and severe bleeding occurring from direct laryngoscopy, endotracheal intubation, or advancing a nasogastric tube.[59]

Breathing (Pulmonary)

The changes that occur in the pulmonary system reflect the following: (1) increased tidal volume (45%) and minute ventilation (40%); (2) decreased functional residual capacity (25%); (3) increased oxygen consumption (60%); differences in ventilation

and lung volumes result in respiratory alkalosis with a metabolic acidosis secondary to compensation.[59] Consequently, the pregnant trauma patient rapidly develops a metabolic acidosis because of hypoperfusion and hypoxia because of the decreased ability to buffer, as well as developingasdecreased functional residual capacity and increased oxygen consumption. The pregnant trauma patient is extremely prone to hypoxia during periods of apnea and needs to consistently be preoxygenated before intubation.[59]

Circulation (Cardiovascular)

Cardiac output increases 30% to 50%, and heart rate increases 15 to 20 beats/min, while the systemic vascular resistance decreases approximately 35%.[56] As the pregnancy progresses, uterine compression of the vena cava may decrease venous return in the supine patients causing a 30% decrease in cardiac output;[56] this is frequently referred to as *aorta compression* or *supine hypotension syndrome*. The nurse should roll the pregnant patient to the left lateral position to improve the perfusion (Fig. 54-1). Depending on the patient's potential spinal injuries, an alternative method of displacing the uterus includes placing the patient on a backboard at a 15-degree angle until the spinal injury has been ruled out.

Gastrointestinal

The following gastrointestinal changes have an important role in the pregnant trauma patient: progesterone slows gastric emptying and decreases the tone in the esophageal sphincter, and the abdominal contents and diaphragm are pushed upward by the gravid uterus, causing the increased risk of aspiration.[56] Finally, the peritoneum and abdominal muscles are stretched over time, causing a decreased sensation to abdominal pain.

Genitourologic

Common urologic changes seen in pregnancy include: upward displacement of the urinary bladder, placing this organ at an increased risk for rupture; dilation of the ureters; urine blood flow increase from 60 to 600 mL/min at term; and widening of the symphysis pubis and the sacroiliac joints by the seventh month of pregnancy.[55] Blunt trauma to the abdomen leads to the potential for massive blood loss as well as placental abruption.[59,60]

Hematologic

The increase in the maternal blood volume increases by approximately 1500 mL or 40% above

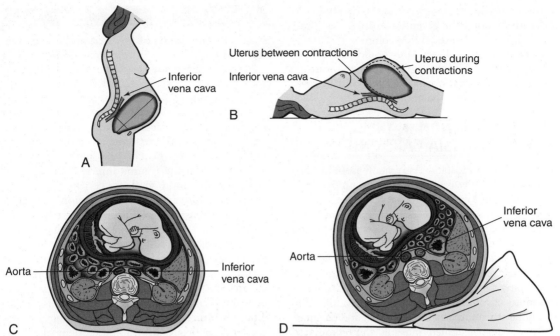

FIG. 54-1 Supine hypotension. Note relationship of gravid uterus to ascending vena cava in standing posture **(A)** and in supine posture **(B)**. **C,** Compression of aorta and inferior vena cava with woman in supine position. **D,** Relieved by use of a wedge pillow placed under woman's right side. (From Lowdermilk DL, et al: *Maternity and women's health care,* ed 10, St. Louis, 2012, Mosby.)

prepregnancy baseline, or approximately 2:1 plasma to red blood cells; this causes the dilutional effect or results in a physiologic anemia.[59] White blood cells may increase to 20,000 to 30,000 cells/mm^3 during the last trimester.[60] The blood has a greater tendency to clot because of the increase in different clotting factors causing an altered clotting cascade. Likewise, there is an increase in fibrinolytic activity with factors VII, VIII, and IX.[59] Consequently, the pregnant trauma patient is susceptible to pulmonary embolus.

Postanesthesia Care Unit Management

The PACU nurse needs to perform systematic primary and secondary postanesthesia assessments on the pregnant trauma patient. The nurse focuses on assessing the mother's airway, breathing, circulation, and neurologic systems first to determine the stability of oxygenation, ventilation, and perfusion of the tissues. High-flow oxygen is a requirement to properly oxygenate the mother and the fetus. According to Tweddale,[51] respiratory changes during pregnancy are comparable to someone exerting

themselves with moderate exercise. As a result, it is prudent to monitor the pulse oximetry closely and to consider providing the trauma obstetric patient with a 100% nonrebreather mask during recovery in the PACU. Remember that the pregnant patient has extra intravascular reserve accumulating and that cardiac output and preload remain constant even in the presence of hemorrhage. It is especially important to remember that fetal survival is dependent on the uterus being adequately perfused and the fetus being well oxygenated.[49] As the uterus becomes more gravid and increases, the inferior vena cava or aorta can become compressed, leading to a decrease in cardiac output, increase in venous perfusion, and decrease in perfusion pressure in the uterus.[51] The PACU nurse should place the pregnant patient on the mother's left side under the right hip. It is important to note that the supine position may compromise the patient's cardiac output by 30%. The neurologic evaluation is also an important component in the primary survey. During the secondary survey, the uterus and fetus are evaluated. Contractions may begin and go unrecognized because of the abdominal wall blunting sensation. Special consideration should be given to limiting vasopressors until adequate fluid volume has been replaced. The fetal heart rate should range from 120 to 150 beats/min. Vigilant cardiac monitoring, fetal heart monitoring, oxygen, and intravenous therapy should be continued.

FAMILY VISITATION IN THE POSTANESTHESIA CARE UNIT

The American Hospital Association is promoting patient- and family-centered care and reuniting families with their loved ones in the hospital setting. A growing body of evidence supports visitation in the PACU.[61] The American Society of PeriAnesthesia Nurses (ASPAN) has promulgated a *Position Statement on Family Visitation in the PACU* (Box 54-1).[61] ASPAN advocates a collaborative inclusive approach to keeping families informed by the PACU nurse. Examples of communication include: (1) notification by phone when the patient is admitted and (2) interaction at regular timed intervals throughout the trauma patient's stay in the postanesthesia unit, which promotes family bonding and coping skills and decreases family anxiety and stress.[61] Although this approach may prove challenging, the benefits to the patient and family are numerous.

SUMMARY

Each year thousands of children and adults have trauma injuries. These injuries may occur within a short time, but if not assessed and treated swiftly they can may have profound long-term effects that affect functional outcomes and quality of life. The PACU nurse must have astute nursing assessments that use critical thinking skills. Furthermore, this specialty nurse must also be cognizant of the MOI and the complex pathophysiologic responses from the trauma injuries. The focus of nursing care is on vigilant, continuous assessments to ensure adequate oxygenation and ventilation and transport (perfusion) of the tissues. The PACU nurse must anticipate and identify the patient at risk of development of shock. Furthermore, prevention and effective management of shock must be the primary goal in care for the trauma patient. In addition, effective management of pain in the trauma patient is foremost. Consequently, the challenge of caring for the complex, critically ill trauma patient demands that the PACU nurse be familiar with current research and evidence-based practice guidelines that provides a framework for understanding and managing these trauma patients in the postanesthesia setting.

Evidence-Based Practice

Spinella and colleagues conducted a retrospective review of 354 combat trauma patients admitted to combat support hospitals in Afghanistan and Iraq by the Joint Theater Trauma Registry maintained at the U.S. Army Institute of Surgical Research (Ft. Sam Houston, Tex.). The researchers compared the use of warm fresh whole blood (WFWB) to the standard transfusion of stored component blood therapy (SCBT) for improved survival of severely injured combat trauma patients. The trauma patients who had received WFWB experienced both a higher 24-hour and 30-day survival compared with the SCBT patients ($p = 0.002$).

IMPLICATIONS FOR PRACTICE

Perianesthesia nurses, who care for massive hemorrhagic and shock in trauma patients in the postanesthesia care unit, need to understand the pathophysiology, implications, and treatment of massive hemorrhage with coagulopathy as the best practice for continued resuscitation of trauma patients.

Source: Spinella PC et al: Warm fresh whole blood is independently associated with improved survival for patients with combat-related traumatic injuries, *J Trauma Injury Infect Crit Care* 66:S69–S76, 2009.

BOX 54-1   ASPAN's Position Statement on Visitation in Phase I Level of Care

The American Society of PeriAnesthesia Nurses (ASPAN) has the responsibility for defining the practice of perianesthesia nursing. An integral part of this responsibility is to promote comfort and satisfaction among patients and families. The specialty of perianesthesia nursing encompasses the care of the patient and family/significant other along the perianesthesia continuum of care.

ASPAN sets forth this position statement to support the needs of both patients and families as it relates to family visitation in the Phase I level of care.

BACKGROUND

Historically, PACUs have been closed units. A patient's family waited anxiously while the patient recovered in the PACU. In recent years, there have been rapid advances in anesthesia management with shorter acting anesthetic agents and increased use of regional anesthetic techniques. There is a growing body of nursing research in support of family visitation and presence at the bedside. ASPAN supports the reevaluation of the needs of both patients and families while striving to maintain quality services across the continuum of care. In response to the concerns of many perianesthesia nurses from around the country, the Standards and Guidelines Committee conducted a review of literature and gathered information from various institutions to identify issues related to visitation in phase I level of care.

A review of current nursing practice revealed a wide range of family visitation practices across the country ranging from no visitation, visitation for intensive care unit (ICU)/overnight patients, and visitation for pediatric patients only, to an open family visitation policy. Perianesthesia nurses also vary in their concerns regarding family visitation as it relates to:

1. Issues of patient confidentially and privacy.
2. Pain and comfort management.
3. Procedures done in phase I level of care.
4. Potential for emergency situations.
5. Unclear family expectations regarding visitation guidelines.

A growing body of research supports the need of both patients and families for increased visitation in the ICUs. In addition, research directly related to the PACU setting reveals that family visitation in phase I level of care benefits both patients and families. The concept of family visitation has gained increased acceptance by nurses when a well-developed visitation program is established.

POSITION

It is, therefore, the position of ASPAN that visitation in the phase I level of care is supported and that perianesthesia nurses develop guidelines within their own settings to incorporate this into their practice.

Guidelines should include the following:

1. Appropriate education for patients and families regarding family visitation to maintain a safe and beneficial experience.
2. The confidentiality and privacy of all patients shall be maintained.
3. The visit will take place at an appropriate time for the patient, visitor, and clinical staff.
4. Perianesthesia nurses should work together with hospital administration to establish a well-organized family visitation program supported by appropriate personnel to meet the needs of families in this unique setting.

EXPECTED OUTCOMES

Perianesthesia nurses need to familiarize themselves with this position statement, current literature and research in support of family visitation.

Perianesthesia nurses should work together with hospital administration to develop organized methods of increasing communication with families throughout the perianesthesia experience and providing appropriate support personnel to establish a visitation program in phase 1 level of care that meets the needs of patients, families, and clinical staff.

ASPAN, as the voice of perianesthesia nursing practice, must externalize this information by sharing this position statement with all disciplines that interface with the practice of perianesthesia patients and families.

APPROVAL OF STATEMENT

This statement was recommended by a vote of the ASPAN Board of Directors on April 5, 2003, and approved by a vote of the ASPAN Representative Assembly on April 6, 2003, in Albuquerque, NM.

From The American Society of PeriAnesthesia Nurses: *A position statement on visitation in phase 1 level of care*, Cherry Hill, NJ, 2011, ASPAN. Reprinted with permission.

SPECIAL CONSIDERATIONS

REFERENCES

1. Spencer BL, Favand LR: Nursing care on the battlefield, *Am Nurse Today* 1:24–26, 2006.
2. Nichols DG, et al: *Golden hour: the handbook of advanced pediatric life support*, ed 3, Philadelphia, 2011, Mosby.
3. Department of Health and Human Services, Centers for Disease Control and Prevention: Surveillance summaries, *Morbidity Mortality Wkly Rep* 59:1–148, 2010.
4. Patel MP, et al: The impact of selected chronic disease on outcomes after trauma: A study from the national trauma bank, *Am J Coll Surg* 212:96–104, 2011.
5. Paulozzi LJ, et al: Recent trends in mortality from unintentional injury in the United States, *J Safety Res* 37: 277–83, 2006.
6. Moore L, et al: Trauma centre outcome performance: a comparison of young adults and geriatric patients in an inclusive trauma system, *Injury*, March 5, 2011 (epub).
7. Chang DC, et al: Undertriage of elderly trauma patients to state-designed trauma centers, *Arch Surg* 243:776–81, 2008.
8. Weigelt JA, et al: Mechanism of injury. In McQuillan KA, et al, editors: *Trauma nursing: from resuscitation through rehabilitation*, ed 4, Philadelphia, 2009, Saunders.
9. Mamaril ME, et al: Care of the orthopaedic trauma patient, *J Perianesth Nurs* 22:184–194, 2007.
10. Emergency Nurses Association: *Trauma nursing core course*, ed 6, Des Plaines, Illinois, 2007, Emergency Nurses Association.
11. American College of Surgeons Committee on Trauma: *Advanced trauma life support for doctors*, ed 8, Chicago, 2008, American College of Surgeons.
12. Von Rueden KT, et al: Shock and multiple organ syndrome. In McQuillan KA, et al, editors: *Trauma nursing: from resuscitation through rehabilitation*, ed 4, Philadelphia, 2009, Saunders.
13. Johnstone RE, et al: Intravenous access. In William CW, et al, editors: *Trauma: emergency resuscitation, perioperative, anesthesia, surgical management, vol. 1*, New York, 2007, Informa Healthcare USA, Inc.
14. DuBose JJ, et al: Clinical experience using 5% hypertonic saline as a safe alternative for use in trauma, *J Trauma, Injury, Infection, and Crit Care* 68:1172–77, 2010.
15. Vencenzi R, et al: Small volume resuscitation with 3% hypertonic saline solution decrease inflammatory response and attenuates end organ damage after controlled hemorrhagic shock, *The Am J of Surgery* 198:407–414, 2009.
16. Scaife ER, Statler KD: Traumatic brain injury: preferred methods and targets for resuscitation, *Surgery* 22:230–245, 2010.
17. Nagele P, et al: Anesthesia and prehospital emergency trauma care. In Miller RD, et al, editors: *Miller's anesthesia*, ed 7, Philadelphia, 2010, Churchill Livingstone.
18. Beekley AC: Damage control resuscitation: a sensible approach to the exsanguinating surgical patient, *Crit Care Med* 36:S267–S274, 2008.
19. Stahel PF, et al: Current trends in resuscitation strategy for the multiply injured patient, *Injury* 4054:S27–S35, 2009.
20. Revell M, et al: Endpoints to fluid resuscitation in hemorrhagic shock, *J Trauma Injury Infect Crit Care* 54:S63–S67, 2003.
21. Bridges E, Biever K: Advancing critical care, *AACN Advanced Critical Care* 21:260–276, 2010.
22. Spinella PC, et al: Warm fresh whole blood is independently associated with improved survival for patients with combat-related injuries, *Journal of Trauma, Injury, Infection, and Critical Care* 66:S69–S75, 2009.
23. Mamaril M: Safety alert: dangerous communication gaps, *Breathline* 26:9, 2006.
24. Smith BP, et al: Review of abdominal control and open abdomen: focus on gastrointestinal complications, *J Gastrointestinal and Liver Diseases* 19:425–435, 2010.
25. Pasero C, McCaffery M: *Pain assessment and pharmacologic management*, St. Louis, 2011, Mosby.
26. Bower TC, Reuter JP: Analgesia, sedation, and neuromuscular blockade in the trauma patient. In McQuillan KA, et al, editors: *Trauma nursing: from resuscitation through rehabilitation*, ed 4, Philadelphia, 2009, Saunders.
27. McGuire JM, Burkhard JF: Risk factors for emergence delirium in U.S. military members, *J Perianesth Nurs* 25:392–401, 2010.
28. Huang YT: Monitoring oxygen delivery in the critically ill, *Chest* 128:554S–560S, 2005.
29. Cottingham CA: Resuscitation of traumatic shock: a hemodynamic review, *AACN Adv Crit Care* 17:317–326, 2006.
30. Scalea TM, Duncan AO: Initial management of the critically ill trauma patient in extremis, *Trauma Q* 10: 3–11, 1993.
31. Alam HB, et al: Combat casualty care research: from bench to battlefield, *World J Surg* 9: S7–S11, 2005.
32. Rice V: Shock, a clinical syndrome: an update: I: an overview of shock, *Crit Care Nurse* 11: 20–27, 1991.
33. Rice V: Shock, a clinical syndrome: an update: IV: nursing care of the shock patient, *Crit Care Nurse* 11:40–51, 1991.
34. Rivers EP, et al: Early and innovative interventions for severe sepsis and septic shock: taking advantage of a window of opportunity, *CMAJ* 173:1–12, 2005.
35. Ozawa K: Energy metabolism. In Cowley RA, Trump BF, editors, *Pathophysiology of shock, anoxia and ischemia*, Baltimore, 1982, Williams & Wilkins.
36. Lee CS: Role of exogenous arginine vasopressin in the management of catecholamine-refractory septic shock, *Crit Care Nurse* 26(6):17–23, 2006.
37. U.S. Department of Health and Human Services: Injury in the United States: 2007. Chartbook, US Department of Health and Human Services, US Government Printing Office: p.49, 2007.
38. Web-based Injury Statistics Query and Reporting System (WISQARS), Centers for Disease Control and Prevention: *Fatal injury reports*, available at www.cdc.gov/injury/wisquars/index.html. Accessed on June 5, 2009.
39. Safe Kids Worldwide: Injury trends fact sheet: trends in accidental injury-related death rates among children, available at www.usa.safekids.org/content_documents/Trends_facts.pdf. Accessed on March 15, 2007.
40. Wilson MH, Levin-Goodman R: Injury prevention and control. In McMillian JA, et al, editors: *Oski's pediatrics principles and practices*, ed 4, Philadelphia, 2006, Lippincott Williams & Wilkins.
41. Mendelson KG, Fallat ME: Pediatric injuries: prevention to resolution, *Surgical Clinics of North America* 87:207–228, 2007.
42. King WK, et al: Child abuse fatalities: Are we missing opportunities for intervention? *Pediatric Emergency Care* 22:211–214, 2006.

43. Karsli C: Airway management. In Mikrogianakis A, et al: *The hospital for sick children manual for pediatric trauma*, Philadelphia, 2008, Lippincott Williams & Wilkins.

44. Schwengal DA, et al: Initial assessment. In Nichols DG, et al: *Golden hour: handbook of advanced pediatric life support*, ed 3, Philadelphia, 2011, Mosby.

45. Schnur M, Mamaril ME: Pediatric patients. In Stannard D, Krenzischek DA: *Perianesthesia nursing care*, Sudbury, Mass, 2011, Jones and Bartlett Learning.

46. Brown HL: Trauma in pregnancy, *Obstetrics & Gynecology* 114:147–160, 2009.

47. Burk Sosa ME: The pregnant trauma patient in the intensive care unit: collaborative care to ensure safety and prevent injury, *J Perinat Neonat Nurs* 22:33–38, 2008.

48. John PR, et al: An assessment of the impact of pregnancy on trauma mortality, *J Surgery* 1016:94–98, 2011.

49. Ruffolo DC: Trauma care and managing the injured pregnant patient, *JOGNN* 38:704–714, 2009.

50. Saunders EE: Screening for domestic violence during pregnancy, *Int J Trauma Nurs* 6:44–47, 2000.

51. Tweddale CJ: Trauma during pregnancy, *Crit Care Nurs Q* 29:53–67, 2006.

52. Ackerson LK, Subramanian SV: Intimate partner violence and death among infants and children in India, *Am J Public Health* 96:1423–1428, 2006.

53. Shah PS, Shah J: Maternal exposure to domestic violence and pregnancy and birth outcomes: a systematic review and meta-analysis, *Journal of Women's Health* 19:2017–2031, 2010.

54. Muench MV, Canterino JC: Trauma in pregnancy, *Obstet Gynecol Clin North Am* 34:555–83, 2007.

55. Hull SB, Bennett S: The pregnant trauma patient: assessment and anesthetic management, *Int Anesthesiology Clinics* 45:1–18, 2007.

56. Criddle LM: Trauma in pregnancy, *AJN* 109:41–47, 2009.

57. El Kady D: Perinatal outcomes of traumatic injuries during pregnancy, *Clin Obstet Gynecol* 50:582–91, 2007.

58. Rudloff U: Trauma in pregnancy, *Arch Gynecol Obstet* 276:101–107, 2007.

59. Shaver SM, Shaver DC: Perioperative assessment of the obstetric patient undergoing abdominal surgery, *J Perianesth Nurs* 20:160–166, 2005.

60. Tsuei BJ: Assessment of the pregnant trauma patient, *Injury* 37:367–373, 2006.

61. American Society of PeriAnesthesia Nurses: *Perianesthesia nursing standards and practice recommendations 2010–2012*, Cherry Hill, NJ, 2010, ASPAN.

55 Care of the Intensive Care Unit Patient in the PACU

Myrna E. Mamaril, MS, RN, CPAN, CAPA, FAAN, and
Mary Beth Flynn Makic, PhD, RN, CNS, CCNS, CCRN

The admission of intensive care unit (ICU) patients to postanesthesia care units (PACUs) is steadily increasing. In addition, the PACU also cares for another type of critically ill surgical patient population: ICU overflow patients, also known as *ICU boarding patients*. This terminology refers to a unique critical care patient population who recovers in the PACU and subsequently meets the PACU discharge criteria. However, these ICU patients are unable to be transferred because of the unavailability of inpatient ICU beds, subsequently they remain in the PACU. This increase reflects a nationwide health care dilemma for emergency department and PACU patients who create a high demand for hospital beds. The American Society of PeriAnesthesia Nurses (ASPAN) Delphi Study identified ICU overflow patients and critical care competencies as the top research clinical, educational, and management priorities.[1] Finally, these national patient safety priorities are strategic for ensuring safe, quality postanesthesia care to ICU patients and to the care environment.

As the science of perianesthesia nursing has evolved and become increasingly more sophisticated, nursing educators, managers, and administrators have realized the importance of an economically sound, evidence-based practice that continuously strives to provide safe quality care to the ICU patient in the PACU. However, recovery of the critically ill postoperative patient in the PACU often poses a myriad of challenges to the postanesthesia nurse and the PACU.

Throughout the United States, divergent postanesthesia practices have existed in the provision of care for the surgical intensive care unit (SICU) patient. Operationally, ICU recovery must occur on a routine basis, regardless of prognosis or acuity in the appropriate care setting. Some PACU care of the postsurgical critical care patient may be sporadic or an exception to the norm. From a clinical and an administrative position, however, the PACU must provide the optimal standard of care to SICU patients.[2] This chapter discusses the historic significance of critical care recovery,

administrative issues in extended ICU care, innovative educational opportunities to ensure competent staff, and clinical strategies in caring for complex, high-acuity, critically ill patients. Because patient safety is essential in providing care to low-volume high-risk patients, complex and highly specialized ICU nursing care concentrates on neurosurgical, burn, and septic management during the postanesthesia period. Ultimately, postanesthesia care must be focused on providing competent care while preventing harm and keeping critically ill patients safe. Finally, when the SICU patient's condition becomes life threatening, family presence during resuscitation is introduced as an end-of-life nursing intervention that promotes patient-family–centered care.

DEFINITIONS

Extended-Stay ICU Patients: Critically ill surgical patients who have recovered from anesthesia but need to stay in the PACU an extended or prolonged period of time because of the severity of illness or the need to be observed for complications.
Family Presence: Families are provided the opportunity to be present in the PACU with their loved one during life-threatening situations or at the end of life during cardiopulmonary resuscitation or codes.
Intensive Care Unit (ICU): A hospital setting where critically ill patients are provided nursing care.
Intensive Care Unit Boarders: Critically ill surgical patients who have recovered from anesthesia in the PACU. These patients have been designated ICU status, but do not have an ICU bed and are boarding in the PACU.
Intensive Care Unit Overflow Patients: Patients who have undergone anesthesia for surgical procedures, have recovered in the PACU, and are awaiting transfer to the ICU or SICU.
Sepsis: A systemic response to infection.
Septic Shock: Sepsis that progresses to a state of inadequate tissue perfusion characterized by persistent hypotension despite adequate fluid resuscitation.
Surgical Intensive Care Unit (SICU): A hospital setting for critically ill surgical patients who need specialized pulmonary, renal, cardiovascular, neurologic, or postoperative monitoring.

Systemic Inflammatory Response Syndrome (SIRS): A systemic response to infection that involves the activation of the inflammatory response to include change in body temperature, elevated heart rate, respiratory rate, and white blood cell count.

HISTORICAL SIGNIFICANCE OF CRITICAL CARE RECOVERY

During the late 1950s and early 1960s, ICUs emerged in hospitals for close monitoring of critically ill patients. Before that time, the critically ill postsurgical patients received care recovery rooms and inpatient wards. Critical care nursing was conceived to provide a setting in which the most acutely ill and injured patients received concentrated nursing care to enhance survival. Fifty years ago, ICUs were composed of a few specialized beds located at the end of or apart from an existing inpatient unit.[3]

Today, the design of the ICU is focused on individual rooms to promote an aesthetic therapeutic environment. The ICU provides patient privacy and is focused on highly technical care that can also be family centered. In comparison, the interior design of the PACU has not changed much in 50 years. It is usually one large room in which individual patient units are separated by curtains.

ADMINISTRATIVE ISSUES

Financial Constraints

The 1990s brought increased financial constraints on hospitals and increased competitiveness among hospitals. The focus in the 1990s on controlling costs led to a dramatic shift in the types of patients who were admitted to hospitals. Only the sickest patients were eligible for admission, and the length of stay was compressed to the shortest possible time.[4] Although hospital population dropped, ICU patient volumes were steadily increasing. Hospital mergers and closings occurred in many cities. During this same time, two significant changes developed: (1) patient acuity of critically ill patients admitted to hospitals increased and (2) the shortage of ICU nurses prompted hospital administrators to close ICU beds. ICU bed closures have had a serious effect on PACUs. PACUs were naturally chosen for critical care overflow because the environment of care included highly technical monitoring and many critical care–educated nursing staff. In addition, the retention of staff in the PACU was much higher with fewer vacancies. This choice seemed

the ideal answer to a complex problem. Consequently, the PACUs were increasingly requested for recovery of SICU patients, and in many hospitals the PACU was designated an ICU overflow unit until an ICU bed became available.

Management Dilemmas

Nurse managers encounter numerous challenges between competing health care providers that relate to patient placement priority for ICU beds. These challenges are affected by decisions of senior administrators (e.g., chief operating officers, chief nursing officers, departmental medical officers of medicine and surgery, emergency or trauma physicians). The dilemmas faced by managers affect ancillary staff, families, patients, and the PACU staff nurses. The PACU manager is obligated to follow hospital policies and protocols. When senior administrators make decisions in the best interest of the hospital to keep the emergency departments and operating rooms open and to perform surgery for elective surgical cases regardless of high hospital population, the PACU becomes the relief valve for medical center admissions. Often the hospitalized patients who occupy beds in the ICU are not ready for transfer to a lower level of care. This gridlock has a domino effect on the PACU beds. Emergency department patients who need critical care may be given priority status for ICU beds, as may "code" call patients from inpatient units. Some ICUs actually hold beds open for potential code call situations. As the inpatient and ICU surgical cases are completed, they too compete for the PACU available beds. Complications arise if the PACU is still holding ICU patients from the day before or from earlier in the morning. Eventually, the operating room (OR) schedule may grind to a halt because of the ensuing gridlocked beds. In some hospitals, the OR continues to perform surgery on critical care patients, with admission of more ICU overflow patients to an already stressed PACU. These SICU patients become known as *boarders, extended stay,* or *ICU overflow.* Patients and families may voice intense dissatisfaction when the PACU is designated for ICU care.[2]

Recovery of the ICU patient who has an extended stay in the PACU may have serious physician repercussions. Anesthesia providers and surgeons become frustrated because they want to complete the elective surgical schedule. At times, their behaviors may strain relationships with the nurse manager. The lost surgical and anesthesia revenue can threaten the viability of the hospital if surgical cases continue to be delayed or cancelled. University hospitals also have graduate medical education and need to perform a required number of surgical or anesthesia cases per year to qualify for accreditation of the programs.

Other challenges encountered by medical staff may be the following issues that place the care of the ICU patient at risk. Medical intensivist management of the SICU patient may be delayed because of the physical location of the PACU or other commitments to patients in the ICU. Confusion may exist regarding whom to contact for medical or surgical problems. Another issue that frequently surfaces is the need to have medical consultations. PACU staff may believe that lack of timely medical care not only increases the stress of the nurse, but ethically affects the professional duty to provide safe timely quality care. Further delays in treatments can critically affect a patient's condition. Finally, the surgeon may become upset with the hospital administration because the order was for the ICU patient to be admitted to the ICU for postoperative care and management.

The physical location of the PACU is always adjacent to the OR; however, the ICU is usually in a different area of the hospital. This situation can create delays in diagnostic care or treatment that otherwise is more expeditious if the patient is in the ICU. For example, respiratory therapy, pulmonary services, blood bank, and the critical care laboratories may be actually located in the ICU. Advanced practice nurses and physician assistants assigned to the ICU may not be available for ICU patients in the PACU. The PACU may have to wait for the hospital's respiratory therapist or laboratory technician to come to the unit. If a computed tomographic scan or magnetic resonance imaging scan is needed, the PACU nurse might not be able to transport the ICU patient in a timely manner because of assigned care of another postanesthesia patient. The ICU patient may need special medications or vasoactive intravenous drips that are not immediately available to the nurse. Ancillary services have a vital role in the care and management of the ICU patient.

ICU patients emerging from anesthetic agents frequently request that their families visit in the PACU. Traditionally, PACUs have been considered large open units in which family visitation is severely limited because of other patients emerging from anesthesia. This type of policy can create intense conflict between the nurse and the family. Family expectations of a private room in which families can visit freely are not met. Furthermore, the family's anxiety increases when the surgeon speaks about the critical nature of the surgery and the need to place the patient in the ICU. Families frequently worry and may perceive the ICU as a sign of impending death, based on past experiences or those of others.[5] Understanding what critical care means to patients and families helps the nurse promote positive coping skills. Depending on the patient's physical condition, effective communication with the ICU patient may be challenging. Barriers to communication can relate to emergence from anesthesia; the patient's physical status; the existence of endotracheal tubes, which inhibit verbal communication; medications; or other conditions that alter cognitive function.[5,6] The critical care patient's anxiety can increase the stress response and further complicate the patient's recovery. Patients may consider that they have a right to see and visit with their family and may find significant emotional support for well-being.

Managing and communicating with the ICU families in the PACU can be challenging. Depending on each patient's diagnosis and acuity, the SICU patient's family may be in crisis. If the patient's condition is critical, the family may exhibit a high degree of stress, anxiety, blame, or other disturbing behaviors. Families may be emotional and act out or exhibit disruptive outbursts. The staff nurse may believe that one's first duty is to provide care to the patient, not to the family. Time can pass quickly for the PACU nurse and not afford the family timely visits. Anxiety and worry mounts for the waiting family as a result of little or no communication and fear of the unknown. The PACU nurse needs to make a conscious effort to effectively communicate with the family in a manner that promotes coping, personal growth, and adaptation to the ICU patient's critical condition (Box 55-1).[7]

STAFFING ISSUES

The PACU nurses may express feelings of inadequacy related to critical care competencies. A PACU nurse may have no ICU nursing experience or outdated critical care experience. The critical care experience may have been generalized and not specific, or new technology may be foreign. Nurse-to-patient ratios may be exceeded for safe care. The PACU nurse may already be assigned one patient with simultaneous care for a newly admitted ICU patient with an unstable condition, and then family members (frequently numerous) want to be present and are upset because visitation is limited or not allowed. PACU nurses may find themselves in the midst of ethical situations that involve conflict between the needs of the ICU patient's family members and the preferences of physicians and other health care providers. Consequently, this PACU environment may be chaotic and not conducive for healing. Visitors may perceive the PACU as a suboptimal

---

BOX 55-1   PACU Nursing Actions for Families in Crisis

- Introduce the PACU Scope of Service.
- Assist the family in defining the SICU problem and condition.
- Aid in identifying sources of support for the family during hospitalization.
- Prepare the family for the PACU care environment, especially the effects of patients emerging from anesthesia, respect for other PACU patients, confidentiality, PACU equipment (e.g., cardiac monitors, ventilators, infusion pumps), and purpose of the equipment.
- Communicate with sincerity and compassion about the critical surgery or illness.
- Avoid false reassurance.
- Express confidence in the family's ability to handle the situation.
- Try to understand the family's perspective about the patient's critical condition.
- Use a "one day at a time" approach and avoid encouraging the family to think of the what-ifs of the patient's long-term outcome.
- Provide opportunities for the patient and family to make choices and feel useful.
- Guide the family in finding therapeutic ways to communicate with the patient.
- Ensure that the family receives information about significant changes in the patient's condition.
- Allow the family the opportunity to call the PACU and speak to the nurse anytime.
- Advocate adjusting visitation hours to accommodate the family's needs.
- Respect the patient's and family's spirituality.

Adapted from Norton C: The family's experience with critical illness. In Morton PG, et al, editors: *Critical care nursing: a holistic approach*, ed 8, Philadelphia, 2005, Lippincott Williams & Wilkins.
PACU, Postanesthesia care unit; *SICU,* surgical intensive care unit.

---

environment for a loved one. When PACU nursing staff members perceive that safe patient care is becoming jeopardized or high risk, they should consult the nurse manager immediately.

As the nursing shortage in the United States has become more severe, placing ICU overflow patients in the PACU has become a standard of practice rather than being a series of isolated incidents.[8] Reports from PACU nurses in different regions of the country have communicated unsafe practices. Postanesthesia nurses turned to their professional organization, the American Society of PeriAnesthesia Nurses (ASPAN), to voice their concerns about serious issues that affected the care they provided to recovering ICU patients in the PACU. The ASPAN Standards and Guidelines Committee conducted a special review of

the evidence to identify current nursing practice issues. The following trends in the care of ICU patients in the PACU were identified:

1. Staffing requirements identified for phase I PACUs may be exceeded during times when PACUs are used for ICU overflow patients.[2,6]
2. The PACU Phase I nurse may be required to provide care to a surgical or nonsurgical ICU patient who has not been properly trained or has not had the required care competencies validated.[2,6]
3. Phase I PACUs may not be able to receive patients normally admitted from the operating room when staff is used to care for the ICU overflow patients.[2,6]
4. When the need to send ICU overflow patients to PACU Phase I does not occur regularly, both the PACU and the hospital management may not be properly prepared to handle the admission and discharge of PACU Phase I and ICU patients.[2,6]

ASPAN invited the American Association of Critical Care Nurses (AACN) and the American Society of Anesthesiologists to address the practice trend of caring for the ICU overflow patient in the PACU and to strategize to promote safe quality care regardless of where the SICU patient recovers from anesthesia. A collaborative position statement was promulgated by these three powerful specialty organizations (Box 55-2).[2]

Critical Care Educational Competencies

The postanesthesia nurse must have in-depth knowledge of anesthesia agents, normal physiology, pathophysiology, and current surgical management to plan appropriate nursing interventions and to care for the postanesthesia patient. Depending on the PACU nurse's critical care experience, competencies, skills, and available medical and nursing resources, the care and management may prove to be frustrating or threatening. However, one should remember that the PACU nurse is recognized for possessing critical care competencies and skills when caring for the vulnerable patient recovering from anesthesia and surgery. Likewise, the challenge of caring for the complex SICU patient can be a rewarding opportunity to use one's critical thinking skills in making a difference in the outcome of the critically ill patient.

Orientation and Basic Critical Care Competencies

The first steps in planning an orientation to the PACU is the interview process and subsequent hiring of the nurse who is motivated to learn

BOX 55-2   Joint Statement on ICU Overflow

ISSUE

A phase I postanesthesia care unit (PACU) is a critical care area that provides postanesthesia nursing care for patients immediately after operative and invasive procedures before discharge to the phase II ambulatory setting, the inpatient surgical unit, or the intensive care unit.

Perianesthesia nurses have identified concerns regarding the increasing use of the phase I PACU for the care of surgical and nonsurgical ICU patients when ICU beds are not available in the facility.

PURPOSE

As professional societies involved in the provision of care for operative and invasive procedures and critically ill patients, the American Society of PeriAnesthesia Nurses (ASPAN), the American Association of Critical-Care Nurses (AACN), and the American Society of Anesthesiologists (ASA) collaborated to develop criteria for the purposes of maintaining quality care in the PACU, ensuring quality care for the intensive care unit patient, and promoting the safe practice of perianesthesia nursing and critical care nursing.

ASPAN exists to promote quality and cost-effective care for patients, their families, and the community through public and professional education, research, and standards of practice. ASPAN has the responsibility for defining the practice of perianesthesia nursing. An integral part of this responsibility involves identifying the educational requirements and competencies essential to perianesthesia practice and recommending acceptable staffing requirements for the perianesthesia environment.

AACN was established to provide the highest quality resources to maximize nurse contributions to care for critically ill patients and their families. AACN provides and inspires leadership to develop standards and guidelines that establish work and care environments that are respectful, healing, and humane.

ASA was established to raise and maintain the standard of the medical practice of anesthesiology and improve the care of the patient during anesthesia and recovery and is involved in the provision of critical care medicine in the intensive care unit.

BACKGROUND

In response to concerns expressed by perianesthesia nurses around the country, the ASPAN Standards and Guidelines Committee conducted a review of current literature and perianesthesia nursing practice to identify issues related to the care of critically ill surgical and nonsurgical patients in Phase I PACUs during

times when all other ICU beds are full. The review identified the following trends:

1. Staffing requirements identified for phase I PACUs may be exceeded during times when PACUs are being used for ICU overflow patients.
2. The Phase I PACU nurse may be required to provide care to a surgical or nonsurgical ICU patient that the nurse has not been properly trained to care for or for which the nurse has not had the required care competencies validated.
3. Phase I PACUs may be unable to receive patients normally admitted from the operating room when staff is being used to care for ICU overflow patients.
4. Because the need to send overflow patients to the Phase I PACU does not occur regularly, both the PACU and the hospital management may not be properly prepared to deal with the admission and discharge of Phase I PACU and ICU patients.

STATEMENT

Therefore, when admission of ICU overflow patients or prolonging the stay of the surgical ICU patient in the Phase I PACU is necessary, ASPAN, AACN, and ASA recommend that the following criteria be met:

1. The primary responsibility for Phase I PACU is to provide the optimal standard of care to the postanesthesia patient and to effectively maintain the flow of the surgery schedule.
2. Appropriate staffing requirements should be met to maintain safe competent nursing care of the postanesthesia patient and the ICU patient. Staffing criteria for the ICU patient should be consistent with ICU guidelines based on individual patient acuity and needs.
3. Phase I PACUs are by their nature critical care units, and as such, staff should meet the competencies required for the care of the critically ill patient. These competencies should include, but are not limited to, ventilator management, hemodynamic monitoring, and medication administration, as appropriate to the patient population.
4. Management should develop and implement a comprehensive resource utilization plan with ongoing assessment that supports the staffing needs for both the PACU and ICU patients when the need for overflow admission arises.
5. Management should have a multidisciplinary plan to address appropriate utilization of the ICU beds. Admission and discharge criteria should be used to evaluate the necessity for critical care and to determine the priority for admissions.

EXPECTED ACTIONS

ASPAN, AACN, and the ASA committees (Anesthesia Care Team, Critical Care Medicine, and Trauma Medicine) recognize the complexity of caring for patients in a dynamic health care environment where reduced

---

BOX 55-2   Joint Statement on ICU Overflow—cont'd

availability of resources and expanding roles for the registered nurse has an impact on patient care. Thus, we encourage all members to actively pursue the education and development of competencies required for the care of the critically ill patient in the perianesthesia environment. We also encourage members to actively identify

strategies for collaboration and problem solving to address complex staffing issues.

This information and position is to be shared with all individuals, organizations, and institutions involved in the care of the critically ill patient in the perianesthesia environment.

From ASPAN, AACN and ASA's Anesthesia Care Team Committee and Committee on Critical Care Medicine and Trauma Medicine: A joint position statement on ICU overflow patients, September 1999, in ASPAN: Perianesthesia nursing standards and practice recommendations 2010-2012, Cherry Hill, NJ, 2010, ASPAN.

many new skills. In addition, the nurse who seeks to be professionally challenged on a daily basis inspires and motivates the critical care preceptor. The PACU should never be viewed as a place to wind down or retire, because nurses with that goal in mind are often immediately disappointed and dissatisfied with their new jobs. Many PACUs prefer to hire nurses with critical care experience. Medical-surgical nurses are also hired, provided that an adequate support system of nursing education exists during orientation and the length of orientation is such that the nurse without prior critical care experience has ample time to master the myriad new skills essential to the new role.

Orientation to the PACU must focus on anesthesia and complications related to anesthetic agents, comorbidities, and surgery, because this subject area encompasses almost the entire patient population in the PACU. But what about the critical care patient? All patients who arrive in the PACU, regardless of invasive lines and mechanical ventilation, must be viewed as having the potential to be a critically ill patient. Even a patient who has had a hernia repair or an appendectomy can become gravely ill. In addition to this fact is the matter of the critically ill patient who arrives in the PACU before the final destination of the ICU. Orientation and education must also focus on the following essentials:

- Cardiac monitoring, rhythm interpretation, electrocardiogram interpretation
- Airway management
  - Bag-mask management
  - Nasal and oral airways
  - Endotracheal tubes
  - Laryngeal mask airways
- Arterial blood gas interpretation
- Mechanical ventilation
  - Modes
  - Appropriate tidal volumes
  - Concept of positive end-expiratory pressure and pressure support

- Adequate rate and methods of delivery
- Assessment of adequate endotracheal tube placement
- Adequate securing of endotracheal tubes per nursing policy
- Invasive monitoring equipment—the care and the assessment of the patient with:
  - Arterial lines
    - Radial
    - Brachial
    - Femoral
  - Central lines
    - Basic multiple lumen
    - Advanced venous access devices (AVA)
  - Pulmonary artery (PA) catheters
    - Assessment of correct placement
    - Ability to perform cardiac outputs
    - Interpretation of cardiac output, cardiac index, stroke volume, systemic vascular resistance, left ventricular stroke work index
    - Titration of medications based on previous values
  - Intracranial access (intracranial pressure [ICP])
    - Drainage
    - Monitoring
  - Pharmacology
    - Anesthetic agents
    - Vasopressors
  - Neurology
    - Neurologic assessments
    - ICP monitoring, cerebral perfusion pressures

Orientation should include the essentials of how to care for the patient who has all or some of the invasive monitoring equipment mentioned previously and how to assemble such equipment in preparation for insertion in the PACU. The PACU should have the necessary equipment readily available in the event that a patient's condition worsens and invasive procedures are to be performed in the PACU.

The main challenge in orienting the newly hired nurse to the critical care element of the PACU is access to these patients. A day in the operating room with an anesthesia provider who inserts a PA catheter and manages a critically ill patient, such as with a cardiac bypass case, can be helpful. An immersion in the ICU is another option, with the PACU registered nurse (RN) spending 1 week or more in the ICU shadowing an ICU nurse. A cardiothoracic ICU is ideal because this type of ICU admits patients frequently, similar to the PACU, and the orientee can learn the tasks of detangling lines, managing the newly ventilated patient, weaning the patient, initiating and titrating vasopressor medications, and other needed skills. The leadership team of the PACU should closely collaborate with the leadership team of the ICU to ensure that the PACU RN has an orientation that is similar or identical to the orientation of the new nurse in the ICU. If the ICU educator or clinical nurse specialist is providing education for the ICU staff members, the PACU RNs should be encouraged to attend as well. Some ICUs use the online orientation program sponsored by the AACN. This program is called *Essentials of Critical Care Orientation,* which is a computer-based standardized orientation of critical care nursing. If the ICUs in the facility use this type of orientation program, the PACU nurse might be helped by using it as well. If the ICU orientation consists of critical care courses, then the PACU trainee should attend as well, after the essentials of perianesthesia nursing and PACU core competencies have been mastered.

But what about the experienced PACU nurse who is suddenly confronted with the increasing volume of critical care patients? Collaboration with the ICU leadership team is helpful, with the possible outcome of an opportunity to shadow an ICU nurse for 1 week or more to learn the basic care and management of the patient with both mechanical ventilation and invasive monitoring equipment that requires vasopressor support.

A competency-based orientation checklist should be completed for the new nurse and the experienced PACU RN who receives any education in critical care. The PACU leadership team must develop a standardized educational process with the requisite paper trail to safeguard the PACU RN, the hospital, and the PACU leadership team in the event of an untoward outcome.

In addition, if the facility sponsors an annual skills fair day, the PACU RN should complete or show similar competencies to the ICU RN, based on the patient population that the PACU cares for, even if that critical care population is rare. The care of a patient who is high risk and low volume is the most challenging for the RN.

The PACU RN should also be expected to complete the same annual competence assessment that is required of the ICU nurses. For example, if a dysrhythmia competency is developed for the ICU RN, the PACU RN should also be expected to complete it, and documentation of completion should be placed in the education folder.

Advanced Critical Care Concepts

Understanding key advanced critical care concepts assists the PACU nurse in refining critical decision-making skills. The ICU patient who remains in the PACU for an extended period of time poses an enormous challenge in many aspects. Both the nursing and physician management of these patients can be difficult. The standards of care that are developed by the ICU and the facility and that are in place in the ICU should be readily available and implemented in the PACU. These standards include:
- Frequency of line and tubing changes
- Frequency of endotracheal tube rotation
- Frequency of ICP and cerebral perfusion pressure (CPP) measurements
- Frequency of measurements (e.g., cardiac outputs and indexes)
- Frequency of weighing the patient
- Frequency of chest radiographs, electrocardiograms, and laboratory studies
- Use of a continuous cardiac output type of PA catheter
- Use of warming devices for intravenous fluids or blood products
- Use of rapid infusers
- Frequency of, and ability to perform and manage, the calculation of oxygen consumption, oxygen demand, oxygen extraction ratios, and other elements of oxyhemodynamic calculations ("oxy-calcs")
- Various modes of mechanical ventilation, including pressure-controlled ventilation
- Use of and care of the patient with continuous infusions of muscle relaxants and twitch monitors
- Competency with protocols in the prevention of ventilatory-acquired pneumonia
- Competency/knowledge of protocols in the prevention of deep vein thrombosis

Creating a Specialized Critical Care Resource for the PACU

Many PACUs across the country care for ICU patients sporadically. This situation occurs when the hospital census is high or when a surgical emergency presents. Specialized critical care educational resources strategically provide the PACU nurse with expert advisors when the critical time arises. This resourceful method can be accomplished in several ways. First, the PACU can recruit expertise from the unit. Second, the nurse manager may elect to request key leadership staff to orient and become competent and proficient in managing the care of specific patient populations.

Another innovative concept to achieving critical resources is cross training the PACU staff to the ICU and critical care nurses to the PACU. When the PACU admits a highly complex high-acuity SICU case and the primary nurse does not possess the knowledge or skill to provide care, an opportunity may exist to exchange nurses rather than patients to appropriately match the patient severity with the nurse's knowledge and competencies.

CLINICAL STRATEGIES FOR THE COMPLEX ICU PATIENT

The PACU nurses are required to use critical decision-making skills in daily practice. Advanced life support competencies are mandated for PACU nurses who care for all vulnerable patients who are emerging from surgery and anesthesia. The foundation of PACU and critical care nursing is an understanding of anesthesia agents and human physiology that guides the postanesthesia nursing assessments and interventions. Foremost, the PACU nurses must ensure that adequate oxygenation, ventilation, transport, and perfusion in the patient occur, regardless of unit: the ICU or the PACU. Impairment in oxygen delivery and utilization at the tissue level leads to global tissue hypoxia. Fundamental to recognition and treatment of global tissue hypoxia is knowledge of the principles of oxygenation, ventilation, transport, and perfusion and their etiologies and how they relate to postanesthesia care. The major differences lie in the complex pathophysiologic disease processes that occur in these critically ill patients. The following section discusses the pathophysiology and clinical strategies in management of the care for three highly specialized high-acuity low-volume populations: the neurosurgical, burn, and septic ICU patients.

COMPLEX SPECIALIZED CRITICAL CARE IN THE PACU

Postoperative Care of the Neurosurgical ICU Patient

The reasons for neurosurgical interventions are numerous. Some of the most common neurosurgical procedures that require intensive care monitoring after surgery include aneurysm clipping or coiling, tumor removal or debulking, lobectomy for seizure management, and cranial surgeries to manage increased ICP. The care of the patient who has had a neurosurgical procedure requires an understanding of the goals for the surgical procedure and continuous focused assessment for the presence of subtle neurologic changes in the patient after surgery. Specifically, the nurse should know: (1) the type of surgical procedure the patient underwent, (2) the length of the operative procedure and any known complications during the surgery, (3) the specific region of the brain in which the operation was performed, (4) the preoperative neurologic examination results to allow comparison with postoperative neurologic assessment results, and (5) the neurologic injury that is considered the primary insult and the negative effects of hypoxemia, hypotension, poor cerebral perfusion, hyperglycemia, hypocapnia, and cerebral edema that are responsible for secondary insults to the brain and further compromise to the patient's recovery.[8-11] Primary goals in the immediate phase of perioperative care of the patient focus on preserving cerebral blood flow through blood pressure management, optimizing tissue oxygenation, maintaining normothermia, and effectively treating cerebral edema.

Brief Review of Intracranial Pressure

One of the greatest risks after surgery is increased ICP. Nurses who provide care to neurosurgical patients must be familiar with the pathophysiology of cerebral edema and interventions to attempt to minimize the negative effects of prolonged increased ICP. Cerebral insult of a variety of mechanisms causes chaos inside the cranial vault.[8,11] Edema and increased ICP are frequently a consequence of injury.

Intracranial pressure is the pressure normally exerted by cerebrospinal fluid (CSF) that circulates around the brain and spinal cord and within the cerebral ventricles.[11] Normal ICP is 0 to 10 mm Hg; however, 15 mm Hg is often considered the high end of the normal range.[8,11] The cranial vault contains three primary elements: brain tissue (80%), CSF (10%), and blood (10%). The Monro-Kellie hypothesis treats the cranial vault as a closed compartment; therefore, if one of these three components increases, reciprocal changes in the other two components must occur to maintain normal ICP.[8,11] For example, if brain tissue swells, CSF production is decreased or displaced into the basal subarachnoid cisterns, and the cerebral vasculature constricts to compensate for brain tissue edema.[11] *Compliance* refers to the ability of these compensatory mechanisms to

SPECIAL CONSIDERATIONS

attempt to maintain a steady relationship between volume and pressure within the cranial vault.[11] Displacement of CSF and vasoconstriction, howeve is limited and when the limit is reached, ICP increases.

Intracranial pressure can be measured with an intraparenchymal catheter bolt or a ventriculostomy (also called an *external ventricular drain* [EVD]). Both devises are surgically placed with sterile technique and should be transduced to a monitor to allow assessment of the ICP waveform. The intraparenchymal catheter displays a continuous ICP reading in addition to the ICP waveform. The ventriculostomy can be used to monitor ICP and evacuate CSF. The pulse wave arises primarily from arterial pulsations and to a lesser degree from the respiratory cycle.[11] Assessment of the ICP waveform provides valuable clinical information regarding cerebral compliance. The ICP waveform has three peaks known as P_1, P_2, and P_3 (Fig. 55-1). P_1 is the percussion wave and originates from pulsations of the arteries and choroid plexus; P_2 is the tidal wave and terminates in the dicrotic notch; and P_3 is the dicrotic wave, which immediately follows the dicrotic notch.[11] The P_2 wave is a reflection of intracerebral compliance; a

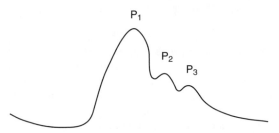

FIG. 55-1 Normal intracranial pressure wave form. (From McQuillan KA, et al: *Trauma nursing: from resuscitation through rehabilitation*, ed 4, St. Louis, 2009, Saunders.)

rise in ICP is reflected by a progressive rise in P_2 and a concomitant rise in ICP numeric reading on the monitor (Fig. 55-2).[11] Analysis of the ICP waveform along with the ICP value and neurologic assessment are used to determine interventions to reduce ICP.

Cerebral edema increases the pressure within the cranial vault, adversely increasing ICP. Cerebral edema may be vasogenic edema, cytotoxic edema, or interstitial edema. Vasogenic edema is an extracellular edema from increased capillary permeability and can develop around tumors or abscesses or with cerebral trauma.[11] Vasogenic edema can be treated with osmotic diuretics or, if the cause is tumors, corticosteroids are usually effective.[11] Cytotoxic edema occurs during states of poor cerebral perfusion, hypoxia, or anoxic states that cause diffuse cerebral edema. Osmotic diuretics or hypertonic saline solution may be beneficial in treating acute states of cytotoxic edema.[10] Interstitial edema occurs with hydrocephalus, and the primary acute intervention is the removal of CSF though an EVD until the condition corrects itself or a surgical shunt is placed.[11]

CSF is a clear colorless fluid that fills the ventricles of the brain and subarachnoid spaces of the brain and spinal cord. Most CSF is produced by the choroids plexus, which are located in the third and fourth ventricles of the brain. CSF is constantly produced at a rate or approximately 25 mL/h or 500 mL/day.[11] When the pressure within the brain exceeds 15 mm Hg, CSF production may slow or the brain displaces CSF to accommodate increases in brain tissue edema. Additional interventions may be the active removal of CSF through an EVD when the ICP exceeds a certain ICP parameter.

Cerebral blood flow (CBF) is the third component of intracranial pressure dynamics. The brain receives approximately 20% of the cardiac

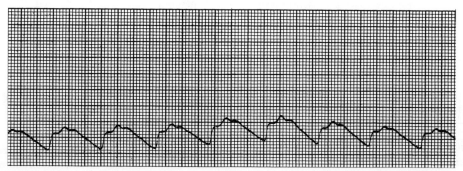

FIG. 55-2 Abnormal intracranial pressure wave form. P_2 is higher than P_3, which is indication of poor cerebral compliance. (From McQuillan KA, et al: *Trauma nursing: from resuscitation through rehabilitation*, ed 4, St. Louis, 2009, Saunders.)

output and consumes 20% of the body's oxygen and 25% of the body's glucose.[8,11,12] When pressures within the cranial vault increase beyond normal ranges, the heart has more difficulty delivering nutrients to the brain. Factors that decrease cardiac output and function, increased blood viscosity, and hypotensive states significantly compromise effective cerebral blood flow. Cerebral vasculature is also influenced by changes in carbon dioxide levels in the blood. High levels of carbon dioxide (i.e., $PaCO_2$) cause cerebral vasculature dilation and increase blood flow, and decreased levels of $PaCO_2$ cause vasoconstriction of cerebral vasculature and decrease blood flow. However, reduction of $PaCO_2$ to less than 35 mm Hg reduces blood flow to the brain tissue and may exacerbate cerebral ischemia, further increasing ICP.[10,11] During states of elevated ICP, $PaCO_2$ may be artificially lowered through mechanical ventilation settings that cause hyperventilation to induce cerebral vasoconstriction. However, caution to avoid hyperventilation that lowers $PaCO_2$ less than 35 mm Hg is warranted to avoid worsening cerebral ischemia causing a secondary cerebral insult.

Autoregulation refers to the ability of the brain to maintain a constant CBF despite changes in the arterial perfusion pressure (systemic circulation). Autoregulation is a protective homeostatic mechanism of the brain that attempts to keep cerebral perfusion constant and generally continues to maintain CBF until the ICP exceeds 40 mm Hg.[11] Autoregulation provides a constant CBF flow by adjusting the diameter of blood vessels based on changes in the intracerebral pressure. It works synergistically with other protective mechanisms of the brain (e.g., reducing $PaCO_2$ and displacing CSF) to maintain CBF. Autoregulation, however, is limited as a compensatory mechanism. A critical point can be reached because of sustained increases in ICP, global or local diffuse injury, cerebral edema, ischemia, or inflammation.[11] If autoregulation is lost, reduced cerebrovascular tone occurs and the CBF becomes dependent on changes in systemic blood pressure. Therefore, a primary goal in management of ICP is effective treatment of the cause of the increase in ICP so that autoregulation is maintained as a compensatory mechanism of CBF.

CPP is a parameter that is calculated from the mean arterial pressure (MAP) minus the ICP and is an indicator of general cerebral perfusion and CBF. Cerebral perfusion pressure becomes increasingly important when the patient loses autoregulatory homeostasis because of sustained increases in ICP. The minimal CPP necessary to maintain adequate perfusion is 50 to 70 mm Hg.[11-15] The optimal CPP remains an area of great controversy, and the mechanism of cerebral injury may influence ideal CPP for brain tissue perfusion. Patients with traumatic brain injury may tolerate a CPP of 50 to 70 mm Hg; however, patients with other etiologies (e.g., cerebral hemorrhage) may require a higher CPP threshold.[11-15] Because CPP is dependent on MAP, interventions to increase MAP may be necessary if ICP cannot be lowered to maintain effective cerebral perfusion during states of increased ICP. Vasoactive agents to support cardiac output and blood pressure are frequently administered to increase CPP to meet cerebral perfusion demands.

Newer technology can be introduced invasively into the brain and cerebral vasculature to measure brain tissue oxygenation ($PtbO_2$). A brain tissue oxygen probe can be inserted through an intracranial bolt or tunneled and provides information that reflects brain tissue oxygenation associated with cerebral oxygen demand and systematic oxygen delivery.[16] A catheter can also be placed in the jugular vein to measure jugular venous oxygen saturation ($Sjvo_2$), which reflects cerebral oxygen demands.[17] Neuromonitoring with microdialysis catheters can be used to identify clinical events that precede clinical examination changes.[18] A cerebral microdialysis catheter can be inserted through an intracranial bolt and allows sampling of cerebral substances within the interstitial fluid to evaluate the brain metabolism markers (e.g., glucose, lactate, pyruvate, glutamate, glycerol). Evaluation of these markers along with clinical assessment can assist with interventions to prevent secondary brain tissue injury from elevated ICP.[18,19]

Transient increases in ICP are dynamic temporary increases in ICP. Transient increases in ICP can be caused by coughing, pain, or excessive stimulation. Transient increases in ICP are associated with cerebral hypoxemic and ineffective cerebral perfusion states.[11] Signs and symptoms of transient increases in ICP of more than 15 mm Hg include headache, aphasia, changes in respiratory pattern (e.g., Cheyne-Stokes), changes in vital signs, decreases or changes in level of consciousness, motor dysfunction (e.g., hemiparesis), visual disturbances, and nausea and vomiting.[11] In addition, sudden diuresis may indicate a dysregulation of antidiuretic hormone related to ICP.

Consequences of increased ICP can be more devastating than the initial neurologic insult.[8,11] Nursing interventions need to focus on assessing risk factors for increases in ICP and implementing and monitoring the effects of interventions to reduce sustained increases in ICP.

SPECIAL CONSIDERATIONS

Postanesthesia Management of the Neurosurgical Patient

Postanesthesia management of the intensive care neurosurgical patient focuses on minimization of increases in ICP and continuous assessment of neurologic status. The goal of nursing care is to minimize secondary insults that are a consequence of ICP. A focused neurologic assessment to include level of arousal, orientation, and motor skills, and a cranial nerve examination should be completed hourly for up to 12 hours or longer depending on the nature of the neurosurgical procedure. The nurse needs to assess for subtle changes in the neurologic assessment rather than looking for gross deviations from normal. Knowledge of the patient's neurologic assessment before surgery is important in establishing a baseline from which to base the immediate postoperative neurologic assessment. Another important variable in neurologic assessment is the nurse. Nurses should validate abnormal findings with each other because subtle changes may be hard to assess. Nurses should also perform a neurologic assessment with each change of shift to ensure maximized consistency in the assessment of the neurosurgical patient. Basic assessments of cerebral dressings after surgery with observation for bleeding or presence of CSF fluid leakage are also part of the immediate perianesthesia nursing assessment. If the neurosurgical procedure was related to spinal pathology, the nursing assessment focuses on motor and sensory function of the patient. Management or prevention of edema and maintenance of body alignment remain the nursing priorities in the immediate postanesthesia period.

Monitoring of ICP, documentation and assessment of the ICP waveform at set intervals, and correlation of the neurologic assessment during elevations in ICP are important nursing assessment interventions. Immediate interventions to reduce ICP include elevating the head of the bed 30 degrees[8,20] and maintaining a neutral neck alignment. If noxious stimuli, environmental stimuli, or nursing activities are the cause of increase in ICP, limiting of noxious events such as venipuncture, suctioning, and nursing cares should be considered.

Maximization of oxygenation and ventilation is an important intervention in the care of neurosurgical patients. Interventions to maximize oxygenation to achieve a PaO_2 greater than 60 mm Hg and normal $PaCO_2$ are important to ensure that cerebral oxygen demands are met and cerebral vasoconstriction from hypocarbia is minimized.

Maintenance of an effective blood pressure and cardiac output to meet cerebral perfusion needs also is a primary nursing intervention.

Medications to lower or raise blood pressure to optimize CPP are ordered for the neurosurgical patient. Immediately after surgery, the physician may want the blood pressure lower to minimize bleeding. If the neurologic examination becomes compromised when the blood pressure is lower, the nurse should notify the physician because this may be an indication of ineffective cerebral perfusion. Depending on the neurologic insult, the nurse either administers medications to lower the patient's blood pressure to prevent further intracerebral bleeding or administers medications to increase the patient's blood pressure to maximize cerebral perfusion and manage cerebral edema. Knowledge of the patient's pathology, neurosurgical procedure, and the neurologic examination results is a crucial assessment variable to help determine optimal blood pressure parameters.

Management of pain and sedation is an important nursing intervention during the perianesthesia care of the neurosurgical patient. Short-acting analgesics and sedation agents should be used to allow continued assessment of the patient's neurologic status. Maintaining normothermia or inducing mild hypothermia (core temperature, 33° to 36° C) has been found to be neuroprotective in patients with cerebral injury.[21] For every decrease in temperature below normal, brain metabolism decreases by 7% to 10%.[11,21] Body temperature can be maintained or lowered with conventional air sources, ice, cooling blankets, or intravascular devices. Regardless of the method used to maintain normothermia or mild hypothermia, interventions should not induce shivering. Shivering can adversely increase metabolic demand and oxygen consumption needs beyond the benefits of lowering the patient's body temperature.

The research on the negative effects of hyperglycemia in critical illness continues to mount. Whereas hyperglycemia can cause adverse patient outcomes, rigorous insulin regimens to maintain tight control of serum glucose can result in hypoglycemia; even transient hypoglycemia can have detrimental effects on patient outcome.[22,23,24] Current guidelines recommend a slightly higher serum glucose during critical illness (140 to 180 mg/dL) as studies have that found attempts for tighter glucose control (e.g., 80 to 110 mg/dL) resulted in transient hypoglycemic events.[24] Critical illness increases the secretion of counterregulatory hormones, such as glucagon, epinephrine, norepinephrine, and growth hormone; it also results in an increase in hepatic glucose production, decrease in peripheral glucose uptake, and induction of a hyperglycemic state. The hyperglycemia of critical illness is initially an adaptive response to stress; however, over time it exacerbates the circulation of abnormal inflammatory mediators and worsens states of tissue ischemia.[23] Glucose is a primary substrate for energy in the brain, and states of both hypoglycemia and hyperglycemia have been found to worsen cerebral perfusion.[22] Therefore efforts to maintain normoglycemic states (serum glucose, 110 to 180 mg/dL) by administering intravenous insulin either intermittently or via continuous infusion are indicated in the management of the critically ill neurosurgical patient.[22]

Care of the critically ill neurosurgical patient after surgical interventions requires that the nurse have a working knowledge of neuroanatomy, the surgical procedure, and monitoring of the patient for subtle changes in neurologic assessment and neurologic hemodynamics. Assessment of subtle changes in the neurologic assessment and correlation of changes to vital sign parameters and neuro-hemodynamics are essential in the treatment of critically ill neuroscience patients. Simple nursing interventions such as maintaining neutral head alignment, preventing shivering, and maintaining the head of the bed at more than 30 degrees are effective first-line interventions in the treatment of patients with altered ICP. Other interventions focus on maximization of oxygenation, cardiac output, blood pressure, and prevention of infection. Technical knowledge related to ICP monitoring and ventriculostomy management is necessary to effectively monitor and treat changes in ICP. Finally, involving the family and ensuring that they understand goals of care and interventions are important so that family-centered care is maximized throughout the patient's acute illness and recovery phase.

Postoperative Care of the ICU Burn Trauma Patient

Unintentional deaths from fire and burns are estimated at 3000 deaths from residential fires and 500 from other sources, including motor vehicle and aircraft crashes and contact with electricity, chemicals, or hot liquids.[25] An estimated 75% of these deaths occur at the scene or during initial transport.[25] Approximately 450,000 burn injuries require medical attention; 45,000 of these individuals need hospitalization.[25] A small percentage of burn-injured patients do not survive (approximately 6%); these patients have associated inhalation injury.[26] However, in the face of these sobering facts, the overall mortality and morbidity rates from burn injury have declined over the years because of advances in burn prevention strategies and medical interventions for this patient population. Elements that have been attributed to patient survival include more rapid response by emergency teams, efficiencies in transport to burn treatment facilities, advances in fluid resuscitation, improvements in

wound coverage, better support of the hypermetabolic response to injury, advances in infection control practices, and improved treatment of inhalation injuries.[27,28]

Patients with burn injury have special needs throughout hospitalization. The American Burn Association (ABA) has established guidelines to determine which burn-injured patients should be transferred to a specialized burn center to maximize treatment and decrease patient morbidity and mortality (Box 55-3).[29] Patients who meet the criteria outlined by the ABA should be transported to the nearest burn center to maximize patient survival and functional outcome.

Brief Review of Burn Injury Pathophysiology

Burn tissue injury is associated with the coagulation of cellular protein caused by exposure or contact with heat produced by thermal, electric, chemical, or radiation energy. The depth of co-agulative tissue necrosis (depth of burn wound) depends on the intensity of the heat and length of time the tissues are exposed to the heat source. Thermal injury from flame, steam, scald, and contact with hot objects is the most frequent cause of burn injury. Inhalation injury is frequently associated with thermal injury when the victim is trapped in an enclosed space during the fire. Electric injury occurs when electric energy is converted into heat and causes tissue destruction as the current flows through the body. Electric current travels through the body along a path of least resistance, such as nerves, blood vessels, and

---

BOX 55-3	Criteria for Burn Center Transfer and Referral

- Partial-thickness burns of greater than 10% total body surface area
- Burns that involve the face, hands, feet, genitalia, perineum, or major joints
- Third-degree burns in any age group
- Electrical burns, including lightning injury
- Inhalation injury
- Burn injury in patients with preexisting medical disorders that could complicate management, prolong recovery or affect mortality.
- Any patients with burns and concomitant trauma
- Burned children in hospitals without qualified personnel or equipment for the care of children
- Burn injury in patients who will require special social, emotional, or rehabilitative intervention

From American Burn Association: From Committee on Trauma: Guidelines for the operation of burn centers, resources for optimal care of the injured patient (excerpted), Chicago, 2006, American College of Surgeons, available at www.ameriburn.org/BurnCenterReferralCriteria.pdf. Accessed May 20, 2011.

muscles, sparing the skin except at the entry and exit points of the current resulting in deep internal tissue damage.[27,28] Chemical injuries from either acidic or alkaline agents cause tissue destruction related to the type, strength, and duration of contact. Radiation burns are infrequent and usually are the result of medical radiation treatments or industrial accidents.

Regardless of what caused the burn injury, the tissue damage can be conceptualized as having three zones that represent the depth of tissue coagulation. Full-thickness burn is the deepest tissue injury in which full coagulation of the tissue proteins has occurred and causes irreversible tissue necrosis. Immediately surrounding the necrotic tissue area is the region or zone of stasis in which blood flow is impaired.[27,28] This region is considered a critical area because it can progress to tissue necrosis if tissue perfusion is inadequate during the burn fluid resuscitation period, which creates a larger burn wound injury. The outer zone of hyperemia has sustained minimal tissue injury and usually heals rapidly. Early goals of burn management focus on stopping the burning process and providing adequate fluid resuscitation to prevent the extension of burn injury from lack of perfusion.

When burn injury occurs, myriad local mediators are released by the body in response to the tissue insult. These mediators—such as histamine, serotonin, prostaglandins, thromboxane A_2, kinins, oxygen radicals, platelet aggregation factor, complement cytokines, interleukins, and catecholamines—cause arteriolar and venules dilation, increased microvascular permeability, and decreased perfusion.[28,30,31] Proteins leak from the intravascular space into the extravascular space and increase tissue oncotic pressure, creating edema.[31] Thromboxane A_2, a mediator that causes vasoconstriction, is also released by the body and may compromise perfusion to the burn injury area and cause extension of the depth of burn tissue injury.[28,31] Concurrently, the coagulation system is activated, which causes platelet aggregation and activation of polymorphonuclear neutrophil leukocytes and macrophages, which are essential to wound healing. The summation of the activation of the body's intense inflammatory response is vascular stasis and rapid formation of tissue edema. Edema places the patient at risk of developing intraabdominal hypertension (IAH) that can progress to life-threatening abdominal compartment syndrome.[28,30,32] Measurement of intraabdominal pressure via, bladder pressure monitoring may be initiated to evaluate the development of IAH.[32] Extensive edema also compromises intravascular fluid volume creating osmotic and hydrostatic pressure changes, often

necessitating continued fluid resuscitation to meet tissue perfusion needs that exacerbates edema formation, creating a clinical challenge for optimal fluid volume replacement that minimizes edema formation.

Effective fluid resuscitation is an initial priority to prevent burn shock and progression of tissue injury. Several formulas can be used to guide fluid resuscitation needs based on the patients total body surface area (TBSA) injured. One of the more common formulas used to calculate fluid volume resuscitation is the Parkland formula (Box 55-4). Regardless of the formula used, the goal is to support the circulatory system throughout the initial 24 to 48 hours following the burn injury.[33] Fluid shifts are significant during early resuscitation, requiring ongoing evaluation of tissue perfusion (e.g., heart rate, blood pressure, urine output, serum lactate levels) and assessment of complications from edema formation (e.g., IAH and compartment syndrome). Optimal fluid for resuscitation remains a topic of significant research. Fluids for resuscitation include crystalloids (typically lactated Ringer solution), hypertonic saline, and colloids (e.g., albumin, fresh frozen plasma).[33] A critical balance is needed to provide optimal fluid resuscitation to meet tissue and organ perfusion needs without inducing secondary complications associated with overresuscitation and edema.

In addition, the extensive loss of tissue and the exaggerated physiologic inflammatory and stress response associated with the burn injury place the patient at risk for infection, hypothermia, hypercatabolism, and development of acute respiratory distress syndrome (ARDS), sepsis, systemic inflammatory response syndrome (SIRS), acute kidney injury (AKI), and multiple organ dysfunction syndrome.[34-36] The intensity of the hypermetabolic changes experienced by burn patients is directly related to the extent of injury.[35] Metabolic demands increase by an estimated 30% in patients with an injury that covers 20% of the TBSA or more and by 100% in patients with

---

BOX 55-4   Parkland Formula for Estimating Adult Burn Patient Resuscitation Fluid Needs

4 mL × patient weight (in kg) × % TBSA
= total volume of fluid to be given in
24 hours

Half of the volume calculated is given in the first 8 hours; the remaining half is given over the following 16 hours.

burns that cover 50% of the TBSA or more.[35,37] Meeting nutritional goals is essential because 10% loss of total body mass leads to immune dysfunction, 30% leads to decreased wound healing, and 40% loss leads to death.[35] Efforts to attenuate the hypermetabolic response in critically ill burn patients may include beta-adrenergic blockage with propranolol.[35] Other pharmacologic anticatabolic therapies include growth hormone, insulin-like growth factor, intensive insulin therapy, and oxandrolone.[35,37]

Primary goals in the management of a patient with burn injury focuses on: (1) providing adequate fluid resuscitation to restore circulating volume and minimize the conversion burn tissue injury to deeper full-thickness tissue injury; (2) optimizing tissue oxygenation and management of associated pulmonary insults; (3) preventing hypothermia; (4) preventing infection though topical antibiotics and excision and coverage of burn wounds; (5) maintaining nutritional support the immune system and maximize wound healing; and (6) effectively treating pain and emotional needs of the patient.

Extent and Depth of Tissue Injury

Burn injuries are described according to the extent and depth of tissue injury. Extent is the TBSA that has been injured, and depth is the severity of tissue necrosis. The rule of nines is a quick and easy method of estimating TBSA (Fig. 55-3). Using this method, the body is divided into seven areas that represent 9% or a multiple of 9% of the body surface area, with the remaining 1% representing the genitalia. This method is most frequently used in the emergency room or upon initial assessment of the burn injured patient to estimate TBSA needed in calculated fluid resuscitation needs for the patient.[27] When the patient is in the acute care setting, the percentage of TBSA is more precisely calculated with the Berkow[38] and Lund-Browder[39] formulas. This assessment tool is used to estimate the amount of tissue injured by the thermal agent. The primary goal in estimating the TBSA of burn injury is to predict: morbidity or survival, physiologic response in relation to fluid shifts, fluid resuscitation requirement, and metabolic and immunologic responses.

Burn wound depth describes tissue damage based on anatomic loss of the layers of the skin. Depth is estimated from the most external layers of the skin to the internal. Fig. 55-4 depicts the anatomic depth and nomenclature used to describe burn wound depth. Deep partial-thickness and full-thickness burn wounds require tissue grafting for effective healing, cosmesis, and prevention of infection with removal of devitalized tissue. Assessment of burn wound depth may occur several times in the initial 48 hours of admission as burn wounds may progress or extend to deeper layers of the skin in the early days post injury.

Surgical and Postanesthesia Management of the Burn-Injured Patient

Current management involves the early excision of eschar (necrotic tissue) of deep partial-thickness and full-thickness burn wounds.[30] Early surgical debridement is thought to decrease bacterial load, release of inflammatory mediators, and lower the risk of SIRS and sepsis complications.[30,40] The goal of surgery is to remove most of the devitalized tissue and cover wounds with either autografts or

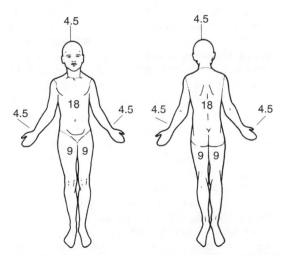

FIG. 55-3 Schematic outline of Rule of Nines. Use of the rule provides a rapid method for determining the percentage of body surface burned, but is of limited accuracy. (From Townsend CM, et al, editors: *Sabiston textbook of surgery*, cd 18, Philadelphia, 2008, Saunders.)

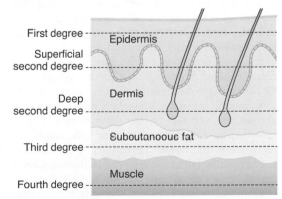

FIG. 55-4 Depth of burn wound injury. (From Townsend CM, et al, editors: *Sabiston textbook of surgery*, ed 18, Philadelphia, 2008, Saunders.)

biologic or synthetic dressings that promote wound healing and closure. The operative plan involves removal of devitalized tissue and an evaluation of the wound bed before application of an autograft or synthetic dressing. If an autograft is used to cover the burn wound, it is important to realize that the donor site for the autograft tissue is also a wound that requires observation after surgery. Physician orders and postoperative notes identify the surgical procedure (e.g., excision, debridement, grafting technique) and type of wound coverage place on the burn wound.

Postanesthesia care of the burn wound (autograft or synthetic dressing) consists of limiting or immobilizing the area of the body where the wound is located. Frequently, the physician splints the wound or sutures the dressing in place to minimize movement of the wound covering off of the fragile burn wound bed. In addition, observations for strikethrough or frank bleeding of the graft or donor site are required during the immediate postanesthesia period. Efforts to prevent friction and motion of the grafted area are necessary in the first 48 hours after surgery to prevent shearing of the graft from the wound bed. Simple interventions such as turning a patient or moving a patient off a stretcher onto a bed require utmost caution to preserve the graft adherence and successful coverage of the burn wound.

Other priorities focus on ensuring adequate fluid perfusion though effective management of intravenous fluids and vasoactive agents as needed. Efforts to maximize perfusion are necessary to enhance effective blood flow to the tissue bed. Evaluation of blood loss from the surgical procedure and insensible loss from the dressings need to be assessed, and blood products or fluids are adjusted to maintain mean arterial pressure greater than 70 mm Hg and urine output greater than 0.5 mL/kg/h.[34] Continuous heart rate monitoring and trends are helpful in monitoring the cardiovascular response after surgery. The heart rate may be falsely elevated from a catecholamine response to the burn injury and surgery; however, changes in heart rate can be used to evaluate effectiveness of fluid replacement interventions.[27] Other invasive parameters such as pulmonary artery wedge pressure, stroke volume assessment, and mixed venous oxygen saturation may also provide helpful assessment data to evaluate effectiveness of tissue perfusion.[33,41,42] Caution should be used in evaluating fluid volume replacement needs based on central venous pressure readings. Current evidence suggests that central venous pressure readings alone might not adequately reflect the vascular volume status (e.g., hypovolemia or hypervolemia) in guiding fluid

resuscitation needs.[42] Acid-base balance and serum lactate levels can also provide valuable information on the effectiveness of fluid resuscitation after surgery and tissue perfusion. A base deficit and elevated serum lactate are markers of metabolic acidosis and corrects to normal with adequate resuscitation. A base deficit of 5 mEq/L or more and serum lactate greater than 2.0 are indicators of shock and have been associated with increased mortality.[41]

Patients with electrical burn injury need additional attention and monitoring of heart rate and rhythm. As voltage passes through the patient's body, damage to the myocardial system is possible. These patients should receive continuous cardiac monitoring for up to 72 hours to assess for conduction disturbances and myocardial damage.[27] Typically, if dysrhythmias occur, they are seen in the first few hours after injury. Myoglobinuria, however, is a serious complication that must be assessed and treated in electrical burn–injured patients. Therefore fluid resuscitation to support the patient's perfusion and additional fluid to clear the kidneys of myoglobin are necessary during the postanesthesia period. Urine output of 75 to 100 mL/h or 1 to 2 mL/kg/h is usually necessary to treat myoglobinuria.[33,34]

Pulmonary assessment involves management of the ventilator to maximize oxygenation and ventilation. Third spacing and edema place the burn patient at risk for ARDS. Nursing interventions that monitor the ventilatory management of the patient, airway pressures, patient's tolerance of the ventilatory mode, and oxygenation parameters are important aspects of nursing care after surgery. The nurse should assess for early signs of ARDS by evaluating the patient's ventilatory airway pressures, changes in tidal volumes, and signs and symptoms of hypoxemia. The patient may need sedation or neuromuscular blocking agents to assist with ventilator efforts as the ARDS progresses. Newer mechanical ventilation modes, specifically high frequency percussive ventilation, may be initiated as a salvage option for refractory ARDS and treatment of inhalation injury. [43] Pneumonia is a serious complication in a burn-injured patient. Nursing interventions to reduce ventilator-associated pneumonia are essential. Nursing interventions include assessment of the head of bed greater than 30 degrees; frequent oral care and toothbrushing with oropharyngeal suctioning; assessment of cuff pressure of the endotracheal tube; and assessment of enteral tube feeding tolerance.[44] Patients with inhalation injury are at greater risk of developing ARDS and pneumonia because of the direct injury to the lung parenchyma. Inhalation injury frequently requires more aggressive fluid resuscitation to support systemic perfusion; however, this may increase pulmonary third spacing. Serial bronchoscopy is frequently performed to evaluate the severity of inhalation injury, and aggressive pulmonary suctioning is usually needed to assist with removal of debris and secretions.

Prevention of hypothermia and adverse effects of hypothermia such as electrolyte imbalances, tissue vasoconstriction, and coagulopathies are additional areas for nursing care focus.[21] Application of convection air heating devices and thermal hats and warming of the patient's room can assist with preventing hypothermia. Care is needed, however, to prevent overshoot that causes hyperthermia. The burn patient cannot effectively regulate body temperature because of the tissue loss; therefore external temperature changes can greatly influence the patient's body temperature.

Maintenance of nutritional management through surgery and after surgery is also a standard of care in the management of the burn patient. Typically the patient has a postpyloric feeding tube in which low-dose continuous tube feeding is provided to the patient, including during the perioperative procedure.[37] Hypermetabolism associated with burn injury requires significant nutritional replacement strategies to meet metabolism demands and provide substrates for tissue healing.

The final nursing priority is effective management of pain. Burn-injured patients have hypermetabolism in response to the injury and ongoing insults with surgical management for burn wound excision and wound coverage. Opioid infusions, usually morphine or fentanyl, are the mainstay for treating pain. The addition of continuous or intermittent (scheduled) anxiolytic agents is also beneficial with pain management.[27,45] Evidence-based pain assessment tools are needed to assess a patient's pain, and the patient may have a difficult time obtaining pain relief during the immediate postanesthesia period. Burn patients frequently have a tolerance to analgesic agents; therefore continuous infusions of analgesics and sedation agents titrated to desired pain and sedation responses for the patient provide optimal management after surgery. Efficacious postanesthesia management of the critically ill, burn-injured patient plays a vital role in the functional outcome and future rehabilitation.

Postoperative Care of the Septic ICU Patient

Patients admitted and treated for sepsis in the emergency department, inpatient medical-surgical unit, or ICU is often transferred to the OR for surgery. The initial presentation is often nonspecific, and the severity may be deceiving. Critical illness may often be accompanied by localized or systemic infection. Patients may arrive with a relatively benign diagnosis, or clinically unapparent infection can progress within hours to a more devastating form of disease.[46] Sepsis is an acute systemic response to a bacteria invasion or to the toxins produced by bacteria (Box 55-5); it is associated with SIRS.[47] Dellinger and colleagues[47] provided clinical definitions of SIRS, sepsis, severe sepsis, and septic shock. Although sepsis can occur from infection by gram-positive or yeast infections, the most common cause is from gram-negative endotoxins. With system infection, myriad cellular, humoral, and immunologic defense systems initiate a cascade of mediator-induced responses. With sepsis, this inflammatory response is exaggerated, creating the complex

---

BOX 55-5   Consensus Definitions

Bacteremia: The presence of viable bacteria within the blood.

Multiple organ dysfunction syndrome (MODS): The presence of altered organ function in a patient who is acutely ill and in whom homeostasis cannot be maintained without intervention.

Sepsis: The presence of infection associated with SIRS. SIRS plus the clinical presence of one manifestation:
- Altered mental state
- Hypoxemia in the absence of pulmonary disease etiology
- Elevated plasma lactate level
- Oliguria; urine output less than 0.5 mL/kg for at least 1 hour

Septic Shock: A state of acute circulatory failure characterized by persistent arterial hypotension despite adequate fluid resuscitation or tissue hypoperfusion unexplained by other causes.

Severe Sepsis: Sepsis complicated by end-organ dysfunction.

Systemic Inflammatory Response Syndrome: Systematic response to infection with the presence of two of the following clinical findings:
- Temperature greater than 38° C or less than 36° C
- Heart rate greater than 90 beats/min
- Respiratory rate greater than 20 breaths/min or arterial CO_2 tension lower than 32 mm Hg
- White blood cell count greater than 12,000 cells/mcL or less than 2000 cells/mcL or 10% immature bands

From Dellinger RP, et al: Surviving sepsis: campaign guidelines for the management of severe sepsis and septic shock, *Crit Care Med* 32:858–872, 2004.

clinical presentation of activation of neutrophil, inflammation, increased vascular permeability, platelet aggregation and destruction, and vasoconstriction. Cellular and humoral mediators such as lipoteichoic acid, leukotrienes, cytokines, tumor necrosis factor-alpha, interleukins, prostaglandins, histamine, serotonin, complement, thromboxane A$_2$, and arachidonic acid metabolites are mediators known to be responsible for the overwhelming systemic response seen with sepsis and SIRS.[48] Research continues to identify additional mediators and their actions. Serum marker of inflammation to include C-reactive protein and procalcitonin are also an area of active research exploring the variation in these markers and a patient's inflammatory responses during sepsis.[49,50]

The key to treating septic patients is early identification and aggressive treatment of the suspected cause.[41] Patients at highest risk of sepsis include very young and older patients and patients with chronic illness, immunosuppression, exposure to infection, and invasive procedures.[51] Implementation of early sepsis recognition and treatment protocols is needed to reduce the morbidity and mortality of patents with sepsis.[52, 53]

Pathophysiology and Management of Sepsis and Septic Shock

The key to understanding septic shock is the profound hemodynamic instability. The nurse may witness two different dysfunctional patterns of the cardiovascular system as a consequence to sepsis. The first is characterized by high cardiac output and low systemic vascular resistance, and the second reveals a more classic shock with low cardiac output and high systemic vascular resistance.[51] These two clinical findings reflect a hyperdynamic or hypodynamic shock state. The hyperdynamic response is termed *early septic shock,* and the hypodynamic response is the late septic shock that indicates a severe septic shock and is not reversible.

Activation of a SIRS and subsequent mediator release creates the complex clinical presentation of profound vasodilation and increased capillary permeability that manifests as hypotension. Activation of the complement cascade causes mast cells to degranulate liberating histamine, resulting in local vasodilation and capillary permeability. Neutrophil activation initiates synthesis of leukotrienes and oxygen free radicals, also increasing permeability and bronchoconstriction. Platelet aggregation in the microvasculature obstructs flow, perpetuating an inflammatory response to injury. Platelet consumption also ensues, causing coagulopathies and ultimately profound thrombocytopenia.[51]

Treatment of hypoperfusion associated with sepsis focuses on aggressive fluid resuscitation and early diagnosis and source identification to include obtaining blood cultures prior to antibiotic administration.[53] Fluid resuscitation with crystalloid or colloid agents should occur as soon as possible in patients with hypotension or elevated serum lactate. A fluid challenge of 1000 mL of crystalloids or 300 to 500 mL of colloids over 30 minutes should be given initially to treat sepsis-induced tissue hypoperfusion.[53] Continued fluid resuscitation goals include: (1) central venous pressure of 8 to 12 mmHg, (2) mean arterial pressure $\geq$65 mmHg, (3) urine output $\geq$0.5 mL/kg/h, and (4) central venous oxygen saturation $\geq$70% or mixed venous oxygen saturation $\geq$65%.[53] Vasopressor agents such as norepinephrine or dopamine centrally administered may need to be added to increase blood pressure. Epinephrine, phenylephrine, or vasopressin should not be administered as the initial vasopressor agent in patients with septic shock.[53] Vasopressin (0.03 units/min) may be added to norepinephrine infusion.[53] Inotropic support may be indicated to augment cardiac function.

Pulmonary Dysfunction

The lung is one of the primary target organs in sepsis. Transport and utilization of oxygen at the cellular and tissue levels are vital for survival (Fig. 55-5). ARDS is associated with an oxygen extraction defect that affects the utilization and delivery of oxygen to the tissues. The subsequent formation of interstitial edema contributes to the inability to extract oxygen. In addition, the release of inflammatory mediators damages the endothelium of the pulmonary vasculature and increases the permeability of the alveolar-capillary defect, resulting in ventilation–perfusion mismatch and impaired gas exchange.[51] Changes in lung compliance and impaired gas exchange are two pathophysiologic abnormalities that can lead to ARDS. Protracted oxygen debt can result in the development of multiple organ dysfunction syndrome and eventual organ death.[54]

The goals of managing septic patients with ARDS are maximizing pulmonary gas exchange, optimizing oxygen delivery to the tissues, and preventing further organ injury. Mechanical ventilation or noninvasive ventilation may be needed to assist with oxygenation and effective ventilation. Positive end-expiratory pressure can be used to avoid extensive lung collapse at end expiration.[53] The PACU nurse's role in ongoing vigilant assessments, interventions, and monitoring that

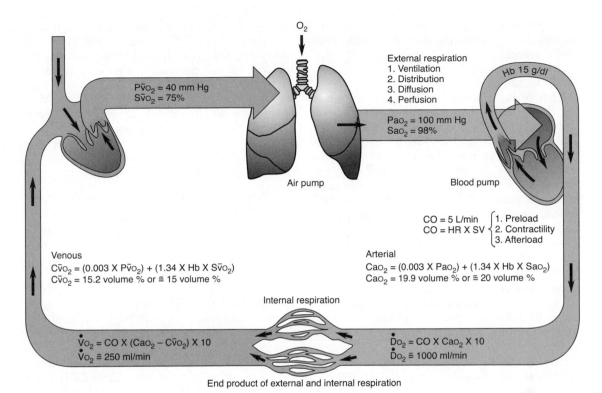

FIG. 55-5 Oxygen transport. (From Copstead LE, Banasik JL: *Pathophysiology*, ed 4, St. Louis, 2010, Saunders.)

help to promote improved gas exchange and reduced oxygen demands provides a crucial key to better survival rates.

Metabolic Dysfunction

The metabolic derangements that accompany septic shock are dependent on the severity and duration of the illness that result in intensified transport and perfusion problems. Some of these abnormalities are manifested by: (1) mechanical obstruction of capillary beds by platelet aggregation, (2) vasoconstriction that causes shunting formation in the organs, (3) inflammatory mediator interaction, and (4) impaired cellular oxidative metabolism or oxygen debt to the tissues.[54] Increased lactic acidosis is persistent even though oxygen consumption is consistently increased. Patients in septic shock need higher oxygen delivery because of the escalating metabolic demand. Sustained proteolysis is evidenced by high urinary nitrogen excretion.[54] Gluconeogenesis is increased; however, concurrent insulin resistance results in hyperglycemia in the hyperdynamic state of septic shock. In late septic shock, a profound hypoglycemia develops as glycogen stores are depleted and are insufficient to supply the body's demands.

Steroid Therapy

In the neurohumoral response to septic shock, many patients have an inadequate adrenal reserve. Although the physiologic mechanism is not fully understood, it is likely caused by the inflammatory cascade that leads to inadequate release of adrenocorticotropin. Intravenous hydrocortisone may be considered in adult septic shock patients when hypotension responds poorly to aggressive fluid and vasopressor support.[53] An adrenocorticotrophin hormone level is not recommended before administering hydrocortisone.[53] The recommended hydrocortisone dose is ≤300 mg/day, and therapy can be weaned when vasopressor agents are no longer needed to support the patient's blood pressure.[53]

Glycemic Control

As discussed previously, tight glycemic control (serum glucose of 80 to 100 mg/dL) is no longer recommended, because hypoglycemic events associated with regulating tight control in critically ill patients have been found to result in adverse patient outcomes.[55] Current evidence suggests maintaining serum glucose between 140 to 180 mg with aggressive insulin therapy and close monitoring indicated in the management of the critically ill septic patient.[24]

Acute Kidney Injury

AKI is often associated with sepsis and septic shock. Generally, two pathophysiologic causes are cellular ischemia related to hypoperfusion and the presence of SIRS. Mediators of inflammation, such as tumor necrosis factor-alpha, interleukin-1, and interleukin-6, influence the perfusion to the kidneys and cause damage to the renal tubules.[54] Because the cause of AKI is inadequate renal perfusion, often related to deficits in intravascular volume, prompt replacement of crystalloids, colloids, and blood is warranted.[41] Low-dose dopamine (1 to 3 mcg/kg/min) does not provide renal protection and should not be administered.[56] Management of acid-base, cardiovascular, and intake and output alterations is vital in preserving kidney function and preventing organ failure in the septic patient.[54]

Postanesthesia Management of the Patient in Septic Shock

Advances continue in early identification and aggressive treatment of patients with sepsis, severe sepsis, and septic shock .The surviving sepsis campaign (www.survivingsepsis.org) provides a comprehensive, evidence-based guideline to assist clinicians in the management of severe sepsis and septic shock.

Postanesthesia care of the patient in septic shock must first focus on fluid resuscitation and identification of possible cause. Peripheral vasodilation, hypotension, and myocardial depression can significantly impede tissue perfusion. End-organ perfusion should be monitored with assessment of skin temperature, color, capillary refill, and peripheral pulses every hour. Because of mediators of inflammation, vasopressor and inotropic agents may be needed, in addition to aggressive fluid resuscitation, to support tissue and end-organ perfusion. Blood product administration may be indicated if the patient has a hemoglobin less than 7.0 g/dL, with a goal of transfusing to a hemoglobin of 9.0g/L.[53] Tachycardia should be assessed, and interventions to keep the heart rate at less than 100 beats/min should be initiated.

Interventions to maximize oxygenation and ventilation are concurrently necessary to ensure that cellular oxygen delivery and consumption needs are being met. The patient may need frequent suctioning to remove secretions and careful monitoring of blood gases. Because ARDS

frequently accompanies sepsis, the patient may need mechanical ventilation. Lower tidal volumes (6 mL/kg of estimated body weight) is the current recommendation for patients requiring mechanical ventilation, because lower tidal volumes result in less barotrauma.[53] The PACU nurse should frequently monitor the septic patient for decreased pulmonary compliance associated with airway hyper-reactivity or pulmonary consolidation, which further impairs ventilation.[57]

Sepsis Management Implications for the PACU Nurse

Management of the septic critically ill patient in the PACU can be challenging, even to the most experienced critical care nurse. The high mortality rate of septic shock emphasizes the importance of preventing and reversing the rapid progression of the disease.[41,51,53] Effective postanesthesia nursing care mandates knowledge of current sepsis research related to pathophysiology and clinical manifestations of SIRS. An understanding of the process of sepsis, severe sepsis, and septic shock sequelae is imperative. The PACU nurse must have a high degree of suspicion when the etiologies that predispose sepsis are seen in the recovering patient. Likewise, monitoring of the ICU patient vigilantly for signs and symptoms of decreased cardiac output and alterations in oxygenation and tissue perfusion provides key assessment information. Furthermore it is necessary to report, in a timely manner, the subtle but significant critical changes in the patient's condition to the surgeon, anesthesia provider, or intensivist. New advancements in sepsis therapies should be used as evidence-based practice guidelines to care.

FAMILY PRESENCE DURING RESUSCITATION

The impressive expertise of postanesthesia nurses is often taken for granted by both the nursing staff members and medical colleagues.[58] The staff members expect the patients under their care to do well. However, what does the staff do when the patient's condition becomes life threatening or even fatal? What happens in the PACU when things go wrong? Are these specialty nurses prepared for end-of-life nursing interventions? PACU nurses must become knowledgeable about the current evidence that emphasizes not only the needs of the patients, but more importantly the needs of the surviving families.

Evidence-Based Practice

In 2001, the Emergency Nurses Association published a position statement encouraging family presence during procedures and resuscitation. Since that sentinel event, the practice of including family during procedures and resuscitation has continued to evolve. Two critical reviews of the literature have been conducted in the space of 6 years (2005 and 2011) examining family presence during resuscitation. Research and other forms of evidence have focused on provider perceptions of family presence, family perceptions, and ethical consideration. Current evidence suggests that family presence fosters trust between the family and provider, increases collaboration, assists families with understanding the patient's condition, enhances collaborative practice of health care providers during a crisis, and assists families in meeting spiritual and emotional needs. Early research found health care providers to be hesitant toward family presence, but the practice has evolved and more current evidence reports increased support and acceptance of family presence by all health care providers. Families report a sense of deeper understanding of the family member's crisis, closure, and engagement in the decision making. Establishing evidence-based protocols and practice guidelines have been found to be helpful as the practice of family presence evolves in a new practice setting.

IMPLICATIONS FOR PRACTICE

Perianesthesia nurses should actively encourage family to be present for procedures, emergencies, and resuscitations that can occur during the postoperative management of a patient. Ideally a protocol is established to provide support to the family member explaining the situation, allowing the health care providers to focus on the immediate needs of the patient. But the focus should be inclusive, welcoming family presence during procedures and resuscitations in the perianesthesia practice environment and creating a holistic patient- and family-centered atmosphere.

Source: Dollin CT, et al: Family presence during cardiopulmonary resuscitation: using evidence-based knowledge to guide the advanced practice nursing in developing formal policy and practice guidelines, *J Am Acad Nurse Pract* 23:8–14, 2011; Halm MA: Family presence during resuscitation: a critical review of the literature, *Am J Crit Care* 14:494–511, 2005.

The presence of a patient's family during resuscitation is emerging as an acceptable practice in the critical care setting. Critical care and emergency department nurses have been leaders in advocating family presence during resuscitation. In the landmark article of 2001 entitled *Family Presence During Invasive and Resuscitation: Hearing the Voice of the Patient*, the authors reported an NBC Dateline poll that showed 74% of 2464 respondents believed family members should be allowed to be in an emergency department during invasive procedures.[59] Current evidence supports the multiple benefits of this practice to patients, families, and health care providers.[58-63] Patients believe that family presence gives them the feeling of support, personhood, connectedness, and advocacy.[61,63] Research has repeatedly revealed that families have specific needs that include: (1) having honest, consistent, and thorough communication with health care providers; (2) being physically and emotionally close to their loved one; (3) feeling that the health care providers care about their loved one; and (4) visiting the patient frequently during a health-related crisis.[64] Both patients and families believe that they have a right to have families present during resuscitation.[65] Health care providers agree that family presence encourages professional behavior of staff at the bedside and facilitates end-of-life closure issues for families.[64-68] The Emergency Nurses Association and the AACN have issued position statements in support of family presence during resuscitation.[69,70] PACU nurses need to expand their knowledge of family presence during resuscitation and adopt a holistic framework that provides the best possible outcomes for patients and families during the end of life.

The PACU nurse must remember the family when resuscitating an ICU patient in the PACU. The benefits far outweigh the risks in implementing family presence in the PACU. Research reveals that families perceive that: (1) they have been supported, (2) everything was done for the patient, (3) patient-family connectedness was maintained, (4) the patient's personhood was respected, and (5) they coped better with death.[61-64]

SUMMARY

The practice of providing postanesthesia care to the ICU patient in the PACU can be challenging and rewarding. Important administrative decisions to care for these critically ill patients must ensure safeguards to provide a comparable level of ICU care in the PACU. Key critical care education and clinical ICU competencies must be maintained. PACU nurses are recognized for their critical care skills and abilities in providing care to the ICU patient. This chapter has provided advanced clinical ICU nursing concepts in managing some of the highest risk, high-acuity, specialized complex cases (e.g., neurosurgery, burn, septic shock). Finally, the introduction of family presence during resuscitation in the PACU advocates the family's right to be with the critically ill patient at the end of life.

REFERENCES

1. Mamaril M, et al: ASPAN's Delphi study on national research: priorities for perianesthesia nurses in the United States, *J Perianesth Nurs* 24:4–13, 2009.
2. American Society of PeriAnesthesia Nurses: *Perianesthesia nursing standards and practice recommendations 2010-2012*, Cherry Hill, NJ, 2010, American Society of Peri-Anesthesia Nurses.
3. Fontaine DK: Impact of the critical care environment on the patient. In Morton PG, et al, editors: *Critical care nursing: a holistic approach*, ed 9, Philadelphia, 2009, Lippincott Williams & Wilkins.
4. Ayres SA, et al: *Care of the critically ill*, ed 3, Chicago, 1988, Yearbook Medical Publishers.
5. Bizek KS: The patient's experience with critical illness. In Morton PG, et al, editors: *Critical care nursing: a holistic approach*, ed 9, Philadelphia, 2009, Lippincott Williams & Wilkins.
6. Norton C: The family's experience with critical illness. In Morton PG, et al, editors: *Critical care nursing: a holistic approach*, ed 8, Philadelphia, 2009, Lippincott Williams & Wilkins.
7. Johannes MS: A new dimension of the PACU: the dilemma of the ICU overflow patient, *J Perianesth Nurs* 9:297–300, 1994.
8. Bader MK: Gizmos and gadgets for the neuroscience intensive care unit, *J Neurosci Nurs* 38: 248–260, 2006.
9. Saiki RL: Current and evolving management of traumatic brain injury, *Crit Care Nurs Clin N Am* 21:549–559, 2009.
10. Inoue K: Caring for the perioperative patient with increased intracranial pressure, *AORN J* 91:511–518, 2010.
11. Hickey J, Olson DM: Intracranial hypertension: theory and management of increased intracranial pressure. In Hickey JV, editor: *The clinical practice of neurological and neurosurgical nursing*, ed 6, Philadelphia, 2009, Lippincott Williams & Wilkins.
12. Bershad EM, et al: Intracranial hypertension, *Semin Neurol* 28:690–702, 2008.
13. Slazinski T: Intracranial bolt and fiber optic catheter insertion (assist), intracranial pressure monitoring, care, troubleshooting, and removal. In Weigand D, editor: *AACN procedure manual for critical care*, ed 6, St. Louis, 2011, Elsevier.
14. Bratton SL, et al: Guidelines for the management of severe traumatic brain injury: a joint project of the Brain Trauma Foundation, *J Neurotrauma* 24(Suppl1):S1–S106, 2007.
15. Li LM, et al: The surgical approach to the management of increased intracranial pressure after traumatic brain injury, *Anesthesia-Analg* 111:736–748, 2010.
16. Maloney-Wilensky E, et al: Brain tissue oxygen monitoring: insertion (assist) care and troubleshooting. In Weigand D, editor: *AACN procedure manual for critical care*, ed 6, St. Louis, 2011, Saunders.
17. Slazinski T: Jugular venous oxygen saturation monitoring: insertion (assist), patient care, troubleshooting, and removal. In Weigand D, editor: *AACN procedure manual for critical care*, ed 6, St. Louis, 2011, Saunders.
18. Presciutti M, et al: Neuromonitoring in intensive care: focus on microdialysis and its nursing implications, *J Neurosci Nurs* 41:131–139, 2009.
19. Timofeev I, et al: Cerebral extracellular chemistry and outcome following traumatic brain injury: a microdialysis study of 223 patients, *Brain* 134:484–494, 2011.
20. Fan J: Effect of backrest position on intracranial pressure and cerebral perfusion pressure in individuals with brain injury: a systematic review, *J Neurosci Nurs* 36:278–288, 2004.
21. Niklasch DM: Induced mild hypothermia and the prevention of neurological injury, *J Infus Nurs* 33:236–242, 2010.
22. Godoy DA, et al: Treating hyperglycemia in neurocritical patients: benefits and perils, *Neurocrit Care* 13:425–438, 2010.
23. Moghissi ES: Revisiting inpatient hyperglycemia: new recommendations, evolving data and practice implications for implementation, *Postgraduate Institute for Medicine LLC, and Global Directions in Medicine, Inc.*, December 2009.
24. Kavanagh BP, McCowen KC: Glycemic control in the ICU, *New England Journal Med* 363:2540–2546, 2010.
25. American Burn Association: *Burn incidence and treatment in the United States: 2011 fact sheet*, available at www.ameriburn.org/resources_factsheet.php. Accessed May 20, 2011.
26. Colohan SM: Predicting prognosis in thermal burns with associated inhalation injury: A systematic review of prognostic factors in adult burn victims, *J Burn Care Res* 31; 529–539, 2010.
27. Makic MBF, Mann E: Burn injuries. In McQuillan K, et al, editors: *Trauma nursing from resuscitation through rehabilitation*, ed 4, Philadelphia, 2009, Saunders.
28. Kramer GC, et al: Pathophysiology of burn shock and burn edema. In Herndon D, editors: *Total burn care*, ed 3, Philadelphia, 2007, Saunders.
29. American Burn Association: *Burn Center Referral Criteria*, available at www.ameriburn.org/BurnCenterReferralCriteria.pdf /. Accessed March 1, 2012.
30. Chipp E, et al: Sepsis in burns, *Annals of Plastic Surg* 65:228–236, 2010.
31. Shupp WJ, et al: A review of the local pathophysiologic basis of burn wound progression, *J Burn Care Res* 31: 849–873, 2010.
32. World Society of the Abdominal Compartment Syndrome: *Consensus definitions and recommendations*, available at www.wsacs.org/consensus.php. Accessed May 20, 2011.
33. Warden GD: Fluid resuscitation and early management. In Herndon D, editor: *Total burn care*, ed 3, Philadelphia, 2007, Saunders.
34. Brusselaers N, et al: Outcome of acute kidney injury in severe burns: a systematic review and meta-analysis, *Intensive Care Med* 36:915–925, 2010.

35. Gauglitz GG, et al: Burns: Where are we standing with propranolol, oxandrolone, recombinant human growth hormone and the new incretin analogs? *Curr Opin Clin Nutr Metab Care* 14:176–181, 2011.

36. Sheridan RL, Tompkins RG: Etiology and prevention of multisystem organ failure. In Herndon D, editor: *Total burn care*, ed 3, Philadelphia, 2007, Saunders.

37. Norbury WB, Herndon DN: Modulation of the hypermetabolic response after burn injury. In Herndon D, editor: *Total burn care*, ed 3, Philadelphia, 2007, Saunders.

38. Berkow SG: A method for estimating the extensiveness of lesions (burns and scalds) based on surface area proportions, *Arch Surg* 8:138–142, 1924.

39. Lund CC, Browder NC: Estimation of areas of burns, *Surg Gynecol Obstet* 79:352–357, 1944.

40. Bessey PQ: Wound care. In Herndon D, editor: *Total burn care*, ed 3, Philadelphia, 2007, Saunders.

41. Funk D, et al: A systems approach to the early recognition and rapid administration of best practice therapy in sepsis and septic shock, *Curr Opin Crit Car* 15:301–307, 2009.

42. Marik PE, et al: Does central venous pressure predict fluid responsiveness? A systematic review of the literature and the tale of seven mares, *Chest* 134:172–178, 2008.

43. Allan PF, et al: High-frequency percussive ventilation revisited, *J Burn Care Res* 31:510–520, 2010.

44. Institute for Healthcare Improvement: *Prevent ventilator associated pneumonia*, available at www.ihi.org/IHI/Programs/Campaign/VAP.htm. Accessed May 20, 2011.

45. Meyer WJ, et al: Management of pain and other discomforts in burned patients. In Herndon D, editor: *Total burn care*, ed 3, Philadelphia, 2007, Saunders.

46. Rivers EP, et al: Early innovative interventions for severe sepsis and septic shock: taking advantage of the window of opportunity, *Can Med Assoc* 173:1054–1065, 2005.

47. Dellinger RP, et al: Surviving sepsis: campaign guidelines for the management of severe sepsis and septic shock, *Crit Care Med*, 32:858–872, 2004.

48. Pinksy MR: Septic shock, *Medscape Drugs, Conditions and Procedures*, available at emedicine.medscape.com/article/168402-overview. Accessed May 20, 2011.

49. Becker KL, et al: Procalcitonin in sepsis and systemic inflammation: a harmful biomarker and a therapeutic target, *Br J Pharm* 159:253–264, 2010.

50. Pierrakos C, Vincent JL: Sepsis biomarkers: a review, *Critical Care* 14:1–18, 2010, available at ccforum.com/content/14/1/R15. Accessed May 20, 2011.

51. Latto C: An overview of sepsis, *Dimension in Critical Care Nurs* 27:195–200, 2008.

52. Westphal GA, et al: Reduced mortality after the implementation of a protocol for the early detection of severe sepsis, *J Crit Care* 26:76–81, 2011.

53. Dellinger RP, et al: Surviving sepsis campaign: intervention guidelines for management of severe sepsis and septic shock 2008, *Intensive Care Med* 34:17–60, 2008.

54. VonRueden K, et al: Shock and multiple organ dysfunction syndrome. In McQuillan K, et al, editors: *Trauma nursing from resuscitation through rehabilitation*, ed 4, Philadelphia, 2009, Saunders.

55. Griesdale DE, et al: Intensive insulin therapy and mortality among critically ill patients: a meta-analysis including NICE-Sugar study data, *CMAJ* 180:821–827, 2009.

56. Rauen C, et al: Evidence-based practice habits: Transforming research into bedside care, *Crit Care Nurse* 29:46–59, 2009.

57. Lee CS: The role of exogenous arginine vasopressin in the management of catecholamine-refractory septic shock, *Crit Care Nurse* 26:17–29, 2006.

58. Iacono M: Critical stress debriefing: application for perianesthesia nurses, *J Perianesth Nurs* 17:423–426, 2002.

59. Eichorn DJ, et al: Family presence during invasive procedures and resuscitation: hearing the voice of the patient, *Am J Nurs* 101:48–53, 2001.

60. Oman KS, Duran CR: Health care providers' evaluations of family presence during resuscitation, *J Emerg Nurs* 36:524–533, 2010.

61. Moreland P: Family presence during invasive procedures and resuscitation in the emergency department: a review of the literature, *J Emerg Nurs* 31(1):58–72, 2005.

62. Clark AP, et al: Family presence during cardiopulmonary resuscitation, *Crit Care Nurs Clin North Am* 17:23–32, 2005.

63. Adridge MD, Clark AP: Making the right choice: family presence and the CNS, *Clin Nurse Specialist* 19:113–116, 2005.

64. Duran CR, et al: Attitudes and beliefs about family presence: a survey of health care providers, families, and patients, *Am J Crit Care* 16(3):270–282, 2007.

65. Halm MA: Family presence during resuscitation: a critical review of the literature, *Am J Crit Care* 14:494–511, 2005.

66. Bradley C, et al: Family presence during resuscitation, *J Pallia Care* 14:97–98, 2011.

67. Bradley C, et al: Implementation of a family presence during resuscitation protocol, *J Pallia Care* 14:98–99, 2011.

68. McGahey PR: Family presence during pediatric resuscitation: a focus on staff, *Crit Care Nurse* 22:29–34, 2002.

69. Emergency Nurses Association: *Position statement: family presence at the bedside during invasive procedures and cardiopulmonary resuscitation*, revised September 2010, available at www.cna.org. Accessed May 30, 2011.

70. American Association of Critical Care Nurses: *Practice alert: family presence during CPR and invasive procedures*, revised April 2010, available at www.aacn.org. Accessed May 30, 2011.

SPECIAL CONSIDERATIONS

56 Bioterrorism and Its Impact on the PACU

Robin Blixt, BSN, MS, RN, CNOR*

Before September 11, 2001, terrorism did not have the full attention of the average American as it does today.[1] However, with our past experience and current knowledge, we must be able to define what bioterrorism is and how it impacts the postanesthesia care unit (PACU).

DEFINITIONS

Aerosolization: A gaseous suspension of organisms that contains minute particles.
CBRNE: Chemical, Biologic, Radiologic, Nuclear, Explosive event.
Cohort: Group together with similar likenesses.
Dirty Bomb: A mix of explosives, such as dynamite, with radioactive powder or pellets. The dynamite explodes and carries material into the surrounding area (e.g., radioactive material, biologic agents).
Empiric Treatment: Broad-based antibiotic treatment based on prior experience with the microorganism.
Sepsis: The body's response to an infection.
Septic Shock: Multiple organ failure resulting from advancement of severe sepsis.
Weapon of Mass Destruction (WMD): A former Soviet Union term that was used to denote nuclear, chemical, and biologic weapons. The term has been broadened to include radiologic weapons. Since the World Trade Center airliner attacks, the term includes any means to cause mass casualties.

The Centers for Disease Control and Prevention (CDC) define *bioterrorism* as the intentional release (or threatened release) of viruses, bacteria, or their toxins for the purposes of harming or killing citizens.[2] Potential vehicles of releasing the biologic agents include aerosolization, insects, and food and water source contamination.[2] As a critical care unit, the PACU will be challenged to adapt usual care to supplement mass casualty victims of bioterrorism. The PACU must prepare immediately for this inevitable role, brainstorming scenarios by participating in mock disaster drills and augmenting staff competencies. The release

*The views expressed in this manuscript are those of the author and do not reflect the official policy or position of the Department of the Army, Department of Defense, or the U.S. Government.

of biologic weapons is specifically designed to promote or spread fear or intimidation upon an individual, a specific group, or the population as a whole for religious, political, ideological, financial, or personal purposes.[3] Overwhelming terror and panic are just two of the psychological goals, with incapacitation and destruction as the ultimate objectives. Deliberate release of biologic agents is a growing and real threat, because the agents are easier to acquire and are more likely to be used. Unlike nuclear, radiologic, or chemical attacks, biologic attacks can be overt or covert and much easier to deploy. Covert attacks offer no immediate effects on victims because of a delay between exposure and onset of illness (incubation period).[4] There are several advantages of covert biologic operations including: biologic agents are easier to hide, decreasing the chance of disclosure; biologic agents are cheaper, allowing small radical groups or single individuals access; and release might not be detected until the incubation period is completed, eliminating the "window of opportunity" for postexposure prophylaxis.[5]

There is a plethora of biologic agents that could be used in bioterrorism. Rapid and accurate diagnosis may be hindered because of the commonality of symptoms (e.g., fever, body aches, lethargy) with other universal illnesses. With a delay in diagnosis, there is a greater the chance of infecting a much larger population. The goal of the perpetrator may include a multitiered reaction, including the initial release of a toxic substance and followed by fear and panic in the populace that could lead to a physical injury in conjunction to exposure to toxic biologic agents. It is critical to remember that when a civilian population is the target of a biologic attack, the diversity in age and health status influences overall outcomes. Victims of bioterrorism rely on health care providers to be cognizant of the rapid detection and proper treatment of exposure to a multitude of items.

HISTORICAL USE OF BIOTERRORISM

Greek history documents one of the earliest written descriptions of biologic weapons being used. In 184 BC, Hannibal used snakes as a biologic weapon by casting pots of poisonous snakes into the midst of the Pergamene forces, ultimately defeating them. In 300 BC, the Greeks used decaying bodies to pollute the water supply of their enemies.[1] In the fourteenth century, bodies infected with plague were catapulted over the walls of cities in an attempt to infect the habitants and attenuate their defenses. Blankets that were once used to wrap smallpox victims were subsequently distributed to Native Americans in an effort to infect and incapacitate them. The use of biologic weapons continued into the 1900s, and stakes became higher as the sophistication of microbiology improved and travel became easier. During World War I, the Germans inoculated horses and cattle with anthrax and glanders before shipping them to France.[6] In 1937, Japan started a biologic warfare program code named Unit 731. An investigation after World War II revealed that the Japanese used prisoners of war as research subjects for aerosolized anthrax and also dropped plague-infected fleas over China and Manchuria.[6]

In 1925, the Geneva Protocol called for the first multilateral agreement for the prohibition of biologic warfare.[1] This agreement served to describe biologic warfare, but did not address the prevention of their use. During World War II, there were accusations that the United States used biologic agents against the Eskimos in Canada and released the Colorado beetles on crops in Germany. In 1942 at a small National Guard airfield (Fort Detrick), the United States began a research and development program on the use of biologic agents. This program produced agents and conducted field testing on biologic agents until 1969, when President Richard Nixon stopped all offensive biologic and toxin weapon research and production by executive order. In 1953, the United States initiated a medical defensive program against biologic warfare at the U.S. Army Medical Research Institute of Infectious Disease that continues today.[7] Over recent decades, the threat has changed from Cold War scenarios to the asymmetric and terrorist threat.[5] In 1978 the toxin "yellow rain," was used in the assassination of a exiled Bulgarian in London.[6] Terrorist plots to use ricin were uncovered in England in January 2003, in a South Carolina postal office, and in the Dirksen Senate Office Building in Washington D.C.[6] Lawmakers were directly affected in October 2001 when an anthrax contamination resulted in the closing the Hart Senate Office Building in Washington D.C. shortly after the terrorist attack on September 11, 2001.[6] Radical groups or individuals can easily gain access to biologic agents. Iraq had a large biologic weapons program, and in 1995 they admitted to producing and deploying bombs, rockets and aircraft spray tanks containing *Bacillus anthracis* and botulinum toxin.[7] In 1995, a cult in Japan released sarin gas in a Tokyo subway, resulting in significant injury. This same group had additional plans for biologic terrorism involving botulinum toxin, anthrax, and drone aircraft carrying spray tanks.[7] They had also traveled to Zaire in 1992 to obtain Ebola virus.[7] It is concerning that access to once highly protected biologic weapons is becoming easier for the highest bidder. In the former Soviet Union, one of the former biologic weapons laboratory facilities, highly protected in the 1980s, was left vulnerable with a few guards who had not been paid in months. The location of the smallpox, Ebola, Marburg, and hemorrhagic fever viruses that were stored there remain unknown.[7] Today's global economy, free and mobile society, instant Internet connectivity, and continued research indicate the most worrisome infections have yet to be recognized.[6]

BIOTERRORISM AGENTS

The Centers for Disease Control and Prevention (CDC) classifies bioterrorism agents into three groups (Table 56-1). Category A includes high-priority agents that could pose a risk to national security because they can be easily disseminated, result in high mortality rates, have the potential for major public health impact, might cause public panic, and require special action for public health preparedness.[8] Category B includes agents that are moderately able to be disseminated, resulting in moderate morbidity and low mortality rates, and require specific enhancements of the CDC's diagnostic capacity and enhanced disease surveillance.[8] Category C is the lowest priority and includes emerging pathogens that could be engineered for mass dissemination in the future because of the availability, ease of production, dissemination, and the high morbidity and mortality rates and major health impact.[8]

Anthrax

In the PACU, patients may exhibit a wide variety of conditions and syndromes. Many are related to the respiratory system. For example, anthrax has three identifiable symptom clusters. *Bacillus anthracis*, a spore-forming bacterium, can lead to inhalational anthrax, which can appear much like a case of influenza, atypical pneumonia, or pneumonic plague. In its classic form, it appears in two phases. The first phase follows an incubation period of up to 6 days and is characterized by a nonspecific syndrome of fever, chills, weakness, muscle pain, headache, dyspnea, nonproductive

Table 56-1	CDC Categories of Bioterrorism Agents and Diseases
CATEGORIES	BIOTERRORISM AGENTS AND DISEASES
Category A	Anthrax (*Bacillus anthracis*)
	Botulism *(Clostridium botulinum* toxin)
	Plague (*Yersinia pestis*)
	Smallpox (variola major)
	Tularemia (*Francisella tularensis*)
	Viral hemorrhagic fevers (e.g., Ebola, Marburg, Lassa)
Category B	Brucellosis (*Brucella* species)
	Food safety threats (*Salmonella* species, *Escherichia coli, Shigella*)
	Glanders (*Burkholderia mallei*)
	Q fever (*Caxiella burnetii*)
	Ricin toxin
	Viral encephalitis (VEE, EEE, WEE)
Category C	Emerging infectious diseases
	Nipah
	Hantavirus
	SARS

From Woods JB: *USAMRIID's medical management of biological casualties handbook*, ed 6, Fort Detrick, Frederick, Md, 2005, U.S. Army Medical Research Institute of Infectious Disease, available at www.usamriid.army.mil/education/bluebookpdf/USAMRIID%20BlueBook%206th%20Edition%20-%20Sep%202006.pdf. Accessed April 10, 2011.
CDC, Centers for Disease Control and Prevention; *EEE,* eastern equine encephalitis, *SARS,* severe acute respiratory syndrome; *VEE,* Venezuelan equine encephalitis; *WEE,* western equine encephalitis.

cough (a diagnostic clue), and abdominal or chest pain. It then progresses to a second phase over 2 or 3 days, with progressive fever, diaphoresis, severe dyspnea, and possibly cyanosis. In 50% of the cases, hemorrhagic meningitis occurs and leads to delirium, meningismus, obtundation, seizures, and coma. An additional diagnostic clue is mediastinal widening, as revealed on chest radiographs or tomographic scan results. The patient may have stridor and subcutaneous edema of the upper thorax or neck. This syndrome can progress to obtundation and coma, with hypothermia, circulatory failure, and death within 2 to 3 days. Prompt treatment with antibiotics may result in survival. Finally, the rarest form of anthrax, gastrointestinal anthrax, occurs when undercooked contaminated meat is consumed. Gastrointestinal anthrax is characterized by acute inflammation of the gastrointestinal tract and can lead to ulcers in the upper tract (oropharynx) or in the terminal ileum or cecum. Presenting symptoms include fever, sore throat, difficulty swallowing, nausea, vomiting, abdominal pain, bloody diarrhea, and total body sepsis. Mortality rates are higher than

50%. The gastrointestinal disease can be confused easily with nonspecific gastroenteritis and other bacterial or viral syndromes.

Pneumonic Plague

Another disease that may be encountered in the PACU is pneumonic plague. One should suspect plague in the patient who has rapid onset of pneumonia, high fever, headache, and chills combined with a history of exposure to possibly infected animals or fleas. The pneumonic form of the disease can spread by the dispersion of *Yersinia pestis* to the bloodstream from infected lymph nodes of the bubonic form through inhalation of the bacilli (so-called primary plague pneumonia). Diagnosis is facilitated by the finding of bipolar or gram-negative coccobacilli on a smear from a lymph node, from aspirate from trachea or lung, or in the blood. The diagnosis can be confirmed with the more specific fluorescent-antibody test.

Botulism

The disease of botulism is caused not by the bacterium itself, but by bacterial toxin produced by *Clostridium botulinum,* a spore-forming organism. The toxin is generally accelerated in anaerobic conditions and results in a syndrome characterized by the triad of descending flaccid paralysis with bulbar palsies, clear sensorium, and no fever. Initial symptoms may include the sudden onset of visual difficulties, which are the result of paralysis of cranial nerves. Paralysis may then progress downward and result in difficulty swallowing, dry mouth, and manifestations of further paralysis of motor and autonomic nerves. The lack of fever and clear mentation are characteristic and frightening aspects of the disease. Most fatalities result from respiratory failure, and those who survive have respiratory residual respiratory symptoms.

The management of cases of botulism consists largely of supportive care, augmented by immunization with botulism antitoxin (available from the CDC). This antitoxin can reduce the severity of symptoms if administered sufficiently early in the course of the disease; however, patients may require weeks or months of respiratory care. Ventilatory support is the key to survival.

Smallpox

In 1977, smallpox was eradicated worldwide with routine vaccination not administered since 1972.[1] Because of this documented eradication, the reappearance of the disease would be highly indicative of a bioterrorism attack. Smallpox is caused by the variola virus and is highly infectious, spreading from person to person primarily via respiratory tract. The virus can spread through oral secretions, drainage from lesions, and direct contact with contaminated items such as blankets. Five clinical syndromes of smallpox can be observed. The initial symptoms of high fevers, headache, backache, malaise, and vomiting closely resemble other acute viral illnesses, including influenza. During the first 2 to 3 days, the maculopapular rash is almost indistinguishable from chicken pox, except for its centripetal evolution. The rash continues to evolve, and by day 8 or 9 the lesions start to crust and scabs begin to develop. The risk of transmission lasts until all the scabs have fallen off. Smallpox can also take on a hemorrhagic form, which is characterized by diffuse hemorrhagic manifestations and a rapid progression to death. The flat type has a fatality rate of 95% and is characterized by a slow evolution of flat soft focal skin lesions and severe systemic toxicity. The nurse in the PACU is unlikely to encounter smallpox because this contagious systemic viral illness with its characteristic skin rash would likely be treated as an international emergency, with mandatory treatment at home in isolation conditions. Within the hospital setting, patients with smallpox would be under strict airborne isolation in a negative-pressure room with high-efficiency particle air filtration. No proven treatment exists for the disease. Supportive therapy includes hydration and electrolyte replacement for hypovolemic shock. Patients with flat and hemorrhagic types may need mechanical ventilatory support, because the incidence of pulmonary edema is higher. Contacts of cases should be vaccinated within 3 to 4 days, because vaccination can decrease the severity of the disease. Cidofovir, an antiviral agent, has shown effectiveness in laboratory cultures when given in the first 1 or 2 days and is a promising research development.

Severe Acute Respiratory Syndrome

Severe acute respiratory syndrome (SARS) is a viral respiratory illness caused by the coronavirus.[9] It was first reported in 2003 in Asia but quickly spread globally. In the following 2 months, the disease spread to more than 24 countries in North America, South America, Europe, and Asia.[9] The World Health Organization acknowledged that approximately 8000 people contracted SARS in 2003, with 774 deaths.[9] The presenting symptoms are usually fever, headache, an overall feeling of discomfort, and body aches. After 2 to 7 days a dry cough develops, and many patients develop pneumonia. Treatment is based on symptoms. If pneumonia develops, antibiotics may prove effective. SARS is spread from person to person through close contact. Contact and droplet precautions should be used to prevent the spread to other patients and staff members.[9]

Viral Hemorrhagic Fevers (Ebola, Marburg, Lasso)

Viral hemorrhagic fever is a group of illnesses caused by distinct families of viruses. In general, the name *viral hemorrhagic fever* is used to describe a severe multisystem syndrome in which the vascular system is damaged.[10] Symptoms include a rapidly escalating illness beginning with fever, fatigue, dizziness, muscle aches, loss of strength, and exhaustion. Severe cases show signs of bleeding under the skin, in internal organs, and from body orifices such as the mouth, ears, or eyes, in addition to nervous system shutdown, shock, coma, and seizure.

Viral hemorrhagic fevers are transmitted to humans from rodents or arthropod vectors. Ebola, Marburg, Lassa, and Crimean-Congo hemorrhagic fever viruses can be transmitted from person to person after the initial person is infected from a rodent or arthropod vector.[10] Other vectors spread the disease to animals or livestock. Humans acquire the disease when they care for or slaughter animals.[10]

For PACU nurses, supportive therapy using advanced trauma life support and Surviving Sepsis Campaign bundles is the only treatment. There is no established cure. Ribavirin, an antiviral drug, has been effective in treating some individuals. Patient isolation and standard precautions will protect against spreading the infection.

PREPAREDNESS

The best preparation for an inevitable attack is knowledge and the sharing of that knowledge. With such repugnant, unconventional choices of biologic weapons, is it possible to prepare? Like any mass casualty events, there will be chaos, but using a standard national emergency plan, the state and county health department levels can provide a local response plan. Each hospital is required by The Joint Commission to have an emergency plan that includes bioterrorism. Because the discovery of a biologic attack might be recognized at the hospital emergency department or a physician's private office, local health care facilities must always maintain an index of suspicion and facilitate quick action. Incidents that would suggest a possible biologic event include: multiple people suddenly becoming ill quickly in a normally healthy population, the epidemic curve rising and falling during a short period of time, an unusual number of people with similar symptoms (especially with fever, respiratory or gastrointestinal complaints), a large number of rapidly fatal cases occurring, or patients exhibiting relatively uncommon symptoms (Table 56-2). The local

Table 56-2	Biologic Agents			
AGENT	**INCUBATION PERIOD**	**EFFECTS**	**PROTECTION**	**TREATMENT/PROPHYLAXIS**
Bacillus anthracis	1-5 days	Mediastinitis, meningitis, multiple organ failure	Isolation, vaccination, standard precautions	Ciprofloxacin 400 mg IV tid; doxycycline 200 mg IV × 1, then 100 mg IV tid, PCN 2 MU IV 2 hourly plus streptomycin 30 mg/kg IM daily
Yersinia pestis (bubonic or pneumonic plague)	2-3 days	Pneumonia, septicemia, multiple organ failure (septic shock)	Isolation, standard precautions, droplet precautions	Streptomycin 30 mg/kg IM every day × 10; doxycycline 200 mg IV, then 100 mg IV tid × 14 days
Viral hemorrhagic fevers	4-21 days	Coagulopathy, edema, multiple organ failure (septic shock)	Isolation, HEPA filter masks, standard precautions	Ribavirin 30 mg/kg × 1, then 15 mg/kg IV daily × 4 days, then 7.5 mg/kg tid × 6 days (immunoglobulin)
Francisella tularensis	2-10 days	Pneumonia, pleural effusions, possible sepsis	Standard precautions	Streptomycin 30 mg/kg IV daily × 10-14 days; gentamycin 3-5 mg/kg IV every other day
Escherichia spp.	1-5 days	Vomiting, diarrhea, renal failure	Barrier nursing	NA
Brucella spp.	5-60 days	Malaise, cough	Barrier nursing	Doxycycline 100 mg PO bid plus rifampin 900 mg tid for 6 weeks
Smallpox (variola)	7-10 days	Rash, secondary pneumonia, possible sepsis and septic shock	Isolation, standard precautions	Cidofovir 5 mg/kg IV once every 2 weeks

From Centers for Disease Control and Prevention: *Severe acute respiratory syndrome fact sheet,* available at www.cdc.gov/ncidod/sars/factsheet.htm. Accessed April 3, 2011.

IV, Intravenous; *IM,* intramuscular; *HEPA,* high-efficiency particulate air; *MU,* million units; *NA,* not applicable, *PCN,* penicillin; *PO,* by mouth.

and state Public Health Departments should be notified immediately.

As with any mass casualty, a single facility might be overwhelmed with patients. The hospital's emergency plan will delegate roles to accommodate the patient load with properly skilled staff. All elective surgeries will be cancelled, and only emergency surgeries will be performed. Because the PACU is also a critical care unit by definition,[11] the perianesthesia nurse's special capabilities may be required to care for ICU overflow patients and provide beds for patients needing mechanical ventilation and one-on-one patient care. The PACU directors need to ensure that their staff receives the competency training needed to provide for this expanded role. Cross training in the ICU could help to maintain those skills needed to care for the critically ill patient. During mass casualty practices, serious and creative role play can assist in problem solving issues

that could be problematic if a real event should occur. Staffing issues, space, and supply acquisition solutions should be considered. The "just in time" mindset for supplies and staff will be a detriment. Minimal staff and supplies will necessitate working with other hospitals and distribution supply houses. All staff members must to be prepared for emergencies and to successfully care for patients. That preparation must occur before a real emergency. The staff members will need to make contingency plans for their own families to decrease the stress during staff recall. Stress will be elevated and workplace violence could be an issue. Staff member concerns for personal safety and that of their family, patients, and family members who are stressed, and lack of preparation and planning can contribute to workplace violence. Recognition and training on workplace violence, "zero tolerance" for workplace violence, and an open door policy for the administration and stress teams will assist to diminish the possibility workplace violence will occur.[12]

Health care workers must always protect themselves first. The use of appropriate personal protective equipment, appropriate patient isolation, and hand washing when dealing with any patient will protect against most biological agents (Table 56-3). It is important for health care workers to maintain a healthy life style that includes current immunization status (e.g., tetanus, diphtheria, influenza vaccine, polio). In the event of an exposure secondary to caring for victims of a biologic incident, rapid postexposure treatment (prophylactic medications or vaccinations) must be started.

RESPONSE

Practice good infection control. The simplest and most effective practice a nurse can have to reduce contamination and spread infection is hand washing. Personal protective equipment (e.g., gown, mask, gloves, hair cover) should be used if an infectious disease is suspected. This is true for any potentially infectious patient or one known to be contaminated with a biologic agent associated with terrorism.[13]

Decontamination of the patient may be required. If the biologic attack is overt, decontamination should occur. Removing all clothes and sealing them in a plastic bag as well as a shower with soap and large amounts of water are important to dilute and remove biologic agents. Bleach kills the anthrax spores on clothes and objects, but it should not be used on skin. In the event of a covert attack, decontamination is not important because of the time from exposure. The medical facility should quickly attempt to make a presumptive diagnosis and not delay treatment awaiting complete test results. Treatment should begin immediately as it is most effective in the prodromal phase. Empiric treatment of respiratory casualties should be used because they might have anthrax, plague, or tularemia.

Table 56-3	CDC Recommendations of Precautions to Prevent Transmission of Infectious Agents		
TYPE OF PRECAUTION	GOAL OF PRECAUTION	ELEMENTS OF PRECAUTION	PREVENT TRANSMISSION OF DISEASES
Standard precautions	Prevent direct contact with body fluids, secretions, excretions, nonintact skin, rashes and mucous membranes	Hand washing, gloves, masks and eye protection, and gowns and safe injection practices, respiratory and cough hygiene, wearing of mask when injecting into epidural or spinal spaces	Tuberculosis, legionnaires disease, Q fever, tetanus, tularemia, botulism, viral hemorrhagic fevers (Ebola, Lassa, Marburg), smallpox, SARS, anthrax, VEE
Airborne precautions	Prevent transmission of agents that remain infectious over a long distance when suspended in air	AIIR, N95 or higher respirator masks for staff before entering room	Smallpox, tuberculosis, SARS, chickenpox, measles
Contact precautions	Prevent direct or indirect contact with patient or patient's environment	Isolation in private room, or cohorting with patients with same diagnosis, spacial separation >3 feet, gown and gloves donned when entering room and removed when leaving	VRE, MRSA, bubonic plague, smallpox, SARS, viral hemorrhagic fevers (Ebola, Lassa, Marburg)
Droplet precautions	Prevent transmission through close respiratory or mucous membrane contact with respiratory secretions	Isolation in private room, or cohorting with patients with same diagnosis and spacial separation of >3 feet, or drawing curtain between beds, mask worn by HCW	Pandemic influenza, pertussis, pneumonic plague, SARS, viral hemorrhagic fevers (Ebola, Lassa, Marburg)

From Siegel JD, et al: *2007 Guidelines for isolation precautions: preventing transmission of infectious agents in healthcare settings,* Healthcare Infections Control Practices Advisory Committee, available at www.cdc.gov/hicpac/pdf/isolation/Isolation2007.pdf. Accessed April 3, 2011.
CDC, Centers for Disease Control and Prevention; *HCW,* health care worker; *SARS,* severe acute respiratory syndrome; *AIIR,* airborne infection isolation room; *VEE,* Venezuelan equine encephalitis; *VRE,* vancomycin-resistant enterococcus; *MRSA,* methicillin-resistant *Staphylococcus aureus.*

Patient treatment should follow the advanced trauma life support protocol, concentrating on airway, breathing, and circulation. New best practice guidelines recommend using the *Surviving Sepsis Campaign* model for improvement of care using bundles.[14] A *bundle* is a group of therapies that, when implemented together, may result in better outcomes for patients with sepsis than if implemented individually. The individual components included in a bundle are built around best evidence-based practices. Use of the Severe Sepsis Bundles can achieve a 25 percent reduction in mortality due to severe sepsis or septic shock. [14]

Evidence-Based Practice

The Surviving Sepsis Campaign is the result of an international guideline-based program to target severe sepsis. In 2003, critical care and infectious disease experts representing 11 international organizations developed management guidelines based on best evidence for severe sepsis and septic shock that would be of practical use for the bedside clinician. The program was a multifaceted intervention to facilitate compliance with selected guideline recommendations in the intensive care unit, emergency department, and wards of individual hospitals.

The process was a modified Delphi method, using a consensus conference, several smaller meetings of subgroups, teleconferences, keynote subject experts, and electronically based discussions between subgroups and the entire committee.

IMPLICATIONS FOR PRACTICE

The mortality rate of severe sepsis is unacceptably high at 30% to 50%. When shock is present, mortality is reported to be even higher (50% to 60%). There are approximately 750,000 new sepsis cases each year, with at least 210,000 fatalities. The analysis of more than 15,000 patient charts showed that the campaign was associated with sustained, continuous quality improvement in sepsis care and a reduction in reported hospital mortality rates. In an effort that spanned three continents, compliance with sepsis bundles increased by 20% over 2 years and was associated with a 7% reduction in hospital mortality. The design was to expedite initial resuscitation, optimize diagnosis pathways, and provide guidelines for supportive and preventative therapies by delineating pathways, guidelines and protocols for sepsis care.

Source: Levy M: *The surviving sepsis campaign*, Society of Critical Care Medicine 2010, available at www.survivingsepsis.org/About_the_Campaign/Pages/CommentaryMitchell MLevy,MD,FCCM.aspx. Accessed April 20, 2011.

As seen in Table 56-2, bacterial infections can lead to sepsis quickly, especially anthrax, tularemia, pneumonic plague. Through evidence-based recommendations for sepsis management and treatment, rapid and clearly articulated strategies help to reduce negative outcomes from sepsis. The intention is to apply the bundles 100% of the time within the first 6 hours of identification of severe sepsis.

Isolation for patients can present a problem. Gathering patients with similar symptoms into a separate room or area of a room and separating the infected persons from postoperative patients solves the problem of isolation needs. Manipulation of ventilation and air pressure within smoke compartments can provide a solution for negative pressure rooms. See Table 56-2 for specific requirements for each agent.

In the event of a death, the body of the deceased will need to be used as evidence and cannot be released to the mortuary without approval from local law enforcement.

COMMUNICATION

Plans for a rapid response to bioterrorism must be communicated to the community at the local, state, and national levels. The PACU must evaluate and define their roles in a bioterrorism event. Communication must exist between the administration, management, and staff members to identify training, staffing, and supply needs to be adequately prepared to respond and meet the challenge of bioterrorism events.

The psychological aspects of terrorism must be anticipated and communicated. Expected responses for health care workers, patients, and their families can include horror, anger, panic, and unrealistic fears about infection, fear of contagion, and social isolation. When developing a facility emergency plan, the following should be addressed: rapid availability of medical evaluation and treatment to reduce panic; availability of educational materials for the public; availability of mental health support personnel for staff members, patients, and families; and provision of care for persons experiencing psychosomatic symptoms.

SUMMARY

Tremendous resources are being injected into bioterrorism response systems. The Federal Bureau of Investigation), Department of Defense, CDC, Federal Emergency Management Agency, and states and municipalities are all receiving funds to develop their responses. Computerized communications systems, large quantities of antibiotic dose-packs, vaccines, decontamination systems, hazardous materials suits, and biosafety laboratories all can be made available on short notice. These vast resources are only called into play if an alert health professional detects an unusual situation and notifies the local health department. That local health department must have the epidemiologic and laboratory support to confirm or deny the possibility of a threat exposure. The keen clinician can alert the authorities and put the appropriate resources into play.

Strong local health departments and health officers are generally not in place in many areas throughout the country. This problem has been widely recognized. The need to upgrade our local health departments becomes obvious when bioterrorism is considered; however, an upgrade would have salutary effects on all of the public health challenges that confront us now and in the future.

Other bacterial and viral agents may be encountered as a result of bioterrorism events, and the critical care unit should have a plan that is both responsive and flexible. In consideration of the large numbers of individuals who may need care, the establishment of temporary care units in various community locations may be necessary, with logistical support from a wide variety of sources. The use of mechanical ventilators can be augmented through manually assisted ventilation if large numbers of victims are identified. PACU nurses should develop plans that include other health professionals and perhaps nonprofessionals who can be given immediate on-the-job training in operation of life-saving techniques. Non–health care workers can supply logistic support, patient data recording and appropriate security and crowd management.

The old adage applies in this case, as in so many others; "If we fail to plan, then we must plan to fail."

REFERENCES

1. Jones R, VanGilder A: Bioterrorism agents: what the anesthesiologist needs to know, *The Internet Journal of Anesthesiology*, available at www.ispub.com/journal/the-internet-journal-of-anesthesiology/volume-16-number-2/bioterrorism-agents-what-the-anesthesiologist-needs-to-know.html. Accessed April 5, 2011.
2. Public Health Response to Biological or Chemical Terrorism: *Interim planning guidance for state public health officials*, U.S. Department of Health and Human Services, available at www.bt.cdc.gov/Documents/Planning/PlanningGuidance.PDF. Accessed April 10, 2011.
3. Abraham RB: Practical guidelines for acute care of victims of bioterrorism: conventional injuries and concomitant nerve agent intoxication, *Anesthesiology* 97(4), 2002.
4. Khan AD, Sage M: *Biological and chemical terrorism: strategic plan for preparedness and response*, 49(RR04):1–14, 2000, available at cdc.gov/mmwr/preview/mmwrhtml/rr4904a1.htm. Accessed April 10, 2011.
5. Bland SA: Chemical, biological and radiation casualties: critical care considerations, *JR Army Med Corps* 155(2):122–174, 2009.
6. Woods JB, editor: *USAMRIID's medical management of biological casualties handbook*, ed 6, U.S. Army Medical Research Institute of Infectious Disease, 2005, Fort Detrick, Frederick, Maryland, available at www.usamriid.army.mil/education/bluebookpdf/USAMRIID%20BlueBook%206th%20Edition%20-%20Sep%202006.pdf. Accessed April 10, 2011.
7. Henderson DA: Bioterrorism as a public health threat, *Emerging Infectious Diseases* 4(3), 1998, available at www.cdc.gov/ncidod/eid/vol4no3/hendrsn.htm. Accessed April 15, 2011.
8. Centers for Disease Control and Prevention: *Bioterrorism agents/disease*, available at www.bt.cdc.gov/agent/agentlist-category.asp. Accessed April 3, 2011.
9. Centers for Disease Control and Prevention: *Severe acute respiratory syndrome fact sheet*, available at www.cdc.gov/ncidod/sars/factsheet.htm. Accessed April 3, 2011.
10. Centers for Disease Control and Prevention: *Viral hemorrhagic fevers fact sheet*, available at www.cdc.gov/ncidod/dvrd/spb/mnpages/dispages/Fact_Sheets/Viral_Hemorrhagic_Fevers_Fact_Sheet.pdf. Accessed April 20, 2011.
11. A Joint Position Statement on ICU Overflow Patients developed by ASPAN, AACN, and ASA's Anesthesia Care Team Committee and Committee on Critical Care Medicine and Trauma Medicine: *Perianesthesia nursing standards and practice recommendations*, available at www.aspan.org/Portals/6/docs/ClinicalPractice/PositionStatement/1012/Pos_Stmt_7_MedSurg_OverflowPts.pdf. Accessed April 20, 2011.
12. A Position Statement on Workplace Violence in the Perianesthesia Settings: *Perianesthesia nursing standards and practice recommendations*, available at www.aspan.org/Portals/6/docs/ClinicalPractice/PositionStatement/1012/Pos_Stmt_13_Workplace_Violence.pdf. Accessed April 20, 2011.
13. Siegel JD, et al: *2007 Guidelines for isolation precautions: preventing transmission of infectious agents in healthcare settings*, healthcare infections control practices advisory committee, available at www.cdc.gov/hicpac/pdf/isolation/Isolation2007.pdf. Accessed April 3, 2011.
14. Levy M: The surviving sepsis campaign, *Society of Critical Care Medicine 2010*, available at www.survivingsepsis.org/About_the_Campaign/Pages/CommentaryMitchellMLevy,MD,FCCM.aspx. Accessed April 20, 2011.

RESOURCES

Arnon SS, et al: Botulinum toxin as a biological weapon: medical and public health management, *JAMA* 285(8):1059–1070, 2001.
Baker D: Chemical and biological warfare agents: the role of the anesthesiologist. In Miller RD, editor: *Miller's anesthesia*, ed 7, Philadelphia, 2010, Churchill Livingstone.
Candiotti KA, et al: Critical care and trauma emergency preparedness for biological and chemical incidents: a survey of anesthesiology residency programs in the United States, *Anesthesia and Analgesia*, 101:1135–40, 2005.

SPECIAL CONSIDERATIONS

Centers for Disease Control and Prevention: *Emergency prepared-ness,* available at www.bt.cdc.gov/. Accessed November 29, 2011.

Clark NP, Rinderknecht JL: Bioterrorism: intentional introduction of animal disease, *Rev Sci Tech* 30:131–138, 2011.

College of Nurses of Ontario: *Infection prevention and control practice standards,* available at www.cno.org. Accessed April 5, 2011.

English JF, et al: *Bioterrorism readiness plan: a template for healthcare facilities,* APIC Bioterrorism Task Force and CDC Hospital Infections Program Bioterrorism Working Group, 2002.

Foster D: Smallpox as a biological weapon: implications for the critical care clinician, *Dimens Crit Care Nurs* 22(1):2–9, 2003.

Heyman DL, editor: *Control of communicable diseases manual,* ed 17, Washington, DC, 2009, APHA.

Inglesby TV, et al: Plague as a biological weapon: medical and public health management, *JAMA* 283(17):2281–2290, 2000.

Inglesby TV, et al: Anthrax as a biological weapon: medical and public health management, *JAMA* 281(18):1735–1745, 1999.

Karwa M, et al: Bioterrorism: preparing for the impossible or the improbable, *Crit Care Med* 33(Suppl 1):S75–95, 2005.

Schwartz MN: Recognition and management of anthrax: an update, *N Engl J Med* 345(22):1621–1626, 2001.

Shafazand S, et al: Inhalational anthrax, *Chest* 116:1369–1376, 1999.

Steinhauer R: Bioterrorism, *RN* 65(3):48–55, 2002.

Switala CA, et al: Bioterrorism—a health emergency: do physicians believe there is a threat and are they prepared for it? *Am J Disaster Med* 6:143–152, 2011.

Thavaselvam D, Vijayaraghavan R: Biological warfare agents, *J Pharm Bioallied Sci* 2:179–188, 2010.

Varkey P, et al: Confronting bioterrorism: physicians on the front line, *Mayo Clinic Proc* 77(7): 661–672, 2002.

57 Cardiopulmonary Resuscitation in the PACU

William Hartland, Jr., PhD, CRNA

Cardiopulmonary emergencies are common in the postanesthesia care unit (PACU). PACU and perianesthesia nurses must keep their cardiopulmonary resuscitation (CPR) skills and knowledge base up to date to most effectively respond to this potentially devastating event. In October 2010, the American Heart Association (AHA) *Guidelines for Cardiopulmonary Resuscitation and Emergency Cardiovascular Care* (ECC) were published in *Circulation*. This CPR update was based on an international evidence-based evaluation process involving hundreds of resuscitation experts.[1]

This chapter looks at cardiopulmonary resuscitation based on the 2010 AHA guidelines for CPR and ECC as it applies to the PACU. Although this chapter highlights the responsibilities of the health care provider during a cardiopulmonary emergency, it is not designed to replace formal training in either basic life support or advanced cardiopulmonary life support as offered through the American Heart Association.

DEFINITIONS

Antiarrhythmics: A group of drugs used to suppress abnormal rhythms of the heart.

Cardiopulmonary Arrest: The cessation of normal circulation of the blood because of failure of the heart to contract effectively.

Cardiopulmonary Resuscitation (CPR): An emergency procedure that is performed in an effort to return life to a person in cardiac arrest.

Chest Compression: An emergency procedure that is performed on a person in cardiac arrest in an effort to create artificial circulation by manually pumping blood through the heart.

Defibrillation: A treatment for the life-threatening cardiac arrhythmias that consists of delivering a therapeutic dose of electrical energy to the heart, which depolarizes a critical mass of the heart muscle, terminates the arrhythmia, and allows normal sinus rhythm to be reestablished via the patient's sinoatrial node.

Differential Diagnosis: A systematic method, essentially a process of elimination, used to identify unknowns.

Vasopressors: Sympathomimetic drugs that mimic the effects of the sympathetic nervous system.

ETHICAL ISSUES RELATED TO CARDIOPULMONARY RESUSCITATION

Many patients are increasingly concerned about the inappropriate use of life-sustaining procedures that can have a dramatic effect on the length and quality of life. Consequently, increasing numbers of patients place limitations on medical treatments that may affect their lives in the future, through the use of living wills, advanced directives, do-not-resuscitate (DNR) orders, and no-CPR programs. Living wills allow a person to express preferences concerning end-of-life medical care. Some states have adopted DNR and no-CPR programs with focus on the use or extent of resuscitation efforts. Advanced directives are usually prepared by the physician attending critically or terminally ill patients who are unable to make decisions for themselves. These directives are based on the patient's living will, if one exists. The patient's right to limit medical interventions is firmly established in modern medical practice.[2,3]

The operating room, however, is one area in which restrictions on cardiopulmonary resuscitation have caused considerable ethical conflicts between patients and health care providers. Approximately 75% of all cardiac arrests in the operating room are related to specific anesthesia or surgical causes, such as an accidental overdose of an anesthetic agent. In these circumstances, resuscitation has been found to be highly successful. As such, many health care providers view honoring a patient's DNR order as failure to treat a reversible process and thus similar to committing murder.[3,4] One could argue that the same ethical dilemma exists in the PACU because it is so closely aligned with surgery. All the various ethical dilemmas concerning DNR orders that may arise in the PACU and other topics related to advanced directives are beyond the scope of this chapter. As such, PACU nurses must be thoroughly familiar with their individual institution's policies and guidelines concerning these issues.

CARDIOPULMONARY RESUSCITATION

Urgency of Cardiopulmonary Resuscitation

During cardiopulmonary arrest, time is a factor that profoundly influences patient outcomes. The probability of survival decreases rapidly with each minute of cardiopulmonary compromise. The survival rate from cardiac arrest caused by ventricular tachycardia decreases approximately 7% to 10% for each minute the patient is deprived of defibrillation.[5] Therefore the PACU nurse must respond quickly and efficiently during all cardiopulmonary emergencies.

Indications for Resuscitation

Numerous precipitating events are associated with cardiopulmonary arrest. These events include respiratory compromise, circulatory or cardiac compromise, metabolic imbalances, medication or anesthetic overdoses or toxicity, and anaphylaxis. All these events have the potential to occur in the PACU.

Respiratory compromise appears to be the primary cause of morbidity in the PACU. Respiratory compromise can result from residual anesthesia, upper airway obstruction, laryngeal edema, laryngospasm, bronchospasm, noncardiogenic pulmonary edema, and aspiration.[6]

One of the most common causes of upper airway obstruction in the postanesthetic patient results from mechanical obstruction from the tongue. This situation occurs when the tongue falls back into a position that mechanically obstructs the pharynx and thus blocks the passage of air to and from the lungs. The underlying cause of this obstruction may be the result of residual anesthetics, opioids, or muscle relaxants administered during surgery. The tongue may also be edematous from surgical manipulation, anatomic deformities, or allergic reaction. Clinical signs of this type of obstruction include snoring, flaring of the nostrils, use of accessory muscles for ventilation, retraction of the intercostal spaces and suprasternal notch, asynchronous movements of the chest and abdomen, tachycardia from hypoxia, and decreased oxygen saturation.[3,6]

Arterial carbon dioxide pressure ($PaCO_2$) increases 6 mm Hg during the first minute of total obstruction, with an additional 3 to 4 mm Hg increase each passing minute.[7] If the obstruction is not corrected, the patient's condition will continue to deteriorate resulting in cardiopulmonary arrest. This occurrence is especially tragic when the obstruction could have been corrected by simply stimulating the patient to take deep breaths or by repositioning the airway via a chin lift or jaw thrust. (These maneuvers will be discussed in more detail later.) Additional techniques include the use of a nasal or oral airway. When deciding which of these two airways to use, the PACU nurse should remember that the nasal airway is usually less stimulating and thus tolerated better in the patient emerging from general anesthesia. The nasal airway should, however, not be used with patients with known or suspected basal skull fractures, because of the possibility of inadvertent intracranial placement of the airway. Nasal airways should also not be used with patients presenting with severe coagulopathy due to the increased incidence of nasal bleeding associated with insertion of the nasal airway.[8]

If the obstruction persists, advanced airway management procedures with the esophageal-tracheal Combitube, Laryngeal Tube or King LT, laryngeal mask airway, or endotracheal tube may be indicated. Obviously, prevention of cardiopulmonary arrest is more desirable than treatment. When a cardiopulmonary arrest does occur, emergency procedures must be administered rapidly and decisively before irreversible damage occurs.[8]

Emergency Equipment

The perianesthesia nurse, faced with a cardiopulmonary event, has an obvious advantage over a layman or health care provider faced with a similar event outside the hospital. This advantage is based on the numerous resources available to the PACU nurse to aid in the diagnosis and treatment of an actual or pending adverse cardiopulmonary event. These resources include the monitoring modalities, medications, essential equipment, and access to the patient's medical history, which can give valuable insight into possible underlying causes and pathology leading up to the adverse event. Another advantage is the availability of assistance and consultation from other health care professionals.

The routine use of various monitoring modalities in the PACU is invaluable for the diagnosis of many developing patient complications that could precipitate a cardiopulmonary arrest. The use of pulse oximetry, for example, can be extremely helpful in the diagnosis of problems concerning patient oxygenation, as in the case of a progressing airway obstruction. The use of a capnograph may be helpful in the early detection of adverse respiratory events such as hypoventilation. The routine use of an ECC monitor assists the nurse in identifying life-threatening arrhythmias such as pulseless ventricular tachycardia (VT), ventricular fibrillation (VF), asystole, and pulseless electrical activity (PEA). These and other monitoring modalities provide the nurse with a more definitive means of diagnosis and opportunity for early intervention.[8]

All advanced cardiac life support equipment should be immediately available to the perianesthesia nurse. This equipment is usually found on a designated code cart or tray that is located in a designated area of the PACU. The cart should contain various emergency items including a defibrillator and monitor; emergency pharmacologic agents; equipment for circulatory, airway, and respiratory management; and specialty trays for various emergency procedures. Usually the individual PACU or health care institution establishes the general setup and contents of the cart. Each PACU nurse must be familiar with the location of the cart, its contents, and their proper use. The immediate availability of emergency equipment and pharmacologic agents is essential for successful cardiopulmonary resuscitation.

Management of Cardiac Arrest

Usually some event occurs that alerts the PACU nurse to the onset of a cardiopulmonary emergency. This event may be in the form of a witnessed collapse of a patient or the onset of a life-threatening arrhythmia such as pulseless VT, VF, asystole, or PEA.

Assess for Responsiveness

At the first sign of potential trouble, the nurse should immediately assess the responsiveness of the patient. The last thing the nurse wants to do is prematurely call a code and start CPR only to find out that the patient had just fallen asleep and one of the electrocardiogram (ECG) leads was loose or disconnected. At the same time the PACU nurse is checking the patient's responsiveness, the patient's breathing status should also be assessed; this should be a visual inspection for abnormal (only gasping) or lack of breathing.[9]

Activation of the PACU Emergency System

When unresponsiveness has been determined, the nurse should follow unit protocol to activate the emergency response system, retrieve a defibrillator, and provide CPR and defibrillation as indicated. In most PACUs, a lone nurse can get another colleague's help by simply calling out for assistance, activating a wall switch, or pushing a button on the telephone in the room. In the unlikely event the PACU nurse is alone, the nurse must activate the emergency response system, retrieve the defibrillator and start CPR. If two rescuers are present, one should begin CPR while another activates the emergency response system

and retrieves a defibrillator. Activation of the emergency response system brings help in the form of necessary emergency equipment and essential personnel to the patient's bedside. Assistance from other health care team members serves many purposes, including the ability to perform many essential tasks simultaneously, availability of various knowledge backgrounds and experience levels for consultation, and overall support. Nursing personnel should be thoroughly familiar with the unit's specific protocols for initiating a code and obtaining needed assistance.

Circulatory Assessment

Once unresponsiveness has been confirmed and the emergency system has been activated, the PACU nurse should immediately precede with the AHA basic life support and advanced cardiac life support protocols. The nurse should now proceed to evaluate the patient's circulatory status. For an adult and child, this assessment is performed by palpating the carotid artery for no more than 10 seconds. If the patient is an infant, the brachial artery should be palpated.[9]

If a pulse is detected, the patient's lungs should be ventilated using one of the unit's readily available bag-mask devices. Respirations should be delivered at a rate of one breath every 5 to 6 seconds or approximately 10 to 12 breaths/min. Each breath should be given over 1 second and cause a visible chest rise. The patient's pulse should be checked every 2 minutes. This process should continue until the emergency response team can determine and correct the underlying cause of the respiratory arrest or initiate more advanced treatment.[9]

If no pulse is detected within 10 seconds, the 2010 AHA Guidelines for CPR and ECC state that cardiac arrest should be assumed and CPR initiated immediately. These guidelines recommend initiating a CPR sequence of (1) chest compressions, (2) airway, and (3) breathing (CAB). Anytime during this sequence, defibrillation should be initiated as soon as a defibrillator is available.[9]

Cardiopulmonary Resuscitation
Chest Compressions

As stated previously, cardiac arrest can be caused by four heart rhythms: VF, pulseless VT, PEA, and asystole. VF consists of disorganized electrical activity in which VT consists of organized electric activity of the ventricular myocardium. The electrical activity exhibited in these rhythms is insufficient to generate enough forward blood flow to sustain life. PEA encompasses a group of organized electrical rhythms with insufficient or absent mechanical ventricular activity. Although this rhythm may generate ventricular electrical activity on the monitor, the ventricle does not mechanically respond, resulting in the absence of a clinically detectable pulse. PEA has previously been referred to as *electromechanical dissociation* or *nonperfusing rhythm*. Asystole, also known as *ventricular asystole*, consists of the absence of detectable ventricular activity with or without atrial electrical activity.[8]

Ventricular Fibrillation and Pulseless Ventricular Tachycardia

During the first few minutes of witnessed VF cardiac arrest, the primary limiting factor for the delivery of oxygen to the heart and brain is blood flow and not arterial oxygen content. As a result, in the initial step of CPR, uninterrupted chest compressions take priority over positive pressure ventilation.[8] External cardiac compression should be performed with the patient in a horizontal position on a firm surface. If a bed board is to be used, care must be taken not to delay the initiation of compressions while one is being retrieved. If the patient is on an air-filled mattress, the mattress should be deflated when performing CPR.[10]

To begin compressions, the rescuer should be positioned at the patient's side. The rescuer should place the heel of one hand on the center (middle) of the chest between the patient's nipples (the lower half of the sternum; Fig. 57-1). The heel of the rescuer's free hand should be placed on top of the hand already positioned on the patient's chest. The rescuer should keep the arms straight with shoulders directly over the adult patient's

sternum. The adult sternum should be depressed at least 2 inches (5 cm; Fig. 57-2). Rescuers should "push hard, push fast" at a rate of at least 100 compressions/min. Evidence appears to support the premise that this rapid compression rate effectively benefits the patient in terms of blood flow and blood pressure. Interruptions to chest compression should always be minimized to as few as possible with each interruption lasting less than 10 seconds. The chest should be allowed to completely recoil after each compression. Incomplete recoil has been associated with high intrathoracic pressures and decreased hemodynamics, including decreased coronary perfusion, cardiac index, myocardial blood flow, and cerebral perfusion. If two rescuers are present, it is recommended that they rotate giving compressions every 2 minutes. This is done to prevent rescuer fatigue, which can lead to decreased compression effectiveness such as insufficient rate, depth of compression, and incomplete recoil of the chest. It has been found that significant fatigue and shallow compressions are common after 1 minute of CPR, although the rescuer might not recognize that fatigue affecting effective compressions is present. Rescuers should consider switching roles during any intervention that is associated with appropriate interruptions in chest compressions such as defibrillation. The rescuers should strive to accomplish this switch in less than 5 seconds.[9] The actual ratio between ventilations and chest compressions will be discussed in the third segment of the CABs, which addresses breathing.

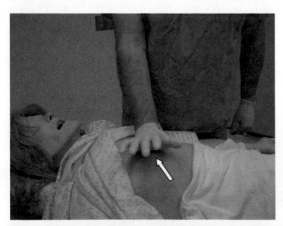

FIG. 57-1 To begin external cardiac compressions, rescuer should place heel of one hand over lower half of patient's sternum, between nipples in center of chest. (Courtesy Department of Nurse Anesthesia, Virginia Commonwealth University, Richmond, Va.)

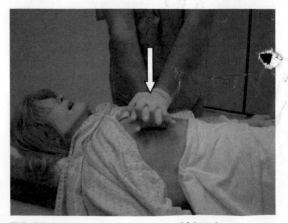

FIG. 57-2 Rescuer's free hand should be placed on top of hand already positioned on patient's chest so that hands are overlapped and parallel. Rescuer should keep arms straight and shoulders directly over adult patient's sternum while pressing down on sternum least 2 inches (5 cm). (Courtesy Department of Nurse Anesthesia, Virginia Commonwealth University, Richmond, Va.)

Evidence-Based Practice

The lack of compression recoil is known to adversely affect hemodynamics in experimental arrest models, but the prevalence of leaning during actual resuscitation is poorly understood. Fried and colleagues evaluated the effectiveness of chest compressions during cardiac arrest, specifically examining the lack of compression recoil ("leaning" or "incomplete recoil"). The authors analyzed 112,569 chest compressions from 108 arrest episodes from May 2007 to February 2009. Leaning was found in 98 of 108 (91%) cases; 12% of all compressions exhibited leaning. Leaning varied widely across cases: 41 of 108 (38%) of arrest episodes exhibited <5% leaning, yet 20 of 108 (19%) demonstrated >20% compression leaning. When evaluating blocks of continuous compressions (>120 s), only 4 of 33 (12%) had an increase in leaning over time, and 29 of 33 (88%) showed a decrease ($p < 0.001$).

IMPLICATIONS FOR PRACTICE

Chest compression leaning was common during resuscitation care and exhibited a wide distribution. Leaning decreased over time during continuous chest compression blocks, suggesting that either leaning is not a function of rescuer fatiguing or that it may have been mitigated by automated feedback provided during resuscitation episodes. In either case, the rescuer must continuously strive for complete chest recoil during the administration of chest compressions during a cardiac arrest.

Source: Fried DA, et al: The prevalence of chest compression leaning during in-hospital cardiopulmonary resuscitation, *Resuscitation* 82(8):1019–1024, 2011.

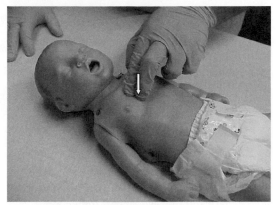

FIG. 57-3 In infants, sternum is compressed with tips of two fingers when only one rescuer is present, which frees rescuer's other hand to open the airway for ventilations. (Courtesy Department of Nurse Anesthesia, Virginia Commonwealth University, Richmond, Va.)

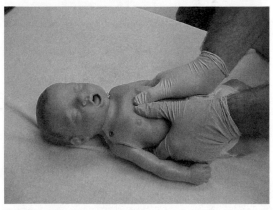

FIG. 57-4 If two rescuers are present, one rescuer can perform compressions with thumbs of encircling hands while other rescuer performs ventilations. (Courtesy Department of Nurse Anesthesia, Virginia Commonwealth University, Richmond, Va.)

In children, the sternum is compressed with the heel of one hand only. In infants, the sternum is compressed with the tips of two fingers for one rescuer or the thumbs of the encircling hands of the rescuer when two rescuers are present (Figs. 57-3 and 57-4).[11] The compression depth for children should be one third the anteroposterior (A-P) diameter of the chest or approximately 2 inches (5 cm). When treating an infant, the compression depth should be one third the A-P diameter or approximately 1.5 inches (4 cm). As in adults, a rate of at least 100 compressions/min is also recommended for children and infants.[9]

The nurse ventilating the patient's lungs should periodically check the patient's pulse during compressions as a guide for their effectiveness. If external cardiac compression is done correctly, systolic blood pressure will reach 60 to 80 mm Hg with a diastolic pressure of zero. Mean blood pressure in the carotid artery will seldom exceeds 40 mm Hg. Cardiac output from chest compression is approximately one fourth to one third of normal. As a result, compressions must be regular, smooth, and uninterrupted.[12]

Airway

After chest compressions have been started, rescue breaths by mouth-to-mouth or bag-mask should be delivered. During the initial evaluation of the patient's responsiveness, the rescuer has already observed the patient's respiratory status and determined that the patient is not breathing. To facilitate ventilations, particular airway maneuvers should be performed. The PACU nurse should use the head tilt–chin lift maneuver to open the patient's airway if no evidence of cervical spine trauma exists. The head tilt maneuver is accomplished by simply tilting the patient's head backward and hyperextending the neck (Fig. 57-5). The chin lift involves placing two fingers under the bony portion of the lower jaw, near the chin, and pushing the patient's chin upward with moderate pressure (Fig. 57-6). The head tilt–chin lift maneuver is simply a combination of both these maneuvers (Fig. 57-7). For patients with actual or possible cervical spine injury, the airway should be opened using only a jaw thrust without the head extension maneuver. To perform the jaw thrust, the rescuer is positioned at the head of the patient. The rescuer places one hand on each side of the patient's head and grasps the angles of the patient's lower jaw and lifts with both hands (Fig. 57-8). If the jaw thrust does not open the airway in a patient with possible cervical spine injury, the head tilt–chin lift maneuver should be used because adequate ventilation is a priority in CPR.[9]

Early in the CPR process, a decision should be made concerning the need for an advanced airway. Because the insertion of an advanced airway may necessitate the interruption of chest compressions for many seconds, the rescuer must weigh the need for compressions against the need for an advanced airway device. Deference of insertion of an advanced airway until the patient fails to respond to initial CPR and defibrillation or shows return of spontaneous circulation is acceptable.[9]

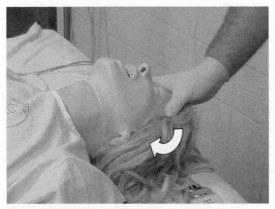

FIG. 57-5 *Head tilt.* Patient's head is tilted backwards and neck is hyperextended. This maneuver is contraindicated in presence of possible cervical injury. (Courtesy Department of Nurse Anesthesia, Virginia Commonwealth University, Richmond, Va.)

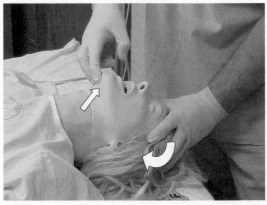

FIG. 57-7 Head tilt and chin lift maneuvers are often done collectively. (Courtesy Department of Nurse Anesthesia, Virginia Commonwealth University, Richmond, Va.)

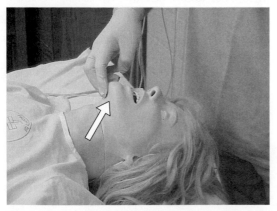

FIG. 57-6 *Chin lift.* Rescuer places two fingers under bony portion of lower jaw, near chin, and pushes patient's chin upward with moderate pressure. (Courtesy Department of Nurse Anesthesia, Virginia Commonwealth University, Richmond, Va.)

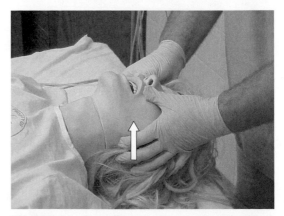

FIG. 57-8 *Jaw thrust.* Rescuer grasps angles of patient's lower jaw and lifts with both hands. Jaw thrust can be done with head tilt (as pictured) or alone without head tilt. Jaw thrust without head tilt is technique of choice for patient with suspected neck injury because it causes least movement of cervical spine. (Courtesy Department of Nurse Anesthesia, Virginia Commonwealth University, Richmond, Va.)

Recommended advanced airway devices include: esophageal-tracheal Combitube, Laryngeal Tube or King LT, laryngeal mask airway, or endotracheal tube. The esophageal-tracheal Combitube, Laryngeal Tube or King LT, laryngeal mask airway are classified as supraglottic airways. Unlike endotracheal intubation, subglottic airways do not require visualization of the glottis. As a result, training and maintenance of skills with these devices are usually easier as compared to endotracheal intubation. In addition, because direct visualization of the glottis is not necessary, a subglottic airway can be inserted without interruption of chest compressions.[8]

When the patient's airway is secured, proper placement of the advanced airway device should be confirmed. This confirmation is especially critical when endotracheal intubation is performed, because of the high risk of tube misplacement, displacement, and obstruction. Confirmation of proper endotracheal tube placement should be assessed with auscultation of the lungs to determine whether breath sounds are present and bilaterally equal in both lungs. Auscultation over the epigastric region is an additional method to confirm misplacement of the endotracheal tube in the esophagus. In addition to auscultation, a confirmation device such as an exhaled CO_2 detector or an esophageal detector device can also be used. If a capnogram is available, the presence of end-tidal carbon dioxide should be confirmed along with oxygen saturation with an oxygen saturation monitor. A continuous wave from capnography in addition to clinical assessments is considered the most reliable method of confirming and monitoring correct endotracheal tube placement. When proper placement has been confirmed, the advanced airway should be secured in place to prevent displacement and dislodgement. This can be accomplished with tape or in the case of an endotracheal tube, with a specially designed endotracheal tube holder.[1]

All four of these advanced airways should be used only by a rescuer who is properly trained and experienced with these devices. In many institutions, endotracheal intubations performed in the PACU are often the responsibility of an anesthesiologist or certified registered nurse anesthetist.

Breathing

Coronary perfusion pressure gradually rises with consecutive compressions; therefore a ratio of 30 compressions to 2 ventilations is recommended for adults, without advanced airways, whether one or two rescuers are present. When the patient is a child or infant, one rescuer should use a 30:2 compression-to-ventilation ratio. If two rescuers

are present, a 15:2 compression-to-ventilation ratio should be used.[9]

When an advanced airway device is in place, a continuous and uninterrupted compression rate of 100 compressions/min should be maintained. Ventilations of 1 breath every 6 to 8 seconds or 8 to 10 breaths/min should be simultaneously delivered without interruption of the compression rate. Each breath should take 1 second to deliverer with a resulting visible chest rise. Studies suggest that a tidal volume of 8 to 10 mL/kg will maintain normal oxygenation and eliminations of carbon dioxide (CO_2). During CPR, oxygen uptake from the lungs and CO_2 delivery to the lungs are reduced because cardiac output is approximately 25% to 33% of normal. Therefore a lower-than-normal minute ventilation can maintain effective oxygenation and ventilation of the patient's lungs. With the adult patient, a CPR tidal volume of approximately 500 to 600 mL should be adequate.[8] Excessive ventilation should be avoided because it has been implicated with gastric inflation resulting in regurgitation and aspiration. Excessive ventilation can also cause increased intrathoracic pressure, decreased venous return to the heart, and decreased cardiac output and survival.[13] The patient should be assessed rapidly for spontaneous breathing and circulation approximately every five cycles (2 minutes) of CPR. During this assessment, chest compressions should be interrupted for no longer than 10 seconds.[1]

The vast majority of patients in the PACU will have intravenous (IV) infusions and will be connected to various monitors including the ECG, pulse oximeter, and other monitors for blood pressure and temperature. If for some reason the patient's IV catheter has been discontinued or not all monitoring devices are in use (as may be the case when preparing a patient for discharge or transfer from the PACU) intravenous access should be secured and the patient should be reconnected to an ECG monitor as soon as possible. Remember, interruptions to chest compressions must be kept to a minimum. Cardiac rhythm analysis should be performed and arrhythmias should be treated with appropriate pharmacologic interventions. Vital signs such as blood pressure, pulse rate, and temperature should also be monitored and assessed.[8]

Defibrillation

As discussed earlier, as soon as lack of responsiveness has been determined, the rescuer immediately activates the PACU emergency response system and retrieves a defibrillator if it is easily available. In the PACU, the code cart with a defibrillator should always be easily available. If on the rare occurrence that the PACU nurse is alone, the defibrillator should be retrieved, connected to the patient, and used as appropriate. The rescuer should then provide high-quality CPR. In the more common PACU scenario, when two or more rescuers are present and unresponsiveness is determined, one rescuer should begin chest compressions while the other activates the emergency response system and retrieves a defibrillator.[9]

Defibrillation is the most important determinant for survival in adult VF and VT. If the patient is not already being monitored, the patient should be connected to an ECG monitor or defibrillator with monitoring capabilities. Rhythm assessment is imperative for the detection of VF or VT. The PACU nurse must remember that for each minute of persistent VF, the patient's chance of survival decreases. Survival rates are highest when immediate CPR is provided and defibrillation is performed within 3 to 5 minutes from the onset of the arrest. After VF or VT have been identified, the defibrillation sequence should start immediately.[1]

Automated external defibrillators (AEDs) are reliable computerized devices that use voice and visual prompts to guide the rescuer to safely defibrillate VF and pulseless VT. Some of the newer AEDs will record information concerning frequency and depth of chest compressions, prompting the rescuer to achieve more effective CPR performance.[5]

Although AEDs are gaining popularity in hospital settings, conventional defibrillators are still used in many PACUs and other hospital specialty areas. PACU nurses must have a working knowledge of all defibrillators available in their respective units whether they are the older monophasic or the newer biphasic models. Although biphasic waveform defibrillators have equivalent or higher efficiency for terminating VF when compared to the monophasic waveform defibrillators, many hospital units still use the older monophasic models.[6]

When the nurse uses the conventional (manual) defibrillator, a basic protocol should be followed. As soon as the defibrillator is brought to the patient's bedside, it should be immediately prepared for use. Uninterrupted CPR should be continued while the defibrillator is charging. When determining the energy settings for the unit's biphasic defibrillator, the nurse should follow the manufacturer's recommendations and the institution's protocol (usually 120 to 200 J). If the rescuer is unaware of the effective dose range for the unit's biphasic defibrillator, the maximum dose of 120 J should be administered. Subsequent energy levels should be equivalent, and higher energy levels considered. If a monophasic defibrillator is being used, a charge of 360 J should be used for the first and all subsequent shocks. AEDs are device specific in the charge they deliver.[5]

Although cardiac arrest is less common in children than adults, VF has been observed in 5% to 15% of pediatric and adolescent arrests. When treating a pediatric patient, it is acceptable to use an initial dose of 2 to 4 J/kg. If refractory VF is encountered, at least 4 J/kg should be used with higher doses considered, not to exceed 10 J/kg or the adult maximum dose. Some AEDs are equipped with pediatric dose attenuator systems that reduce the delivered energy to a dose suitable for a pediatric patient who is 1 to 8 years old. If a dose attenuator AED is not available, then a regular AED should be used. For infants younger than 1 year, a manual defibrillator should be the rescuer's first choice, with the dose attenuation AED second. Units that provide care to pediatric patients who are at risk for cardiac arrest should have immediate access to a manual defibrillator that is capable of dose adjustment.[5]

When a manual defibrillator is being used, the lead selection switch should be switched to "paddles" or "pads." If monitor leads are used, then lead I, II, or III should be selected. Paddles should have specific defibrillation gel or paste applied to them before they are positioned on the patient's chest. This gel or paste maximizes current flow by reducing transthoracic impedance between the paddles and the patient's chest. If the defibrillator uses adhesive conductor pads instead of paddles, they should be positioned on the patient's chest at this time. Four pad or paddle positions—anterolateral, anterior-left infrascapular, anteroposterior, and anterior–right-infrascapular, are equally effective in treating atrial and ventricular arrhythmias. For ease of placement, the anterolateral position is the most common. With this position, one paddle or pad should be positioned just to the right of the patient's upper sternal border, below the clavicle. The second paddle or pad should be placed on the left side of the patient's chest slightly to the left of the nipple, with the center of the electrode in the midaxillary line (Fig. 57-9). Often the defibrillator's manufacturer marks the paddles or pads to designate position on the patient. Next, the monitor display should be visually checked for rhythm assessment. If VF or VT are present, the operator should announce to all team members that the defibrillator is being charged and everyone should stand clear. The charge button on the

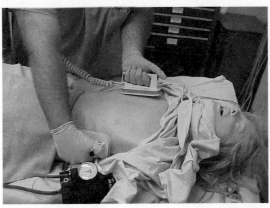

FIG. 57-9 During defibrillation, operator should apply approximately 25 lbs of pressure on paddles while simultaneously pressing both paddle discharge buttons with rescuer's thumbs. Courtesy Department of Nurse Anesthesia, Virginia Commonwealth University, Richmond, Va.)

defibrillator or apex paddle should be pressed. As soon as the defibrillator is charged, the operator should firmly announce to all present that the patient is about to be shocked. No one should be in direct or indirect contact with the patient during defibrillation, which means that no one is touching the patient or any item or apparatus in contact with the patient, including the stretcher or bed. If the rescuer is in direct or indirect contact with the patient during defibrillation, the electric shock may pass through the patient to the rescuer, resulting in a potential second arrest scenario. To alleviate this danger, the AHA suggests the following chant be used. First, the defibrillator operator states loudly and clearly, "I am going to shock on three. One, I'm clear." At this time, the operator checks to be sure he or she is clear of any contact with the patient. Next, the operator states, "Two, you're clear," and makes a visual check to ensure that no one else is touching the patient or any item that is in contact with the patient. Finally, the operator announces, "Three, everybody's clear." At this point, the operator checks everyone, including himself or herself, one last time before administering the shock to the patient. If pads are used instead of paddles, pressing the defibrillator discharge button discharges the defibrillator. With paddles, the operator should apply approximately 25 lb of pressure on the paddles while simultaneously pressing both paddle discharge buttons.[14]

After the charge has been delivered to the patient, CPR should be resumed immediately and continued for five cycles, after which the patient's rhythm should be again evaluated.[1] As long as VF or VT persist, attempts to defibrillate must continue. The PACU nurse must remember that as long as the patient's myocardium has the energy to produce VF or VT, it should also have the energy to produce a perfusing rhythm.[8]

In the case of VT or VF, as soon as the defibrillator is available one shock is delivered. Immediately after this shock, CPR is continued for five cycles (approximately 2 minutes), at which time the patient's rhythm is evaluated. If the VT or VF persists, the patient should be shocked once again with CPR immediately following. As soon as IV or intraosseous (IO) access is available, a vasopressor (epinephrine, 1 mg IV or IO) repeated every 3 to 5 minutes or one dose of vasopressin (40 units IV or IO to replace the first or second dose of epinephrine) should be given during CPR before or after the shock.[1] Additional pharmacologic interventions that may be considered include the administration of amiodarone, lidocaine, and magnesium. Magnesium is considered in the case of magnesium deficiency or for the treatment of torsades de pointes.[1] A summary that compares resuscitation interventions across age groups is presented in Table 57-1.

Differential Diagnosis

The differential diagnosis consists of determining the underlying cause of the arrest. The primary purpose of the differential diagnosis is identification of reversible causes that have a specific therapy. For the PACU nurse, this diagnosis may involve reviewing the patient's preoperative history and physical condition, preoperative and postoperative laboratory values, postoperative diagnosis, surgical procedure performed, and condition on arrival into the PACU. It should also involve the patient's intraoperative course, including unexpected surgical events such as excessive blood loss, fluid replacement, pharmacologic management, and any other intraoperative surgical or anesthetic events. Any of these factors may add some insight into the underlying question of why the patient has suffered a cardiac arrest. Potentially reversible causes of an arrest include hypovolemia, hypoxia, acidosis, hypokalemia, hyperkalemia, hypoglycemia, hypothermia, drug overdoses, cardiac tamponade, tension pneumothorax, coronary or pulmonary thrombosis, and trauma. The PACU nurse should remember that successful resuscitation outcomes usually depend on the discovery and treatment of these or other reversible underlying causes.[8]

Table 57-1	Summary of Key Resuscitation Interventions across Age Groups		
INTERVENTION	**ADULT**	**CHILD**	**INFANT**
Identification	Unresponsive No breathing or not normal breathing No palpated pulse within 10 sec	Unresponsive No breathing or only gasping No palpated pulse within 10 sec	Unresponsive No breathing or only gasping No palpated pulse within 10 sec
CPR Sequence	C-A-B	C-A-B	C-A-B
Compressions	At least 100 per min Minimize interruptions (limit <10 sec)	At least 100 per min Minimize interruptions (limit <10 sec)	At least 100 per min Minimize interruptions (limit <10 sec)
Compression depth	At least 2 in (5 cm) Complete chest recoil	At least ⅓ A-P diameter (≈2 in or 5 cm) Complete chest recoil	At least ⅓ A-P diameter (≈1.5 in or 4 cm) Complete chest recoil
Compression-to-ventilation ratio, no advanced airway	30:2 (1 or 2 rescuers)	30:2 (1 rescuer), 15:2 (2 rescuers)	30:2 (1 rescuer), 15:2 (2 rescuers)
Ventilations with advanced airway	1 breath every 6-8 sec (8-10 breaths/min) Asynchronous with compression rate of at least 100 per min	1 breath every 6-8 sec (8-10 breaths/min) Asynchronous with compression rate of at least 100 per min	1 breath every 6-8 sec (8-10 breaths/min) Asynchronous with compression rate of at least 100 per min
Defibrillation	Use defibrillator as soon as available	Use defibrillator as soon as available	Use defibrillator as soon as available

A-P, Anteroposterior.

Asystole and Pulseless Electrical Activity

Thus far, the discussion of managing cardiac arrest has focused on pulseless VT and VF. The following sections will examine two other life threatening arrhythmias: asystole and PEA. Looking at the patient's monitors, the PACU nurse may observe that the patient's rhythm on the ECG monitor is flat or straight-line. The nurse should remember that asystole is a specific diagnosis, but that a flat line is not. Many nonphysiologic reasons could explain why the monitor may be flat or straight-line. One of the most common causes is that one of the monitor leads becomes disconnected or unplugged. A change in lead selection may also assist the nurse in identification of a disconnected lead. Monitor failure or an insufficient gain setting may also cause a straight-line wave.[2]

A straight-line ECG rhythm may also indicate that the patient is in cardiopulmonary arrest. The PACU nurse should approach this situation in the same way as other potential cardiopulmonary emergencies. The first step to be taken is to assess patient consciousness. If the patient is awake and talking, without any distress, true asystole is unlikely. While assessing consciousness, the nurse may discover that the patient was merely sleeping and inadvertently became disconnected from one of their monitor leads. If, however, the nurse confirms that the patient is unconscious and unresponsive the, unit's emergency response system should be immediately activated. The nurse should then immediately follow with the CPR sequence of CAB. Asystole is commonly considered an end-stage rhythm that usually follows VF or PEA, resulting in a generally poor prognosis.[8] If the patient is confirmed to be in asystole, defibrillation is not recommended.[1]

During asystole, shocks may be harmful by producing a "stunned heart" and profound parasympathetic discharge. As a result, the AHA considers the practice of empiric shocking of asystole to have no evidence of support and to be harmful to the patient.[14]

With asystole, uninterrupted CPR should continue. As soon as IV or IO access is available, epinephrine (1 mg intravenous push IV or IO) should be administered every 3 to 5 minutes. Vasopressin (40 units IV or IO) can be given as a replacement for the first and second doses of epinephrine. Drugs should be delivered immediately after rhythm assessments without interruption of CPR. After drug administration and approximately five cycles of CPR, the patient's rhythm should be reassessed. During this time, the rescuers should be continuously searching for and treat identified reversible causes of the arrest as presented in the differential diagnosis. Evidence suggests that the routine use of atropine during asystole has little therapeutic benefit.[8]

PEA is a little deceptive in its presentation in that it mimics an organized perfusing rhythm on the monitor, but no perfusing pulse is present when the pulse is palpated. As with asystole, the CPR sequence of CAB should be followed without defibrillation. Epinephrine (1 mg IV or IO push) should be administered every 3 to 5 minutes. Vasopressin (40 units IV or IO) may be given as a replacement for the first and second doses of epinephrine. As with asystole, the routine use of atropine has little therapeutic benefit. Drugs should be delivered immediately after rhythm assessments without interruption of CPR. After drug administration and approximately five cycles of CPR, the patient's rhythm should be reassessed. During this process, the rescuers must always remember to continuously search for and treat identified reversible causes of the arrest as presented in the differential diagnosis. This is especially the case with PEA. PEA is frequently caused by reversible conditions that may have caused the arrest or are complicating the resuscitation efforts such as hypoxemia and hypovolemia. Correction of these reversible conditions often leads to a successful patient recovery.[8]

Recovery

If adequate spontaneous circulation returns without spontaneous breathing, rescue breathing should continue but compressions should be terminated. Hyperventilation should be avoided because of the potential for increasing intrathoracic pressure and decreasing cardiac output. Hyperventilation also has the adverse potential to decrease cerebral blood flow. Ventilation may be started at 10 to 12 breaths/min and titrated to achieve a partial pressure of end-tidal CO_2 of 35 to 40 mm Hg as monitored by capnometry.[15]

If the patient is attempting to breathe but spontaneous ventilations are inadequate, the nurse can assist the patient with the bag-mask device. This assistance is performed by manually ventilating the patient's lungs each time the patient attempts to inhale. Depending on the adequacy of the patient's own ventilations, the rescuer can assist with every breath, every other breath, or as needed. When the patient's spontaneous ventilations are adequate, positive pressure ventilation can be discontinued, but supplemental oxygen should be continued via a mask or nasal cannula.

As recommended by the AHA, the initial objectives of postcardiac arrest care are:
- The optimization of cardiopulmonary function and perfusion of vital organs

- The transport of the postcardiac arrest patient to an appropriate critical care unit capable of providing comprehensive postcardiac arrest care
- The identification and treatment of all precipitating causes of the arrest and the prevention of recurrent arrest

Subsequent objectives include:
- Body temperature control to optimize survival and neurological recovery
- Identification and treatment of acute coronary syndromes.
- Optimization of mechanical ventilation to minimize lung injury
- Decreased risk of multiorgan injury and support of organ function as required
- Objective assessment of the patient's prognosis for recovery
- Assisting the survivors with required rehabilitation services[14]

PHARMACOLOGIC THERAPY

The following short summary is based on the AHA recommendations concerning various drugs that are commonly used during cardiovascular resuscitation.[5] The PACU nurse should have a thorough understanding of every drug found in the PACU code cart, including indications, contraindications, interactions, dosage, and adverse reactions.

Vasopressors
Epinephrine

The adrenergic effect of epinephrine increases myocardial and cerebral blood flow and may improve return of spontaneous circulation during CPR. The recommended dose of epinephrine hydrochloride is 1.0 mg (10 mL of a 10:000 solution) IV every 3 to 5 minutes during adult cardiac arrest. Epinephrine can also be administered via the endotrachea tube at a dose of 2 to 2.5 mg. if IV or IO access has not been secured.[8]

Vasopressin

Vasopressin is a naturally occurring antidiuretic hormone. In high doses, higher than those needed for antidiuretic effects, vasopressin acts as a nonadrenergic peripheral smooth muscle vasoconstrictor. Vasopressin has been found useful as an alternative to epinephrine for the treatment of adult shock-refractory VF and increase recovery of spontaneous circulation in the event of asystole or PEA. For patients in pulseless arrest, the recommended one time adult dose of vasopressin is 40 units IV/IO, which can be given to replace the first or second dose of epinephrine.[8]

Antiarrhythmics

Amiodarone

Amiodarone affects potassium, sodium, and calcium channels. It has both alpha and beta adrenergic blocking properties. Amiodarone may be considered for VF, pulseless VT that is unresponsive to CPR, defibrillation, and vasopressor therapy. The initial dose of amiodarone is 300 mg IV, which can be followed by one additional dose of 150 mg IV.[8]

Lidocaine

Lidocaine can be considered if amiodarone is not available. During cardiac arrest, it is administered as a bolus of 1.0 to 1.5 mg/kg IV. If pulseless VT persists, additional doses of 0.5 to 0.75 can be administered IV push at 5 to 10 minute intervals to a maximum dose of 3 mg/kg. Side effects include slurred speech, muscle twitching, altered consciousness, respiratory compromise, seizures, and tachycardia.[1]

Magnesium

Magnesium is used during a cardiac arrest when the arrhythmia is suspected of being caused by magnesium deficiency or the presence of torsades de pointes. When VF or pulseless VT cardiac arrest is associated with torsades de pointes, magnesium sulfate can be administered slowly IV at 1 to 2 g diluted in 10 mL of 5% dextrose in water.[8]

Atropine Sulfate

Available evidence suggests that the use of atropine sulfate during PEA or asystole has little if any therapeutic benefit and is no longer recommended by the AHA for this use. As an anticholinergic agent, it remains the first line of treatment for symptomatic sinus bradycardia. Atropine sulfate should not be used when Mobitz type II block is suspected. It should always be used with caution in a patient with an acute myocardial infarction since acceleration of the patient's heart rate may increase ischemia. The recommended dose of atropine sulfate in the presence of bradycardia is 0.5 mg IV every 3 to 5 minutes up to a maximum total dose of 3 mg.[8]

Sodium Bicarbonate

Hyperventilation corrects respiratory acidosis by removing carbon dioxide. Acidemia during cardiac arrest and resuscitation primarily results from a low blood flow. For the maintenance of acid base balance, adequate alveolar ventilation and tissue perfusion must be maintained. Clinical and laboratory data have not conclusively shown that acidosis interferes with defibrillation, restoration of spontaneous circulation, or short-term survival. Most data indicate that the use of buffers does not improve outcomes. Present data do, however, indicate that bicarbonate can compromise coronary perfusion pressure and induce hypernatremia. In addition, it can exacerbate central venous acidosis and cause adverse effects from extracellular alkalosis.[1]

Sodium bicarbonate can be beneficial in patients with hyperkalemia, tricyclic antidepressant overdose, or preexisting metabolic acidosis. If used, bicarbonate should be administered at an initial dose of 1 mEq/kg. Administration of bicarbonate should be guided by blood gas analysis and laboratory measurements.[1]

SUMMARY

A cardiopulmonary emergency is not an event that any health care provider looks forward to facing. It is, however, an event that is more common in highly specialized acute nursing units, such as the PACU. Every nurse working in the PACU has the responsibility to be prepared for catastrophic emergencies.

REFERENCES

1. Travers AH, et al: Part 4: CPR overview: 2010 American Heart Association guidelines for cardiopulmonary resuscitation and emergency cardiovascular care, *Circulation* 122(Suppl 3):S676–S684, 2010.
2. Morrison LJ, et al: Part 3: ethics: 2010 Amercian Heart Association guidelines for cardiopulmonary resuscitation and emergency cardiovascular care, *Circulation* 122(Suppl 3): S665–S675, 2010.
3. Barash P, et al: *Clinical anesthesia*, ed 6, Philadelphia, 2009, Lippincott Williams & Wilkins.
4. Walker R: DNR in the OR: resuscitation as an operating room risk, *JAMA* 266:2407, 1991.
5. Link MS, et al: Part 6: electrical therapies: automated external defibrillators, defibrillation, cardioversion, and pacing: 2010 American Heart Association guidelines for cardiopulmonary resuscitation and emergency cardiovascular care, *Circulation* 122(Suppl 3):S706–S7196, 2010.
6. Odom J: Airway emergencies in the post anesthesia care unit, *Post Anesth Care Nurs* 28:483–491, 1993.
7. Nagelhout J, Plaus K, editors: *Nurse anesthesia*, ed 4, Philadelphia, 2010, Saunders.
8. Neumar RW, et al: Part 8: adult advanced cardiovascular life support: 2010 American Heart Association guidelines for cardiopulmonary resuscitation and emergency cardiovascular care, *Circulation* 122(Suppl 3):S729–S767, 2010.
9. Berg RA, et al: Part 5: adult basic life support: 2010 American Heart Association guidelines for cardiopulmonary resuscitation and emergency cardiovascular care, *Circulation* 122(Suppl 3):S685–S705, 2010.
10. Perkins GD, et al: Do different mattresses affect the quality of cardiopulmonary resuscitation? *Intensive Care Med* 29:2330–2335, 2003.

11. Hazinski MF, editor: *PALS provider manual*, Dallas, 2002, American Heart Association.

12. AHA: Part 4: adult basic life support: 2005 American Heart Association guidelines for cardiopulmonary resuscitation and emergency cardiovascular care, *Circulation* 112(Suppl 4): 19–24, 2005.

13. Aufderheide TP, et al: Hyperventilation-induced hypotension during cardiopulmonary resuscitation, *Circulation* 109:1960–1965, 2004.

14. American Heart Association in collaboration with the International Liaison Committee on Resuscitation: Guidelines 2000 for cardiopulmonary resuscitation and emergency cardiovascular care: international consensus on science, *Circulation* 102(Suppl 1):8, 2000.

15. Pederdy MA, et al: Part 9: post-cardiac arrest care: 2010 American Heart Association guidelines for cardiopulmonary resuscitation and emergency cardiovascular care, *Circulation* 122(Suppl 3):S768–S786, 2010.

RESOURCES

Graham-Garcia J, et al: Defibrillation and biphasic shocks: implications for perianesthesia nursing, *J Perianesth Nurs* 20(1):23–33, 2005.

SPECIAL CONSIDERATIONS

Index